S0-AEA-093

Pediatric Orthopaedics

Volume Two

Volume Two

Pediatric Orthopaedics

Second Edition

edited by

Wood W. Lovell, M.D.
Medical Director
Nemours Children's Hospital
Jacksonville, Florida

and

Robert B. Winter, M.D.
Professor of Orthopaedic Surgery
University of Minnesota Medical School
Minneapolis, Minnesota
Chief of Spine Service
Gillette Children's Hospital
St. Paul, Minnesota

with 45 contributors

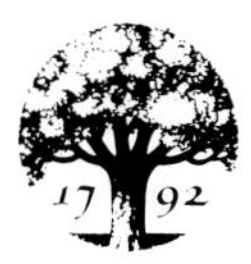

J. B. LIPPINCOTT COMPANY
Philadelphia
London Mexico City New York St. Louis São Paulo Sydney

Sponsoring Editor: Delois Patterson
Manuscript Editor: Linda Fitzpatrick
Indexer: Angela Holt
Art Director: Tracy Baldwin
Design Coordinator: Earl Gerhart
Cover Design: Anthony Frizano
Production Supervisor: J. Corey Gray
Production Coordinator: Barney Fernandes
Compositor: Monotype Composition
Printer/Binder: Halliday Lithograph

2nd Edition

Printed in the United States of America. For information write J. B. Lippincott Company, East Washington Square, Philadelphia, Pennsylvania 19105.

6 5 4 3 2 1

Library of Congress Cataloging in Publication Data
Main entry under title:

Pediatric orthopaedics.

Includes bibliographies and index.
1. Pediatric orthopedia. I. Lovell, Wood W., 1915– . II. Winter, Robert B., 1932– .
[DNLM: 1. Orthopedics—in infancy & childhood.
WS 270 P371] RD732.5.C48P43
1985 617.3 85-4529
ISBN 0-397-50706-2 (set)

The authors and publisher have exerted every effort to ensure that drug selection and dosage set forth in this text are in accord with current recommendations and practice at the time of publication. However, in view of ongoing research, changes in government regulations, and the constant flow of information relating to drug therapy and drug reactions, the reader is urged to check the package insert for each drug for any change in indications and dosage and for added warnings and precautions. This is particularly important when the recommended agent is a new or infrequently employed drug.

Contributors

Behrooz A. Akbarnia, M.D.

Associate Professor of Orthopaedic Surgery and Pediatrics, and Director, Orthopaedic Surgery, Cardinal Glennon Children's Hospital, St. Louis, Missouri

Loui G. Bayne, M.D.

Clinical Professor of Orthopaedics, Emory University, and Director, Hand Clinic, Scottish Rite Hospital, Atlanta, Georgia

Anthony J. Bianco, Jr., M.D., M.S.

Professor of Orthopaedic Surgery, Mayo Medical School, Rochester, Minnesota

Walter P. Bobechko, M.D.

Assistant Professor of Surgery, University of Toronto, and Chief of Orthopaedic Surgery, Hospital for Sick Children, Toronto, Ontario

Joyce Brink, M.D.

Associate Clinical Professor of Pediatrics, University of Southern California School of Medicine, Los Angeles, California, and Chief, Department of Pediatrics, Rancho Los Amigos Hospital, Downey, California

Wilton H. Bunch, M.D., Ph.D

Dean of Medical Affairs, and Professor, Department of Surgery (Orthopaedics), University of Chicago, Chicago, Illinois

William P. Bunnell, M.D.

Assistant Medical Director and Director of Orthopaedics, Alfred I. duPont Institute, Wilmington, Delaware, and Associate Professor of Orthopaedic Surgery, Jefferson Medical College of Thomas Jefferson University, Philadelphia, Pennsylvania

Jonathan Cohen, M.D.

Professor of Orthopaedic Surgery, Tufts University School of Medicine, Senior Orthopaedic Surgeon, Children's Hospital Medical and Kennedy Memorial Hospital for Children, and Deputy Editor, Journal of Bone and Joint Surgery, Boston, Massachusetts

Sherman S. Coleman, M.D.

Chief of Staff, Shriner's Hospital for Crippled Children, and Professor of Orthopaedic Surgery, University of Utah College of Medicine, Salt Lake City, Utah

Henry R. Cowell, M.D., Ph.D

Surgeon-in-Chief, Alfred I. duPont Institute, Wilmington, Delaware, and Editor, Journal of Bone and Joint Surgery, Boston, Massachusetts

Alvin H. Crawford, M.D.

Chief of Orthopaedics, Cincinnati Children's Hospital, Cincinnati, Ohio

Jose de la Garza, M.D.

Orthopaedic Surgeon, University of Monterrey, Nuevo Leon, Mexico

F. Denis, M.D., F.R.C.S. (C)

Assistant Professor of Orthopaedic Surgery, University of Minnesota, Minneapolis, Minnesota, Staff, Spine Service, Gillette Children's Hospital, St. Paul, Minnesota, and Staff, Spine Service, Shriner's Hospital, Minneapolis, Minnesota

Samuel H. Doppelt, M.D.

Assistant in Orthopaedic Surgery, Massachusetts General Hospital, and Assistant Professor of Orthopaedic Surgery, Harvard Medical School, Boston, Massachusetts

James C. Drennan, M.D.

Assistant Professor, Department of Orthopaedic Surgery, University of Connecticut School of Medicine, Farmington, Connecticut, Assistant Clinical Professor, Department of Orthopaedic Surgery, Yale University School of Medicine, New Haven, Connecticut, and Director of Orthopaedics, Newington Children's Hospital, Newington, Connecticut

J. William Fielding, M.D.

Clinical Professor of Orthopaedic Surgery, Columbia University College of Physicians and Surgeons, and Director of Orthopaedic Surgery, St. Luke's Hospital, New York, New York

Robert E. Florin, M.D.

Assistant Professor of Neurological Surgery, University of Southern California School of Medicine, Los Angeles, California, and Consulting Neurological Surgeon, Rancho Los Amigos Hospital, Downey, California

Paul P. Griffin, M.D.

Professor of Orthopaedic Surgery, Harvard Medical School, and Orthopaedic Surgeon-in-Chief, Children's Hospital, Boston, Massachusetts

Richard J. Hawkins, M.D.

Clinical Assistant Professor of Orthopaedic Surgery, University of Western Ontario Faculty of Medicine, St. Joseph's Hospital, London, Ontario

Robert Hensinger, M.D.

Professor, Department of Surgery, Section of Orthopaedics, University of Michigan Medical School, Ann Arbor, Michigan

M. Mark Hoffer, M.D.

Professor and Chief of Orthopaedics, University of California at Irvine, Irvine, California, and Chief, Children's Orthopaedic Surgery, Rancho Los Amigos Hospital, Downey, California

Linda Krach, M.D.

Staff Physician, St. Paul-Ramsey Medical Center, and Medical Director, St. Paul Rehabilitation Center, Attending Staff, Codirector of Head Injury Services, and Medical Director of Rehabilitation, Gillette Children's Hospital, St. Paul, Minnesota, and Instructor, Physical Medicine and Rehabilitation, University of Minnesota, Minneapolis, Minnesota

Henry LaRocca, M.D.

Associate Professor of Orthopaedic Surgery, Tulane University School of Medicine, New Orleans, Louisiana

Wood W. Lovell, M.D.

Medical Director, Nemours Children's Hospital, Jacksonville, Florida

Newton C. McCollough III, M.D.

Professor and Chairman, Department of Orthopaedics and Rehabilitation, University of Miami School of Medicine, and Chief, Orthopaedics and Rehabilitation, Jackson Memorial Hospital, Miami, Florida

G. Dean MacEwen, M.D.

Medical Director, Alfred I. duPont Institute, Wilmington, Delaware, and Professor of Orthopaedic Surgery, Jefferson Medical College of Thomas Jefferson University, Philadelphia, Pennsylvania

Henry J. Mankin, M.D.

Orthopaedist-in-Chief, Massachusetts General Hospital, and Edith F. Ashley Professor of Orthopaedic Surgery, Harvard Medical School, Boston, Massachusetts

John S. Marsh, M.D.

Assistant Clinical Professor of Neurological Surgery, University of Southern California School of Medicine, Los Angeles, California

Peter L. Meehan, M.D.

Director of Pediatric Orthopaedic Education, Scottish Rite Hospital, Atlanta, Georgia

Lyle J. Micheli, M.D.

Director of Sports Medicine, and Professor of Orthopaedic Surgery, The Children's Hospital, Boston, Massachusetts

Colin F. Moseley, M.D., C.M., F.R.C.S. (C)

Assistant Professor of Surgery, University of Toronto, and Orthopaedic Surgeon, Hospital for Sick Children and Ontario Crippled Children's Centre, Toronto, Ontario

Audrey M. Nelson, M.D.

Assistant Professor of Internal Medicine, Mayo Medical School, and Consultant in Rheumatology and Pediatric Rheumatology, Mayo Clinic, Rochester, Minnesota

Kurt M.W. Niemann, M.D.

John D. Sherill Professor of Orthopaedic Surgery, and Director, Division of Orthopaedic Surgery, University of Alabama School of Medicine, Birmingham, Alabama

Hamlet A. Peterson, M.D.

Professor of Orthopaedics, Mayo Medical Center, Rochester, Minnesota

Charles T. Price, M.D.

Pediatric Orthopaedic Surgeon, Orlando Regional Medical Center, Orlando, Florida

Paul L. Ramsey, M.D.

Former Associate Surgeon, Alfred I. duPont Institute, Associate Professor of Pediatric Orthopaedics, Indiana University, Past Chief of Surgery, St. John's Medical Center, Anderson, Indiana, and Past Chief of Staff, Community Hospital, Anderson, Indiana

Mercer Rang, M.D., F.R.C.S. (C)

Associate Professor, University of Toronto, Orthopaedic Surgeon, Hospital for Sick Children, and Orthopaedic Surgeon, Hugh MacMillan Medical Centre, Toronto, Canada

Daniel C. Riordan, M.D.

Professor of Clinical Orthopaedics, Tulane University School of Medicine, Professor of Clinical Orthopaedics, Louisiana State University School of Medicine, New Orleans, Louisiana, and Consultant in Hand Surgery, Shriner's Hospital for Crippled Children, Shreveport, Louisiana

Marvin B. Rothenberg, M.D.

Director, Growth and Metabolic Clinic, Scottish Rite Hospital, Atlanta, Georgia

Ronald Silver, M.D.

Director of Sports Medicine and Attending Orthopaedic Surgeon, Michael Reese Medical Center, Chicago, Illinois

Frank H. Stelling, M.D.

Associate Clinical Professor of Orthopaedic Surgery, Medical University of South Carolina College of Medicine, Charleston, South Carolina, Assistant Clinical Professor of Orthopaedic Surgery, Duke University School of Medicine, Durham, North Carolina, and Chief Surgeon, Shriners Hospital for Crippled Children, Greenville, South Carolina

Robert E. Tooms, M.D.

Professor, Department of Orthopaedics, University of Tennessee Center for the Health Sciences, and Active Staff, Campbell Clinic, Memphis, Tennessee

Chester M. Tylkowski, M.D.

Associate Professor of Pediatric Orthopaedics and Pediatrics, Department of Orthopaedics, and Director, Gait Analysis Laboratory, University of Florida, Gainesville, Florida

Robert B. Winter, M.D.

Professor of Orthopaedic Surgery, University of Minnesota Medical School, Chief of Sp[illegible]rvice, Gillette Children's Hospital, St. Paul, Min[illegible]ta

David J. Zaleske, M.D.

Assistant in Orthopaedic Surgery, Massachusetts General Hospital, and Instructor of Orthopaedic Surgery, Harvard Medical School, Boston, Massachusetts

Contents

Volume One

1 **Embryology of the Neuromusculoskeletal Apparatus**
Henry LaRocca **1**

The Process of Ontogeny *1*
The Nervous System *7*
The Muscular System *13*
The Skeletal System *16*
The Axial Skeleton *17*
The Limbs *19*

2 **Growth**
Colin F. Moseley **25**

Patterns of Growth *25*
Mechanisms of Bone Growth *29*
Mechanisms of Soft-Tissue Growth *37*

3 **Bone Dysplasias**
Frank H. Stelling and *Marvin B. Rothenberg* **41**

Classification *41*
Achondrogenesis *44*
Thanatophoric Dwarfism *45*
Achondroplasia *45*
Chondrodysplasia Punctata *47*
Metatropic Dwarfism *48*
Kniest Syndrome *49*
Diastrophic Dwarfism *50*
Chondroectodermal Dysplasia *52*
Asphyxiating Thoracic Dysplasia *53*
Mesomelic Dwarfism *53*
Cleidocranial Dysplasia *54*

Metaphyseal Chondrodysplasia *56*
Multiple Epiphyseal Dysplasia *59*
Hereditary Arthro-Ophthalmopathy *61*
Dysplasia Epiphysealis Hemimelica *61*
Multiple Cartilaginous Exostoses *61*
Enchondromatosis *64*
Osteopoikilosis *65*
Osteopathia Striata *65*
Melorheostosis *65*
Diaphyseal Dysplasia *66*
Ribbings Disease *67*
Osteodysplasty *67*
Osteo-Onychodysostosis *68*
Mucopolysaccharidosis *69*
Spondyloepiphyseal Dysplasias *75*

4 Metabolic and Endocrine Abnormalities of the Immature Skeleton
David J. Zaleske, Samuel H. Doppelt, and *Henry J. Mankin* **81**

Introduction *81*
Mineral Phase *84*
Organic Phase *110*

5 Genetic Aspects of Orthopaedic Conditions
Henry R. Cowell **147**

The Spectrum of Genetic Diseases *147*
Congenital Disorders *148*
The Sporadic Incidence of Genetic Diseases *150*
The Molecular Basis of Inheritance *150*
Conditions Not Noticed at Birth *151*
Mendelian Disorders *153*
Chromosome Abnormalities *166*
Multifactorial Conditions *172*
Genetic Counseling *172*
Summary *177*

6 Diseases Related to the Hematopoietic System
Kurt M. W. Niemann **181**

Gaucher's Disease *181*
Niemann-Pick Disease *185*
Leukemia *186*
Hemoglobinopathies *188*
Hemophilia *195*
Acquired Immunodeficiency Syndrome *210*

7 Bone Tumors
Jonathan Cohen **217**

Classification *217*
Significance *218*

Critical Bibliography *220*
Diagnosis *221*
Specific Lesions *226*

8 Neuromuscular Disorders
James C. Drennan **259**

Diseases of the Muscle and Peripheral Nerves *259*
Evaluation of Muscular Disorders *260*
Progressive Muscular Dystrophy *263*
Congenital Myopathies *275*
The Inflammatory Myopathies *277*
Systemic Lupus Erythematosus *279*
Scleroderma *280*
Myositis Ossificans *280*
Progressive Contracture of the Quadriceps Muscle *282*
Myasthenia Gravis *282*
Poliomyelitis *283*
Acute Idiopathic Postinfectious Polyneuropathy (Guillain-Barré-Strohl Syndrome) *317*
Spinal Muscular Atrophy *317*
Arthrogryposis Multiplex Congenita *318*
Hereditary Neuropathies and Peripheral Nerve Lesions *328*
Congenital Indifference to Pain *332*

9 Cerebral Palsy
Mercer Rang, Ronald Silver, and *Jose de la Garza* **345**

Prevalence *345*
Etiology *346*
Prevention *346*
Classification *346*
Assessment *347*
Making a Diagnosis *347*
Examination for Planning Treatment *350*
Basic Science *355*
Treatment *361*
Problems and Options *368*
Aphorisms *392*

10 Myelomeningocele
Wilton H. Bunch **397**

Pathology *397*
Embryology *397*
Classification and Pathology *398*
Natural History *400*
Selection for Treatment *402*
Effect of Myelomeningocele on the Developmental Sequence *402*
Genetics *403*
Treatment *404*
Habilitation *430*

11 Infections of Bones and Joints
Walter P. Bobechko **437**

General Features *437*
Acute Hematogenous Osteomyelitis *439*
Septic Arthritis *448*
Granulomatous Infections of the Bone and Joint *452*
Problems and Pitfalls Relating to Bone Infection *453*

12 Juvenile Arthritis and Ankylosing Spondylitis
Anthony J. Bianco and *Audrey M. Nelson* **457**

Juvenile Arthritis *457*
Ankylosing Spondylitis *474*

13 Head Injuries
M. Mark Hoffer, Joyce Brink, John S. Marsh,
and *Robert E. Florin* **479**

Initial Evaluation *479*
Long-Term Neurologic Management *487*
Acute and Long-Term Orthopaedic Measures *489*
Other Causes of Acquired Cerebral Spastic Disability *495*
Conclusion *495*

14 Spinal Injuries in the Growing Person
F. Denis and *Linda Krach* **499**

Rationale for Classification of Spinal Injuries *501*
Classification of Neural Injury *502*
Acute Spinal Injury Approach *503*
Acute Cervical Spine Injuries *504*
Acute Thoracolumbar Injuries *508*
Spine Deformities Secondary to Spinal Cord Injuries *509*
Rehabilitation *515*

15 The Cervical Spine
J. William Fielding, Robert Hensinger,
and *Richard J. Hawkins* **531**

Basilar Impression *531*
Klippel-Feil Syndrome (Congenital Synostosis
of the Cervical Vertebrae, Brevicollis) *535*
Congenital Anomalies of the Odontoid (Dens) *545*
Occipitocervical Synostosis *552*
Congenital Muscular Torticollis (Congenital Wryneck) *555*
Torticollis Due to Bony Anomalies *559*

INDEX

Volume Two

16 Spinal Problems in Pediatric Orthopaedics
Robert B. Winter **569**

Classification *569*
Terminology *570*
Glossary *571*
Evaluation of the Patient *571*
The Adult Sequelae of Untreated Spinal Deformity *576*
Nonstructural Scoliosis *578*
Idiopathic Scoliosis *580*
Congenital Spine Deformity *604*
Neurofibromatosis *617*
Neuromuscular Scoliosis *617*
Postural Kyphosis *619*
Scheuermann's Disease *619*
Post-Laminectomy Kyphosis *635*
Post-Radiation Spine Deformity *635*
Back Pain in Children *637*
Spondylolysis and Spondylolisthesis *638*

17 The Upper Limb
Daniel C. Riordan and *Loui G. Bayne* **649**

Classification of Upper Limb Malformations *649*
Congenital Amputations *650*
Phocomelia *651*
Congenital Absence of the Radius *652*
Congenital Absence of the Ulna *656*
Hypoplastic Thumb *662*
Congenital Absence of the Thumb *664*
Lobster-Claw Hand *664*
Congenital Dislocation of the Shoulder *666*
Congenital Pseudarthrosis of the Clavicle *667*
Congenital Radioulnar Synostosis *671*
Congenital Radiohumeral Synostosis *672*
Congenital Dislocation of the Radial Head *673*
Congenital Dislocation of the Elbow *673*
Pterygum Cubitale (Congenital Webbing of the Elbow) *675*
Arthrogryposis *676*
Syndactyly *678*
Camptodactyly *680*
Clinodactyly *681*
Trigger Thumb *683*
Triphalangeal Thumb *683*
Delta Phalanx *685*
Congenital Clasped Thumb *686*
Polydactyly *687*
Gigantism of the Fingers *690*

Constricting Bands *691*
Madelung's Deformity *692*
Sprengel's Deformity (Congenital Elevation
of the Scapula) *693*
Birth Injuries of the Brachial Plexus (Obstetric Paralysis) *696*
Osteochondritis Dissecans of the Elbow *698*

18 The Hip
G. Dean MacEwen, William P. Bunnell, and *Paul L. Ramsey* **703**

Congenital Dislocation of the Hip—Evaluation
and Treatment Before Walking Age *703*
Congenital Dislocation of the Hip—Evaluation
and Treatment After Walking Age *717*
Coxa Vara *736*
Congenital Short Femur with Coxa Vara *739*
Slipped Capital Femoral Epiphysis *741*
Legg-Calvé-Perthes Syndrome (Coxa Plana) *750*
Transient Synovitis *770*

19 Lower Limb Length Discrepancy
Sherman S. Coleman **781**

Normal Growth and Behavior of a Long Bone *781*
Factors Governing the Decision for Equalization *784*
Methods of Equalization of Limb Lengths *808*

20 The Lower Limb
Paul P. Griffin **865**

Tibial Torsion *865*
Genu Valgum *866*
Physiologic Genu Varum *869*
Tibia Vara (Blount's Disease) *869*
Congenital Angular Deformities of the Tibia *875*
Recurrent Subluxation and Dislocation of the Patella *878*
Congenital and Habitual Dislocation of the Patella *882*
Congenital Dislocation and Subluxation of the Knee *882*
Bipartite Patella *886*
Discoid Meniscus *887*
Osteochondritis Dissecans *887*
Osgood-Schlatter Disease *890*
Popliteal Cyst *891*

21 The Foot
Wood W. Lovell, Charles T. Price, and *Peter L. Meehan* **895**

Structure and Function *895*
Equinovarus Deformities *901*
Flatfoot Deformities *919*
Pes Cavus *942*
Osteochondroses *951*

Forefoot Deformities *954*
Abnormalities of Skin and Nails *966*

22 The Amputee
Robert E. Tooms **979**

Acquired Amputations *980*
Limb Loss from Malignancy *998*
Congenital Limb Deficiencies *998*

23 Orthotic Management
Newton C. McCollough III **1031**

Orthotic Terminology *1031*
Rationale for Orthotic Prescription *1031*
Advances in Orthotics *1032*
Philosophy of Orthotic Prescription *1033*
Lower Limb Orthotics *1033*
Upper Limb Orthotics *1053*
The Spine *1059*

24 Assessment of Gait in Children and Adolescents
Chester M. Tylkowski **1061**

Kinematics *1061*
Muscle Activity *1070*
Kinetics *1071*
Development of Mature Gait *1076*
Interpretation of Normal Gait *1077*
Methods of Gait Assessment *1078*
Conclusion *1079*

25 Partial Growth Plate Arrest and Its Treatment
Hamlet A. Peterson **1083**

Evaluation *1085*
Treatment *1089*

26 Overuse Injuries in Children
Lyle J. Micheli **1103**

Etiology: Risk Factors *1104*
Types of Injury *1106*
Sites of Overuse Injury *1109*
Prevention *1119*

27 Neurofibromatosis
Alvin H. Crawford **1121**

Historical Comments *1121*
Diagnostic Problems in Neurofibromatosis *1122*
Genetics *1124*
Clinical Findings *1124*

Skeletal Manifestations *1127*
Miscellaneous *1141*

28 The Role of the Orthopaedic Surgeon in Child Abuse
Behrooz A. Akbarnia **1147**

History *1147*
Definition *1148*
Prevalence *1148*
Diagnosis *1148*
Clinical Manifestations *1149*
Skin Lesions *1149*
Head Injuries *1150*
Internal Injuries *1150*
Orthopaedic Manifestations *1151*
Management *1154*

INDEX

16

Spinal Problems In Pediatric Orthopaedics

Robert B. Winter

Deformity of the spine was probably the most neglected area of orthopaedics during the first half of this century. In the past 35 years, there has been tremendous progress in this field. New approaches and devices have made possible better operative correction of advanced deformities and better nonoperative treatment of the lesser deformities. Despite all these new advances, the basic fundamentals remain much the same. The care of the patient with a spine deformity must be approached with thoughtfulness and attention to small details. There is no easy "cookbook" solution.

CLASSIFICATION

The following classification is that which has been endorsed by the Scoliosis Research Society. It is a "fluid" classification, that is, one that is constantly undergoing revision and alteration according to new advancements in the basic sciences.

CLASSIFICATION OF SCOLIOSIS

- Idiopathic
  - Infantile—0–3 years
    - Resolving
    - Progressive
  - Juvenile—4 years–puberty onset
  - Adolescent—puberty onset to epiphyseal closure
  - Adult—epiphyses closed
- Neuromuscular
  - Neuropathic
    - Upper motor neuron lesion
      - Cerebral palsy
      - Spinocerebellar degeneration
        - Friedreich's
        - Charcot-Marie-Tooth
        - Roussy-Lévy
      - Syringomyelia
      - Spinal cord tumor
      - Spinal cord trauma
      - Other
    - Lower motor neuron lesion
      - Poliomyelitis
      - Traumatic
      - Spinal muscular atrophy
      - Myelomeningocoele (paralytic)
    - Dysautonomia (Riley-Day)
    - Other
  - Myopathic
    - Arthrogryposis
    - Muscular dystrophy
      - Duchenne (pseudohypertrophic)
      - Limb-girdle
      - Facio-scapulohumeral
    - Congenital hypotonia
    - Myotonia dystrophica
    - Other
- Congenital
  - Congenital scoliosis

- Failure of formation
  - Wedge vertebra
  - Hemivertebra
  - Failure of segmentation
    - Unilateral bar
    - Bilateral ("fusion")
  - Mixed
- Associated with Neural Tissue Defect
  - Myelomeningocele
  - Meningocele
  - Spinal dysraphism
    - Diastematomyelia
    - Other

Neurofibromatosis
Mesenchymal
- Marfan's
- Homocystinuria
- Ehlers-Danlos
- Other

Traumatic
- Fracture or dislocation (nonparalytic)
- Postirradiation
- Other

Soft Tissue Contractures
- Postempyema
- Burns
- Other

Osteochondrodystrophies
- Achondroplasia
- Spondyloepiphyseal dysplasia
- Diastrophic dwarfism
- Mucopolysaccharidoses
- Other

Tumor
- Benign
- Malignant

Rheumatoid Disease
Metabolic
- Rickets
- Juvenile osteoporosis
- Osteogenesis imperfecta

Related to Lumbosacral Area
- Spondylolysis
- Spondylolisthesis
- Other

Thoracogenic
- Post-thoracoplasty
- Post-thoracotomy
- Other

Hysterical
Functional
- Postural
- Secondary to short leg
- Due to muscle spasm
- Other

CLASSIFICATION OF KYPHOSIS

Postural
Scheuermann's Disease
Congenital
- Defect of segmentation
- Defect of formation
- Mixed

Paralytic
- Polio
- Anterior horn cell
- Upper motor neuron

Myelomeningocele
Post-traumatic
- Acute
- Chronic

Inflammatory
- Tuberculosis
- Other infections
- Ankylosing spondylitis

Postsurgical
- Postlaminectomy
- Post body excision (e.g., tumor)

Postirradiation
Metabolic
- Osteoporosis
  - Senile
  - Juvenile
- Osteogenesis imperfecta
- Other

Developmental
- Achondroplasia
- Mucopolysaccharidoses
- Other

Tumor
- Benign
- Malignant
  - Primary
  - Metastatic

Postural
Congenital
Paralytic
- Neuropathic
- Myopathic

Contracture of Hip Flexors
Secondary to Shunts

TERMINOLOGY

A glossary of terms has been developed by the Scoliosis Research Society so that a working set of words is understood by everyone. In the past, there was much confusion between the terms *major, primary, secondary, compensatory, structural, nonstructural, postural, functional*. Hopefully, these terms are better defined and better understood now. The following list has been slightly modified from the original.

GLOSSARY

Adolescent scoliosis. Spinal curvature developing after onset of puberty and before maturity.

Adult scoliosis. Spinal curvature existing after skeletal maturity (closure of epiphyses).

Apical vertebra. The vertebra most deviated from the vertical axis of the patient.

Cervical curve. Spinal curvature that has its apex between C2 and C6.

Cervicothoracic curve. Spinal curvature that has its apex at C7 and T1.

Compensation. Accurate alignment of the midline of the skull over the midline of the sacrum.

Compensatory curve. A curve (which can be structural) above or below a major curve, that tends to maintain normal body alignment.

Congenital scoliosis. Scoliosis due to congenitally anomalous vertebral development.

Double structural curve (scoliosis). Two structural curves in the same spine, one balancing the other.

Double thoracic curve (scoliosis). Two structural curves, both having their apex within the thoracic spine.

End vertebra. The most cephalad vertebra of a curve whose superior surface or the most caudad one whose inferior surface tilts maximally toward the concavity of the curve.

Fractional curve. A curve that is incomplete because it returns to the erect position. Its only horizontal vertebra is its caudad or cephalad one.

Full curve. A curve in which the only horizontal vertebra is at the apex.

Gibbus. A sharply angular kyphos.

Infantile scoliosis. Spinal curvature developing during the first 3 years of life.

Juvenile scoliosis. Spinal curvature developing between the skeletal ages of 4 years and the onset of puberty.

Kyphos. An abnormal kyphosis.

Kyphoscoliosis. Lateral curvature of the spine associated with either increased posterior or decreased anterior angulation in the sagittal plane in excess of the accepted normal for that area.

Lordoscoliosis. Lateral curvature of the spine associated with an increase in anterior curvature or a decrease in posterior angulation in the sagittal plane in excess of normal for that area.

Lumbar curve. Spinal curvature that has its apex from L2–L4.

Lumbosacral curve. Spinal curvature that has its apex at L5 or below.

Major curve. The most apparent curve, and usually the most structural curve.

Nonstructural scoliosis. Spinal curvature without structural characteristics. (See structural curve.)

Pelvic obliquity. Deviation of the pelvis from the horizontal in the frontal plane.

Primary curve. The first or earliest of several curves to appear. Usually, but not necessarily, the most structural curve.

Structural curve. The segment of spine with a fixed lateral curvature. It is not necessarily the major or primary curve. Radiographically, it is identified in supine lateral side-bending or traction films by the failure to demonstrate normal flexibility.

Thoracic curve (scoliosis). Curve with the apex between T2 and T11.

Thoracolumbar curve. Spinal curvature that has its apex at T12 or L1 or at the interspace between these.

EVALUATION OF THE PATIENT

HISTORY TAKING

As in all fields of medicine, the taking of an adequate history is important. Quite frequently, this seems to be ignored in the field of scoliosis and other spine deformities. Important clues for both diagnosis and treatment can be derived from the taking of a good history.

The following questions are important: When did the deformity first appear? In what manner did it come to attention (pain, elevated shoulder, prominent hip, and so on)? Is the deformity progressive? Is there pain? Is there any family history of spine deformity? Is there any weakness, numbness, tingling sensation, or awkwardness of gait? Is there any family history of neurologic disease? Have there been any past illnesses? Has radiation been given? Is there any shortness of breath, either with or without exertion?

One of the most important aspects of spinal problems is growth. It is of the utmost importance to determine the status of growth. Therefore we ask: Is there still active growth? Have the menses begun? When? Has pubic hair development begun? Has breast development begun? In boys one asks about the onset of pubic hair development, change of voice, and onset of facial hair.

It is also important to ask about other observations or treatment. Has the patient seen another doctor? What was that doctor's opinion? Was treatment given? Was an x-ray taken? Were chiropractic treatments given? Was a brace applied? Was surgery done? What kind of surgery? Has the patient had surgery elsewhere than on the spine? Was a cast applied? What type? For how long? Were there any complications?

PHYSICAL EXAMINATION

Physical examination of the patient with spine deformity involves far more than the spine alone. The patient who presents with a scoliosis who has, on further examination, dislocation of the lenses of the eye, a heart murmur, and long thin fingers has Marfan's syndrome *with* scoliosis, not just scoliosis alone.

It must, therefore, always be remembered that scoliosis, kyphosis, and lordosis are only *symptoms* of an underlying disease process. It is unfortunate that the etiology of the most common cause of scoliosis (idiopathic) remains unknown. It is easy to fall into the habit of calling all scolioses "idiopathic," but one can easily have a spinal cord tumor, or a syringomyelia, or a Friedreich's ataxia, or any number of diagnoses that may first present with a scoliosis.

Examination of the Spine

Physical examination of the spine includes noting the area of the curve (*e.g.*, right thoracic, or double right thoracic and left lumbar), the magnitude of the curve, the amount of deviation of a plumb line from the occiput or from the seventh cervical vertebra (measured in centimeters), and the presence or absence of shoulder elevation (also measured in centimeters). The presence or absence of the flank crease is noted. The prominence of one hip should be noted, if present. Are the hips (iliac crests) level? Any deviation should be measured.

On forward bending *toward* the observer, the presence or absence of rib hump should be noted. A high left thoracic curve may show a slight hump on forward bending but can usually be seen more easily by noting prominence in the trapezius area at the base of the neck. The typical thoracic rib hump may be very mild or very severe. The quantity of rib hump should be measured in centimeters or in degrees of deviation from the horizontal. A level is placed at the point of maximal deformity. A vertical ruler is placed on the concave side at a point that is an equal distance from the midline as the point of maximal rib hump is from the midline on the convex side. This quantitates the rib hump deformity (it really measures the amount of "hump" plus the amount of "valley").

In forward bending away from the examiner, persistent deviation to one side suggests cord or cauda equina irritation. A bone scan and myelography are indicated in such patients to rule out tumors.

Anteriorly, one should note the presence or absence of rib flare on one side, asymmetry of breast development, the presence or absence of pectus excavatum or carinatum, and the state of breast development in the female.

It should be noted whether there is pure scoliosis, pure kyphosis, pure lordosis, or a combination of the above. The term *kyphoscoliosis* must be reserved for those patients with *both* kyphosis and scoliosis. A rib hump due solely to rotation should never be called kyphoscoliosis. Most patients with adolescent idiopathic scoliosis have *lordosis* of the throacic spine, not kyphosis.

Examination of Other Areas

The skin should be examined for the presence or absence of abnormal defects in the spine area such as lipomas, dermal sinuses, hairy patches, hemangiomas, or nevi. One should then look for generalized skin abnormalities, especially café-au-lait spots (a sign of neurofibromatosis). Hyperelasticity of the skin suggests Ehlers-Danlos syndrome.

The ears should be examined for congenital abnormalities, such as preauricular skin tags, a sign of Goldenhar's syndrome (oculoauriculovertebral dysplasia).

The palate should be examined. A high-arched palate is suggestive of Marfan's syndrome. A cleft palate suggests a congenital deformity.

The hands should be examined for congenital anomalies, for joint hyperelasticity (Ehlers-Danlos and Marfan's syndromes), and muscle weakness (e.g., clawing of the fingers in syringomyelia).

The hips should be examined for range of motion, especially for contractures. In paralytic disorders, look for tightness of the extensors, flexors, adductors, abductors, and the iliotibial bands. (See the section about neuromuscular spine deformity).

The feet can reveal much, especially in the diagnosis of neuromuscular problems. High arches suggest Friedreich's ataxia or Charcot-Marie-Tooth syndrome. Clubfeet, vertical tali, or heel varus suggests spinal dysraphism. The presence of both a foot deformity and a spine deformity in the same patient suggests either a generalized neurologic disorder or spinal dysraphism (e.g., diastematomyelia, intraspinal lipoma, filum terminale).

Neurologic examination should include biceps, triceps, and patellar- and Achilles-tendon reflexes. The Babinski's reflexes should be tested in all patients. A basic motor and sensory examination of the extremities is important. A Romberg test and finger-to-nose examination should be done for any existent or suspected neuromuscular problem. Straight-leg raising should always be done to look for cauda equina irritation or tight hamstrings (Fig. 16–1).

RADIOLOGIC EVALUATION

Measurement of Curvature

One of the greatest advancements in the field of scoliosis and other spine deformities was the development of techniques for accurate measurement of the quantity of deformity. All techniques suffer from certain inadequacies, particularly in that most spine deformities are three-dimensional and the measurement techniques are only two-dimensional. Nevertheless, by measuring both the anteroposterior and lateral projections, the physician can document well the quantity and pattern of deformity. Several techniques for measurement have been developed, but the most widely accepted and the one officially recommended by the Scoliosis Research Society is the *Cobb technique*.

This technique must be learned well and applied precisely; otherwise, major errors in treatment will result. It may be absolutely critical whether a curve is progressive or not. Only precise measurement can provide the answer. It is impossible to compare two x-rays accurately without measurement.

In the Cobb technique, first select the end vertebrae of the curve. *The end vertebrae are those vertebrae that are the most tilted from the horizontal.* By convention, the upright x-ray (usually standing, but sitting for those with leg paralysis) is used for this determination. A line is drawn along the upper end-plate of the upper end vertebra and along the lower end-plate of the lower end vertebra. Perpendiculars are erected from these two lines. The angle of intersection of these perpendiculars is the angle of the curvature.

If there is difficulty in determining which is the end vertebra, lines can be drawn along the end-plate of *every* vertebra and projected out to the edge of the x-ray. It will then be noted that those lines from the vertebrae in the curve will converge in the concavity of the curve. Those vertebrae outside the curve being measured will diverge.

When there is a double curvature, both curves should be measured. There is one vertebrae that will be the upper end vertebra for the lower curve and the lower end vertebra for the upper curve. This is called the *transitional* vertebra. It is necessary to place only one line on this vertebra, because usually the upper and lower end-plates are parallel.

Once these end vertebrae have been established, measurement should always be from the same vertebrae. The supine x-ray and the bending x-ray should also be measured from the *same* end vertebrae as chosen on the erect film, even though they may not be the maximally tilted vertebrae on these other films.

Occasionally, one will see a curve in which the end vertebra is difficult to determine because two or more vertebrae are parallel. In such a case, select the parallel vertebra *furthest* from the apex of the curve.

Usually the end-plates are clearly seen and the line along the end-plate can be drawn with great precision. Independent observers should be able to measure the same x-ray within 1 or 2 degrees. One some occasions, the end-plate cannot be clearly defined (especially in congenital scoliosis), in which case it is permissible to use a line drawn along the lower border of each pedicle. The same points of reference should then be used on subsequent films (Fig. 16–2).

Measurement of Kyphosis and Lordosis

The measurement of the lateral x-ray has largely been ignored but is just as important as the anteroposterior x-ray. The Cobb technique can be readily applied to the measurement of both kyphosis and lordosis. The same basic principles apply, that is, the selection of end vertebrae based on the maximally tilted vertebrae as seen on a lateral upright x-ray, preferably with the patient standing. Considerable variation of measurement of sagittal curves can occur as a result of the patient's position and muscle tone at the moment that

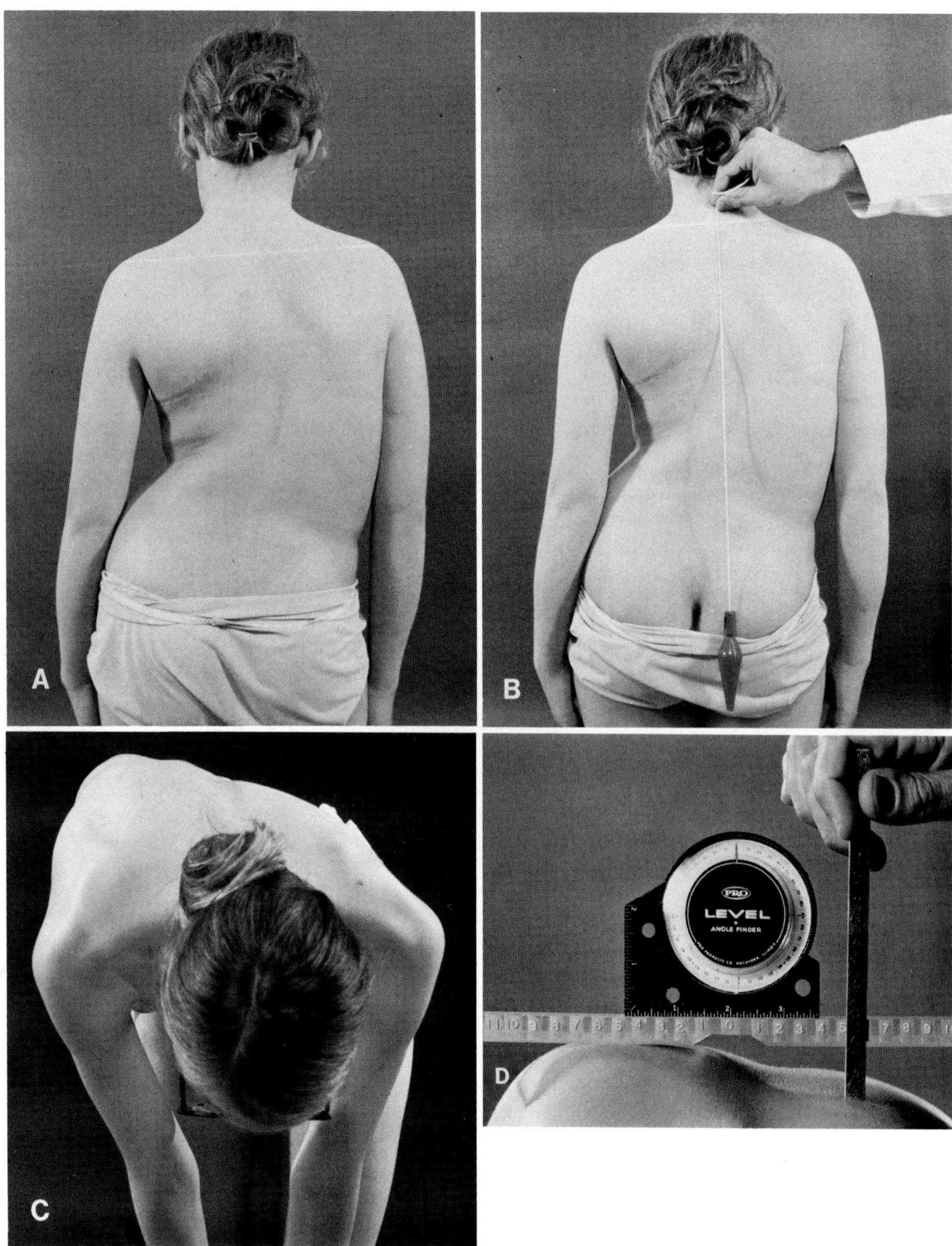

FIG. 16-1. Physical examination. *(A)* Back view of a patient. *(B)* Back view of patient with a plumb line. *(C)* Forward bending view from the head to show the thoracic rotation. *(D)* The thoracic bending as measured by a standardized technique. The center of the level is placed over the midline spinus processes. The level is placed at the zero mark. The maximal prominence is noted to be at 5 cm lateral to the midline and, therefore, 5 cm to the opposite side. A ruler is dropped and the distance is measured. This technique measures both the hump and the valley, as a single figure. In this case, it is 2.4 cm.

the x-ray is taken. The most reliable films are obtained with the patient standing in a normal tone with the arms *forward and resting on a pole or frame* (Figs. 16–3 and 16–4).

Other Radiologic Examinations

Laminography (Tomography). Laminograms are useful for special problems. The most common use is in the better definition of congenital anomalies. It may be difficult to determine the exact nature of a jumbled mass of abnormal bones on a routine film, but the laminogram can distinguish the exact anomaly. Laminograms are also useful for the detection of osteoid osteomas, which, if present in the spine, usually produce scoliosis, and for the better definition of certain fracture problems.

Myelography. Myelography is also useful in certain complex problems. A myelogram is always indicated if there is *any suspicion* of a spinal cord tumor, *any suspicion* of a spinal dysraphism, or any neurologic problems secondary to the curvature. Myelography, if done, should always examine the entire spinal canal, never just the lower spine. If there is kyphosis, the patient will require either a high-volume myelogram or supine positioning in order to adequately visualize the cord at the apex of the curve.

Water-soluble myelographic techniques are rapidly replacing the oil-based dyes. For good definition in the lumbar area, especially for dysraphic lesions, water-soluble techniques are virtually mandatory (see Fig. 16–31).

Computed Tomography (CT Scan). This advanced technique is seldom useful in the evaluation of ordinary curvature problems but is highly useful for bone tumors, infections, spinal stenosis, and some fractures. It can be combined with water-soluble myelography, a technique particularly useful for dysraphic problems, tumors, and cystic lesions.

Evaluation of Rotation

It is important to be able to recognize rotation on the x-ray, because the length of the arthrodesis is partly determined by the appreciation of rotation. The quantity or amount of rotation can be measured and graded, but, at the present time, it seems to be of little practical value.

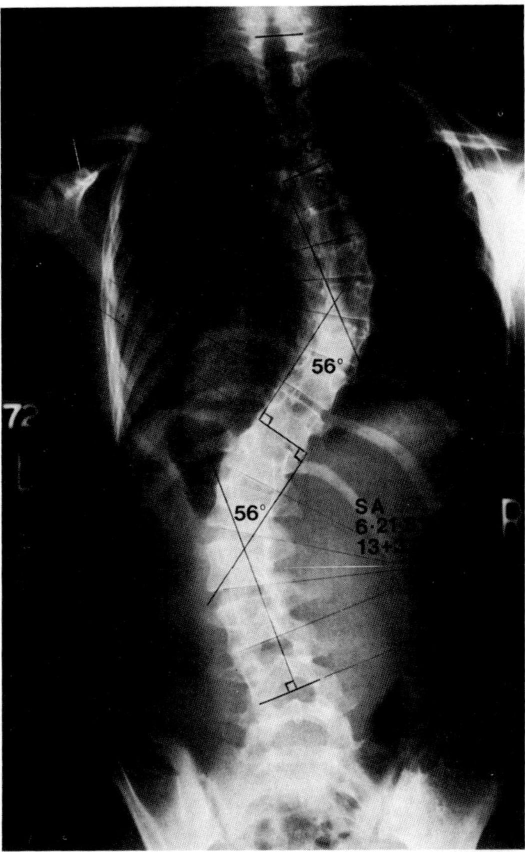

FIG. 16-2. A typical scoliosis with a line drawn along the lower end-plate of each vertebra. Note that the lines converge to the left for the right thoracic curve and to the right for the left lumbar curve. The most tilted vertebrae are the end vertebrae of the curve. At the junction of the two curves, one vertebra is the end vertebra of both curves (the "transitional" vertebra).

After selection of the lower end vertebra of the curve (the vertebrae most tilted from the horizontal), a line is placed along the end-plate of this vertebra, and a perpendicular is erected from that. Similarly, the upper end vertebra is selected, a line is drawn along its upper end-plate, and a perpendicular is erected that crosses the first one drawn. The angle of intersection is the angle of the curvature (Cobb-Lippman technique of scoliosis measurement).

The proper measurement of the double major curve pattern is shown here. One line on the transitional vertebra serves for measurement of both the upper and lower curves.

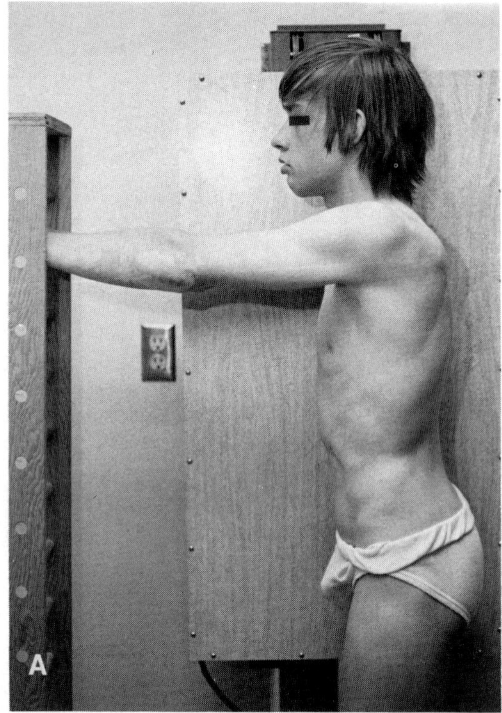

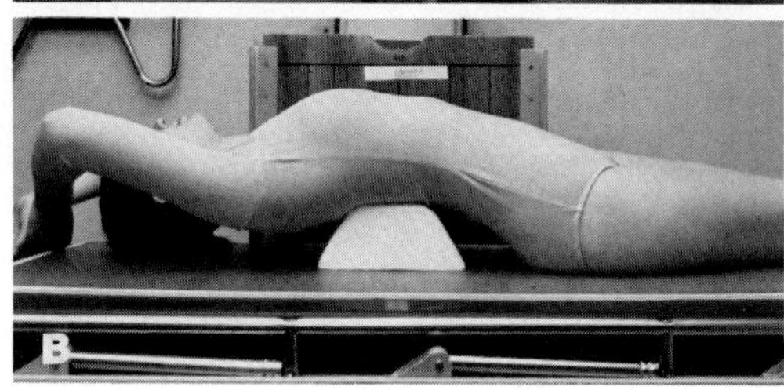

FIG. 16-3. Positioning for lateral roentgenograms. *(A)* The proper position for obtaining a lateral standing roentgenogram. Note that the patient's arms are resting on a ladder at 90° to the torso. The patient is standing in a neutral posture (*i.e.*, neither attempting to stand slouched or "super" straight). *(B)* To obtain a hyperextension roentgenogram to test the flexibility of a kyphosis, the patient is hyperextended over a firm plastic block placed at the apex of the kyphosis. A cross-table lateral roentgenogram is then obtained.

PULMONARY FUNCTION TESTING

The major reason for treating scoliosis, especially thoracic scoliosis, is preservation of lung capacity. Thus, it can be quite important to know whether or not pulmonary function has been affected by the curve. In the patient with significant deformity, it is important to know how much damage has been done, because this can materially affect the risks of surgery and, thus, the technique of surgical management.

In borderline situations when a decision must be made as to whether or not the patient should have surgery, pulmonary function testing should be used to assist in the decision. If there is decrease in the lung function, surgery should be done. If the lung function is normal, perhaps surgery is not needed.

When performing pulmonary function tests in scoliotic patients, serious errors can occur if the patient's *actual* height is used for calculation. The scoliosis causes loss of height, and a falsely high value will be obtained. Always correct for true height. We use arm span with a conversion factor to eliminate this problem.

Both volume analysis, including flows, and blood gases are necessary for the evaluation. The blood gases are more reliable than the volumes, because they are independent of true height and independent of voluntary action and cooperation.

Beware of patients with thoracic lordosis. These patients have a far greater loss of pulmonary function than one would expect from their anteroposterior x-ray. The presence of thoracic lordosis significantly alters the indications for surgery.

THE ADULT SEQUELAE OF UNTREATED SPINAL DEFORMITY

What happens to scoliotic patients who receive no treatment during the growing years? How do they function as adults? Do they have problems related to their spine? These are all very pertinent questions and must be answered before undertaking the active treatment of the growing child. If, indeed, there were no problems in the adult scoliotic, we would be hard pressed to justify the stresses, anxieties, and problems encountered in treating the child.

One way to best answer these questions would be to document the actual natural history of a group of untreated patients who have gone many years into adult life. Such documentation is available in several studies. The best study was done by Nilsonne and Lundgren,[60] in which 113 patients with idiopathic scoliosis were reviewed an average of 50 years after being seen at a scoliosis clinic from 1913 to 1918. Ninety percent of the patients were located. Forty-five percent were dead, twice

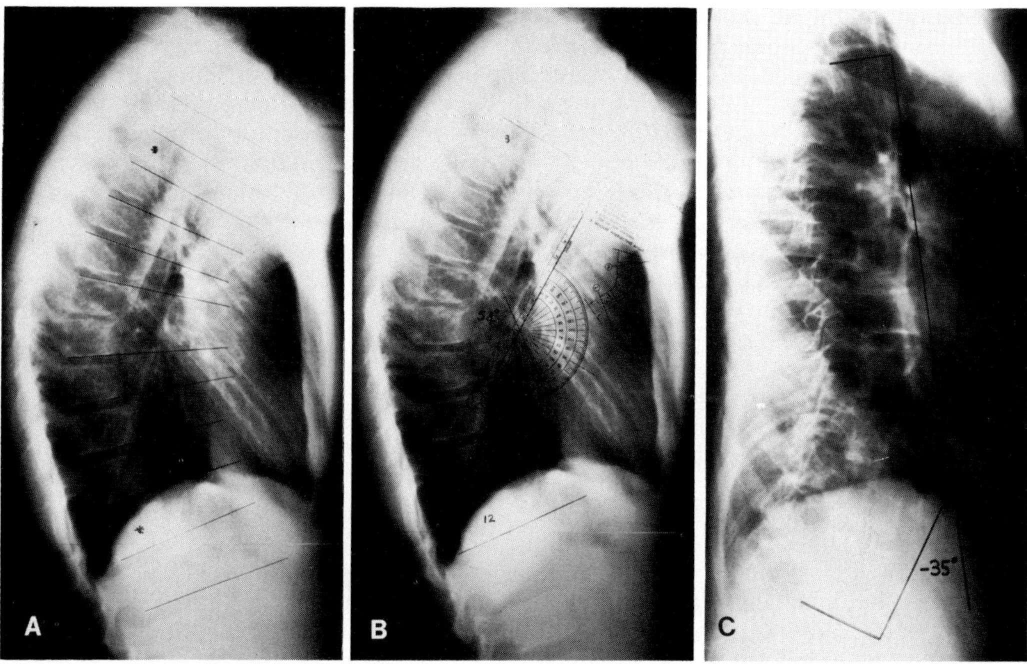

FIG. 16-4. Measurement of roentgenograms for kyphosis and lordosis. *(A)* A standing lateral roentgenogram with lines drawn along the end-plate of all the vertebrae. Note that T3 and T12 are the vertebrae most tipped from the horizontal and are thus the end vertebrae. *(B)* By the same technique as is used for scoliosis, perpendiculars are erected from the lines along the end-plates, and the angle of intersection defines the angle of the curvature. In this case, the patient exhibits a 54°T3–T12 thoracic kyphosis. *(C)* This patient exhibits thoracic lordosis. The same technique of measurement is used. Any lordotic measurement less than 0° is recorded as a negative number, in this case −35°.

the expected mortality rate for the age. Most of the deaths were a result of cardiac or pulmonary disease. There was a noticeable increase in mortality after age 45 years. Of the females, 76% had never married. No one was engaged in heavy labor, and 47% were on disability pensions, 30% specifically because of their spinal deformities. Ninety percent had symptoms of a bad back.

In a very similar article in the same journal issue, Nachemson[58] reviewed 130 patients with various types of scoliosis, again 90% being located for follow-up an average of 35 years later. Again the mortality rate for the group as a whole was twice that of the population in general. If only thoracic curves were considered, the mortality rate was four times that of the general population. The mortality rate was higher in paralytic and congenital curves. Forty percent of the patients noted backache, 30% were disabled (the expected rate of disability was 15%). No one was employed in heavy labor.

A third study of the long-term results of untreated idiopathic scoliosis was done by Collis and Ponseti.[15] They attempted to locate the 353 patients reviewed in 1950 by Ponseti and Friedman.[62] This study is the only one in the world with both original and current x-rays. They located and personally examined 105 patients, and an additional 100 patients were reviewed by questionnaire only. The average follow-up was 24 years. Most curves increased after skeletal maturity. Thoracic curves of 60° to 80° progressed the most, an average of 28°. Thoracic curves less than 60° showed an average of only 9° of progression. Lumbar curves of more than 30° progressed an average of 18°, whereas those less than 30° did not progress.

The mortality rate was less than that seen in the two Swedish series noted above, but the length of follow-up was shorter and there was a much lower percent of deaths at follow-up. Decreased vital capacity was noted in all thoracic curves over 60°. Dyspnea was noted in 40% of patients, usually in those with thoracic curves of 85° or more. Although 54% of the patients had backache complaints, the authors did not think that this incidence was higher than that of the population as a whole. Only 8 of the 205 patients had been hospitalized for back pain. It is unfortunate that 148 (42%) of the original patients could not be located.

The great lesson of these studies is that scolioses are not always static once growth ceases. Some progress, especially thoracic curves of 60° or more, and will cause decreased pulmonary function and a significant likelihood of premature death due to respiratory failure. The question of lumbar curves is less obvious. Undoubtedly, lumbar curves over 50° do tend to progress, but whether there is higher likelihood of back pain is unknown.

Another way to determine the presence or absence of adult problems in the scoliotic patient is to examine the files of those physicians who might have contact with the scoliosis patient in adult life. If no adults came to these physicians, one could safely say that adults do not have significant problems. However, such is not the case. Many patients go to internists and pulmonary physicians because of respiratory failure with or without secondary right heart failure. The pathodynamics of "scoliotic heart failure" were well outlined by Bergofsky and associates[5] in 1959.

Similarly, the orthopaedic surgeon interested in scoliosis sees many adult scoliotics for a variety of problems. Several series of patients treated in adult life have been reported. The most common complaint is pain, especially in lumbar curves. Some patients come to the orthopaedic surgeons because of dyspnea. They are hopeful that the curve can be straightened and their breathing improved. Some are concerned about the cosmetic disfigurement of their "hump."

Finally, there is a small group of patients who come because of paralysis due to the spine deformity. They are more likely to be patients with severe kyphosis.

It can thus be stated with certainty that scoliosis is not necessarily a benign condition. Early death from respiratory failure is likely in thoracic curves over 60°, if they are left untreated. Lumbar curves, especially those over 50°, are likely to progress in adult life. These patients have a high likelihood of degenerative disc disease and pain. Therefore, even if cosmetic and emotional factors are not taken into account (and they may be of considerable importance), aggressive treatment of the child with a spinal deformity is justified (Figs. 16-5 and 16-6).

NONSTRUCTURAL SCOLIOSIS

Postural Scoliosis

Although the normal spine is perfectly straight in the frontal plane, there are certain children who do not voluntarily stand perfectly straight. They may slouch and cause one or more curvatures to be present. Usually these are thoracic kyphosis and lumbar lordosis, but there may also be a scoliosis of mild degree. It is usually easy to detect the difference between postural and structural scoliosis by a careful physical and x-ray examination. Postural scoliosis is not associated with a rib hump on forward bending. It disappears in the prone position and when the child is asked to stand in a very straight position. On the x-ray, the curves are different from a structural scoliosis. There is a long curve, usually extending from one end of the spine to the other, and it is not associated with rotation. The supine x-ray is usually perfectly straight and bending films show no areas of contracture. Such curves do not progress nor do they become structural.

Leg Length Discrepancy

A difference in the length of the legs will result in a curvature of the spine in the standing position. This is a functional or nonstructural curve in that there is no intrinsic stiffness of the curve in the spine. When the patient is sitting or lying down, the curve disappears. When the difference in leg length is corrected, the curve disappears. One is frequently asked whether the presence of a leg length discrepancy for a long period of time will result in a functional curve becoming structural. This is highly doubtful, because we spend so little of our time standing on our two feet with even weight. When we walk, we shift weight from one leg to the other. When we sit, the discrepancy disappears and we usually spend a great deal of time lying down. Thus, the inequality of leg length does not act on the

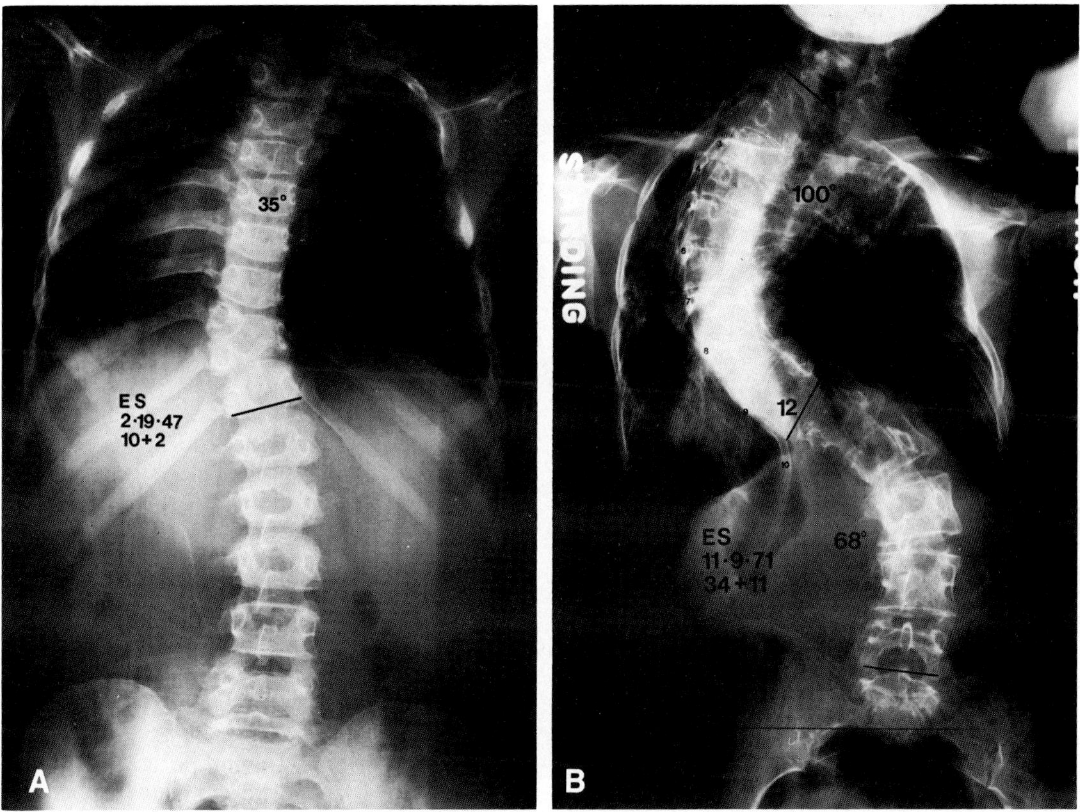

FIG. 16-5. *(A)* A 10-year-old girl with a congenital scoliosis of 35° as measured from T1–T12. She has an obvious hemivertebra at T10 on the left and a second one at T2 also on the left. There are only nine ribs on the right. This curve was thought to be benign and no treatment was recommended. *(B)* The same patient 25 years later when she presented to the author with cor pulmonale and a scoliosis of 100°. She died soon after this.

spine more than a small percentage of each day. People with leg length discrepancies over a long period of time do not usually have any fixed scoliosis (*e.g.,* hemihypertrophy). Neuromuscular conditions that may result in leg length discrepancy (*e.g.,* poliomyelitis) can also cause a structural scoliosis so that the two may coincide because of the common etiology (Fig. 16-7).

Hysterical Scoliosis

Hysterical scoliosis has been reported by Blount.[6] It is certainly possible for some emotionally disturbed teenagers to develop a curvature of the spine. This is constant in the upright position, usually constant in the sitting position, but may or may not be present in the prone or supine position. It is always absent while sleeping and will disappear under an anesthetic. It is characterized by curvatures that have a long, sweeping, bizarre pattern not associated with rotation on the x-ray or true rib hump on forward bending. There may be considerable contortions of the torso during the examination process, which may confuse the examiner as to the presence or absence of thoracic deformity. X-rays taken in the supine or prone position may demonstrate the absence of any fixed curve. If necessary, x-rays can be obtained under heavy sedation or even under an anesthetic. Before labeling a child as hysterical, one must be absolutely sure that there is no spinal cord tumor or other neurologic pathology present. Consultation is strongly recommended. Hysterical scoliosis should not be treated by orthopaedic methods (*e.g.,* exercises, braces, or casts) and certainly never by surgery. This is a psychiatric problem and

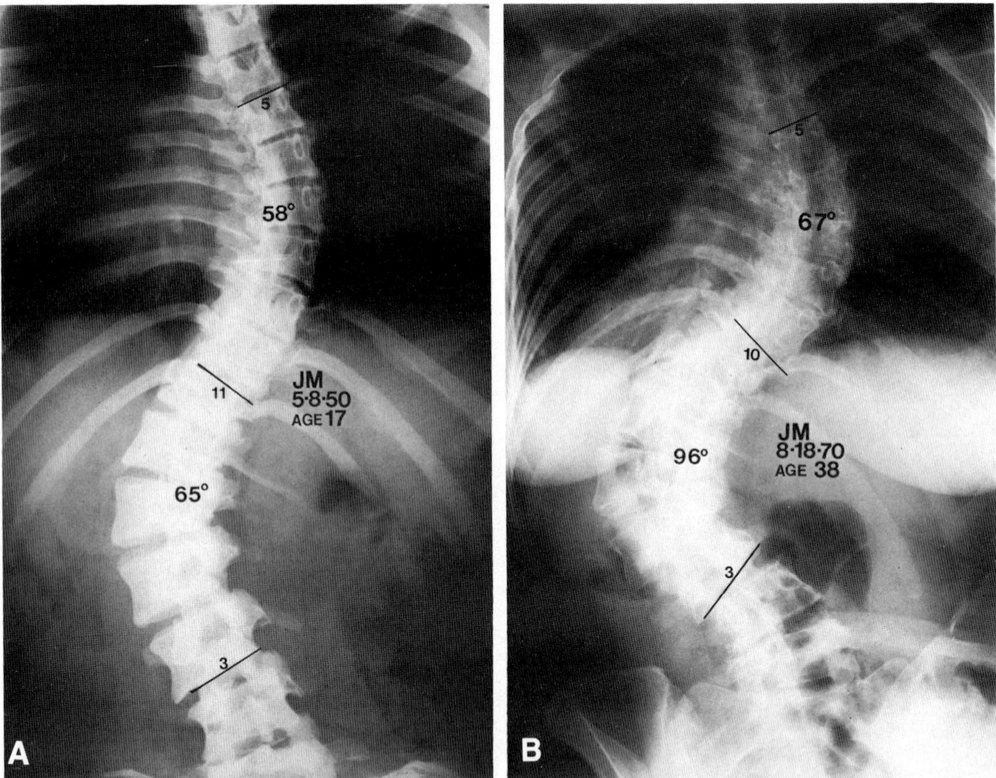

FIG. 16-6. *(A)* A double structural idiopathic scoliosis in a 17-year-old girl with a Risser sign of 4+. The thoracic curve measures 58°, and the lumbar curve 65°. She was told at this time that she had "nicely balanced curves that should give her no problem in the future." *(B)* The same patient at age 38 years, when she presented to the author with severe back pain and severe sciatica in the left leg. This type of progression is common with lumbar curve greater than 60°.

should be dealt with promptly by specialists in this field. Continued orthopaedic treatment will only lead to a greater degree of fixation of the hysteria (Fig. 16-8).

IDIOPATHIC SCOLIOSIS

Introduction

Idiopathic scoliosis is the most common form of scoliosis. Unfortunately, there is no concrete evidence as to the cause of this problem. The child is usually perfectly healthy, has a normal spine at birth and develops a curvature at some time during growth, usually between the ages of 9 and 12 years. The incidence of idiopathic scoliosis is slightly more common in females, but the female has a far greater tendency to progression of the curve to the point where treatment is required. There is certainly a genetic pattern, but the exact nature of the genetics is unknown. Cowell and colleagues[16] believe that it is an autosomal dominant trait, but Wynn-Davies[90] believes that it is a multifactoral trait. Recent studies have confirmed a malfunction of the vestibular balancing system.[68,69]

INFANTILE IDIOPATHIC SCOLIOSIS

Infantile idiopathic scoliosis is a definite entity, most commonly seen in Great Britain, but also to a lesser extent in other parts of Europe. In this condition, the scoliosis appears some time between birth and age 3 years.

Infantile idiopathic scoliosis is more common in the male than in the female and usually produces a curve to the left; the curve is thoracolumbar. Fortunately, approximately 85% of the time, the curve spontaneously disap-

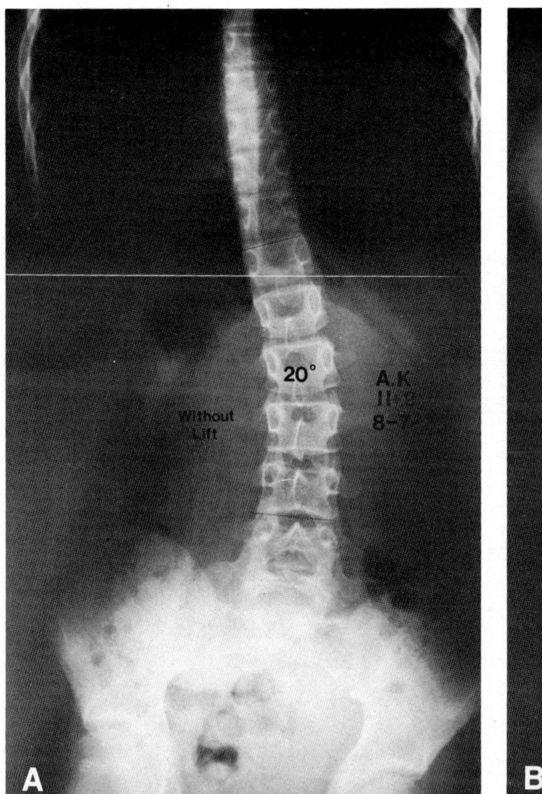

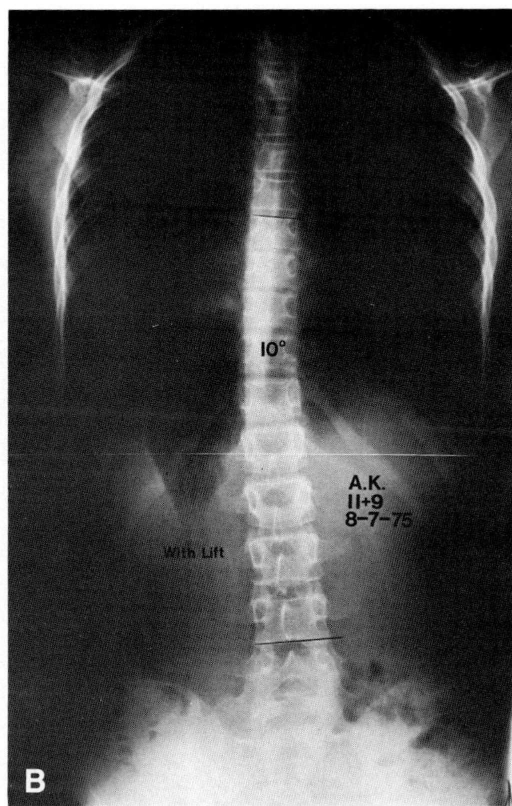

FIG. 16-7. *(A)* This 11-year-old girl was seen for a finding of scoliosis. She has a 20° right lumbar scoliosis from T11–L3, but there is no rotation of the vertebrae in the curve. This is a standing roentgenogram, and the significant leg length discrepancy can easily be seen. *(B)* The same patient on the same day but with the film taken with a 2.5-cm lift under the right foot. The scoliosis has disappeared.

pears. The work of Lloyd-Roberts and Pilcher[44] has shown that this spontaneous regression of the curve occurs without any treatment.

The 15% of curves that are not self-resolving are progressive. They lead to very severe deformities. These have been well documented by James.[37] Thus, it is important to note carefully whether or not an infantile idiopathic scoliosis is progressive. This can be determined only by careful serial examination and serial roentgenograms. Mehta[54] developed a method for measurement of the difference in the angle at which the rib meets the spine at the apex of the curve. This measurement is called the "rib-vertebral angle difference," or "RVAD." If the angle is greater than 20°, it is likely that the child will have a progressive infantile idiopathic scoliosis. This has proven to be helpful, but not absolutely reliable, in determining the curve potential.

Treatment

No treatment is necessry for the nonprogressive type. It spontaneously resolves without treatment; to apply treatment is to deceive both the physician and the family. Progressive curves must be treated and treated vigorously. Generally speaking, the patient with nonprogressive infantile idiopathic scoliosis does not have a curve greater than 35°. Thus, the easiest rule is to apply orthopaedic treatment to those curves that are shown to be progressive, to have a magnitude of 35° or more, or a rib-vertebral angle difference of 20° or more (Fig. 16-9).

The treatment of choice for the progressive curve is serial casting followed by a Milwaukee brace. It is difficult to make a good brace for a child of 1 year of age, but with care, it can be done. The model for the pelvic section is taken under an anesthetic to obtain a decent

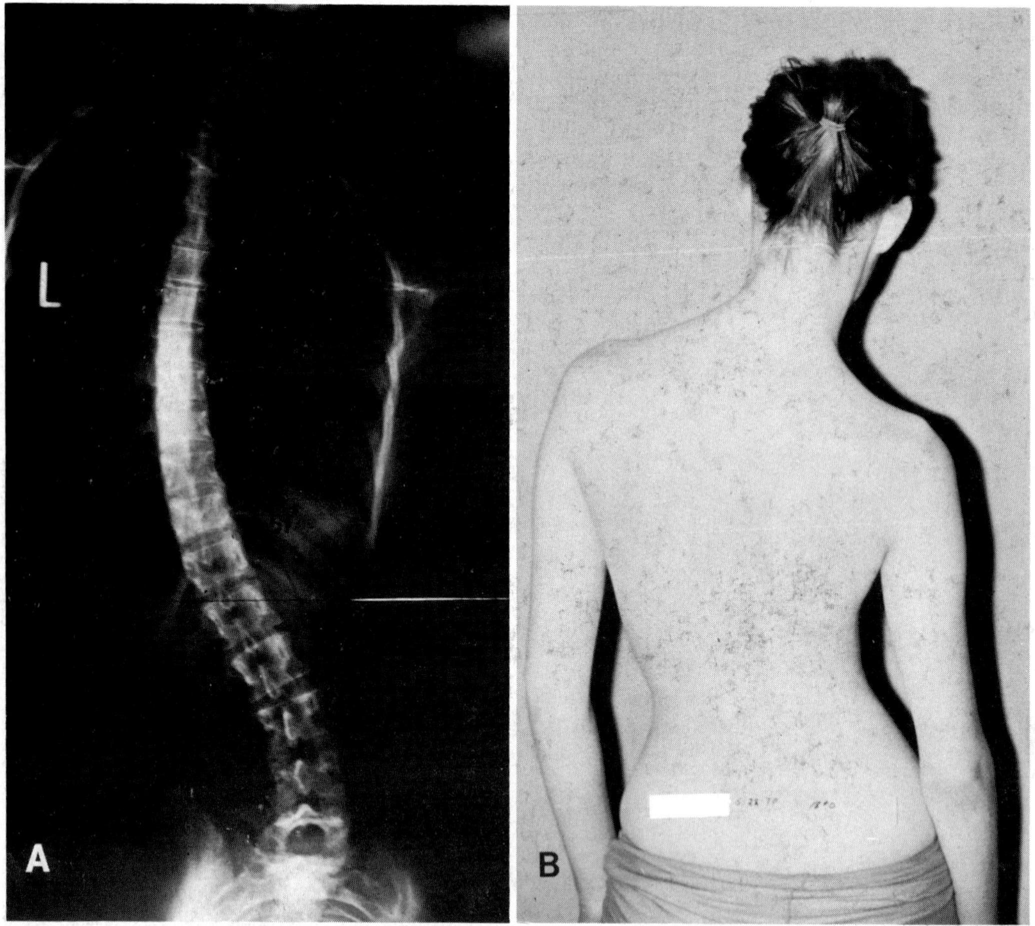

FIG. 16-8. *(A)* A long, sweeping nonrotated scoliosis. This particular pattern of curvature does not resemble any of the usual types of scoliosis. *(B)* A photograph of the patient, taken at the same time as the roentgenogram, demonstrates the clinical appearance. This patient had a purely hysterical scoliosis. The curve eventually disappeared after 3 years of psychiatric treatment.

molding about the hips. A lateral holding pad should be applied. The brace should be maintained on a full-time schedule, removing it only for bathing purposes. Usually the brace will successfully manage the curve for many years. Some patients (''benign progressive type'' of Mehta) can be cured of the scoliosis. The more severe patient (''malignant progressive type'') will usually require fusion at a later time.

Milwaukee brace treatment must continue until the curve is maximally and permanently corrected or until the curve progresses in the brace and demonstrates a need for surgery. The curve must never be allowed to go beyond 60°. If, in a good Milwaukee brace, the curve is still progressing, application of a Risser localizer cast will usually maintain a better improvement than in the brace. If the curve progresses despite all nonoperative measures, instrumentation without fusion should be instituted. By this technique, arthrodesis can be delayed until a more optimal time, preferably age 12 in girls and age 14 in boys (Fig. 16-10).

JUVENILE IDIOPATHIC SCOLIOSIS

By definition, juvenile idiopathic scoliosis is that type of idiopathic scoliosis occurring after the age of 3 years but before the onset of puberty. The age difference between late onset of juvenile idiopathic scoliosis and early onset of adolescent idiopathic scoliosis is not

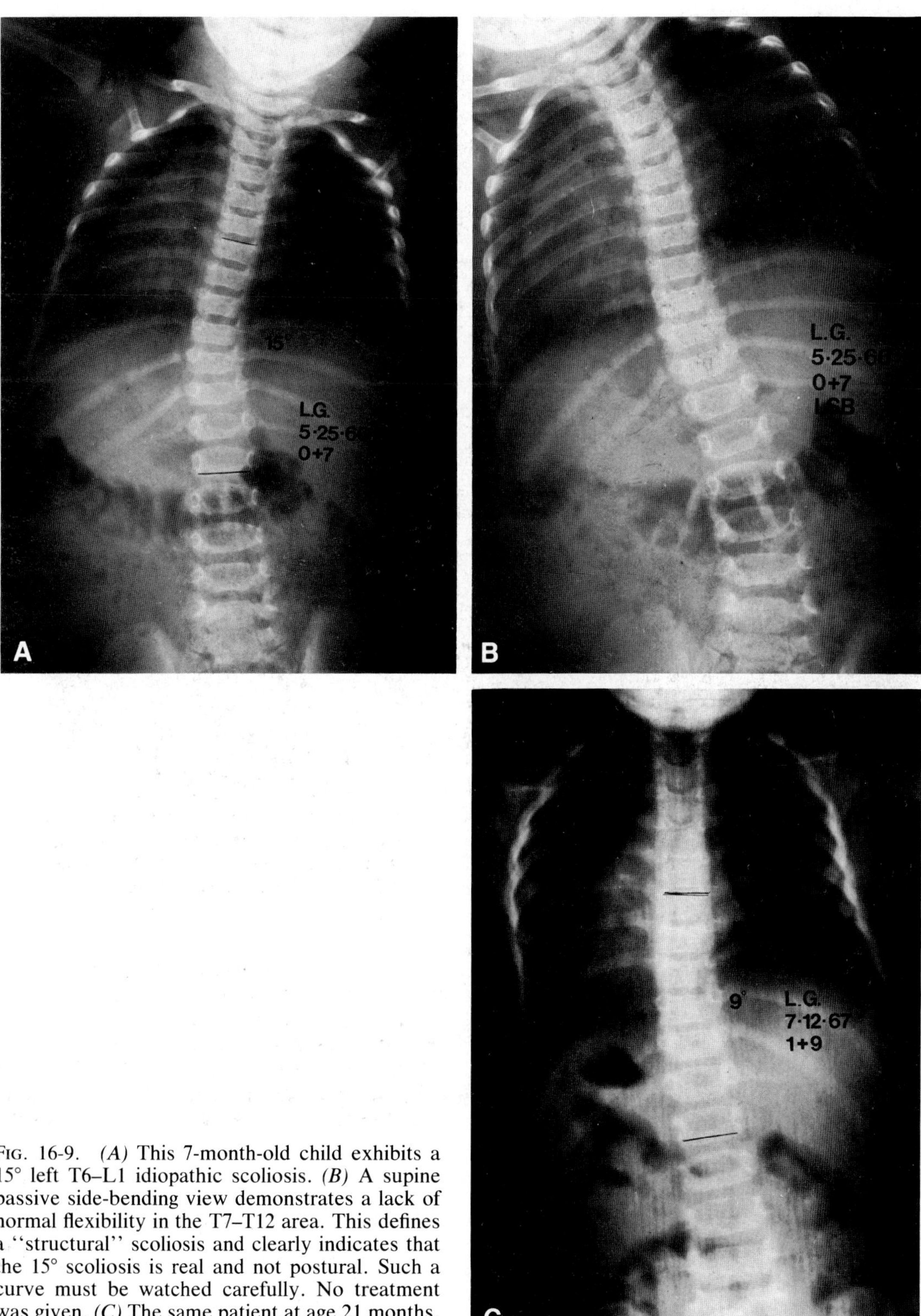

Fig. 16-9. *(A)* This 7-month-old child exhibits a 15° left T6–L1 idiopathic scoliosis. *(B)* A supine passive side-bending view demonstrates a lack of normal flexibility in the T7–T12 area. This defines a "structural" scoliosis and clearly indicates that the 15° scoliosis is real and not postural. Such a curve must be watched carefully. No treatment was given. *(C)* The same patient at age 21 months. The scoliosis is spontaneously resolving.

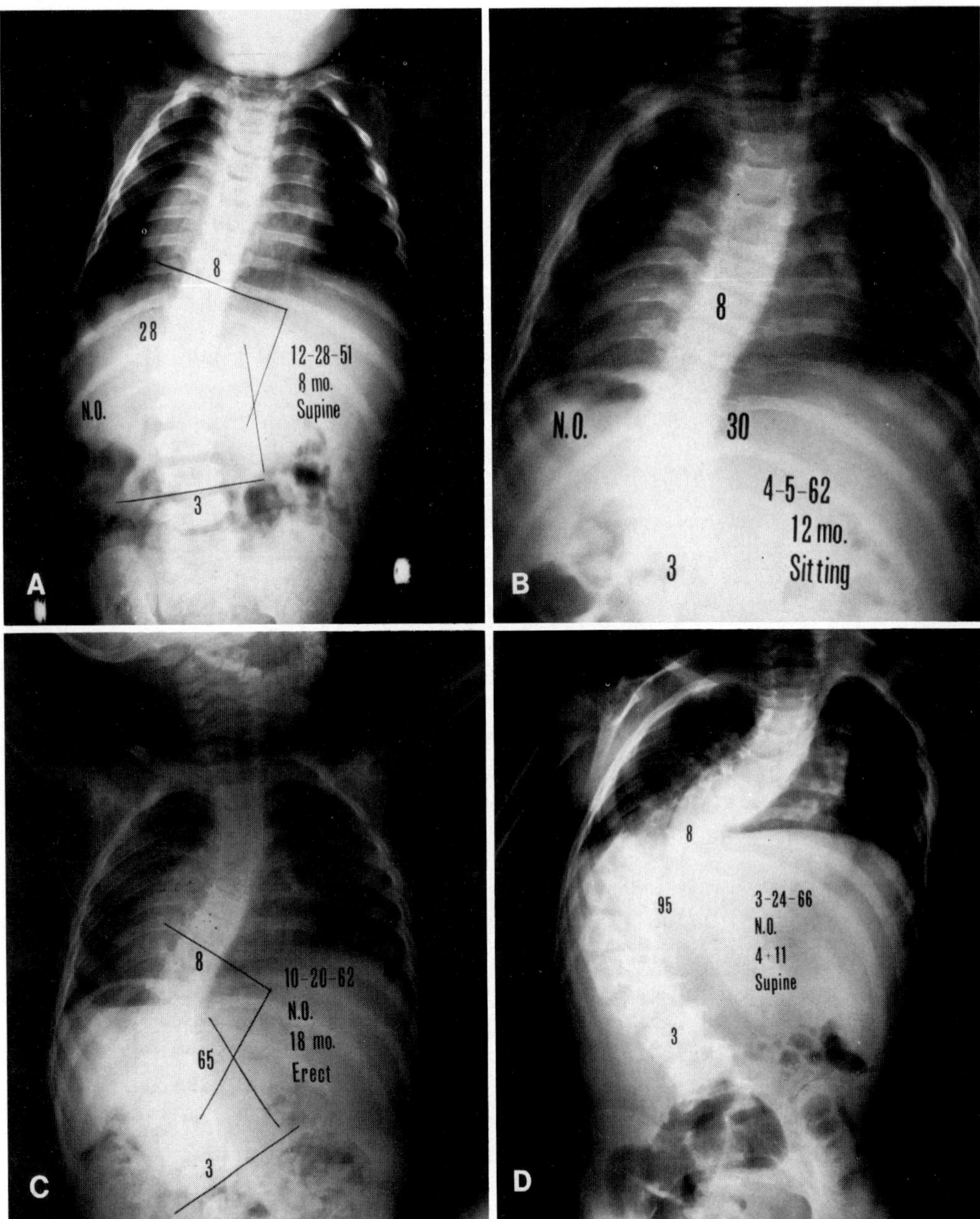

FIG. 16-10. *(A)* An 8-month-old girl with a 28° left thoracolumbar infantile idiopathic scoliosis. *(B)* The patient, sitting, at age 12 months. The curve measures 30°. *(C)* The patient at age 18 months. In a sitting roentgenogram, the curve now measures 65°, indicating a rapidly progressive curvature. The curve should not have been allowed to deteriorate to this degree without treatment. *(D)* The patient at age 4 years 11 months. A supine roentgenogram shows the curve to have increased to 95°. This progression represents a tragic delay in treatment. (Photographs kindly donated by Dr. John A. Moe)

a sharp line, and the two blend into one another. Nevertheless, there is a significant difference between a deformity appearing at age 6 or 7 years and one beginning at age 10 or 11 years. Juvenile idiopathic scoliosis is quite different from infantile idiopathic scoliosis in that the curvatures usually do not resolve spontaneously. The curves usually progress steadily for many years and may produce extremely severe deformities, very similar to infantile idiopathic scoliosis. A few curves may remain relatively small and rather static for several years and then progress at a later time. Thus, any patient with progressive juvenile idiopathic scoliosis must be treated. Any patient with a curve of 20° or more should also be treated, because the likelihood of progression is so high. It is not wise to watch curves greater than 20° without treatment. A golden opportunity to achieve permanent correction of the curve will have been lost.

The best treatment for curves of less than 60° is the Milwaukee brace. In the juvenile years, the spine is more flexible and more correctable than it is later. The results of Milwaukee brace treatment are excellent, even though many years of brace treatment are necessary. Sometimes permanent correction can be achieved during growth, and the brace can be completely or partially discontinued before the end of growth. Quite often such a stable correction can be achieved that part-time wearing is possible, even though the patient is still growing. A minimum of 2 years of full-time use is necessary. The brace should never be completely discontinued while the child is still growing.

Progressive juvenile idiopathic scoliosis despite brace or cast treatment should have instrumentation without fusion. The author uses a Harrington rod protected by a Milwaukee brace. The rod is lengthened or replaced every 6 months. Arthrodesis is done at age 12 in girls and at age 14 in boys or sooner if the curve deteriorates despite the rodding and bracing.[39]

ADOLESCENT IDIOPATHIC SCOLIOSIS

Adolescent idiopathic scoliosis is the most common cause of spinal deformity. Approximately 80% of all children coming to any scoliosis clinic will have this condition. By definition, the onset is at or just after puberty. In actual practice, the age of onset is very difficult to determine. Several curve patterns may occur, the most common being right thoracic. The second most common is right thoracic and left lumbar; the third most common is thoracolumbar, the fourth most common is double thoracic, (left thoracic-right thoracic); and the least common is an isolated left lumbar curve. Rarely, one sees a right lumbar curve or a right thoracic and left thoracolumbar double pattern.

As stated previously, the etiology of this condition is not known at this time. Many speculations have been offered, but definite proof is lacking. There is a strong genetic tendency, and females are more likely to have the progressive type of curve requiring treatment. Most series of spine operations for idiopathic scoliosis show a female to male ratio of 8 to 1, but school screening surveys show a female to male ratio of 1.5 to 1.0.

The curves usually begin early, at age 10 or 11 years. At this point in time, they are very small and not easily detected. Mass screening techniques have, however, shown the existence of these curves at this time; thus, we know that the curves are usually present just prior to puberty. At the time of puberty, an increase in the curvature takes place in certain patients. Thus, during the growth spurt, we see the appearance of a number of significant curves. As stated previously, these patients usually are perfectly healthy and have no other medical problems. Careful history and physical examination must be carried out to ensure that other conditions that may mimic idiopathic scoliosis are not missed. Syringomyelia is probably the most likely condition to go undetected, because it often produces a curve that mimics idiopathic scoliosis precisely. Neurologic changes early in syringomyelia are quite subtle. Spinal cord tumors may also simulate idiopathic scoliosis.

The natural history of adolescent idiopathic scoliosis is quite varied. Some patients never progress at all. They may have a 10° curve at age 10 years, which may remain constant, may totally disappear, or may progress. At the present time, there is no way to distinguish in the 10-year-old child whether or not the curve is going to progress, resolve, or remain static. Thus, the physician is obligated to observe this situation carefully and to note whether or not progression occurs. Progression indicates the need for treatment.

The possibility of progression varies with

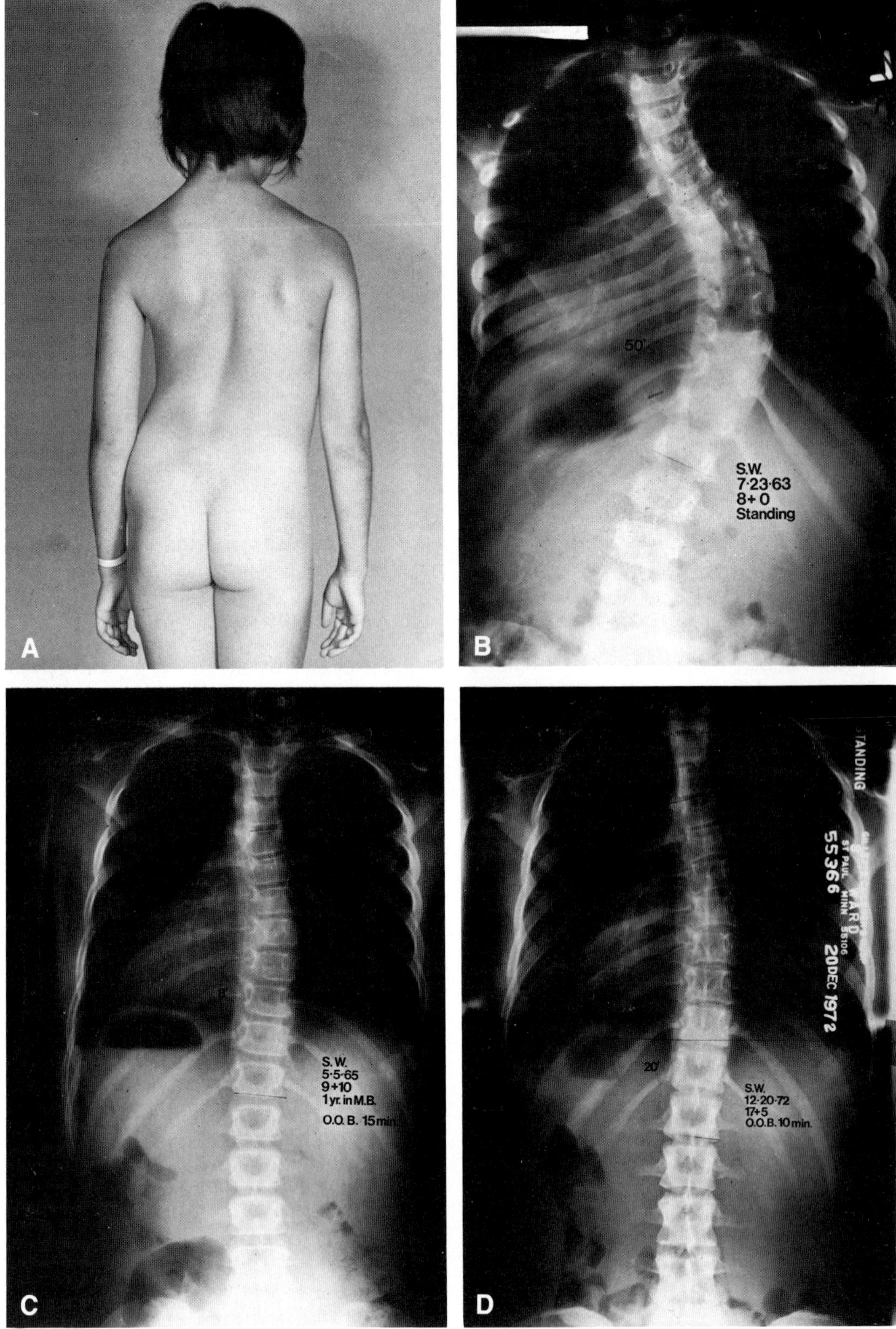
A
50°
S.W.
7·23·63
8+0
Standing
B
S.W.
5·5·65
9+10
1 yr. in M.B.
O.O.B. 15 min.
C
20°
S.W.
12·20·72
17+5
O.O.B. 10 min.
D

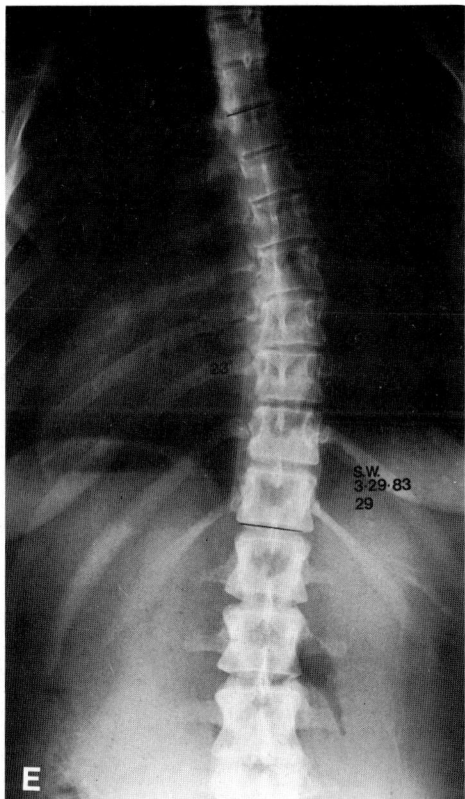

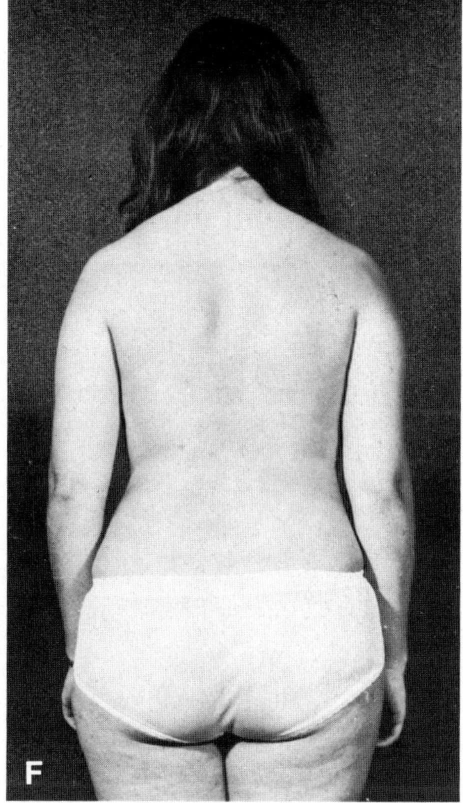

FIG. 16-11. *(A)* The clinical photograph of an 8-year-old girl presenting with a right thoracic scoliosis. *(B)* She has a 50° right thoracic, T5–L1 scoliosis with no congenital anomalies. This is a classic example of a juvenile idiopathic scoliosis. *(C)* After 1 year of Milwaukee brace treatment, her curve measured only 8°. Repeated attempts to treat her with part-time bracing failed. *(D)* After 9 years of orthotic treatment, her curve measured 20°. Weaning was *begun* at this time. She had no psychologic problems from 9 years of full-time brace use. *(E)* At age 29, 11 years out of the orthosis and after having three children, her curve measured 23°. *(F)* Her clinical appearance several years after brace removal.

several factors. Gender, skeletal age, curve location, and curve magnitude are correlated with progression, whereas family history, compensation, and quantity of lordosis or kyphosis do not correlate. A girl with a thoracic scoliosis of 20° to 29° and who has a Risser sign of 0 or 1 has a 68% chance of progression, whereas a boy with a lumbar curve of 10° to 19° and a Risser sign of 2, 3, or 4 has only a 2% chance of progression (Figs. 16-13 and 16-14).[12,47]

Treatment

The treatment of adolescent idiopathic scoliosis is by braces, electronic stimulators, or surgery. There are no other available treatment methods. Exercises do not influence the curves unless they are combined with brace treatment. Exercises or manipulation have not been demonstrated to even stop the progression of curve, much less improve them. Exercises have been attempted with thousands of patients. No series of patients has ever been reported to have improved by exercises. Clinical research studies comparing exercise-treated groups with nontreated groups showed no differences.[77]

Milwaukee Brace. The Milwaukee brace is the standard orthosis for the treatment of adolescent thoracic idiopathic scoliosis. This brace was developed in Milwaukee in 1945 by Drs. Blount and Schmidt and has subsequently been further refined and developed and is used

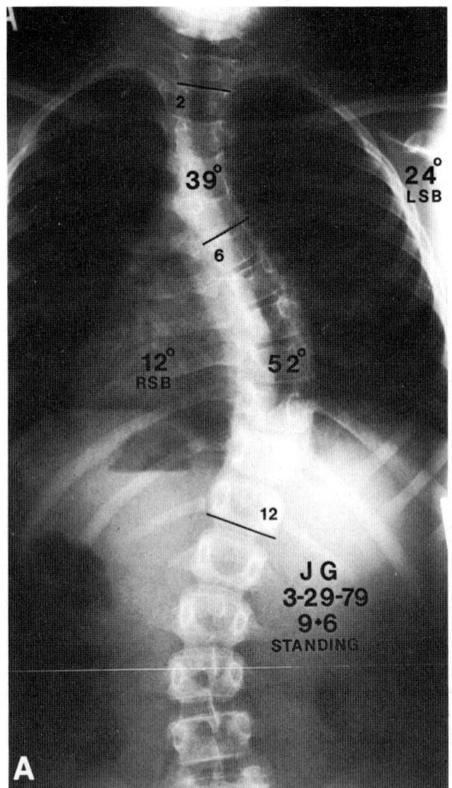

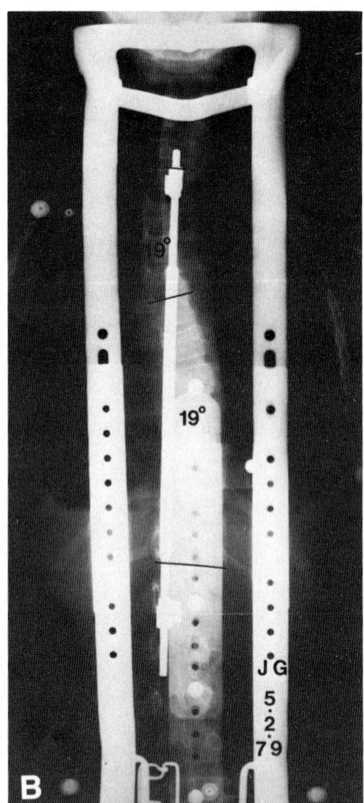

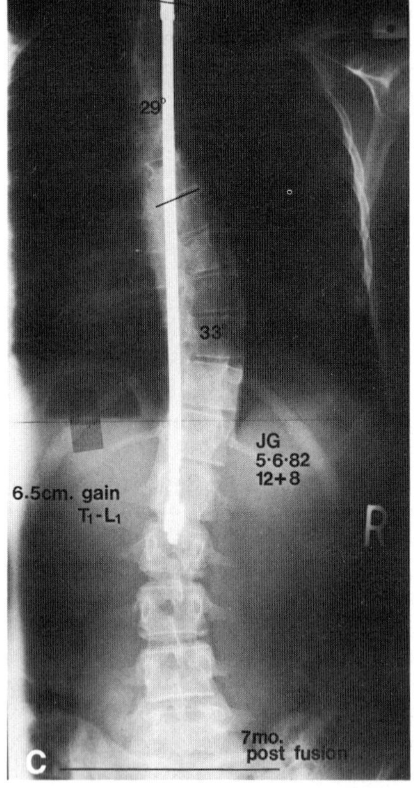

FIG. 16-12. *(A)* This 9-year-old girl presented with a double thoracic curve pattern, a 39° T2–T6 left curve, and a 52° T6–T12 right curve. The lumbar scoliosis was purely compensatory. *(B)* She was treated by subcutaneous Harrington instrumentation without fusion and Milwaukee brace external support. The curves were corrected to 19° each. The rod was lengthened every 6 months. *(C)* This film was taken at age 12, 7 months after her final instrumentation and fusion. The curves are 29° and 33°. There was 6.5 cm of height gain in the T1–L1 area during the 3 years of periodic rod lengthening.

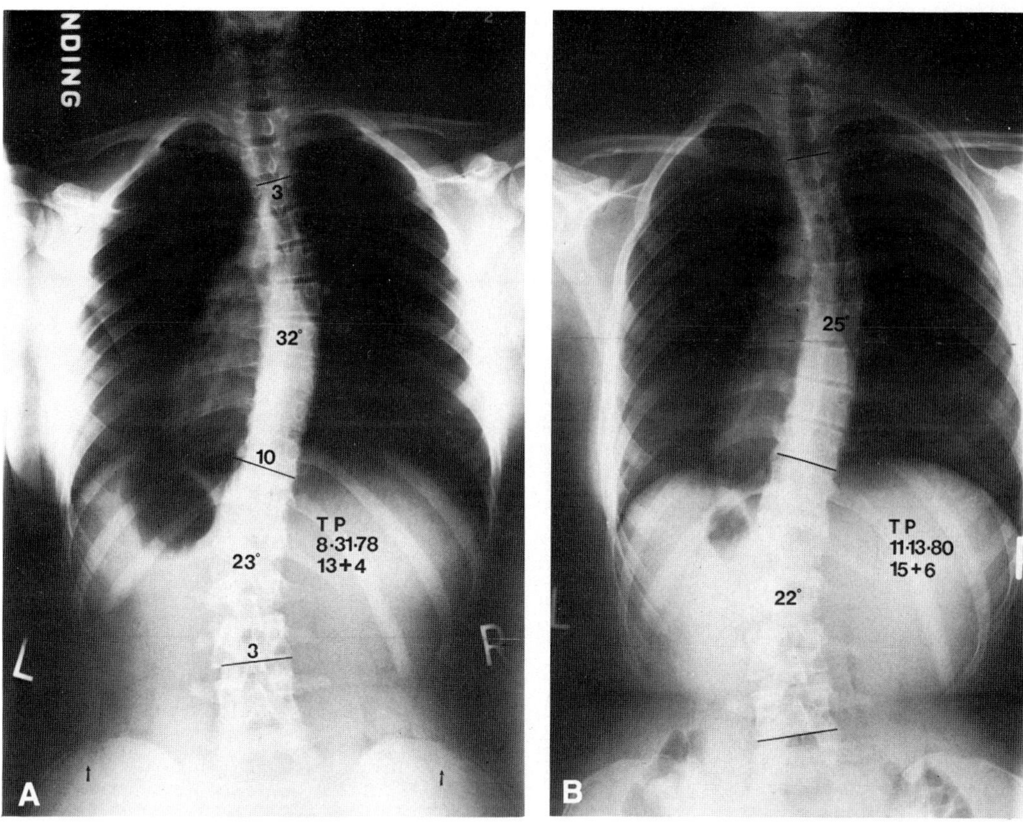

FIG. 16-13. *(A)* This 13-year-old girl presented with a 32° right thoracic idiopathic scoliosis. The Risser sign (iliac crest epiphysis) was 2. A Milwaukee brace was recommended but was refused by the patient. *(B)* After years of observation and no treatment of any kind, the major thoracic curve measures 25°.

throughout the world.[6] Various types of holding pads can be added to the basic Milwaukee brace to provide treatment of the various curve patterns. The basic Milwaukee brace must have a very well-formed pelvic girdle, deeply indented above the iliac crests to maintain a solid foundation. This is the most critical part of the brace. There are two posterior uprights and a single anterior upright. There is a neck ring at the upper end, with a throat mold anteriorly and two occipital pads posteriorly. For a right thoracic curve, an L-shaped thoracic pad is positioned on those ribs leading to the apex of the curve. For the lumbar component of a couple curve pattern, a lumbar pad is applied to the transverse process area above the iliac crest and below the lowermost ribs. It is usually best to fit this pad to the inside of the pelvic girdle with velcro. For high curves involving the upper thoracic area, a shoulder ring or trapezius pad should be used. The pelvic section is usually made of plastic material, which is heated and then shaped from a model of the patient's waist and hip line. Sometimes prefabricated pelvic sections can be used if the patient's shape fits a standard model. Some orthotists prefer to use leather for the pelvic section with metal bands in the iliac crest area. It is not important whether the brace is made of plastic or leather, but it is important that the girdle fits precisely.

The Milwaukee brace is effective for mild to moderate curves. It is not a device that can effectively correct or even control severe curves. The optimal range for the use of the orthosis is for curves between 20° and 45°. Below 20°, many curves are nonprogressive or even spontaneously resolving, and thus, the orthosis is unnecessary. On the other hand, curves above 45° tend to respond poorly to the orthosis, particularly if the child has reached the later stages of puberty. Thus, the orthosis

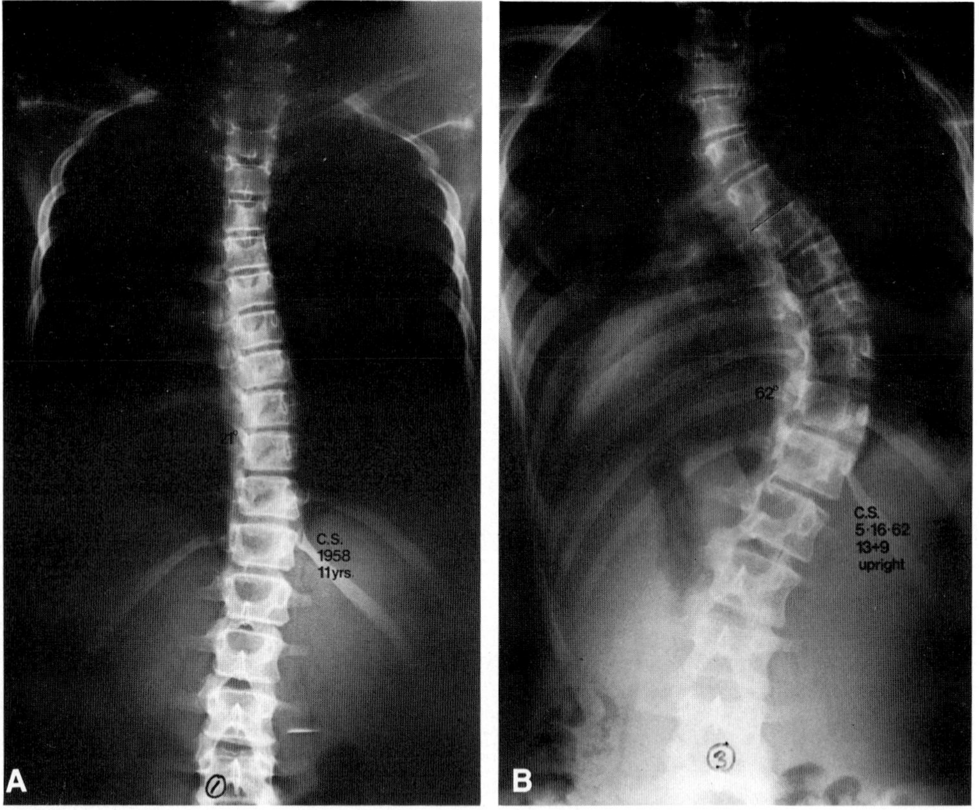

FIG. 16-14. *(A)* This 11-year-old girl was seen elsewhere with a 21° right thoracic idiopathic scoliosis. Her Risser sign was 0 and her menses had not yet begun. *(B)* The same patient after 2½ years of periodic observation but no treatment. Her curve is now 62°.

becomes ineffective when the curves become excessively large. Therefore, if the treatment is to be effective, it is important that the orthosis be applied when the curve is small and flexible. Thus, from a particular point of view, *the Milwaukee brace is ideal for growing children with curves between 20° and 40°.* Curves between 20° and 29° are usually not treated until progression has been documented. Treatment of curves between 30° to 45° is started immediately. Children who have already reached a Risser sign of 4 are seldom treated due to their skeletal maturity.

Curves above 45° can be treated in a Milwaukee brace, but the results are not as good and the physician should warn the family and the patient that results cannot be as reliable. Thus, such treatment should be approached on a trial basis. If an adequate improvement is not obtained during the first 6 months, surgery should be considered without excessive delay.

Management of the patient in a Milwaukee brace is not easy. The patient should be seen as frequently as necessary to maintain a quality fitting and quality maintenance of the orthosis and control of the curvature. In our own clinics, we find that every 3 to 4 months seems appropriate. Other centers require more frequent visits for better emotional reinforcement of the patient. More frequent visits are necessary early in the course of management and less frequent later when growth is slower and the patient is more accustomed to the device.

At the time that treatment is started, the orthosis should be checked by the physician responsible to be sure that it fits well. At this point, treatment should be started on a full-time basis. The patient should not be "weaned" into the brace. Under this program, there is usually a period of approximately 1 week when the child will not be very happy, may often cry, and will not sleep well the first night or two. Nevertheless, this period of adjustment passes and a happy and outgoing patient will soon emerge. A slow weaning into the orthosis will only prolong the period of adjustment and does the patient no benefit. After the patient has worn the brace for 2 or 3 weeks, he or she should be seen for further adjustments of the orthosis, because it may need to be lengthened due to correction of the curve. At this point, there will be many questions about which activities can or cannot be carried out in the orthosis, and the patient will need verbal support. X-rays should be obtained to check the response of the curve. After this, the patient can usually be seen at intervals of 3 to 4 months. An x-ray should be obtained either every visit or every other visit and should be carefully measured.

It is very important to recognize whether or not control is being maintained. The patient who progressively loses control while wearing the device is either cheating, has an orthosis that does not fit well, or has a curve that is simply beyond the ability of the orthosis to control. Providing there is a good orthosis and it is being worn full-time, a loss of control usually means a difficult curve problem. Under such circumstances, a curve progressing beyond 45° should have surgical correction and fusion. As long as the curve can be maintained under 35° with the orthosis, surgery is probably not justified.[14]

It is foolish to allow a curve to progress to 60° or 70°, because a golden opportunity will be lost for ideal surgical correction. It is senseless to ask a child to wear an orthosis when it is obviously doing no good (Figs. 16-15 and 16-16).

The Lumbar Orthosis in Idiopathic Sco-

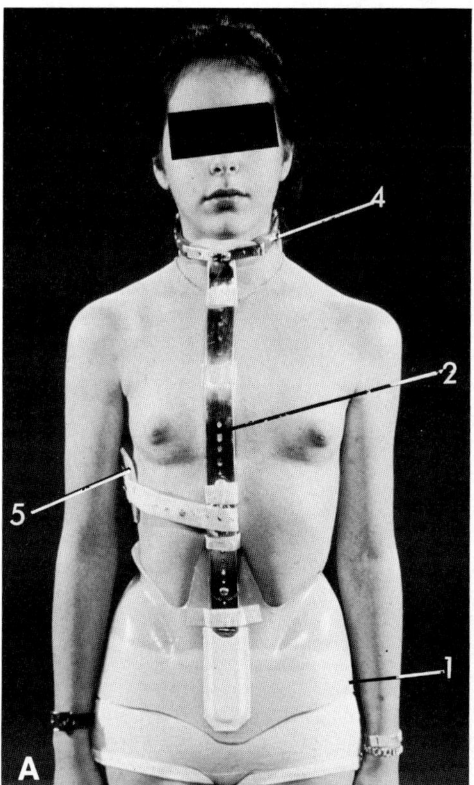

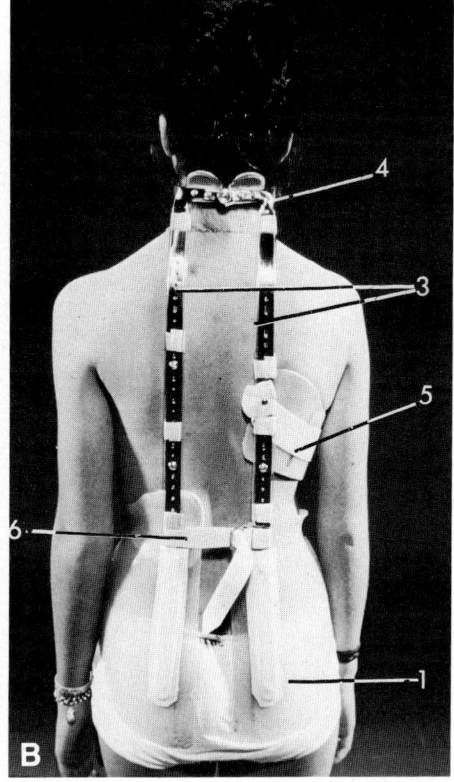

FIG. 16-15. *(A and B) 1,* The pelvic girdle is closely contoured to the pelvis, being deeply indented at the waistline, cut higher in the front to permit hip flexion to 100°, and kept low posteriorly to control lumbar lordosis. *2,* The anterior upright is well centered. *3,* The posterior uprights are parallel. *4,* The neck ring tilts forward from front to back and supports the suboccipital pads and throat mold. Note that the throat mold does *not* touch the chin. *5,* A thoracic pad for the typical right thoracic curve. *6,* The posterior strap connecting the pelvic section. This should be kept quite snug. Beneath it on the left side is a lumbar pad.

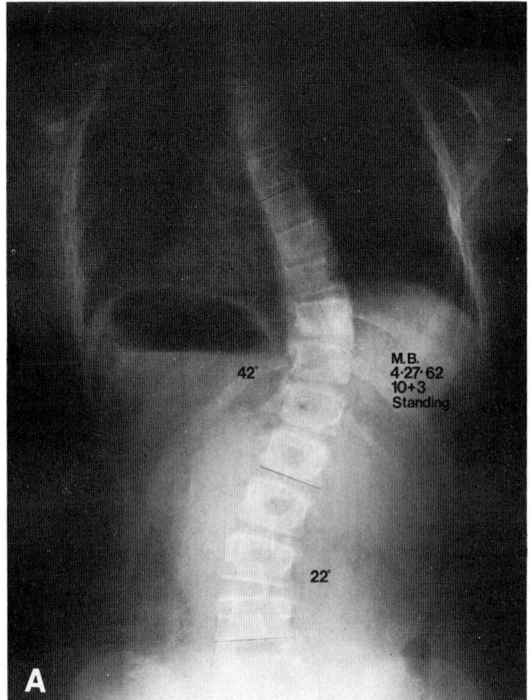

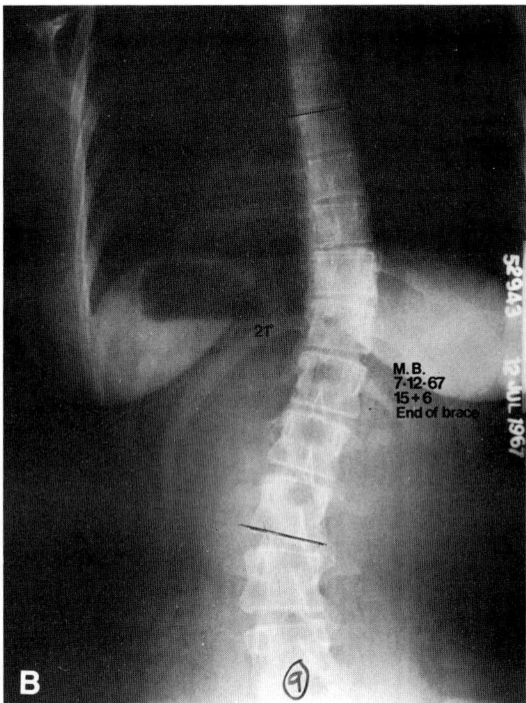

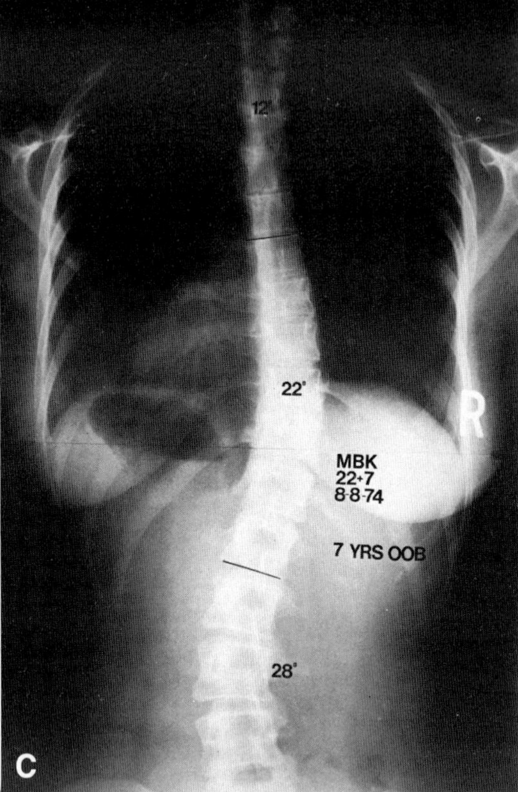

FIG. 16-16. *(A)* A 10-year-old girl with a 42° right thoracic T7–L1 idiopathic scoliosis. Menses had not yet begun and the Risser sign was 0. Milwaukee brace treatment was begun immediately. *(B)* The same patient at age 15, at the completion of orthotic treatment. The curve measured 21°. *(C)* Seven years out of the orthosis and after two pregnancies, her curve measured 22°.

liosis. During the past 10 years, excellent underarm orthoses, both custom-made and prefabricated, have been developed. The advent of thermoplastic materials has stimulated this reactivation of an old idea.

The lumbar orthosis is effective only for flexible curves of less than 40°. It is effective only in curves with the apex at T12 or lower. It is *not* designed nor intended for thoracic curves.

The orthosis is made from a cast of the patient taken in the corrected position. Lumbar lordosis must be reduced. The orthosis provides a basic three-point holding system. The brace must be worn 23 of each 24 hours and removed on the same schedule as a Milwaukee brace (Fig. 16-17 and 16-18).[52]

Weaning From an Orthosis. Total nonoperative treatment with an orthosis demands that the treatment continue until the end of growth. Otherwise relapse will occur. There has, however, been considerable controversy as to just when growth ceases and just when the orthosis should be discontinued. To obtain optimal results, the orthosis should be maintained on a full-time schedule until (1) full vertical height has been achieved as determined by serial height measurement, and (2) the Risser sign shows full capping (Risser IV). In girls, these factors usually coincide, but in boys, there is customarily another 2 cm of vertical growth after full capping of the iliac epiphysis.

Once vertical growth has ceased to increase and full capping has occurred, weaning can *begin*. This progresses slowly, usually increasing at about 1 hour more each day per month. It thus requires 1 year to go from full-time use to "nights only" use. The patient should wear the orthosis at night only for at least 1 year. This is a stringent schedule, but experience as well as clinical research studies have shown that lesser schedules produce inferior results.

Treatment of Thoracic Curves With Underarm Orthoses. This remains a controversial topic in spinal deformity. Advocates of this technique state that results equivalent to the Milwaukee brace can be achieved, but the data available at this writing is meager. Improvement of x-rays at the expense of pulmonary function must be avoided. Compliance with underarm orthoses is no better than with Milwaukee braces.

Nonoperative Treatment With Electrical Stimulators. The past 10 years have seen the development of electronic devices that provide an electrical stimulus to the muscles on the convexity of the curve. Originally, these were implanted, but recently most of the devices have been external with surface electrodes. These devices are used for the nonoperative treatment of idiopathic scoliosis, and the general indications for their use are quite similar to the indications for orthotic treatment. They are used only at night, with no treatment during the day.

The exact mechanism by which these work is unknown. Theoretically, the convex musculature is strengthened and is thus better able to combat the tendency for increased curvature.

Analysis of the first 500 patients treated has shown that approximately 70% of *progressive* curves between 20° and 40° were arrested, that is, no further progression took place. The device is not designed to correct curves, only to halt their progression. Results in curves above 40° have been very poor. Several more years of experience will be necessary before the true efficacy of these devices will be known.[2]

SURGICAL TREATMENT OF IDIOPATHIC SCOLIOSIS

With modern techniques, the surgical approach to idiopathic scoliosis has become a safe and reliable procedure. It should not be viewed as a "last ditch" measure and should not be avoided when it is clear that the patient would benefit by such a procedure.

At the same time, it is a surgical procedure of significant magnitude that should never be entered into lightly. There are several basic components to the surgical program: (1) selection of the patient for surgery, (2) selection of the exact area to be fused, (3) the actual fusion procedure itself, (4) the instrumentation procedure, (5) the immediate postoperative management, and (6) the postoperative immobilization.

Selection of the Patient for Surgery

The indication for surgery is based on the magnitude of the deformity and the problems that it has caused or may cause in the future. Over the years, a solid, rational basis for the selection of the patient for surgery has evolved.

(*Text continues on page 596*)

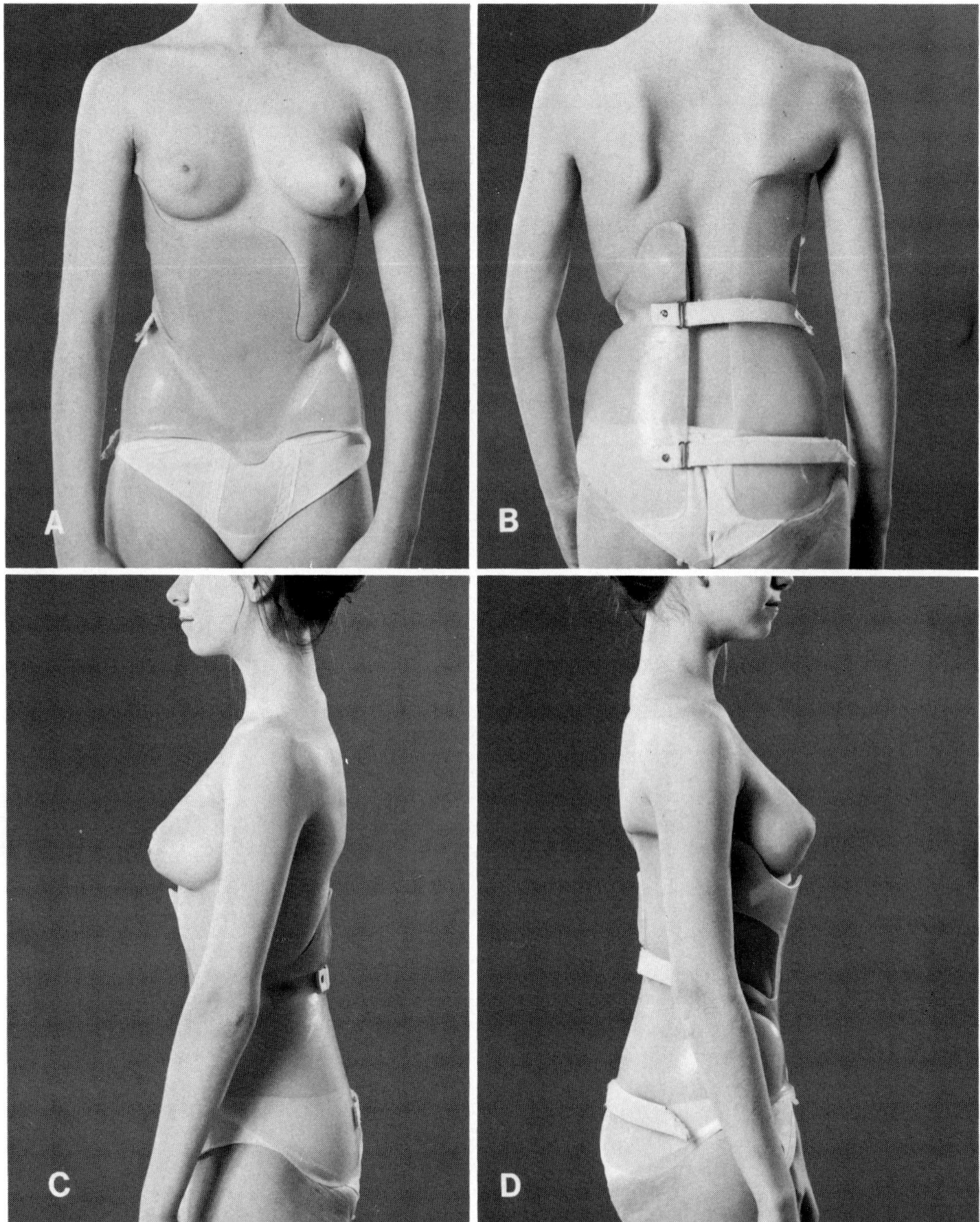

FIG. 16-17. *(A)* A thoracolumbar sacral orthosis for the treatment of a lumbar idiopathic curvature, front view. *(B)* The same brace, as viewed posteriorly. She has a left lumbar curve. *(C)* The patient as viewed from the left side. *(D)* The patient as viewed from the right side. Note that the brace is cut high in the front for sitting, kept low in the back to control lumbar lordosis, and kept below the breast area to avoid compression.

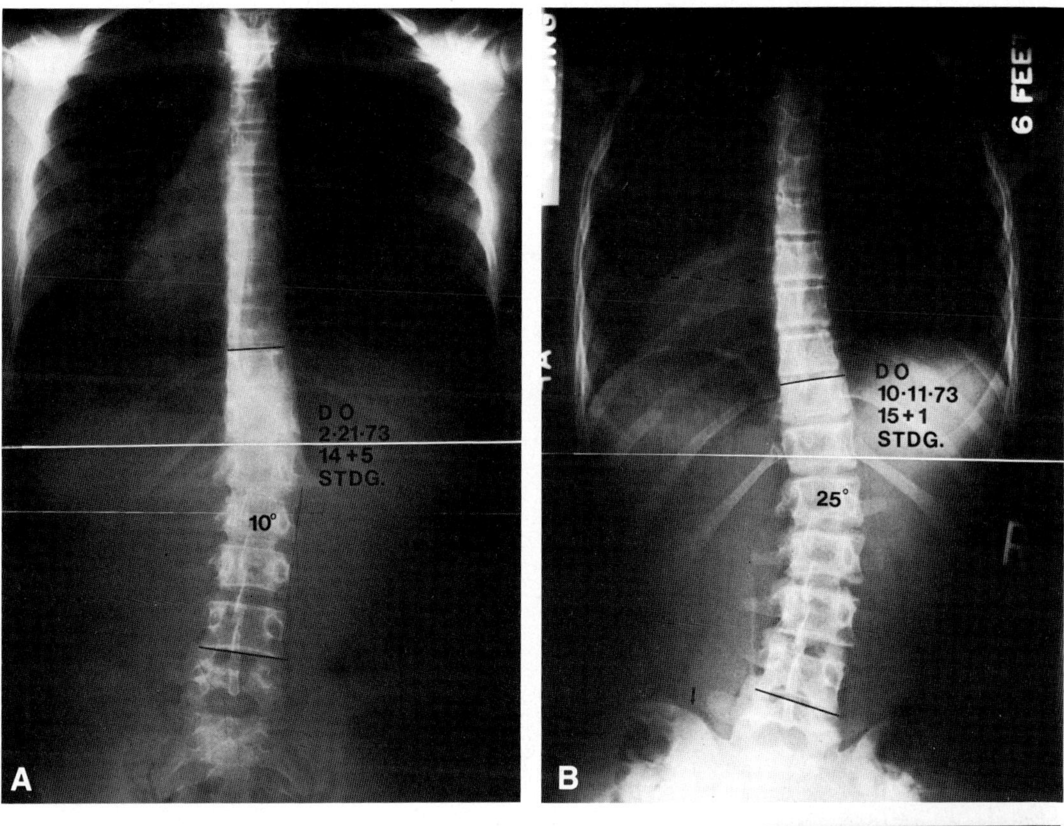

FIG. 16-18. *(A)* A 14-year-old girl with a 10° right lumbar idiopathic scoliosis. Her Risser sign was 0 and her menses had not yet begun. No treatment was given. *(B)* After a year of periodic observation, it was obvious her curve was progressing, now measuring 25°. The Risser sign was 3+, but her menses had not yet appeared. She was placed in a TLSO of the type seen in Figure 16-17. *(C)* She was treated from ages 15 to 17 full-time, and then on a gradually decreasing scale from ages 17 to 19. This film was taken at age 24, 5 years after completion of orthotic treatment and after one pregnancy; it shows maintenance of the curve at 8°.

Based on the Cobb measurement system, adolescent curves beyond 50° are best treated by surgery. This is true regardless of the curve pattern present. The use of 50° as a baseline for making this decision is a result of long-term studies of untreated patients. As was noted in the section on natural history, patients with curves of greater than 50° at the end of growth usually have progression of their curves during adult life and will end up 20 or 30 years later with curves of 75° to 80°. With curves of this magnitude, symptoms are so apparent that it is obviously better to take care of the situation in childhood rather than allowing the adult to deteriorate to a point of malfunction. Thus, the recommendation for surgery is based on the *predictability* of complications in adult life.

The most important indication for fusion is the *prevention* of respiratory insufficiency. Thoracic curvatures above 60° are definitely associated with an increase in curvature and with a progressive decline in pulmonary function. Correction of curvatures in adults seldom provides signficant improvement of respiratory function. Therefore, it is best to prevent a patient from ever having a respiratory insufficiency rather than to wait for insufficiency to develop and then try to correct it.

The use of the 50° baseline is not a magic figure below which surgery must never be done and above which surgery must always be done. It is intended merely as a guideline. It must always be remembered that scoliosis is a three-dimensional deformity and that the anteroposterior x-ray is only a two-plane evaluation. The prudent physician must look at the lateral x-ray and especially at the patient and put all the factors together to make a determination. Thus, some patients with 40° curves will require surgery. These are patients who have a considerable structural deformity of their thorax, particularly if they have thoracic lordosis or a larger than average rib hump. Other patients with 40° curves may require fusion because of pain. Some patients with 55° curves have virtually no deformity at all and on testing of pulmonary function are entirely normal. These patients do not require surgery but should be periodically observed for progression.

Selection of Fusion Area

Improper selection of the fusion area will lead to many tragedies. It is wrong to either fuse too much of the spine or not enough of the spine. The question of exactly what area to fuse is a constant problem. One should fuse the structural (major) curve or curves and avoid fusion of the compensatory (secondary) curves. The determination of whether a curve is major or compensatory is based on analysis of traction and/or bending films. It is also determined upon examination of the patient, because the absence of significant rotation is usually a sign of a secondary curve and the presence of significant rotation indicates a structural curve.

One must never fuse less than the measured curve. This should be considered a minimal fusion area. Thus, if the measured curve is T5 to T12, the fusion must never be less than T5 to T12. Usually this is not enough, and one vertebra above and one vertebra below the measured area should be included. Thus, the rule that "one above and one below the measured curve is the area for fusion" is a practical rule and is used by many surgeons.

Even this rule, however, is not totally adequate. There are certain curves in which the fusion will still be too short. The curve will lengthen after the cast is removed. Careful analysis of these complications has lead to the use of verebral rotation as a guideline for selection of the fusion area. With this rule one should include in the fusion area *all of the vertebrae rotated in the same direction as the vertebra at the apex of the curve, and the fusion should extend to the first vertebra that is not rotated*. Thus, if the end of the measured curve is L1, but L2 and L3 are both rotated in the same direction as the apical vertebra, and L4 is the first neutral vertebra in terms of rotation, the fusion should extend to L4. The fusion may stop at L3 if on the supine x-ray film L3, rather than L4, would be the neutral vertebra on rotation. If the child still has more than a year of growth remaining, it is better to select the longer vertebra than the shorter one. If, however, the patient has completed growth, lengthening of the curve is less likely and the slightly shorter area can be chosen. King and associates,[40] in a comprehensive review of a large number of idiopathic scolioses with a major thoracic curve, showed that a line erected vertically from the center of S1 can provide an excellent reference for the fusion area; both ends of the fusion should lie on this "central gravity line" (Fig 16-19).[40]

If the patient has a double major curve

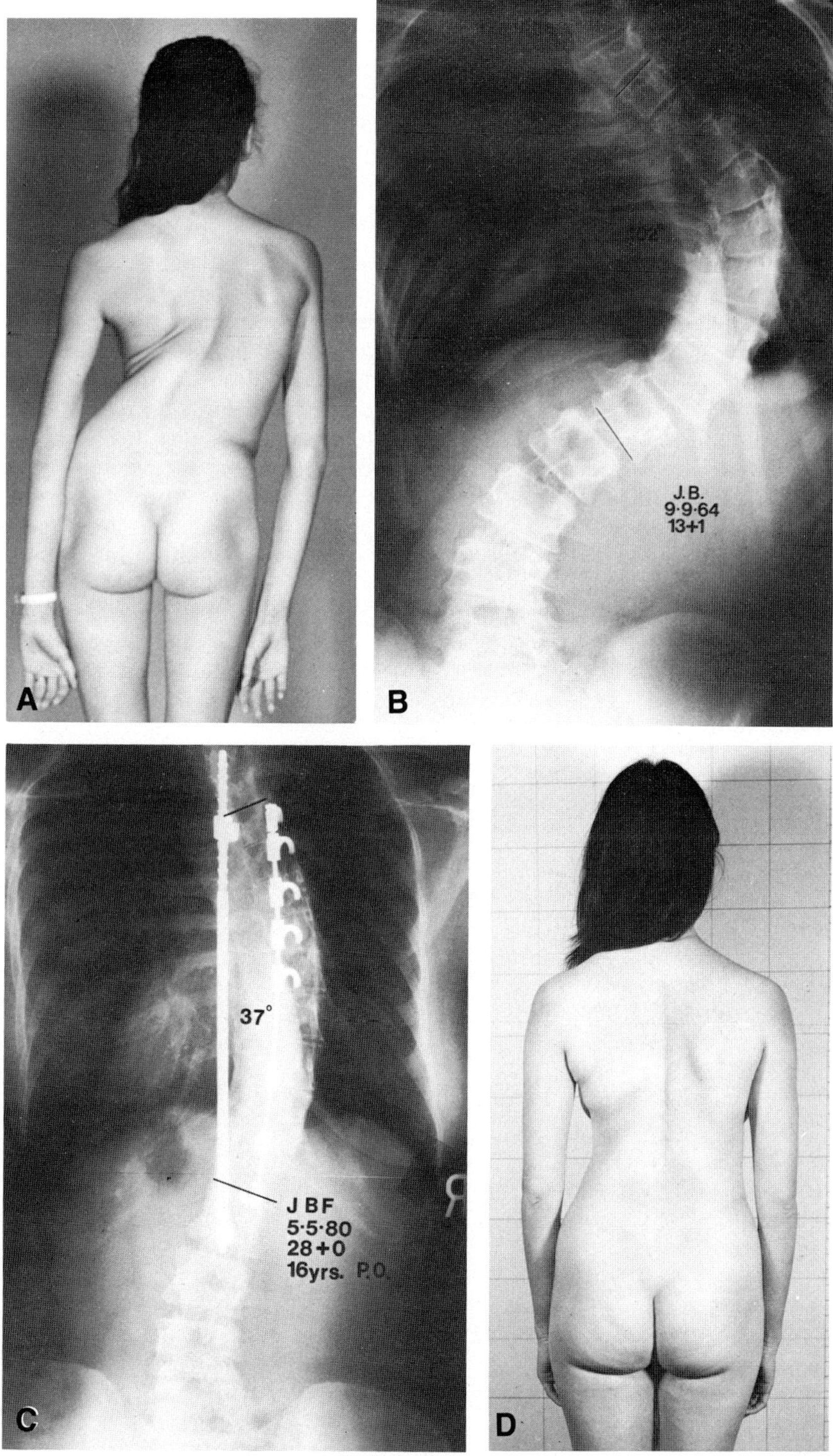

FIG. 16-19. *(A)* The clinical appearance of a 13-year-old girl with severe right thoracic idiopathic scoliosis. *(B)* Her roentgenogram shows a 102° T5–L1 scoliosis. The Risser sign is still 0. *(C)* A roentgenogram 16 years after surgical correction and fusion to 37°. (Surgery at Gillette Children's Hospital by Dr. John H. Moe) *(D)* A posterior photograph several years after the surgery. She is married, has had four children, and has no back pain.

pattern, both curves must be fused. It is useless to fuse only one curve, because the second curve will progress and a second fusion will be necessary at some other time. Fusion of two curves is a more involved procedure than that of a single curve, but, with care, it is possible to accomplish both at one time.

There is much controversy about the proper level for fusion of lumbar curves. The rule that the fusion must extend to the first neutrally rotated vertebra does not hold when the vertebra is L5. In lumbar curves, the fusion should stop at L4 even though L4 is still rotated in the same direction as the apical vertebra. Fusion to L5 is not necessary. (Fig. 16-20).

It is never necessary to fuse a child with idiopathic scoliosis to the sacrum unless there is a coincident and symptomatic spondylolisthesis.

Patients undergoing fusion to L4 must have a careful physical examination and radiologic evaluation of the lumbosacral area to ensure there is no spondylolysis or spondylolisthesis. It is safe to extend a fusion to L4 if there is a nonsymptomatic and nondisplaced spondylolysis at L5.

Patients with idiopathic scoliosis do not have curves that extend into the cervical spine. Thus, the uppermost vertebra that should be included in the fusion area for idiopathic scoliosis is T1. Any curve extending into the cervical spine must be suspected of being a condition other than idiopathic scoliosis.

One of the common mistakes has been the failure to fuse the high left thoracic curve in the double major thoracic curve pattern. It is sometimes difficult to decide whether or not this upper curve requires fusion.

If on erect films the upper curve has the same magnitude at the right thoracic curve, if on bending films it has the same quantity of rigidity, and if on x-rays the uppermost ribs on the left side are higher than the uppermost ribs on the right side, this upper curve must be included in the fusion area (Fig. 16-21).

One of the most difficult problems in all of

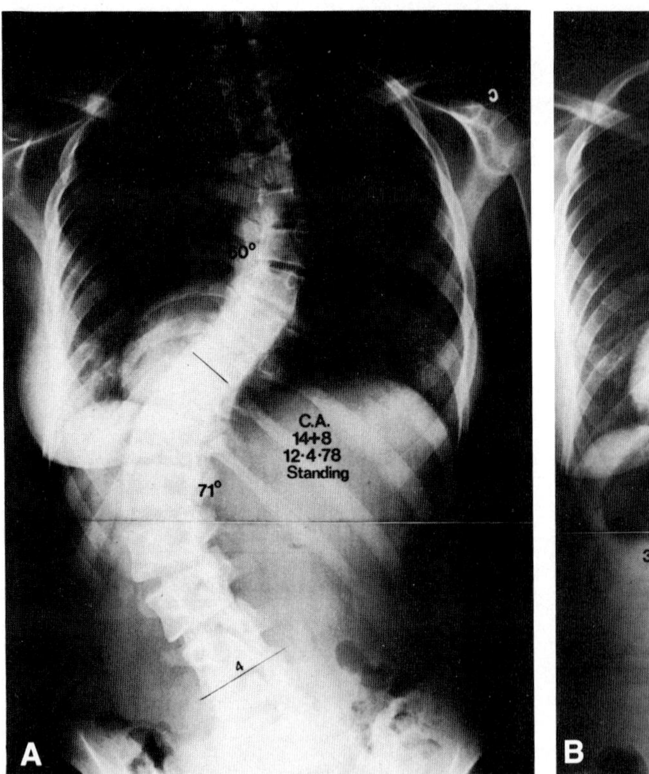

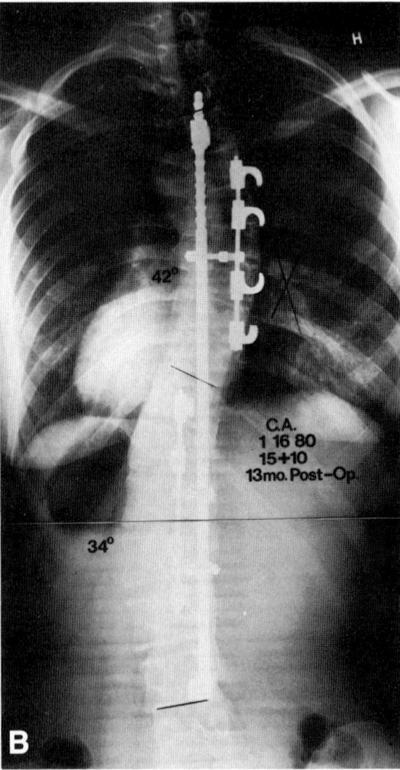

FIG. 16-20. *(A)* A 14-year-old girl with a double major, right thoracic (60°) and left lumbar (71°) idiopathic scoliosis. *(B)* One year after surgical instrumentation and fusion from T4–L4. The curves measure 42° and 34°. Fusion below L4 is not necessary. The rods should be bent into lordosis in the lumbar spine.

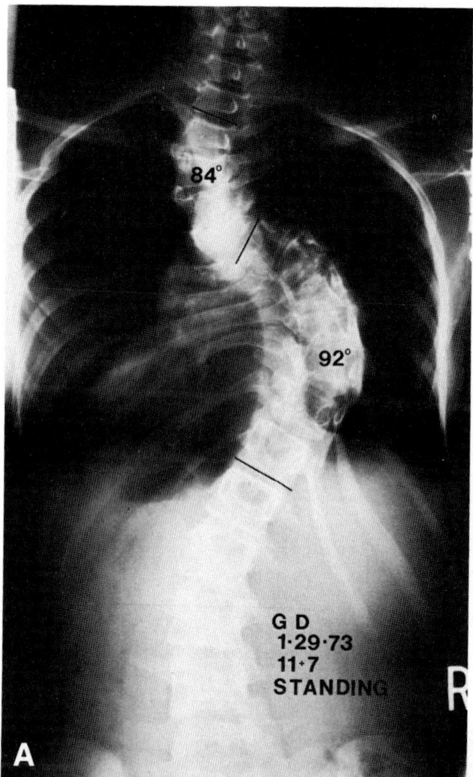

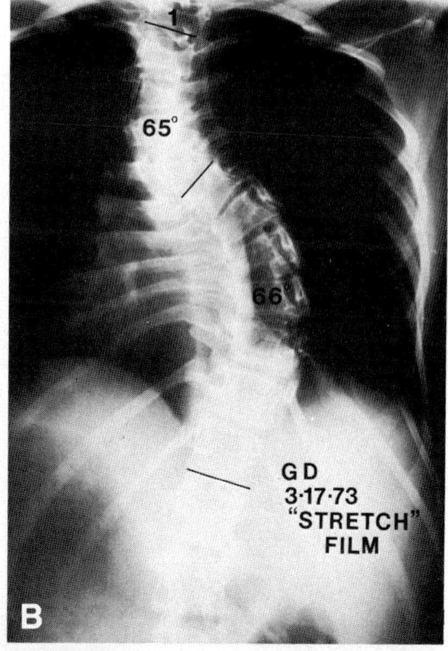

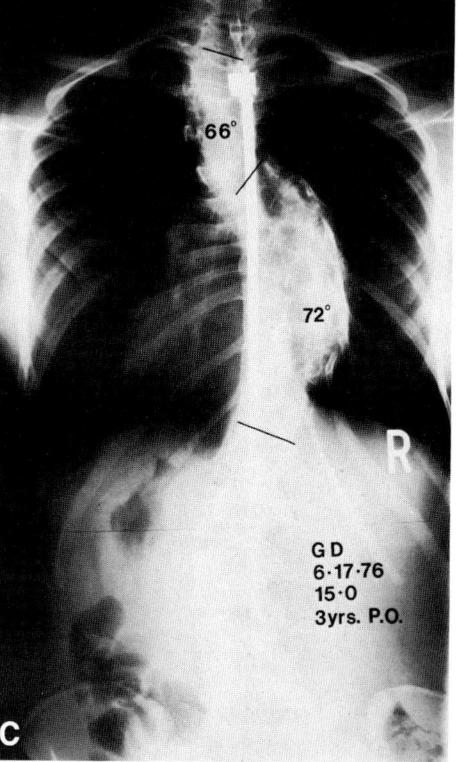

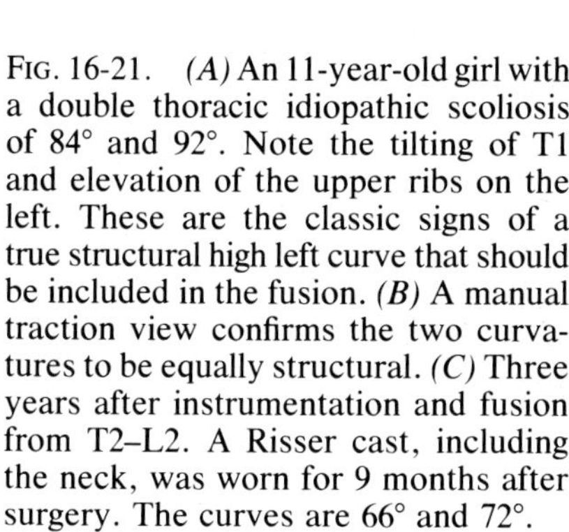

FIG. 16-21. *(A)* An 11-year-old girl with a double thoracic idiopathic scoliosis of 84° and 92°. Note the tilting of T1 and elevation of the upper ribs on the left. These are the classic signs of a true structural high left curve that should be included in the fusion. *(B)* A manual traction view confirms the two curvatures to be equally structural. *(C)* Three years after instrumentation and fusion from T2–L2. A Risser cast, including the neck, was worn for 9 months after surgery. The curves are 66° and 72°.

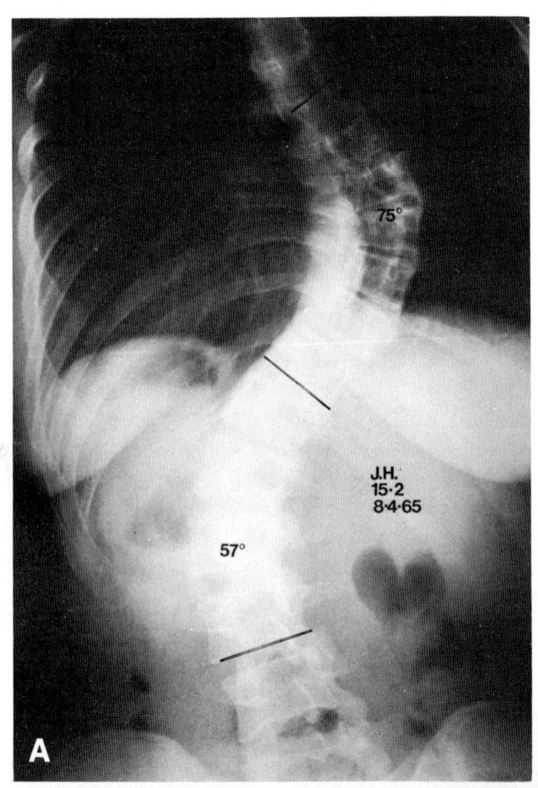
75°
J.H.
15·2
8·4·65
57°
A

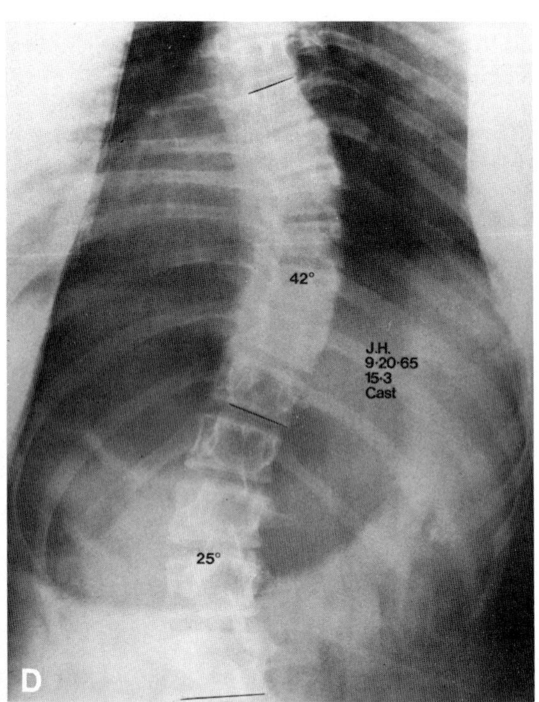
42°
J.H.
9·20·65
15·3
Cast
25°
D

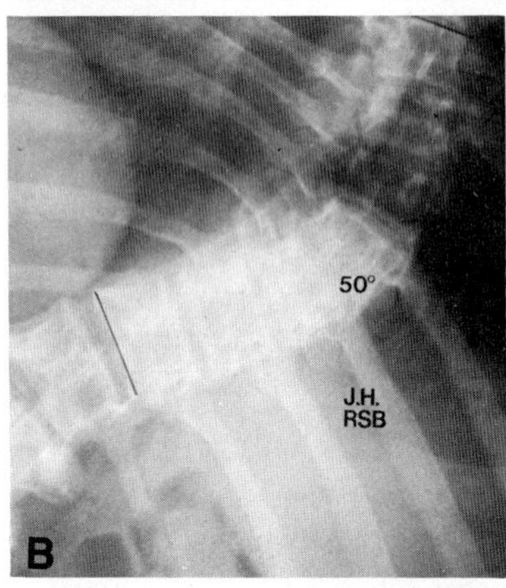
50°
J.H.
RSB
B

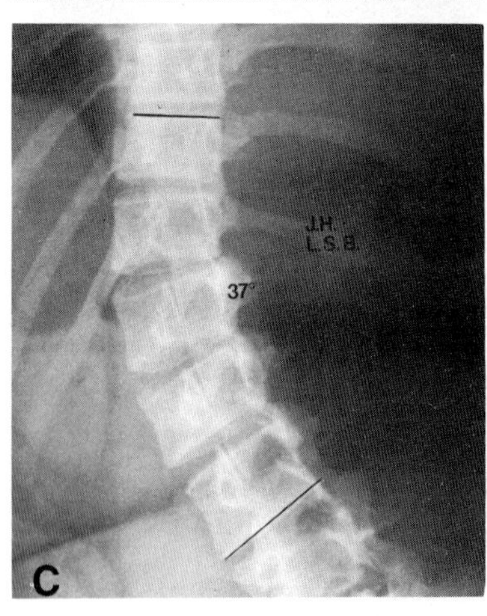
J.H.
L.S.B.
37°
C

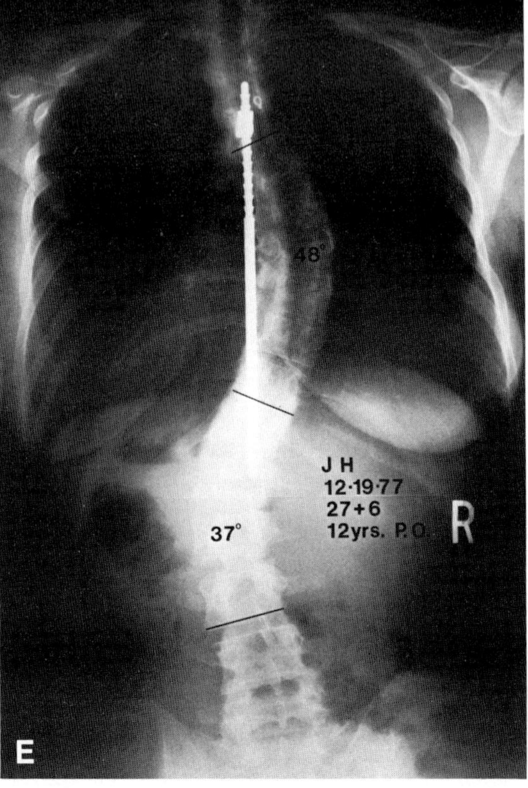
48°
J H
12·19·77
27+6
12yrs. P.O.
R
37°
E

scoliosis is the decision whether to fuse the lumbar curve in patients with right thoracic, left lumbar double structural curve patterns in which the lumbar curve is not as structural as the thoracic curve. These patients have curves that are usually of equal or almost equal magnitude on the standing film, but on the supine and bending films, the lumbar curve is of less magnitude and is more flexible than the thoracic curve. Here the decision-making becomes quite difficult. As stated previously, if the two curves are of equal magnitude on the standing film, of equal magnitude on the supine film, and of equal structural quality on the bending films, both curves *must* be fused. If, however, the lumbar curve is considerably more flexible than the thoracic curve and if the lumbar curve on voluntary supine side-bending corrects to a degree equal to or better than the *expected* correction of the thoracic curve, it is satisfactory to fuse only the thoracic curve and not the lumbar curve. The lumbar curve must be carefully followed, and, if it progresses beyond that value in the fused thoracic spine, it also must be fused at a later time.[40]

It is a nuisance to the patient to have a second fusion at a later time, but this is sometimes preferable to a single procedure in which a lumbar curve is fused unnecessarily (Figs. 16-22 and 16-23).

Surgical Technique

The reader is referred to standard texts and references on fusion technique; it is beyond the scope of this chapter to provide details on technique procedures.[57] The author stresses the importance of (1) complete facet joint excision on both sides (concave and convex), (2) replacement of the facet joint area by a plug of iliac cancellous autogenous bone, (3) complete decortication of all exposed laminae and transverse processes, and (4) the routine addition of fresh autogenous iliac bone graft. When these components are religiously applied to each and every case, consistently good results can be obtained. Surgeons who try to "get by" without excising the facet joints or using extra bone have much poorer results than those surgeons who use the preferable procedure.

Surgical technique must be learned in the operating room from a skilled surgeon. It is simply not possible to review a textbook, slides, or movie and then perform this type of procedure.

Instrumentation. Harrington instrumentation has become almost standard throughout the world for the surgical treatment of idiopathic scoliosis. It must be remembered that the Harrington instruments are an *adjunct* to the fusion technique and never replace fusion. Therefore, the instrumentation is only a device that will give internal correction and internal stabilization of the area to be fused. There has been a tendency for surgeons to depend too much on instrumentation and not perform an adequate fusion. This has been proved over and over again to lead to bad results. Scoliosis surgery was done for many years prior to the invention of the Harrington instruments, and very good results were obtained and are still obtained in cases without instrumentation.

Bending of the distraction rod is frequently necessary and should not be avoided when the indication arises. This is usually necessary to fit a distraction rod to the normal roundness of the thoracic spine, particularly when dealing with double thoracic curves. Failure to bend the rod in these circumstances may result in hook dislocation. The rod should be bent only in the nonracheted portion.

The Harrington distraction system is customarily inserted under the lamina at the upper

◀ FIG. 16-22. *(A)* This 15-year-old girl presented with a 75° right thoracic curve and a 57° left lumbar curve. On clinical examination, her right thoracic prominence was 3 cm and the left lumbar prominence was 1 cm. Should both curves be fused or only the thoracic? *(B)* A supine right side–bending view shows correction of the thoracic curve to 50°. *(C)* A supine left side–bending view shows correction of the lumbar curve to 37°. *(D)* A supine view in a preoperative cast shows correction of the thoracic curve to 42° and the lumbar to 25°. Putting together the information gained from the clinical examination as well as all the radiologic evaluation, it is evident that she has a primary right thoracic scoliosis and that the lumbar is not a primary curve and fusion can be done only of the thoracic curve. *(E)* A film of the patient at age 27, 12 years after surgery and after three pregnancies. (Decision and surgery by Dr. John H. Moe)

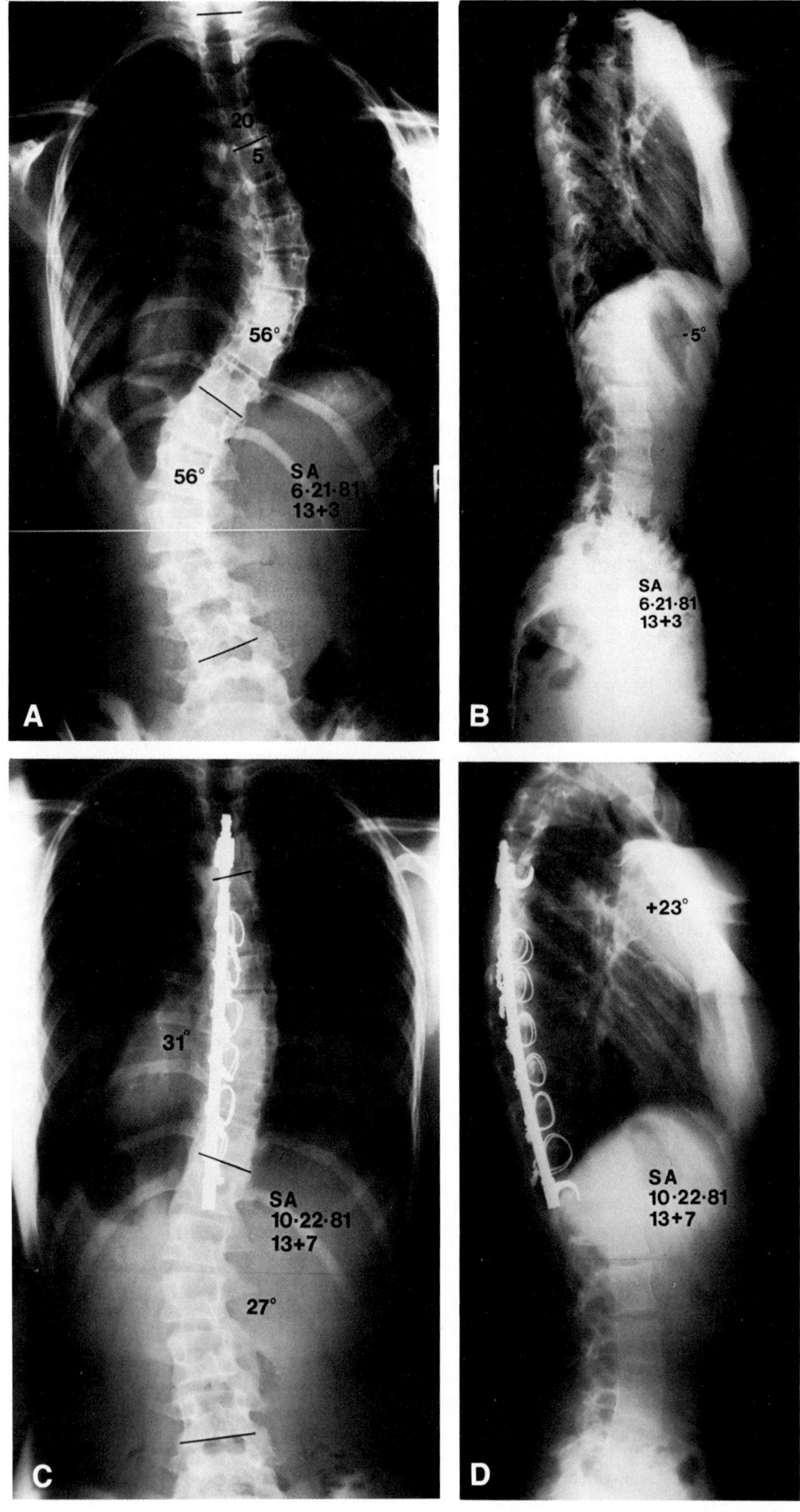
20°
5
56°
56°
SA
6·21·81
13+3
A
-5°
SA
6·21·81
13+3
B
31°
SA
10·22·81
13+7
27°
C
+23°
SA
10·22·81
13+7
D

end using a No. 1262 or 1253 hook. The lower insertion is underneath the lamina of the lowermost vertebra to be included in the fusion area. A small window is made in the ligamentum flavum, and a No. 1254 hook is placed in this area. All the facet joint fusion and decortication fusion on the concave side should be done prior to the insertion of the rod. The rod is distracted to the comfortable limit. The amount of force used can be learned only in the operating room. It cannot be verbally described. Certainly it is possible to overstretch the tissues. Overstretching can cause fractures of the lamina and can produce paraplegia.

The Harrington compression system is particularly useful for the kyphotic component of a kyphoscoliosis. It can also be used as a convex stabilizer and can be brought toward the distraction rod by a "DTT" device or twisted wire loops. The compression assembly tends to aggravate thoracic lordosis.

For thoracic lordoscoliosis, the best results have been attained by Luque sublaminar wires brought to a Harrington distraction rod (square-ended) bent into normal kyphosis.

After insertion of all the rods to the desired tension, it is our custom to awaken the patient to a lighter level of anesthesia and command the patient to move the hands and then the feet. When the patient has demonstrated the *voluntary* ability to move the feet, he or she is placed back to a deeper level of anesthesia. With good anesthetic control, this is easily performed and provides a simple and immediate knowledge of the neurologic status. Electronic cord monitoring is being used in many centers but is still in the research and development stage.

The Zielke device has been advocated for treatment of lumbar and thoracolumbar curves. Orthotic treatment, however, is so successful that the author has found it necessary to use only one Zielke device in an adolescent in the past 10 years.

After surgery, the patient is nursed in a regular bed and turned with a careful log-rolling technique. If the rod is well inserted dislocation of the rod is most unusual. At the end of 5 to 7 days, the patient will be able to apply the postoperative cast or brace. We apply a Risser-Cotrel cast, with a small amount of padding around the hips and no padding elsewhere except for two layers of stockinette. The cast is applied with traction, and a localizer force is created by a Cotrel derotation lateral-flexion strap. After the cast has dried for 2 or 3 hours, the patient can be started on ambulation and should be fully ambulatory by the time of discharge from the hospital.

This early ambulation program is possible provided that there has been (1) proper and precise insertion of the Harrington rods, and (2) proper and precise application of the Risser-Cotrel cast or brace. Provided that these conditions are met, a loss of correction by early ambulation can be limited to no more than 5° or 6°.

Well-made braces can be used after surgery in place of casts, provided that the patient can be trusted to keep the brace on.

Duration of Immobilization. The duration of postoperative support varies from center to center and from surgeon to surgeon. Like all other bone healing processes, it should be individualized according to the patient's healing capacity. Generally speaking, most scoliosis fusions require 6 to 9 months of external support time to become sufficiently solid, with good vertical trabeculation of the fusion mass to tolerate being without support. Some surgeons remove the cast in as short a time as 4 months, but this is the bare minimal requirement. The most important factor is that good-quality x-rays must demonstrate a solid fusion with good vertical trabeculation of the fusion mass. In our experience, this is seldom present at 4 months; it is usually present at 6 to 8 months in the usual adolescent patient with idiopathic scoliosis.

◀ FIG. 16-23. (*A*) This 13-year-old girl presented with two 56° curves, right thoracic and left lumbar. Although the two curves were equal on the standing view, the lumbar curve was much more flexible on bending films (12° versus 34° for the thoracic curve), and the lumbar prominence was much smaller on clinical examination. (*B*) Her lateral view shows a thoracic lordosis of −5°. (*C*) Treatment consisted of posterior instrumentation from T4–T12 with a kyphotically bent, square-ended Harrington rod and multiple sublaminar wires in order to "pull out" the thoracic lordosis. The lumbar spine was not touched. A brace was used for 4 months to support the operated area and to treat the lumbar curve. (*D*) A lateral view at the same time showing correction of the hyperlordosis to +23°.

Luque instrumentation has also been advocated by its designer for use in idiopathic scoliosis. Dual L-shaped rods are appropriately bent (to the degree of curve as noted on the bending film), and each laminae is wired to the rod on both sides. The facet joints are excised, and bone graft should be added.

At the time of this writing, the Luque system is highly controversial, especially for idiopathic curves. The advantages of ambulation without external support are outweighed by an increased neurologic risk. For this reason, most surgeons do not use the Luque system for idiopathic scoliosis (Figs. 16-24 and 16-25).

Pseudarthrosis. Pseudarthrosis is a recognized problem in the surgical treatment of any type of scoliosis, including idiopathic scoliosis. The incidence of pseudarthrosis has decreased steadily as better surgical techniques and postoperative immobilization have developed. It is the author's opinion that early ambulation promotes healing and that the pseudarthrosis rate has been reduced in our hands by early ambulation.

If at the time of cast or brace removal a definite pseudarthrosis is noted, the patient should be scheduled for pseudarthrosis repair without further delay. It is unwise to "observe" the pseudarthrosis and allow any loss of correction to take place. Harrington rods do not ordinarily break, but they can break with the repeated stresses of a pseudarthrosis.

CONGENITAL SPINE DEFORMITY

Congenital spine deformities are those curvatures in which the curve is due to anomalous development of the vertebra. A curve in a very young child without congenital anomalies is usually an infantile idiopathic scoliosis or some other type but should not be referred to as congenital. Because these anomalies are present at birth, children with congenital scoliosis tend to have a curvature either at birth or developing much earlier in life than the typical idiopathic scoliosis or paralytic patient.

This early development has resulted in a tendency for the young child with a congenital scoliosis to receive less than optimum care. The curves are all too frequently allowed to progress to a serious degree. There is a tendency for congenital curves to be very rigid and very resistant to correction. Thus, these curves must not be allowed to progress. Early fusion is necessary in a large number of cases, and is far preferable to allowing severe curves to develop. Usually early fusion will not stunt the potential growth, because the area of the anomalies and the area that needs to be fused cannot grow in a normal vertical manner due to the undeveloped growth plates.

There are many different types of congenital spine deformity, and they are customarily classified first as to whether they are scoliotic, kyphotic, lordotic, or a combination thereof.

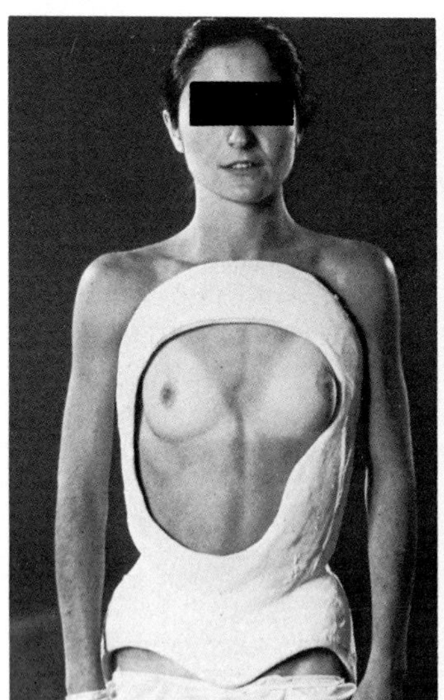

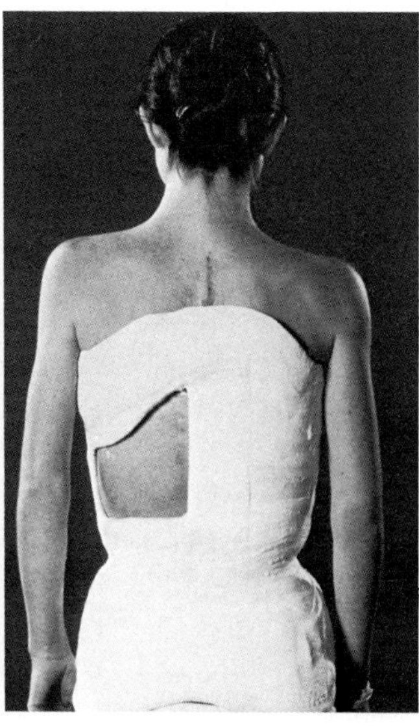

FIG. 16-24. Photographs of a typical underarm cast used after Harrington instrumentation and fusion for idiopathic scoliosis.

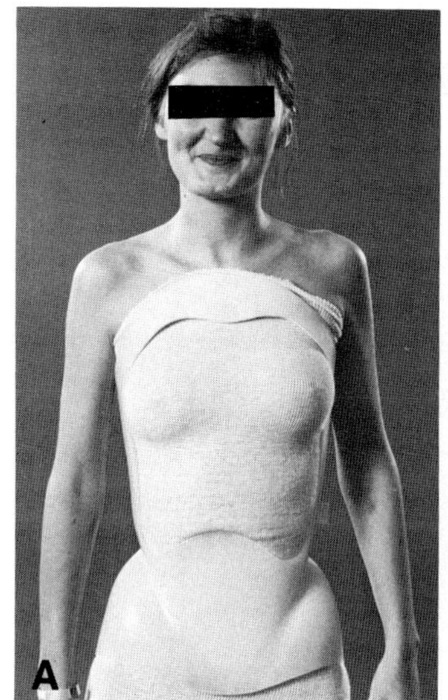

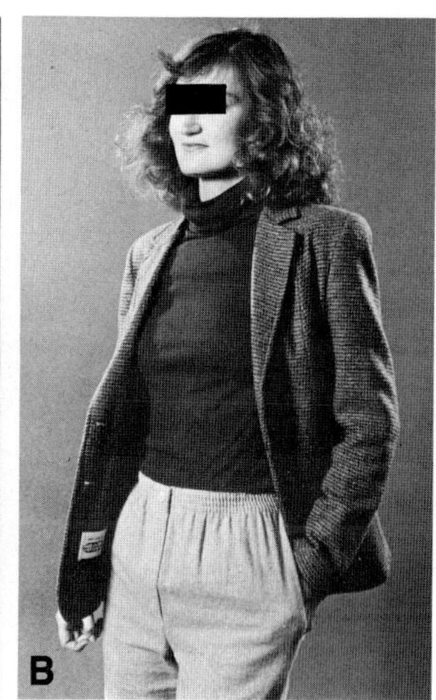

FIG. 16-25. (*A*) Photograph of a postoperative patient in a custom-molded polypropylene brace (8th postoperative day). (*B*) The same patient with ordinary clothes. (Photographs reproduced with permission of the CV Mosby Company. Reproduced from AAOS Instructional Course Lectures, Vol 32, 1983, p 181)

Next, the type of congenital anomaly present must be determined. This often provides useful clues as to the prognosis of the deformity (Fig. 16-26).

CONGENITAL SCOLIOSIS

Classification of Congenital Scoliosis

- Failure of Formation
  - Partial unilateral failure of formation (wedge)
  - Complete unilateral failure (hemivertebra)
    - Fully segmented
    - Semi-segmented
    - Nonsegmented
- Failure of Segmentation
  - Unilateral failure of segmentation (unilateral unsegmented bar)
  - Bilateral failure of segmentation (bloc vertebrae)
- Miscellaneous
- Mixed

Although one would theoretically like to associate a certain prognosis with a certain anomaly, this is not always possible. It is best to consider the curve in its general character and to see what problem it produces and whether or not it is progressive, regardless of the specific type of anomaly. Thus, careful documentation of the quantity of the curve by high-quality x-rays and photographs is necessary on the first examination. Subsequently, serial photography and serial radiology are important. Children should be followed at 6-month intervals and must be followed until the end of their growth. Many patients have mild curves that are very stable for many years and then suddenly become severe at the time of the adolescent growth spurt.

Some patients curves never progress at all and, after being followed for many years, do not show any significant deformity or change in their condition. These patients, of course, do not require any treatment, and it is foolish to apply an orthosis or perform a fusion for a condition that is not progressive and not disabling (Fig. 16-27).

Statistically, about 25% of patients with congenital scoliosis in the average clinic do not show any progression and do not need any treatment. Conversely, about 75% will show some progression, and approximately 50% will progress significantly and will require treatment.[87]

Certain anomalies are associated consistently with progression, especially the unilateral unsegmented bar. This anomaly is so reliably malicious that the patient with this anomaly should have a fusion immediately and not wait for progression. The unilateral segmented bar causes a total lack of growth on the concave side of the curve, and, if growth

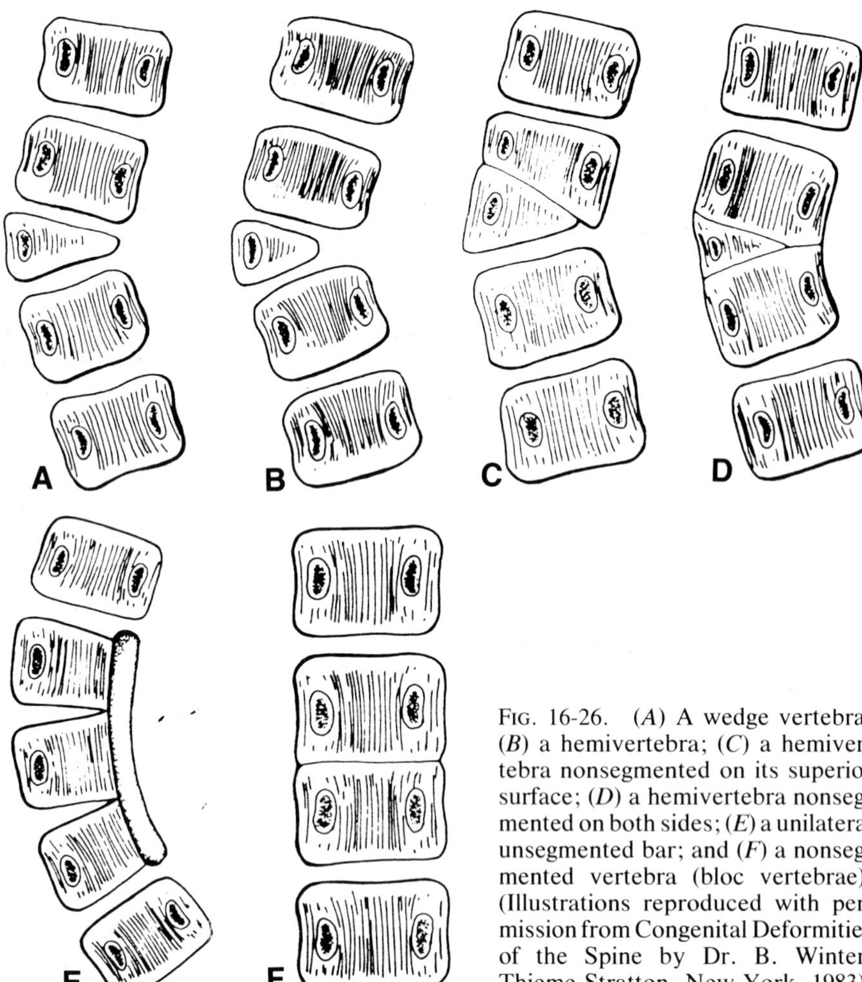

FIG. 16-26. (*A*) A wedge vertebra; (*B*) a hemivertebra; (*C*) a hemivertebra nonsegmented on its superior surface; (*D*) a hemivertebra nonsegmented on both sides; (*E*) a unilateral unsegmented bar; and (*F*) a nonsegmented vertebra (bloc vertebrae). (Illustrations reproduced with permission from Congenital Deformities of the Spine by Dr. B. Winter, Thieme-Stratton, New York, 1983)

continues on the convex side, the patient will grow into severe deformity. Naturally, this deformity is extremely rigid and virtually impossible to correct except by extraordinary and difficult surgery. Therefore, it is far better to prevent an increase in the deformity than to correct it once it has become severe (Fig. 16-28).

Hemivertebrae may be single or multiple and balanced or unbalanced. Balanced hemivertebrae often may not progress and not require treatment. Contralateral hemivertebrae when separated by several segments, will often produce a double curve, and both curves may progress. In such cases, both curves require fusion. A single hemivertebra may or may not cause deformity; this is very difficult to predict. The patient must be followed carefully, and, if deformity occurs, fusion should be performed. A single hemivertebra at the lumbosacral level produces a significant decompensation of the patient, because there is no room below the hemivertebra for natural compensation to occur. These patients may develop a severe list to one side, which is progressive with growth. This produces a rigid deformity that is extraordinarily difficult to correct.[83]

Evaluation of the Patient with Congenital Scoliosis

Patients with congenital anomalies of the spine quite frequently have congenital anomalies involving regions other than the spine. It is extremely important that these patients receive a complete evaluation.

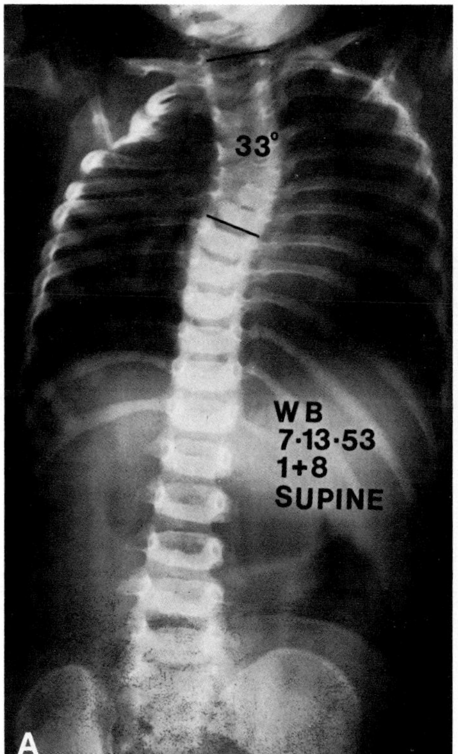

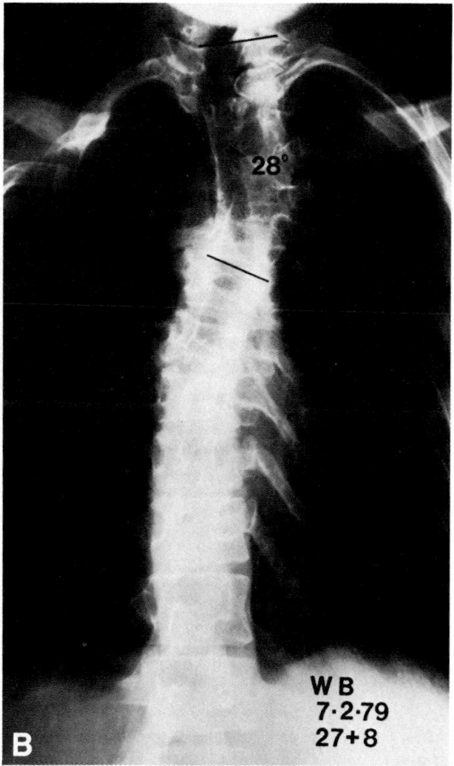

FIG. 16-27. (*A*) A 20-month-old boy with a 33° upper thoracic congenital scoliosis. There are multiple rib synostoses on the left. Is this a unilateral defect of segmentation with a bad prognosis or a bilateral defect of segmentation with a good prognosis? No treatment was given. (*B*) The same patient 26 years later, with a 28° curve. No treatment was ever given. (Illustrations reproduced with permission from Congenital Deformities of the Spine by Dr. B. Winter, Thieme-Stratton, New York, 1983)

The most frequent associated congenital anomaly is found in the genitourinary tract. Studies of patients with congenital scoliosis by MacEwen and associates[50] revealed an incidence of 20% having anomalies of the urinary tract on routine intravenous pyelography. This is not surprising from an embryologic point of view in that the same undifferentiated block of mesenchyme will differentiate medially into the vertebra and ventrolaterally into the mesonephros, which subsequently becomes the kidney and the urinary tract. Many of the anomalies noted are not demanding of urologic treatment (*e.g.*, unilateral kidney with good function or a crossed-fused ectopia with good function). However, in the study by MacEwen and colleagues,[50] 6% of the patients were noted to have a life-threatening urologic problem, usually obstructive uropathy. If such obstructive uropathy is detected during screening of the scoliotic patient, appropriate urologic procedures should be carried out before instituting orthopaedic treatment of the scoliosis.

A second area of great concern is cardiac anomalies. As many as 10% to 15% of patients with congenital scoliosis have been noted to have congenital heart defects. These may have previously been undetected. Murmurs should never be attributed to the scoliosis alone and must be thoroughly evaluated. It is tempting to blame murmurs on distortion of the thorax due to the scoliosis, but, in actuality, scoliosis does not produce murmurs. Therefore, any murmur must be considered as intrinsic in the heart until proven otherwise (Fig. 16-29).

Examination of the back and extremities for any evidence of hidden neurologic disorder is very important. There is a fairly high frequency of spinal dysraphism in patients with congen-

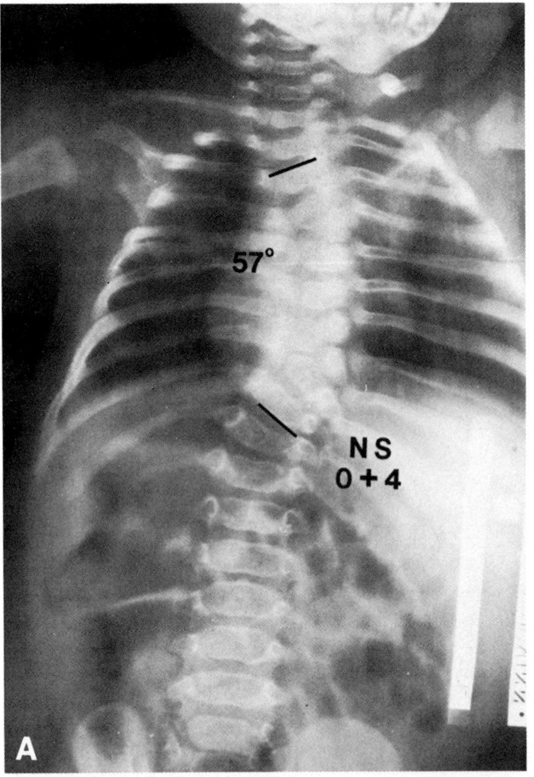

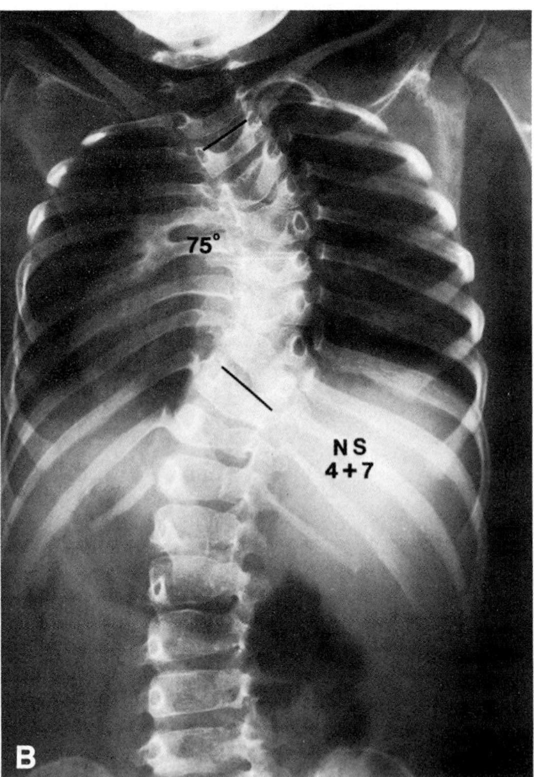

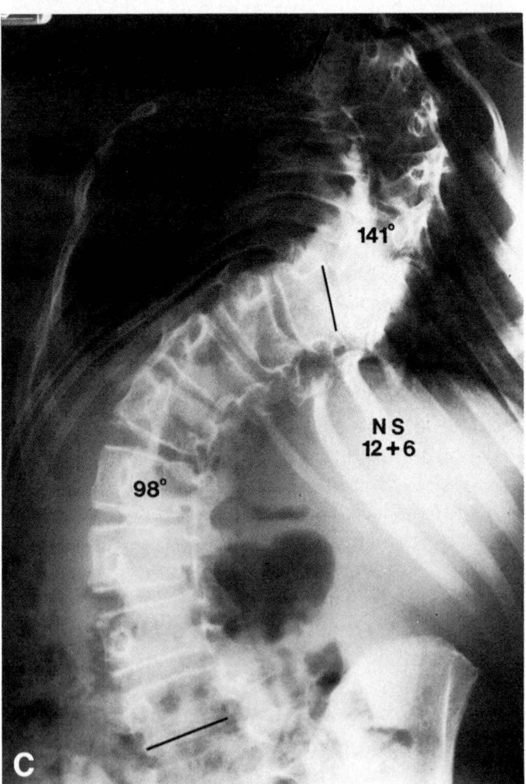

FIG. 16-28. (*A*) A 4-month-old girl with a 57° congenital thoracic scoliosis. There are hemivertebrae on the right and segmentation defects on the left, the most likely of all congenital curves to progress. No treatment was given. (*B*) The same patient at age 4 years. The curve has progressed to 75°. The segmentation defect on the left is more obvious now. (*C*) By age 12, her curve had increased to 141°. A highly structural secondary lumbar curve of 98° had also appeared. Such progression should not be allowed to happen. (Illustrations reproduced with permission from Congenital Deformities of the Spine by Dr. B. Winter, Thieme-Stratton, New York, 1983)

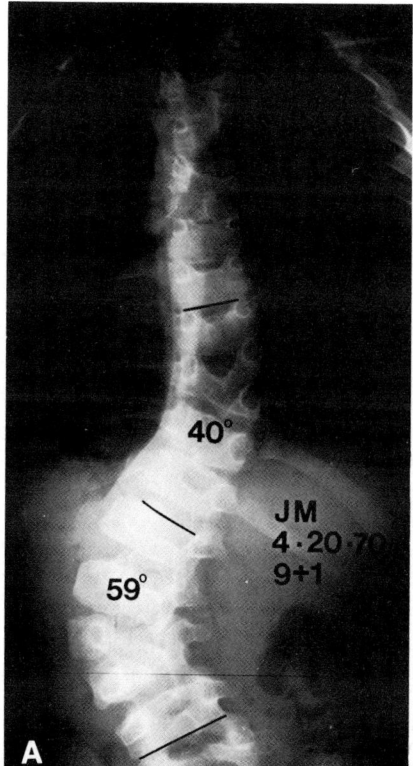

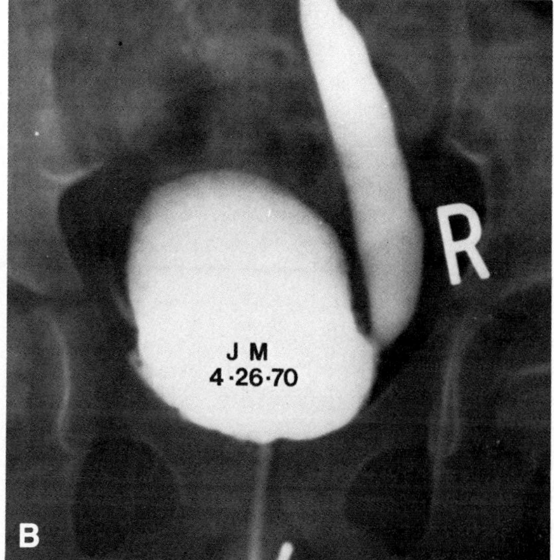

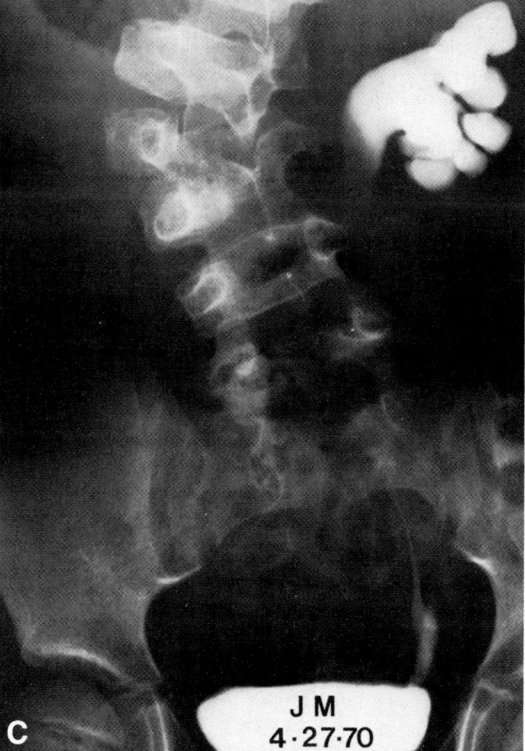

FIG. 16-29. (*A*) A 9-year-old boy with a 59° lumbar congenital scoliosis with a mid-lumbar hemivertebra. A second hemivertebra on the right at T10 is also noted. (*B*) Urographic studies demonstrated a ureterovesical obstruction with hydroureter. There were no urinary symptoms. (*C*) Marked hydronephrosis of the right kidney is noted. (Illustrations reproduced with permission from Congenital Deformities of the Spine by Dr. R. Winter, Thieme-Stratton, New York, 1983)

ital scoliosis. Winter and associates[84] reported that approximately 5% of their patients with congenital scoliosis had a diastematomyelia and another 5% can be presumed to have some other form of dysraphism such as a tethered spinal cord, fibrous dural bands, intradural lipoma, and so on. These are frequently associated with hair patches on the back, dimples, hemangiomata, and various abnormalities on the examination of the lower extremities. These abnormalities include flat feet, cavus feet, vertical tali, clubfeet, and more subtle afflictions such as slight atrophy of one calf, a slightly smaller foot on one side, and asymmetry of the reflexes. It is possible for a patient to have diastematomyelia and have none of these associated findings. The physician must be very astute to evaluate the x-rays for interpedicular widening or midline bony spicules (Figs. 16-30 and 16-31).

Orthotic Treatment

Because the primary deformity in congenital scoliosis is in the bones rather than in the soft tissues, the curves tend to be rigid; thus, are not as amenable to orthotic treatment as are idiopathic and paralytic curves. Nevertheless, there are definite indications for orthotic treatment of congenital spine deformities.

A study by Winter and colleagues[88] indicated that certain patients did well in the Milwaukee brace for many years, and a few could even permanently be treated in an orthosis, avoiding surgery. The patients who did well had very flexible curves. These were patients in whom the curvature was primarily in noncongenital vertebrae. There were three or four patterns in which this occurred. In the first pattern, the congenital anomalies might be at the proximal end of the curve, because the major portion of the curve was below the nonanomalous vertebrae. In the second pattern, there were instances in which the anomalies were at the lower end, below an area of curvature, and most of the curve was in nonanomalous vertebrae. In the third pattern, there were situations in which the apex of the curve contained anomalous vertebrae, but the totality of the curve was far longer than just the area of the anomalies, and the areas above and below the apex were not involved by anomalous vertebrae and, thus, had correctability. The fourth pattern in which the brace helps were those situations in which there were a few anomalies scattered up and down the spine, with normal segmented and mobile vertebrae between them. These authors believed that it was useless to

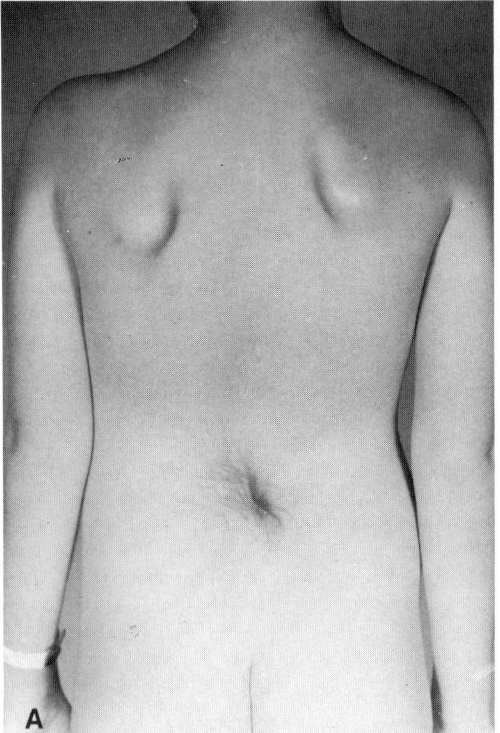

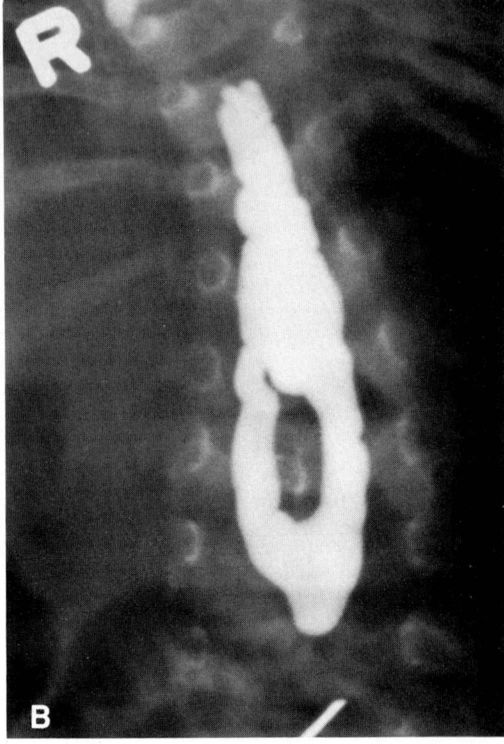

FIG. 16-30. (*A*) This patient presented with thoracic scoliosis (no prominence of the right scapula) and a hairy patch in the low back. One foot was smaller than the other, and there was an absence of the ankle reflex on the side of the smaller foot. (*B*) A myelogram demonstrating a classic diastematomyelia.

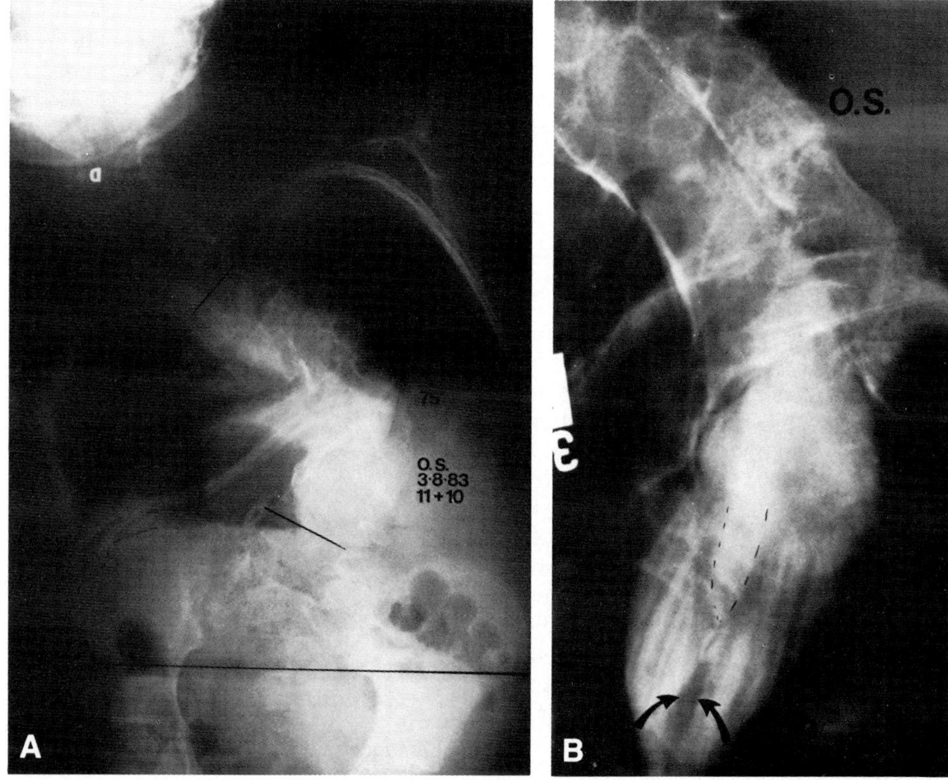

FIG. 16-31. (*A*) An 11-year-old boy with a severe congenital scoliosis of 75°. He also had bilateral talipes equinovarus. (*B*) A water-soluble myelogram shows a split spinal cord (diastematomyelia), a low-lying conus, and a tight filum terminal (*arrows*).

attempt to treat rigid curves with a Milwaukee brace.

It is important that the physician recognize that the orthosis must accomplish its goal. That is, it must control the curve in an acceptable alignment. It is doing the patient no service to try to put a 90° curve in an orthosis. The main indication for bracing appears to be the delay of surgery until a more optimal age. This is particularly true of a long curve in which a long fusion at a very early age would be less preferable than at a later age. This delay in fusion can be accomplished with a Milwaukee brace in a few selected patients. If the patient's curve progresses despite the orthosis, fusion must be done without further delay. It is only if the orthosis successfully holds the curve that it can be continued.

The most common error seen in the treatment of congenital scoliosis by a Milwaukee brace is the attempt to treat with an orthosis a curve that requires surgery. The second most common mistake is the failure to recognize that the orthosis is not doing an adequate job of controlling the curve. It is imperative that the physician carefully monitor the progress of the patient while in the device; he must not delegate this responsibility to anyone else, and he must be prepared to admit that it is not working and to proceed to a fusion.

Surgical Treatment

Surgery is the most customary treatment of severe or progressive congenital scolioses. Several different types of operative procedures can be applied. Thus, there emerge two fundamental questions: What is the best procedure? and What is the best time for the procedure?

The nature of the procedure depends on the nature of the problem. The fundamental procedure is posterior spine fusion without instrumentation. Posterior fusion can also be done with instrumentation, but the risks of neurologic damage are higher. Hemivertebra excision can be done, but this is not necessary for all hemivertebra problems. Epiphyseodesis and arthrodesis done both anteriorly and posteriorly on the convex side has begun to emerge as another valid method of treatment.

Progressive curves should be treated surgically, especially if they do not respond to orthotic treatment. If a 25° curve in a 3-year-old child progresses to 35° by age 6 years, the curve requires surgical treatment. There is a tendency to avoid surgery at this age for fear of "stunting the child's growth," but, in reality, the child will grow taller if the curve is fused than if progressive deformity occurs.

Posterior fusion must cover the entire measured curve and extend to the "central gravity line." Correction is best obtained with a carefully molded Risser cast. Abundant bone graft should be added, because a thick fusion mass is necessary to avoid bending of the fusion by the intact anterior growth plates (Figs. 16-32 and 16-33).

Anterior and posterior convex hemiarthrodesis and hemiepiphyseodesis was designed to arrest progressive deformity and to prevent bending of the fusion mass. If concave growth persists, progressive improvement of the curve can occur (Fig. 16-34).[82]

Hemivertebra excision is difficult and can be dangerous to spinal cord or nerve root function. It appears to be most useful in those patients who have severe decompensation due to lumbosacral area hemivertebrae. It must be remembered that hemivertebra excision is a wedge osteotomy at the apex of a curve, and the whole curve must always be fused.

Harrington distraction rods have been dangerous in congenital scoliosis, mostly due to dysraphic problems. Distracting a tethered cord is very likely to produce paralysis. Shortening of a long (convex) side of the curve is preferable to lengthening of a short (concave) side.

MARFAN'S SCOLIOSIS

Scoliosis is a common manifestation in the patient with Marfan's syndrome. The reported incidence of scoliosis in this condition ranges from 30% to 70%.[65] Patients with Marfan's syndrome have a defect of the connective soft tissues. Therefore, it is not surprising that deformity of the spine should occur. Scoliosis may appear at a young age, particularly in the more florid cases of Marfan's syndrome, or it may occur in the adolescent ages, particularly in the less obvious forms of Marfan's syndrome.

Clinical Features

The scoliosis in Marfan's syndrome has some typical characteristics. The curvatures are usually those same patterns seen in idiopathic scoliosis. Pelvic obliquity, commonly seen in neuromuscular diseases, is not seen in Marfan's syndrome. Patients usually have double structural right thoracic, left lumbar curves; a right thoracic curve; or a thoracolumbar curve, all of which are radiologically similar to idiopathic scoliosis. Double curve patterns seem to be more frequent in Marfan's syndrome, whereas single curve patterns are more common in idiopathic scoliosis.

The quantity of curvature varies from very mild to extremely severe. Because of the high incidence of scoliosis in patients with Marfan's syndrome, all patients with this syndrome should have regular spine examinations. The physician must look for scoliosis in these patients, seeking such classic manifestations as dislocation of the lens of the eye, heart murmurs, and arachnodactyly. Echocardiography should be done in all true Marfan's patients as well as all borderline suspected cases. A very high frequency of valve prolapse has been detected.

Treatment

The treatment of the scoliosis of Marfan's syndrome is very similar to that for most idiopathic scolioses. Very mild curves of 15° or less need no treatment but must be very carefully followed to ensure they do not progress into more serious curves.

Orthotic Treatment. This is appropriate for moderate curves of less than 40°, particularly in the younger child. Orthotic treatment has not been as effective in Marfan's syndrome as in idiopathic scoliosis, apparently due to the inability of the soft tissues to "stabilize." Because of the great flexibility of the curve in Marfan's syndrome, particularly early in the course of the disease, excellent realignment can be obtained in the brace. However, despite 2 or more years of full-time brace wearing, it is not unusual to see a patient relapse to the original deformity or worse after removal of the brace. A few patients have been success-

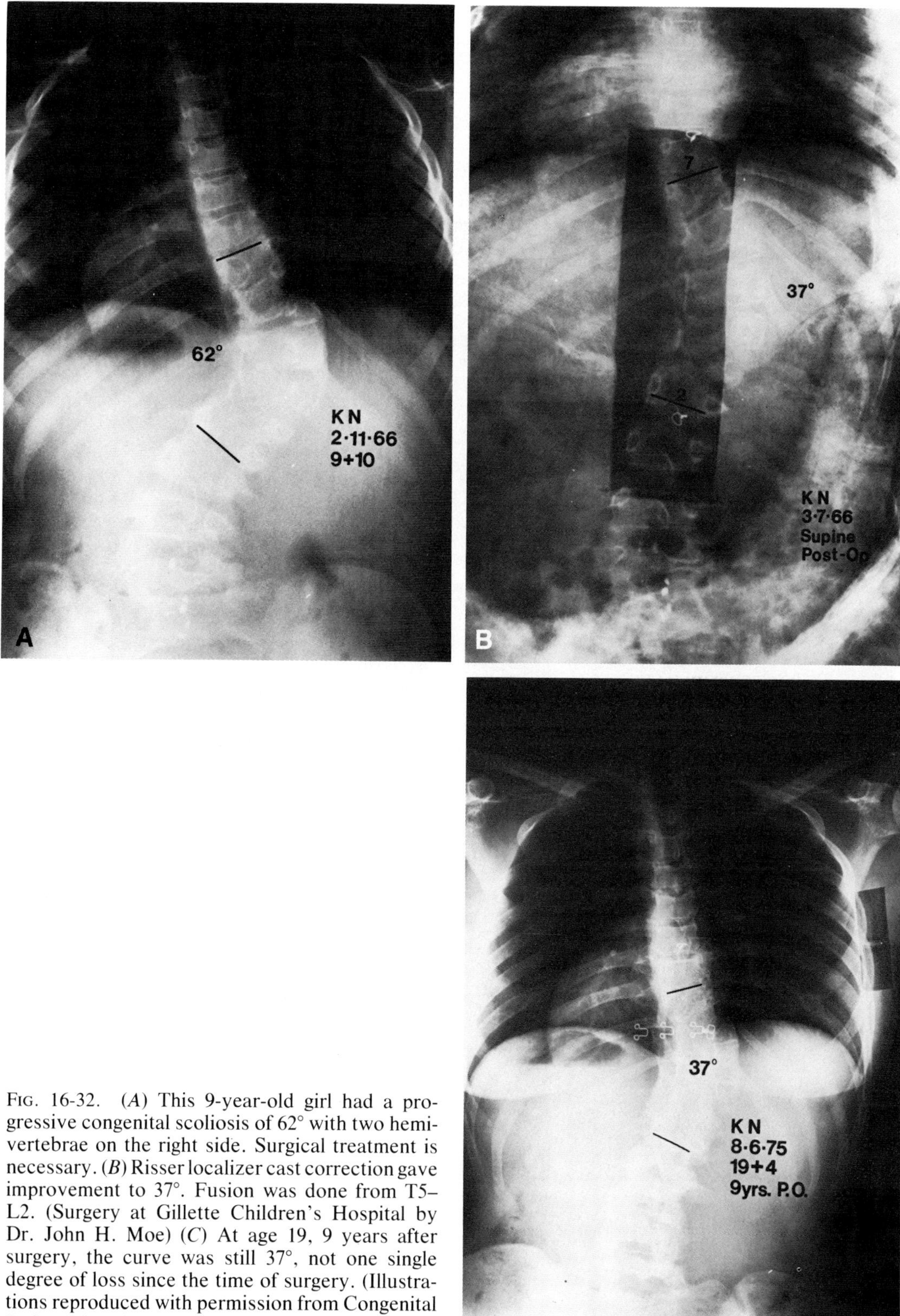

FIG. 16-32. (*A*) This 9-year-old girl had a progressive congenital scoliosis of 62° with two hemivertebrae on the right side. Surgical treatment is necessary. (*B*) Risser localizer cast correction gave improvement to 37°. Fusion was done from T5–L2. (Surgery at Gillette Children's Hospital by Dr. John H. Moe) (*C*) At age 19, 9 years after surgery, the curve was still 37°, not one single degree of loss since the time of surgery. (Illustrations reproduced with permission from Congenital Deformities of the Spine by Dr. B. Winter, Thieme-Stratton, New York, 1983)

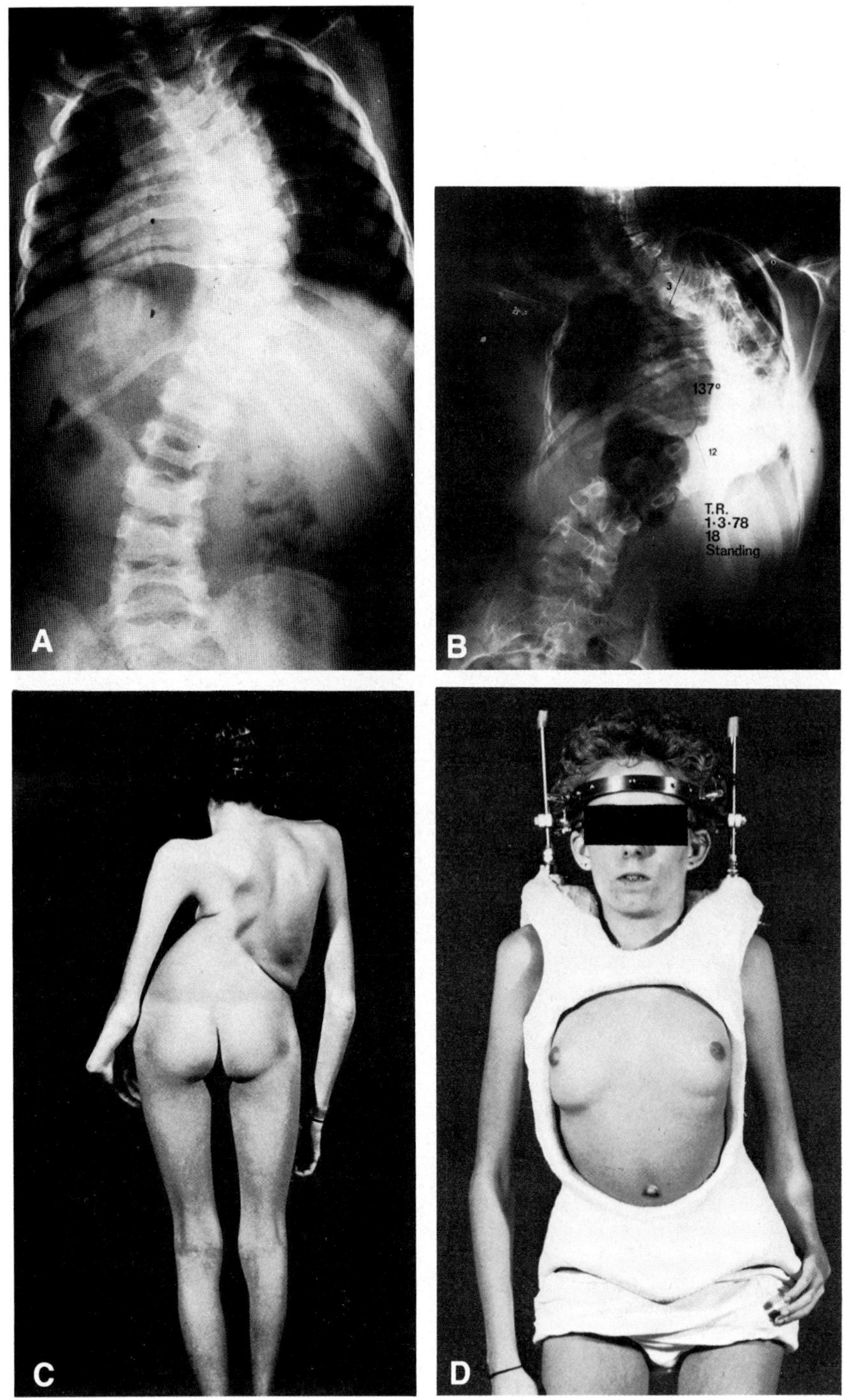
A
3
137°
12
T.R.
1·3·78
18
Standing
B
C
D

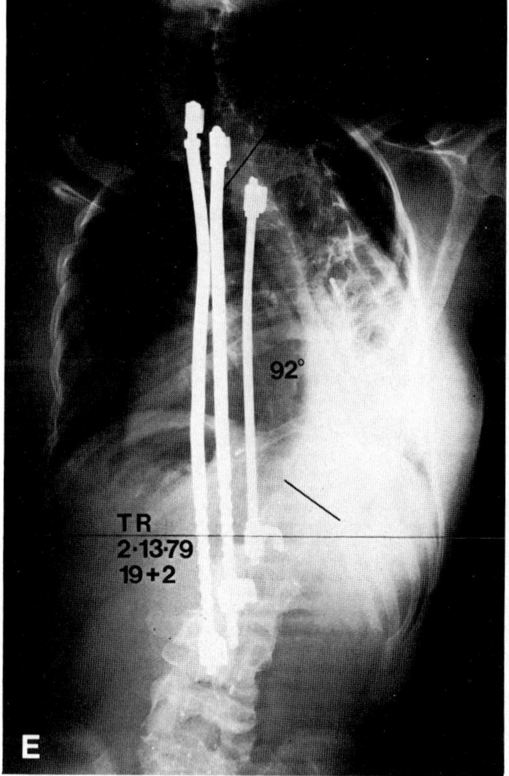

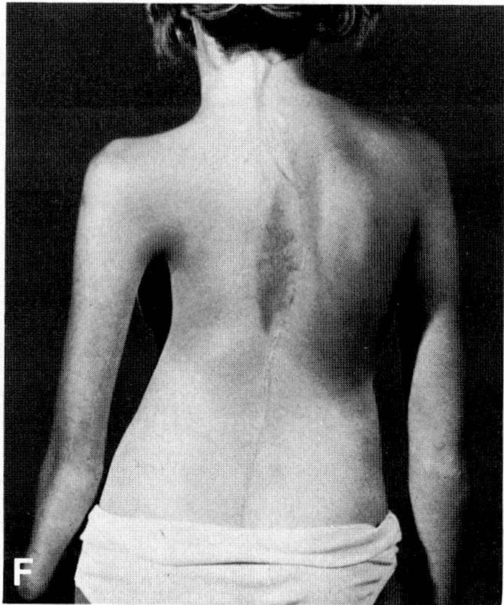

FIG. 16-33. (*A*) At age 8, this girl had a 60° congenital scoliosis with two hemivertebrae on the convex side. Note the rib gap on the left at T10 and T11. No treatment of her spine was given, although she was under the care of an orthopaedist for a congenital clubfoot and radial clubhand. (*B*) By age 18, her scoliosis had increased to 137°. (*C*) Her clinical appearance at age 18. (*D*) In a postoperative halo-cast. (*E*) A radiograph 1 year after surgery showing correction to 92° with three distraction rods. (*F*) A postoperative photograph. She gained 11 cm in height and increased her vital capacity by 750 ml. (Illustrations reproduced with permission from Congenital Deformities of the Spine by Dr. B. Winter, Thieme-Stratton, New York, 1983)

fully managed with an orthosis, but the incidence of relapse is certainly much higher than it is in idiopathic scoliosis.

Surgical Treatment. Most patients with Marfan's scoliosis of moderate to severe degree should be considered as surgical candidates. The only contraindications to surgery are known cardiac decompensation or aortic aneurysm. Because of the high incidence of cardiac and aortic defects in this disease, all patients considered for scoliosis surgery must have a very thorough cardiovascular evaluation. Aortic insufficiency and mitral insufficiency are about equally common. Echocardiography has been greatly helpful in the evaluation of these patients.

The moderately advanced curve (40° to 70°) can usually be corrected by direct surgical instrumentation and fusion. Patients with more severe curves, particularly those with curves of 90° or more should have preliminary discectomy followed by instrumentation and fusion. The fusion area encompasses the same limits as for idiopathic scoliosis; the reader is referred to that section for selection of the fusion area.

The healing time appears to be reasonably normal in these patients, and usually 6 to 9 months of immobilization is sufficient. With good internal fixation by Harrington instruments and good cast or brace fixation externally, early ambulation is very practical for

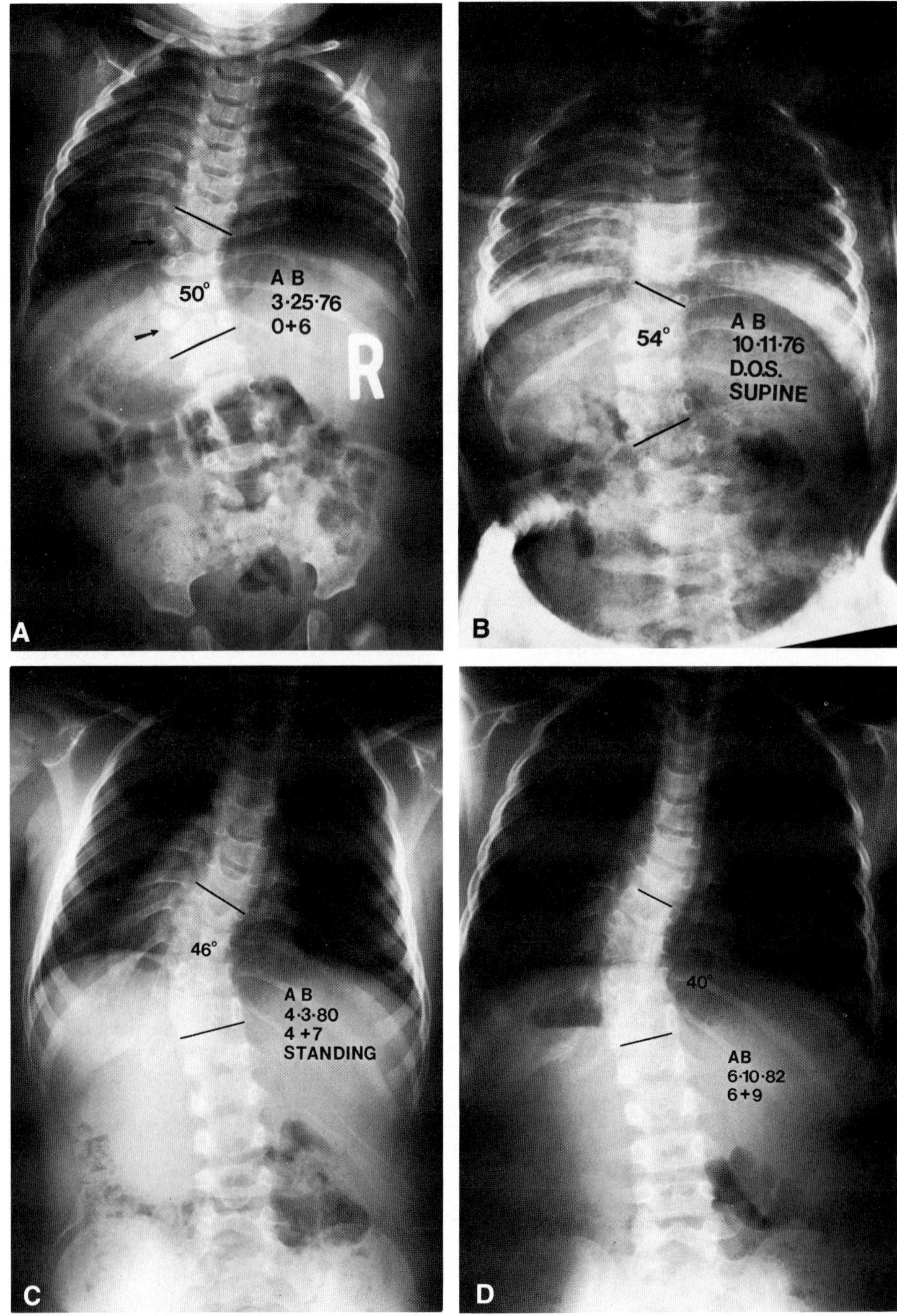
50°
A B
3·25·76
0+6
R
A
54°
A B
10·11·76
D.O.S.
SUPINE
B
46°
A B
4·3·80
4 +7
STANDING
C
40°
AB
6·10·82
6+9
D

these patients. Prolonged bed rest is not necessary. Surgical treatment should not be denied to the patient with Marfan's syndrome because of the fear of creating an aortic aneurysm or because of the expectation of early death.

NEUROFIBROMATOSIS

See Chapter 26.

NEUROMUSCULAR SCOLIOSIS

There are a multitude of diseases that fall into this category. Some general principles apply to almost all neuromuscular problems, and there are some specific principles within each category.

Almost all children who suffer from some type of neuromuscular disorder have a tendency for scoliosis or some other type of spine deformity. The severity of the deformity depends on the severity of the weakness, as well as the pattern of weakness and the patient's age at the time that the paralysis develops.

Neuromuscular curves tend to be long and sweeping, usually involving many more vertebrae than those of idiopathic scoliosis. There are fewer compensatory curves. There may be a pelvic obliquity, which is never seen in idiopathic scoliosis. The cervical spine may also be involved, again a finding never seen in the idiopathic patients. Pulmonary function can be quite severely involved due to intercostal muscle weakness; thus, the patients are at a higher risk for pneumonia and atelectasis.

Orthotics can be used for patients with neuromuscular deformities but usually only as a delaying tactic until there is a more optimal time for surgery. Milwaukee braces are seldom used; molded body jackets provide better support and better patient function.

When fusion is necessary, the area of fusion is longer, the bones are more osteoporotic, the blood loss is higher, and the postoperative complication rate is worse. Surgery is performed to achieve stability and balance, not to correct the deformity by a certain number of degrees or percentage.

UPPER MOTOR NEURON LESIONS

Cerebral Palsy

Most upper motor neuron lesions are due to cerebral palsy. The incidence of scoliosis in cerebral palsy varies according to the pattern and severity of neuromuscular involvement. Ambulatory patients with mild involvement, such as a spastic hemiparesis, seldom have a curve of more than 10°. On the other hand, severely involved, nonambulatory spastic quadriplegics have a high incidence of curves.

Mild but progressive curves in ambulatory patients can be treated in conventional orthoses but should be fused if the curves progress beyond 50°. Structural curves in the more severely involved patients should also be fused, preferably before horrendous deformity develops. Some physicians believe that retarded patients should not have surgery, but most believe that these patients should have surgery to help them function better.

Many children with cerebral palsy have hypotonic, collapsing spines, tending to slump into a long postural kyphosis. These patients are unable to sit well and benefit from seating devices that permit supported sitting in a wheelchair. These devices can be pads added to the chair or molded plastic supports made from an impression of the patient (Fig. 16-35).

Patients who progress on to surgery tend to fall into two groups: (1) the lesser involved patient with a thoracic or thoracolumbar curve and no pelvic obliquity, and (2) the more severely involved group, with lumbar or thoracolumbar curves accompanied by pelvic obliquity.[46]

The lesser involved group can be readily treated by standard techniques of posterior fusion and instrumentation and do not require fusion to the sacrum. The most severely involved group definitely requires fusion to the sacrum and may require both anterior and

◀ Fig. 16-34. (*A*) A 16-month-old child with a 50° scoliosis due to two hemivertebrae on the left. She progressed to 62° by age 12 months. (*B*) Treatment consisted of combined anterior and posterior hemiepiphyseodesis and hemiarthrodesis from T9–T12 on the left with cast correction to 54°. (*C*) By age 4, the curve was 46°. (*D*) By age 6, she had improved to 40°. (Illustrations reproduced with permission from Journal of Pediatric Orthopaedics, Vol 1:361–366, 1983)

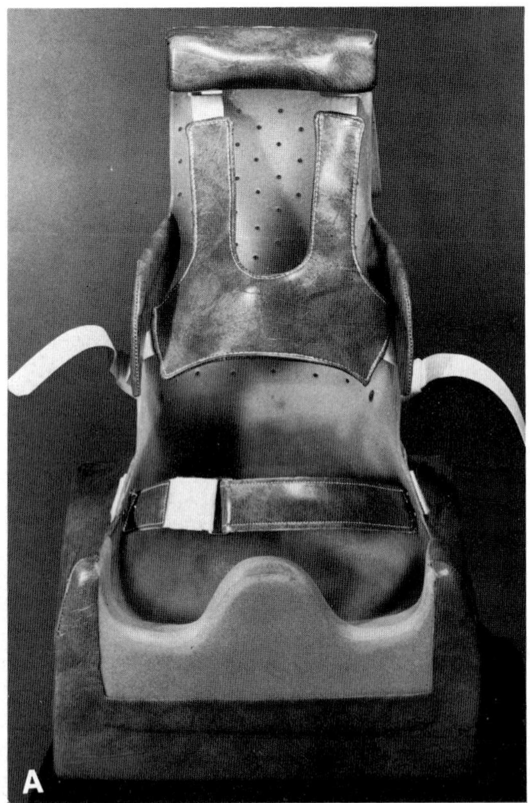

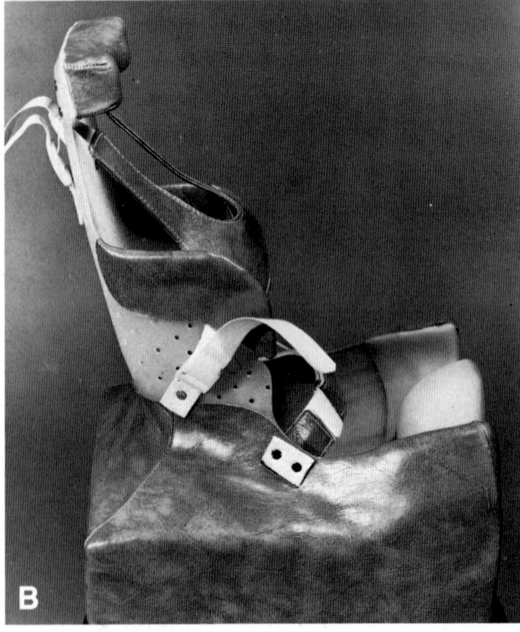

FIG. 16-35. (*A and B*) A sitting support orthosis used for providing a sitting alignment for the seriously handicapped child.

posterior surgery. The goal of the surgery is to achieve a *vertical torso centered over a level pelvis* (Figs. 16-36–16-38).

LOWER MOTOR NEURON LESIONS

Prior to the advent of poliomyelitis vaccines, the most common cause of paralytic scoliosis was poliomyelitis. Many of the understandings of the treatment of all neuromuscular problems developed from the treatment of poliomyelitis curves. Unfortunately, there are still some parts of the world where this condition persists. In North America, the only children presenting with this problem are those coming from other countries.

Spinal muscle atrophy has emerged as one of the leading causes of paralytic spinal deformity. (See Chapter 8 for a general discussion of this condition.) Many severe curves have been allowed to develop with the mistaken thought that the child was inevitably going to die. This is not the case, and there is no justification for allowing severe curves to develop. Many of the deaths were due to the untreated scoliosis, not the primary disease itself (Fig. 16-39).

Orthotic support should begin at the first sign of a structural curve (a curve present on a supine film) and should be continued as long as the curve remains controlled. If the orthosis fails to control the curve, surgery is indicated. Children younger than 10 years of age who need surgery can be treated by instrumentation without fusion, the fusion being done at about age 12 in girls and age 14 in boys.

Patients presenting with severe curves require prompt surgical treatment. These are high-risk patients, requiring major intensive care units and physicians with highly expert anesthesia and surgical skills. The Luque procedure appears to be the best form of surgery for these patients. It provides a reasonable correction, excellent stabilization, and no need for a postoperative cast or brace. Rapid (within 2 to 3 days) return to the upright position is mandatory. The cervical spine is often weak and should not be made weaker by bed rest, or casts or braces extending to the neck (Fig. 16-40).

DUCHENNE MUSCULAR DYSTROPHY

The most common myopathic disease to cause scoliosis is Duchenne (pseudohyper-

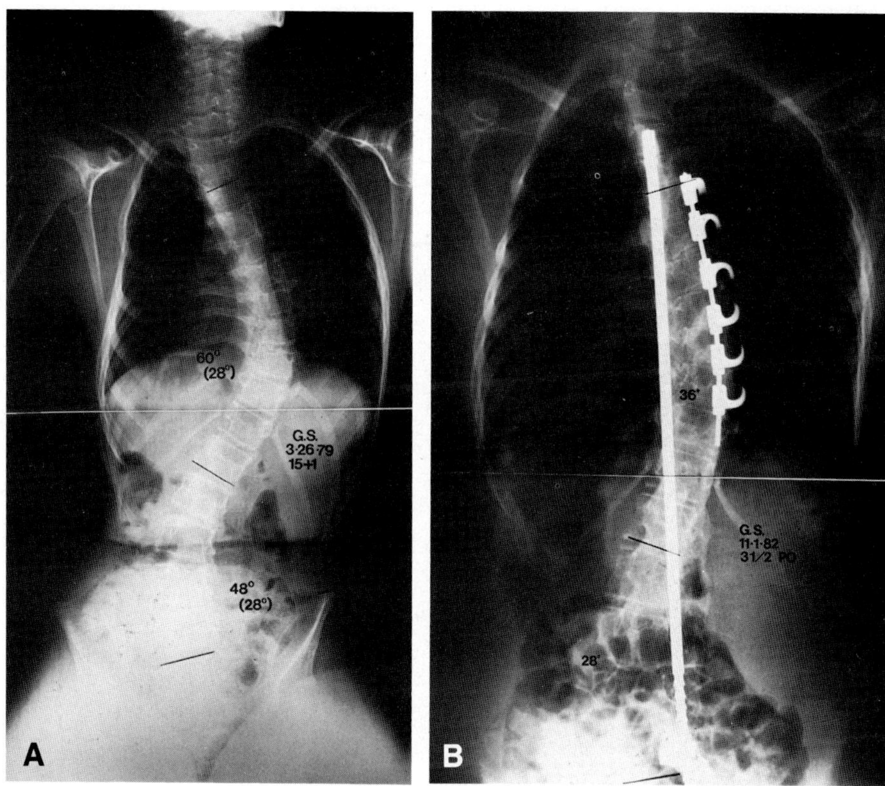

FIG. 16-36. (*A*) A 15-year-old girl with a 60° T4–L1 right thoracic scoliosis associated with cerebral palsy. There is no pelvic obliquity. (*B*) Three and one-half years after posterior fusion from T3–L4.

trophic) muscular dystrophy. Scoliosis as a result of Duchenne muscular dystrophy is unusual until after the child has stopped walking. About 80% of the patients then show serious scoliosis progression; this is always associated with decreasing pulmonary function. Part of the pulmonary function decrease is due to the scoliosis itself, and part is due to the weakened intercostal muscles.

Bracing is not effective for curve control, and surgery is becoming the optimal treatment for those curves showing serious progression relatively early in the disease. The Luque technique is best, because rapid (2 to 3 days) return to upright activities is mandatory (Fig. 16-41).

POSTURAL KYPHOSIS

"Bad posture" is a common presenting problem in the orthopaedist's office, but fortunately, it is not a major problem. Postural kyphosis is diagnosed by the ability of the child to voluntarily correct the roundness in the standing position and to demonstrate reversal of the thoracic spine to lordosis by hyperextension in the prone position. X-ray examination demonstrates no abnormalities of the vertebrae. There may be increased kyphosis, but a supine hyperextension film will show the complete correctibility. It is the child's responsibility to stand correctly, and it is foolish to treat such an entity with casting, orthotics, or stimulators. The physician's most important function is to rule out more significant pathology.

SCHEUERMANN'S DISEASE

Scheuermann's disease is a common problem affecting the spines of adolescents. It occurs approximately equally among males and females, and, second to idiopathic scoliosis, it is the most common cause of patients coming to spine deformity clinics.

(*Text continues on page 623*)

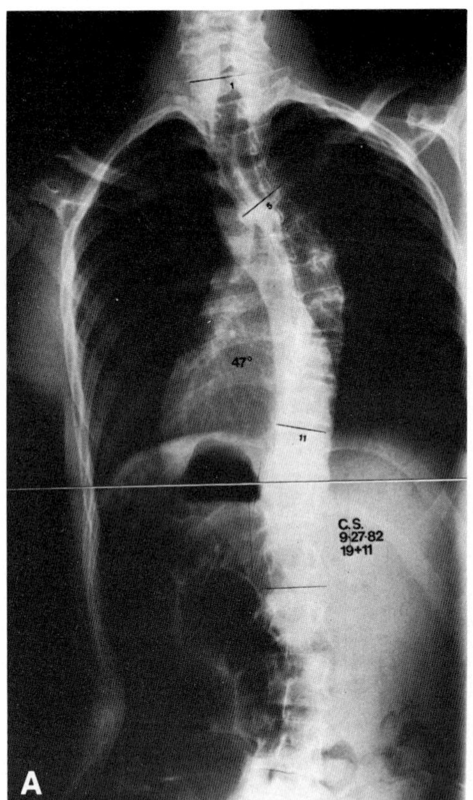

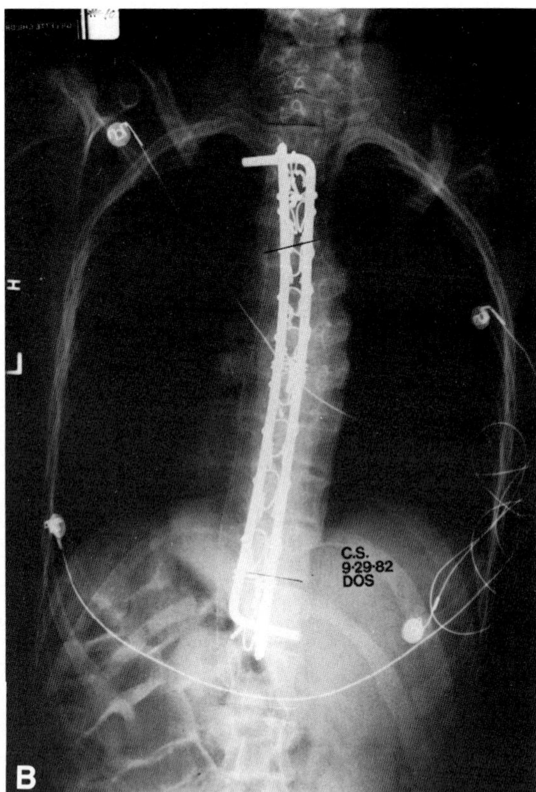

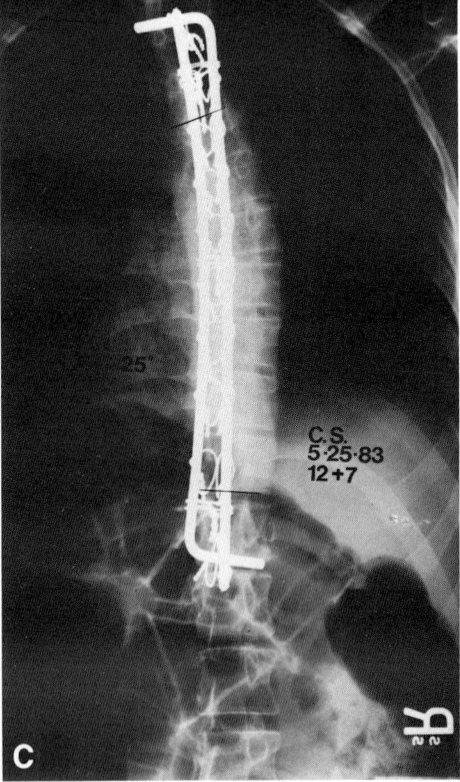

FIG. 16-37. (*A*) A male with cerebral palsy and mild mental retardation. The scoliosis is purely thoracic. (*B*) After Luque instrumentation and fusion, the curve has been corrected from 48° to 24°. One year later, his curve is still 24°. No cast or brace was used.

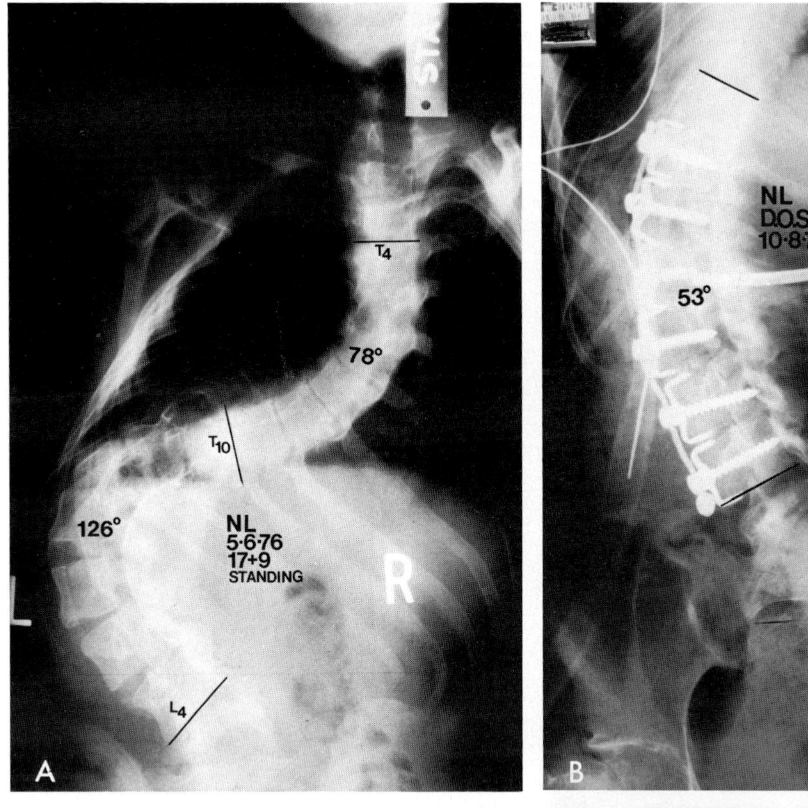

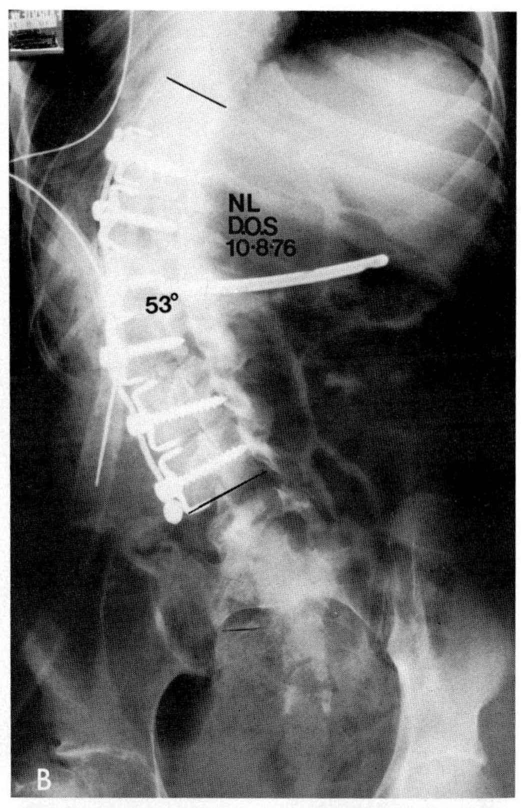

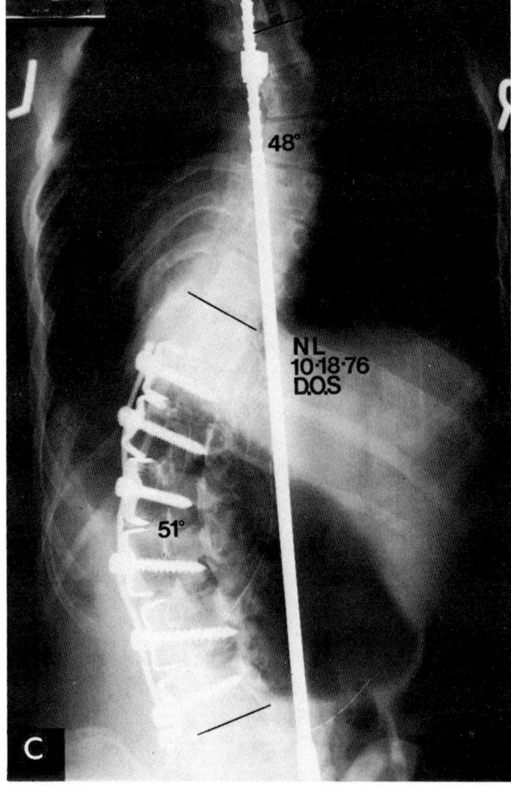

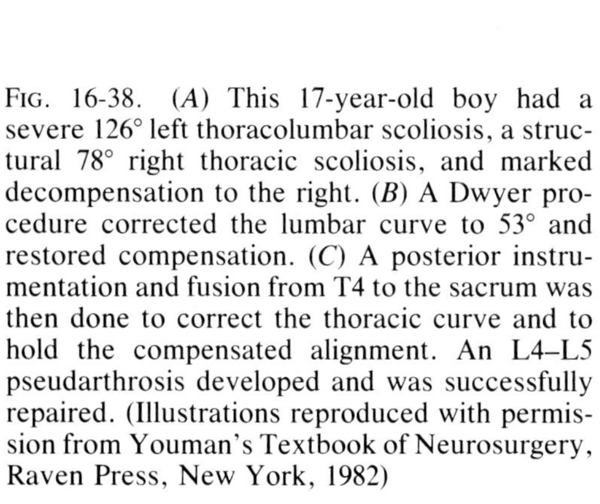

FIG. 16-38. (*A*) This 17-year-old boy had a severe 126° left thoracolumbar scoliosis, a structural 78° right thoracic scoliosis, and marked decompensation to the right. (*B*) A Dwyer procedure corrected the lumbar curve to 53° and restored compensation. (*C*) A posterior instrumentation and fusion from T4 to the sacrum was then done to correct the thoracic curve and to hold the compensated alignment. An L4–L5 pseudarthrosis developed and was successfully repaired. (Illustrations reproduced with permission from Youman's Textbook of Neurosurgery, Raven Press, New York, 1982)

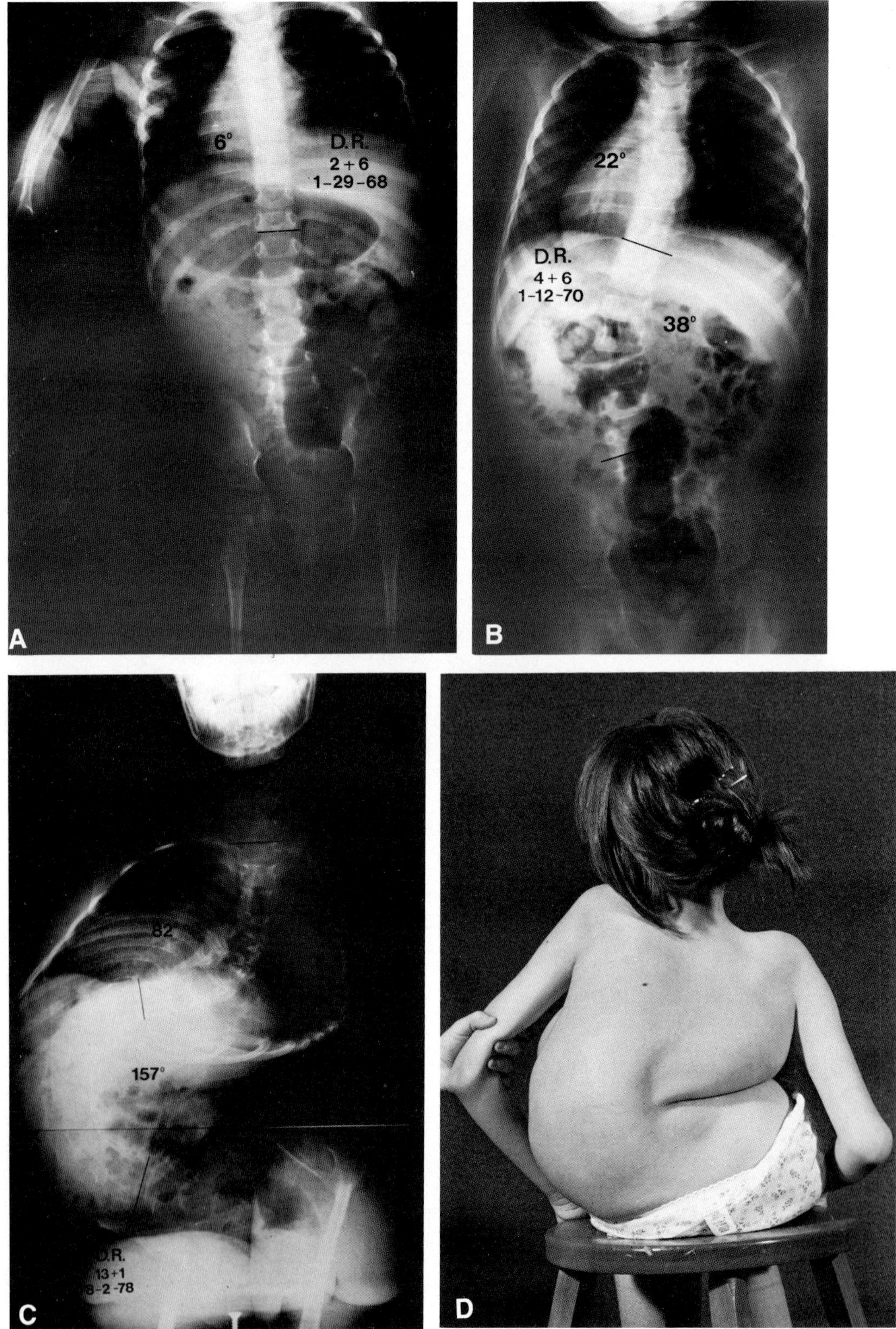
6°
D.R.
2+6
1-29-68
A
22°
D.R.
4+6
1-12-70
38°
B
82°
157°
13+1
C
D

Etiology

The cause of Scheuermann's disease is totally unknown. In the past, it has been called an "epiphysitis," but there is no evidence of any inflammatory changes. Histologic examination of disc and end-plate material removed at surgery has revealed only marked irregularity of the end-plates and frequent perforations into the vertebral body of nuclear material.

Scheuermann's disease is a hereditary condition, but the hereditary patterns have not been clearly defined. As stated previously, males and females appear to be affected equally. It is quite common to see several children in one family with the condition, as well as one or both parents.

Diagnosis

The typical patient is between the ages of 12 and 15 years of age, with a round-shouldered appearance. The patient may or may not have pain of the thoracic spine.

The differential diagnosis is usually a problem of distinguishing Scheuermann's disease from postural roundback, although other conditions causing kyphosis as idiopathic juvenile osteoporosis, congenital kyphosis, and infectious disorders of the spine may occasionally cause diagnostic confusion.

Scheuermann's disease can usually be readily distinguished from postural kyphosis by basic physical and x-ray examinations. Patients with true postural roundback can readily assume a very straight spine position if they are correctly encouraged. The patient with Scheuermann's disease and fixed spine deformity cannot truly correct the kyphosis, either in the standing position or in the prone hyperextended position. When viewed from the side while bending forward, the patient with Scheuermann's disease will show an area with acute angulation, usually at about T7. The patient with postural roundback shows a smooth, symmetrical contour. Most patients with Scheuermann's disease have a fixed or relatively fixed kyphosis. These two simple clinical tests will usually distinguish structural kyphosis from postural roundback (Fig. 16-42).

X-ray examination will provide the final diagnosis. The classic findings include narrowing of the disc spaces, increased anteroposterior diameter of the apical thoracic vertebrae, loss of normal height of the involved vertebra, and irregularity of the end-plates and there may or may not be Schmorl's nodes. On the supine hyperextension x-ray, loss of the normal flexibility of the spine will be noted, and, in addition, there is usually wedging of one or more apical vertebrae (Fig. 16-43).

Some investigators believe that Scheuermann's disease cannot be correctly diagnosed without there being three consecutive vertebrae with wedging of at least 5°.[75] The author does not believe that this wedging is necessary for diagnosis and thinks that the presence of other signs, particularly relatively fixed deformity, is sufficient to make the diagnosis.

Natural History

Scheuermann's disease may exist in the spine without causing either pain or deformity. It can thus run its natural course without creating any clinical problem. Often, however, it creates either pain or deformity or both. A slight scoliosis is quite common, but the main problem is kyphosis, usually in the midthoracic spine. There is one variety of Scheuermann's disease involving the thoracolumbar area in which the kyphosis is less prominent, but pain is more prominent and of a longer duration.

Most adolescents outgrow the pain at the conclusion of growth and are left with only the fixed deformity. Only a few have chronic

(*Text continues on page 626*)

◀ FIG. 16-39. (*A*) A 2-year-old girl with infantile onset spinal muscle atrophy. (*B*) By age 4, she had a 22° thoracic curve and a 38° lumbar curve. Brace treatment was refused by the family. (*C*) By age 13, her lumbar curve was 157°. Such progression should not be permitted. The pessimistic predictions of her neurologists that death by age 6 was inevitable were obviously incorrect. (*D*) Her clinical appearance at age 13. Such a severe collapsing spine deformity contributes a major part of her decreased vital capacity, due also to intercostal muscle weakness. (*A, B, and C* reproduced with permission of Spine, Vol 7, pp 476–483, 1982, Spinal deformities in patients with spinal muscle atrophy by M. F. Riddick, R. B. Winter, and L. D. Lutter.

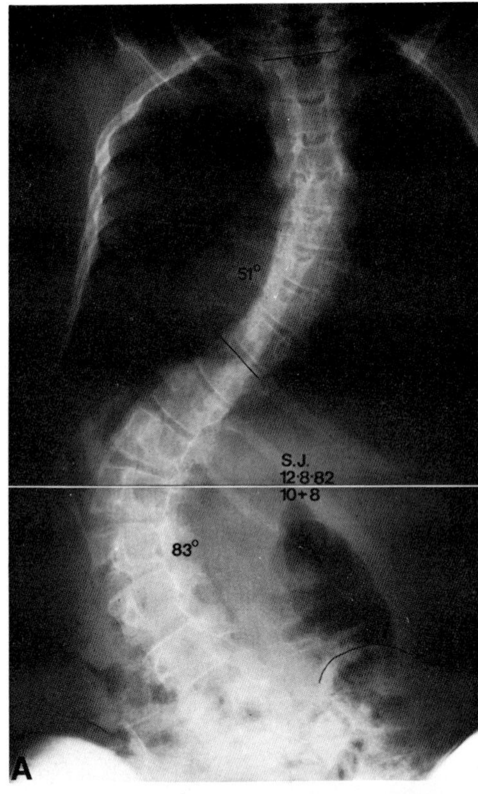

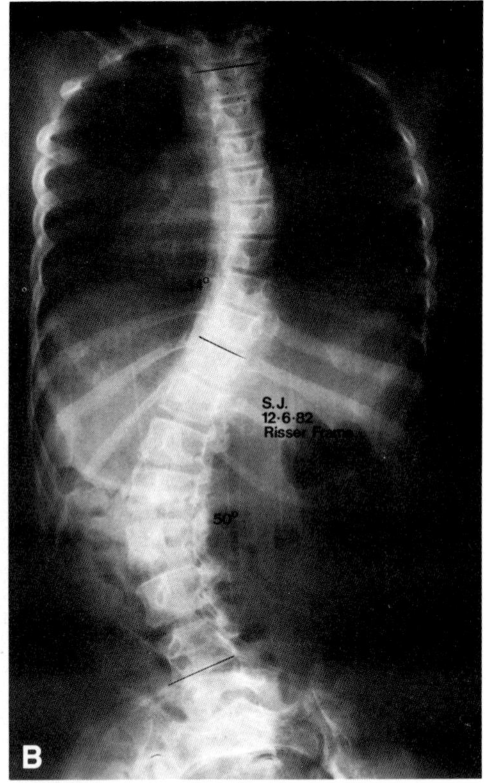

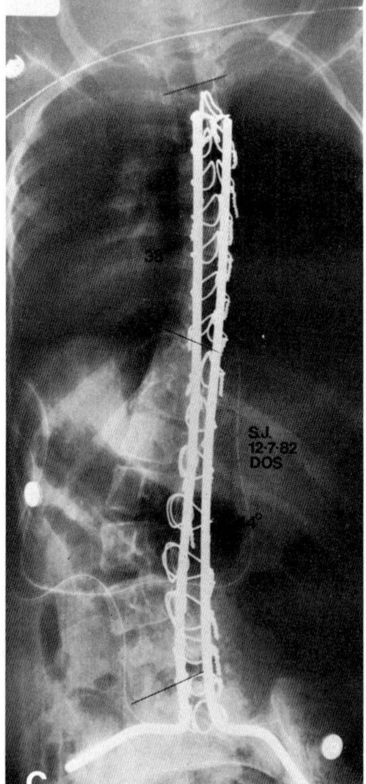

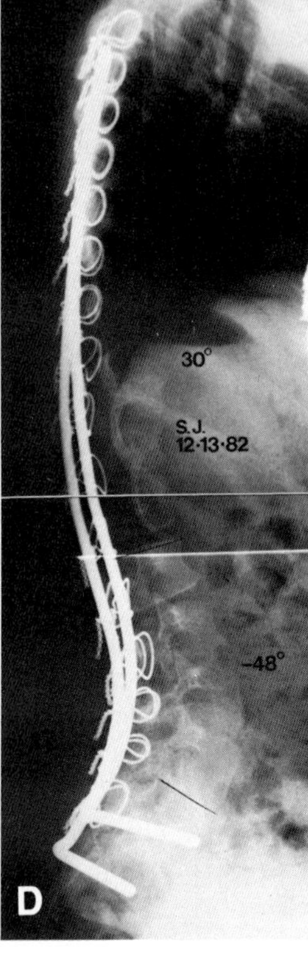

FIG. 16-40. (*A*) This 10-year-old girl had progressive deformity due to spinal muscle atrophy with a thoracic curve of 51° and a lumbar curve of 83°. She was a wheelchair ambulator with excellent general health. Such deformities should be surgically stabilized to maintain sitting balance, to free her hands for activities other than support, and to preserve respiratory capacity. (*B*) On a Risser table in traction and with localizers, her curves were 34° and 50°, and the pelvis was leveled. (*C*) At surgery, using Luque instrumentation and fusion with "Galveston" pelvic fixation, the curves were stabilized at 38° and 44° with a level pelvis. (*D*) In the sagittal plane, normal thoracic kyphosis and lumbar lordosis are preserved. Bank bone was used for grafting.

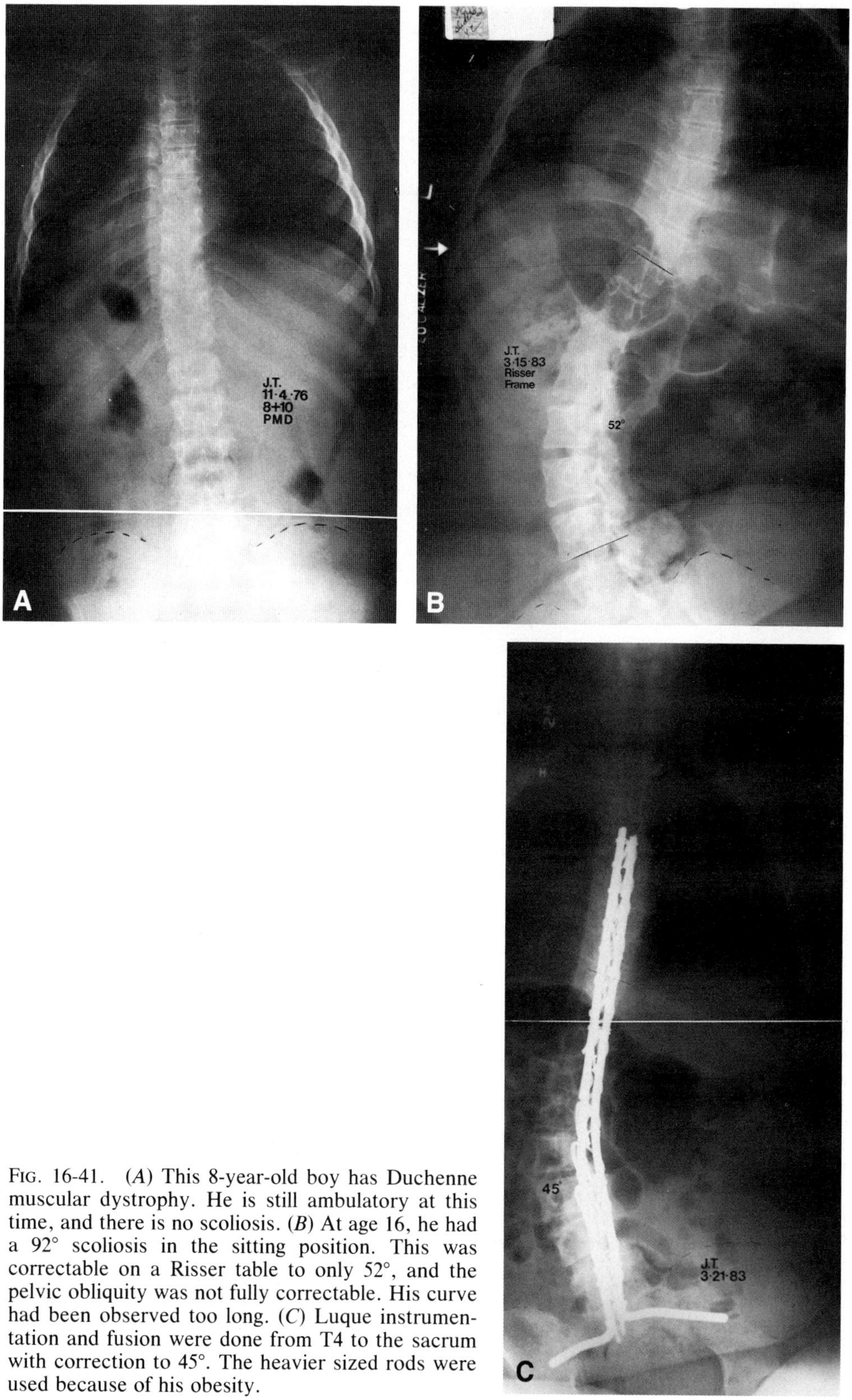

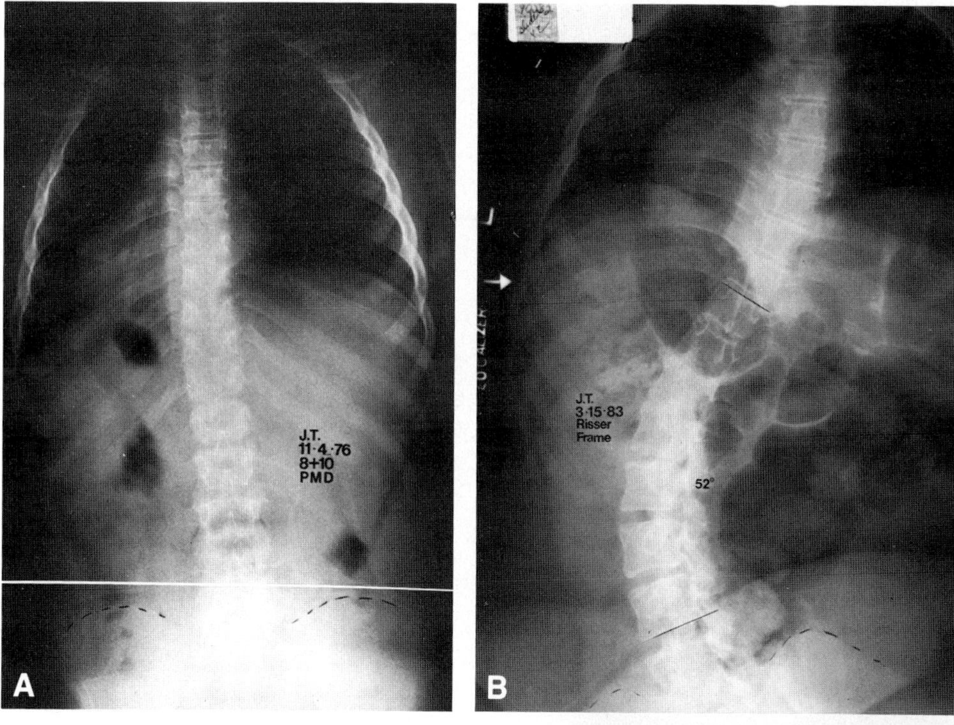

FIG. 16-41. (*A*) This 8-year-old boy has Duchenne muscular dystrophy. He is still ambulatory at this time, and there is no scoliosis. (*B*) At age 16, he had a 92° scoliosis in the sitting position. This was correctable on a Risser table to only 52°, and the pelvic obliquity was not fully correctable. His curve had been observed too long. (*C*) Luque instrumentation and fusion were done from T4 to the sacrum with correction to 45°. The heavier sized rods were used because of his obesity.

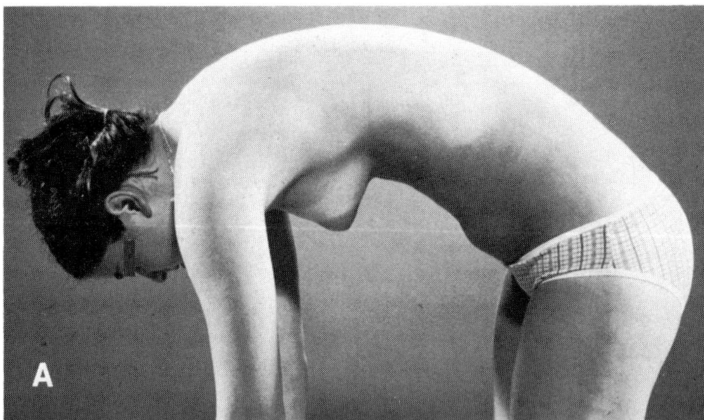

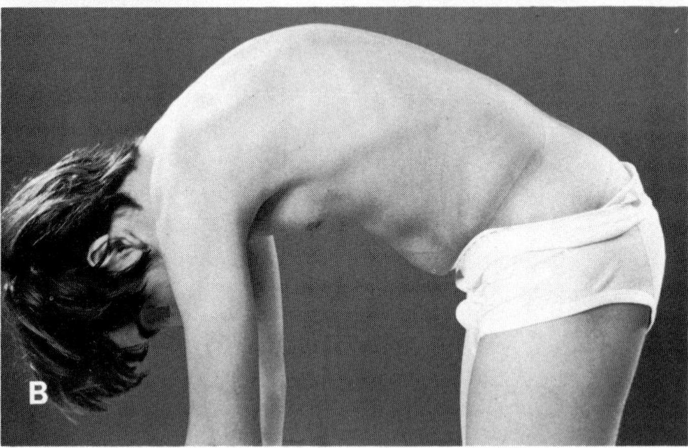

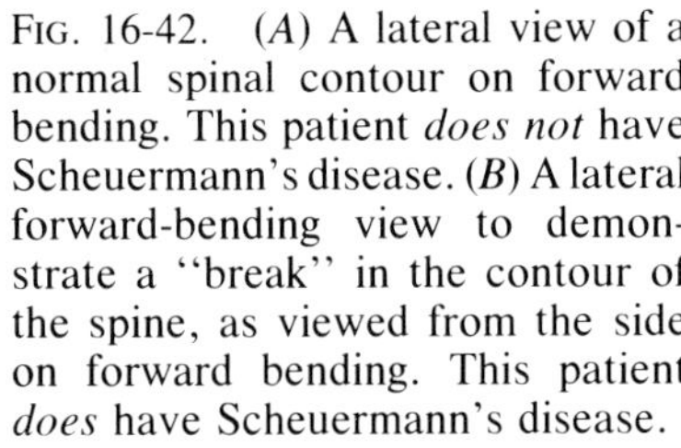
FIG. 16-42. (*A*) A lateral view of a normal spinal contour on forward bending. This patient *does not* have Scheuermann's disease. (*B*) A lateral forward-bending view to demonstrate a "break" in the contour of the spine, as viewed from the side on forward bending. This patient *does* have Scheuermann's disease.

pain into adult life. These are usually the patients with more marked kyphosis or those with lumbar involvement. The cosmetic aspect of kyphosis considerably bothers some adults, others it does not.

Treatment

The question then arises as to whether treatment is appropriate, and, if treatment is to be instituted, what is the best treatment.

Exercises. Postural exercises have been tried for many years but have never been demonstrated to cause any significant improvement in any documented series of structural kyphoses. Exercises in conjunction with orthotic or cast treatment are important.

Nonoperative Treatment. There are only two documented methods of nonoperative treatment that have proved to be beneficial: corrective plaster casts, and the Milwaukee brace. Plaster casts have been used by European physicians, and if they are maintained for at least 1 year and are followed by an exercise program, they will, in most patients, effect and maintain a satisfactory correction. A few (15% to 20%) may relapse and require a second period of casting. The author prefers to use a Milwaukee brace, which is usually less objectionable to the patient than a plaster cast. It is certainly cooler and can be removed daily for bathing and other activities. A patient can be "weaned" from a brace, but a cast is an "all or nothing" device. Orthoses other than the Milwaukee brace have not been demonstrated to be successful for thoracic disease. Some of the thoracolumbar types of roundback can be managed in hyperextension underarm braces, but the majority of patients with Scheuermann's disease have the apex at about the T7 and T8. At this level, only the Milwaukee brace has been demonstrated to be beneficial. Most patients with Scheuermann's disease have a forward jutting head, and only the Milwaukee brace will get the head back above the hips.

A good Milwaukee brace for the patient with Scheuermann's disease maintains pelvic tilt to eliminate lumbar lordosis. It has two posterior kyphosis pads and a neck ring that is centered above the thorax. The most frequent mistake is to have the neck ring forward, perpetuating the forward jutting of the head and thus perpetuating the kyphosis.

The patient who is placed in a Milwaukee brace and who is put on an exercise program will experience a 1- to 2-week period of adjustment after which the pain disappears and significant height is gained, requiring adjustment of the orthosis. Usually within 4 to 6 weeks, the deformity has been corrected if it is of the flexible type. After this, it is only a problem of maintaining the correction and allowing the soft tissues and the vertebrae to readjust and grow more normally. The typical patient requires a year of full-time brace wearing (23 out of 24 hours), coupled with a supervised physical therapy program to maintain and improve thoracic extensors and to eliminate the lumbar lordosis. At the end of 1 year, if the deformity has been kept fully corrected during that time, weaning can gradually be instituted, even though full growth may not have been reached. Patients with Scheuermann's disease usually require less intensive Milwaukee brace treatment than patients with idiopathic scoliosis. For weaning, usually a minimum period of 1 year is necessary. If there is loss of correction at any time during the weaning process, a return to full-time wearing is necessary, with weaning resumed 6 to 12 months later.

Some patients, particularly those with the more structural types of Scheuermann's disease with marked wedging, cannot achieve correction with this minimal type of orthotic program. These patients require full and intensive orthotic treatment, including exercises until growth has been completed. Weaning is to be done only after the closure of the ring apophyses of the involved vertebral bodies.

The age at which treatment can be started with an orthosis depends on the maturity of the vertebrae in the area of the disease. Bone age, as determined by the hand film and the status of the iliac epiphyses, is of less importance than the degree of growth in the area of the disease. Growth appears to be delayed in many patients. The author has seen successful brace treatment started as late as age 17 in males and 15 in females.

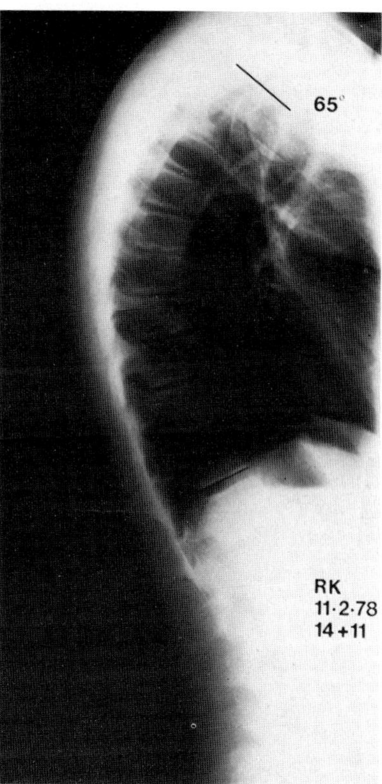

FIG. 16-43. The classic radiologic features of Scheuermann's disease include disc space narrowing, and end-plate irregularity, apical vertebral body wedging. Schmorl's nodes are commonly seen as is increased antero-posterior vertebral body diameter.

The results of brace treatment are usually excellent. Bradford and associates[10] demonstrated in a series of 75 patients who had completed Milwaukee brace treatment that good correction could be obtained in most patients. The average correction of the kyphosis was 40%, and the average correction of the vertebral wedging was 41%. Patients with more severe and rigid deformities, especially when more advanced in growth, had the least improvement, but all groups had some improvement (Figs. 16-44 and 16-45).

Surgical Treatment

Surgical treatment in Scheuermann's disease is rarely necessary. It is indicated only for those patients who have completed growth, who have a significant deformity (greater than 60°), and who have chronic pain in the curve

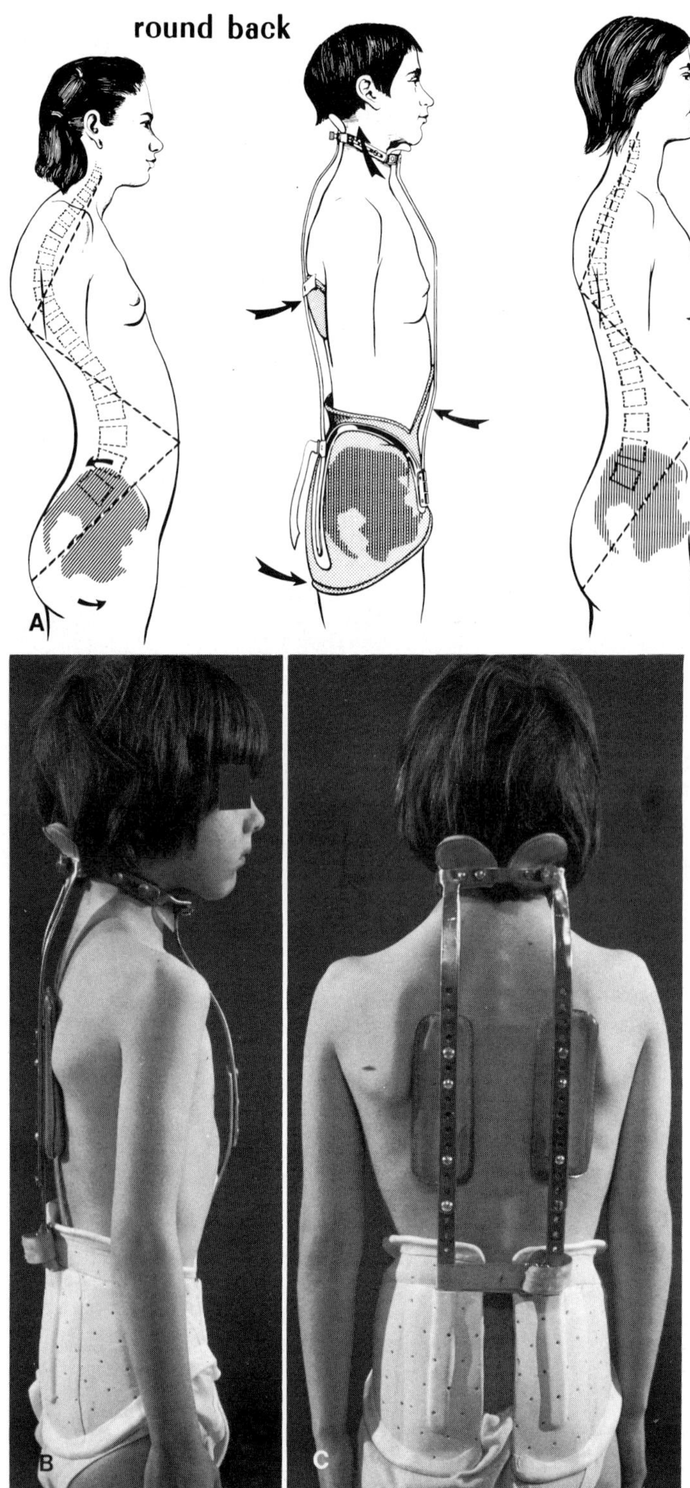

FIG. 16-44. (*A*) Diagrams of lateral views, illustrating both the deformity of the Scheuermann's disease and its correction by the multiple forces of a Milwaukee brace. (From Blount WP, Moe JH: The Milwaukee Brace. Baltimore, Williams & Wilkins, 1973) (*B*) A patient fitted with a Milwaukee brace for kyphosis. The posterior uprights are kept close to the body, the occipital pads are below the occiput and the throat mold is kept fairly high under the chin to encourage posterior displacement of the head. The anterior upright is sufficiently far from the chest to permit full and complete inspiration, along with correction of the curve. The patient's ear is directly above the shoulder and the hip line, showing satisfactory total body alignment. (*C*) A posterior view of the patient, showing the brace for Scheuermann's kyphosis. In this illustration, the pads are too large and they encroach upon the scapular wing. To be properly applied, the pad should be quite narrow and should not extend lateral to the posterior upright.

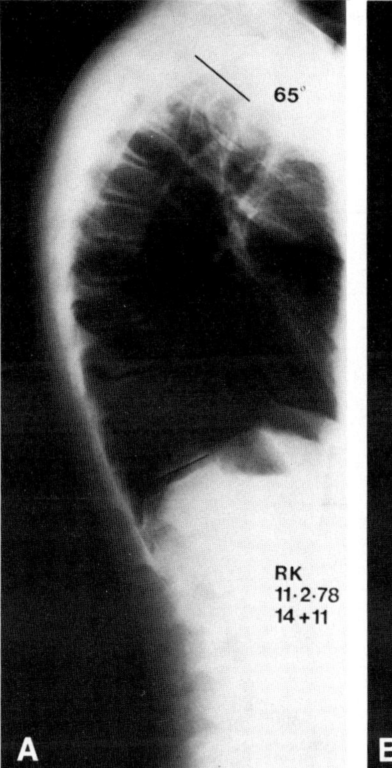

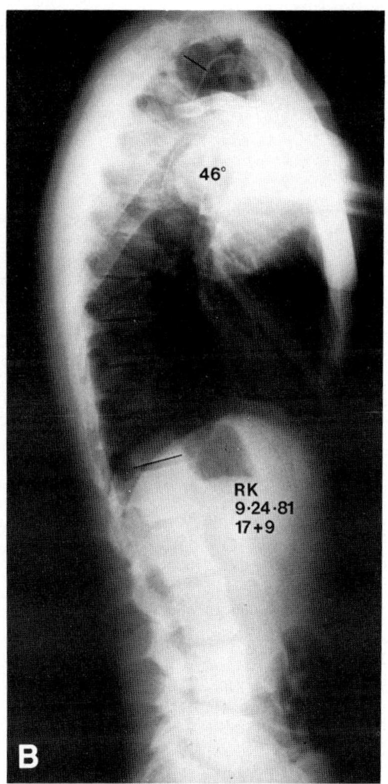

FIG. 16-45. (*A*) A 15-year-old boy with a 65° Scheuermann's kyphosis. A Milwaukee brace was started immediately. (*B*) At age 17 years and 9 months, 1 year after brace removal, his kyphosis measures 46°.

area. Thus, of hundreds of patients seen with Scheuermann's disease, the author has found it necessary to operate on only a few.

Initially, surgeons at our center were pleased with the correction obtained by posterior Harrington instrumentation and spine fusion. Satisfactory correction was obtained, and the patients were relieved of their discomfort. Unfortunately, many of these patients lost their correction, particularly those with curves greater than 70°.[10a]

At the present time, if a patient with Scheuermann's disease requires fusion, (as stated above, this situation is rare), both anterior and posterior arthrodeses are necessary. The patient with kyphosis of this degree does not obtain a posterior fusion sufficiently solid to withstand the tension forces placed upon it. It is only by anterior surgery that adequate correction is obtained and maintained. An anterior approach is first performed, usually through a left thoracotomy. The five apical discs are removed, and the anterior longitudinal ligament is either excised or incised transversely at each disc level. The anterior longitudinal ligament has been found to be quite thickened and hypertrophied in these patients and is certainly responsible for limiting correction. Thus, the release of the anterior longitudinal ligament and annulus is important. The discs are thoroughly removed back to the posterior longitudinal ligament, leaving the posterior annulus and posterior longitudinal ligament intact. The end-plates are perforated into cancellous bone. The rib removed for the thoracotomy is then broken up into tiny pieces, and the disc are packed with fragments of this autogenous bone. If there is not enough bone obtained from the single rib, iliac crest bone should be obtained. On rare occasions, a strut graft has been used, but the segmental small grafts have been quite satisfactory for most cases of Scheuermann's disease and appear to heal more rapidly.[9]

A posterior arthrodesis encompassing the entire kyphotic curve is performed 1 to 2 weeks later. Harrington instrumentation should be used, usually two heavy compression instruments, but, occasionally one bent distraction rod and one compression rod can be used

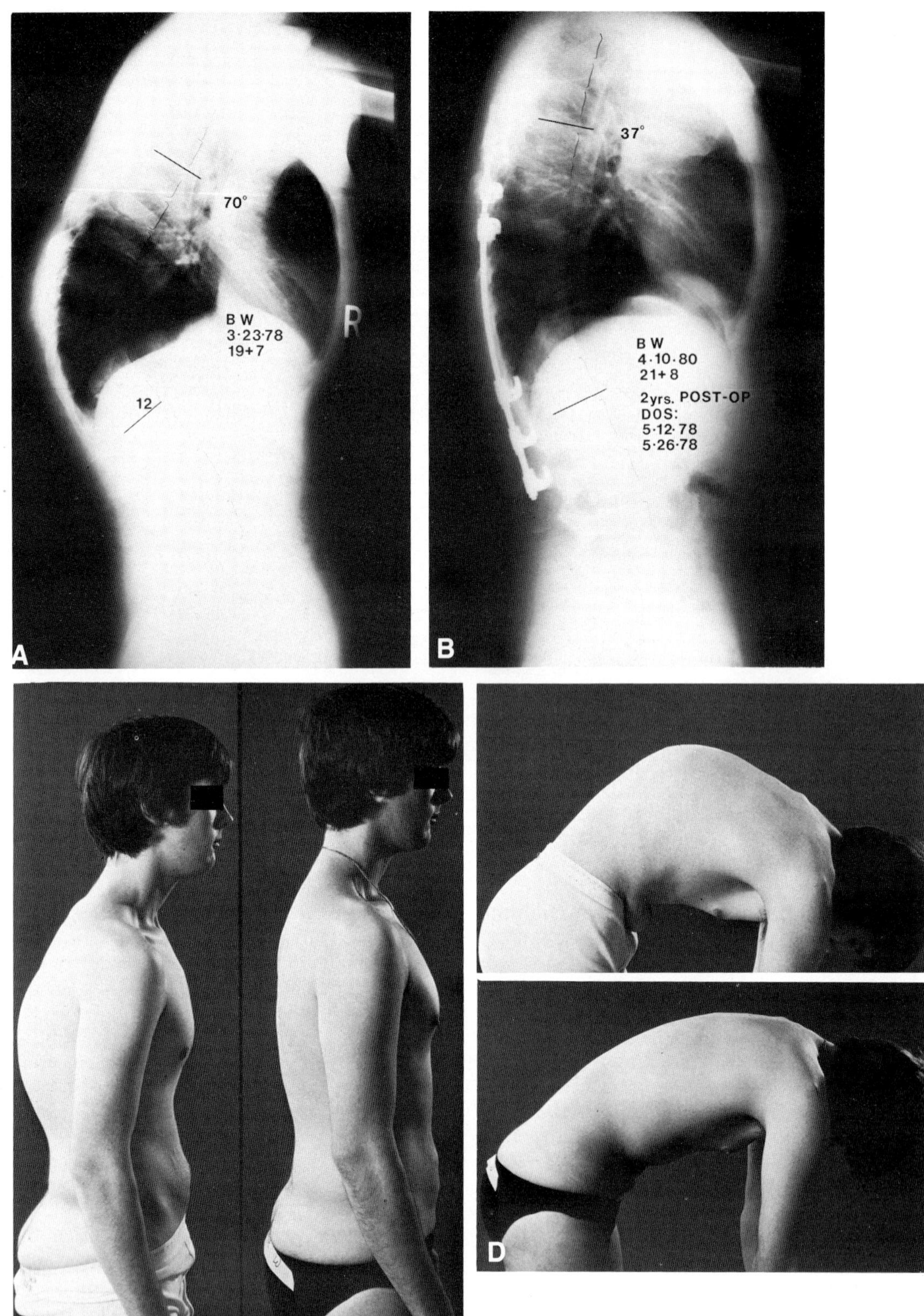

70°
B W
3·23·78
19+7
12
R
A
37°
B W
4·10·80
21+8
2yrs. POST-OP
DOS:
5·12·78
5·26·78
B
C
D

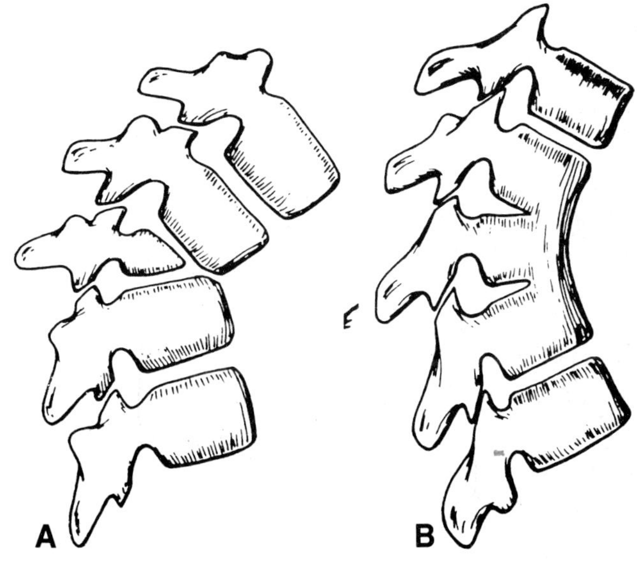

FIG. 16-47. (*A*) A congenital kyphosis due to failure of formation of the vertebral body. (*B*) Congenital kyphosis due to anterior failure of segmentation (anterior unsegmented bar). (Illustrations reproduced with permission from Congenital Deformities of the Spine by Dr. B. Winter, Thieme-Stratton, New York, 1983)

when there is some scoliosis. Use of the thinner type of compression rod usually results in more loss of correction. Recently, dual ¼-inch Luque rods have been used by some, and dual ¼-inch Harrington distraction rods with segmental wiring have been used by others.

Approximately 1 week following the second procedure, a hyperextension type of cast or brace is applied. The patient is then allowed to ambulate but remains in the cast or brace for approximately 9 months (Fig. 16-46).

CONGENITAL KYPHOSIS

Congenital kyphosis is a kyphotic deformity due to congenitally anomalous vertebra. There are two basic types: The first (Type I) is caused by a congenital failure of formation of all or part of the vertebral body. This may range from the absence of two or even three vertebral bodies, with the preservation of the posterior element in which a severe deformity is produced, to only a very partial absence of a vertebral body with a less severe deformity. The second (Type II) is due to congenital failure of segmentation of the vertebral body anteriorly, producing an "anterior unsegmented bar." In both situations, progressive deformity occurs as a result of nongrowth anteriorly and persistent growth posteriorly.

The more severe deformities may be manifest at birth and may progress steadily thereafter. The less obvious deformities may not appear until years later and tend to have accentuation of deformtity at the time of the adolescent growth spurt (Fig. 16-47).

Once progression begins, it does not cease spontaneously, but progresses until the end of growth. The more severe types of kyphotic problems may progress even after growth is complete.

Progression can take place due to not only growth differential but also because of actual erosion of the vertebral body from mechanical pressure related to the disturbance of biomechanics of the kyphosis. Studies of the natural history of progression revealed very severe deformity to occur, particularly with congenital failure of formation of one or more vertebral bodies.

Paraplegia can result from progressive kyphotic deformity, particularly when the kyphosis

◀ FIG. 16-46. (*A*) This 19-year-old male had a painful 70° low thoracic Scheuermann's kyphosis. This was treated by anterior ligament release and interbody fusion followed 2 weeks later by posterior instrumentation and fusion. (*B*) Two years after surgery, the kyphosis is within normal limits at 37°. (*C*) Standing photographs before and 2 years after surgery. (*D*) Forward-bending photographs before and 2 years after surgery.

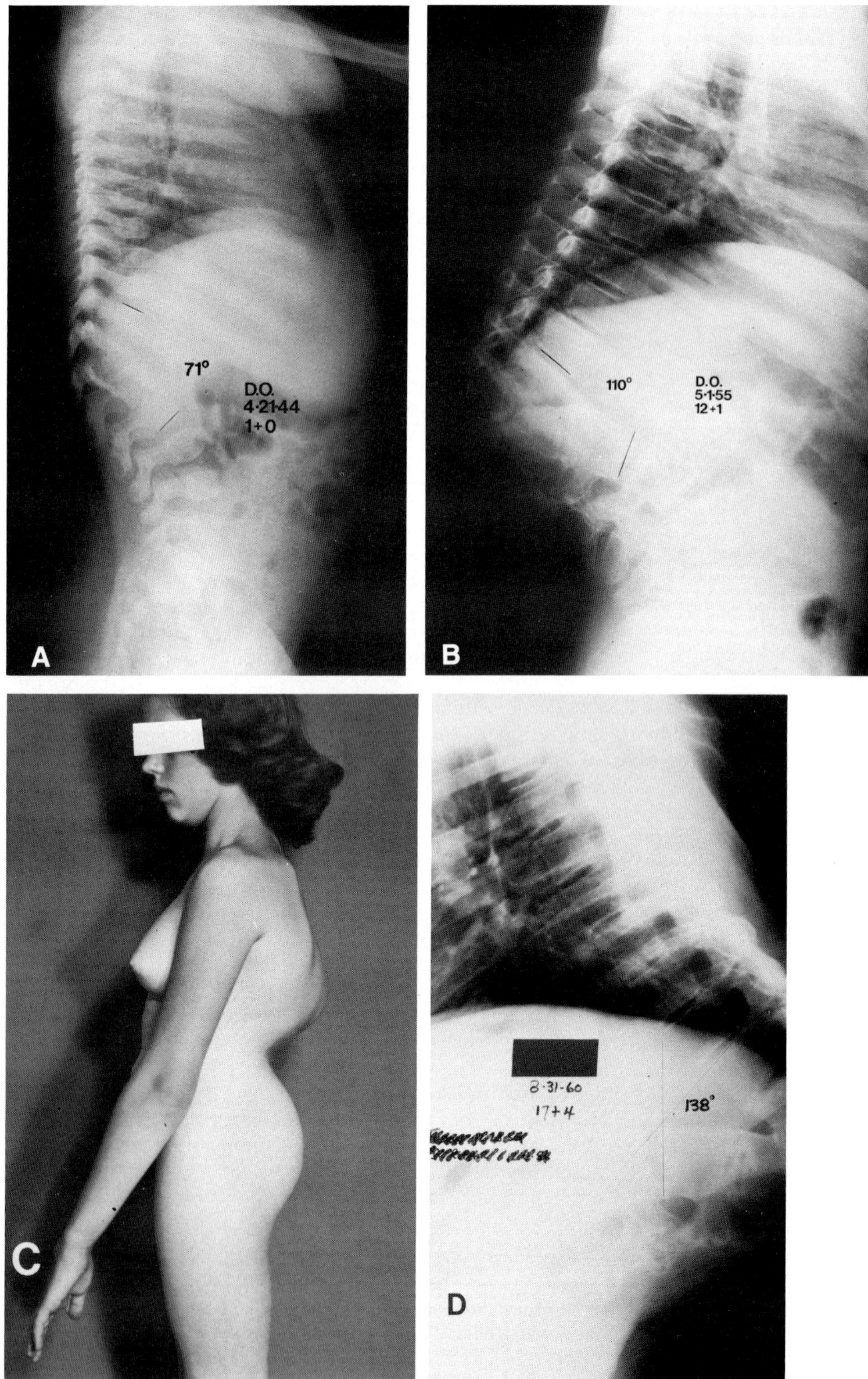
71°
D.O.
4·21·44
1+0
A
110°
D.O.
5·1·55
12+1
B
C
8·31·60
17+4
138°
D

is in the thoracic spine. Paraplegia is associated with Type I deformities, but it has not been described in Type II deformities. Partial paralysis can be present even at birth, or the onset of paralysis may not occur until adult life. Congenital kyphosis is the most common noninfectious spine deformity to cause paraplegia (Fig. 16-48).

Nonoperative Treatment

There is no nonoperative treatment. Orthoses have never been shown to be effective.

Surgical Treatment

The ideal treatment for congenital kyphosis is early detection and early posterior fusion. As shown by Winter and Moe,[86] the best results obtained are in those patients who had posterior fusion prior to age 3 years. Fusion can be done as early as 6 months of age, if necessary. A strong posterior fusion will stop the asymmetric growth and appears to allow growth to take place anteriorly where there are viable growth plates.

Posterior fusion is often inadequate to stabilize the spine in the patient with significant kyphosis. The posterior fusion mass is under a distraction force and does not develop strongly. The pseudarthrosis rate is extremely high, and, beyond a certain point, posterior fusion cannot be accomplished. Thus, if posterior fusion is to be attempted for these problems, the fusion mass must be thickened at the apex; the best way to achieve this is by concentrating the bone graft material in this area on the first operation. Six months later, the incision is intentionally reopened, and the fusion mass is stimulated by "feathering" the graft and adding additional autogenous bone. The fusion mass takes a long time to develop vertical trabeculation sufficiently strong to withstand gravity and flexion forces. Therefore, a period of at least 1 year in a cast is necessary. Protection in an orthosis for 1 or 2 more years thereafter is strongly recommended (Fig. 16-49).

Anterior and posterior fusion has become the treatment of choice for the more severe congenital kyphosis problems. In essence, patients with kyphosis of greater than 50° who are 5 years of age or older will require anterior fusion.[89] If anterior fusion is performed, posterior fusion must be done also, usually one more level above and below the anterior fusion. This allows the fusion mass to develop some degree of lordosis with time.

The surgical treatment of a well-established and severe kyphosis is one of the greatest challenges to the orthopaedic surgeon. Preliminary traction should be avoided. The anterior surgery should be done first. An anterior transthoracic exposure is made, the anterior longitudinal ligament is excised, several discs are removed, and a strong anterior strut graft operation is performed using rib or fibular bone plus additional rib or iliac bone. Correction is obtained manually or by the use of an anterior distractor (not an implant).

One to 2 weeks following the initial procedure, the patient is returned to the operating room where a posterior fusion of adequate length is performed supplemented by Harrington compression instrumentation (if the patient is 10 years of age or older). One week following the second operation, a snug cast is applied, using either a halo cast or Risser-Cotrel type of hyperextension cast. The patient can be ambulated if there is adequate internal fixation, or a period of 6 months of bed rest may be necessary if there is any question about the ability to control the deformity in the upright position. A period of 1 year in this type of cast is necessary to achieve total and complete healing.

The patient with a severe angular kyphosis in the thoracic area, with the apex in the T3 to T8 area, is in great jeopardy of paraplegia, both with and without treatment. Traction should be avoided. Anterior fusion without traction is the procedure of choice. Posterior fusion without instrumentation should follow 2 weeks later (Fig. 16-50).

For severe Type II deformities, anterior

◀ FIG. 16-48. (*A*) A 1-year-old girl with a 71° congenital kyphosis. No treatment was given. (*B*) Current 16-7 A. Her clinical appearance at that time. By age 12, her kyphosis was 110°. (*C*) Paraplegia is common in such severe kyphoses. (*D*) At age 12, the patient has marked increase in her kyphosis.

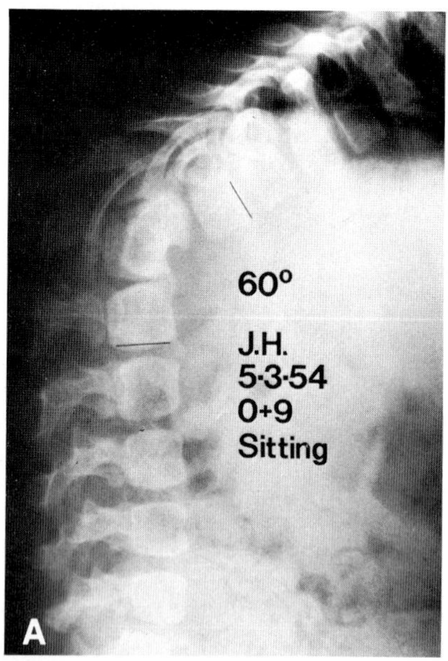

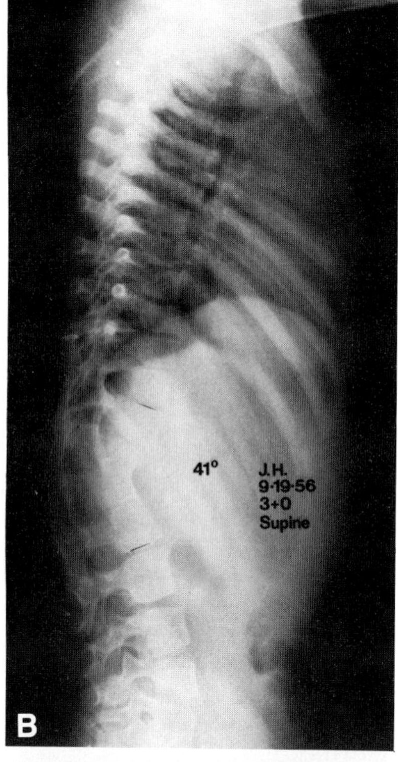

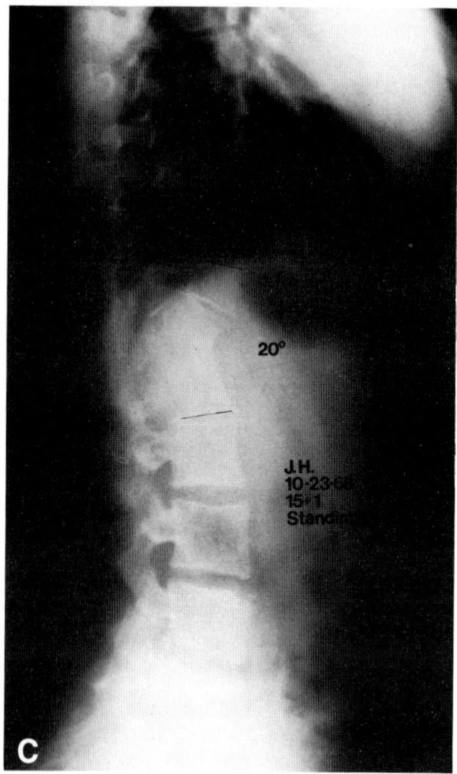

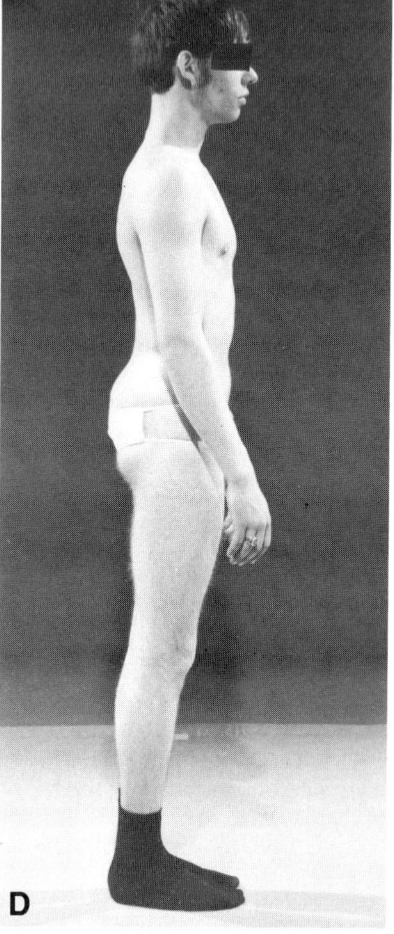

FIG. 16-49. (*A*) A 9-month-old boy with a 60° congenital kyphosis. A posterior fusion was done at age 16 months by Dr. John H. Moe at the Gillette Children's Hospital. (*B*) At age 3, his kyphosis was 41°. (*C*) By age 15, his kyphosis had spontaneously (due to the posterior growth arrest) decreased to 20°. (*D*) A clinical photograph at age 15. (Illustrations reproduced with permission from Congenital Deformities of the Spine by Dr. B. Winter, Thieme-Stratton, New York, 1983)

osteotomy of the unsegmented bar, disc excision, and anterior bone grafting followed by posterior fusion with Harrington compression rods is recommended. It is obvious that a correction cannot be obtained unless the anterior osteotomy is performed first. It is desirable to detect these problems early and to perform a simple posterior fusion, preventing the need for such complex surgery.

POST-LAMINECTOMY KYPHOSIS

In the thoracic and thoracolumbar spine, the forces of gravity have a natural tendency to produce kyphosis. In the normal spine, these gravity forces are counteracted by the posterior ligament complex, including the interspinous ligament, the ligamentum flavum, and the facet joint ligaments. A radical laminectomy, regardless of the cause for such, will result in the removal of some or all of these supporting structures. When the laminectomy is sufficiently extensive to result in removal of facet joints bilaterally, a kyphotic deformity will inevitably occur in the growing child. The more radical the laminectomy and the younger the child at the time of laminectomy, the more severe the deformity is likely to become.[45]

In most situations, laminectomy is absolutely necessary because of the original diagnosis, usually a spinal cord tumor. Under such circumstances, it is important to recognize that the facets have been removed and that a deformity will develop if the child survives the tumor. Therefore, it is pertinent that the potential of the deformity be recognized, that the child be followed on a regular basis by an orthopaedic surgeon familiar with spine problems, and that early bracing be instituted if a deformity develops. Most postlaminectomy spine deformities do not respond well to the orthosis, and fusion may be necessary. Fusion usually has to be performed through an anterior interbody route, because there are no laminae or bony structures posteriorly to support a posterior fusion. In some circumstances, it may be wise to perform a prophylactic anterior spine fusion following the laminectomy if the general prognosis of the tumor is known to be good.

Certainly, if a child develops a progressing deformity, the necessary steps to correct and stabilize the spine should be undertaken without delay. It is tragic to see a child progress severely without the institution of adequate spine surgery.

Many times there is a lack of understanding of the basic nature of the original tumor process. All too often, the physicians believe the child has a doomed prognosis from the spinal cord tumor and will die at a young age. Thus, the spine deformity is ignored. However, the child may live for many years or even have a normal life span, despite the original diagnosis, and a valuable opportunity to correct and stabilize the spine will have been lost.

Neurosurgeons must learn that these deformities can develop and that the amount of bone removed should be minimized if at all possible. Especially important is the preservation of the facet joint complex (Fig. 16-51).

POST–RADIATION SPINE DEFORMITY

Radiation of the young child can produce deformity of the spine due to the effect of the radiation on the growth plates of the vertebra and upon the soft tissues. The usual problems requiring radiation of young children are Wilms' tumor and neuroblastoma. With the increased survival rate of these tumors under modern medical treatment, there is an increased number of patients at risk for spine deformity. Quite often, the scoliosis does not manifest itself until many years after the radiation. Therefore, it is mandatory that these children be followed until their growth is completed if the radiation has been given at a young age.[51]

Treatment of the radiation deformity may be either by orthosis, if the curve is mild, or by surgery, if the curve has reached significant levels. Recently, we have seen cases with kyphosis following radiation, which appears to be a problem probably due to symmetrical anterior radiation of the vertebral bodies and also secondary effects of the radiation on the anterior abdominal wall, producing shortening, particularly in the rectus abdominus and its fascia. The soft tissues show considerable atrophy in patients who have had radiation, and the apparent deformity may be more severe than is actually seen on the x-ray, due to the hypoplasia of the soft tissues of the flank and particularly of the iliac wing.

Healing following surgery may be significantly delayed due to the radiation effect. The patient should be warned that the cast or brace will probably have to remain on for a longer period of time than would be expected for a patient with a nonradiation problem. Anterior and posterior fusion is necessary if there is significant kyphosis (greater than 50°).

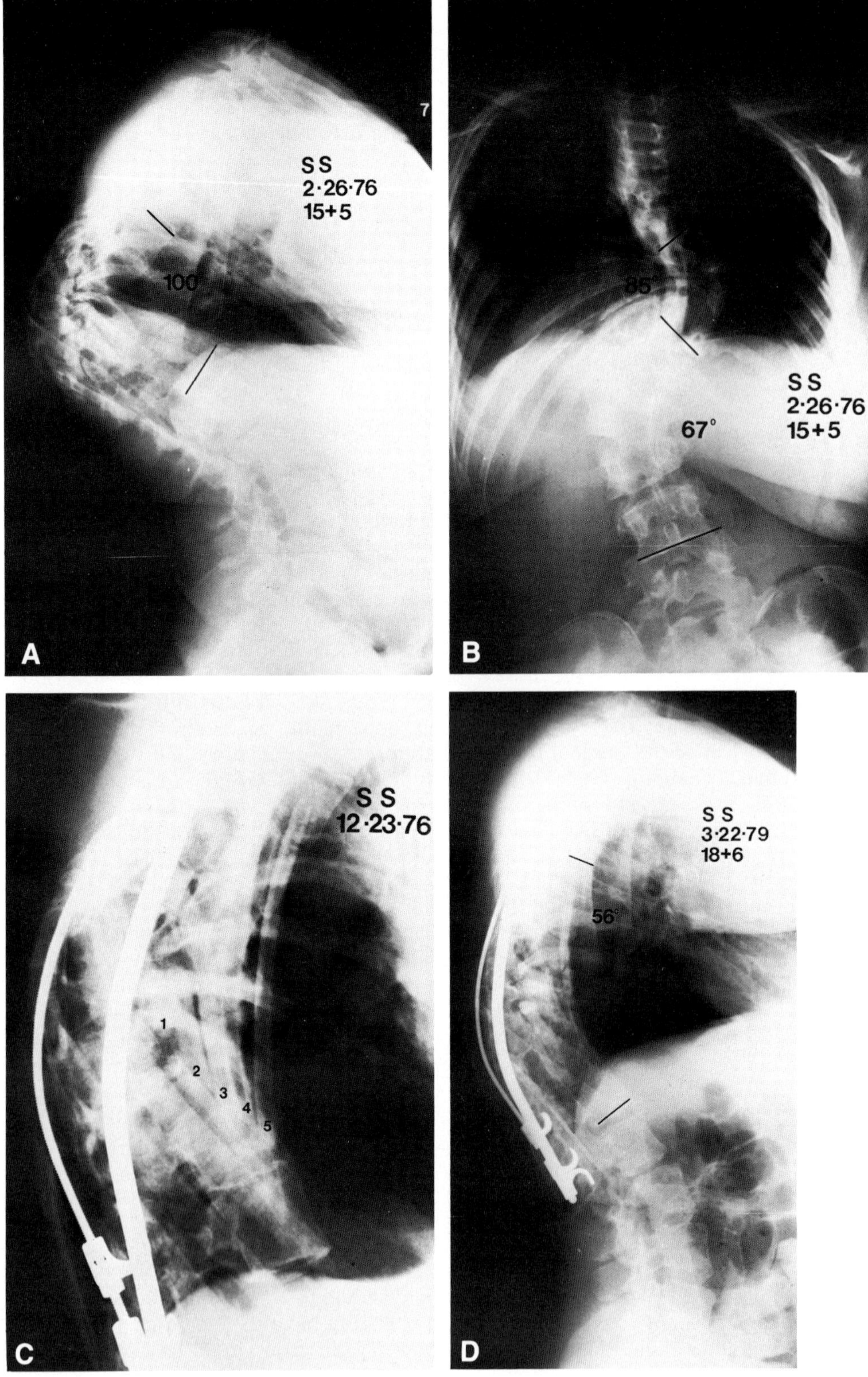
7
SS
2·26·76
15+5
100°
A
85°
SS
2·26·76
15+5
67°
B
SS
12·23·76
1
2
3
4
5
C
SS
3·22·79
18+6
56°
D

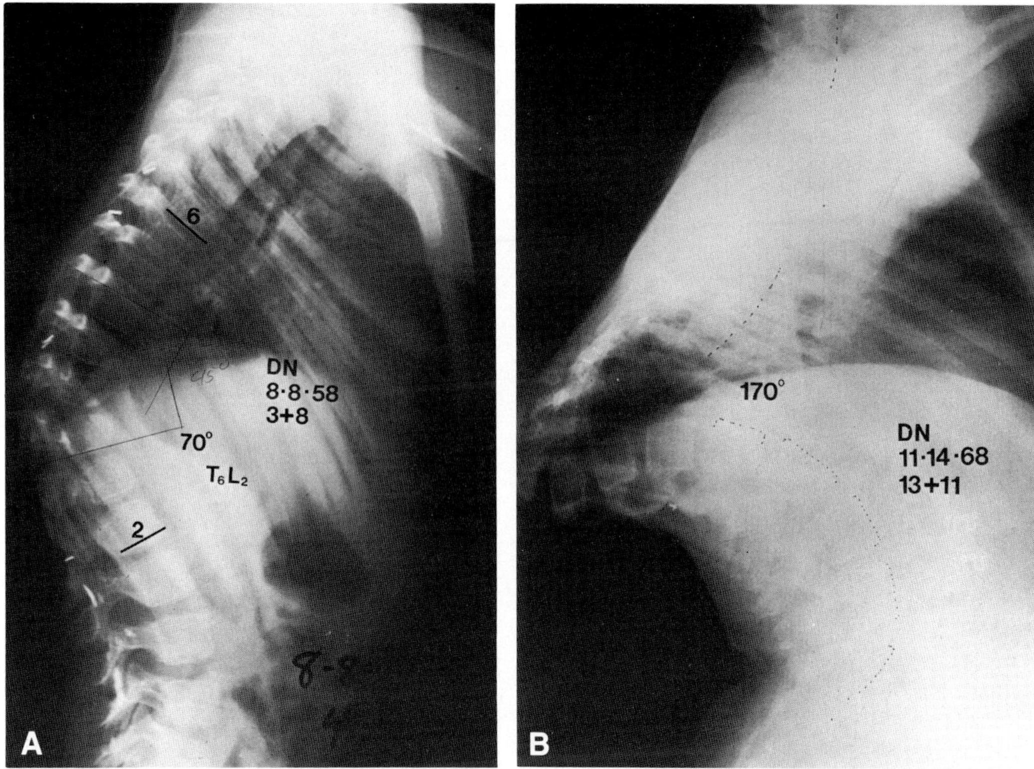

FIG. 16-51. *(A)* A 3-year-old girl with a 70° T6–L2 kyphosis secondary to a laminectomy for an astrocytoma at age 2. *(B)* By age 14, she had a 170° kyphosis and was totally paraplegic due to her deformity.

BACK PAIN IN CHILDREN

Contrary to adults in whom back pain is common and there is a high association of back pain with psychosomatic disturbances, back pain in children is unusual and when present is virtually always due to specific organic (nonpsychosomatic) causes. Back pain in a child that lasts more than a few days should be viewed with concern and investigated thoroughly.

There are many causes of such pain, including the general categories of developmental abnormalities (spondylolysis, spondylolisthesis, and Scheuermann's), traumatic (acute or stress fracture of the pars interarticularis, or ruptured disc), infectious (disc space infection or tuberculosis), and neoplastic (benign or malignant spinal cord or bone tumors).

Spondylolysis or spondylolisthesis is the most common cause of low back pain. Diagnosis is by good-quality x-rays of the lumbosacral area, including spot lateral and oblique views. Treatment is discussed elsewhere.

Scheuermann's disease is most common in the thoracic spine but can occur in the thora-

◀ FIG. 16-50. *(A)* A 15-year-old girl with a 100° thoracic congenital kyphosis. She was neurologically normal. *(B)* Her anteroposterior film shows an 85° scoliosis. *(C)* A slightly oblique view 10 months after surgery shows the five strut grafts necessary to stabilize this severe kyphosis. *(D)* A true lateral view 3 years after surgery shows the solid kyphosis and correction to 56°. (Illustrations reproduced with permission from Congenital Deformities of the Spine by Dr. B. Winter, Thieme-Stratton, New York, 1983) columbar region or even lumbar area. Pain is more common in these lower lesions than in the thoracic area. The pain lessens with rest and becomes worse with activity. It is non-radicular. Bone scans are normal.

Disc herniation in children can occur and must always be considered in the differential diagnosis of low back pain, especially if there was a traumatic or lifting episode. Metrizamide myelography and/or CT scans assist in the diagnosis.

Disc space or vertebral body infections are associated with back pain and can occur in perfectly healthy children without other infectious processes. Temperature elevation, sedimentation rate elevation, and positive bone scans are the keys to diagnosis. See Chapter 11 for details about this problem.

Bone tumors are frequently the cause of painful scoliosis. The child has a "tight" back and will tend to deviate to one side while bending forward. There is local tenderness in the area of the tumor. Pain may be present night or day and is not fully relieved by bed rest. The most common tumors are osteoid osteoma, osteoblastoma, and aneurysmal bone cyst. See Chapter 7 for further details.

Spinal cord tumors may also express themselves as back pain, either with or without neurologic deficit.[78] Again, there tends to be back spasm and tightness, with deviation to one side on forward bending. Because of the slow-growing nature of these tumors, the spinal cord accommodates to the pressure and remarkably normal neurologic examinations can occur in the presence of large tumors. One should not hesitate to do a spinal tap and myelography if there is the slightest possibility of a spinal cord tumor, *even if the neurologic examination is totally normal*.

In summary, back pain in children is almost always due to a specific organic cause. Psychosomatic causes are very rare and should be placed at the bottom of a differential diagnosis list. A complete workup includes routine x-rays, oblique x-rays, sedimentation rate, bone scan, EMG, and myelography. Adequate consultations should also be obtained (Fig. 16-52).

SPONDYLOLYSIS AND SPONDYLOLISTHESIS

Spondylolysis means the presence of a lysis or defect in the pars interarticularis. Spondylolisthesis refers to the presence of a slipping or displacement of one vertebra in relation to another. The classification of spondylolisthesis is listed below:

Classification of Spondylolisthesis

- Dysplastic
- Isthmic
  - Pars defect
  - Pars elongation
- Degenerative
- Traumatic
- Pathologic

Degenerative spondylolisthesis is a problem related to disc degeneration in older adults and is not relevant to this textbook. Traumatic spondylolisthesis refers to acute traumatic events with fracture-dislocation and is thus also not relevant to this text. Pathologic spondylolisthesis refers to tumors or other bone processes resulting in bone weakness and can therefore occur in children, but they are rare.

This, types I and II, the dysplastic and isthmic, are the problems of daily concern. Dysplastic spondylolisthesis refers to a congenital inadequacy of the facet joints and disc complex, resulting in displacement without a defect or elongation of the pars interarticularis. It is rare and of concern mainly because of the high frequency of nerve root pressure due to the intact lamina of L5 being pulled against the dural sac. Significant neurologic impairment can thus occcur in the presence of only minor degrees of slip.

Isthmic spondylolisthesis is by far the most common type seen in children and young adults. It is very common, occurring in 5% of the population. Studies by Baker, and McHollick[3] have shown that the lesion is *not* present at birth but is present in 5% of children by age six. There are important genetic considerations as shown by Wiltse and associates.[81]

Children involved in certain sports (*e.g.*, gymnastics) have a much higher incidence than those in the normal population. This appears to be especially related to repetitive hyperextension stresses.

Results of many studies suggest that there exists a genetically determined tendency to develop stress fractures of the pars interarticularis during the first few years of upright existence. Most people with these defects have

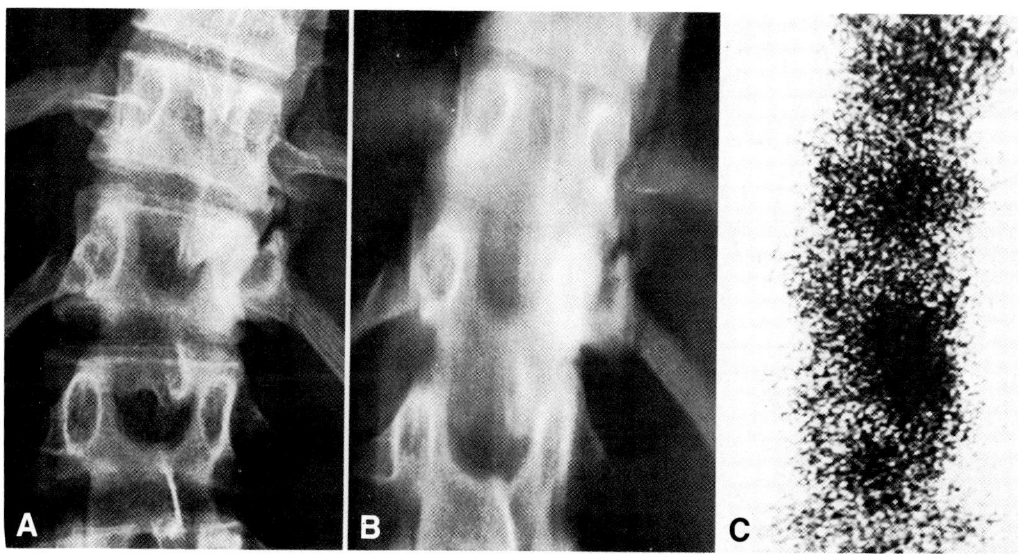

FIG. 16-52. *(A)* A 15-year-old male presenting with a painful scoliosis. Note the sclerotic right pedicle of T12. *(B)* An anteroposterior tomogram more clearly shows the same findings. *(C)* A bone scan shows increased activity at that level.

no slipping of the vertebrae and no pain and can be detected only on routine x-ray surveys.

A few people do develop problems, either pain or progressive slipping or both. Those with more severe degrees of slipping early in life are most often female, and it is most often associated with spina bifida occulta of L5 and S1.[33]

Evaluation

Good patient evaluation should include history-taking and physical and x-ray examinations. The history should include questions as to family history, presence or absence of pain, location of pain, any radicular pain, bowel or bladder malfunction, numbness, tingling, weakness of the legs or feet, or change of gait.

Physical examination of the back should include general alignment, posture, presence or absence of scoliosis, muscle spasm, localized tenderness, localized "step-off" at the lumbosacral area, and position of the sacrum (*i.e.*, ? vertical, ? normal).

Examination of the legs should include gait pattern, presence or absence of tight hamstrings, calf circumference, reflexes at the knee and ankle, and a full motor and sensory evaluation (Fig. 16-53).

Radiologic examination should include a spot standing lateral view of the lumbosacral area and supine oblique and anteroposterior views of the lumbosacral area. If there is an associated spinal deformity or malalignment, full-length spine views, both anteroposterior and lateral, should be obtained.

Myelography should be done in those patients having neurologic signs in order to rule out other reasons for neurologic deficit, such as a cauda equina tumor. Myelograms are not of any value in displaced lesions without neurologic deficits, because dural indentation and malalignment are customary findings (Fig. 16-54).

Treatment

The form of treatment given depends on many factors, including the age of the patient, type of defect, degree of slipping, degree of slip angle (sagittal rotation), and especially the nature of the symptoms. The treatment of children with spondylolisthesis is considerably different than that of adults.

Treatment of Spondylolysis Without Slip. Patients with nonsymptomatic spondylolysis but with no slipping require no active treatment. They should, however, be followed periodically to see whether a slip develops (Fig. 16-55).

Patients with painful spondylolysis, but with no slip, should be treated by bracing for 6 to

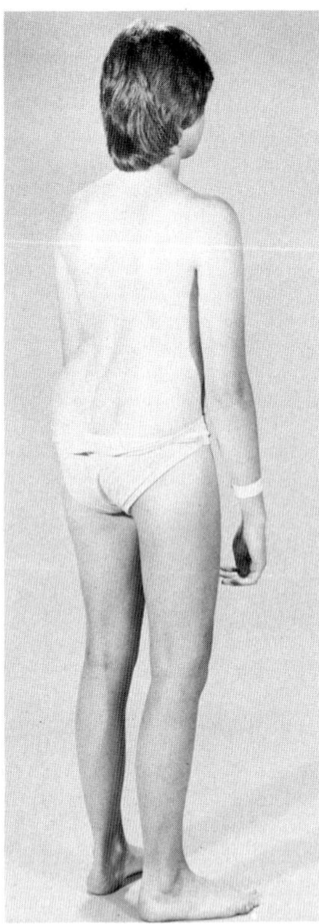

FIG. 16-53. A clinical photograph showing the typical findings of spondylolisthesis. There is flattening of the buttocks, a lumbosacral kyphosis, and increased lumbar lordosis.

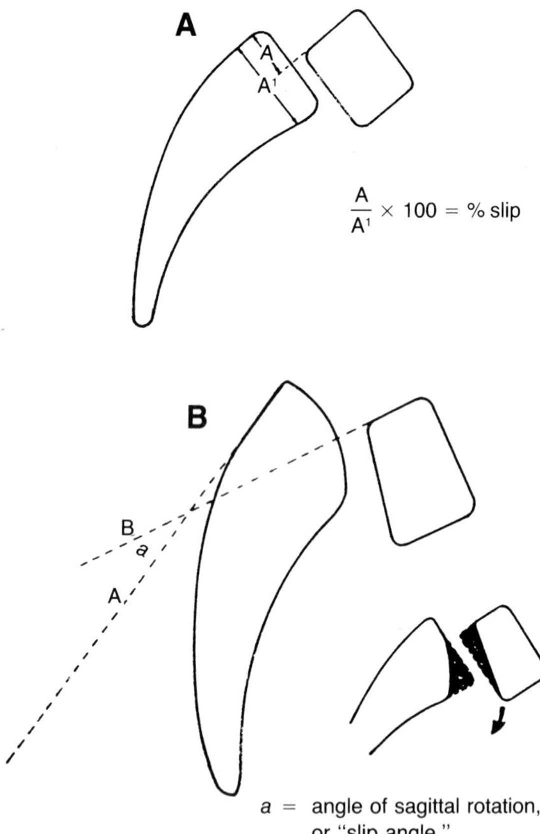

FIG. 16-54. *(A)* Proper measurement of the percentage of slip or displacement of L5 relative to S1. *(B)* Measurement of the angle of sagittal rotation of "slip angle." This angle measures the kyphotic relationship of L5–S1. As the vertebrae gradually slip, there is abnormal growth (pressure inhibition) of the anterior lip of S1 and the posterior lip of L5. Due to the malformation of these end-plates, using the top of S1 or the bottom of L5 does not allow accurate measurement of the angular deformity.

8 months and then gradual brace removal. The patient should be followed until growth is completed to ensure that there is no slipping. Periodic episodes of pain may require repeat bracing.

Painful spondylolysis not responding to brace treatment should have surgical treatment. If there is an L5 pars defect, an L5–S1 arthrodesis should be done. Care should be taken *not* to include L4 in the fusion area.

A chronically painful L4 pars defect without displacement is probably best treated by a direct repair of the lesion. This preserves good lumbar spine motion and is much preferable to an L4–S1 arthrodesis. The author prefers the Scott technique.[72]

Treatment of Spondylolisthesis. Considerable controversy exists as to the proper management of these problems, but a rational approach has gradually emerged from the many conflicting opinions.

Grade I slips (0% to 25%) need not be fused unless there is a problem of chronic pain despite adequate conservative (brace) treatment. Treatment of a painful slip by exercises is not appropriate, because exercises tend to increase pain rather than decrease it. If fusion is necessary, a good-quality alar-transverse (posterolateral) fusion is preferred. Postoperative support in an orthosis appears to be adequate support.

Grade II slips (25% to 50%) should be more aggressively treated. This is where the difference between adults and children is most notable. In younger children (ages 6 to 12

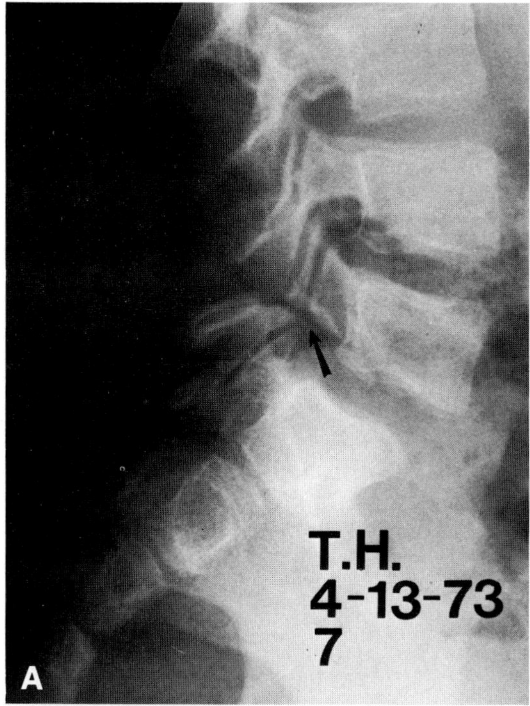

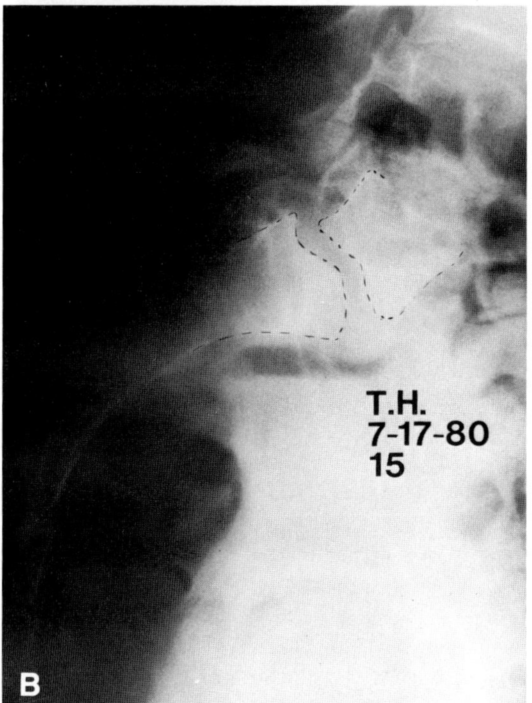

FIG. 16-55. *(A)* This 7-year-old male was seen for swayback but had no back pain symptoms. He was periodically observed. *(B)* At age 15, he was still asymptomatic, and was an outstanding high-school athlete.

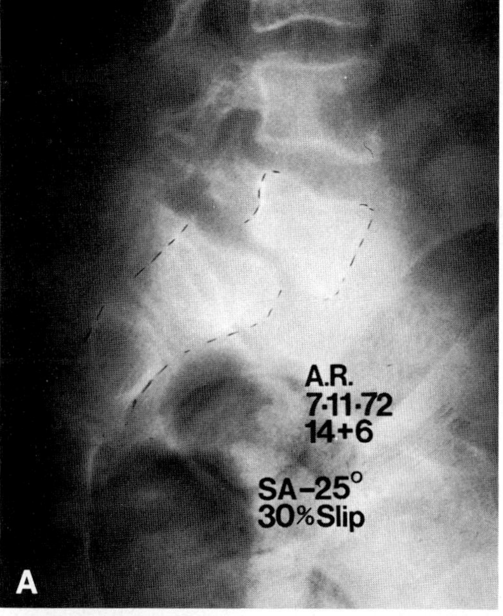

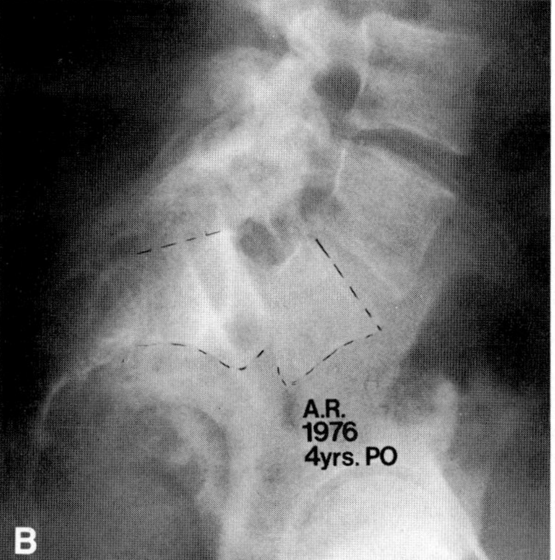

FIG. 16-56. *(A)* A 14-year-old boy with a 30% displacement and a −25° slip angle. Although nonprogressive, his significant chronic lumbosacral pain problem indicated the need for fusion. *(B)* A solid lumbosacral fusion is noted at a 4-year follow-up. He had complete pain relief. This is a good example of fusion *in situ*.

years), a slip of this degree is quite significant and highly likely to progress during the remaining growth years. Fusion should thus be done, even if the patient has no symptoms. It is the surgeon's responsibility to prevent the catastrophy of total spondyloptosis by such early fusions. An L5–S1 fusion is usually adequate.

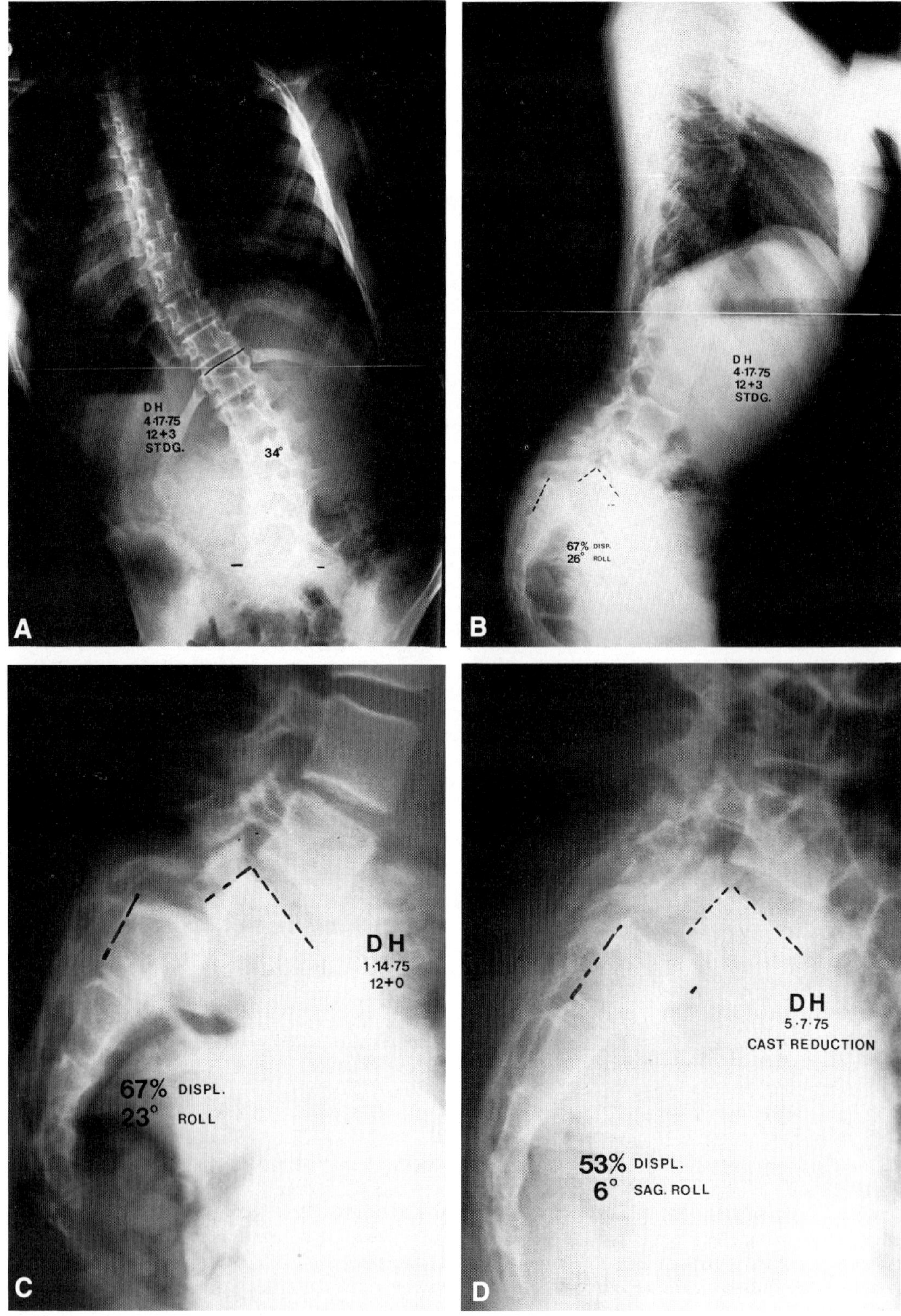
A
DH
4·17·75
12+3
STDG.
34°
B
DH
4·17·75
12+3
STDG.
67% DISP.
26° ROLL
C
DH
1·14·75
12+0
67% DISPL.
23° ROLL
D
DH
5·7·75
CAST REDUCTION
53% DISPL.
6° SAG. ROLL

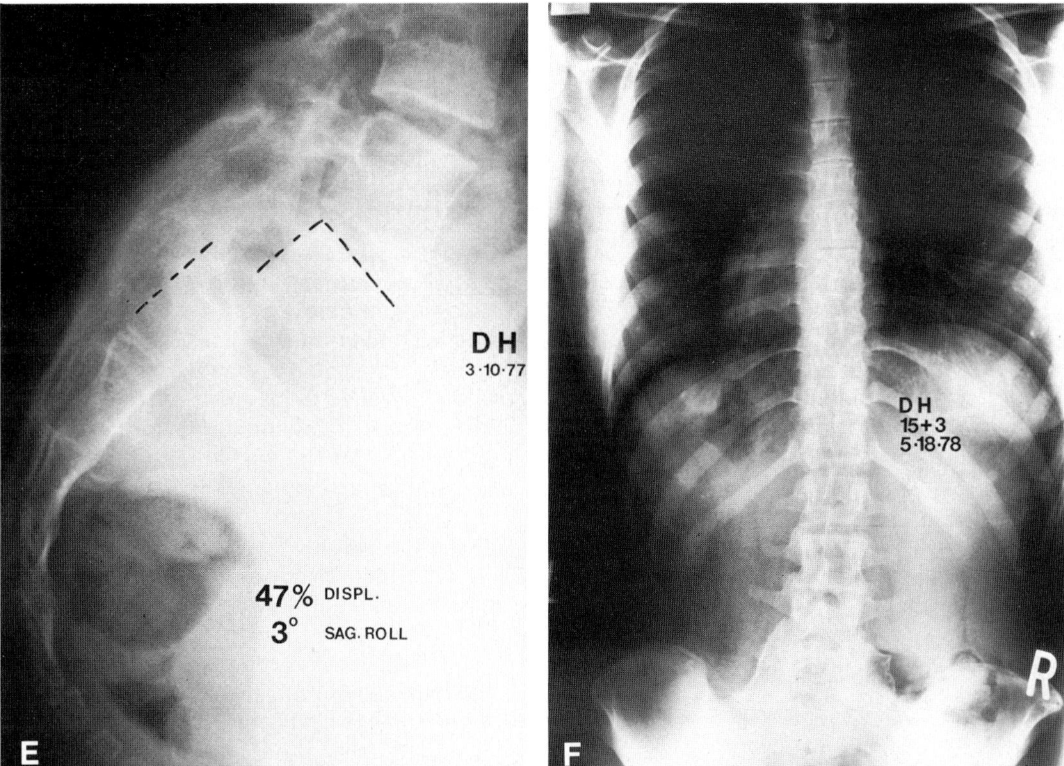

FIG. 16-57. *(A)* This 12-year-old girl presented to the author with a "spasm" type of scoliosis, lumbosacral pain, and sciatica. *(B)* Her lateral standing film shows a relatively vertical sacrum, a 67% displacement, a 26° slip angle (sagittal roll), and total lordosis from L5–T1. Note how the torso is displaced forward relative to the pelvis. *(C)* This detailed view of the lumbosacral area shows an elongated pars of L5 with a pars defect near the pedicle. *(D)* She was treated by nerve root decompression, L4–S1 transverse process fusion, and partial reduction by cast application (double pantaloon) in a hyperextended position. The percentage of slip was reduced from 67% to 53%, but, more importantly, the slip angle was reduced from 23° to 6°. *(E)* At a 2-year follow-up, her fusion is solid, and there has been no loss of correction. All pain was gone. *(F)* An anteroposterior view 3 years after surgery shows the solid L4–S1 fusion and total correction of her scoliosis.

A slip in a mature adolescent is a somewhat different situation, because the risk of progression is far less. Symptomatic slips of 25% to 50% should be fused, but asymptomatic slips can be periodically checked.

Grade III (50% to 70%) and Grade IV (75% to 100%) slips in children and adolescents should always be fused. Contrary to the lesser degrees of slip, these usually require L4–S1 fusion. The best technique appears to be the posterolateral alar-transverse fusion, with special attention given to a thorough cleaning-out and bone grafting of the L5 transverse process—alar interval. Often, the inexperienced surgeon will find a transverse process and think it is that of L5, when in reality it is that of L4.

With such significant degrees of slipping, a higher pseudarthrosis rate has been reported, and thus, a more vigorous immobilization is necessary if a solid fusion is to be anticipated. The author prefers cast immobilization with one or both thighs included (Fig. 16-56).

Treatment of Spondylolisthesis With Nerve Root Involvement. True evidence of nerve root compression is seen by motor weakness and sensory deficit. If these factors are present, nerve root decompression should be added to the fusion described previously. In a child, adolescent, or young adult, nerve root decompression without fusion should never be done.

The nerve root involved is almost always L5, and the compression takes place by the proximal part of the pars interarticularis as it is carried forward by the slipping body of L5. Thus, removal of the loose element of the L5 lamina will not by itself decompress the root. Further dissection is always necessary (Fig. 16-57).

On the rare occasion when the sacral roots are involved (bladder weakness), removal of the prominent portion of the body of S1 anterior to the dural sac is necessary.

Are tight hamstrings a sign of nerve root compression? This frequent question was addressed by Boxall and colleagues[8] in their discussion of severe slips. They found no correlation between tight hamstrings and objective neurologic findings such as motor deficits, sensory deficits, or reflex changes. Many patients at our center have been fused *in situ* without root decompression, even when the hamstrings were quite tight. This tightness resolved with time. Late root decompression to solve tight hamstrings (in the presence of a solid fusion) has not been necessary (Fig. 16-58).

Treatment of Severe Spondylolisthesis With Lumbosacral Kyphosis (Severe Sagittal Rotation). Recently, there have been many procedures published by a large number of surgeons from many different countries. All these procedures deal with the "reduction and fusion" of severe (or not so severe) spondylolisthesis. Most reports are of a small number of patients with a short follow-up period.

The concept of hyperextension in the treatment of severe lordosacral spondylolisthesis was first demonstrated by Taillard[79] in 1954, using leg and cranial skin traction in the prone position. Italian opthopaedists followed with cast reductions using hyperextension and elongation forces.[71] Daymond first used halo-femoral traction for the partial reduction of spondylolisthesis in 1969 and reported his work in 1975.[18]

Anterior fusion for spondylolisthesis was first described by Burns in 1933.[13] European surgeons have tended to use anterior fusion more often than North American surgeons during the past 20 years.

Patients with high degrees of lumbosacral kyphosis have significant deformity. They have

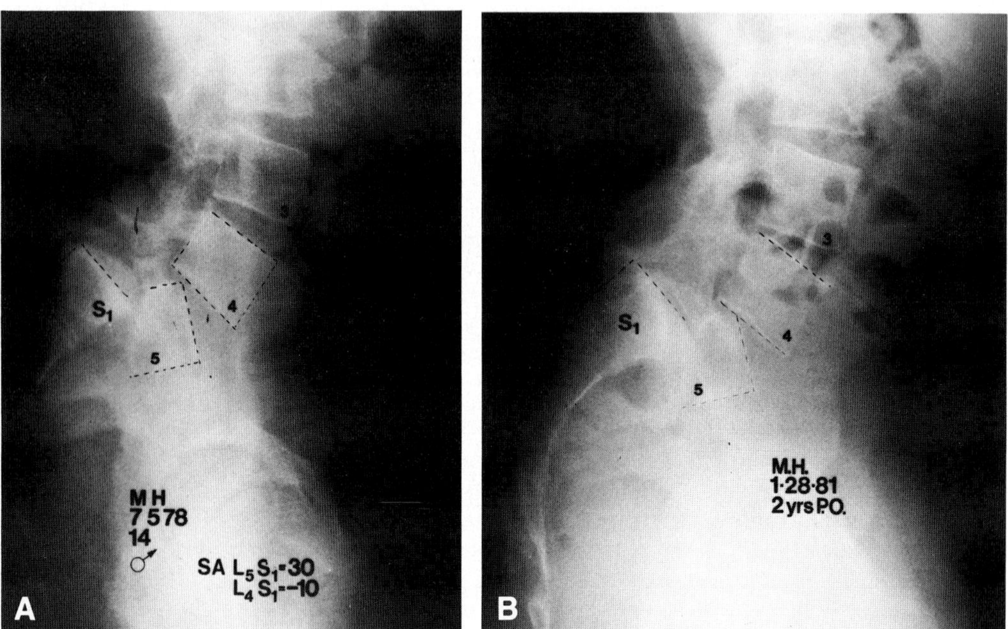

FIG. 16-58. *(A).* This 14-year-old male presented to the author with severe low back pain but no sciatica. Although he has a 100% slip and a 30° L5, S1 slip angle, there is a retrolisthesis of L4 on L5 so that the L4–S1 relationship is a −10° slip angle. An L4–S1 fusion is all that is necessary. Attempts to "reduce" L5 are *not* indicated. *(B)* Two years following L3–S1 fusion, his pain was gone and he had become an outstanding high-school athlete. Except for slight shortening of the waistline, his clinical appearance was normal.

FIG. 16-59. *(A)* This 16-year-old male with Marfan's syndrome presented to the author with severe low back pain and sciatica. His straight–leg–raising test was positive at 10° bilaterally. *(B)* A lateral tomogram of the lumbosacral area demonstrates a 100% slip and a 55° slip angle. There were bilateral pars defects of both L5 and L4. Both partial reduction and combined anterior and posterior fusion were thought to be necessary. *(C)* Treatment consisted of posterior L3–S1 fusion with root decompression at L5 bilaterally. This was followed by halo-femoral traction, anterior fusion, and double pantaloon casting. He is solid and pain-free 2 years after surgery. (Illustrations reproduced with permission of Journal of Pediatric Orthopedics, Vol 2, 51–55, 1982)

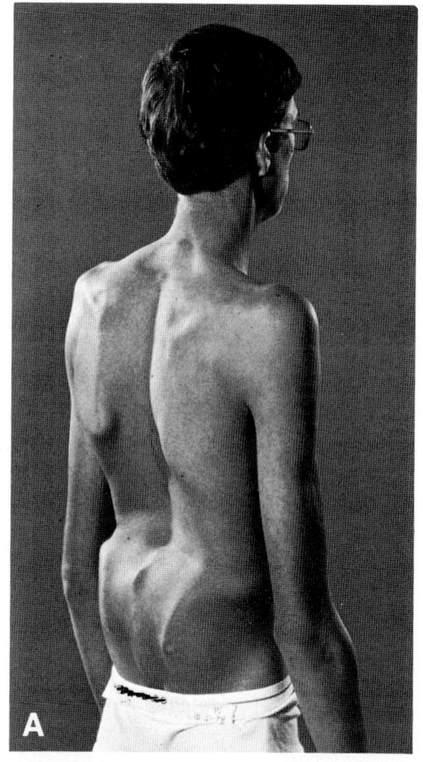

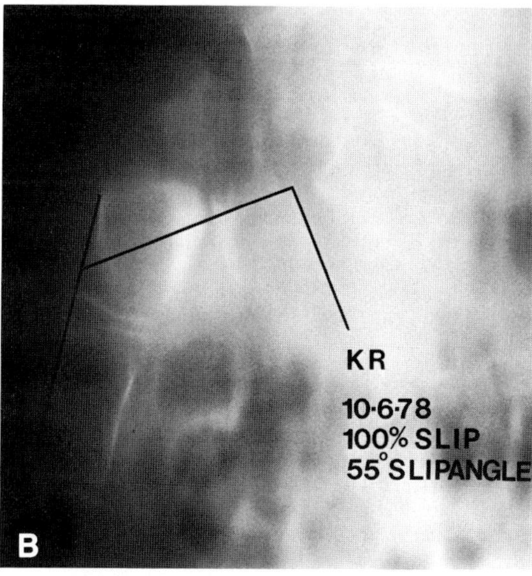

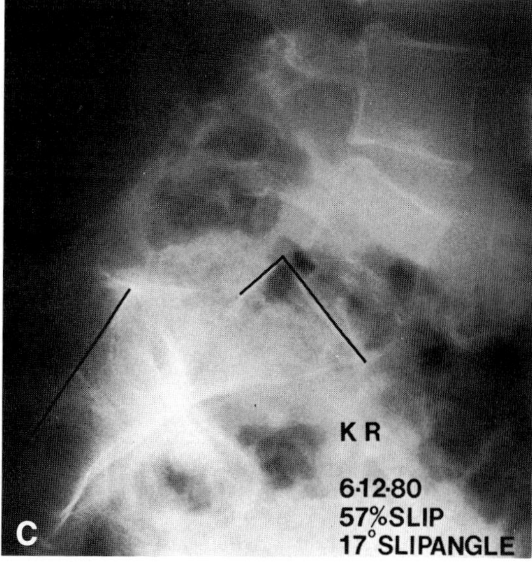

a vertical sacrum with absence of the buttock contour. There is marked shortening of the waistline and severe lumbar lordosis (which is the *compensatory* curve). These patients are highly gratified if this ugly deformity can be corrected and if that correction can be maintained.

For children and adolescents, the author believes that an alar-transverse and midline posterior fusion (L4–S1) should be done first, followed by 2 to 4 weeks of halo-femoral traction in mild hyperextension, followed by 4 to 6 months of bed rest in a double pantaloon cast. No internal fixation is used, although a supplementary exploration and compression rod fixation at 6 months is sometimes beneficial. Occasionally an anterior L5–S1 fusion is also needed.

Most children and adolescents with Grade III and even Grade IV slips do *not* require "reduction." They can almost always be managed successfully by posterior-posterolateral fusion of L4–S1 and cast immobilization (Fig. 16-59).[34]

REFERENCES

1. Anderson M, Hwang SC, Green WT: Growth of the normal trunk in boys and girls during the second decade of life. J Bone Joint Surg 47A:1554, 1965
2. Axelgaard J, Brown JC: Lateral electrical surface stimulation for the treatment of progressive idiopathic scoliosis. Spine 8:242, 1983
3. Baker DR, McHollick W: Spondyloschisis and spondylolisthesis in children. J Bone Joint Surg 38A:933, 1956
4. Balmer, GA, MacEwen GD: The incidence and treatment of scoliosis in cerebral palsy. J Bone Joint Surg 52B:134, 1970
5. Bergofsky EH, Turino GM, Fishman AP: Cardiorespiratory failure in kyphoscoliosis. Medicine 38:263, 1959
6. Blount WP: Use of the Milwaukee brace. Orthop Clin North Am 3:3, 1972
7. Blount WP, Moe JH: The Milwaukee Brace. Baltimore, Williams & Wilkins, 1973
8. Boxall D, Bradford D, Winter R, Moe J: Management of severe spondylolisthesis in children and adolescents. J Bone Joint Surg 61A:479, 1979
9. Bradford DS, Ahmed K, Moe J, Winter R, Lonstein J: The surgical management of patients with Scheuermann's disease: A review of 24 cases managed by combined anterior and posterior spine fusion. J Bone Joint Surg 62A:705, 1980
10. Bradford DS, Moe JH, Montalvo FJ, Winter RB: Scheuermann's kyphosis and roundback deformity—results of Milwaukee brace treatment. J Bone Joint Surg 56A:740, 1974

10a. Bradford DS, Moe JH, Montalvo FJ, Winter RB: Scheuermann's kyphosis—results of surgical treatment by posterior spine arthrodesis in 22 patients. J Bone Joint Surg 57A:439, 1975

11. Brooks HL, Azen SP, Gerberg E, Brooks R, Chan L: Scoliosis: A prospective epidemiologic study. J Bone Joint Surg 57A:968, 1975
12. Bunnell W: A study of the natural history of idiopathic scoliosis. Orthop Trans 7:6, 1983
13. Burns BH: An operation for spondylolisthesis. Lancet 1:1233, 1933
14. Carr W, Moe J, Winter R, Lonstein J: Treatment of idiopathic scoliosis in the Milwaukee brace. J Bone Joint Surg 62A:599, 1980
15. Collis DK, Ponseti IV: Long-term follow-up of patients with idiopathic scoliosis not treated surgically. J Bone Joint Surg 51A:425, 1969
16. Cowell HR, Hall JN, MacEwen GD: Genetic aspects of idiopathic scoliosis. Clin Orthop 86:121, 1972
17. Dandy DJ, Shannon MJ: Lumbosacral subluxation (group I spondylolisthesis). J Bone Joint Surg 53B:578, 1971
18. Daymond K: Adolescent spondylolisthesis. J Bone Joint Surg 57B:118, 1975
19. dePeloux J, Fauchet R, Faucon B, Stagnara P: Le plan d'election pour l'examen radiologigue des cypho-scolioses Rev. de chir, orthop. e repar. de l Appareil Motor 51:517, 1965
20. Dommissee GF: The blood supply of the spinal cord, a critical vascular zone in spinal surgery. J Bone Joint Surg 56B:225, 1974
21. Dubousset J, Guillaumat M, Méchen JF: Retentissement rachidjen des laminectomies, les compressions medullaires non-traumatiques de l'enfant. J Rougerie, Mason et Cie, Chapitre XI, Paris, 1973
22. Duval-Beaupere G: Pathogenic relationship between scoliosis and growth. In Zorab PA (ed): Scoliosis and Growth. London, Churchill Livingstone, 1971
23. Ferriera JH, James JIP: Progressive and resolving infantile idiopathic scoliosis—differential diagnosis. J Bone Joint Surg 54B:648, 1972
24. Garrett AL, Perry J, Nickel V: Stabilization of the collapsing spine. J Bone Joint Surg 43A:474, 1961
25. Ghavamian T: The future of minor scoliotic curves of the spine. J Bone Joint Surg 57A:134, 1975
26. Goldstein LA: Treatment of idiopathic scoliosis by Harrington instrumentation and fusion with fresh autogenous iliac bone grafts. J Bone Joint Surg 51A:209, 1969
27. Goldstein LA: The surgical treatment of idiopathic scoliosis. Clin Orthop 93:131, 1973
28. Goldstein LA, Waugh TR: Classification and terminology of scoliosis. Clin Orthop 93:10, 1973
29. Guthkelch AN: Diastematomyelia with median septum. Brain 97:729, 1974
30. Hall JE: The anterior approach to spinal deformities. Orthop Clin North Am 3:81, 1972
31. Harrington PR: Treatment of scoliosis—correction and internal fixation by spine instrumentation. J Bone Joint Surg 44A:591, 1962
32. Harrington PR: Technical details in relation to the successful use of instrumentation in scoliosis. Orthop Clin North Am 3:49, 1972
33. Hensinger R: Spondylolysis and spondylolisthesis in children. Am Acad Orthop Surg Inst Course Lect 32:132, 1983
34. Hensinger RN, Lang JR, MacEwen GD: Surgical management of spondylolisthesis in children and adolescents. Spine 1:207, 1976
35. James JIP: Idiopathic scoliosis, the prognosis, diagnosis, and operative indications related to curve patterns and the age of onset. J Bone Joint Surg 36B:36, 1954
36. James JIP: Kyphoscoliosis. J Bone Joint Surg 37B:414, 1955
37. James JIP: Infantile idiopathic scoliosis. Clin Orthop 77:57, 1971
38. Johnson BE, Westgate HD: Methods of predicting vital capacity in patients with thoracic scoliosis. J Bone Joint Surg 52A:1433, 1970
39. Kharrat K, Moe JH, Winter RB: Subcutaneous Harrington instrumentation without fusion for treatment of scoliosis in young children. Clin Orthop [In press].
40. King H, Moe J, Bradford D, Winter R: Selection of fusion levels in thoracic idiopathic scoliosis. J Bone Joint Surg 65A:1302, 1983

41. Kuhns JG, Hormel RS: Management of congenital scoliosis. Arch Surg 65:250, 1952
42. Leatherman KD: The management of rigid spinal curves. Clin Orthop 93:215–224, 1973
43. Lindh M, Bjure J: Lung volumes in scoliosis before and after correction by the Harrington instrumentation method. Acta Orthop Scand 46:934, 1975
44. Lloyd-Roberts GC, Pilcher MF: Structural idiopathic scoliosis in infancy—a study of the natural history of 100 patients. J Bone Joint Surg 47B:520, 1965
45. Lonstein JE: Postlaminectomy kyphosis. Clin Orthop 126:93, 1977
46. Lonstein JE, Akbarnia BA: Operative treatment of spinal deformities in patients with cerebral palsy or mental retardation. J Bone Joint Surg 65A:43, 1983
47. Lonstein JE, Carlson M: Prognostication in idiopathic scoliosis. Orthop Trans 5:22, 1981
48. Lonstein JE, Winter RB, Moe JH, Chou S, Pinto WC: Spinal cord compression due to spine deformity. Reconstr Surg Traumatol 13:58, 1972
49. MacEwen GD, Bunnell WP, Sriram K: Acute neurologic complications in the treatment of scoliosis. (A report of the Scoliosis Research Society). J Bone Joint Surg 57A:404, 1975
50. MacEwen GD, Winter RB, Hardy JH: Evaluation of kidney anomalies in congenital scoliosis. J Bone Joint Surg 54A:1451, 1972
51. Mayfield J: Postradiation spinal deformity. Orthop Clin North Am 10:829, 1979
52. McCullough N, Schultz M, Javech H, Latta L: The Miami TLSO in the management of scoliosis: preliminary results in 100 cases. J Pediatr Orthop 1:141, 1981
53. McKee BW, Alexander WJ, Dunbar JS: Spondylolysis and spondylolisthesis in children, a review. J Can Assoc Radiol 22:100, 1971
54. Mehta MH: The rib-vertebra angle in the early diagnosis between resolving and progressive infantile scoliosis. J Bone Joint Surg 54B:230, 1973
55. Moe JH: A critical analysis of methods of fusion for scoliosis. An evaluation in 266 patients. J Bone Joint Surg 40A:529, 1958
56. Moe JH, Kettleson DN: Idiopathic scoliosis—analysis of curve patterns and the preliminary results of Milwaukee brace treatment in 196 patients. J Bone Joint Surg 52A:1509, 1970
57. Moe JH, Winter R, Bradford D, Lonstein J: Scoliosis and Other Spinal Deformities. Philadelphia, WB Saunders, 1978
58. Nachemson A: A long-term follow-up study of non-treated scoliosis. Acta Orthop Scand 39:466, 1968
59. Newman PH: The etiology of spondylolisthesis. J Bone Joint Surg 45B:39, 1963
60. Nilsonne U, Lundgren KD: Long-term prognosis in idiopathic scoliosis. Acta Orthop Scand 39:456, 1968
61. Nordwall A: Studies in idiopathic scoliosis—relevant to etiology, conservative and operative treatment. Acta Orthop Scand [Suppl] 150, 1973
62. Ponseti IV, Friedman, B: Prognosis in idiopathic scoliosis. J Bone Joint Surg 32A:381, 1950
63. Reckles LN, Peterson HA, Bianco AJ, Weidman WH: The association of scoliosis and congenital heart defects. J Bone Joint Surg 57A:449, 1975
64. Riseborough EJ, Wynn-Davies R: A genetic survey of idiopathic scoliosis in Boston, Mass. J Bone Joint Surg 55A:974, 1973
65. Robins PR, Moe JH, Winter RB: Scoliosis in Marfan's syndrome. Its characteristics and results of treatment in 35 patients. J Bone Joint Surg 57A:358, 1975
66. Robson P: The prevalence of scoliosis in adolescents and young adults with cerebral palsy. Dev Med Child Neurol 10:447, 1968
67. Rosenthal RK, Levine DB, McCarver CL: The occurrence of scoliosis in cerebral palsy. Dev Med Child Neurol 16:664, 1974
68. Sahlstrand T, Ortengren R, Nachemson A: Postural equilibrium in adolescent idiopathic scoliosis. Acta Orthop Scand 49:354, 1978
69. Sahlstrand T, Petruson B, Ortengren R: Vestibulospinal reflex activity in patients with adolescent idiopathic scoliosis. Postural effects during caloric labyrinthine stimulation record by stabilometry. Acta Orthop Scand 50:275, 1979
70. Samilson R, Bechard R: Scoliosis in cerebral palsy: incidence, distribution of curve patterns, natural history, and thoughts on etiology. Curr Pract Orthop Surg 5:183, 1973
71. Scaglietti O, Frontino G, Bartolozzi P: Technique of anatomical reduction of lumbar spondylolisthesis and its surgical stabilization. Clin Orthop 117:164, 1976
72. Scott JC: Figure 16.15, page 319. In Roof R (ed): Spinal Deformities, 2nd ed. Tunbridge Wells, Kent, England, Pitman Medical Ltd., 1980
73. Scott JC, Morgan TH: Natural history and prognosis of infantile idiopathic scoliosis. J Bone Joint Surg 37B:400, 1955
74. Shannon DC, Riseborough EJ, Valenca LM, Kazeuri H: The distribution of abnormal lung function in Kyphoscoliosis. J Bone Joint Surg 52A:131, 1970
75. Sörenson KH: Scheuermann's Juvenile Kyphosis. Copenhagen, Munksgaard, 1964
76. Stagnara P, Fauchet R, Boulliat G, dePeloux J, Mazoyer D, et al: A propos de 17 observations de paraplegies par deformations vertebrales traites par redressment partiel. Revd Chir Orto e Repar Appar Moteur 54:623, 1968
77. Stone B, Beckman C, Hall V, Guess V, Brooks H: The effect of an exercise program on change in curve in adolescents with minimal idiopathic scoliosis. Phys Ther 59:759, 1979
78. Tachdjian MO, Matson DD: Orthopaedic aspects of intraspinal tumors in infants and children. J Bone Joint Surg 47A:223, 1965
79. Taillard W: Le spondylolisthesis chez l'enfant et l'adolescent. Acta Orthop Scand 24:115, 1954
80. Turner RH, Bianco AJ: Spondylolysis and spondylolisthesis in teenagers and children. J Bone Joint Surg 53A:1298, 1971
81. Wiltse LL, Widell EH, Jackson DW: Fatigue fracture: The basic lesion in isthmic spondylolisthesis. J Bone Joint Surg 57A:17, 1975
82. Winter R: Convex anterior and posterior hemiarthrodesis and epiphyseodesis in young children with congenital scoliosis. J Pediatr Orthop 1:361, 1981
83. Winter R: Congenital Deformities of the Spine. New York, Thieme-Stratton, 1983
84. Winter RB, Haven JJ, Moe JH, Lagaard SM: Diastematomyelia and congenital spine deformities. J Bone Joint Surg 56A:27, 1974
85. Winter RB, Lovell WW, Moe JH: Excessive thoracic lordosis and loss of pulmonary function in patients with idiopathic scoliosis. J Bone Joint Surg 57A:972, 1975

86. Winter R, Moe JH: The results of spinal arthrodesis for congenital spine deformity in patients younger than 5 years old. J Bone Joint Surg 64A:419, 1982
87. Winter RB, Moe JH, Eilers VE: Congenital scoliosis—a study of 234 patients treated and untreated. J Bone Joint Surg 50A:1, 1968
88. Winter R, Moe J, MacEwen GD, Peon-Vidales H: The Milwaukee brace in the nonoperative treatment of congenital scoliosis. Spine 1:85, 1976
89. Winter RB, Moe JH, Wang JF: Congenital Kyphosis. Its natural history and treatment as observed in a study of 130 patients. J Bone Joint Surg 55A:223, 1973
90. Wynn-Davies R: Familial (idiopathic) scoliosis—a family survey. J Bone Joint Surg 50B:24, 1968

17

The Upper Limb

Daniel C. Riordan
Loui G. Bayne

CLASSIFICATION OF UPPER LIMB MALFORMATIONS

It is difficult to discuss congenital anomalies of the upper extremity without some way of classifying them so that everyone will know exactly what defect is being discussed. In the past, the use of various Greek and Latin names to describe common deficiencies has only served to confuse many conditions. The classification submitted here has been adopted by the American Society for Surgery of the Hand, the International Federation of Societies for Surgery of the Hand, and the International Society of Prosthetics and Orthotics. This classification groups similar patterns of deficiencies according to the parts that have been primarily affected by a certain embryonic failure, whether the insult involves a total part (skeletal and soft tissues) or only the dermal myofascial structures. The main categories of this classification are

- Failure of formation of parts (arrest of development)
- Failure of differentiation of parts (separation of parts)
- Duplication
- Overgrowth (gigantism)
- Undergrowth (hypoplasia)
- Congenital constriction band syndrome
- General skeletal abnormalities

A detailed explanation of these classifications can be found in an article by Swanson.[1]

Failure of Formation of Parts (Arrest of Development)

This category consists of a group of deformities that are distinguished by failure, or arrest, of formation of the limb, either complete or partial. There are two subcategories: transverse and longitudinal. Transverse defects include all congenital amputation–type conditions, ranging from aphalangia (absence of the fingers) to amelia (complete absence of the entire upper extremity). Longitudinal deficiencies include all the other deficiencies in this category that occur along the longitudinal axis of the extremity. Longitudinal deficiencies are subdivided into segmental, preaxial (radial), postaxial (ulna), and central (hand and wrist). In previous classifications, segmental deficiencies were listed under intercalary deficiencies. Examples of segmental deficiencies include phocomelias, in which the hand is attached to the shoulder, eliminating one whole segment of the upper extremity. Preaxial deficiencies include the absence of any of the structures on the radial side of the forearm, such as the radial clubhand. Postaxial deficiencies include the deficiencies that occur on the ulna aspect of the forearm, such as congenital absence of the ulna. Central deficiencies are primarily associated with the hand and wrist, with absence of the central segments. Central deficiencies include the second, third, and fourth rays of the hand. An example is the lobster-claw hand, with the deficiency involving either the second, third, or fourth rays.

Failure of Differentiation of Parts

The anomalies in this category are those in which the basic units have developed but the final form is not complete. Examples of this category would be synostosis, syndactylies, and contractures secondary to failure of differentiation of soft parts, including arthrogryposis and camptodactyly.

Duplication of Parts

Duplication of parts is thought to be an injury to the ectodermal cap of the limb bud, producing a splitting of the original embryonic part.

Duplication can occur anywhere along the upper extremity, but it seems to occur more often in the fingers and thumb. Examples of this category would be duplication of the thumb or the little finger, which are probably the most common.

Overgrowth (Gigantism)

The terms *overgrowth* and *gigantism* describe those conditions in which either part or all of the limb is disproportionately large. Overgrowth may occur in a digit, hand, or forearm or in the entire limb. Probably the most common example of this category is the macrodactyly involving one or more fingers.

Undergrowth (Hypoplasia)

The term *hypoplasia* was used earlier to describe the condition of skeletal elements that persist after some failure of formation of parts (Category I). However, because of their prevalence in the absence of other skeletal involvement, hypoplastic defects are represented separately in this classification system. Hypoplasia may involve the entire upper extremity or any of its parts. Brachydactyly is probably the most common hand malformation seen in association with this category.

Constriction Band Syndrome

Constriction bands, annular bands, and Streeter's bands, as they are sometimes referred to, occur so frequently without other limb deficiencies that a separate category is necessary. The actual cause of this deformity has not been determined. Constriction bands are more likely to involve the distal parts of the extremity, especially the hand and foot. The constriction, however, may be so severe as to produce amputation of the part.

Generalized Skeletal Abnormalities

Defects in the hand may be a manifestation of a generalized skeletal defect, such as dyschondroplasia, achondroplasia, and osteocartilaginous exostosis. These deformities are unique to each syndrome and are placed in this category.

CONGENITAL AMPUTATIONS

Congenital amputations can occur at any level of the upper extremity. However, they most frequently involve the hand or wrist. The deforming factor affects the limb bud transversely, and growth does not occur distal to the insult.

The incidence of such conditions varies but forearm amputations have been reported to occur in 1 in 20,000 live births, and upper arm amputations in 1 in 27,000 live births.[3] Amputation of the upper extremity is seen with constriction band syndrome; however, the stumps are bulbous and usually associated with constriction bands involving other parts. The structures proximal to the amputation are usually normal. The stumps in congenital amputation vary. They are usually well rounded and covered with a well-padded end. In the forearm, they can be tapered, and, when they occur at the hand level, they may have some vestigial nubbings on the terminal end. Moderate proximal atrophy and hypoplasia of the extremity is common (Fig. 17-1).

Treatment

The treatment of congenital amputation is divided into surgical and prosthetic fittings. There are few indications for surgical treatment. Terminal digital remnants are usually of no benefit. They can be removed to give a more pleasing appearance or to provide a better stump for prosthetic fitting. Some patients become attached to them and do not want them removed, and, if there is no beneficial reason to have them removed, they should be left.

Prosthetic Fittings. Prosthetic fitting as early as possible is indicated in these patients. Usually, the best time to begin fitting with the prosthesis is when the patient attempts to crawl. It is vital that the prosthesis be fit before the child begins ambulation. It is important for the infant to become accustomed to the device and to integrate it into his activities. Instruction in simple maneuvers is useful throughout childhood, particularly when new terminal devices or controls are introduced. The initial prostheses are simple devices and are upgraded as the child gets older. Myoelectric systems, sensory feedback systems,[4] and other more complex prostheses may or may not be instituted when the child gets older, and only if the child shows some desire for continuing use of the prosthesis.

Operative Procedures. Excision of the vestigial digits is accomplished by simple wedge resection. Occasionally, the angulatory osteotomies of the humerus in above-elbow amputations are necessary to provide a slight anterior bow, 20° to 30° of flexion, to aid in the fitting of a prosthesis. A closing wedge–type osteotomy is usually sufficient.

In bilateral upper extremity amputees who have visual impairment, a Krukenberg's procedure can be considered. This converts the forearm to a pair of opposing prehensile digits. For details of and indications for this procedure, the reader is referred to the article by Swanson.[7]

A few congenital amputations of the fingers will leave a portion of the finger present. This can also be a result of constriction bands. If these remaining digits contain the base of the proximal phalanx with its epiphysis, bone can be implanted in the remnant cutaneous sleeves to increase length. The proximal phalanx of the second toe serves as a good source of bone for this type of procedure.

PHOCOMELIA

The term *phocomelia* means seal limb, derived from the two Greek words, *phobe*, meaning seal, and *melos*, meaning limb.[10] This deformity is an extreme example of a Category I, longitudinal deficiency. The typical deformity is characterized by the hand attaching to the shoulder with the absence of the arm and forearm (Fig. 17-2).

Birch-Jensen[9] estimated that a radioulnar defect occurred once in about 75,000 births. The deformity occurs infrequently, however, it became more frequent in the 1950s and

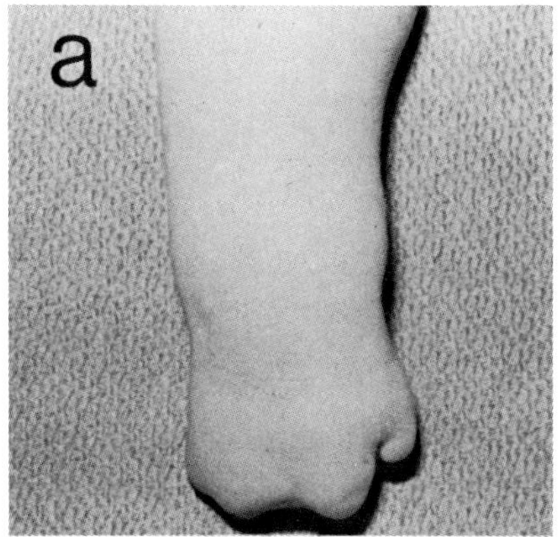

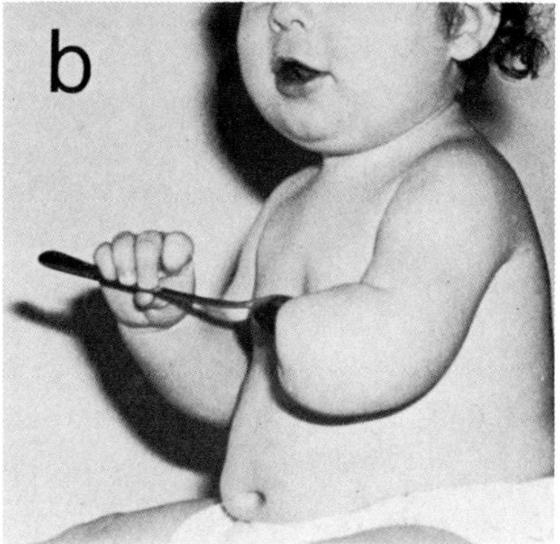

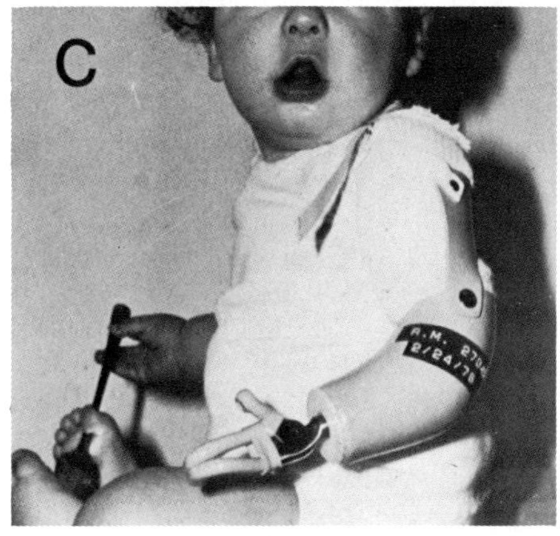

FIG. 17-1. *(a)* Congenital amputations occur at any level along the upper extremity. Amputation of the fingers with the thumb may occur (as here), but frequently, small nubbing will be present. (*b*) Amputation at the forearm level. B.E. amputations are most common. (*c*) A prosthetic device can be helpful if applied early, usually when the infant begins to pull up or use the hand in space.

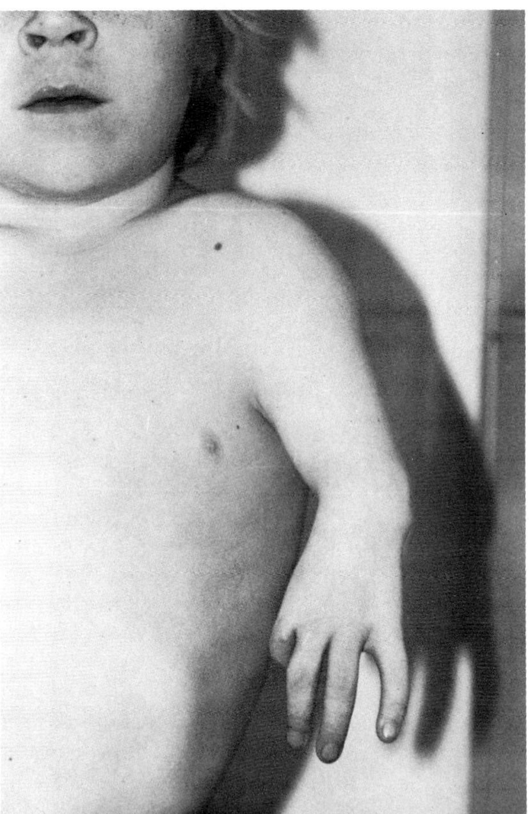

FIG. 17-2. This figure shows a patient in whom there is a failure of formation of an intermediate portion of the upper extremity. The hand and forearm appear to be attached to the shoulder, with a missing humerus.

1960s, when it affected about 60% of infants born to mothers who had taken thalidomide during their first trimester of pregnancy. However, cases can also occur sporadically.

Phocomelias can be associated with other congenital defects as well as syndromes. Clinically, they are associated with cleft palate and scoliosis but can be associated with Holt-Oram syndrome. Cardiac anomalies are frequent and may be due to the fact that the cardiac structures are formed at the same time that the limb structures are formed in the embryo.

Treatment

There are few indications for surgery in phocomelia. Most of the surgery performed in these patients is designed to aid in the fitting of a prosthetic device. If a tubular bone is present, lengthening may be indicated. If no bone is present, the bone from the fibula or clavicle can be used. Digital function may be improved by web space deepening or by correction of contractures that may facilitate the use of a prosthetic device. Treatment is mainly the devising of a prosthetic supplement to aid the patient in the use of the remaining part.

CONGENITAL ABSENCE OF THE RADIUS

Clinical Features

Congenital absence of the radius is characterized by radial deviation of the hand, marked shortening of the forearm, and general underdevelopment of the upper extremity. There are two types: one in which there is total absence of the radius, and one with only partial absence of the radius. The most common manifestation of this type is absence of the distal half of the radius. There may also be absence of only the central segment or absence of the proximal segment of the radius. Approximately 50% of the reported cases are bilateral. There may or may not be associated anomalies, and there does not seem to be any pattern of these anomalies.

The lack of the support of the radius to the carpus results in radial deviation of the hand and carpus. This may vary from a mild radial deviation of the hand if the radius is only mildly shortened to more than 90° of deviation if the radius is totally absent. The greater the radial deviation, the less effective are the forearm muscles, due to the greater relaxation and proportionate loss of strength (Fig. 17-3*A–C*).

In addition to the radial deviation of the hand, the forearm is shortened. The ulna is usually short, hypertrophied, and, in most cases, curved, with the concavity toward the radial side. In unilateral cases, the hand, forearm, upper arm, and shoulder girdle are usually underdeveloped in comparison to the normal arm and shoulder. At maturity, the total length of the upper extremity is between one half and two thirds the length of the normal extremity.

As is true in other congenital anomalies, there may be associated deformities. There is no set pattern of associated anomalies and no relationship to a partial or complete absence of the radius. The list of associated anomalies includes hairlip; cleft palate; clubfoot; hydrocephalus; hernia; kyphosis; scoliosis; hemivertebrae; rib deformity, including fusions; and aplasia or absence of a lung.

The skeletal changes that occur in this deformity may involve any bone of the upper extremity. The scapula is commonly reduced in size, and the clavicle may be shortened and more curved. The humerus is usually shorter than normal, and either end may be deformed. The carpal bones are rarely complete in number. The scaphoid is the bone most frequently absent, and, occasionally, it is fused to the lunate. The trapezium is the next most commonly absent. The capitate, hamate, triquetrum, and pisiform bones are usually present. The first metacarpal may be absent, whether or not the thumb is present. Varying degrees of floating thumb result, depending on whether all or only the proximal part of the metacarpal is absent.[12]

The muscles are frequently involved in the deformity. The pectoralis major may have an abnormal insertion, or either the clavicular or costal part may be absent. The pectoralis minor and deltoid are usually present but may have abnormal insertions. The biceps may be absent. If it is present, it inserts into the lacertus fibrosis or may be fused to the brachialis. The brachialis is usually present. The brachioradialis is usually present and may insert into the carpus, acting as a tether. The extensor carpi radialis longus and brevis are usually present or may be fused together. The extensor digitorum communis is usually present and is fairly normal. The supinator is usually absent unless the proximal radius is present, as is the pronator. If the thumb is present and is fully developed, its extensor is usually normal, but the flexor pollicis longus may or may not be present, depending on whether the distal radius is present or absent. The interosseous, lumbrical, and hypothenar muscles are usually present and normal.

The nerve supply of the brachial plexus and upper arm is usually normal. The radial nerve sensory branch may not extend below the elbow, and the median nerve then gives off a branch to the dorsal surface of the hand and may unite with the dorsal branch of the ulnar nerve. If this is the case, the median nerve is the most superficial nerve found on the radial side of the forearm (Fig. 17-3*D*). It must be looked for in any surgical approach from the radial side. The ulnar nerve is usually normal and supplies its normal flexors of the ring and little fingers, the interosseous and hypothenar muscles.

Fanconi's syndrome, a hypoplastic anemia, should be sought in any child with this anomaly or multiple anomalies involving the bones. This syndrome is characterized by a severe, progressive, refractory, macrocytic anemia, with neutropenia and thrombopenia and hypoplastic bone marrow. This condition may be fatal, and the extent of the hypoplastic factors must be determined before any surgical reconstruction is undertaken.

Treatment

Casting. Treatment for congenital absence of the radius should be started as soon as possible after birth if the condition of the child permits.[13] If seen shortly after birth, plaster cast correction of the deformity should be undertaken (Fig. 17-3*E*). Like a cast for a clubfoot, the cast should be put on in three parts, with only one part of the deformity being corrected with each section of the cast. A hand piece, leaving the fingers free, is applied first. The elbow is then flexed to 90°, allowing relaxation of the forearm muscles, and traction is applied to the hand to move the carpus as far distally as possible in relation to the distal end of the ulna. The plaster is then applied to the forearm and is joined to the hand section, with the hand in neutral rotation. The cast should be trimmed out over the anterior aspect of the elbow so that there is no pressure exerted anteriorly when the third part is applied. The third part of the cast is then applied, while the hand-forearm is held in neutral rotation and the elbow is flexed to 90°, and the upper section is joined to the forearm section. As with a clubfoot cast, unless this technique is followed every time, satisfactory correction is not obtained. If the cast is applied within the first few days of life, a great deal of correction can be obtained quickly. If not started until 2 years or later, casting does not achieve much correction.[14]

Surgery. If there is no contraindication for surgery, such as Fanconi's syndrome or heart anomalies that preclude surgery, the surgical correction can be started as early as 2 or 3 months. Historically, the surgical treatment of this deformity has been by osteotomy of the ulna, leaving the hand and distal ulna alone, to bone grafting (tibial, fibular, ulnar, and epiphyseal graft), to centralization of the hand over the ulna by a number of methods (Fig. 17-3*F–I*). In the past 80 years, treatment methods have made a full circle. The treatment recommended by most orthopaedists actively

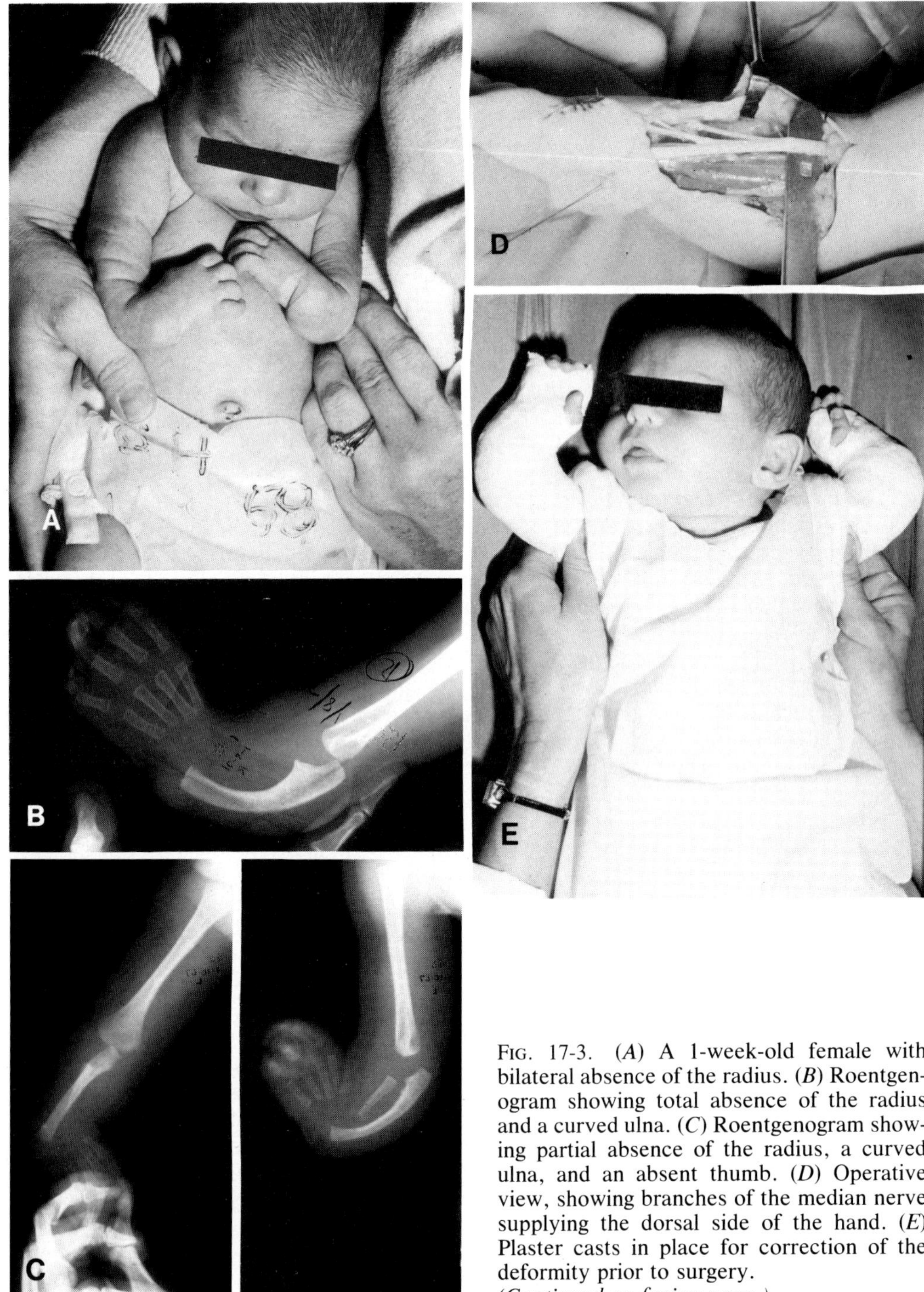

FIG. 17-3. (*A*) A 1-week-old female with bilateral absence of the radius. (*B*) Roentgenogram showing total absence of the radius and a curved ulna. (*C*) Roentgenogram showing partial absence of the radius, a curved ulna, and an absent thumb. (*D*) Operative view, showing branches of the median nerve supplying the dorsal side of the hand. (*E*) Plaster casts in place for correction of the deformity prior to surgery.
(Continued on facing page.)

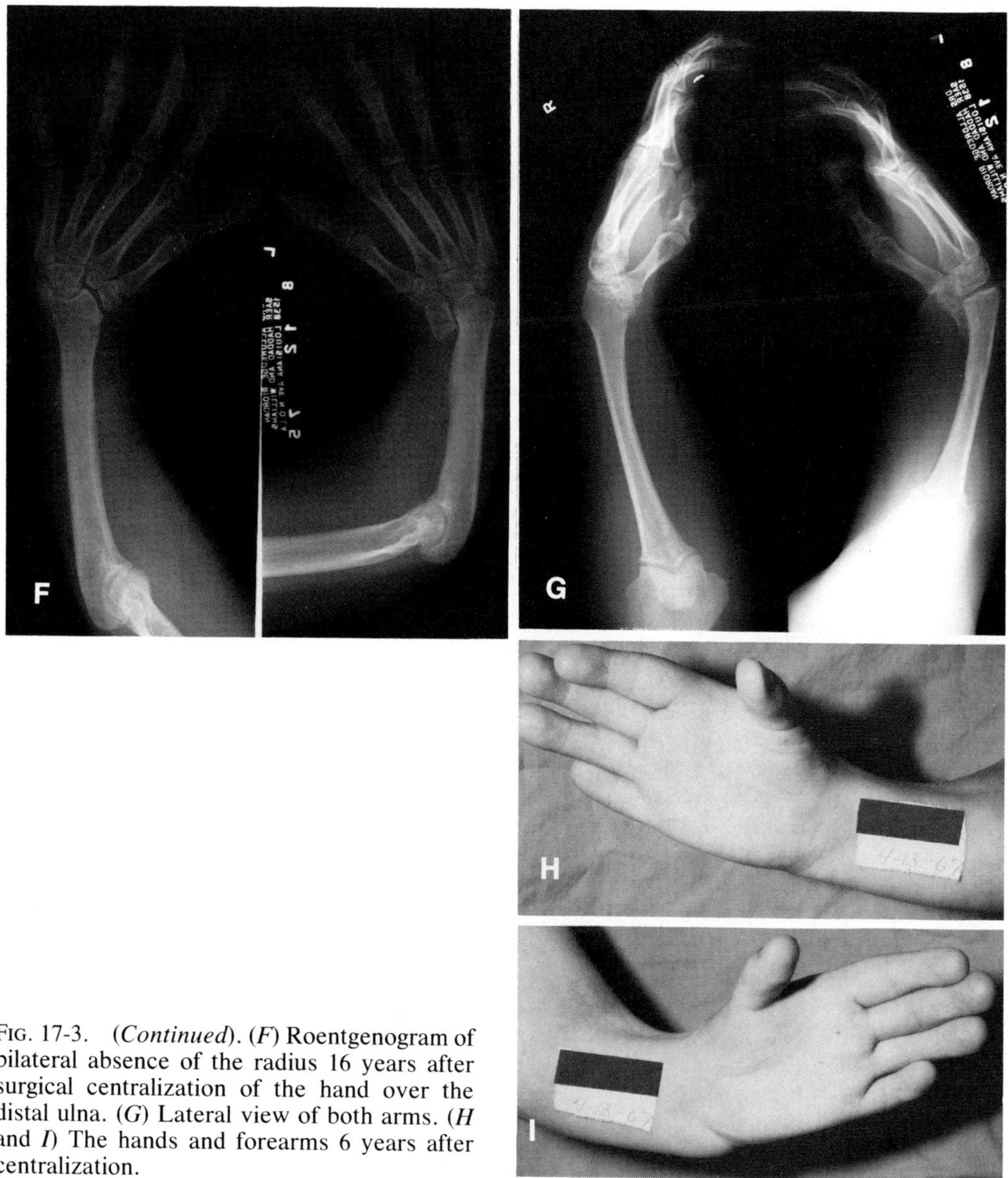

FIG. 17-3. (*Continued*). (*F*) Roentgenogram of bilateral absence of the radius 16 years after surgical centralization of the hand over the distal ulna. (*G*) Lateral view of both arms. (*H* and *I*) The hands and forearms 6 years after centralization.

engaged in managing this condition today is centralization of the hand over the distal end of the ulna, coupled with osteotomy of the ulna if it is curved. Internal fixation for 8 to 10 weeks with a pin no larger than a 0.062 Kirschner wire is recommended. The pin is then removed to prevent damage to the distal ulnar epiphysis. Short-arm splints are used to maintain correction and to keep the hand over the distal ulna. The splints must be worn 24 hours a day until the child is 6 years old, removing them only for bathing. After the child reaches school age, the splints may be left off during the day and worn at night until full maturation is achieved. This allows the distal ulna full enlargement, with the hand centralized. The ulna frequently becomes almost as large as the distal radius would have been. Arthrodesis of the wrist is rarely necessary except in a few patients, usually those in whom treatment was started after age 4 years, so that full development of the distal ulna could not take place.

The surgical approach varies from surgeon

to surgeon. Some recommend an approach from the radial side, coupled with a Z-plasty and an ulnar approach for the osteotomy, if necessary. This author prefers to use an ulnar approach, transversely oriented at the distal ulna, excising a football-shaped wedge of skin and fat, thus removing excess skin and fat that would give a cosmetically poor result if allowed to remain. The dorsal branch of the ulnar nerve is identified and protected. The extensor ulnaris and extensor digiti quinti are freed from their compartment, and the distal ulna is then exposed. This bone should not be widely exposed, so as to preserve as much of the blood supply of the distal epiphysis as possible. Then, by increasing the deformity, the proximal end of the proximal row of carpal bones can be exposed, the capsule freed from the inner side of the ulna, and, by flexing the elbow, the hand carpus can usually be brought over the distal end of the ulna to the centralized position. If the structures are still too tight on the radial side and if there is no need for a Z-plasty, the central carpal bone (lunate) can be partially or wholly removed.[16] This shortens the bone length without interfering with growth and usually allows the hand to be centralized on the distal ulna. If successful, the hand is then moved out of the way, the distal ulna is exposed, and a Kirschner wire is drilled through the ulna and made to come out the forearm (if the ulna is bowed) or out of the olecranon process (if the ulna is not bowed). This does not interfere with growth. The drill is then placed on the proximal end of the wire, and it is drilled into the carpus and third metacarpal, after recentralizing the hand over the distal ulna. The wire is not drilled across the metacarpal epiphysis but is stopped short of it. Long-arm splints over adequate padding are used to assist the fixation. After 1 or 2 weeks, a long-arm cast can be applied for 8 to 10 weeks, followed by a short-arm plastic splint. This method has given good results, but it is dependent upon the complete cooperation of the parents, since the splints must be continuously worn if Wolff's law is to prevail and the distal end of the ulna is to enlarge sufficiently to support the hand.

If the treatment is started within the first year of life, the ulna develops into a bone large enough to support the hand by the time the child is 6 or 7 years old. At that time, the splint may be left off during the day while the child is at school, but it should be worn at night. It is essential that the splint be kept on until full development of the hand and forearm has occurred. If this is done, the hand remains corrected and a wrist stabilization procedure does not have to be done.

If splinting is discontinued and the deformity recurs, it is necessary to do another centralization procedure or, perhaps, an osteotomy at the distal end of the ulna. The distal ulna frequently has a curvature within the distal inch or so, and an osteotomy at this level, leaving the carpus in its relation with the distal end, repositions the hand and corrects the distal curve. After the osteotomy has healed, splinting can be resumed until growth is complete (Fig. 17-4).[17–19]

CONGENITAL ABSENCE OF THE ULNA

Clinical Features

Congenital absence of the ulna is characterized by ulnar deviation of the hand, radial bowing of the radius with concavity toward the ulna, and dislocation of the head of the radius, when present. This deformity is about one third as common as congenital absence of the radius. It may be seen with other deformities but usually only on the involved extremity. It may be unilateral or bilateral (Fig. 17-5).

There are three types of congenital absence of the ulna. The rarest type is that with complete and total absence of the ulna. The child has an unstable elbow, because there is no ulna present to give stability at the elbow. Because there is no distal cartilaginous ulnar anlage to tether the wrist, the radius is usually straight. In the second type, there is absence of the distal or middle third of the ulna and the proximal third has an articulation with the humerus. The radial head may be articulating with the capitellum, or it may be dislocated laterally and displaced posteriorly. In the third type, the radius is fused with the humerus in flexion or extension. Even though there is no elbow joint, there is usually a cartilaginous anlage. Because this cartilaginous anlage has no longitudinal growth, the distal radial epiphysis is compressed on its ulnar side, and the wedge-shaped epiphysis produces further ulnar deviation of the hand with growth. The longitudinal growth of the radius occurring while the distal radial epiphysis is tethered by

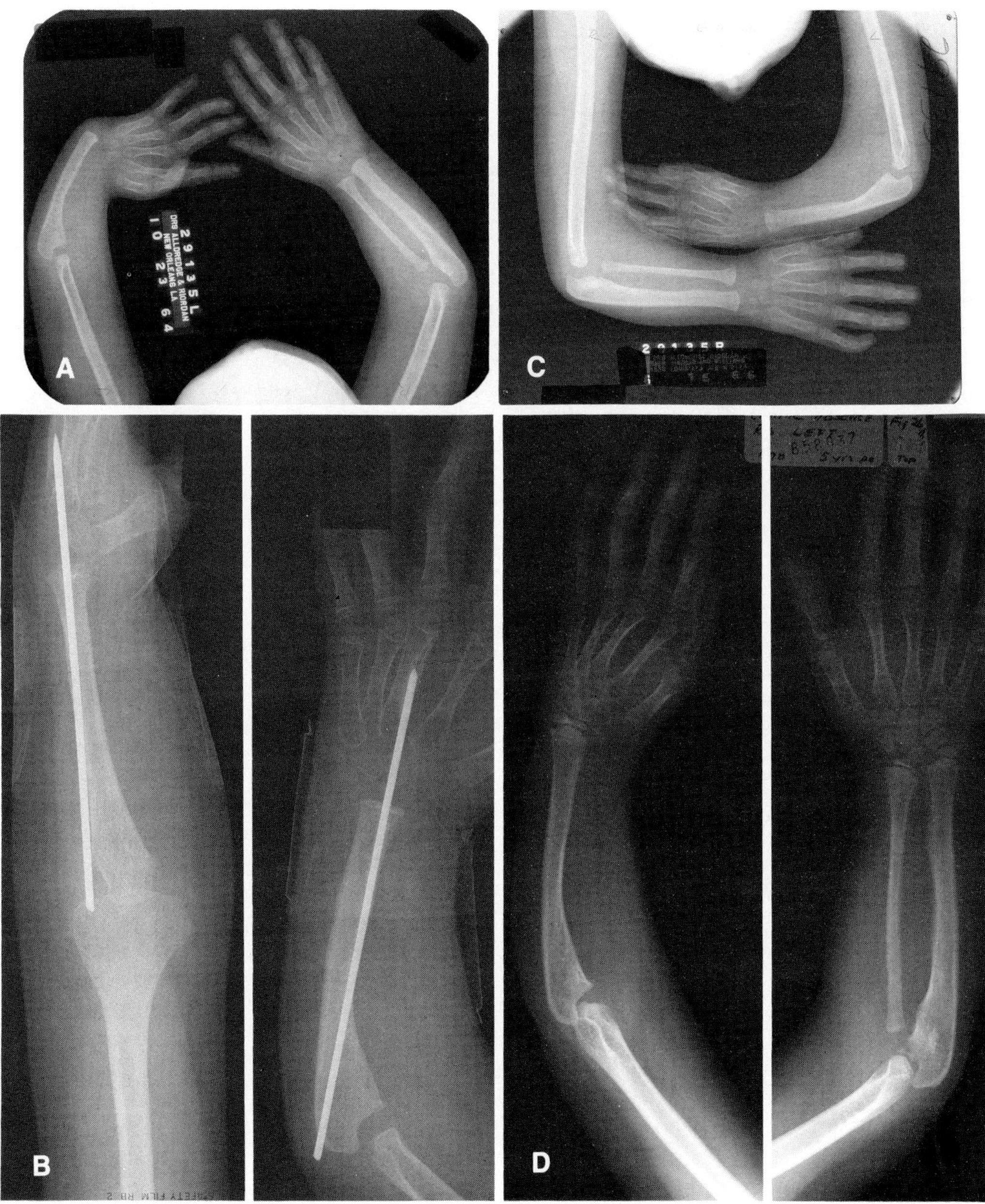

FIG. 17-4. (*A*) Roentgenogram of both arms of a 5-year-old male with an absent radius on the left and a slightly small radius on the right. (*B*) Roentgenographic view 3 months after surgical centralization of the left hand. (*C*) Seventeen months after centralization. (*D*) Five years after centralization. (*Continued on next page.*)

the anlage results in a radial bowing of the radius. If the radial head is articulating with the humerus at birth, the combination of radial bowing and ulnar anlage tethering result in eventual dislocation of the radial head on the humerus. If the ulnar anlage tether is not released early by excision of the anlage, ulnar deviation of the hand increases with growth, and the radial head slides posteriorly past the humerus, thus wasting longitudinal growth.

Occasionally, there may be a fibrous band from the distal end of the short ulna attaching

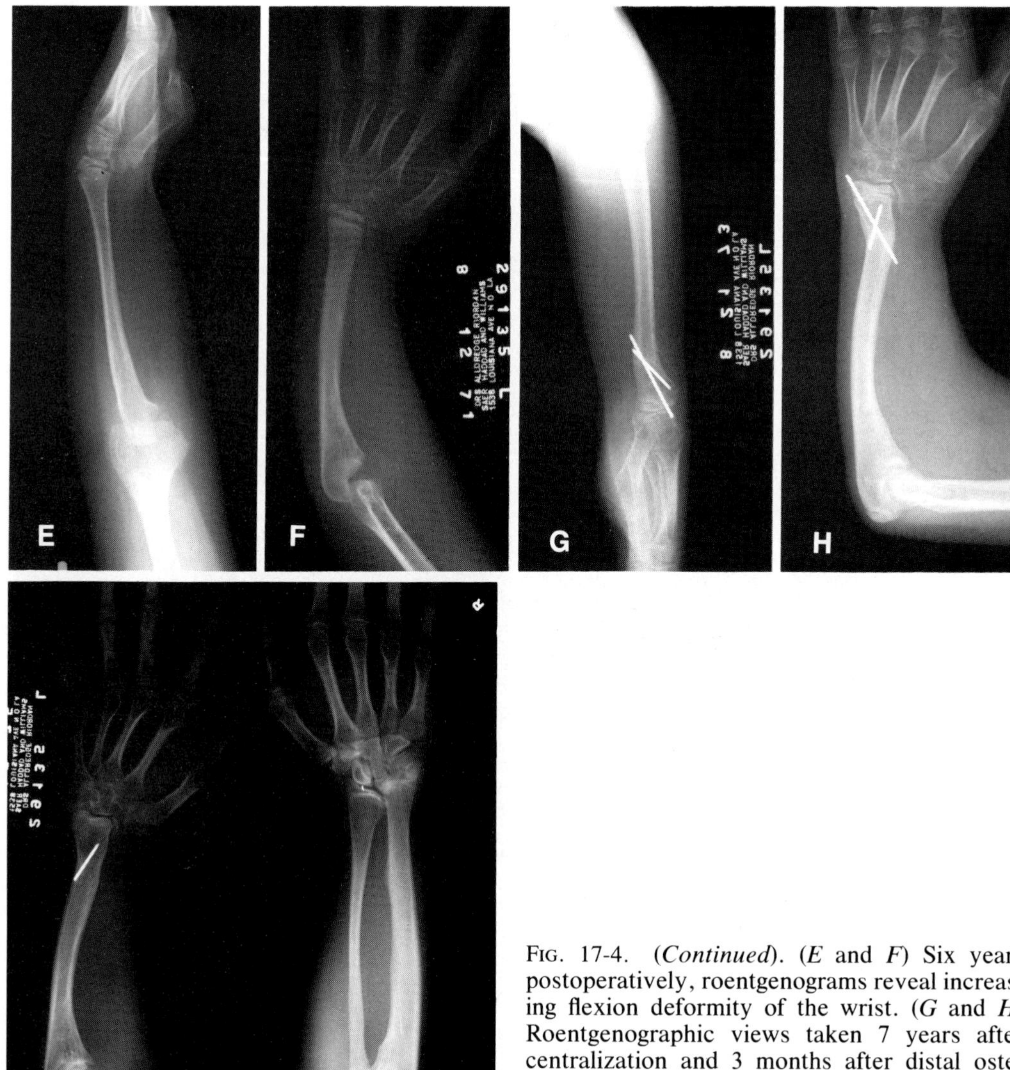

FIG. 17-4. (*Continued*). (*E* and *F*) Six years postoperatively, roentgenograms reveal increasing flexion deformity of the wrist. (*G* and *H*) Roentgenographic views taken 7 years after centralization and 3 months after distal osteotomy to correct the flexion deformity. (*I*) Ten years after centralization and 2 years after distal osteotomy.

to the ulnar border of the distal radial epiphysis. Because the continuation of the ulnar anlage does not attach to the carpus or hand, the hand will not be markedly ulnar deviated. However, with growth, the hand will tether the ulnar side of the distal radial epiphysis and cause a wedge-shaped distal radial epiphysis, which will tilt the hand toward the ulnar side because of the unequal growth. This band should be recognized and removed early.

In the third type, the proximal radius is fused with the distal humerus. Thus, there is no distal humeral epiphysis, and there is no proximal radial epiphysis. Even though there is fusion of the radius and humerus, there is a proximal ulnar anlage, which extends distally and attaches to the carpus. Even though there is a fusion of the radius and humerus, there may be a proximal ulnar anlage. This fibrocartilage also tethers the distal radius and causes it to bow, and the distal radial epiphysis grows in a wedge shape. As with the other types, this anlage should be excised early to lessen the tendency for the radial bowing and to lessen the wedging of the distal radial epiphysis.

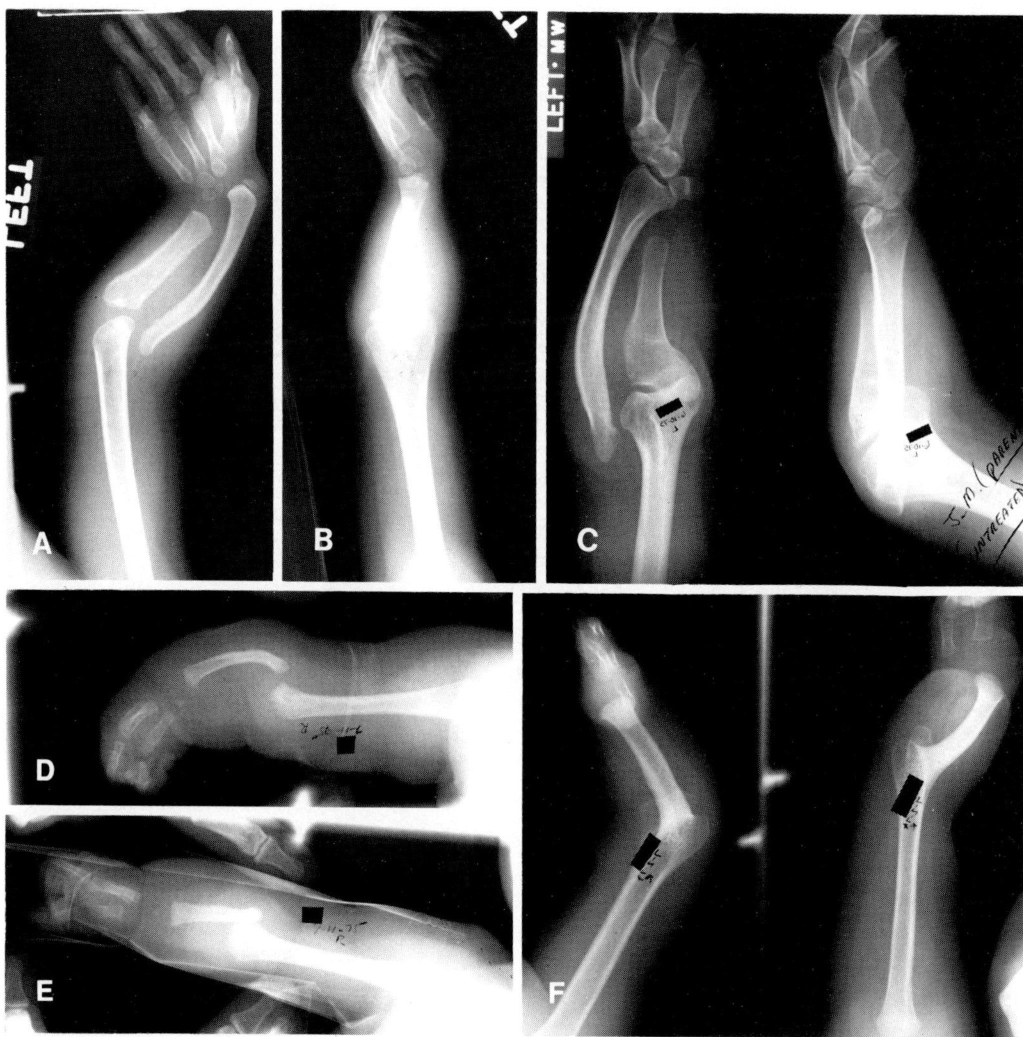

FIG. 17-5. (*A* and *B*) Anteroposterior and lateral roentgenograms of a child with partial absence of the distal ulna, showing the dislocation of the radial head and marked ulnar drift of the hand. (*C*) Roentgenogram showing the arms of the 34-year-old father of the child in *A*. The father was untreated. (*D* and *E*) Roentgenogram of a 3-month-old male with absence of the ulna and the fourth and fifth rays of the hand. (*F*) Roentgenogram of a 2-year-old male with synostosis of the humerus and radius and partial absence of the ulna.

Treatment

If the anomaly is detected at birth, plaster casts should be used to prevent increasing deformity. If the child has no other congenital anomalies preventing surgery, the ulnar anlage should be excised early, perhaps at 6 months. When there is marked radial bowing and dislocation of the radial head, an osteotomy of the radius and creation of a one-bone forearm can be done at the same time. With care, the osteotomy can be done from the ulnar side, after excision of the ulnar anlage. The removal of the anlage gives adequate exposure through the interosseous membrane to osteotomize the radius from the ulnar side. The radial osteotomy is done as close to the elbow as possible, and the distal radial shaft is brought into alignment with the remaining proximal ulna. This can be done even if the ulna is still cartilaginous. Intramedullary fixation with a 0.062 Kirschner wire is used to affix the radius to the ulna. The proximal part of the neck of the radius and radial head are left alone at this

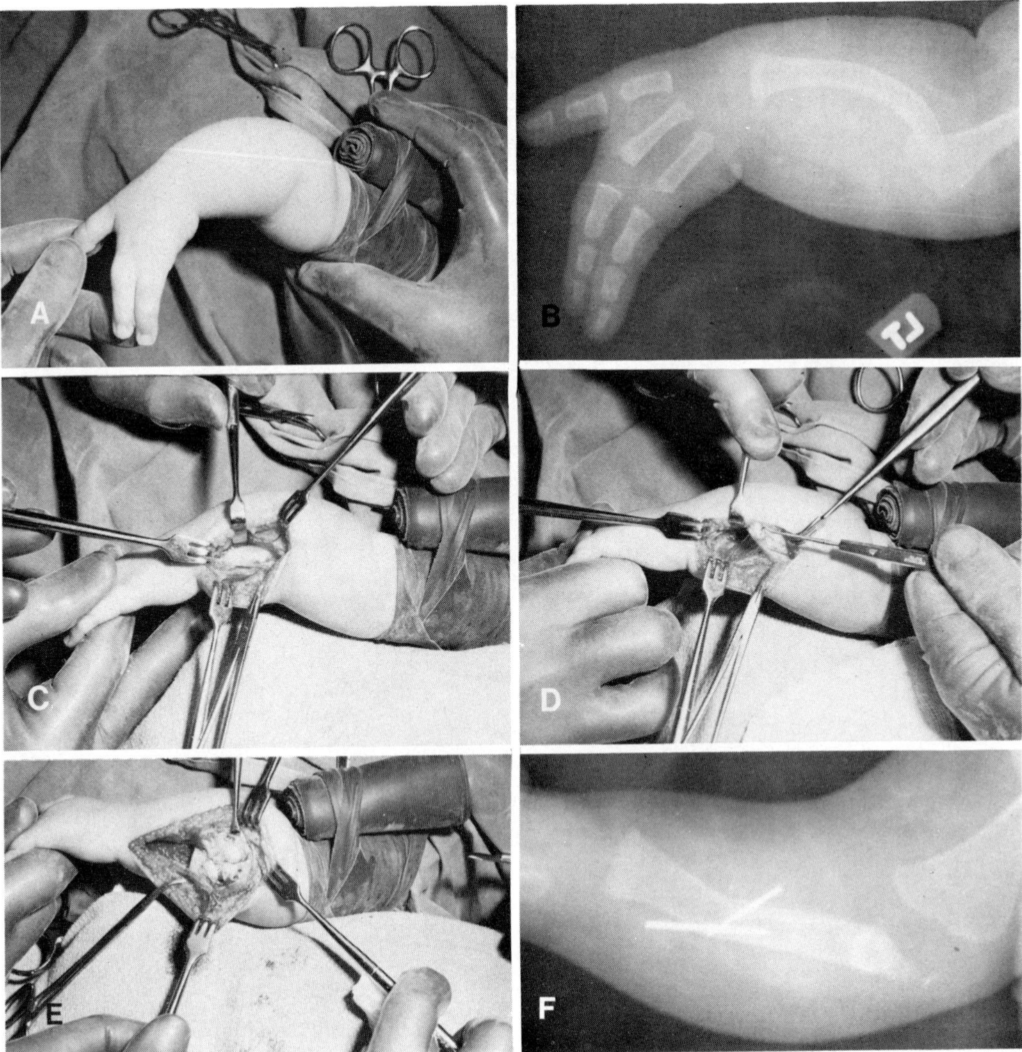

FIG. 17-6. (*A*) A 6-month-old female at surgery, showing ulnar deformity of hand, radial bowing, and absence of the fourth and fifth rays. (*B*) Roentgenogram of the arm at age 6 months. (*C*) View at surgery, with the ulnar anlage exposed. (*D*) The ulnar anlage is detached and is pulled upward by a hook. (*E*) The anlage is excised to the point just distal to the joint. The capsule is opened to show the capitellum of the humerus. (*F*) The postoperative roentgenogram, showing pins in the osteotomy site of the radius. Wire sutures were used to connect the cartilaginous ulna with the radius as close to the joint as possible. (*Continued on facing page.*)

time unless they are interfering with motion. It is safest to wait some months before removing the proximal radius, because the combined procedures are extensive. Occasionally, the radial bowing is so great that several osteotomies of the radius are necessary to straighten the curve, and the intramedullary pin is used to skewer the multiple fragments. Thus, the ulnar anlage can be excised, a one-bone forearm can be made, and the radius can be straightened at one operation.

As with absence of the radius, the initial immobilization is with a plaster cast, followed in 2 months by splints (usually short-arm splints), until the child reaches school age. This 24-hour wearing of the splint is continued until school age, and if conditions are satisfactory, the splint can be left off while the child is at school and worn the rest of the day and night. Once full growth has been achieved, splinting can be discontinued. The total length of this forearm will be about two thirds the

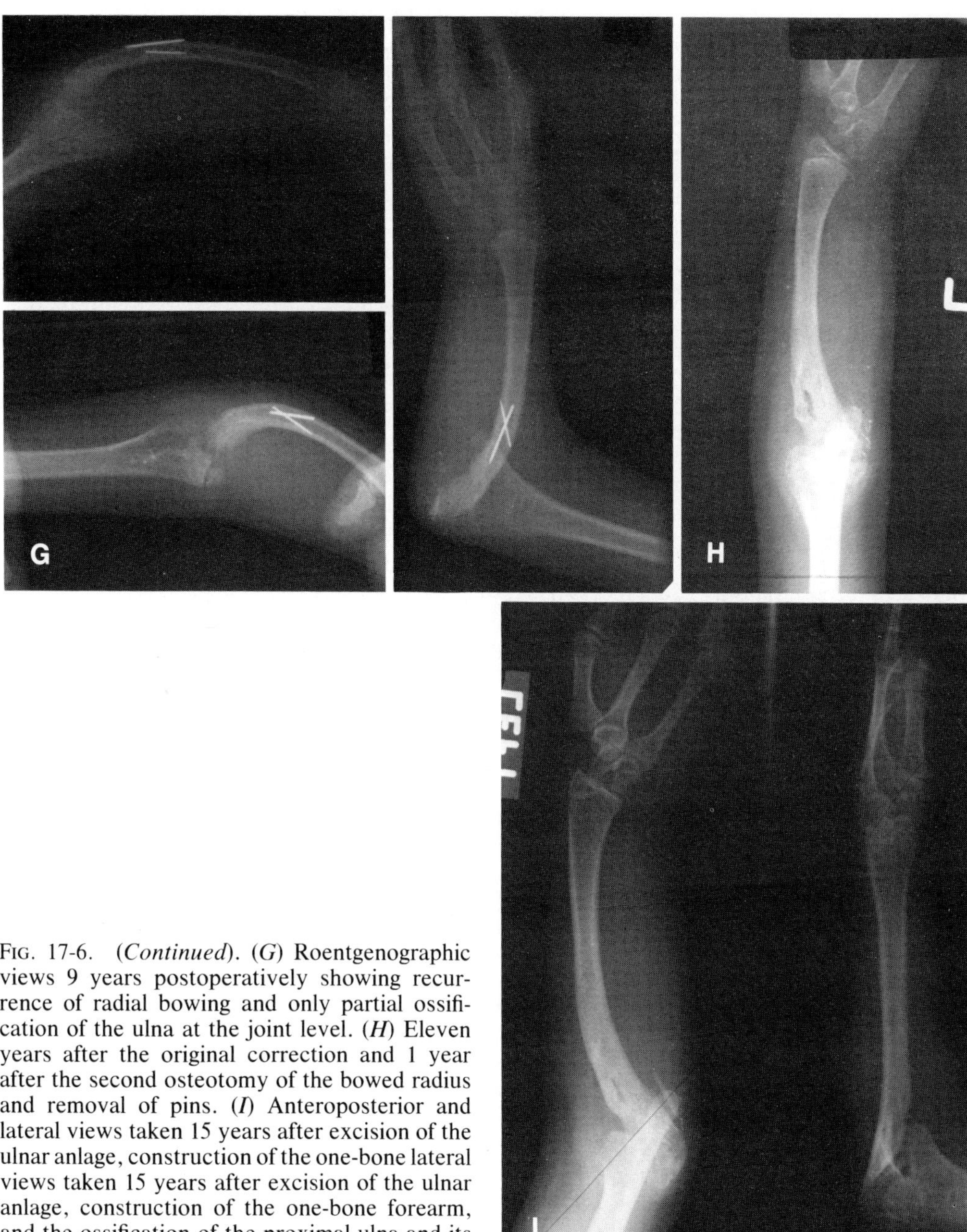

FIG. 17-6. (*Continued*). (*G*) Roentgenographic views 9 years postoperatively showing recurrence of radial bowing and only partial ossification of the ulna at the joint level. (*H*) Eleven years after the original correction and 1 year after the second osteotomy of the bowed radius and removal of pins. (*I*) Anteroposterior and lateral views taken 15 years after excision of the ulnar anlage, construction of the one-bone lateral views taken 15 years after excision of the ulnar anlage, construction of the one-bone forearm, and the ossification of the proximal ulna and its union with the radius.

length of a normal arm on thc same child (Fig. 17-6).

There are many different hand deformities associated with absence of the ulna. The most common deformity is presence of a thumb and an index and long finger, with the fourth and fifth rays being absent. However, a normal five-ray hand may be present. The thumb and index ray may be absent, and the third, fourth, and fifth rays may be present. The fingers may be webbed in varying combinations. The hand problems should be solved after the arm deformity has been corrected. If there is webbing and the bones are fused distally, this must be corrected as early as possible to prevent the shorter finger from causing a deformity of the longer finger. It must be emphasized that the earlier the deformity is corrected, the greater the growth potential of the arm.

HYPOPLASTIC THUMB

The hypoplastic thumb is a defective digit, incomplete in its development. The degree of hypoplasia can range from minimal deficiency to complete absence of the thumb. The soft tissues are involved, and the deficiencies of the intrinsic and extrinsic structures contribute to the disability of the thumb. Grasp and prehension may be normal or may be sufficiently decreased, depending on the extent of the defect. The defective thumb can occur individually or in association with other skeletal defects.

The hypoplastic thumb can be divided into five separate groups, determined by the various structures that are deficient: (1) short thumb, (2) adducted hypoplastic thumb, (3) abducted hypoplastic thumb, (4) floating thumb, and (5) absent thumb.

Short Thumb

In the short thumb (Fig. 17-7*B*), the hypoplasia is primarily osseous. Functional loss is slight except for that due to the shortening *per se*. These thumbs are frequently associated with other congenital anomalies and syndromes. The shape and size of the metacarpal and phalanx correspond to certain anomalies and syndromes. When the metacarpal is short and slender, it can be associated with various anomalies of the spine, the cardiac system, and the gastrointestinal system. It can also be associated with Fanconi's syndrome, Holt-Oram syndrome, or Juberg-Hayward syndrome.[33] When the metacarpal is short but broad, it can be associated with Cornelia de Lange's syndrome, hand-foot-uterus syndrome, dystrophic dwarfism, and myositis ossificans progressiva.[33] When the proximal phalanx is short and broad, it is usually associated with brachydactyly. When the distal phalanx is short and broad, it can be associated with Rubinstein-Taybi syndrome, Apert's syndrome, and Carpenter's syndrome.[26]

The short thumb rarely requires any treatment. The hand defect is due to shortness with very little functional loss. However, if the degree of shortening is extensive, lengthening of the metacarpal can be contemplated.[30]

Adducted Hypoplastic Thumb

The adducted hypoplastic thumb (Fig. 17-7*A*) lies close to the radial side of the hand. There is a deficiency of the thumb-index web space. The web space is usually extended distally. There is usually a deficiency or absence of the thenar muscles. Active flexion of the distal joint is frequently decreased or absent to abnormal insertion of the flexor pollicis longus tendon. The flexor pollicis brevis is present to give active flexion of the metacarpophalangeal (MP) joint. The radial collateral ligament is defective to varying degrees. Extensor function is usually adequate.

The principal functional loss is the inability to abduct the first metacarpal due to (1) the web space deficiency, and (2) absent defective thenar musculature.

The treatment of these thumbs primarily concerns the correction of the thumb-index web space contracture, replacement of thenar muscle function, and stabilization of the radial collateral ligament of the MP joint.

Abducted Hypoplastic Thumb

In the abducted hypoplastic thumb (Fig. 17-7*C*), there is a complete instability of the MP joint, which is markedly abducted. However, the first metacarpal is in an adducted position and the thumb web space is narrowed, as in the adducted hypoplastic thumb. The thenar muscles are frequently absent or defective, and flexion of the distal joint of the thumb is also impaired. Dissection in these thumbs has shown that the flexor pollicis longus tendon is joined to the extensor mechanism over the proximal segment of the thumb by tendinous commissures, limiting the function of the distal joint. Surgical treatment for correction of these thumbs requires deepening and broadening of the web space, correction of the adduction contracture of the first metacarpal, stabilization of the MP joint, and restoration of opposition of the thumb. Details of this technique can be found in Dobyns, Wood and Bayne, *et al.*

Floating Thumb (Pouce Flottant)

The Pouce flottant, or floating thumb (Fig. 17-7*D*), is slender and quite unstable at its base. It appears to be attached simply to the radial surface of the hand by a slender pedicle, usually containing a single neurovascular bundle. This is sometimes referred to as a thumb

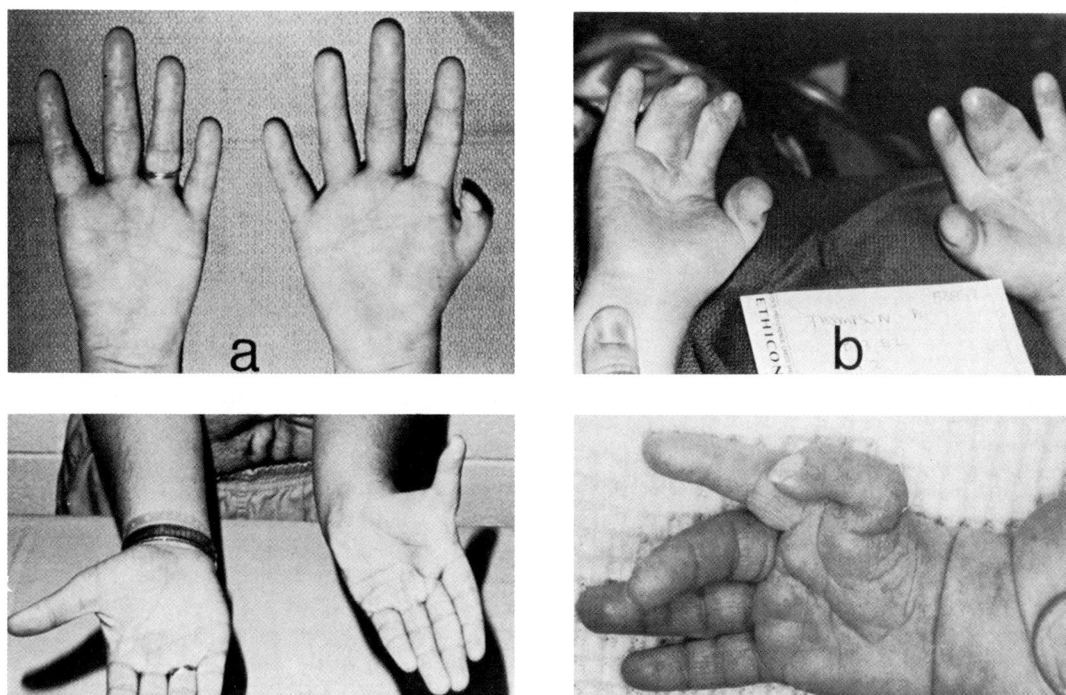

FIG. 17-7. (*a*) Thumb hypoplasia varies from hypoplastic thumb to absence of the thumb. (*b*) Short stubby thumbs are frequently related to various syndromes—acrocephalosyndactyly, Cornelia de Lange's syndrome, hand-foot-uterus syndrome. (*c*) The abducted thumb is defective at the metacarpal phalangeal joint, being extremely unstable. (*d*) The floating thumb is an extremely deficient thumb lacking a skeletal stability and tendons.

with no visible means of support (vagrant thumb). The distal phalanx is present with a fingernail. The proximal phalanx is present and forms the interphalangeal metacarpal joint. The proximal one half of the first metacarpal is usually absent. All these structures are hypoplastic. There is no skeletal support to the base of the thumb. The intrinsic and extrinsic structures are absent. Because of the above deficiencies, most surgeons believe that reconstruction is futile.

Stabilization by using toe proximal phalanges, along with the epiphysis, or with a free transfer using microvascular techniuqes, has been tried with varying success. The thumb is usually placed too far distally and radially to provide reasonable opposition. With further development of microsurgical techniques, transfer of skin, bone, and joint, as well as tendons from a unit in the foot to replace the entire bone of the thumb, may become feasible. At present, in bilateral cases, pollicization of the index finger seems to give the best functional and cosmetic result.

Absent Thumb

The most severe form of hypoplasia of the thumb is complete absence of the thumb (Fig. 17-7*A*) and may be associated with a normal hypoplastic or absent radius, ring D chromosome abnormalities, Holt-Oram syndrome, trisomy-18 syndrome, Rothmud-Thompson syndrome, and thalidomide embryopathy.[33] Patients born without one or both thumbs are usually seen by the orthopaedist soon after birth, and, at the present time, the parents can be reassured that surgical reconstruction can usually provide significant functional improvement. Pollicization of the index finger has probably been the most successful and cosmetically pleasing procedure developed in the last few years through the efforts of Littler,[29] Riordan,[32] and Buck-Gramco,[20] to mention only a few. However, patients with unilateral involvement who have already attempted to pollicize the index finger by continuous abduction of the finger may be very pleased with an abduction, pronation, and recession procedure described by Hentz and Littler.[27] With the continued development and success of microvascular transfers, toes and other digits may be used successfully in the future.

CONGENITAL ABSENCE OF THE THUMB

Clinical Features

Congenital absence of the thumb may involve a total absence, partial absence, or perhaps only a slight underdevelopment of the thumb (Fig. 17-8). Total absence of the thumb is usually associated with other deformities of the hand or forearm. The deformity may be unilateral or bilateral. In some cases, the remainder of the hand and forearm may be practically normal except for some mild shortening of the radius. There may be incomplete development of the proximal part of the first metacarpal, so that there is instability of the thumb at the carpometacarpal joint. There may be a partial or total absence of the first metacarpal, which leaves the proximal and distal phalanx with only flail motion. Partial absence of the thumb is frequently associated with defects of the radius, ranging from a partial absence or total absence of the radius. Rarely, the absence of the thumb is associated with partial or complete absence of the ulna and its attendant deformities.

Treatment

Reconstruction of the thumb depends on the type of deformity present. The thumb that has only slight underdevelopment of the proximal end of the first metacarpal may be stabilized by reconstructing ligaments, giving some stability between the trapezium and the loose base of the first metacarpal. If this is done in a young patient, it should be remembered that the growth center for the first metacarpal is the proximal end, and no drilling of the bone should be done at this point. The cartilaginous part of this first metacarpal may be sutured, but no holes should be drilled in this bone until the child is old enough so that the epiphysis is visualized on roentgenogram. If there is absence of the proximal half of the first metacarpal, with a distal metacarpal and thumb of reasonable size with tendons, it may be possible to do a proximal reconstruction of this bone by transplanting the distal one third of the fourth metatarsal. In this case, the entire joint surface is taken with the attendant collateral ligaments, so that stability can be obtained when grafting this part of the bone. As is usual with the transplant of non-vascularized epiphyses in growing children, this graft should not be expected to grow. Unless the first metacarpal has an anomalous distal epiphysis, the thumb at full maturation will be a very short digit. Some authors have recommended repeated bone grafting to lengthen these thumbs.[38] In some conditions, this is warranted. If the entire first metacarpal is absent, it is recommended that an early amputation of the floating thumb be done. If the condition is unilateral, it is not recommended that pollicization of the thumb be carried out. If the condition is bilateral, it is recommended that reconstruction of the thumb by pollicization of the index finger be done bilaterally. If reconstruction of the thumb is carried out by pollicization of the index finger, it is recommended that the principles outlined by Littler[37] and Buck-Gramcko[35] be used. The technical details of this procedure can be obtained from the original articles. The preferred age for pollicization, as recommended by Buck-Gramcko, is at least 4 years.[36] This author performs pollicization on patients between the ages of 6 and 12 months and finds that satisfactory development of the thumb can be achieved even when the procedure is done at this early age. It is recommended that if pollicization is carried out, the techniques of using the second metacarpal head and its ligaments as the trapezium and advancing the interossei to the middle joint of the index finger establish a much better functioning thumb and a better appearing thumb (Fig. 17-9).

LOBSTER-CLAW HAND

Clinical Features

Unfortunately, this term is widely used to describe what is actually a clefting of the hand. This widely varying deformity is hereditary, is frequently bilateral, and may also involve the lower extremities.

The term *lobster claw* is used to describe the absence of the central ray of the hand. The index finger may also be absent, as may be the thumb. Many combinations have been

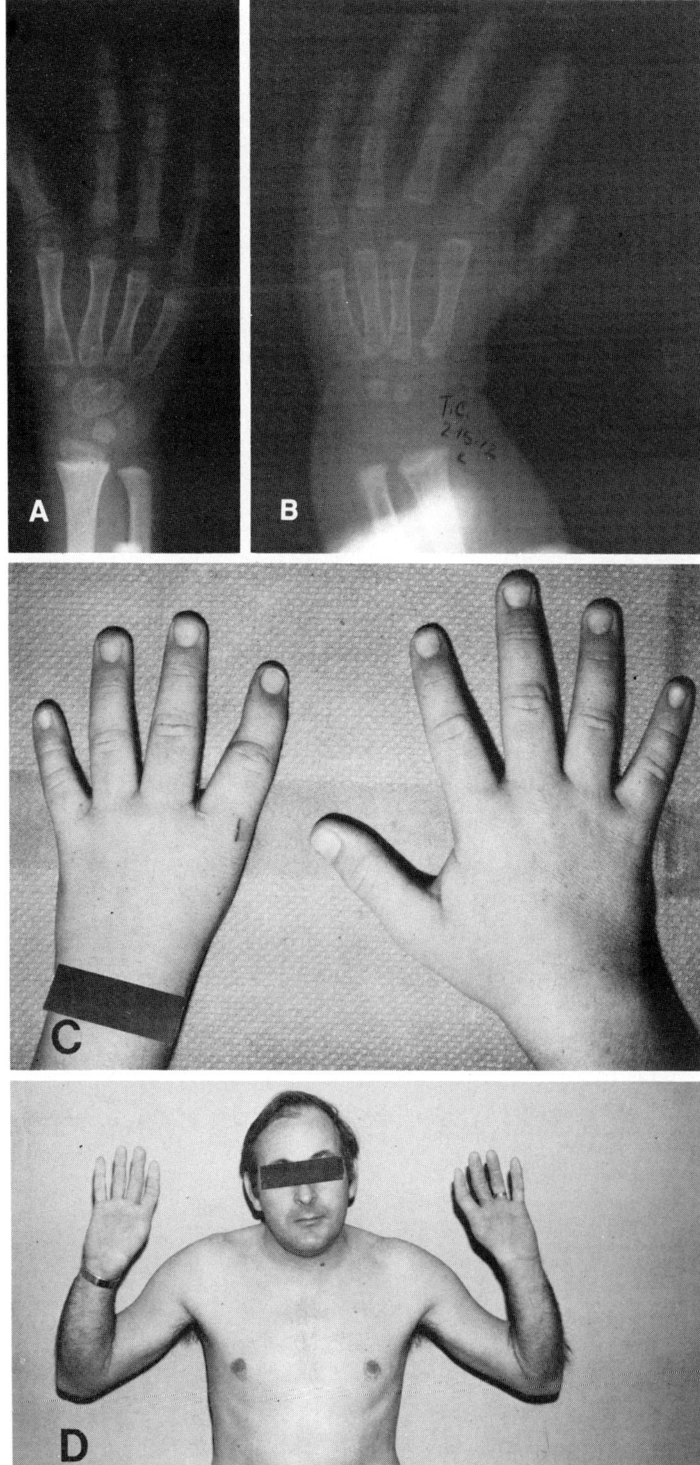

FIG. 17-8. (*A*) Anteroposterior roentgenogram, showing total absence of the thumb with a delta middle phalanx of the index finger and fusion of capitate and hamate. (*B*) Partial absence of the first metacarpal. (*C*) An absent thumb with a normal hand; no other deformities are present. (*D*) Bilateral absence of the thumbs in an adult.

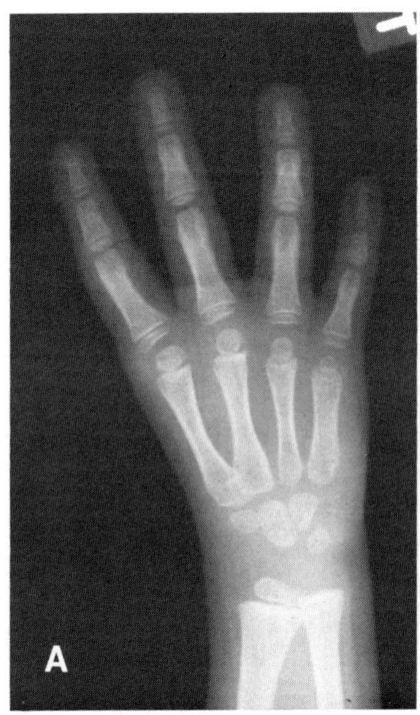

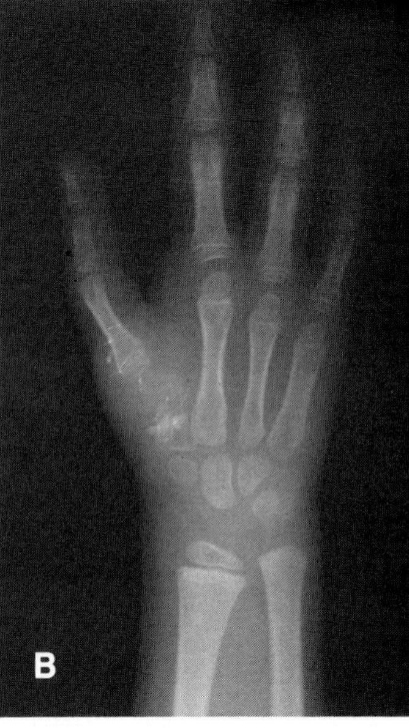

FIG. 17-9. (*A*) Preoperative view of a hand with absence of the thumb. (*B*) The thumb as it appears 1 year after pollicization.

described, with absence of the central ray or rays and preservation, either partial or complete, of the border rays being the most common. Roentgenograms show which bones are absent or which parts of the osseous structures are present. There may be a simple absence of a central ray, or there may be complex anomalies with transverse phalanges or metacarpals and absence of the central finger. There are many variations of the tendon, vessel, and nerve involvement, and these are only identifiable at surgery (Fig. 17-10).

Treatment

The treatment of choice is surgery. Early treatment between the ages of 6 and 24 months is recommended. In the absence of the central metacarpal and long finger, surgery must provide skin cleft closure and web reconstruction between the index and ring fingers. Realignment of the second and fourth metacarpals to a parallel position is essential and may require osteotomy of one or both metacarpals. This necessarily means construction of a transverse metacarpal ligament between the second and fourth metacarpal heads to prevent recurrence of the deformity. The excess skin resulting from the closure between the second and fourth metacarpals gives adequate skin for widening of the web between the thumb and index fingers, if this web is contracted. In this latter condition, the index finger must be shifted ulnarward to take the place of the third metacarpal, and the surrounding skin is shifted into the thumb web (Fig. 17-11).

In the more complicated cases with other deformities, metacarpal osteotomies are usually necessary to realign the fingers or the thumb, for example, in cases where there are transversely oriented phalanges. Closure of the central defect is essential in all cases, probably combined with osteotomies of the metacarpals or phalanges, if necessary.

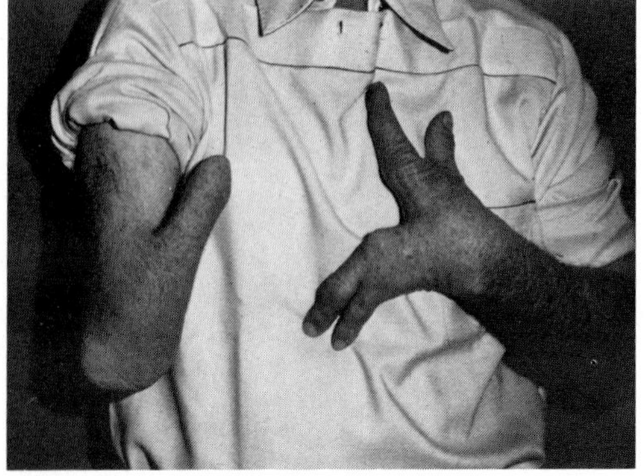

FIG. 17-10. In this patient, there is no hand on the right and a lobster-claw hand on the left.

CONGENITAL DISLOCATION OF THE SHOULDER

Clinical Features

Congenital dislocation of the shoulder is usually seen only when there are other asso-

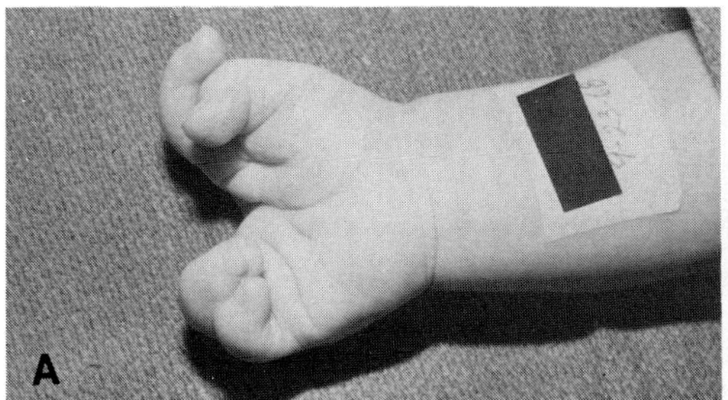

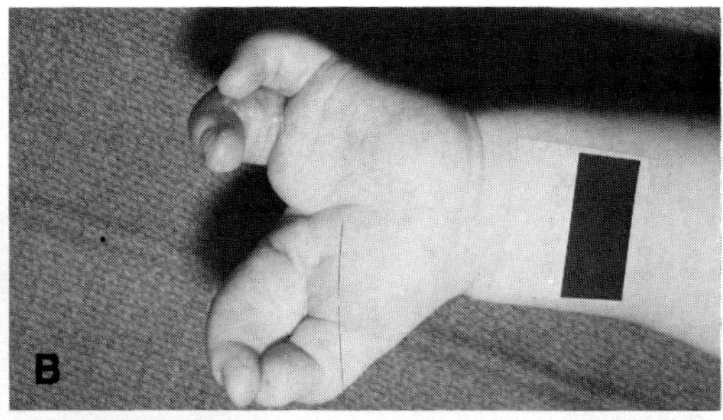

Fig. 17-11. (*A*) A 1-year-old male with a cleft hand and syndactyly of the ring and little fingers. (*B*) The hand as it appeared 2 months after separation of the ring and little fingers. (*C*) The hand as it appeared after completion of closure of the central cleft and reconstruction of the thumb web.

ciated deformities of the upper extremity. It is seen in general underdevelopment of the upper extremity, in absence of the radius, and in arthrogryposis in varying degrees. The shoulders are small in appearance, and the humerus is unstable in all directions, but its instability does not produce pain. The deltoid, pectorals, and other periscapular muscles are deficient or absent. The proximal, central, or distal humerus may be deficient, or it may be totally absent. Roentgenograms show a small scapula in normal position, an undeveloped glenoid, and a small or absent one third of the humerus. If the condition is associated with arthrogryposis, the biceps or triceps, or both, may be absent or markedly underdeveloped.[39]

Diagnosis

Diagnosis is made by observation of a small shoulder and an unstable shoulder joint, and the diagnosis is confirmed by roentgenograms. The physical examination shows a more or less unstable, paralyzed shoulder, as seen in poliomyelitis. Motion is attained by contortions of other body parts and gravity.

Treatment

No satisfactory surgical treatment is available at this time. In rare instances, shoulder fusion may offer some functional improvement if there is sufficient bone present to achieve fusion and sufficient muscular support of the scapula to achieve control (Fig. 17-12).[40]

CONGENITAL PSEUDARTHROSIS OF THE CLAVICLE

Clinical Features

The term *congenital pseudarthrosis of the clavicle*[41] implies the presence of a proximal and distal clavicle, with an absent central section. This is more common than total absence of the clavicle. A partial absence of the clavicle may be seen. This may be an absence of the lateral half of the clavicle and may be unilateral or bilateral.

In true pseudarthrosis of the clavicle, there is usually a deficient central one third of the clavicle (Fig. 17-13), or absence of the lateral half (Fig. 17-14). Occasionally, it is present at birth but is overlooked. It may also exist as a thinned, central portion of the clavicle, which may be fractured by lifting the infant or child or by the child's falling. When this occurs, the area is painful when the shoulder is moved. Consequently, this type of defect is often diagnosed by the presence of pain and shoulder instability, and the diagnosis is confirmed by roentgenogram. Lack of callus and failure to heal means that surgery is necessary.

Treatment

The best treatment is early operation, at age 3 to 6 years (Fig. 17-15). Internal fixation is achieved with an intramedullary pin, the type being dependent upon the size of the child. Multiple bone grafts are taken from the ilium;

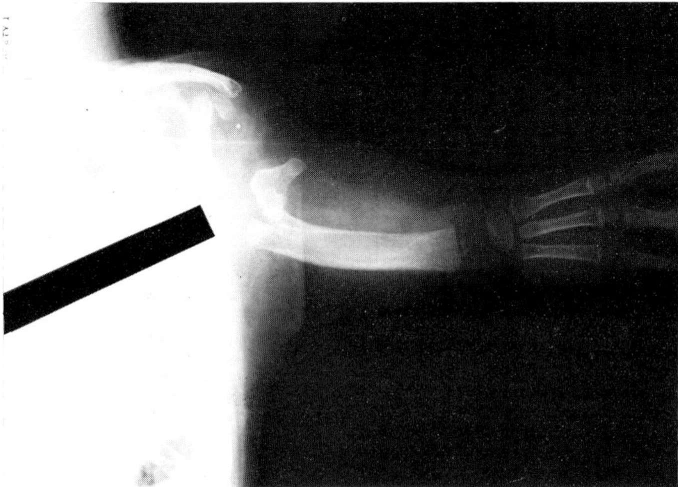

FIG. 17-12. Anteroposterior roentgenogram of congenital dislocation of the shoulder due to the incomplete formation of the scapula and humerus.

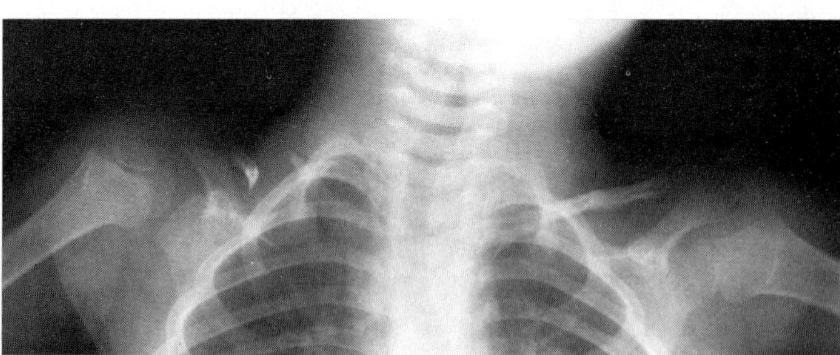

FIG. 17-13. Anteroposterior roentgenogram of pseudarthrosis of the right clavicle, the central portion being defective.

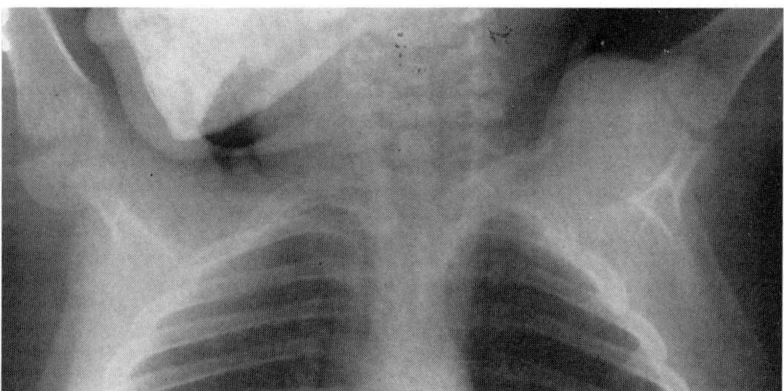

FIG. 17-14. Anteroposterior roentgenogram of congenital absence of the lateral half of both clavicles.

the bone grafts are fixated to the site by sutures placed like bands around barrel staves. The graft should be long enough to bridge the defect between the proximal and distal fragments and to fill the intervening spaces in the medullary canal with cancellous bone. If good technique is used, adequate fixation is obtained, and if an adequate amount of bone is used, union should result. The symptoms of pain and instability disappear. Fixation of grafts with screws, such as on a double onlay graft, is not recommended because of the proximity of the brachial artery and plexus.

Cleidocranial Dysostosis

Absence of the clavicle associated with cranial deformation is known as cleidocranial dysostosis.[42] In this condition, there may be a total absence of the entire clavicle, absence

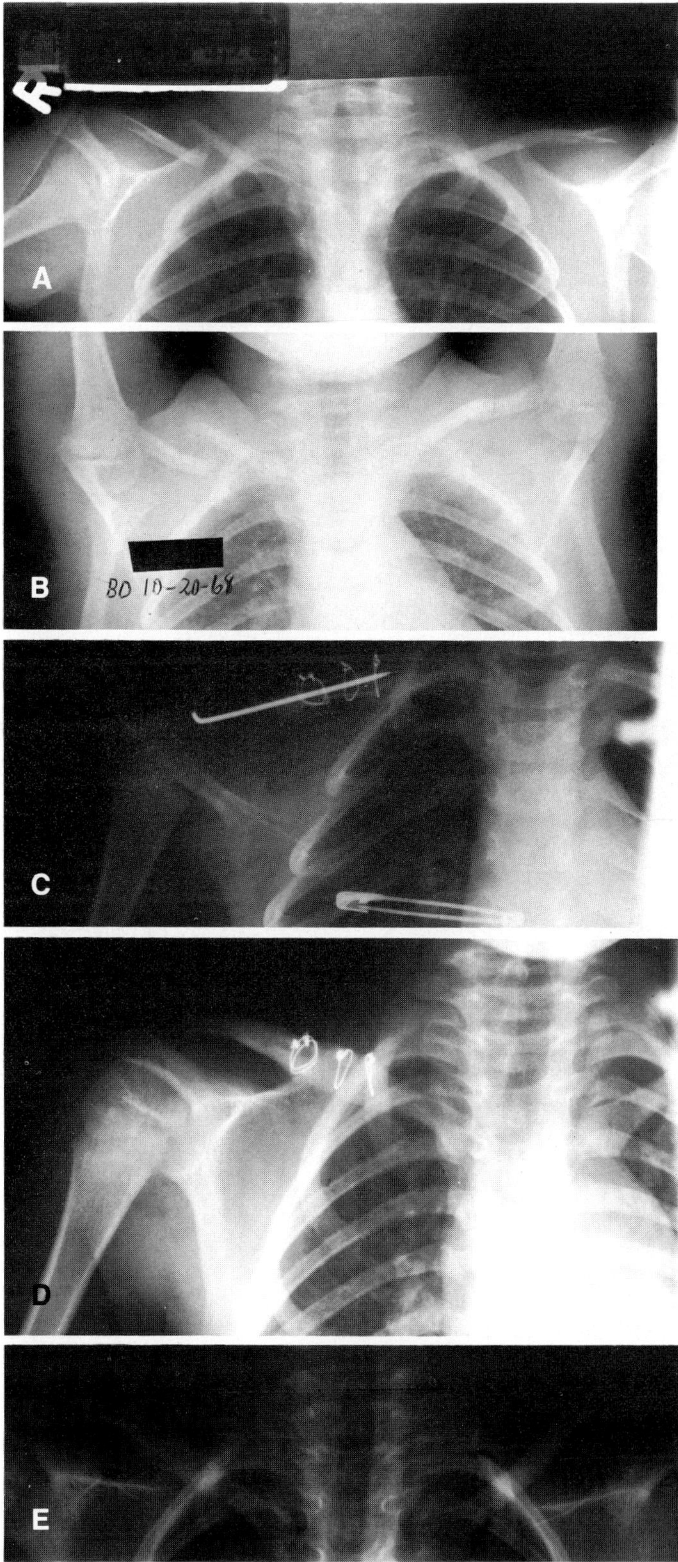

Fig. 17-15. (*A*) Anteroposterior roentgenogram of congenital pseudoarthrosis of the right clavicle, which was painful. (*B*) Roentgenogram of the same patient with the arms elevated, showing motion at the pseudoarthrosis. (*C*) Roentgenogram of the patient 2 months later after iliac segmental grafting. Barrel-stave grafts were fixed with an intramedullary 0.062 Kirschner wire and wire loops. (*D*) Roentgenogram of the patient 5 months after grafting and after removal of the intramedullary pin. (*E*) A roentgenogram of the patient taken 1 year postoperatively.

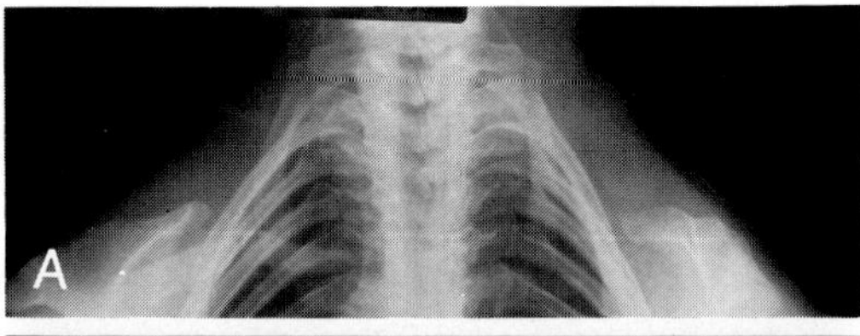

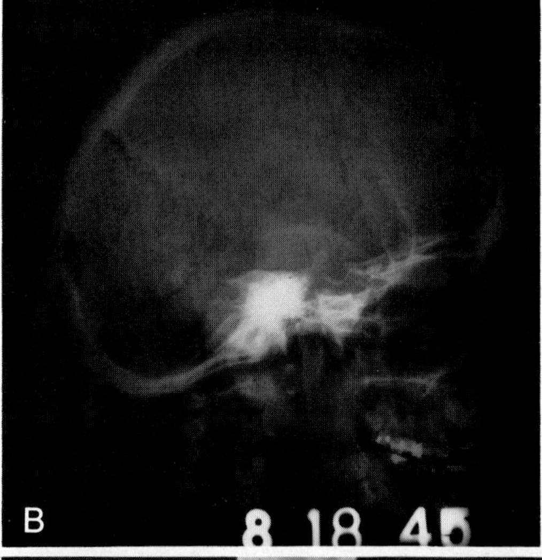

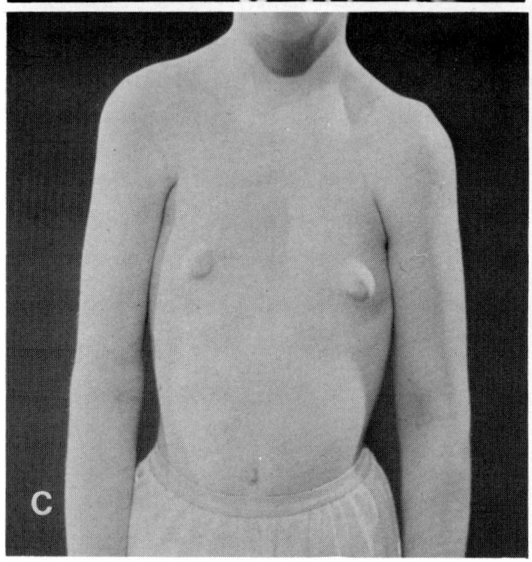

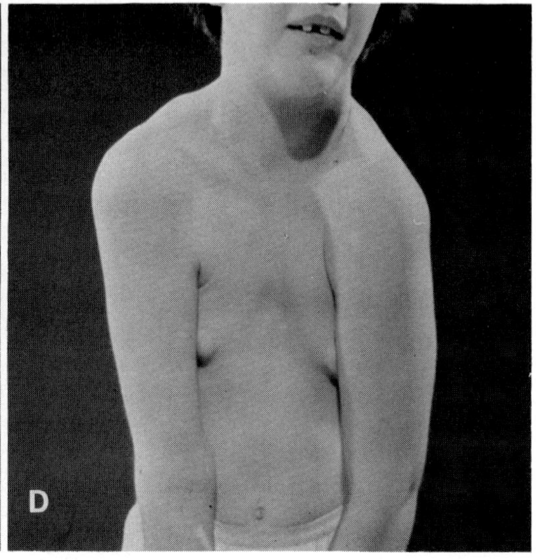

FIG. 17-16. (*A*) This roentgenogram, although marred, shows a 25-year-old adult with cleidocranial dystosis, showing absence of proximal third of both clavicles and pseudarthrosis of both clavicles. (*B*) Lateral view of the skull, showing open suture lines and frontal bossing. (*C*) A child with cleidocranial dystosis, showing drooping shoulders. (*D*) The same child, showing the left shoulder swinging anteriorly.

of all but a small bony remnant of the distal or proximal ends, or both (Fig. 17-16*A*). The skull is broad, with an increased transverse diameter and widely opened fontanelles due to the delayed or absent ossification of the skull (Fig. 17-16*B*). The clinical appearance of the absence of the clavicle is that of drooping shoulders (Fig. 17-16*C*). This is usually bilateral, and the neck is quite wide at its base, giving the appearance of a web between the neck and shoulders. With the total absence of the clavicles, the patient usually has the ability to bring the shoulders together anteriorly (Fig. 17-16*D*). The muscles attaching to the clavicle are anomalous or absent. The patient usually has no symptoms except that the adult may occasionally have difficulty carrying heavy weights due to the traction on the brachial plexus. Treatment for this condition is not indicated. There are few or no symptoms.

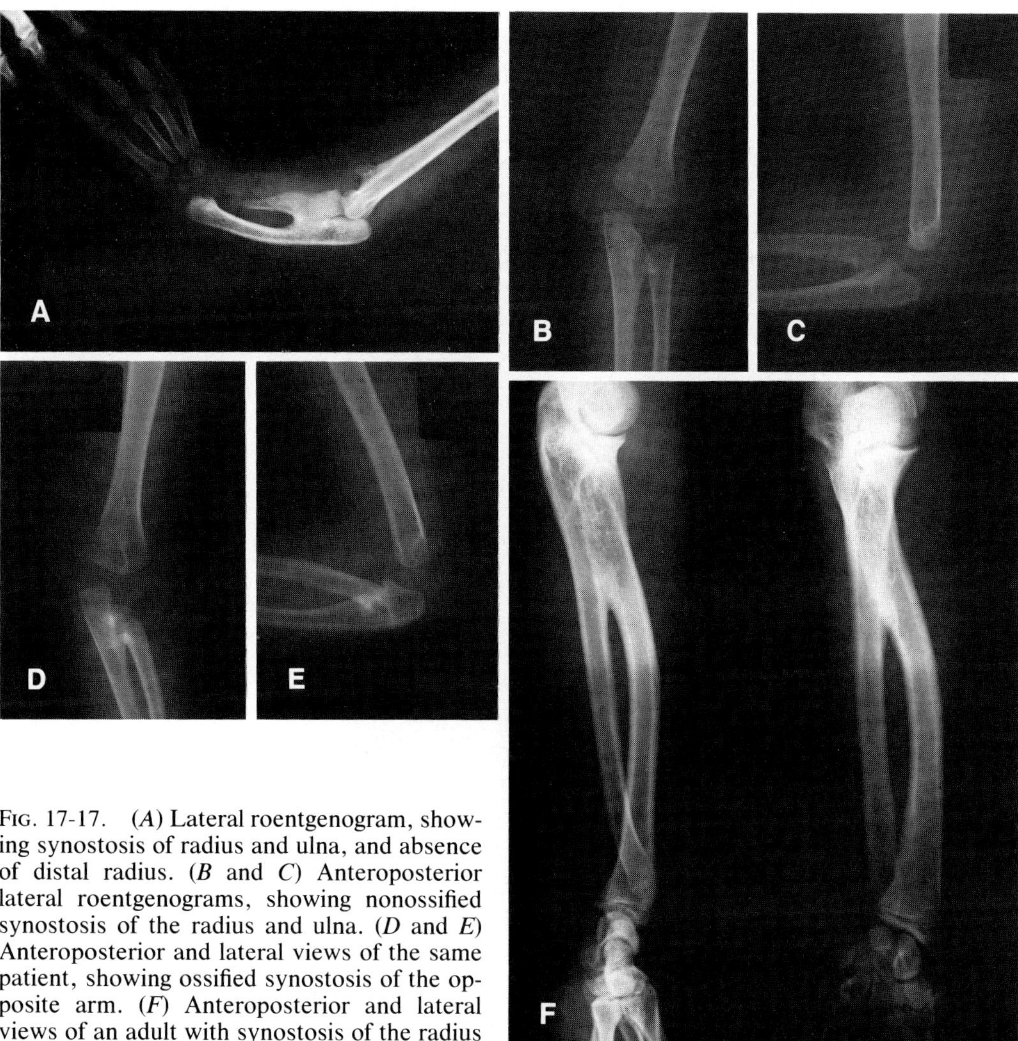

FIG. 17-17. (*A*) Lateral roentgenogram, showing synostosis of radius and ulna, and absence of distal radius. (*B* and *C*) Anteroposterior lateral roentgenograms, showing nonossified synostosis of the radius and ulna. (*D* and *E*) Anteroposterior and lateral views of the same patient, showing ossified synostosis of the opposite arm. (*F*) Anteroposterior and lateral views of an adult with synostosis of the radius and ulna.

CONGENITAL RADIOULNAR SYNOSTOSIS

Congenital radioulnar synostosis is present at birth and may be bilateral. It occurs in the proximal one third of the forearm (Fig. 17-17). The lack of rotation may be the only finding in a newborn or very young infant, because roentgenograms of children this young do not show the synchondrosis, which later becomes the osseous bridge between thc radius and ulna. The joining of the marrow cavities of the radius and ulna may not be evident on roentgenograms at birth and may only appear after the age of 1 year, when more ossification has occurred. In some cases, the elbow may be dislocated anteriorly or posteriorly. Because of the lack of rotation, there is usually an absence of the supinator brevis muscle and underdevelopment or absence of the pronator teres and pronator quadratus. The forearm is usually in pronation and occasionally may be so pronated that derotational osteotomy is indicated on one arm if the condition is bilateral. Other surgical procedures, such as resection of the synostosis or resection of the radial head and arthroplasty of the synostosis by insertion of a swivel type of joint, have been uniformly unsuccessful and are not recommended. Generally this condition produces no symptoms except for the inability to supinate. This loss of function is usually not too much of a handicap except if it is bilateral, in which case the person is usually unable to

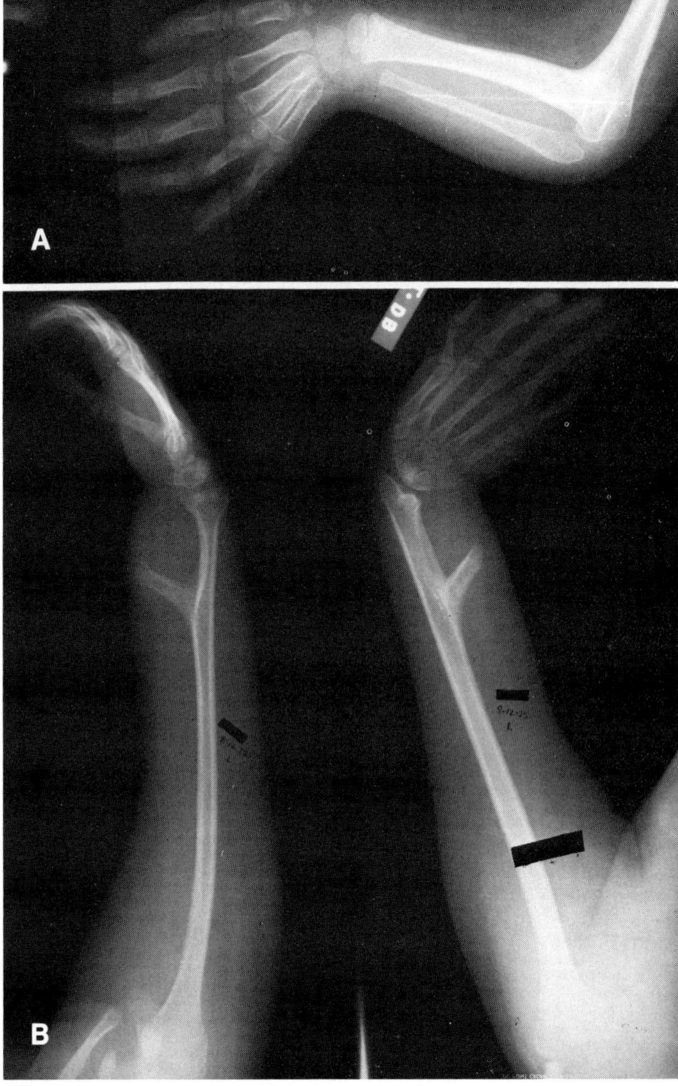

FIG. 17-18. (*A*) Anteroposterior roentgenogram, showing synostosis of humerus and radius, with partial absence of distal ulna and ulnar defects of the hand and wrist. (*B*) Anteroposterior and lateral views of synostosis of the humerus and radius in a straight line, with the ulna appearing as a supracondylar bone.

supinate the forearm and cup the palm, as for receiving change. If osteotomy for derotation of the forearm is contemplated, it is usually believed that it should be done on the minor arm rather than on the major arm, because the position of the function is usually considered to be in mild to moderate pronation, the usual position of most cases of synostosis.

CONGENITAL RADIOHUMERAL SYNOSTOSIS

Clinical Features

Congenital radiohumeral synostosis is rarely seen except in association with other deformities of the forearm and hand. The most commonly associated deformity is partial or complete absence of the ulna. In this condition (Fig. 17-18*A*), there is failure of segmentation of an elbow joint during development, so that the distal humeral epiphysis and proximal radial epiphysis are not formed, and there is fusion of those two bones. There may be partial or complete absence of the ulna. Most commonly, the absence is in the distal half of the ulna, with only a small cartilaginous anlage present at the elbow region. This results in considerable shortening of the upper extremity, because growth attributable to the distal humeral epiphysis and the proximal radius and ulna is absent (Fig. 17-18*B*). There is usually deformity of the forearm, with the radius being markedly bowed, and frequently the hand points toward the posterior aspect of the body, rather than the anterior aspect.

Treatment

Surgical treatment of the elbow joint is not recommended unless the forearm is pointed posteriorly. The absence of the elbow joint is usually accompanied by absence or deficiency of the muscles associated with flexion of the elbow or rotation of the forearm. Surgical attempts to provide motion of the elbow joint are not recommended, because the deformity results in severe shortening of the forearm. It is thought that if osteotomy is done to correct the posterior angulation of the arm, the anterior angulation accomplished by the osteotomy should be not more than 25° of flexion. This puts the hand into a range of function, avoiding its being so acutely flexed that the person is unable to take care of normal toilet needs because of the shortness of the extremity. Arthroplasty performed in an attempt to establish motion is not advised.

CONGENITAL DISLOCATION OF THE RADIAL HEAD

Clinical Features

Congenital dislocation of the radial head (Fig. 17-19*A*) may occur as an isolated deformity with no other deformity of the extremity. It is probably due to a malformed capitellum, which leads to a dome-shaped rather than a cup-shaped radial head, thus resulting in instability. The radial head may be dislocated at birth, or dislocation may occur shortly after birth. The head may dislocate anteriorly, posteriorly, or posterolaterally. The anterior dislocation is not obvious clinically at birth and may not be diagnosed early. The posterior or posterolateral dislocation causes a prominence at the elbow and is usually more easily recognized. Therefore, it may be diagnosed at birth or shortly thereafter. The anterior dislocation may not be evident for some months until it is noticed that the patient is unable to fully flex the elbow. Roentgenograms of both elbows taken shortly after birth reveal the dislocation of the radius, even though there is not full ossification of the proximal end of this bone at birth. There may be some limitation of flexion or extension, depending on the direction of the dislocation of the radius. There is usually loss of rotation, with supination usually being the motion lost.

Treatment

There are usually few symptoms associated with the congenital form of this condition, and the need for surgical correction is not usually great. Traumatic anterior dislocation of the head of the radius from traction on the forearm may be difficult to differentiate from congenital dislocation, although this condition is usually seen in a child of 2 years or older, as it is usually associated with a child who is walking. The radial head is dome-shaped, not cup-shaped (Fig. 17-19*B*).

If the dislocation of the radius is diagnosed at or shortly after birth, it may be possible in some cases to reduce the dislocation, but it is usually quite difficult to maintain the reduction. Even if an open surgical procedure should be done to accomplish the reduction and reconstruct the ligaments around the radial head and the capitellum, the success rate of maintaining the reduction is usually not very high. The capitellum is usually deformed and rather flat, and the radial head is dome-shaped, so that the dislocation frequently recurs within a short period of time. Resection of the radial head is not advised on growing children, because it usually produces considerable disturbance of the distal radioulnar articulation and results in proximal migration of the radius, increasing the shortening of the forearm. Late complications usually can be expected at the distal articulation if the radial head is resected in a growing child. This approach to the treatment of the condition is not recommended.

Congenital dislocation of the radial head can also be seen in association with partial or complete absence of the ulna (Fig. 17-19, *C* and *D*), and this was discussed in that section. Resection of the radial head can be done after growth is complete if the problem is symptomatic.

CONGENITAL DISLOCATION OF THE ELBOW

Clinical Features

Congenital dislocation of the elbow is a rare condition as an isolated deformity. If the dislocation is posterior, there is limitation of flexion. Most commonly, deformity of the forearm bones is the cause for the dislocation

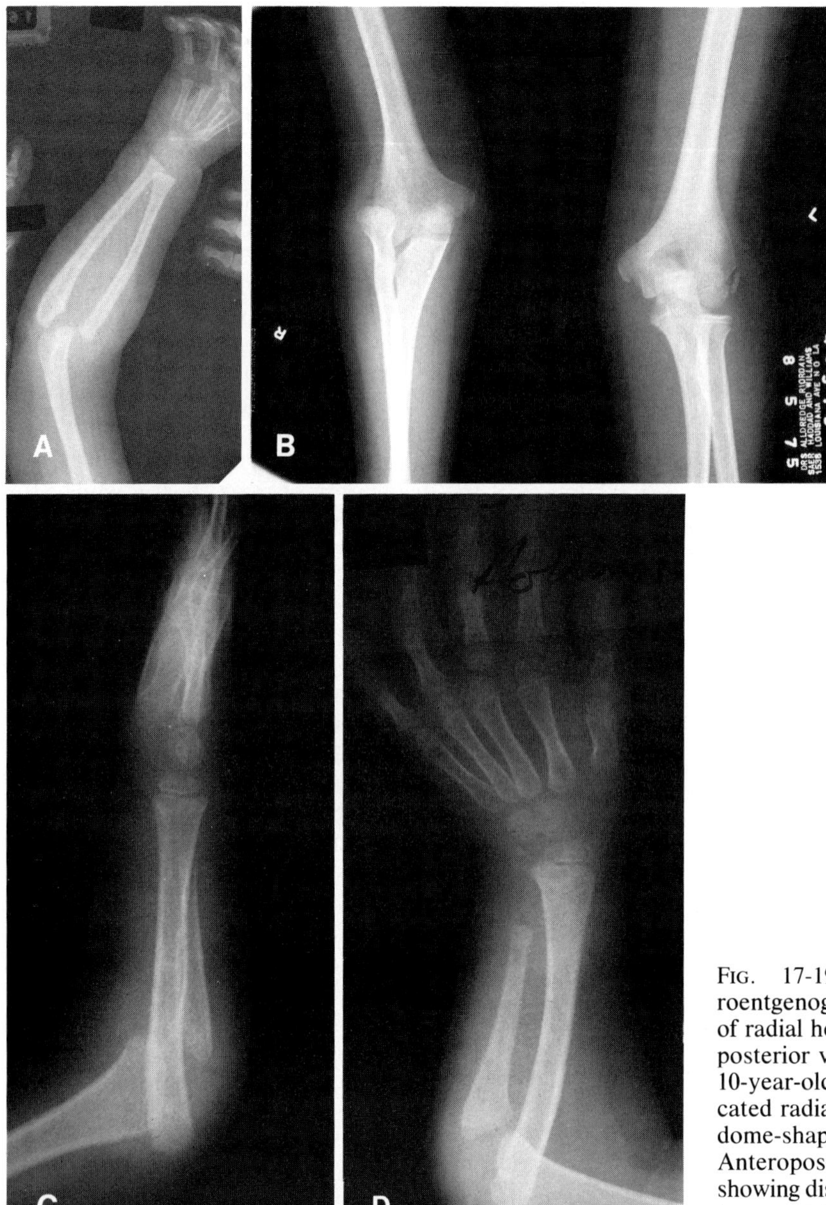

FIG. 17-19. (*A*) Anteroposterior roentgenogram, showing dislocation of radial head at elbow. (*B*) Anteroposterior views of both elbows of a 10-year-old child, showing a dislocated radial head on the right and a dome-shaped radial head. (*C* and *D*) Anteroposterior and lateral views, showing dislocation of the radial head in association with partial absence of distal ulna.

of the elbow. It is either incomplete formation of the distal humerus or incomplete formation of the proximal ulna that results in an unstable or dislocated elbow. In contrast to a traumatic dislocation of the elbow, the congenitally dislocated elbow is usually not painful (Fig. 17-20).

Treatment

The dislocation is usually obvious at birth, and, if treated then, a reduction can usually be obtained and should be immobilized in plaster. The treatment should be similar to the type of treatment used for a congenital clubfoot, with frequent cast changes to obtain the reduction and maintain the reduction, gradually bringing the elbow into flexion in a normally articulated position between the humerus and ulna. In the rare case in which an open reduction of the elbow may be necessary, it is usually difficult to maintain the reduction. Short-term pinning with Kirschner wires is

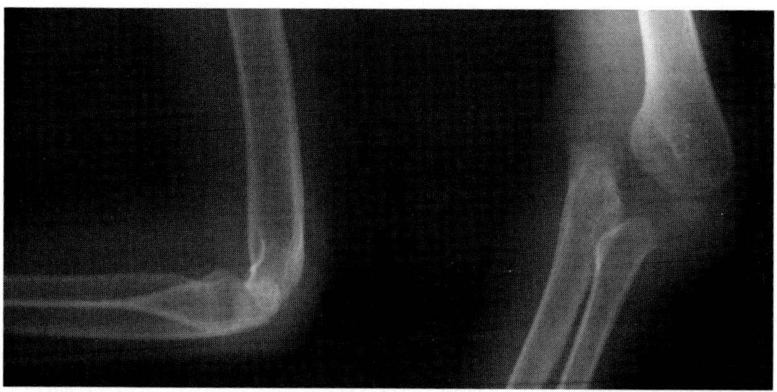

FIG. 17-20. Anteroposterior and lateral views of a dislocated elbow.

recommended to maintain the reduction until ligament reconstruction is given a chance to heal. Immobilization should probably not exceed 2 months, and efforts should be made to establish motion early, so that the motion will help in the formation of a proximal ulna and distal humerus.

PTERYGIUM CUBITALE (CONGENITAL WEBBING OF THE ELBOW)

The most prominent feature of this deformity is the broad web of skin that spans the elbow joint, extending from the mid arm, across the antecubital space, to the forearm. The elbow is usually flexed 90°, and extension is limited. The deformity is placed in Category II, failure of differentiation (separation of parts), due to failure of differentiation of the soft parts of the elbow, although the failure may also involve the osseous structures. The deformity is not common, and most of the reported cases have a familial basis. They are most frequently reported to be transmitted by an autosomal dominant gene. Some cases have been reported in recessive pedigree patterns.[45] Several patients who have been seen at the Scottish Rite Clinic have no familial history. The deformity can be part of a generalized webbing deformity, multiple generalized pterygia, with webbing of the neck, axilla, popliteal fossa, and all flexed areas.[44] It can be associated with nail-patella syndrome, Cornelia de Lange's syndrome, Mobius' syndrome, ulnar hypoplasia, radial hypoplasia, and arthrogryposis.[43] Associated anomalies of the cardiovascular and urogenital systems are frequently found occurring in this deformity. Disturbance of the muscles supplied by the oculomotor and facial nerves have also been observed in these patients.

Clinical Picture

Webbing of the elbow most frequently occurs bilaterally. The arm is usually short; the web begins well up on the arm and extends across the antecubital space to the mid forearm. The elbow appears thick, and the degree of flexion deformity of the elbow can vary but is usually 90°. There is no extension past the degree of flexion deformity, but flexion is seldom limited. The forearm is usually in a position of pronation; however, pronation is more restricted than is supination. The wrist and hand motion is not restricted. Atrophy of the soft tissue of the upper part of the arm is apparent or is made more apparent by the webbing (Fig. 17-21*A*). These patients function quite well with very little apparent handicap. Their main difficulty is reaching high places and lifting heavy objects.

Radiographic Findings

The humerus is short. The radial head may be subluxed or dislocated posteriorly, and the olecranon fossa may be shallow or elongated. The author has seen several cases in which the epiphyseal segment of the elbow has been deformed. The trochlea and medial epicondyle have been defective, and the ulnohumeral joint has been displaced (Fig. 17-21*B*). The distal forearm, wrist, and hand are not affected.

Abnormal Anatomy

The failure of the formation of the proximal skin fold in the antecubital fossa is most apparent in the anomaly. The underlying soft-tissue structures may be defective. The biceps may have an abnormal insertion or may be fibrotic, contracted, or absent. The origin of the brachioradialis may be fibrous or thickened. The brachioradialis, as well as the capsule, may be defective or tensely contracted.

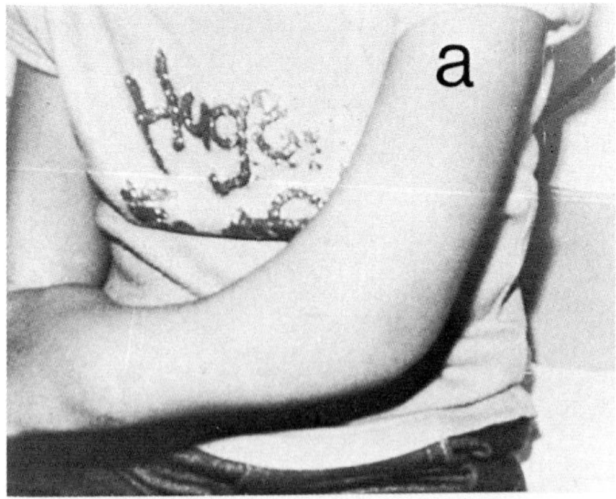

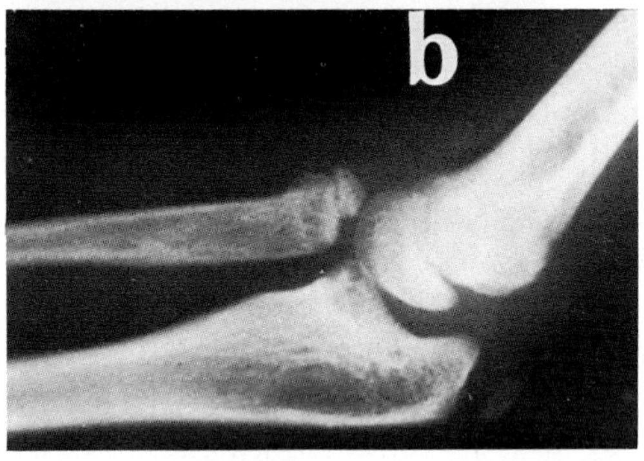

FIG. 17-21. Pterygium cubitale. (*a*) The elbow shows excessive webbing, and no antecubital crease is present. The motion is usually restricted in extension. (*b*) Frequently the radial head will be dislocated and the biceps will be contracted as well as all the soft tissues.

The neurovascular structures are present but are frequently bound in the adjacent contractured structures. The fibrous septa and aponeurotic bands contained in the web are usually hypertrophic. All these factors make correction of this deformity treatment hazardous and difficult. Very little is recorded in the literature as to the treatment of this deformity. Reported cases in which surgical correction has been attempted have not been gratifying. Most patients gained very little motion. Release of the soft-tissue contractures frequently reduced the active range of useful motion and decreased power. Limitation of correction has been determined by the neurovascular structures. Z–plasty and skin grafts can improve the cosmetic appearance but will yield little in functional improvement.

ARTHROGRYPOSIS

Arthrogryposis multiplex congenita has many synonyms.[48] The term *arthrogryposis* is derived from the Greek word meaning curved joint.[55] Arthrogryposis is a syndrome of persistent joint contracture, which is always present at birth.[56] Fortunately, it is not progressive. However, contractures are persistent and will recur following correction if not splinted.

The exact cause of the syndrome is not known at this time. It was first thought to be a disorder of joints and ligaments, but later it was thought to be primarily an affliction of muscles. Recently, it has been suggested that arthrogryposis is due to defective formation or degeneration of the anterior horn cells of the spinal cord.[48,52,53]

The striated muscles and the central nervous system seem to be the primary sites of involvement. The joint contractures are secondary to development. The affected joints are contracted due to marked thickening and fibrosis of the capsule. The cartilage and joint configuration is altered due to long-standing contractures.

Clinical Features

Patients with arthrogryposis are usually easy to diagnose. Their shoulders are abducted and externally rotated. They are thin, and very little girdle musculature is noted (Fig. 17-22*A*). The elbows and knees are flexed or fixed in either flexion or extension. The hands and wrists are usually clublike (Fig. 17-22*B*). The wrist is flexed and slightly deviated ulnarward. The hands are slender and shiny, the fingers are gathered together, and the thumb is usually abducted. Joint contractures are present at birth and are usually multiple and symmetrical. The extremities appear atrophic, and there is marked limitation of active and passive motion. The involvement of the lower extremities corresponds to the upper extremities. There are variable degrees of involvement. Some patients may have only involvement of the feet, but this will be symmetrical.

Treatment

Treatment should begin in the neonatal period, with range-of-motion exercises, casts, stretching of the various contractures, followed by splinting. The lower extremities are usually given the first surgical priority, because it is important that the child have lower extremity support by the age of 18 months. However, during this period, valuable passive motion can be obtained in the upper extremities. If the newborn's upper extremities are

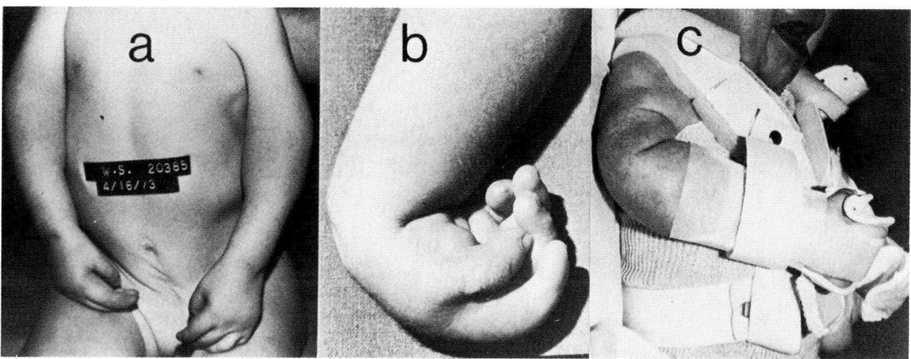

FIG. 17-22. Arthrogryposis. (*a*) Arthrogryposis involving both the upper and lower extremities. The shoulder girdle is frequently involved as shown, with marked atrophy of the upper arm and shoulder. (*b*) Frequent contracture of the wrist and fingers is seen. Often there will be no flexion crease in the palm and absence of intrinsic musculature. (*c*) This is a splint frequently used to aid flexion of the elbow; splints on the hands are used to stretch the contracture.

untreated, they will function as scissors, clamping objects between the hands.

There is usually very little active abduction of the shoulders, but they do have adductor function. Treatment is designed to mobilize the shoulders through active and passive stretching. If this is not significantly successful to allow significant external rotation, to place the elbows in a plane that when flexed will enable the hand to meet the mouth, an osteotomy of the upper one third of the humerus will have to be done. Fusion of the shoulder has been performed by Hansen,[55] but I found it unnecessary. The elbow is usually fixed in extension. There is always some passive motion present, although this varies from patient to patient. Cast wedging can be done until there is 40° to 50° of passive motion, then active stretching and mobilization can be initiated, along with passive splinting. As the patient gets older, 2 years of age and up, the elastic harness is applied (Fig. 17-22*C*). This gives active assist to flexion. This also allows the patient to bring his hands to his mouth and to use the hands in a flexed position, which helps to develop a normal use pattern. Quite often these patients will have active triceps function, but very few have biceps function. In more resistive patients, in whom passive elbow flexion cannot be obtained, surgical release may be necessary. This should be done on one extremity only. The child will need one straight extremity to push up from the sitting position. Active-elbow flexion can be provided in several ways, depending on the structures that are present. The triceps, when functioning, can be brought forward around the lateral border of the elbow and sutured into the biceps tendon, as described by Carroll.[49] Bilateral tricep transfers are never done. One functioning tricep is necessary for toilet care and assistance when rising from the chair. The procedure is usually contraindicated in those patients who need to use crutches.

Biceps function has been restored more frequently by the use of the pectoralis major muscle. The pectoralis muscle is almost always present and has good power. The method used by Lloyd-Roberts and Lettin[57] and Carroll and Hill,[50] in which the attachment of the biceps is placed more distally on the ulna to give it a better advantage, has been used successfully in some cases.

The wrist is usually flexed and somewhat ulnarly deviated. Fixed forearm pronation may prevent getting the hand to the mouth.

Persistent wrist flexion contracture can be aided by volar capsulotomy and can be relieved by volar capsulotomy and occasionally by tendon transfer from the volar to the dorsal wrist. Pronator release may also be necessary in order to get the hand to the mouth.

The most common finger contracture is flexion of the proximal interphalangeal (PIP) joints. Casting and splinting are the initial treatment modalities, followed by active exercises. The patients develop an uncanny skill in manipulating stiff fingers so that they can perform many tasks. Surgery will seldom improve the function of these hands and has too often caused great harm.

Even after correction of the deformity has

been accomplished by casting and surgery, the extremities have to be splinted at night until growth maturity to prevent recurrence.

The goal in treating the upper extremity deformity in arthrogryposis is to provide one extremity that can be brought to the mouth for feeding and to provide one extremity that can be used to push up from the sitting position or to use with a crutch if necessary and for toilet care.

SYNDACTYLY

Clinical Features

Syndactyly is one of the most common hand anomalies and is seen most often between the long and ring fingers. The next most common area is between the ring and little fingers. It occurs slightly more often in males than in females. It is frequently accompanied by syndactyly of the feet. It is also associated with a number of syndromes with multiple anomalies, such as Apert's syndrome (acrocephalosyndactyly). Different degrees of webbing may occur. The simplest is for the fingers to be joined only by a skin bridge, each finger having its own tendons, nerves, and bone structures, which are essentially normal.

Treatment

Treatment requires reconstruction of the skin web and skin grafting at the bases of the adjoining fingers and, in varying amounts, on the contiguous sides of the involved fingres (Fig. 17-23). The distal phalanges may be joined by fusion, and they usually have a common nail. If the fingers are of equal lengths, the need for surgical separation is not urgent. If the fingers are of different lengths, the fingers should be separated in the period between 6 months and 1 year; otherwise, the shorter finger causes curved growth of the longer finger.[61] Treatment in these cases requires web reconstruction and skin grafting of the contiguous sides, including grafting directly on the bone laid bare by the separation of the fused distal phalanges. In some cases, the bones are fused the full length of the fingers, which

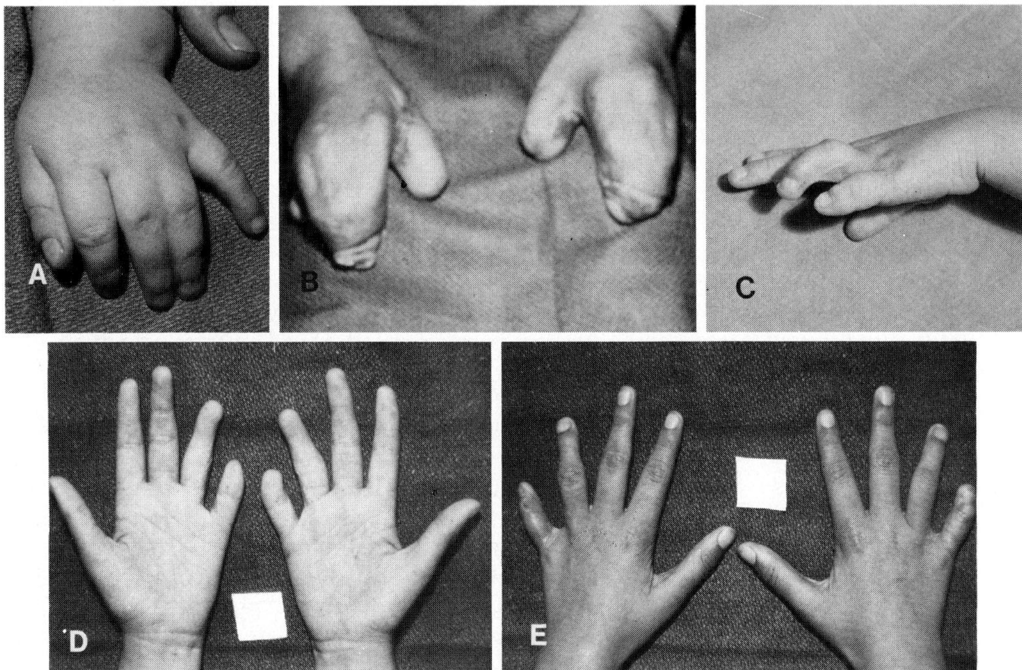

FIG. 17-23. (*A*) Simple syndactyly between the long and ring fingers. (*B*) Complex syndactyly of Apert's syndrome, with partially separated thumbs. (*C*) Lateral view of a hand 4 years after separation and grafting of the ring and little fingers, showing residual curvature of ring finger. (*D*) The hands of the patient in *C* 13 years after operation for separation of both ring and little fingers. (*E*) Dorsal view of the hands of the same patient.

requires splitting of the bone of all three phalanges. Skin grafting is necessary to a greater degree. In this type of case, the flexor and extensor tendons may be Y-shaped, with a single tendon at the metarcarpal head level, or the tendons may be broad and flat, necessitating the splitting of the tendons along the full length of the fingers. In this case, there are no collateral ligaments of the interphalangeal joints and no pulleys for the flexor tendon. Usually, however, the joint motion is so poor that a fibrous ankylosis usually results, and the fingers are best immobilized in the position of some flexion during the healing phase. There is some disagreement as to when separation of the fingers should be done. The best rule to follow is to separate the fingers early, between the ages of 6 and 12 months if the distal bones are fused, and certainly by age 1 or 2 years if only a skin bridge exists. If a web is properly constructed with a flap of skin and subcutaneous fat, the tissues usually remain where they are placed during growth. Occasionally, they may have to be revised if they migrate distally during the rapid growth period of adolescence. When separating the skin of these fused fingers, surgical incisions should be zig-zagged or S-shaped to prevent longitudinal scars from contracting at a later time and leading to late deformities.

If more than two fingers are included in the syndactyly, it is not recommended that both sides of the finger be operated on at the same time. If the index, long, ring, and little fingers are all joined, it is best to separate the border fingers (the index and little) first, separating the central fingers after an interval of approximately 3 months (Fig. 17-24). Nerves can be split and made to go to individual fingers, but vessels cannot. It requires some care and demands proper spacing of procedures if all four fingers are to be separated safely.

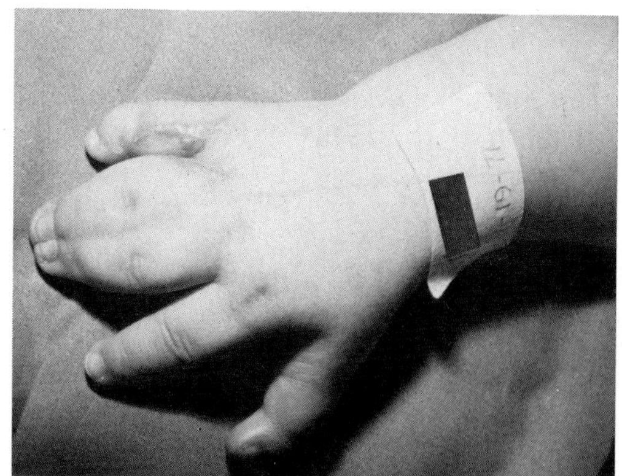

FIG. 17-24. In this hand, separation of the border fingers was the first operation.

Apert's Syndrome

Complicated syndactylies are seen in syndromes such as Apert's achrocephalosyndactyly.[62] In this condition, the facies is characterized by a high broad forehead, wide-set eyes with the outer canthus lower than the inner, a prominent lower jaw and a sunken, small maxilla (Fig. 17-25 *A*). The teeth are crowded, and the hard palate is high and arched and may be cleft posteriorly. The hand deformities are usually symmetrical, and there

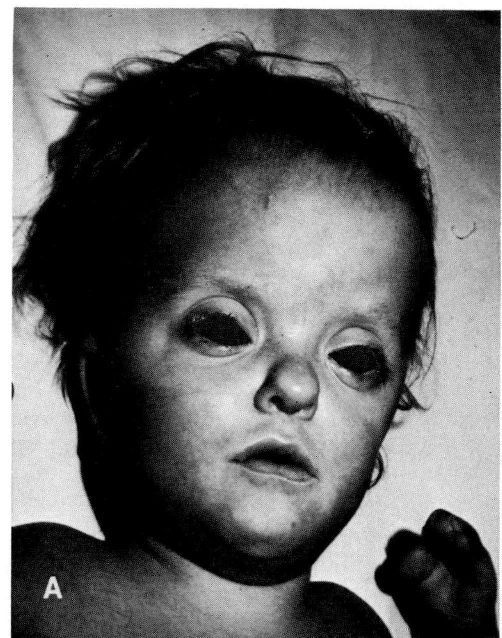

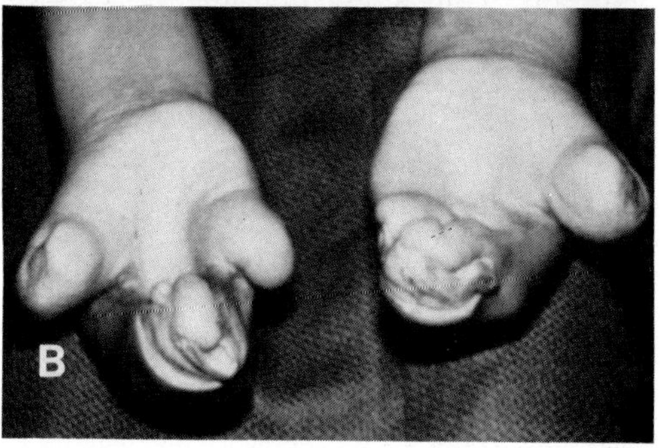

FIG. 17-25. (*A*) A child with Apert's syndrome, showing the typical facies. (*B*) The fused nails and distal phalanges of Apert's syndrome.

is complicated syndactyly of the long, ring, and little fingers. There is little or no interphalangeal joint motion. The fingers are shorter than normal. The syndactyly is usually complete, with bone fusion of the distal phalanges of the central fingers (Fig. 17-25 *B*). The fingernail may be a broad sheet covering all distal phalanges. The different finger lengths combined with the distal fusion results in a diamond-shaped configuration of the fingers and their metacarpals. The little finger is not usually fused at the distal phalanx. The thumb is usually separate and short and may have a single phalanx, although the thumb metacarpal is usually normal.

The finger metacarpals are short. The bases of the fourth and fifth metacarpals may be fused. If separation of the bony fusion of the distal phalanges of the index, long, ring, and fifth fingers is not done early, the third and fourth metacarpals are forced to diverge because of differential growth and distal tethering. A roentgenographic appearance of diamond-shaped, longitudinally arranged fusions is a characteristic feature. The surgical treatment of Apert's syndrome is difficult because of the complex syndactylies present. It is recommended that the separation of the border digits—the thumb and little finger—be done before the age of 1 year. Separation of the central fingers can be delayed until sufficient ossification has occurred to determine which bones belong to which fingers. Because of the complex syndactyly involving the bones, there is usually insufficient skin to provide adequate coverage for all four fingers, and it is wiser to produce a hand containing a thumb and three fingers (Fig. 17-26 *A*). Generally, separation of the thumb and index fingers and the ring and little fingers is done before 1 year, and separation of the remaining fingers is usually best accomplished by amputation of the central or long finger, making two fingers out of the three. Because of the marked bony involvement, there is usually marked limitation of motion of the interphalangeal joints. When the fingers are separated, it is best to place the interphalangeal joints in some degree of flexion when doing the skin grafting. This is most easily accomplished by using Kirschner wires to maintain bone position during the healing phase of the skin graft. This may prevent a second operative procedure for fusion of the interphalangeal joints in flexion at a later date. Late surgery is frequently indicated in these unfortunate children because of the lack of interphalangeal joint motion and the need to place the fingers in a more curved position to allow better grasping of medium-sized objects.

CAMPTODACTYLY

Clinical Features

This term means "bent finger." There is much confusion concerning the definition condition, but strictly speaking, it means a bent little finger. Primarily, the flexion contracture occurs at the middle joint or the PIP joint. It is usually hereditary, appearing in early childhood, and gradually increases in severity. When it first appears, it is correctable with passive extension, but, with growth, there is secondary shortening of the skin, tendons, and joint, and the bend eventually becomes a fixed deformity that is not correctable by splinting.[63]

The early roentgenograms are normal, but roentgenograms taken at puberty or later show notching of the fossa at the neck of the proximal phalanx because of the acute flexion of the middle phalanx. The bone structure is otherwise normal.

Treatment

The treatment in the early stages is dynamic splinting in the daytime and fixed extension splinting at night. Fixed deformities may be prevented with prolonged diligent splinting. Splinting should begin as soon as the deformity is noticed. Frequently, however, late fixed deformity does not respond well to splinting.[64]

The surgical treatment, therefore, requires correction of all the involved tissues. This means a shift of a lateral skin flap to cover the short volar skin surface and skin grafting of the donor area on the lateral and dorsal side of the finger. If the sublimis tendon is short, it may be lengthened at the wrist level if surgery is performed when the patient is still quite young. If the extensor central slip is attenuated, sublimis slips may be used as an intrinsic central slip replacement. If the joint capsule is contracted, it usually requires capsulotomy. If these surgical procedures are carried out, prolonged follow-up treatment and splinting are necessary. Even with the best efforts at treatment, prolonged splinting, and follow-up care, the result is usually incomplete correction. In late untreated cases with severe flexion deformities, arthrodesis of the middle joints in 30° to 35° of flexion is indicated.[65]

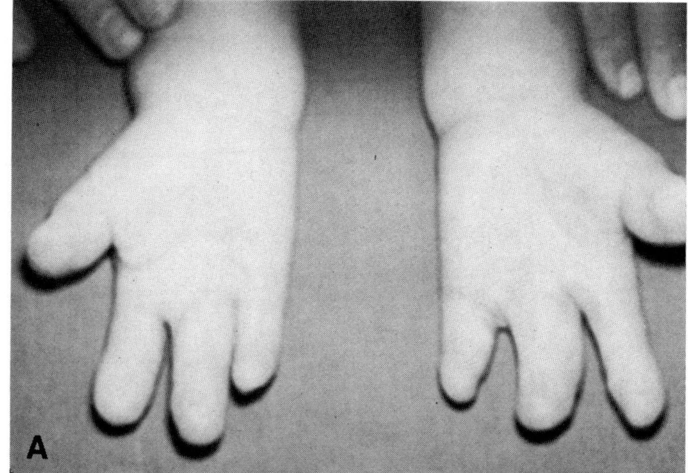

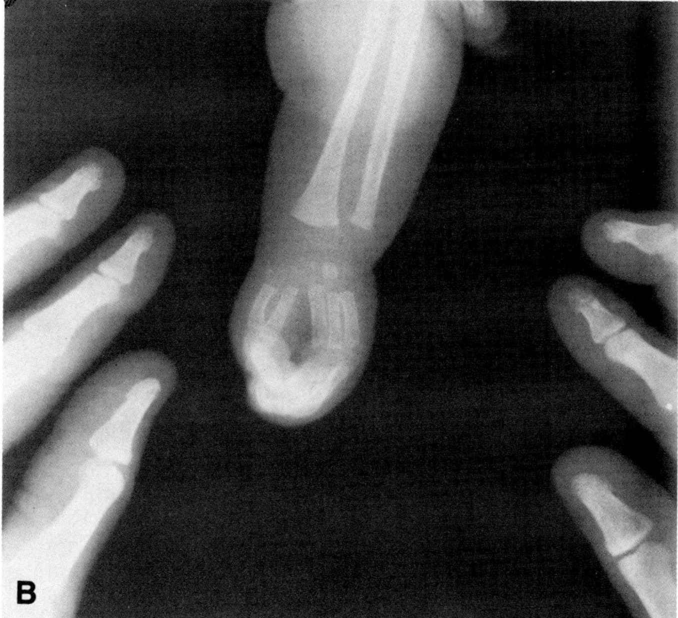

FIG. 17-26. (*A*) Palmar view of the hands of a child with Apert's syndrome after separation and construction of the thumb and three fingers. (*B*) Anteroposterior x-ray showing fused tips of fingers and diamond shape of metacarpals.

CLINODACTYLY

Clinodactyly means bent finger. A better definition would be curved finger. The finger is actually angulated in the plane of the fingers. This is in contrast to camptodactyly, which means bent finger but also signifies a flexion deformity of the finger. In clinodactyly, the finger or fingers can be angulated in either radial or ulnar direction. It occurs in any finger but is most common in the little finger. It occurs quite commonly bilaterally. Clinically, the finger is usually short and the degree of curvature varies from patient to patient (Fig. 17-27 *A*). Function is seldom impaired unless the curvature is severe. Several patients have complained of difficulty in writing, typing, or playing the piano. However, these complaints are seldom verified as a functional defect, and it appears that the complaints are based primarily on cosmetic sensitivity. Most patients who seek treatment are young adolescents who have become sensitive to their deformity. Clinodactyly is frequently seen in the young child who has numerous syndromes,[71] but it plays such an insignificant part in the overall problem of the child that it is often overlooked. Clinodactyly is important because it is frequently associated with mongoloid children with mental retardation.[69] The incidence of

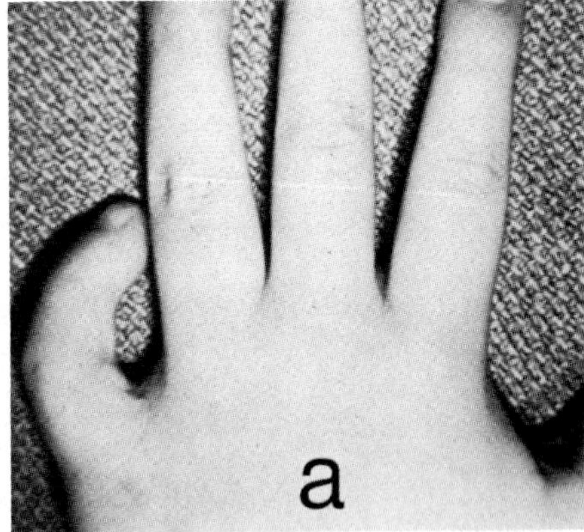

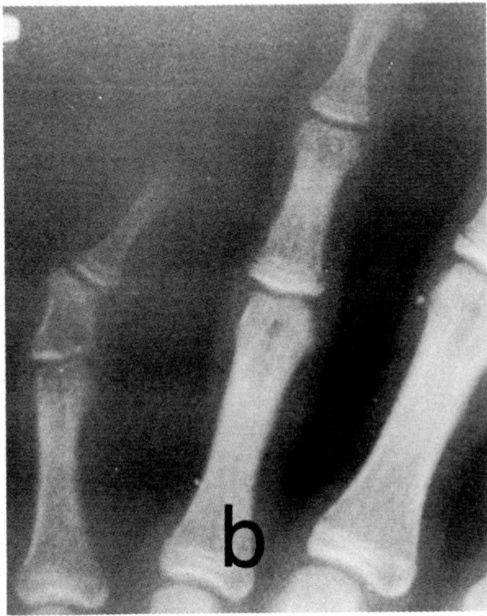

FIG. 17-27. Clinodactyly. (*a*) This usually involves the fifth digit. The finger is curved laterally toward the thumb. (*b*) The middle phalanx is deformed. It is short and the radial cortex is shorter than the ulnar cortex, causing the articular surface to be divergent rather than parallel.

clinodactyly in the mongoloid has been reported between 35% and 79%. In normal children, the incidence is between 1% and 19%.

Crooked little fingers are frequently thought of as a family trait.[71] Pedigree analysis has shown that it is usually a dominant trait of inheritance, with variable expressivity, and that it is usually bilateral. Sporadic cases are frequently seen and may or may not be bilateral. The cause of the angulation is due to maldevelopment in the middle phalanx (Fig. 17-27 *B*). The phalanx is short on one side and longer on the other, giving it a trapezoid shape. This causes the alignment of the articular surface of the distal joint to deviate from the normal perpendicular alignment with the longitudinal axis of the finger. Some orthopaedists believe that because the middle phalanges ossify last,[68] there is a greater tendency for shortening and deformity to occur in this area. The deformity may be mild at birth or in the young child and is hardly noticed. However, the deformity will increase during rapid growth spurts and will be especially noticeable in the young adolescent.

Treatment

When the deformity is seen at an early age, splinting has been recommended by some orthopaedists.[68] This has not been found to be an effective method of treatment. The growth pattern of the middle phalanx seems to be set, and sufficient external forces cannot be maintained effectively to alter this pattern. The preferred treatment is to recommend that nothing be done, and, when the child nears skeletal maturity, if the deformity is severe and causing some functional handicap, surgical correction can be done. Surgical correction carries with it the possibility of complication of nonunion, loss of correction, infection, tenodesis, and loss of function. These possible complications should be explained to the patient and the parents.

Correction of the angulation can best be accomplished by a closing wedge osteotomy. The fingers are approached by a mid lateral incision on the side of the convexity of the deformed phalanx. The extensor mechanism is not violated. The periosteum is incised longitudinally, and extreme care is taken not to tear it or rip it when elevating it from the bone. The bone should not be cut with a power saw for fear of damaging the periosteum or extensor tendon. A sharp osteotome is used to cut the bone. After the wedge has been removed, the osteotomy is closed and the alignment is rechecked. Rotation, as well as longitudinal alignment, should be corrected before pinning the osteotomy. Two Kirschner-wires placed parallel across the osteotomy site are used to prevent rotation and malalignment. After fixation, the finger is flexed and extended to ensure that there is no residual deviation of the finger. The wound is closed and dressed, and the splint is applied. Immobilization usually requires 4 weeks. The pins are removed when evidence of union can be seen on the radiograph.

TRIGGER THUMB

Clinical Features and Diagnosis

Congenital trigger thumb, sometimes called *clasped thumb,* is easily misdiagnosed or unrecognized at birth, due to the clenched-fist attitude of the newborn hand. It can be easily diagnosed at birth if the obstetrician or pediatrician passively extends the fingers and thumb as a part of the initial physical examination.

Treatment

If the diagnosis is made at birth and if the thumb can be passively extended, splinting in extension for 6 to 8 weeks may overcome the triggering; however, even some cases that are diagnosed at birth do not allow passive extension, and splinting does not correct the condition. Occasionally, continuous splinting or casting, as for a clubfoot, gradually produces full extension of the thumb.[73]

Mechanically, the annular ligament at the metacarpal head is too tight or too small for the flexor pollicis longus. The distal swelling of the tendon may result in formation of a nodule or enlargement of the tendon. This can be palpated and causes the triggering. If this goes untreated, the fibrosis in the swollen area of the tendon progresses to a permanent nodule on the flexor tendon. If the trigger thumb cannot be extended by splinting with 6 or 8 weeks of treatment, surgical correction is recommended. It can be done under premedication and local anesthesia, but it is more commonly done under general anesthesia if there are no contraindicating physical conditions of the newborn. If surgery is necessary, resection of the small pulley at the metacarpal head is recommended. The more distal cruciate or oblique ligament is preserved to prevent marked bowstringing of the flexor pollicis longus.[74]

TRIPHALANGEAL THUMB

The term *triphalangeal thumb* encompasses a broad spectrum of clinical entities. The extra phalanx varies from a small triangular bone to a normal phalanx in what appears to be a thumbless five-fingered hand (Fig. 17-28). Triphalangeal thumbs are divided into three types: (1) thumbs with a delta or abnormally shaped phalanx, (2) thumbs with three normal phalanges in excessive length, and (3) those hands with five normal fingers and no thumb.

The first type of triphalangeal thumb includes all abnormally shaped extra phalanges, whether triangular, trapezoidal, or rectangular. The distal interphalangeal joint is often incongruous and stiff, especially in the adult. The thumb deviates ulnarward in most cases, only rarely to the radial side.[89] The delta phalanx is located between the distal and proximal phalanges; the more triangular the phalanx, the greater the angulation. The angulation is secondary to the unequal growth of the delta phalanx as well as the abnormal pressure exerted by the phalanx of the normal phalangeal epiphysis.[84,89]

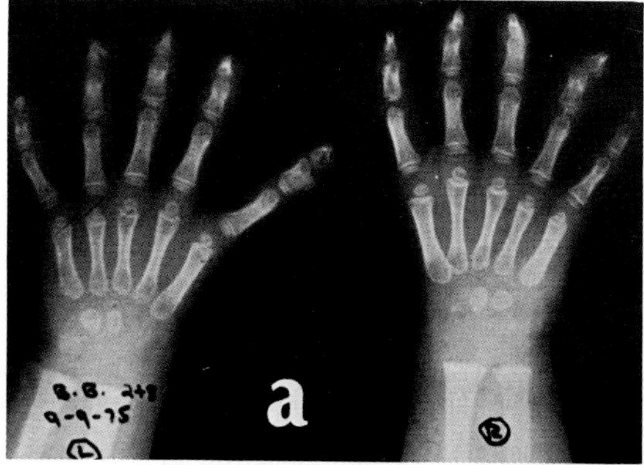

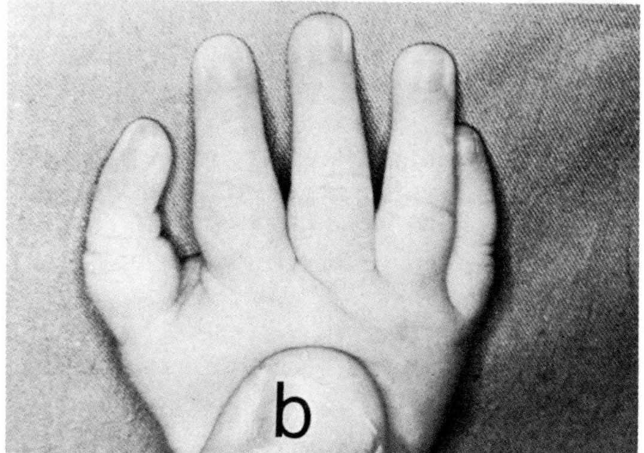

FIG. 17-28. Triphalangeal thumb. (*a*) The thumb has three phalanges. The thumb metacarpal is in the same plane with the fingers. (*b*) The clinical picture of a triphalangeal thumb. Note the increased length and the attempt to rotate toward the fingers.

The second type of triphalangeal thumb is excessively long but retains its normal proximal location and rotation, which distinguishes this from type III. These thumbs present with increased length. When the normal thumb is adducted to the index finger, its tip normally reaches the middle third of the proximal phalanx. In this type of triphalangeal thumb, the tip may reach beyond the proximal interphalangeal joint.

Most patients will deny that their abnormally long thumb presents a problem. Careful observation will reveal that the extra long thumb interferes with precision pinch and is cosmetically unappealing.

Over half of these patients will have contracted first web spaces.[89] This presents a functional deficit, decreasing opposition, and grasp is limited to small objects.

The third type of triphalangeal thumb is actually a misnomer. The hand has five normal appearing fingers and no apparent thumb. More than 50% of all triphalangeal thumbs fit into this category.[89] All the fingers are aligned in the same plane. The joints of the radial-most finger may be stiff.

Pinch is accomplished between the adducted fingers in a clawlike manner. Pinch is quite weak, and many patients will develop a widened first web space and rotate the first finger in an attempt at pollicization. Palmar grip is also weak, and the hand serves only as an aid in picking up objects. Most patients in this category have absence of the thenar musculature.[76,78,85,89]

The triphalangeal thumb is inherited as an autosomal dominant trait, and this has been well documented in the literature.[75,79,80,88] It has also been associated with maternal thalidomide ingestion during pregnancy.[83]

Numerous associated anomalies and syndromes are noted. Triphalangeal thumb is commonly found in polydactyly,[80,82] central deficiencies of the hands and feet, congenital tibial defects,[86] and absence of the pectoral muscles.[86] It can also be part of Holt-Oram syndrome, Fanconi's aplastic anemia, Backfand-Diamond syndrome,[77] trisomy 13, and Juberg-Hayward syndrome.[83]

Conservative treatment has no role in the triphalangeal thumb. Milch[84] believed that the pressure from splinting merely aggravated the epiphyseal imbalance, causing angulation.

In general, surgery should be performed before the child is 6 years of age. The pattern of thumb and hand use rapidly develop between the third and fifth year, and it is best to complete surgery before this time. The child's skeleton achieves a suitable size, making surgery easier to perform. The treatment of each type of triphalangeal thumb is different.

The approach to the delta phalanx thumb should be cautious. Surgery is performed only if severe angulation is present, interfering with normal thumb function. If seen before the child is 1 year of age, Flatt[78] recommends excision of the delta phalanx. He strongly emphasizes the need for adequate collateral ligament reconstruction and Kirschner wire fixation for a prolonged period, approximately 8 weeks. If this point is not carefully attended, an unstable angulated distal phalanx will result, often worse than the original problem. The earlier this operation is performed, the greater the chances for a good result. Many orthopaedists have found this technique to be disappointing in older persons.[76,78,85,89] Several factors are responsible. Joint stiffness and incongruency often prejudice the outcome. Ligament reconstruction frequently fails because of the stresses involved with everyday thumb use. This has led to the conclusion that it is best to excise the distal phalanx and fuse the distal interphalangeal joint, taking appropriate wedges to correct angulation.

The goal of surgery in the type II triphalangeal thumb is the reduction of excessive length. First, web space contracture, if present, is also addressed. Two methods can be used to reduce the length of the triphalangeal thumb. Both are accomplished by dorsal extensor hood–splinting incision. The first includes excision of the entire middle phalanx. The collateral ligaments are left attached to the proximal phalanx for insertion into the distal phalanx. The possibility of joint incongruency is present, and only in the very young should biologic remodeling be relied on for a good result.

An alternate approach maintains joint integrity. Appropriate lengths of the proximal middle phalanges, as well as the PIP joint, are resected. The extensor mechanism must be reefed, and bone must be fixed by one or two Kirschner wires. The long flexor tendon will adjust unless excessive length has been removed. Redundant skin is excised after 3 months if necessary.

If the first web space contracture is present, a four-flap Z-plasty or large dorsal rotational flap, as described by Strauch and Spinner[87] is used. The five-fingered hand requires the reconstruction of the thumb. Recession, abduction, and pronation of the first metacarpal are often adequate in most five-fingered hands. This is the procedure as described by Hertz and Littler.[81]

A large number of five-fingered hands lack

thenar musculature, and, if opposition is ineffective, an opponenoplasty is performed. The author's preference is the ring finger sublimis tendon transfer, using a strip of flexor carpi ulnaris tendon as a pulley.

DELTA PHALANX

The delta phalanx is a triangular, oval, or trapezoidal bone with an abnormal epiphyseal plate. Jones[92] first used this term when he described five cases with angular deformities of the finger, secondary to an abnormally shaped bone, resembling a Greek letter. Other terms, such as congenital triangular bones of the hand[91,98] and longitudinal bracketed diaphysis[96] have been suggested as general descriptions, because these deformities have also been described in metacarpals.

The abnormality is characterized by a triangular bone with a C-shaped epiphysis, usually oriented in a semicircular direction. The triangular or trapezoidal shape often causes angulation of the distal portion of the finger or thumb (Fig. 17-29). The aberrant epiphysis ossifies from proximal to distal, causing unequal longitudinal growth and angulation.

The etiology of the delta phalanx is unknown. Watson and Boyes[97] stated that the delta phalanx was a polydactyly manifestation. They believed that the epiphysis was the site of origin of an extra phalanx and that the delta phalanx is abnormally shaped because the epiphysis is tethered by the extra digit. Very commonly, the phalanges distal to the delta phalanx are duplicated, either completely or in part. Theander and Carstam[96] explained the abnormality as the result of a bony bracket at both ends of the epiphysis, causing unequal epiphyseal growth. They suggested the term longitudinal bracketed diaphysis.

An epiphyseal dysplasia has been mentioned as a possible etiology. Maternal thalidomide ingestion during pregnancy has been reported as a cause of delta phalanx.[91] More than half the reported cases of delta phalanx are bilateral, and review of the literature reveals that the proximal phalanx of the thumb is the most frequent site of the delta phalanx. This is followed by the proximal phalanx of the little finger. Hoover, Flatt, and Weiss[91] noted the middle phalanx of the triphalangeal thumb to be the most common site. The middle phalanx of the little finger was the second most frequent site.

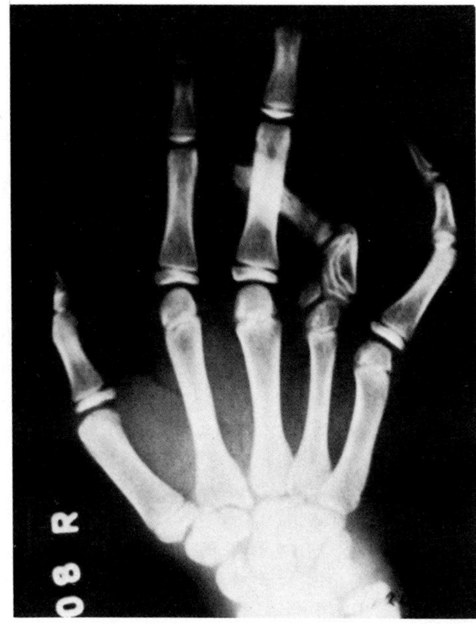

FIG. 17-29. Delta phalanx. The proximal phalanx of the fourth digit is deformed. There is a semicircular epiphyseal plate that forms the shape of the Greek letter delta.

Delta phalanx is found in association with Apert's syndrome,[91] most commonly affecting the index finger. Triangular bones causing angulatory deformities have been noted in dystrophic dwarfs.[90,94,95] In the Holt-Oram syndrome, central deficiencies, polydactyly, symphalangism, and syndactyly are frequently found in association with delta phalanx, especially if more than one triangular bone is present in the hand.

Wood and Flatt[98] have studied the natural course of the delta phalanx. The long and ring fingers were affected by this abnormality, which rarely deviated to any significant degree, because these fingers are internally splinted by the adjacent fingers. Border digits deviate to the greatest degree. The thumb has a classic ulnar deviation, and the little finger frequently angulates toward the hand.

Treatment

Watson and Boyes[97] thought that the main skeletal ray was well united with the extra ray longitudinally. The finger might be larger than normal, but it may retain acceptable function and alignment. However, conservative treatment to the delta phalanx has been universally unsuccessful.

The author agrees with Wood and Flatt[98] in that surgery should be undertaken only in cases in which significant deviation is present and when this interferes with the development of the normal pattern of use of the finger. Surgery should be delayed as long as possible to allow the child to mature and the skeletal elements to attain greater size. The goal of surgery should be a narrow well-aligned functional digit with an intact horizontal epiphysis. Numerous procedures have been described for correction of this deformity, including opening wedge and closing wedge osteotomies. Probably one of the most interesting surgical techniques has been described by Smith,[93] in which the attempt to realign the abnormal epiphyseal plates in a perpendicular alignment with the longitudinal axis of the finger is carried out. The most important factors in the treatment of the delta phalanx, when it is necessary, are to separate the proximal and distal plates from their longitudinal connecting epiphyseal segment and to correct the alignment of the distal and proximal plates by wedge osteotomy, realigning the epiphyseal plates perpendicular to the longitudinal axis of the digit.

CONGENITAL CLASPED THUMB

Clasped thumb is a descriptive term for the position of the thumb in relation to the hand. Another term used is congenital flexion contracture of the thumb. The clasped thumb deformity, however, has been shown to be the result of multiple defects in the extensor and flexor mechanisms, as well as skin contractures and joint instability (Fig. 17-30). Classification of clasped thumb, based on the various causes, is described by Weckesser and associates.[108] In their group, one of the deformities, which was the most common, included all cases with the deformity due only to the failure of the differentiation in formation of the extensor tendons. The Group II deformities included cases in which the flexion contractures of other fingers were combined with the severe flexion contracture of the thumb and deficient extension of the thumb. Group III deformities included the cases in which there were diffuse alterations in all structures of the thumb, including hypoplasia of the extensor, flexor, and thenar muscles, as well as osseous components of the thumb. Group IV deformities included all cases that did not fall into the other categories.

Group I deformities are the most frequently encountered. The diagnosis is hard to make in the first 3 months of life, because the normal infant holds the thumb clasped in the palm most of the time. Careful observation is necessary during this period to establish the fact that adequate extension is present. Group I deformities should not be confused with a trigger thumb. In trigger thumb deformities, the flexion deformity is at the distal joint, and a palpable nodule is noted on the volar surface on the MP joint of the thumb. In Group I deformities, the principal defect involves the extensor pollicis brevis muscle, with a flexion deformity of the MP joint. However, defects in the extensor pollicis longus and abductor pollicis muscle and tendons have been found. When there is a combination of extensor pollicis brevis and extensor pollicis longus defects, both the MP and the distal phalangeal joints are usually flexed in the palm. When the abductor pollicis longus is also involved, all three segments of the thumb are adducted into the palm. Treatment of Group I deformities can be divided into early and late treatment. If the diagnosis is made within the first 3 months of life, a short-arm splint or cast holding the thumb in abduction and extension can be effective. The thumb at this stage is not contracted, and proper positioning can be accomplished easily. Splinting is continuous for the first 3 months. If extensor tendons are hypoplastic or attenuated, splinting allows the musculotendinous units to become functional, being protected against the powerful flexor forces. If at this point extension of the thumb is present, intermittent splinting can be instituted for another 3 months. A good result can be expected in more than two thirds of these cases. Splinting in patients older than 2 years of age does not yield as consistent a result as that in infants, but it certainly merits attempt. Some patients will improve to the point where adequate function is maintained, and, even if they do not, splinting is a good preoperative measure to soften up the contractures.

Surgical treatment is usually reserved for clasped thumb patients older than 2 years of age, and these cases are complicated by secondary contracture of the joint and overlying skin. Z-plasty release or skin grafting may be necessry to release the skin contracture. The extensor hood may be attenuated, and the lateral expansion is displaced volarly or distally, contributing to the flexor force acting on

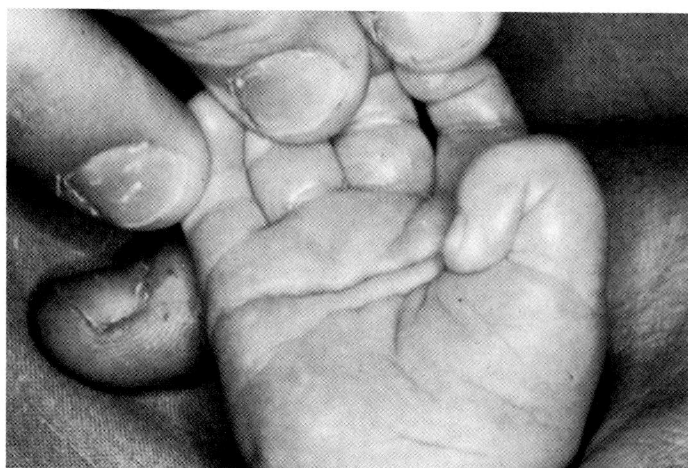

FIG. 17-30. Congenital clapsed thumb. The thumb may be extremely contracted as shown in this figure, or it may be flexed at the metacarpophalangeal (MCP) joint only.

the MP joint. Freeing up the lateral expansion and centralizing the extensor tendons will increase the extensor function. In patients in whom the extensor pollicis brevis and longus are absent, function can be restored by tendon transfers.

The extensor indicis proprius would be an ideal tendon to replace function of the extensor pollicis longus. However, when the extensor pollicis longus is absent, the extensor indicis proprius will also frequently be absent, because both arise from adjacent muscle masses in the forearm. It is best to demonstrate, prior to surgery, that adequate independent function of the index finger is present. Flatt[103] suggests that the common extensor tendon to the index finger can be used to replace the faulty extensor to the thumb, provided that the extensor indicis proprius is adequate. He will also use the brachial radialis, prolonged with tendon graft or attached directly to remnants of the extensor tendon. Crawford and colleagues[101] recommend using the flexor superficiales tendon to replace the extensor pollicis longus function. This type of transfer has the advantage of not requiring a graft. The bradioradialis can also be used to replace abductor pollicis function when it is absent. The transfer of the extensor carpi ulnaris longus can be prolonged by dividing a portion of the tendon proximally and then turning it back on itself and weaving it through the distal stump, thus obtaining sufficient length to attach it to the insertion of the extensor pollicis brevis.

Detailed corrections for Groups II, III, and IV clutch thumb deformities are rather extensive and the author refers the reader to the discussion of treatment in Dobyns, Wood, and Bayne, *et al.*

POLYDACTYLY

Polydactyly has been noted as one of the most common congential anomalies, rivaling syndactyly.

This deformity falls into Category IV, duplication. Polydactyly results when some stimulus causes the embryonic limb bud to duplicate itself. The stage at which this stimulus occurs determines the amount of the digit that is duplicated. Stelling[116] and Turek[118] have classified polydactyly into three main types, basically describing the extra digit. Type I is an extra soft-tissue mass, usually connected to the hand by a pedicle of soft tissue. No skeletal continuity is present. Type II represents a partial duplication of the digit or part of the digit, involving the phalanges or proximal phalanges. The metacarpal head may be enlarged or bifid. Type III is rare and involves a complete duplication of the ray with a separate metacarpal.

The polydactyly is further subdivided into preaxial and postaxial subclassifications. Postaxial, or ulna, polydactyly refers to duplications of the fifth finger (Fig. 17-31*A*). Preaxial polydactyly includes duplication of the thumb (Fig. 17-31*B*). Duplication of the index, long,

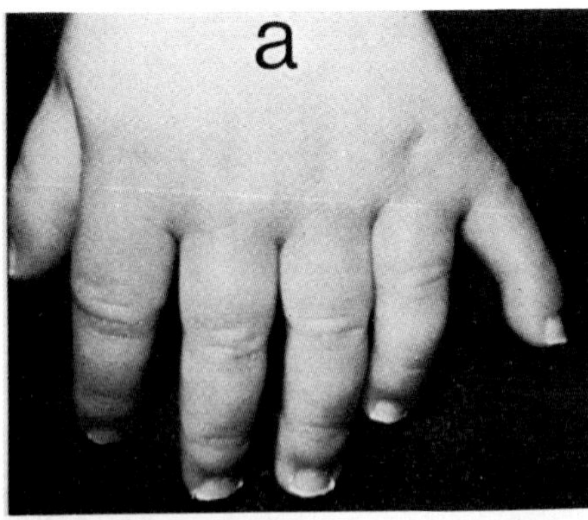

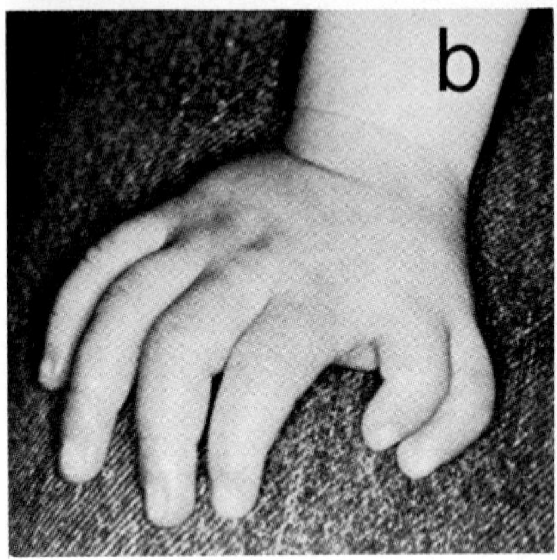

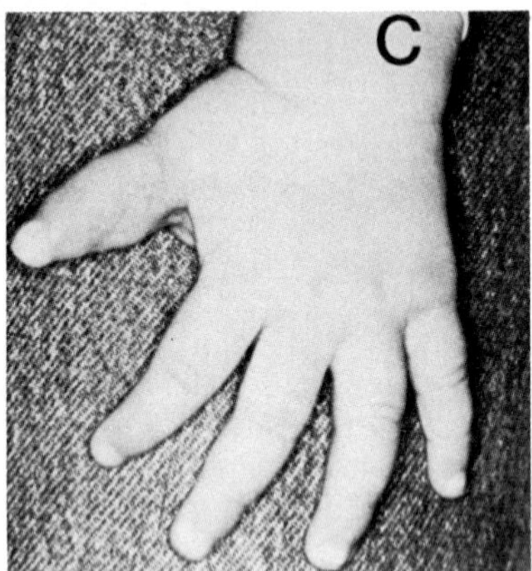

FIG. 17-31. Polydactyly occurs more frequently at the border digits. (*a*) This figure represents a complete duplication of the fifth digit. (*b*) Duplication of the thumb occurs frequently. This represents a complete duplication of all three segments of the thumb. (*c*) This is a postoperative picture of *b*, showing removal of the least complete thumb.

and ring finger can also be termed central polydactyly.

Polydactyly most frequently affects the border digits of the hand.[110] The thumb and little fingers are by far the most commonly duplicated.[110] Blacks demonstrate polydactyly in the fifth finger 10 times more commonly than do Caucasians.[111] Duplication of the thumb occurs more often in Caucasians. The anomalies associated with polydactyly are discussed briefly. Polydactyly is often the most obvious sign of a syndrome in which other serious defects are present. This is especially true in postaxial polydactyly in Caucasians. When present, the child should be thoroughly examined for associated cardiovascular or other anomalies.

Polydactyly of the thumb will be discussed separately from polydactyly of the fingers.

Polydactyly of the Thumb

Polydactyly of the thumb, duplicate thumb, and accessory thumb are frequent terms used to describe duplication of the thumb. Duplication of the thumb can be either complete or incomplete. Occasionally, especially in the distal phalanx, triplication can occur. The following simple classification of duplication of the thumb is treatment oriented and is grouped by levels of duplication.[115] Delta phalanx and triphalangeal thumb are excluded. Group I is duplication of the distal phalanx which includes all types, including triphalangeal distal phalanx. Group II is duplication of the proximal phalanx. Group III is duplication of the metacarpals. Group IV is a mixed quality of duplication.

Treatment. Because functional patterns of the thumb do not appear until the child is 2 ½ to 3 years of age, correction of polydactyly should be accomplished before the child is 3 to 3 ½ years of age.[114]

Surgical treatment is based on anatomic variations and the level of duplication and consists of removal of the least functional part with reconstruction of the remaining components. If function of the two components is equal, the appearance of the digits is the deciding factor as to which should be removed.

The various tissues must be corrected. Incisions must conform to general principles and may also involve Z-plasties or local flap closures. Linear scar formation must be prevented. Flexor and extensor tendons should be centralized to avoid creation of dynamic forces causing subsequent deformity. Collateral ligaments attached to the lateral portions of the corresponding phalanges must be transferred to the remaining phalanx to provide joint stability. The alignment of joints and angulatory deformity of the fingers, with their corresponding epiphysis, must be corrected by wedge osteotomies proximal to the deformity. If this is not done, the joint functions in an improper access, and the epiphyseal growth and angular deformity are accentuated. When duplication occurs at a joint, the head of the proximal phalanx of the metacarpal will be abnormally large to accommodate the double articulation, and partial excision of the head may be necessary to reduce the bulk. When there is duplication of the proximal phalanx or any part of the metacarpal, most of the intrinsic muscles attach to the radial component. These muscles must be transferred to the remaining component to provide proper function. In Group I duplication, with symmetrical parallel duplication of the distal phalanx, a Bihout Colquett procedure, consisting of central wedge resection of the distal phalanx, has been described by Barsky.[110] The technique presents several problems. It is difficult to take out significant bone to reduce the thumb to normal size. Approximating the distal phalanges is difficult, because the head of the proximal phalanx is broad and the collateral ligaments are tight. The slanted epiphysis may or may not accommodate as growth proceeds. The nail bed and matrix require accurate repair. This procedure appears simple upon initial evaluation but is not easy.

Asymmetrical duplication of the distal phalanx, also Group I, requires removal of the least normal-appearing component. The collateral ligament from the outer side of the amputated phalanx should be preserved and transferred to the remaining phalanx to afford joint stability. The extensor tendon and flexor tendon should be centralized. The angular deformity of the interphalangeal joint and distal phalanx is corrected with an osteotomy at the distal end of the proximal phalanx. Fixation is obtained using a Kirschner wire. With correction of the angulatory deformity, the flexor and extensor tendons will usually shift into the longitudinal axis of the thumb.

In Group II, with duplication of the proximal phalanx, the radial component is usually not developed as well as the ulnar component. Extensor tendons are bifurcated with a common hood. The flexor tendons are also bifurcated at the level of the duplication. This is usually a more severe angulatory deformity, with the proximal phalanges deviating outward and the distal phalanges deviating inward. Treatment consists of excising the less dominant thumb, decreasing the size of the distal articular surface of the metacarpal head, transferring the collateral ligaments to the remaining phalanx, and reattaching the intrinsic muscles to the extensor hood. Osteotomy of the metacarpal, as well as the distal phalanx, may be necessary to obtain correct longitudinal alignment of the digit, where the epiphyses are perpendicular to the longitudinal alignment of the thumb. A single intermedullary Kirschner wire can be used to secure both osteotomies. In Group III, the thenar muscles may be duplicated, with each set attaching to their respective digits; the muscles attached to the radial digit are the least hypoplastic. Both sets are preserved and reattached to the extensor mechanism or to the remaining digit. The base of the metacarpal is not reconstructed. As one example of Group IV deformity, the metacarpal or the radial deformity is defective at the proximal end and the ulna component is defective at the distal end. Both components will have adequate tendons, but the intrinsic and extrinsic structures are attached to the well-developed metacarpal. Reconstruction requires transposition of the distal radial component to the proximal ulna component, establishing proper length to provide balanced tension for the multi-tendinous structures (Fig. 17-31*C*). Inadequate web space is dealt with in the same manner as discussed previously. For complete operative details see Marks and Bayne.[115]

Polydactyly of the Fingers

The most common duplication of the fingers is the fifth digit. Duplication of the fifth digit can range from an extra soft-tissue mass, connected only by soft-tissue pedicle, or partial duplication of the digit involving the phalanges or proximal metacarpal. When the extra digit is attached only by a soft-tissue pedicle, simple excision is all that is necessary. However, when the duplication is more complicated, involving the metacarpals and phalanges, the abnormal anatomy must be considered. Neurovascular aberrancies are common. A single flexor tendon may be found to bifurcate at various levels, supplying the parent and duplicated digit. However, in most instances, the bifurcation of the flexor extensor tendons will occur at the point of duplication. Neurovascular structures were also bifurcated at the point of duplication. Central polydactyly frequently presents with associated complex syndactyly. Cases have been described in which an extra finger is hidden in the syndactylized mass. In these particular fingers, the joints are stiff and incongruous. Tethering of the epiphysis causes deviation of the phalanges. Frequently, one or more digits have decreased longitudinal growth potential.

Treatment. Recommended treatment of polydactyly is said to require no ingenuity and creates no problem; one is merely to remove an extra digit and soft tissue. Such a relaxed attitude toward polydactyly can lead to significant complications. Duplication of digits must be thoroughly examined for functional capacity. X-rays often make the selection of the dominant finger obvious, yet a hypoplastic digit with better motion is more valuable to a hand than a normal-appearing finger that has no function. In general, extra digits present a psychological handicap to a child, and parents are usually quite anxious for their removal. The presence of duplicated digits will cause growth disturbances, resulting in angulation.

Surgical correction in polydactyly should be completed by the time that the child is 3 or 4 years of age, if possible. Treatment of postaxial polydactyly depends on the structures duplicated. The most functional of the two digits is selected. Exposure and ablation are gained through a racket-type incision. Skin coverage is always adequate when ablation is considered. In designing skin flaps, longitudinal straight scars are avoided. Remember that excess skin can always be trimmed. Collateral ligaments and flexor and extensor tendons are identified. The extra digit is excised, carefully preserving the collateral ligament or reconstructing one from the periosteum and capsule. The extensor tendon is examined, and the bifurcated portion of the ablated digit is removed, saving a portion of the tendon to act as a retinacular ligament. The articular surface of the enlarged proximal phalanx, or metacarpal head, is examined. A ridge is invariably present, separating the individual articular surfaces. The metacarpal head and a portion of the shaft are reduced by osteotomizing the metacarpal or phalanx parallel to the ridge and the articular surface. If necessary, an osteotomy of the metacarpal is performed for better longitudinal alignment of the digit. Collateral ligaments are reattached, as are the hypothenar muscles. Kirschner wires are necessary to hold the digit in proper alignment and to protect the collateral ligament repair. The Kirschner wires are usually removed at 3 weeks, and the finger is then started on mobilization.

Surgery for central polydactyly is challenging, and results are less satisfying. Many patients present with complex syndactyly. Aberrant neurovascular structures must be delineated. Wood[120] and Flatt[112] recall many surgical disasters in their attempts to maintain a four-fingered hand. They found that frequently the three-fingered hand was more functional than one with four digits, requiring multiple procedures. The most useful parts are salvaged, and heroic attempts to save functional digits are avoided.

GIGANTISM OF THE FINGERS

Clinical Features

Gigantism in fingers may also be termed *macrodactyly*. It is characterized by an increased size of all structures of a finger, including the bony phalanges, tendons, nerves, blood vessels, fat, fingernails, and skin. Macrodactyly must be distinguished from other causes of finger enlargement, such as neurofibroma, hemangioma, lymphangioma, arteriovenous fistula, fibrous dysplasia, and lipoma.[121]

In true macrodactyly, there is usually no family history of the condition. It is more common in males than females. One type usually stops growing at puberty, whereas the second type continues to enlarge the soft tissues after bony growth ceases, resulting in a tremendously large finger. The most frequently involved single finger is the index finger, followed closely by the long finger (Fig. 17-32) and then the thumb and ring fingers, in decreasing occurrence. Some cases show multiple finger involvement, usually two fingers. The most common pair of involved fingers are the index and long fingers; the thumb and

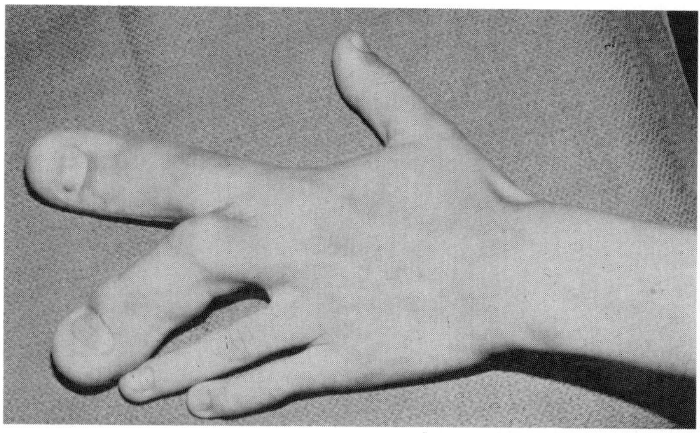
FIG. 17-32. Dorsal view of gigantism of the index and long fingers.

index finger are almost as commonly involved. Slightly less frequently, the long and ring fingers are involved. The little finger seems to be strangely free of this type of involvement. Of the cases of gigantism with multiple digital involvement, about 10% also have syndactyly of the fingers. Syndactyly involving the index and long fingers is probably the most common, followed closely by the syndactyly of the long and ring fingers.

About 5% of the patients with macrodactyly have bilateral involvement. There may occasionally be pedal gigantism along with the hand involvement. Associated systemic anomalies are uncommon. The roentgenogram shows larger-than-normal bones of the involved finger or fingers. The metacarpals are moderately enlarged, but the phalanges are markedly enlarged. In some patients at the age of 7 or 8 years, the finger or fingers are already of adult size.

Treatment

If untreated, these hands acquire a cosmetically unsatisfactory appearance. At cessation of growth, the involved fingers are one and one half to two times the normal circumference and about one and one half times as long as the other fingers. Cosmesis becomes an increasingly important factor as the child gets older. If seen early, no treatment is indicated. The child should be followed at regular intervals until age 7 or 8 years, and then, if the involved digit or digits are of a size comparable to that of the fingers of the parents, epiphysiodesis of the metacarpal and all three phalanges is performed. If the child is not treated until he is 9 or 10 or more years, the involved fingers will be too large for the other fingers to catch up with them. The affected fingers therefore require some sort of bone shortening, at one or more levels, and narrowing of the bone structure, defatting of the finger, and narrowing of the nail and the terminal phalanx. Cosmetically, the child treated late in childhood incurs poor results, whereas the child treated at age 7 or 8 years shows considerably less difference in finger size when fully grown.[122]

The treatment of gigantism due to neurofibroma requires the same bone treatment, but, in addition, defatting, partial nerve resection, and carpal tunnel release are needed to allow for the usually marked enlargement of the median nerve. Gigantism due to hemangiomas or arteriovenous fistulas requires the appropriate treatment for these respective conditions, which is limited resection of the involved tissues. Occasionally, amputation is necessary in conditions in which there is erosion of the skin and the life-endangering episodes of hemorrhage.

CONSTRICTING BANDS

Clinical Features

Much confusion exists as to the cause of this condition. Constriction by the umbilical cord or amniotic bands is frequently mentioned, and the common association of shortened or partially absent phalanges suggests that there must be a common cause. Recent experimental work tends to show that this may be due to an injury to the fetal extremity in early stages of gestation.

The constricting band may be a partially or completely encircling ring or band. There may

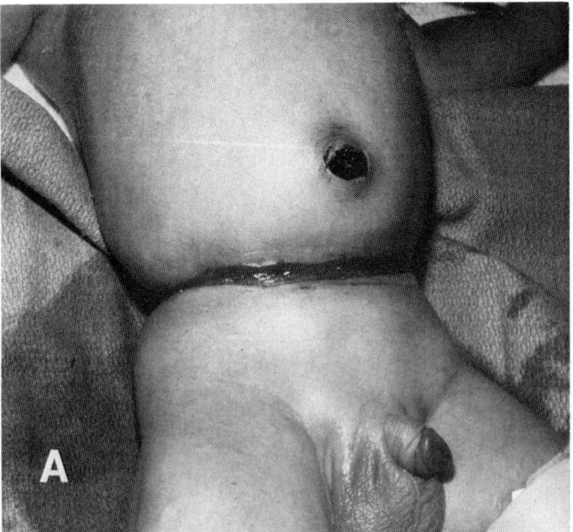

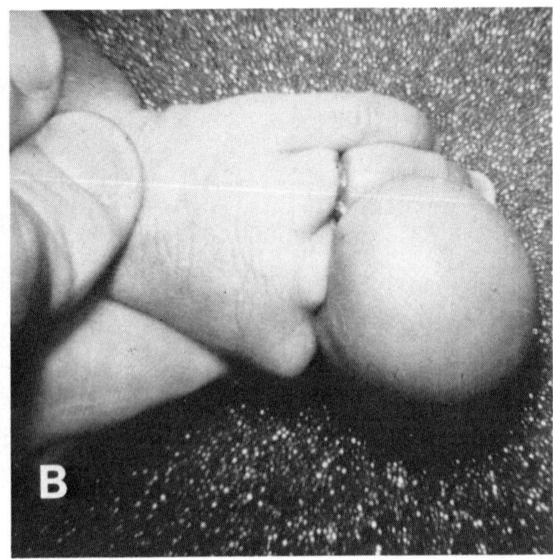

FIG. 17-33. (*A*) A newborn with a constricting band encircling the body at trunk level, with loss of skin and fat at the level of band. (*B*) Dorsal view of an edematous long finger from a constricting band on long finger. There is amputation of the index finger, and another band is present on the ring finger.

be single or multiple bands involving single or multiple fingers. They may also be associated with similar bands involving the hand, forearm, or upper arm and may be accompanied by similar bands around the toes, feet, lower leg, or thigh. The abdomen and thorax are also occasionally encircled by constricting bands. The depth of the constricting bands varies, and the bands may be deep enough to result in circulatory embarassment and, occasionally, to late nerve involvement.

Some bands seem to slowly deepen with growth, which probably indicates lack of growth at the area of the band, and, therefore, there is a slowly increasing tourniquet effect. Edema and a fluid-filled distal part may result. Gangrene may occur if release of the constriction is not done early. This type of involvement is usually seen in the newborn or very young and demands release of the constricting band, because the increasing edema tends to further constrict circulation to the finger.

The relation between constricting bands and ainhum is not clear, but they are probably different conditions. The latter condition is not present at birth and appears at a later time. Constricting bands are probably not inherited, although there are some reports of a recessive inheritance. The most severe form of constricting bands may be associated with the absence of a phalanx or phalanges, and the associated metacarpals may also be absent (Fig. 17-33).

Treatment

Constricting bands as severe as those shown in Figure 17-33*B* should be operated on within 24 hours if the baby's condition warrants it in order to save the finger or fingers. The usual surgical treatment is delayed until age 2 years or later, unless interference with circulation is noted. Multiple Z-plasties are necessary in most cases; at least two Z-plasties are needed for a completely encircling band. Constricting bands at the proximal phalanx, near the metacarpal head, are probably better treated with a Y-V procedure. The Y-V procedure can also be combined with a Z-plasty, if necessary. The Y-V procedure on the dorsal surface over the metacarpal head or base of the proximal phalanx yields a less obvious scar than a Z-plasty at this level. Correction of one half of the circumference at a time is recommended for safety.

MADELUNG'S DEFORMITY

Clinical Features and Diagnosis

This is probably not a true congenital deformity, because it is not present at birth. It is, however, known to be inherited as an autosomal dominant condition. It is more common in females than in males (4:1), and it is frequently bilateral (2:1).

Roentgenograms reveal that the changes begin to appear at age 2 years. The ulnar and volar half of the distal radial epiphysis does

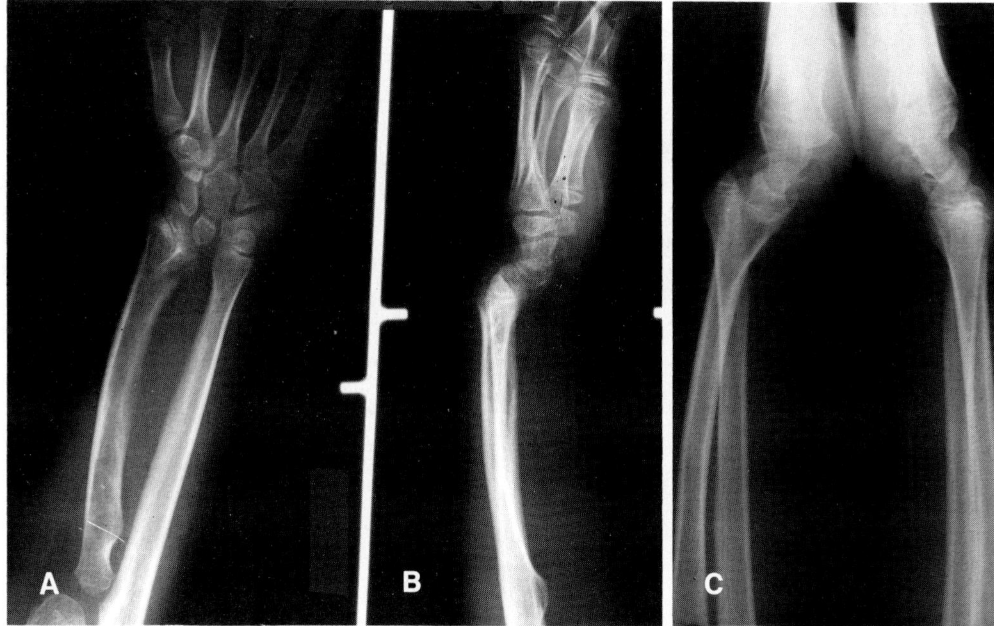

FIG. 17-34. (*A*) Anteroposterior roentgenogram of Madelung's deformity of the left wrist. (*B*) One year and 4 months later, there is a worsening of the deformity. (*C*) Lateral view showing overgrowth and prominence of the distal ulna as compared to the normal wrist (*right*).

not grow as rapidly as the radial half. This results in a radius whose ulnar half is shorter than the radial half, and there is a curving toward the ulnar side. The volar part of the ulnar half of the epiphysis is also involved in the delayed growth, so that the radius curves volarward and ulnarward, simultaneously. This results in dorsal prominence of the distal ulna and, subsequently, greater ulnar length (Fig. 17-34). The combination of these factors leads to limited dorsiflexion of the wrist, with resultant loss of supination. The proximal end of the radius is usually normal but may occasionally be somewhat deformed. There are many other bony anomalies frequently associated with this condition, and there are many reports concerning their relationships, including such anomalies as scoliosis, cervical ribs, defects of the humerus, and many types of bony anomalies of the lower extremities. In recent years, deformities of Hurler's and Morquio's syndromes and the association of these with mucopolysaccharidosis have been studied and compared with Madelung's deformity.

Treatment

Occasionally a patient with Madelung's deformity may be diagnosed at age 8 or 9 years. The epiphyses are still open, and the central volar tethering of the distal radial epiphysis can be excised. The epiphyseal plate is elevated, and a piece of silastic or liquid silastic can be inserted after lifting up or levering the joint surface into a more normal position. This may prevent such severe volar angulation of the distal joint surface and allow more longitudinal growth. After closure of the epiphyses, osteotomy of the radius to correct the volar and ulnar angulation can be done, as can a limited resection of the distal ulna. Resection of the extra length of the ulna must be accompanied by reconstruction of the ulnar carpal ligament and the ulnar radial ligaments to prevent the distal radial ulnar instability so commonly seen when excessive bone is removed. There is rarely a great degree of loss of function of the fingers in this condition. Most of the lost function is in dorsiflexion of the wrist; there is usually good residual supination and finger function.

SPRENGEL'S DEFORMITY (CONGENITAL ELEVATION OF THE SCAPULA)

Clinical Features

This condition was described by Eulenberg[125] in 1863. It is an uncommon congenital anomaly characterized by elevation and medial rotation of the inferior pole of the scapula. The elevation may vary from 2 cm to 10 cm. The deformity is usually unilateral but may be bilateral. It is frequently associated with other deformities of the cervical and thoracic spine, such as hemivertebrae[127] and fusion or absence of the ribs.

Congenital elevation of the scapula occurs as a result of interruption of the normal caudal migration of the scapula, probably occurring between the 9th and 12th week of gestation. There have been several theories to explain the apparent arrest in development, the most comprehensive of which are those of Horwitz[127] and Engel.[124]

There is also an arrest in development of bone, cartilage, and muscle. The trapezius, rhomboids, or levator scapulae muscles may be absent or hypoplastic, or they may contain multiple fibrous adhesions. The serratus anterior muscle may be weak, leading to winging of the scapula. Other muscles, such as the pectoralis major, may also be absent or hypoplastic.

The affected scapula is usually small, with a decreased vertical length and anterior bending of the upper portion. There may be a bony, cartilaginous or fibrous connection to the cervical or upper thoracic spine.[128] The connection may be to the lamina, to the transverse process, or to the spinous process of the vertebrae and may be single or multiple. Occasionally, the connection is by bone, and, if so, this bone is known as the omovertebral bone.[126]

Diagnosis

Roentgenograms are necessary to determine the degree of development of the scapula, the degree of angular deformity, the presence or absence of a connection to the cervical or thoracic spine, and the presence or absence of an omovertebral bone (Fig. 17-35).

The clinical examination shows the amount of elevation and the presence or absence of

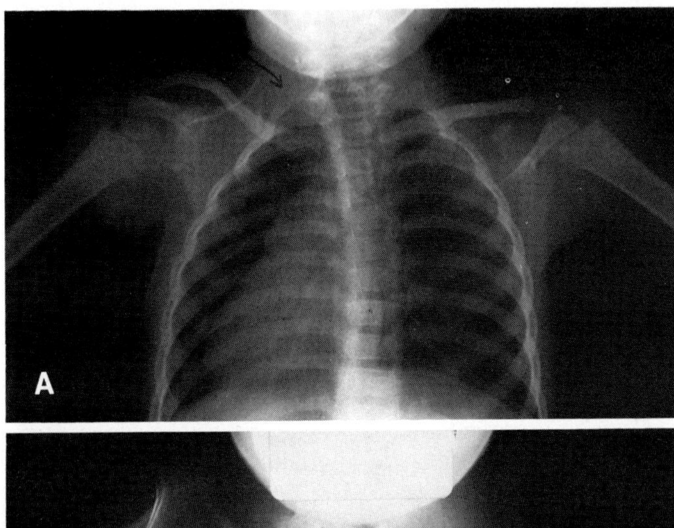

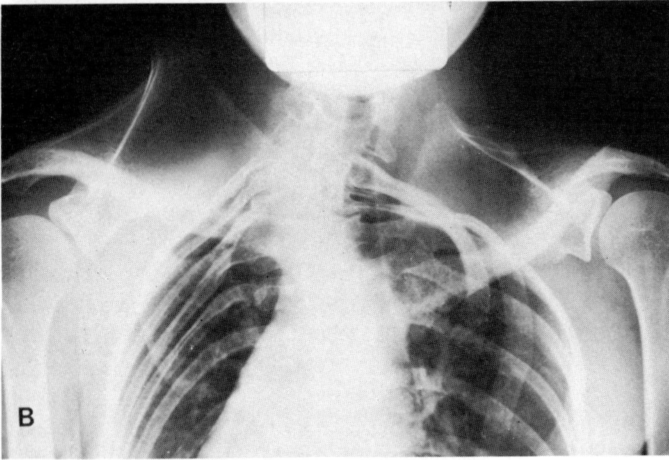

FIG. 17-35. (*A*) Anteroposterior roentgenogram of a unilateral Sprengel's deformity, showing an elevated and slightly rotated left scapula. The arrow points to the region of the tethering. (*B*) Bilateral Sprengel's deformity. The right scapula is severely rotated, the left moderately so. Note the scoliosis, a condition frequently concomitant with Sprengel's deformity.

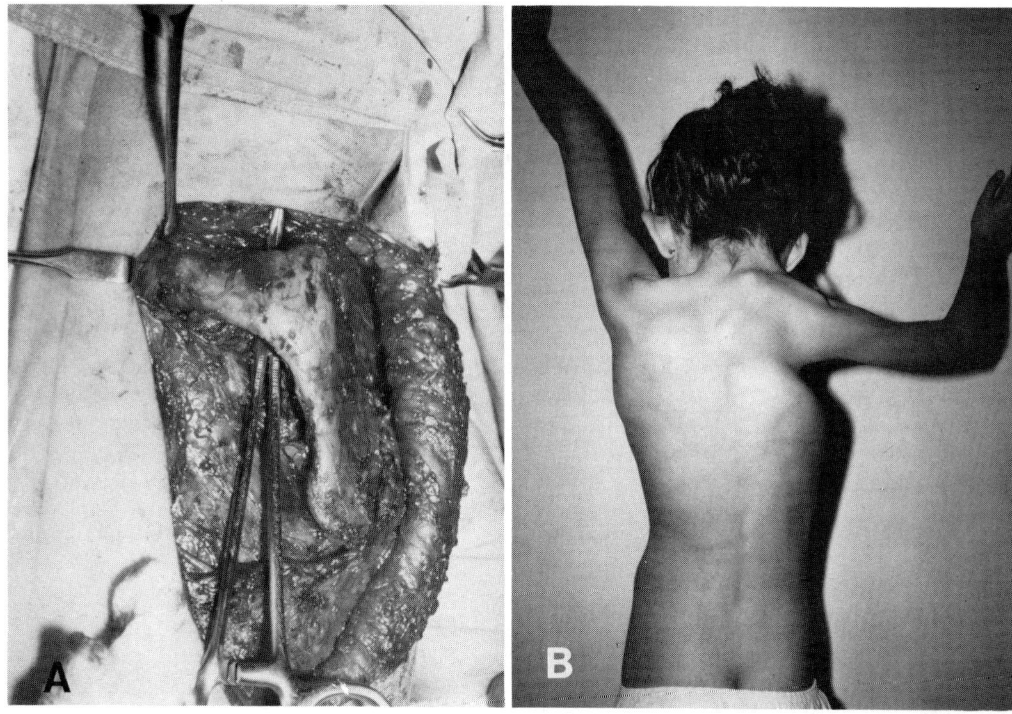

FIG. 17-36. (*A*) In this patient, there is an omovertebral bone connecting the cervical spine and the scapula. (*B*) Posterior view of a patient with a right Sprengel's deformity, showing the typical loss of shoulder abduction and elevation.

an associated torticollis,[129] with or without muscle contraction. The limitation of abduction of the shoulder is generally proportional to the severity of angulation and elevation of the scapula (Fig. 17-36). For differential diagnosis, the muscle examination should rule out paralysis of the serratus anterior muscle and obstetric or birth paralyses. The degree of fixation of the scapula should be determined, as well as the quantity of malrotation and malposition. The muscles about the shoulder should be tested as thoroughly as possible, which may be quite difficult with the fixed position of the scapula.

Treatment

The treatment of choice is surgery. The deformity does not progress, but it does not spontaneously improve without surgery. Conservative treatment does not result in any improvement. Physical therapy is also not helpful.

Numerous surgical treatments have been described. The basic goal of surgery is to lower the scapula to a more normal position and to decrease its fixation or, conversely, to increase its mobility. The Schrock[128] procedure was used in the past, but it involved only excision of the upper portion of the scapula; it neither lowered the body of the scapula nor increased mobility. This procedure is not recommended.

The two procedures that have had the best results are the Green[126] and Woodward[129] procedures. The Green procedure consists of an extraperiosteal dissection of the muscles from the scapula, resection of the upper corner of the scapula, which is affixed over the upper aspect of the first rib, insertion of a pull-out wire to pull the scapula down, resuturing of the scapula at a lower level, and reattachment of the muscles in a more anatomic position. This is followed by a period of traction, in which the scapula is gradually pulled down by rubberband traction attached to the wire. The rubberband is attached to a hip spica.

The Woodward procedure uses somewhat of a different approach. A midline incision is made rather than a scapular incision as in the Green procedure. Basically, in the Woodward procedure, the trapezius and rhomboid muscles are released at their point of origin along the spinous processes. After division of the levator scapula from the scapulae, the scapula is then lowered and derotated, and the previously detached muscle sheet is attached to the spinous process in a more inferior position. However, the caudal displacement of the scapula is preceded by resection of any prominent superiomedial border, anterior curved supraspinatus portion, or ulnovertebral connection, as well as the clavicular osteotomy. Details of this procedure may be obtained from the original description by Woodward;[129] however, several technical points should be emphasized. In their review of cases treated by the Woodward procedure, Carson, Lovell, and Whitesides,[123] pointed out that prior to the scapula exposure, the patient should be placed in the supine position and an osteotomy of the middle third of the clavicle should be performed first to prevent undue compression of the neurovascular structures at the thoracic outlet when the scapula is lowered. They noted that care must be taken to ensure that the correct fascial plane be entered, because an intact aponeurosis or muscle sheet is essential for the success of the operation. They also noted that the spinal accessory nerve on the under surface of the trapezius and the transverse cervical artery on the superiomedial border of the scapula must be avoided. They believe that an adequate release of all binding structures must be accomplished. If the supraspinatus portion of the scapula is curved anteriorly over the upper part of the thorax, it must be resected so that it will not impair downward displacement. They also stated that preoperative scapular winging is a relative contraindication to the Woodward procedure.

Carson, Lovell, and Whitesides[123] believe that the ideal surgical candidate is a child with congenital elevation of the scapula, between 3 and 8 years of age, with a moderate to severe cosmetic deformity and a moderate to severe functional impairment of the shoulder abduction (usually less than 120°), whose associated congenital anomalies are not contraindications to operation.

In general, this combined procedure of clavicular osteotomy coupled with the Woodward procedure has given consistently good results, in terms of the cosmetic appearance of the scapula, as well as providing improved motion, particularly in elevation. Only those patients with severe deficits of motor muscle function to the shoulder girdle have not benefited functionally from this operation. The ideal age for surgery is between 4 and 7 years, but it has been done in both younger and older children.

BIRTH INJURIES OF THE BRACHIAL PLEXUS (OBSTETRIC PARALYSIS)

Paralysis of the upper extremity is not a congenital defect, but because it occurs at birth, it was thought necessary to include this subject in the discussion of the upper limb. The paralysis of the upper extremity that occurs during birth is produced by excessive stretching or contusion of the brachial plexus. The injury most frequently occurs when there is a prolonged or difficult delivery, complicated by a large fetus and narrow pelvis.

The incidence of obstetric parralysis has steadily decreased with the improvement in obstetric management. Adler and Patterson[30] noted in their study, which was conducted at the Hospital of Special Surgery in New York, that the incidence of this complication had decreased from 1.56 per 1000 live births in 1938, to 0.38 per 1000 live births in 1962.

The diagnosis of brachial plexus injury in the newborn is not difficult. The extremity is noted to lie lifelessly by the side of the infant, and passive range of motion is equal on both sides (Fig. 17-37*A*). If active and passive range of motion is restricted, injury to the humerus or clavicle should be suspected. Radiographs of the upper extremity of all infants with suspected paralysis should be obtained routinely.

In the older child, with varying degree of recovery, diagnosis can be made by the findings of residual deformity due to muscle imbalance. The patient will usually be seen to hold the elbow away from the side of the body and partially abducted (Fig. 17-37*B*). There will also be a notable loss of the humeral scapular rhythm (Fig. 17-37*C*). In the older child with a long-standing deformity, it may be noted that the humerus will be short, and the radiographic findings may show the acromion to be hooked or elongated and pointing inferiorly. Shoulder subluxation, or dislocation, has been noted in patients with long-standing deformity. Radial head displacement can also be noted in patients with residual contractures of the elbow. X-rays should always be taken when severe contractures are present. Also, in patients with long-standing contracture about the shoulder, radiographs

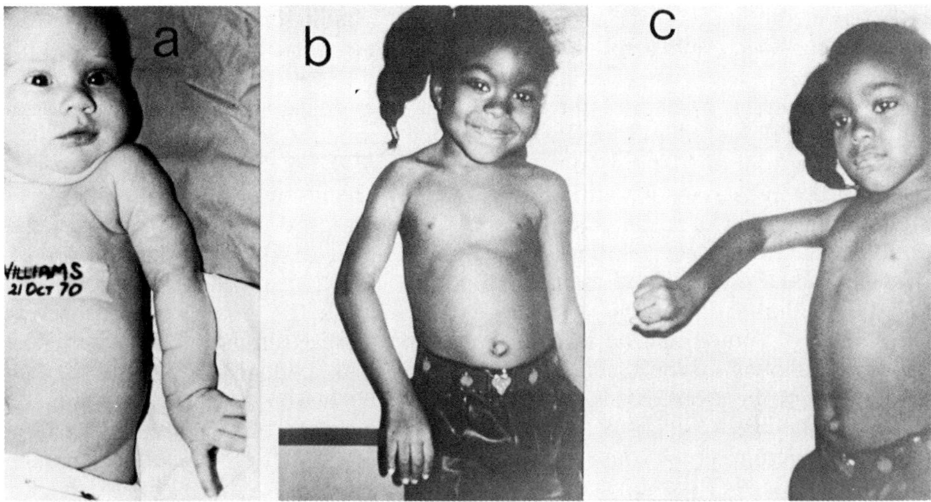

FIG. 17-37. Obstetric paralysis. (*a*) When obstetric paralysis is seen early, the hand lies lifeless beside the infant, internally rotated and extended. (*b*) In the older child, the attitude of the affected extremity is shown. The arm is abducted and internally rotated. (*c*) Contracture of the shoulder and absence of shoulder abductor are the frequent residual.

may show a flattening of the head of the humerus and a shallowing of the glenoid cup.

It is extremely difficult to accurately localize the anatomic lesions in the newborn and in the older patients due to the overlap and innervation of muscles by different trunks of the brachial plexus. However, as recovery progresses, definite areas of involvement can be determined, and these have been classified as to the area of the extremity involvement, as well as to the area of plexus involvement.

The Upper Plexus, or Arm (Erb-Duchenne–Type), C4, C5, and C6

When the primary involvement is confined to the shoulder and the arm, the lesion most likely involves the C4, C5, and C6 cervical root. These lesions are characterized by adduction internal rotational contractures of the shoulder and loss of the extension of the elbow. Where there is mild involvement, the suprascapular nerve may be the only area of injury that would result in paralysis of the supraspinatus and infraspinatus muscles. When there is more extensive involvement of this area, the deltoid and the external rotators of the shoulder, as well as the flexors of the elbow and brachioradialis may be involved. Wickstrom[138] found in his review of cases that the predominant number of patients were in the upper arm category.

The second type is the whole plexus or arm type (the Erb-Duchenne-Klumpke's–type). This category represents the more severe involvement of the upper extremity, with both sensory and motor paralysis, and is usually due to a severe injury to the roots of the brachial plexus. Wickstrom[138] noted that 22 of his 87 cases were in this category.

The third category is the lower plexus, or arm type (Klumpke's). The muscles of the forearm and hand, together with parts of the cervical sympathetic system, are paralyzed and represent an injury to the C8, T1 root area. When the first thoracic root is involved, usually a Horner syndrome will be present. Eleven of the 87 cases reviewed by Wickstrom[138] were in this category.

Treatment

The main aim of treatment is to prevent contracture of the upper extremity while awaiting neurologic recovery. Treatment can be divided into early or late, depending on the stage at which the patient is first seen. In the early paralysis stage, positional splinting is indicated during the normal rest periods; otherwise, range-of-motion exercises are carried out at each diaper change. Continuous splinting is contraindicated, because it may cause positional contractures and may promote subluxations and dislocations of the shoulder and radial head. Splinting of the wrist, elbow, and shoulder in an Orthoplast splint, similar to that described by Wickstrom,[138] is carried out for the first 3 months. The splint places the shoulder in 90° of abduction, 45° of flexion, and 45° of external rotation. The elbow is flexed at 80°, and the wrists are flexed in slight extension, with a platform for the fingers. The abduction and external rotation of the shoulders is gradually decreased at monthly intervals. The splint is discontinued in the daytime at the end of 3 months and is used only for nighttime splinting for the succeeding 3 months. Range-of-motion exercises are carried out through this entire period of time. Most patients will begin to show some recovery, starting at 2 weeks. As function returns, the splint is deleted. At 6 months, the patient is maintained on range-of-motion exercises only. Recovery can be expected, however, up to 18 months of age. Humeral scapular motion should be encouraged during range-of-motion exercises by stabilizing the scapula and actively and passively abducting the humerus.

Surgical treatment may be indicated to restore lost function in the older patient. The timing of surgery should be delayed until the patient is 4 years of age unless the deformity is increasing rapidly despite conservative treatment. Surgery is primarily directed toward increasing the functional level of the upper extremity. In most instances, surgery has been directed toward increasing abduction and external rotation of the shoulder, and in the more severely involved cases, simple osteotomy has been performed to place the extremity in a more functional position. Fairbanks[131] and Sever[137] describe procedures that essentially release the contracting forces about the shoulder when function could be demonstrated in the external rotators and abductors of the shoulder. Operation, however, did not improve strength of the shoulder or increase function to an appreciable degree. L'Episcopo[134] combined the Fairbanks-Sever procedure with a transfer of the released latissimus dorsi and teres major muscles at their insertions and converted them to external rotators by passing them around the outer border of the upper humerus and reattaching them to the divided stump of the subscapularis muscle. Hoffer, Wickenden, and Roper[133] reported a modification of the L'Episcopo procedure, dividing the teres major and latissimus dorsi tendons through a posterior approach and reattaching them through the rotator cuff as near to the attachment of the supraspinatus tendon as possible. They thought that this procedure had the advantage of being easily performed and increased active external rotation. They also thought that it enhanced the stabilizing effect of the rotator cuff and increased glenohumeral abduction, because it enabled the deltoid to be more effective. They reported an average gain of 64° of abduction and 45° of external rotation in the 11 patients they treated by this method. Treatment of lower plexes, or arm type (Klumpke's), is primarily directed toward increasing extension of the wrist and elbow flexion. Various tendon transfers are used to increase wrist extension, as well as elbow flexion. For explanation and discussion of these procedures, the reader is referred to the review article by Leffert.[135]

In general, the prognosis of birth-induced palsy of the brachial plexus is not as severe as previous reviews have indicated. Most recent studies have shown that a considerable number of these patients will recover completely. One series showed that approximately 80% of the children were completely recovered by 13 months of age, and none of those with significant residual defects had any sensory or motor deficits in the hand.[132] Therefore, it would seem that an approach of cautious optimism should be taken in discussing the prognosis of this lesion with the parents in the neonatal period.

The development of microsurgical techniques on peripheral nerves offers new possibilities. Epineurectomy and internal neurolysis in cases of interfascicular fibrosis are possible by this technique without the risk of damage to intact fascicles in patients with partial lesions or lesions of different degrees of damage. Nerve grafting can be used to bridge large defects, and transfer of intercostal nerves to imposter trunks of the plexus are possible in supraganglionic lesions. The work of Millesi[136] and others may improve the function of the more severely involved patients.

OSTEOCHONDRITIS DISSECANS OF THE ELBOW

Clinical features

Osteochondritis dissecans of the elbow (Fig. 17-38) is probably not a congenital lesion, but it is seen predominantly in adolescent males.[139,140] Although trauma is frequently blamed, it has not been definitely linked to this condition. Clinically, the onset is insidious

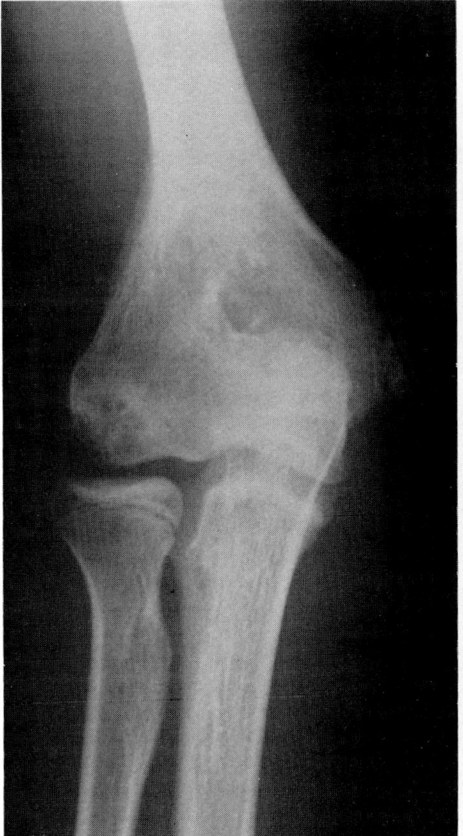
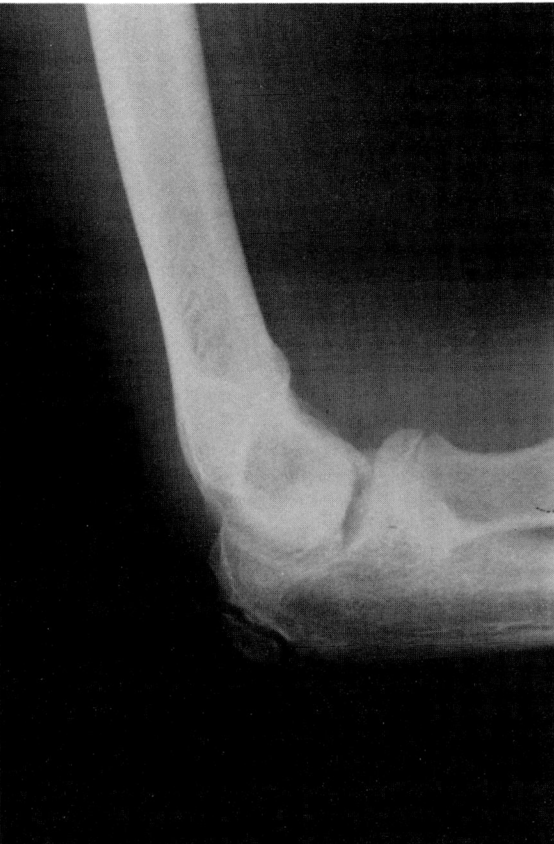

FIG. 17-38. Osteochondritis of the elbow.

and may be manifested by a dull aching pain and slight limitation of motion. Occasionally a loose body may separate and cause locking of the elbow, followed by pain and effusion. It may be a silent lesion, which is discovered only accidentally on a roentgenogram taken for another condition. The radial head may become enlarged clinically, and this is confirmed by roentgenogram. The early roentgenographic changes are rarefaction of a small area in the capitellum and, later, separation of a small fragment, leaving a small punched-out cavity. This usually results in a loose body that locks the elbow.

Treatment

Treatment should not be surgical unless locking occurs or the presence of loose body can be proved by roentgenogram. Conservative treatment, consisting of rest and limited activities, including the use of a sling or posterior splint, if necessary, can result in healing of the bone lesion if treatment is undertaken before separation of the fragment occurs. The radial head should not be resected in children with this condition.[141] Resection should be reserved for adults, but only after marked degenerative changes and limitation of motion has resulted.

REFERENCES

Classification of Upper Limb Malformations

1. Swanson AB: A classification for congenital limb malformations. J Hand Surg 1(1):8–21, 1976

Congenital Amputations

2. Barsky AJ, Kahn S, Simon BE: Congenital anomalies of the hand. Reconstr Plast Surg Philadelphia, WB Saunders, 1964
3. Birch-Jensen A: Congenital deformities of the upper extremities. Andelsbogtrykkeriet and Det Danske Forlag, Odense, Denmark, pp 15–26, 1949
4. Clippinger FW, Avery R, Titus BR: A sensory feedback system for an upper limb amputation prothesis. Bull Prosthet Res 10:247, 1974
5. Kelikian H: Congenital Deformities of the Hand and Forearm. Philadelphia, WB Saunders, 1974

6. Kritter AE: The bilateral upper extremity Amputee. Orthop Clin North Am 3:419, 1972
7. Swanson AB: The Krukenberg procedure in the juvenile amputee. J Bone Joint Surg (Am) 46A:1540–1548, 1964
8. Temtamy SA, McKusick VA: Birth Defects 14:73, 1978

Phocomelia

9. Birch-Jensen A: Congenital Deformities of the Upper Extremities. Andelsbogtrykkeriet, Odense, Denmark, 1949
10. Flatt AE: The Care of Congenital Hand Anomalies. St Louis, CV Mosby, p 41, 1977
11. Kelikian H: Congenital Deformities of the Hand and Forearm. Philadelphia, WB Saunders, pp 891–901, 1974

Congenital Absence of the Radius

12. Buck-Gramcko D: Pollicization of the index finger. Method and results in aplasia and hypoplasia of the thumb. J Bone Joint Surg 53A:1605, 1971
13. Lamb DW: The treatment of radial club hand. Absent radius, aplasia of the radius, hypoplasia of the radius, radial paraxial hemimelia. Hand 4:22, 1972
14. Lamb DW: Radial club hand. A continuing study of 68 patients with 117 club hands. J Bone Joint Surg 59A: 1977
15. Littler JW: The neurovascular pedicle method of digital transposition for reconstruction of the thumb. Plast Reconstr Surg 12:303 1953
16. O'Rahilly R: Radial hemimelia and the functional anatomy of the carpus. J Anat 80:179, 1946
17. Riordan DC: Congenital absence of the radius. J Bone Joint Surg 37A:1129, 1955
18. Riordan DC: Congenital absence of radius: A 15-year follow-up study. [Proc Am Orthop Assoc] J Bone Joint Surg 45A:1783, 1963
19. Tachdjian, MO: Pediatric Orthopedics. Philadelphia, WB Saunders, 1972

Hypoplastic Thumb

20. Buck-Gramco D: Congenital malformations of the hand: Indications, operative treatment, and results. Scand J Plast Reconstr Surg 9:190–193, 1975
21. Buncke H: Toe digital transfer. Clin Plast Surg 3:49–57, 1976
22. Carroll RE: Insertion of toe phalangeal grafts in hypoplastic digits. In Flatt AE, (ed): The Care of Congenital Hand Anomalies. St Louis, CV Mosby, 1977
23. Carroll RE, Green DP: Reconstruction of hypoplastic digits using two phalanges. J Bone Joint Surg 57A:727, 1975
24. Clarkson P: Reconstruction of hand digits by toe transfers. J Bone Joint Surg 37:270–276, 1955
25. Cowen NJ, Loftus JM: Distraction, augmentation, manoplasty: Technique for lengthening digits for the entire hand. Orthop Rev 7(6):45–53, 1978
26. Flatt AE: The Care of Congenital Hand Anomalies. St Louis, CV Mosby, 1977
27. Hentz VR, Littler JW: Adduction, pronation, and recession of the second metacarpal in thumb agenesis. J Hand Surg 2:113, 1977
28. Kessler I, Baruch A, Hecht O: Experience with distraction lengthening of distal rays in congenital anomalies. J Hand Surg 2(5):394–401, 1977
29. Littler JW: Introduction to surgery of the hand. Reconstr Plast Surg 4:1543–1546, 1964
30. Matev IB: Thumb reconstruction in children through metacarpal lengthening. Plast Reconstr Surg 64(5):665–669, 1979
31. O'Brien BM, Franklin JD, Morrison WA, MacLeod AM: Replantation and revascularization surgery in children. Hand 12(1):12–24, 1980
32. Riordan DC: Pediatric Orthopaedics, Vol II, pp 708–714. Philadelphia, JB Lippincott, 1978
33. Temtamy SA, McKusick VA: Birth Defects 14: 1977
34. Van Beek AL, Wavak PW, Zook EG: Microvascular surgery in children. Plast Reconstr Surg 63:457–462, 1979

Congenital Absence of the Thumb

35. Buck-Gramcko D: Operativer Daumener—staz bei Aplasia und Hypoplosie. Verh Dtsch Orthop Ges 55:417, 1968
36. Buck-Gramcko D: Pollicization of the index finger. Method and results in aplasia and hypoplasia of the thumb. J Bone Joint Surg 53A:1065, 1971
37. Littler JW: The neurovascular pedicle method of digital transposition for reconstruction of the thumb. Plast Reconstr Surg 12:303, 1953
38. Littler JW: Principles of reconstructive surgery of the hand. In Converse JM (ed): Reconstructive Plastic Surgery, Vol 4. Philadelphia, WB Saunders, 1964

Congenital Dislocation of the Shoulder

39. Cozen L: Congenital dislocation of the shoulder and other anomalies. Arch Surg 35:956, 1937
40. Whitman R: The treatment of congenital and acquired luxations at the shoulder in childhood. Ann Surg 42:110, 1905

Congenital Pseudarthrosis of the Clavicle

41. Alldred AJ: Congenital pseudarthrosis of the clavicle. J Bone Joint Surg 45B:312, 1963
42. Fitzwilliams DCL: Hereditary craniocleidodysostosis. Lancet 2:1,466, 1910

Pterygium Cubitale

43. Aarskog D: Pterygium syndrome. Birth Defects 7:232, 1971
44. Emed A: Pterygium syndrome. J Pediatr 73, 1978
45. Norum RA, James VL, Mabry CC: Pterygium syndrome in three children in a recessive pedigree pattern. Birth Defects 2:233, 1969
46. Scott CI: Pterygium syndrome. Proceedings of the First Conference on Clinical Delineation of Birth Defects. Part II: Malformation syndromes. Bergsma D (ed): Birth Defects. The National Foundation, NW, 1969
47. Warkany J: Congenital Malformations. Chicago, Year Book Medical Publishers, Inc, 1971

Arthrogryposis

48. Banker BQ, Victor M, Adams RD: Arthropgryposis multiplex due to congenital muscular dystrophy. Brain 80:319–334, 1957

49. Carroll RE: Restoration of flexor power to the flail elbow by transplantation of the triceps tendon. J Surg Gynecol Obstet 95:685–688, 1952
50. Carroll RE, Hill NA: Triceps transfer to restore elbow flexion. J Bone Joint Surg 52A:239–244, 1970
51. Clark JMP: Reconstruction of biceps brachia by pectoral muscle transplantation. Brain J Surg 34:180–181, 1946
52. Drachman DB, Banker BQ: Arthrogryposis multiplex congenita. A case due to disease of the anterior horn cells. Arch Neurol 5:77–93, 1961
53. Ferguson AB, Jr: Orthopaedic Surgery in Infancy and Childhood, pp 438–441. Baltimore, Williams & Wilkins, 1957
54. Friedlander HL, Westin GW, Wood WL: Arthrogryposis multiplex congenita. J Bone Joint Surg 50A:89, 1968
55. Hansen OM: Surgical anatomy and treatment of patients with arthrogryposis. J Bone Joint Surg 43B:855, 1961
56. Lewin P: Arthrogryposis multiplex congenita. J Bone Surg 7:630–638, 1925
57. Lloyd-Roberts GC, Lettin AWF: Arthrogryposis multiplex congenita. J Bone Joint Surg 52B:494–508, 1970
58. Mayer L, Green W: Experiences with the Steindler flexorplasty at the elbow. J Bone Joint Surg 36A:775–789, 1954
59. Mead NG, Lithgow WC, Sweeney HJ: Arthrogryposis multiplex congenita. J Bone Joint Surg 40A:1285, 1958
60. Sedon HJ: Transplantation of pectoralis major for paralysis of the flexors of the elbow. Proc R Soc Med 42:837–838, 1949

Syndactyly

61. Flatt A: Treatment of syndactylism. Plast Reconstr Surg 29:336, 1962
62. Kahn A Jr, and Fulmer J: Acrocephalosyndactylism. N Engl J Med 252:379, 1955

Camptodactyly

63. Iselin F, Levame J, Afanassief A: Les camptodactylies congenitales. [Soc Med Chir des Hôpitaux libres de Fourier, 1966] Arch Hôp 5:1, 1966.
64. Shaff B, Schafer PW: Camptodactyly. Arch Surg 57:633, 1948.
65. Smith RJ, Kaplan EB: Camptodactyly and similar atraumatic flexion deformities of the proximal interphalangeal joints of the fingers. J Bone Joint Surg 50A:1187, 1249, 1968

Clinodactyly

66. Barsky AJ: Congenital Anomalies of the Hand and Their Surgical Treatment. Springfield, Il, Charles C Thomas, 1958.
67. Doege TC, Thuline HC, Priest JH, Bryant JS: Studies of a family with the oral-facial-digital syndrome. N Engl J Med 271:1073, 1964
68. Flatt AE: The Care of Congenital Hand Anomalies. St Louis, CV Mosby, 1977
69. Hefke HW: Roentgenologic study of anomalies of hands in 100 cases of mongolism. Am J Dis Child 60:1319, 1940
70. McKusick VA: Heritable Disorders of Connective Tissue, 3rd ed. St Louis, 1966
71. Poznanski AK: The Hand in Radiologic Diagnosis, Vol 4 Philadelphia, WB Saunders, 1974
72. Warkany J: Congenital Malformations. Chicago, Year Book Medical Publishers, Inc, 1971

Trigger Thumb

73. Broadbent TR, Woolf, RM: Flexion-adduction deformity of the thumb—congenital clasp thumb. Plast Reconstr Surg, 34:612, 1964.
74. White JW, Jensen WE: The infant's persistent thumb-clutched hand, J Bone Joint Surg 34A:680, 1952

Triphalangeal Thumb

75. Barsky AJ: Congenital anomalies of the thumb. Clin Orthop 15:96, 1959
76. Cotta N, Jaeger M: The familial triphalangia of the thumb and its operative treatment. Arch Orthop Unfallchir 58:282, 1965
77. Diamond LR, Allen DB, Magill FB: Congenital (erythroid) hypoplastic anemia: A 25-year study. Am J Child 102:403, 1961
78. Flatt A: The Care of Congenital Hand Anomalies. St Louis, CV Mosby, 1977
79. Gates RR: Human Genetics, 1st ed. New York, Macmillan, 1946
80. Haas SL: Three-phalangeal thumb. Am J Roentgenol Radium Ther Nucl Med 42:677, 1939
81. Hertz VR, Littler JW: Adduction, pronation, and recession of the second metacarpal in thumb agenesis. J Hand Surg 2:113, 1977
82. Jaeger M, Refior HJ: The congenital triangular deformity of the tubular bones of the hand and foot. Clin Orthop 81:139, 1971
83. Juberg CC, Hayward JR: A new familial syndrome of oral, cranial, and digital anomalies. J Pediat 74:755, 1964
84. Milch Jr: Triphalangeal thumb. J Bone Joint Surg 33A:692, 1951
85. Miura T: Triphalangeal thumb. Plast Reconstr Surg 58:587, 1976
86. Polinelli U: A case of familial hyperphalangia of the thumbs. Minerva Nipiol 12:373, 1962
87. Strauch B, Spinner M: Congenital anomaly of the thumb: Absent intrinsics and flexor pollicis longus. J Bone Joint Surg 58A: 115, 1976
88. Swanson AB, Brown KS: Hereditary triphalangeal thumb. J Hered 53:259, 1962
89. Wood VE: Treatment of the triphalangeal thumb. Clin Orthop 120:188, 1976

Delta Phalanx

90. Amuso SJ: Diastrophic Dwarfism. J Bone Joint Surg 504:113, 1968
91. Hoover GH, Flatt AE, Weiss NW: The hand in Apert's syndrome. J Bone Joint Surg 524:878, 1970
92. Jones GB: Delta phalanx. J Bone Joint Surg 46B:226, 1964
93. Smith RJ: Osteotomy for "delta phalanx" deformity. Clin Orthop 123:91, 1977
94. Stover CN, Hayes JT, Holt JF: Diastrophic dwarfism. Am J Roentgenol Radium Ther Nucl Med 89:914, 1963
95. Taybi H: Diastrophic dwarfism. Radiology 80:1, 1963
96. Theander G, Carstam J: Longitudinally bracketed diaphysis. Ann Radiol 17:355, 1974

97. Watson HK, Boyes JH: Congenital angular deformity of the digits. J Bone Joint Surg 49A:333, 1967
98. Wood VE, Flatt AE: Congenital triangular bones in the hand. J Hand Surg 2:193, 1977

Congenital Clasped Thumb

99. Barsky AJ: Congenital Anomalies of the Hand and Their Surgical Treatment, Fig 60, p 112. Springfield, IL, Charles C Thomas, 1958
100. Broadbent TR, Woolf RM: Flexion-adduction deformity of the thumb—congenital clasped thumb. Plast Reconstr Surg 34:612, 1964
101. Crawford HH, Horton C, Adamson J: Congenital aplasia or hypoplasia of thumb and finger extensor tendons. J Bone Joint Surg 48A:82, 1966
102. Crenshaw AH (ed): Campbell's Operative Orthopedics, Vol 1, 5th ed. St Louis, CV Mosby, 1971
103. Flatt AE: The Care of Congenital Hand Anomalies. St Louis, CV Mosby, 1977
104. Loomis LK: Congenital "clasped thumb." J LA State Med Soc 110:23, 1958
105. Matev I: Surgical treatment of spastic "thumb-in-palm" deformity. J Bone Joint Surg 45B:703, 1963
106. Namba K, Muda Y, Hachiguchi T: Congenital clasped thumb. Orthop Surg (Tokyo) 16:1031, 1965
107. Neviaser RJ: Congenital hypoplasia of the thumb with absence of the extrinsic extensors, abductor pollicis longus, and thenar muscles. J Hand Surg 4:301, 1979
108. Weckesser EC, Reed JR, Heiple KG: Congenital clasped thumb (congenital flexion-adduction deformity of the thumb). J Bone Joint Surg 50A:1417, 1968
109. Zadek I: Congenital absence of the extensor pollicis longus of both thumbs. Operation and cure. J Bone Joint Surg 16:432, 1934

Polydactyly

110. Barsky AJ: Congenital Anomalies of the Hand and Their Surgical Treatment. Springfield, IL Charles C Thomas, 1958
111. Flatt AE: Problems in polydactyly. In Cramer LM Chase RA (eds): Symposium on the Hand. St Louis, CV Mosby, 1971
112. Flatt AE: The Care of the Congenital Hand Anomalies. St Louis, CV Mosby, 1977
113. Flatt AE: Problems in polydactyly in Cramer LM, Chase RA (eds): Symposium on the Hand (pp 150–167). St Louis, CV Mosby, 1971
114. Gesell A: The First Five Years of Life. New York, Harper & Row, 1940
115. Marks TW, Bayne LG: Polydactyly of the thumb: Abnormal anatomy and treatment. J Hand Surg 3(2): 107–116, 1978
116. Stelling F: The upper extremity. In Ferguson AB (ed): Orthopedic Surgery in Infancy and Childhood, 2nd ed, p 282 Baltimore, Williams & Wilkins, 1963
117. Temtamy, McKusick VA: Synopsis of hand malformations with particular emphasis on genetic factors. Birth Defects 3:25, 1969
118. Turek SL: Orthopedic Principles and Their Application. Philadelphia, JB Lippincott, 1967
119. Wassel HD: The results of surgery for polydactyly of the thumb. Clin Orthop 64:175–193, 1969
120. Wood VE: Treatment of central polydactyly. Clin Orthop 74:196, 1971

Gigantism of the Fingers

121. Barsky AJ: Macrodactyly. J Bone Joint Surg 49A:1255, 1967
122. Thorne F, Posch, JL, Mladick RA: Megalodactyly. Plast Reconstr Surg 41:232 1968

Sprengel's Deformity

123. Carson WG, Lovell WW, Whitesides TE Jr: Congenital elevation of the scapula. J Bone Joint Surg 63A:1199–1207, 1981
124. Engel D: The etiology of the undescended scapula and related syndromes. J Bone Joint Surg 25:613–625, 1943
125. Eulenberg M: Casuistis Mittheilungen aus dem Begiete der Orthopädie. Arch Klin Chir 4:301, 1863
126. Green WT: The surgical correction of congenital elevation of the scapula (Sprengel's deformity). [Proc Am Orthop Assoc] J Bone Joint Surg 39A:149, 1957
127. Horwitz AE: Congenital deviation of the scapula—Sprengel's deformity. Am J Orthop Surg 6:260, 1908
128. Schrock RD: Congenital abnormalities at the cervicothoracic level. AAOS Instr Course Lect 6: 1949
129. Woodward JW: Congenital elevation of the scapula. Correction by release and transplantation of muscle origins. J Bone Joint Surg 43A:219, 1961

Brachial Plexus

130. Adler JB, Patterson RL Jr: Erb's palsy: Long-term results of treatment in eighty-eight cases. J Bone Joint Surg 49A:1052–1064, 1967
131. Fairbanks HAT: Birth palsy: Subluxation of the shoulder joint in infants and young children. Lancet 1:1217–1223, 1913
132. Hardy AE: Birth injuries of the brachial plexus. J Bone Joint Surg 63B(1):98–101, 1981
133. Hoffer M, Wickenden R, Roper B: Results of tendon transfers to the rotator cuff. J Bone Joint Surg 60A(5):691–695, 1978
134. L'Episcopo JB: Restoration of muscle balance in the treatment of obstetrical paralysis. NY J Med 39:357–363, 1939
135. Leffert RD: Brachial plexus injuries. N Engl J Med 291:1059–1067, 1974
136. Millesi H: Surgical management of brachial plexus injuries. J Hand Surg 2(5):367–379, 1977
137. Sever JW: Obstetric paralysis: Report of eleven hundred cases. JAMA 85:1862–1865, 1925
138. Wickstrom J: Birth injuries of the brachial plexus. Treatment of defects in the shoulder. Clin Orthop 23:187–196, 1962

Osteochrondritis Dissecans of the Elbow

139. Heller CJ, Wiltse LD: A vascular necrosis of the capitellum humeri (Panner's disease). J Bone Joint Surg 42A:513, 1960
140. Panner HJ: An affection of the capitulum humeri, resembling Calvé-Perthes disease of the hip. Acta Radiol 8:617, 1927
141. Smith MGH: Osteochondritis of the humeral capitellum. J Bone Joint Surg 46B:50, 1964

18

The Hip

G. Dean MacEwen
William P. Bunnell
Paul L. Ramsey

CONGENITAL DISLOCATION OF THE HIP—EVALUATION AND TREATMENT BEFORE WALKING AGE

Early diagnosis of a congenitally dislocated hip (CDH) is essential in preventing the infant from experiencing a prolonged and involved course of treatment. The main problem in obtaining an early diagnosis is that generations of students, residents, and practitioners have been taught to examine the hips for clicks, limited abduction, asymmetrical skin creases or femoral shortening. All these methods for determining the presence of congenital dislocation of the hip, with the possible exception of asymmetrical skin folds, are essentially inadequate for examination of newborns, and even asymmetrical skin folds can be misleading, because they are often present when a hip is normal.

Furthermore, the large series reported in the literature demonstrate that the diagnosis of CDH cannot always be established at the time of initial examination. Repeat examination should be performed by the pediatrician or family physician at every opportunity during the first several months of life.[6] All these factors, combined with the fact that the individual practitioner rarely encounters a child with a congenital hip dislocation, account for the frequent delays in diagnosis.

EMBRYOLOGY AND ANATOMY

At 4 to 5 weeks of gestation, bulges representing the extremities develop on the anterolateral aspect of the embryo. Development of the future hip joint is demarcated by a line of increased density,[84] which is saucer-shaped. The cleavage of the joint cavity starts at the peripheral margins and progresses inward. Because the femoral head and acetabulum are formed from a single block of tissue, a dislocation is impossible during early developmental stages.

The blood supply to the femoral head is critical. The femoral artery gives off the profunda femoris artery, which in turn gives the lateral and medial circumflex arteries. Both are important to the circulation to the proximal femur. The lateral circumflex artery passes underneath the rectus femoris, giving off muscular branches, but, most important, a major branch supplies the anterolateral proximal femur. The medial circumflex artery passes between the iliopsoas and adductor muscles, turns across the posterior aspect of the iliopsoas to reach the medial side of the femur, and passes along the femoral neck. There are two methods of extra-articular vascular compromise. With a forced positioning of the proximal femur, there is occlusion of the vessels as the acetabular rim is pressed into the intertrochanteric groove, and occlusion as the vessel passes between the muscle bellies. The anatomic path[4] of the major vessels is significant, because arterial occlusions can occur with either the frog-leg or the abduction-internal rotation positions.

Ogden[58] has reported that at birth the blood is supplied to the femoral head by multiple small vessels arising from both the lateral and medial circumflex vessels. With growth, this pattern changes. The lateral circumflex system recedes as a contributor to the femoral head and supplies the anteromedial metaphysis. At the same time, the medial circumflex artery changes from multiple small vessels to two larger branches called the *posterior-inferior* and *posterior-superior* vessels, which together supply most of the femoral head. As the pattern is changing to become more dependent upon fewer but larger vessels, the amount of tissue to be supplied increases and becomes more distant because of femoral neck growth, thus maintaining the risk of avascular necrosis if the individual vessel is placed under pressure or is slightly stretched.

The anatomic changes associated with dislocation represent a spectrum of abnormalities. Stability is lost when the femoral head begins to migrate laterally. An important adjunct to stability is the vacuum normally created by the snug fit of the femoral head in the acetabulum.[8] The labrum also adds stability by increasing acetabular depth. The anatomic abnormality that allows the dislocation to occur also increases the difficulty of regaining stability. Initially, a lax acetabular labrum loses the vacuum, and the femoral head can be easily provoked to dislocate over the posterior acetabular rim. In the next stage, the acetabular labrum (limbus) is further deformed, and the capsule and ligamentum teres are stretched. In addition, the femoral head begins to lose its spherical shape as it lies in the dislocated position. The limbus may become inverted, and there are secondary acetabular deformities. This degree of deformity is unusual at such an early stage of development. Most congenital dislocations of the hip occur during the perinatal period. However, if the dislocation is present over a long period of intrauterine development, the soft tissues become contracted, preventing relocation of the femoral head; this accounts for the rare teratologic dislocation.

ETIOLOGY

The factors that predispose a hip joint to dislocation are genetic, hormonal, and mechanical. The genetic influence has been demonstrated by studies of families in which more than one child has a dislocated hip. A dislocation in a second child occurs in approximately 22 to 50 per 1000 live births,[12,58] which is at least 10 times the usual risk for dislocation. Andren and Borglin[1] reported an increase in uterine estrogen and content in newborns with dislocations. They postulated that failure of the liver to inactivate estrogen contributes to hormonally induced laxity of the hip capsule. Contrary to this theory, a later investigation[86] found no significant hormonal difference between controls and 16 patients with dislocation. However, animal studies have indicated that estrogen may in fact be a predisposing factor.[103]

It is our clinical experience that newborns may have relative joint laxity for as long as 10 days after birth. During this time, a dislocation that is present at birth often becomes stable. This is supported by Barlow's[4] study, in which 58% of newborns with unstable hips developed stability spontaneously by 3 1/2 days of age.

Mechanical factors also influence the occurrence of dislocation. The incidence of dislocation is greatly increased by breech position.[71] However, passage through the birth canal in the breech position does not seem to influence the dislocation, because breech-position infants delivered by cesarean section are also prone to dislocation. This implicates intrauterine position rather than birth position as a critical factor.[97] In 1941, Chapple and Davidson[12] linked fetal positions to newborn extremity malpositions. They showed that with breech positions, the knees are frequently in hyperextension. Wilkinson[102] reported that full knee extension adds to hip instability, and a delay in assuming the flexed-knee position is a critical factor. The studies in which the knees of rabbits were held in extension are experimental evidence that prolonged knee extension may contribute to dislocation.[54]

The mechanical factors associated with breech malposition seem to be twofold. First, the extended knee and its associated hamstring tightness, combined with hyperflexion of the hip, may increase maldirection of the forces at the hip joint. Second, the hyperflexed hip allows an iliopsoas contracture to develop, so that hip extension following birth promotes instability. Why the left hip should be more frequently involved than the right is unknown. However, it may be due to the more common positioning of the left side of the fetus adjacent to the prominent spine, causing adduction of the left thigh.

Forced post–delivery hip extension may add

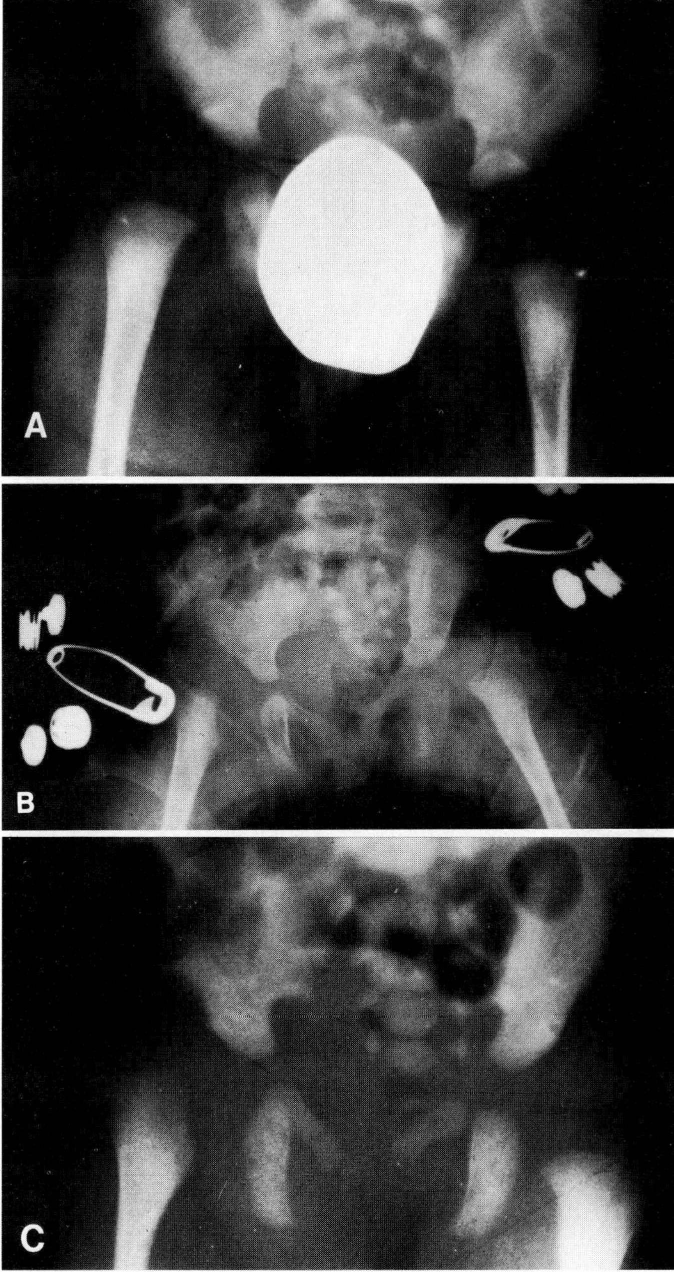

FIG. 18-1. Three types of dislocated hips recognized at birth. (*A*) Lateral displacement occurring at birth reduces easily and responds well to simple treatment. There is only lateral displacement of the femur with no proximal displacement. (*B*) Dislocation due to neuromuscular origin reduces easily but tends to redislocate due to muscle imbalance. (*C*) Teratologic dislocation occurs *in utero*. There is frank dislocation with lateral and proximal migration of the femur at birth, and the femoral head will not reduce into the acetabulum. A false acetabulum has developed.

to hip instability.[73] This probably accounts for the frequent occurrence of dislocations in newborns in societies where infants are bundled with the hips in extension and adduction.

TYPES OF DISLOCATIONS

There are three types of dislocated hips that may be detected in infants (Fig. 18-1). The first type includes dislocations that occur at or near the time of birth, reduce easily, and respond to simple treatment. The second type are those of neuromuscular origin. These usually reduce easily, but, because of the pelvic muscular imbalance, they redislocate with little provocation. Teratologic dislocations are the third type, with secondary adaptive changes of the soft tissue and bone present at birth.

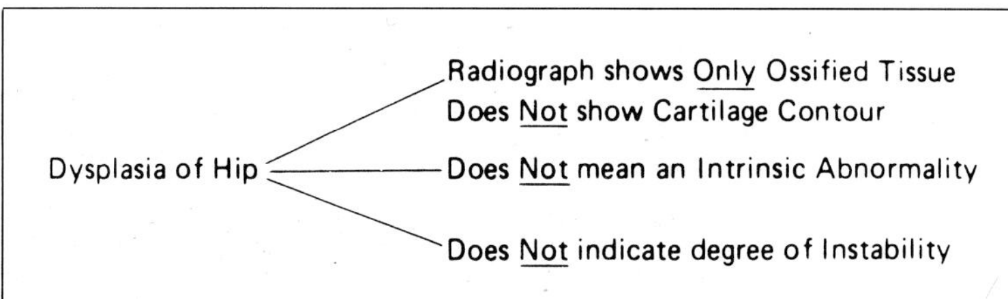

FIG. 18-2. See text.

The clinical characteristics of teratologic dislocations are the absence of the Ortolani sign and the inability to relocate the femoral head without traction. These dislocations are often best diagnosed by roentgenograms.

TERMINOLOGY

The terms used to describe a dislocation can lead to misinterpretation of the anatomic deformity or the degree of instability. For example, the terms *dislocation, dislocatable, subluxatable, lax, unstable,* and *dysplastic* do not have the same meaning to all clinicians. A newborn with a *dislocated* hip has the femoral head completely displaced from the acetabulum, and active reduction is required. A *dislocatable* hip exists when the femoral head is in the acetabulum, but, with a provocative maneuver, it can be completely displaced. Once the leg is released, the femoral head usually moves spontaneously back into the acetabulum. A *subluxatable* hip is the most difficult to detect. Subluxation occurs when the femoral head can be moved significantly, but not completely, out of the acetabulum. Such terms as *lax* or *unstable* are confusing because they imply that the femoral head can be moved away from the depths of the acetabulum. However, the degree of displacement is left to the imagination. Indeed, "unstable" can imply anything from minimal displacement to complete dislocation, and the term should be avoided.

A *dysplastic* hip is characterized by abnormal development of tissue. Because the hip forms from one cartilaginous block as a spherical head and an acetabulum, "dysplasia" does not mean a primary abnormality of the developing tissue, but rather a secondary response to the dislocation. Dysplasia is a term commonly used to describe a greater-than-normal slope of the superior bony portion of the acetabulum. However, this finding is only a roentgenographic description and does not outline the contour of the cartilaginous acetabulum (Fig. 18-2). In fact, the underlying cartilage model may or may not be distorted. Dysplasia can also indicate that the femoral head on the involved side is smaller than that of the uninvolved side. Again, as with the acetabulum, one should remember that only the bony portion of the femoral head is visible and that a large cartilaginous layer surrounds it. Therefore, abnormal roentgenograms, especially in the prewalking child, really represent secondary changes of bone development but do not provide information regarding the contour of the cartilage.

INCIDENCE

The incidence of dislocated hips per 1000 live births is 1.3; dislocatable hips, 1.2; and subluxatable hips, 9.2. Thus, with every 1000 live births, a total of 11.7 newborns have some degree of hip instabillity. The left hip is involved in about 60% of patients, the right hip in 20% and both hips in approximately 20%. Seventy percent of dislocated hips are in girls, and dislocation occurs much more frequently in Caucasians than in Blacks. About 20% of all dislocations occur with breech presentations, whereas the incidence of breech presentation in the general population is about 4%. Females born in breech presentation are therefore categorized as a very high-risk group for CDH, because both their sex and their breech position predispose them to dislocations. In fact, in a study of 25,000 newborns at our Institute, this combination resulted in a true dislocation in 1 of every 35 births. The association of torticollis with hip problems has also been recognized. It was shown that 20% of children with torticollis also have an abnormal hip.[33]

DIAGNOSIS

The diagnosis of congenital dislocation in newborns is based on the clinical examination. The infant should be lying quietly on his back with the pelvis stabilized by one hand as the

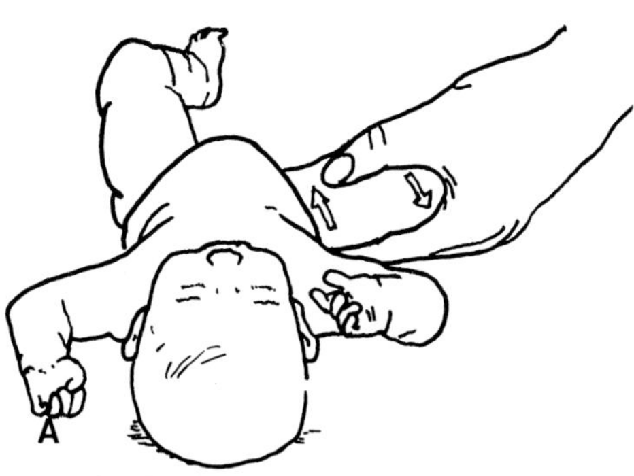

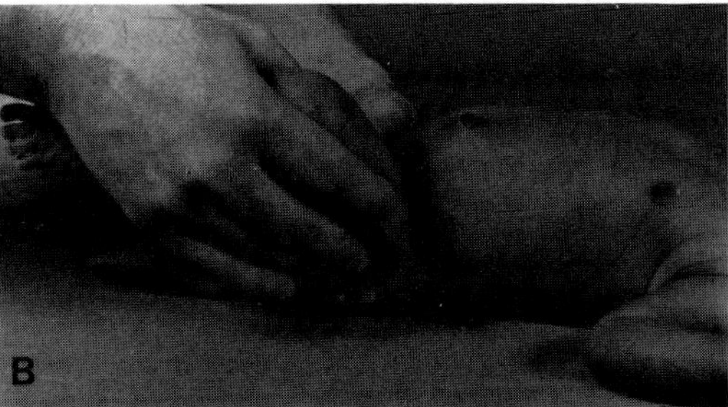

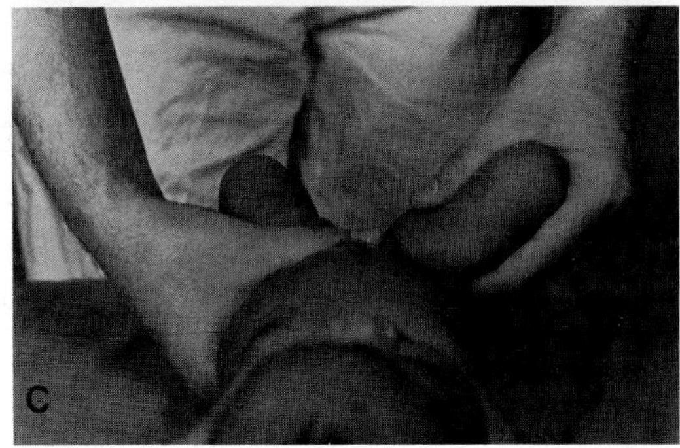

FIG. 18-3. The Ortolani maneuver. In this technique, the hip is gently abducted and the thigh is raised with the fingers to gently reduce the hip. When performing the test, one hand should always be used to stabilize the pelvis; therefore, only one hip at a time can be examined.

examining hand flexes the thigh to 90°. The knee is flexed to an acute angle (Fig. 18-3), and the fingers are placed over the lateral aspect of the thigh, with the finger tips at the level of the greater trochanter and the thumb across the angle of the knee. The thumb should not be placed into the femoral triangle area, because pressure at this point is painful. The maneuver is performed by gently lifting the trochanter toward the acetabulum as the leg is abducted. With this motion, a proprioceptive sensation of the femoral head sliding into the acetabulum is present. The classic jerk sign of reduction is unusual, although it is present in some newborns.

The Barlow[4] examination is a provocative test of dislocation. The extremity is grasped gently in the manner just described, but the leg is adducted slightly past the midline (Fig. 18-4), and gentle downward pressure is placed against the inner thigh with the thumb. A dislocatable hip then becomes completely displaced, but, when the leg is allowed to abduct freely, the hip reduces. These two maneuvers alone can almost always establish the diagnosis of a dislocation or a dislocatable hip in newborns.

A screening program in which all newborns are examined in the nursery is an efficient method to establish this diagnosis. At birth, the normal infant has a hip flexion contracture and extension to within 15° or 20° of the table top. The classic clinical signs of a dislocation

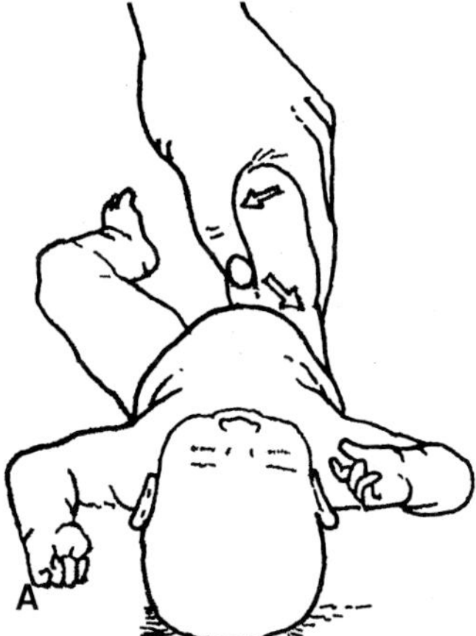

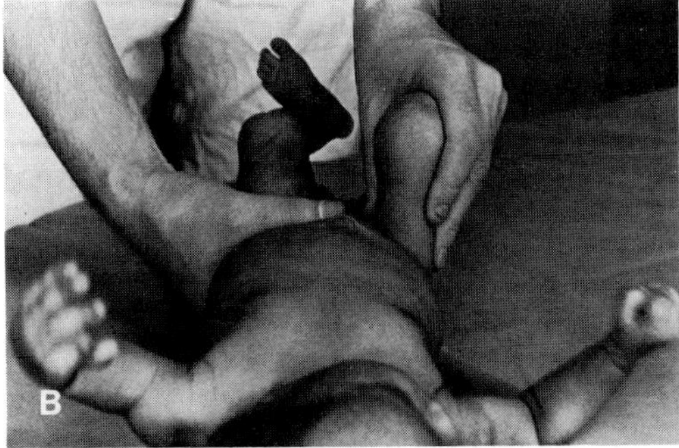

FIG. 18-4. The Barlow test. The thumb is placed on the inner aspect of the thigh and the hip is adducted, with longitudinal pressure exerted on the thigh, pushing it toward the table. The examiner again uses one hand to stabilize the pelvis, testing one hip at a time.

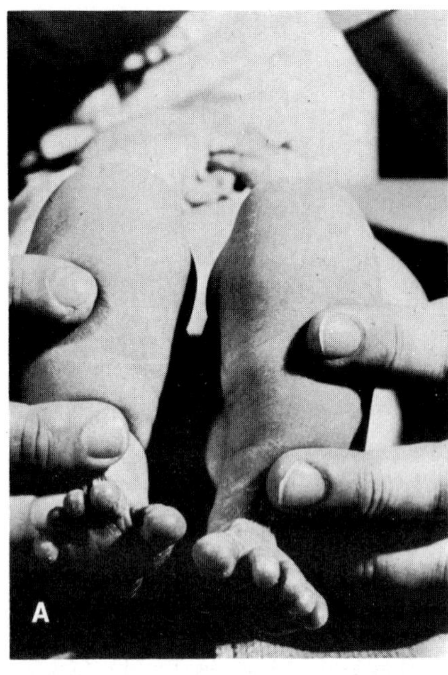

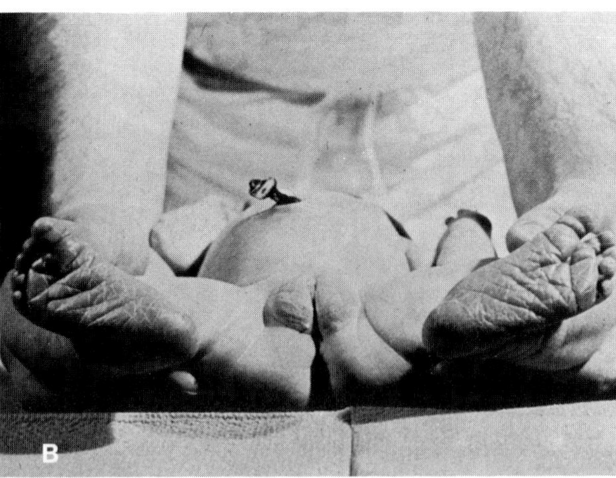

FIG. 18-5. (*A*) Newborn examination to detect limited abduction, asymmetrical thigh folds, and relative femoral shortening. (*B*) There is no limitation of abduction in this newborn, in spite of dislocation.

in an older child include limited abduction, asymmetrical thigh folds, and relative femoral shortening.[62] Contrary to popular belief, the newborn with a dislocation has a remarkably normal examination by these criteria (Fig. 18-5). A dislocation does not demonstrate significant femoral shortening, because dislocation has happened at or near birth, and the femur is slightly lateral to the acetabulum but has not migrated proximally to any degree. Adductor tightness is also absent. Asymmetrical thigh folds are usually present if a dislocation exists; however, a large number of infants with normal hips also have asymmetry, making this method unreliable in detecting a dislocation.

Roentgenographic Studies of the Newborn

Roentgenograms play only a minor role in the diagnosis of newborns with congenital dislocation. In this group, the films are often misleading, because the dislocation occurred at or near birth, and the secondary changes have not occurred (Fig. 18-6). Shenton's line need not be broken, and there is usually no false acetabulum. In addition, ossification of the innominate bone, which outlines the superior acetabulum, is indistinct. Therefore, the established criteria, such as the acetabular index and Hilgenreiner's line, are difficult to identify.[10] Even pelvic positioning on the film makes a vast difference in the acetabular and femoral head contour and relationship. Side-to-side rotation can cause the appearance of an uncovered femoral head or abnormal acetabular index. Also, anterior or posterior pelvic rotation can cause the indices to appear either increased or decreased, even when they are actually within the normal range.[80] This is particularly true with newborns, because their flexion contractures cause the pelvis to rotate forward when the thighs are pressed against

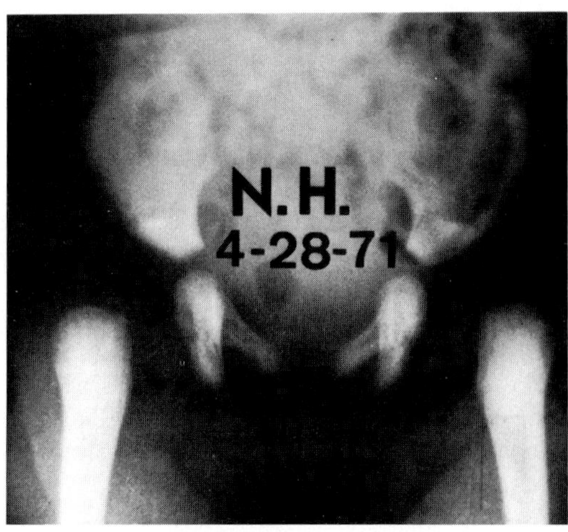

FIG. 18-6. Roentgenograms are not very helpful in detecting the newborn with congenital hip dislocation, because secondary changes have not yet occurred.

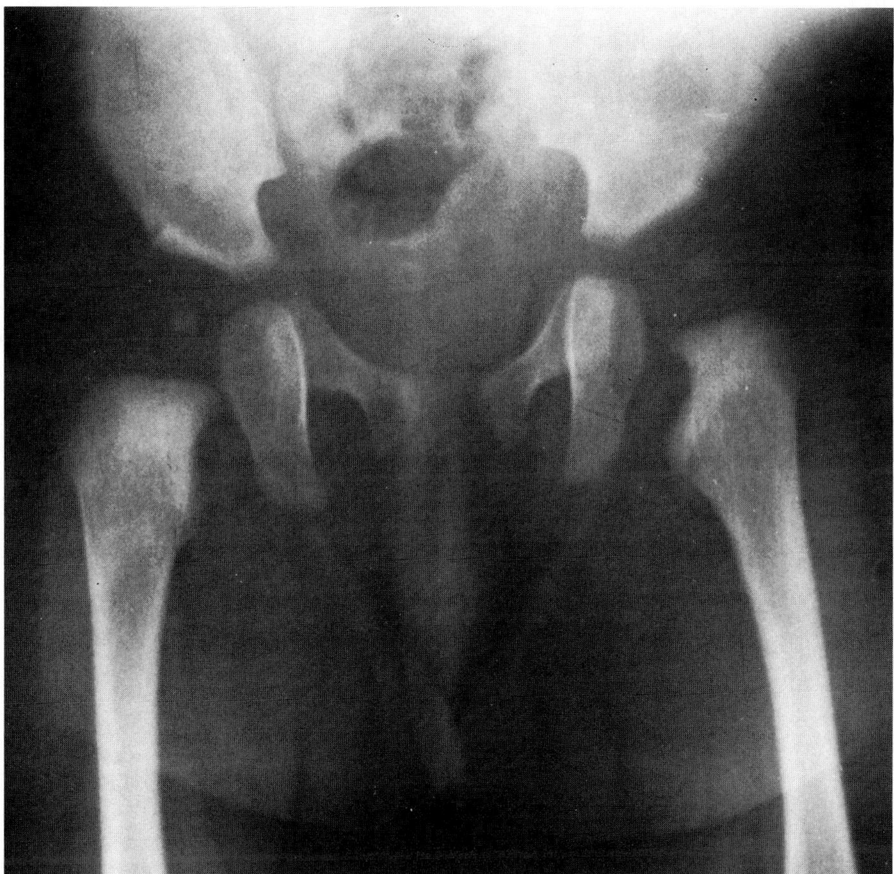

FIG. 18-7. Failure to properly position the infant for roentgenograms may obscure the anatomic landmarks. Marked external rotation of the thighs, as evidenced by prominence of the lesser trochanters, and rotation of the pelvis, as demonstrated by asymmetry in the shape of the sciatic notches and the obturator foramina, make accurate interpretation impossible.

the roentgenography plate. A common error when taking a roentgenogram is failing to position the legs at all, allowing the hips to roll into external rotation, which disrupts the roentgenographic landmarks (Fig. 18-7). The von Rosen[93] view, taken with the legs in abduction and internal rotation, is supposed to direct the femoral metaphysis above the acetabulum when a dislocation is present. However, this is also one of the positions that reduces a hip. Thus, in newborns whose hips are lax and can be placed in and out of the acetabulum with ease, this position often reduces the hip when the hip is actually dislocated in the neutral position. The frog-leg position is popular to attain reduction, yet frequently, a frog-leg view is obtained to determine whether a dislocation is present. This is inconsistent, because the roentgenogram will show an apparently normal hip if the frog-leg position temporarily reduces it, when, in fact, the hip may be dislocated in other positions. Another subtle but important aspect that is often forgotten is the ability of newborns to spontaneously reduce the hip by tightening the pelvic girdle musculature, which can also give a false impression of a normal hip. (Because of the difficulties in positioning and the lack of ossification of the pelvis in newborns, one should not rely on roentgenograms for the diagnosis. A positive roentgenographic study can be helpful in the diagnosis of CDH, but a normal roentgenogram must be overruled by positive clinical findings of instability.) When the infant reaches the age of 4 to 6 weeks, roentgenograms are usually more helpful. At

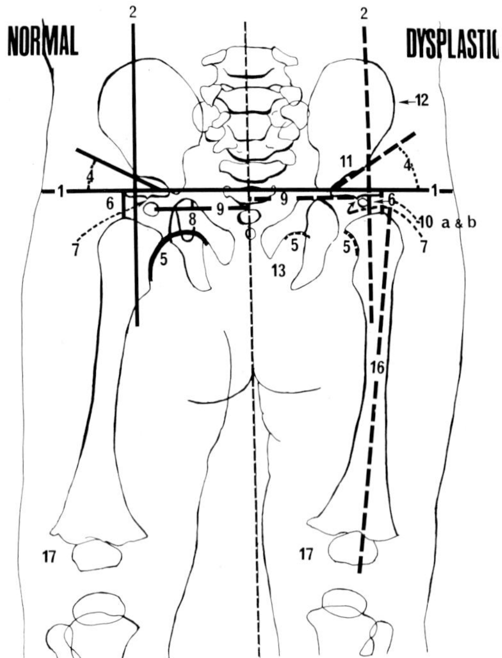

FIG. 18-8. Roentgenographic signs of congenital hip dislocation. (*1*) Horizontal Y line (Hilgenreiner's line); (*2*) vertical line (Perkins' line); (*3*) quadrants (formed by lines 1 and 2); (*4*) acetabular index (Kleinberg and Lieberman); (*5*) Shenton's line; (*6*) upward displacement of the femoral head; (*7*) lateral displacement of the femoral head; (*8*) U figure of teardrop shadow (Kohler); (*9*) Y coordinate (Ponseti); (*10*) capital epiphyseal dysplasia: (*a*) delayed appearance of the center of ossification of the femoral head, (*b*) irregular maturation of the center of ossification; (*11*) bilification (furrowing of the acetabular roof in late infancy—Ponseti); (*12*) hypoplasia of the pelvis (ilium); (*13*) delayed fusion (ischiopubic juncture); (*14*) absence of a shapely, defined, well-ossified acetabular margin, caused by delayed ossification of the roof of the socket; (*15*) femoral neck-shaft angle; (*16*) adduction attitude of the extremity; (*17*) development of the epiphyses of other joints (knees, wrists, and lumbosacral spine); (*18*) radiolucent acetabular roof, limbus, joint capsule (arthrographic studies). (From Hart V: Congenital Dysplasia of the Hip Joint and Sequelae. Springfield, Il, Charles C Thomas, 1952)

this time, the proximal femur has noticeable lateral and proximal displacement. Usually, a false acetabulum is apparent, and Shenton's line is broken. There are numerous roentgenographic signs associated with CDH,[31] as illustrated in Figure 18-8, but it is important to remember that these are usually absent in the newborn.

Recently, we have begun to use ultrasonography in the examination of infants with CDH.[16] The ability to clearly visualize the cartilaginous femoral head by ultrasonography enhances the understanding of the anatomic structures and their relationships. The technique used allows for the hip joint to be imaged in two different planes. This method has been used to identify both frank dislocations and subluxations, as well as to follow patients who are being treated in the Pavlik harness. Our early experience with this technique suggests that it is a reliable, accurate, and useful adjunct to roentgenography.

Change of Clinical Signs

Except for the ability of the examiner to reduce or displace the femoral head, the examination of newborns is normal. However, between 1 and 3 months, secondary changes become readily apparent. It is at this time that the classic signs of adduction contracture and femoral shortening develop.

There is much confusion about the sign that Ortolani described in 1937.[60,61] In his original publication, he described a jerk or sudden movement as the flexed hip is abducted and the femoral head is reduced. Unfortunately, this sign is now commonly referred to as a "hip click," leading to questions such as: "Are hip clicks felt or heard," and "Are there differences in the quality of the clicks?" There are many high-pitched clicks or sounds about the hip and knee that are due to myofascial or ligamentous sources and are not secondary to a dislocated hip (Fig. 18-9). Although the reduction can occasionally be heard, it is far more common for it to be felt. In Ortolani's original description, he stated that his sign was not present in infants younger than 3 months of age. In the newborn, a laterally displaced femoral head is subtly replaced into the acetabulum without a jerk. Vitally important is the concept that reduction is associated with a proprioceptive sensation on the part of the examiner. The misunderstandings of this proprioceptive concept and the extension of the jerk sign to newborns, when it was originally described as a useful sign *only* for older infants, all contribute to undetected dislocated hips in newborns. This is not to say that Ortolani's sign is never present in newborns, because occasionally it is detectable. Thus, the Ortolani sign really has two different presentations: one early and one late. First, in newborns, it is a

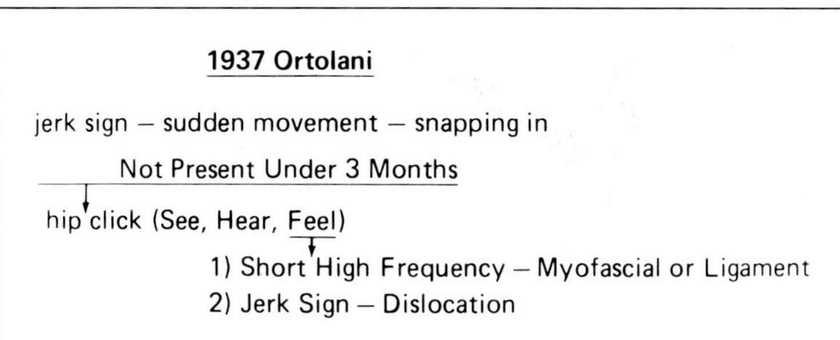

FIG. 18-9. See text.

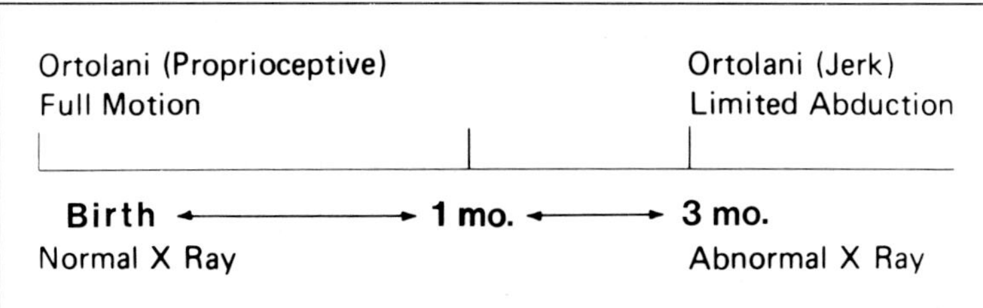

FIG. 18-10. See text.

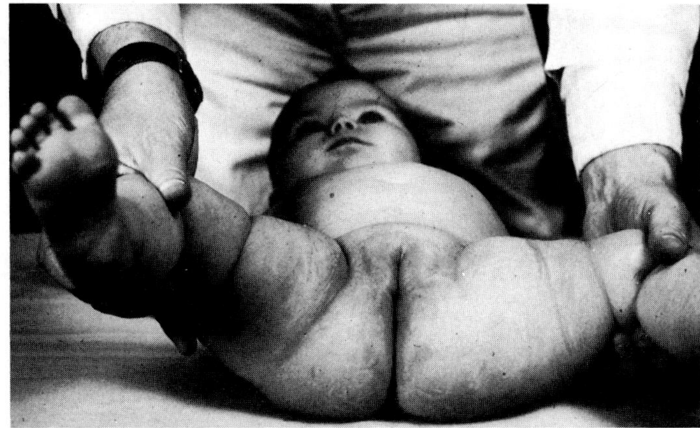

FIG. 18-11. By the age of 3 to 6 months, thigh shortening is apparent, as is tightness of the adductors, on the dislocated right side.

proprioceptive sensation of reduction. Second, in infants between 1 and 3 months of age with hip dislocation, the classic Ortolani jerk sign is common (Fig. 18-10), because the soft tissues demonstrate more resistance to reduction than in the newborn period.

Between 3 and 6 months of age, the contractures progress until thigh shortening becomes easily detectable and tightness of the adductors is obvious (Fig. 18-11). The mother may begin to recognize difficulty with diaper changes because of an inability to spread the infant's legs, especially if the dislocation is bilateral. Bilateral dislocations are often overlooked at this stage, because the infant is symmetrically abnormal. At 3 months of age, the occurrence of the Ortolani sign decreases, because most dislocations become persistently stable in the dislocated position. As the infant becomes older, this trend continues, so that the Ortolani sign becomes a rare occurrence by walking age.

EARLY TREATMENT

Orthotic Devices

Treatment of the newborn is quite different from treatment of the older child, because the newborn has capsular laxity and a mildly eccentric limbus but no abnormality of the femoral head or acetabulum. There are many

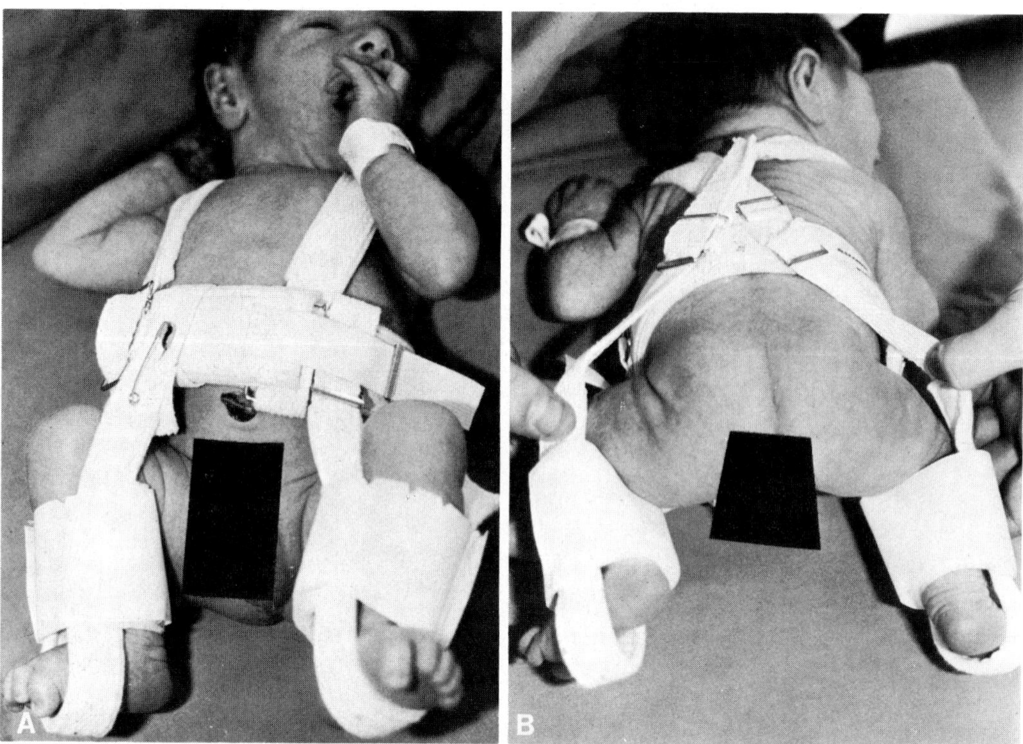

FIG. 18-12. (*A*) The Pavlik harness is applied so that baby's hips are in flexion without force. With 90° of flexion, the hips fall into abduction. (*B*) The prone position encourages gentle abduction.

devices available to facilitate reduction, most of which are based on abduction. In newborns, full abduction is not as risky as it is in older infants, because newborns do not have adduction contractures; however, avascular necrosis can occur. Often, abduction devices do not direct the femoral head toward the triradiate cartilage but, instead, leave it pointing superiorly. A good method for treatment is the use of a Pavlik harness, which was described in 1957 by Professor Pavlik.[62] This harness encourages both flexion and free abduction. Flexion begins to stabilize the hip by directing the femoral head toward the acetabulum. Also, as the hip is flexed, the head-neck axis begins to align with the acetabular axis. Once the flexion range is adjusted (full flexion should not be allowed), the hip is allowed to fall freely into abduction by the weight of the thighs. If the child sleeps in this device in the prone position, gradual abduction is also encouraged. In this way, the femoral head is not locked in any one position. In fact, a controlled activity program is encouraged. The Pavlik harness consists of an abdominal strap, two shoulder harnesses, and two leg stirrups. Each stirrup has a strap that fastens to the abdominal strap, both anteriorly and posteriorly. The posterior strap should not be pulled so tight as to force the legs into abduction (Fig. 18-12), but should be loose enough to allow the knees to be brought within 5 cm of the midline. Once the harness is applied, the position of the hip should be examined. Occasionally, a stable reduction is not attained, and, if the head remains dislocated, a prominence of the trochanter can be palpated in the buttock of the dislocated side. A roentgenogram should be obtained with the infant in the harness. The most common error in applying the harness is to have the hips flexed less than 90° (Fig. 18-13). This may allow the femoral head to point toward the roof or the corner of the acetabulum. Once the harness is properly adjusted, the stirrups are marked at the buckles, as are the shoulder straps, so that the harness can be removed to bathe the child and then reapplied in the same position. However, the device should not be completely removed until the hip is known to be stable (*i.e.*, at least

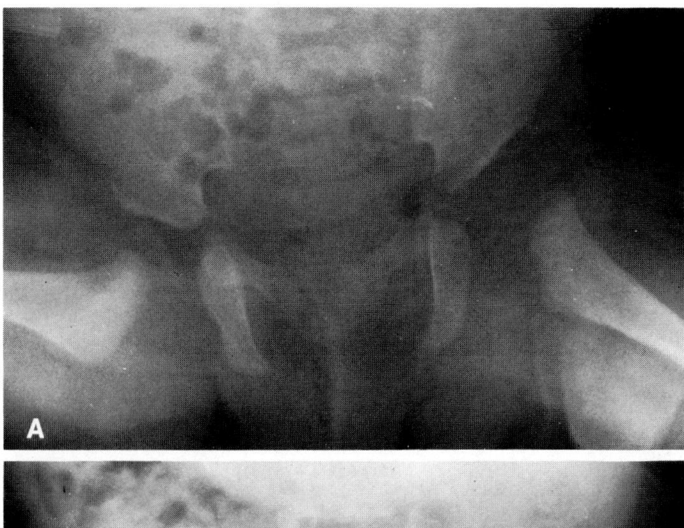

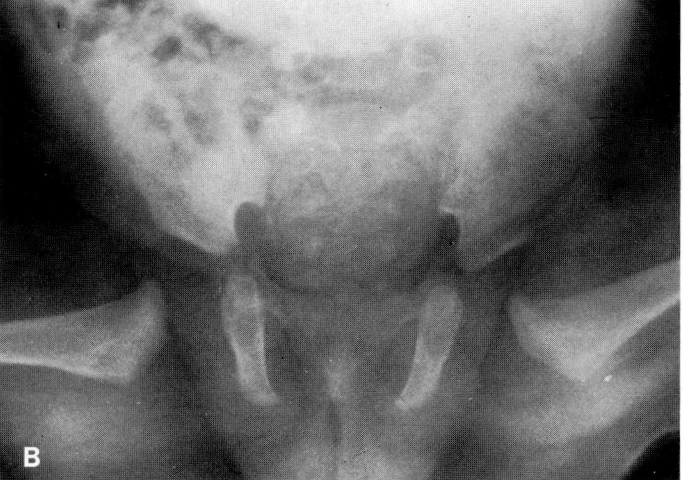

FIG. 18-13. Roentgenograms are taken with the child in harness to ensure that the hips are flexed to at least 90°. (*A*) If this degree of flexion is not obtained, the femoral head may point to the roof or the corner of the acetabulum. (*B*) Further flexion without changing abduction corrects this problem.

until the first follow-up visit). The abdominal strap can be expanded to allow for abdominal growth.

There are many types of devices for treating CDH that are based upon maintaining the hip in a modified frog-leg position. The Frejka pillow, the von Rosen splint, and other similar devices are effective in treating newborns. Their success is based on the fact that newborns lack both adduction contractures and secondary bone and cartilage changes; therefore, there is no increased pressure on the femoral head.

Once any device is applied, an anteroposterior roentgenogram should be taken to determine that the femoral head has been redirected into the acetabulum and not pushed above and against the side of the pelvis.

The anatomic deformity is more pronounced in the child older than 3 months of age. At this stage, contractures are beginning to develop, roentgenograms show a slope of the bony acetabulum, and the cartilaginous portion of the acetabulum that cannot be seen on the film may also have an abnormal slope. Therefore, the reduction in this age group is usually more unstable than in the newborn group. Whatever method is used to treat the child at this stage, these anatomic deformities must be taken into consideration, and the leg must be positioned so that the femoral head remains stable without force. At this stage it is very tempting to abduct the femur against the tight adductors to secure the reduction. However, this *must* be avoided because of the risk of avascular necrosis.

The "safe zone" concept (Fig. 18-14) helps to gain reduction with minimal risk of avascular necrosis. The safe zone margins are a few degrees within the range of motion between

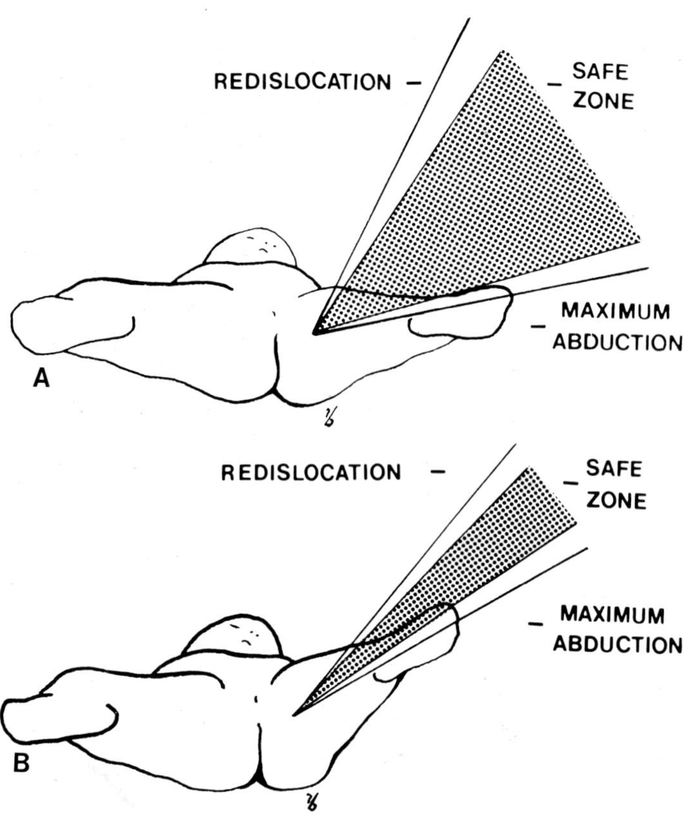

Fig. 18-14. The "safe zone" concept. (*A*) Considerable range between maximum abduction and redislocation. (*B*) Inadequate range suggesting the need for an adductor tenotomy. (From Ramsey PL, Lasser S, MacEwen GD: Congenital dislocation of the hip. J Bone Joint Surg 58A:1000, 1976)

maximum abduction and the point of redislocation as the leg is brought back to the midline. The Pavlik harness allows the femoral head to be stabilized, while at the same time allowing for motion within this guided range. Occasionally, the femoral head points toward the triradiate cartilage with slight lateral displacement. In these cases, it is tempting to tighten the posterior strap of the Pavlik harness to bring the femoral head into a more secure, deeper position. Again, this should be avoided because of the risk of producing avascularity of the femoral head. Occasionally, an adductor tenotomy may be required. When an adduction contracture is present, it will stretch out in about 2 weeks if the femoral head is reduced (Fig. 18-15). Continued contractures are reason to suspect persistent dislocation. The Pavlik harness is left on full time, and the infant is examined after a few days to ensure that there are no complications. The clinical stability is assessed at weekly intervals until stability is achieved. The harness is then removed for 2 hours each day. The time out of the harness is gradually increased by 2- to 4-hour increments if a neutral anteroposterior roentgenogram demonstrates reduction and if the acetabular index is stable or improving.

All children up to 6 months of age may be treated by this method without risk if the thighs are not pulled into abduction. If the femoral head does not become centered after 2 to 3 weeks, the child may be treated by traction and reduction methods.

Clinical stability in newborns is usually attained in 2 to 4 weeks. After the newborn period, the total length of treatment is approximately 1 to 2 times the age at which initial treatment was started.

Diapers

Diapers have no place in the treatment of a true congenital dislocation of the hip. Although multiple diapers have been used, they do not keep the hip in flexion (Fig. 18-16). In fact, the hip is in a great deal of extension most of the time. We have seen a large number of children who were treated with diapers at birth with complete failure.

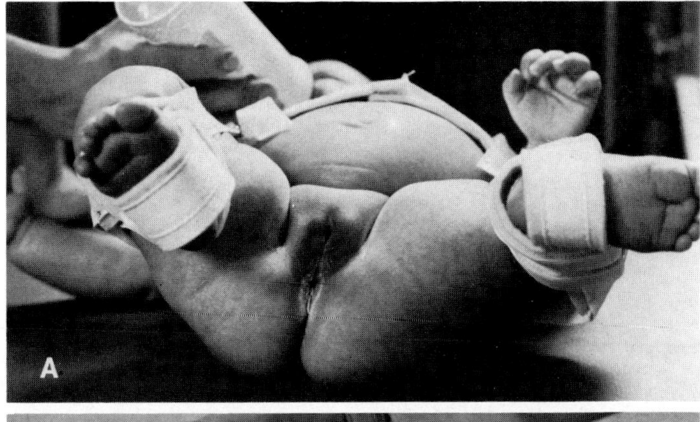

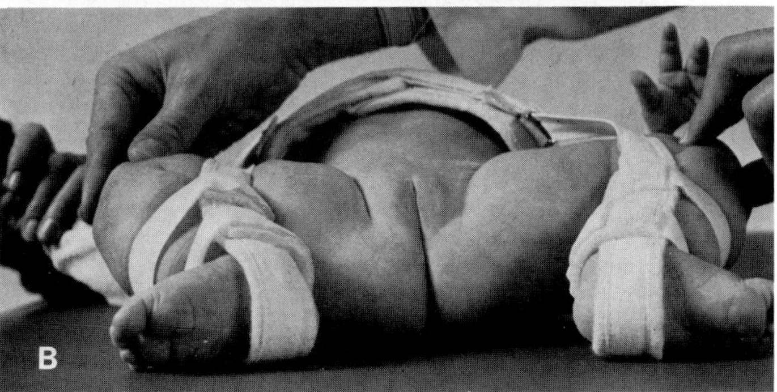

FIG. 18-15. (*A*) The appearance of an infant with adduction contractures immediately after application of the harness. (*B*) After 3 weeks of continual wear, the adduction contractures have stretched out.

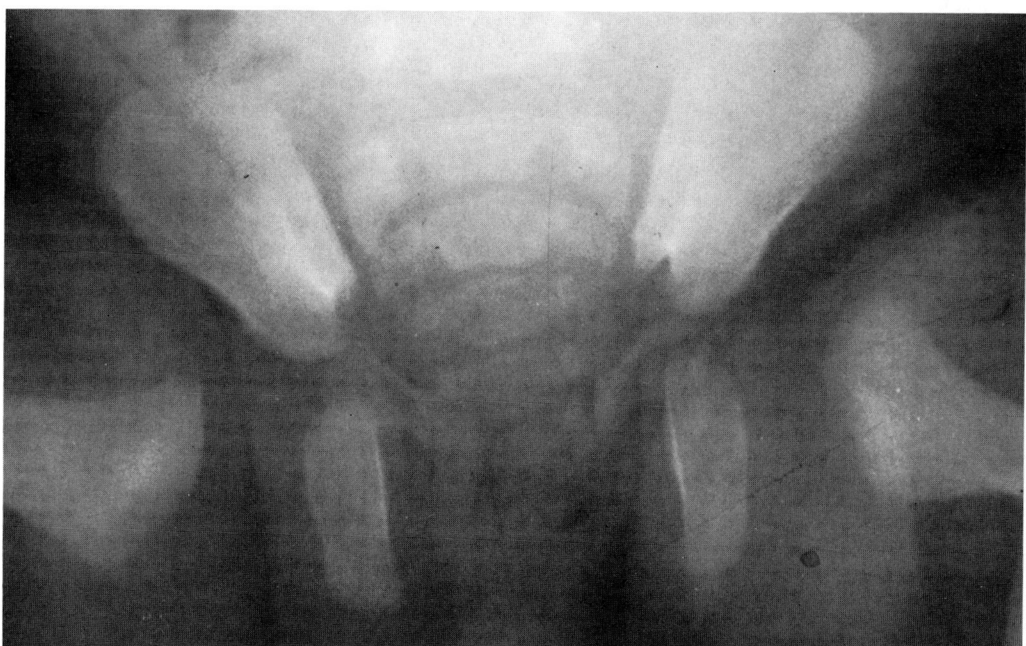

FIG. 18-16. Roentgenogram of an infant being treated with double diapers shows that the hip is not kept in proper position and the femoral head is not directed toward the acetabulum.

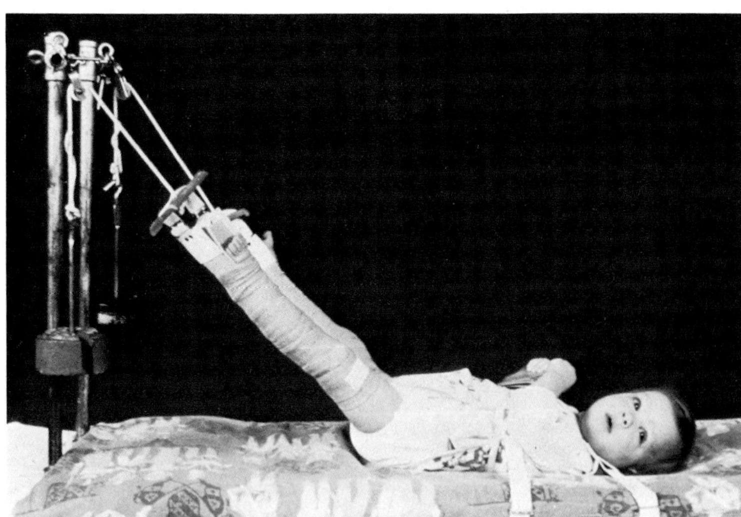

FIG. 18-17. The portable frame used for home traction.

Traction

When the femoral head does not reduce into the acetabulum with flexion or when the patient is older than 6 months of age, a period of traction may be necessary. Skin traction is preferable to skeletal traction, and the hips and knees are maintained in a flexed position to decrease hamstring tightness. Experience has shown that gradual, continuous traction over a period of approximately 3 weeks is the best way to stretch the soft tissues and allow for reduction of the hip without producing avascular necrosis of the femoral head. Thus, whenever possible, a program of home traction, as described by Joseph and associates[35] and Wagner[95] should be considered. The home traction program allows for gradual stretching while at the same time avoiding the psychological and financial burdens imposed upon a family by the extended hospitalization of a young child. In some patients, traction may be initiated in the hospital until both family and child are familiar enough with the setup and the care routine to continue treatment at home.

The basic traction method consists of elastic bandages, which are used to maintain nonadhesive foam strips on the lower limbs; these wrappings should extend from the medial and lateral malleoli to the groin, ending in spreaders, which protect the integrity of both skin and circulation in the area of the ankle (Fig. 18-17). Initially, 1 kg of traction weight is applied to each leg, with increments of 0.5 kg added gradually. The maximum weight that should be applied to an extremity is usually 2.5 kg, in order to avoid excessive risk of skin breakdown.

Whether the traction is being carried out in the home or in the hospital, radiographs should be obtained at weekly intervals. Clinical assessment should be made to determine whether there is an increase in the laxity or reducibility of the hip. The duration of traction treatment will of course vary with individual patients. The goal of traction is to bring the femoral head down to a level below that of the acetabulum so that reduction may safely be attempted. If the radiographs show that there is no improvement or only minimal distal migration of the femoral head or metaphysis, pin traction may be considered.

Cast Application

Once the femoral metaphysis has been pulled well below the level of the acetabulum, the child is taken to the operating room, and, under general anesthesia, an attempt at closed reduction is made. If the hip does reduce, the most stable, yet safe, position must be found to hold it in reduction. With the hip reduced and flexed to at least 90°, the leg is allowed to fall freely into abduction, and the degree of abduction is recorded. The leg is then gradually adducted back toward the midline. The point at which the hip redislocates is identified as the instability point. The hip should then be stabilized midway between the *fully* abducted position and the instability point. Using this degree of abduction, the complication of avascular necrosis can usually be avoided.

To test whether a dislocated hip has been reduced, the knee is extended. If the hip is reduced, the knee cannot be fully extended without a redislocation. Another method of testing for reduction is to palpate the ischium and the greater trochanter, which should be approximately on the same level; if the greater trochanter is posterior to the ischium, the hip has not been reduced. In such cases, a subcutaneous adductor tenotomy is performed in conjunction with the reduction. Most hips reduce by a closed method in children of this age. The reduction of the femoral head into the acetabulum should be confirmed by roentgenogram before application of the cast. Arthrography is rarely helpful in this age group.

The application of a cast is rather complicated. Once the child is placed on the cast table, there should be one person responsible for maintaining the reduction. This may cause difficulties, because the anesthesiologist is trying to maintain the airway while an assistant is pulling at the hip to hold it in a stabilized position. Often, this results in the child sliding cephalad off the post of the table, with the hips coming down into extension, which may render the previously reduced hip unstable. The knee should be in a 45° flexed position, but it must be kept in mind that the knee cannot be fully extended; if so, the hamstrings tighten and produce pressure on the femoral head. We have also found it to be helpful to apply shoulder straps with the cast. This prevents the child from sliding up in the cast and extending the hips, which would increase the risk of redislocation. Once the cast is applied, it is very important that the child be comfortable during the next 6 to 12 hours. If the child should fuss and cry uncontrollably, the cast should be removed immediately. The most frequent cause of pain in the immediate postcasting period is impending avascular necrosis of the femoral head.

Some of the most severe deformities secondary to avascular necrosis occur following cast application without preliminary traction and without general anesthesia. This is not to say that all children need to have general anesthesia for cast application. However, usually it is difficult to apply the cast with the child awake and agitated. There is a temptation to hold the hips very snugly into place and, thus, to risk a very severe avascular necrosis. Therefore, in an unstable hip that requires closed reduction, our approach is to apply the cast under general anesthesia.

Open Reduction

Except for the teratologic type of dislocation, very few children younger than walking age require open reduction, because almost all of these hips can be reduced by closed positioning or reduction methods.

If open reduction is required, the classic anterolateral Smith-Petersen approach should be the standard technique.

The medial adductor approach of Ludloff is appealing because blood loss can be minimized, and it allows for an easy release of the constricted lower portion of the capsule. However, the incidence of avascular necrosis associated with the medial approach is unacceptable.[38,89] The redislocation rate is also higher than with the standard anterolateral approach, because reefing of the superior aspect of the capsule is not possible.

If a child requires an open reduction before he is 1 year of age, secondary procedures on the acetabulum or proximal femur are not required to maintain stability. The acetabular changes are reversible, and anteversion is not a contributing factor to instability in the prewalking child.

Residual Subluxation

If subluxation persists after any of the previously mentioned treatment programs, a few months of abduction therapy, using an Ilfeld or abductor brace with a pelvic band and thigh cuff, will usually produce stability. A roentgenogram should be obtained when the child is first placed in the device to ensure that the femoral head is properly directed and the subluxation is reduced.

CONGENITAL DISLOCATION OF THE HIP—EVALUATION AND TREATMENT AFTER WALKING AGE

Once the child with an untreated congenital dislocation of the hip reaches walking age (regardless of the subsequent treatment), a complete recovery should not be expected. At least some stigmata will be seen in the roentgenograms of the involved hip.

The aims of treatment at this stage should be to re-establish the mechanics of the hip joint, thus delaying the development of osteoarthritis, and, hopefully, avoiding complications so that the patient may reach at least middle age before serious degeneration of the hip joint begins.

PATHOLOGY

In contrast to the pathology of the newborn, which is directly attributable to increased laxity of the joint capsule, the pathology in the walking child shows that all soft tissues and bony parts are distorted to some degree.

Acetabulum

The ossification of the roof of the acetabulum is delayed and can be recognized in a roentgenogram. The acetabular labrum (limbus) may be folded into the posterosuperior lip of the acetabulum as a minor invagination, or, in some patients, it may form an almost complete diaphragm covering the acetabulum. The fat and fibrous tissue in the depths of the acetabulum may be enlarged (pulvinate), thereby obstructing reentry of the femoral head. A false acetabulum may be present and, to the less experienced surgeon, may appear to be the true acetabulum. The proximal location and the absence of an attached ligamentum teres should indicate the difference.

Capsule

The capsule may be constricted between the acetabulum and the femoral head to produce an hourglass deformity. This shape mainly results from the tight iliopsoas tendon indenting the capsule. The inferior surface of the capsule is stretched across the lower half of the acetabulum and, together with the intact transverse acetabular ligament, it may act as a barrier to full reduction of the femoral head below the superior acetabular roof and acetabular labrum. This is probably the most overlooked problem in relation to reduction. The capsule may also adhere to the cartilage of the femoral head and prevent reduction.

Ligamentum Teres

The ligamentum teres may be normal, absent, or enlarged. If enlarged, it may be a relative obstruction to reduction. In the first few years of life, it is not an important source of blood supply to the hip, and, therefore, it can be sacrificed at the time of open reduction.

Femoral Head and Proximal Femur

The femoral head may lose its conical form and become flattened. This change of shape is often exaggerated when the femoral head has been maintained against the side of the pelvis during an unsuccessful treatment program. The proximal femur usually demonstrates an increase in anteversion. This increase can be most accurately determined clinically by the number of degrees above the normal 45° of internal rotation required to produce a concentric repositioning of the femoral head.

ROENTGENOGRAPHIC EVALUATION

Roentgenographic review is most helpful in the follow-up of CDH, because most patients have few, if any, clinical symptoms in adolescence and young adult life. Evaluation of the three dimensions around the hip joint is ideal, but most critical—and most reliable—is the anteroposterior view. Special views for anteversion have been described but are not of much help in the evaluation of an individual patient. A repeat roentgenogram with the thigh in varying degrees of internal rotation may demonstrate subluxation resulting from anteversion of the femur (Fig. 18-18). A cross-table lateral roentgenogram may demonstrate an uncovered anterior aspect of the femoral head; this is best seen when compared with a normal contralateral hip.

Acetabular Index

The acetabular index is determined by first drawing a line across the triradiate cartilage (Hilgenreiner's line).[32] This line intersects with a line drawn from the lateral edge of the acetabulum to the triradiate cartilage. The acetabular index is the angle formed by the intersection of these two lines. In the past, the acetabular index has often been considered the absolute criterion in determining the shape of the developing acetabulum; however, this index represents only the bone formation. Arthrography, however, demonstrates that the acetabulum maintains a normal cartilaginous contour much longer than was formerly believed (Fig. 18-19). Therefore, reconstructive procedures that were once performed on children 3 to 4 years of age can now be safely delayed until they are 6 to 7 years of age if there is no evidence of subluxation, even if the bony outline of the acetabulum appears to be deficient.

Center-Edge (CE) Angle

The center-edge (CE) angle is determined by finding the center of the femoral head and marking the lateral corner of the acetabulum. A horizontal line connects the two femoral head centers, and perpendicular lines are drawn from each center. A line is drawn from the acetabular edge to the center of the femoral head, and the angle formed is known as the *center-edge angle* (Fig. 18-20). The CE angle should be at least 20° (preferably 25°) to ensure normal seating of the femoral head.

After the femoral head has been reduced, the CE angle should be measured to ensure that full reduction has been achieved and that the hip is not subluxated. This evaluation is relatively simple in the normal hip, because the corner of the normal acetabulum can be fully visualized. An acetabular dysplasia makes the evaluation difficult, because the landmarks are less distinct, but this is still the best method to detect a slight degree of subluxation. A computed tomography (CT) scan may occasionally be helpful in distinguishing between dysplasia and subluxation.

REDUCTION OF THE DISLOCATED HIP

A controversy still exists as to the relative merits of closed and open reduction in the treatment of a child who has reached walking age. Primary treatment of a dislocated hip in this age group is becoming increasingly rare, so that in many parts of the world, surgeons are involved in the treatment of relatively few children. Of all the standard operative procedures on the hip joint, an accurate open reduction in a child of any age is probably the most difficult. Therefore, it should not be taken lightly. For most surgeons, in a child up to 3 years of age, a careful closed reduction following a period of traction is the most successful form of treatment. This results in the least amount of stiffness and involves only a minor risk of avascular necrosis. The downward displacement of the femoral head is verified by radiographs before attempting closed reduction. If the initial reduction is successful, redislocation is not likely to occur.

The home traction program has been just as successful in this age group as in infants and has again managed to reduce both the length of hospitalization and the cost of treatment. The home traction period is much less disturbing to the child and is usually less disruptive of family life.

Skin traction is preferable to skeletal traction. If a pin is used, it should be placed in the distal femur instead of the tibia, just above the level of the proximal pole of the patella, and with the knee in extension. Once the femoral head reaches the level of the triradiate cartilage and remains there for several days, it is desirable to remove the pin and return to skin traction before reducing the hip. The reestablishment of skin traction allows the pin-tract to heal and decreases the risk of infection, if an open reduction is necessary.

Closed Reduction

For *gentle* closed reduction or repositioning of a dislocated hip, the child should be anesthetized to allow full muscle relaxation. The child lies in a supine position with the pelvis flat on the table and the opposite extremity flexed, abducted, and stabilized by an assistant. The thigh on the affected side is flexed and adducted to relax the capsule and the adductor muscles. Gentle manual traction is applied to the thigh while the surgeon guides the femoral head into the socket; pressure is applied over the greater trochanter with the opposite hand, while the thigh is gradually abducted 50° to 60° (*never* approaching 80° to 90°). The thigh is then gradually adducted until the femoral head again drops out of the acetabulum. This redislocation gives an indication of the potential stability of the joint and the likelihood of achieving success by closed reduction. This maneuver is also used to determine the safety zone, as previously described.

All maneuvers must be done as gently as possible and carried out as "positioning" the leg rather than forcing a reduction. The procedure is actually similar to the Ortolani maneuver for the infant. If any tightness is demonstrated in the adductors, a subcutaneous adductor tenotomy should be done. This procedure is necessary in almost all children in this age group. If the arc of motion between reduction and dislocation is less than 25°, successful maintenance of reduction is most unlikely and redislocation is to be expected. An open reduction should then be undertaken.

Roentgenograms are taken to confirm the

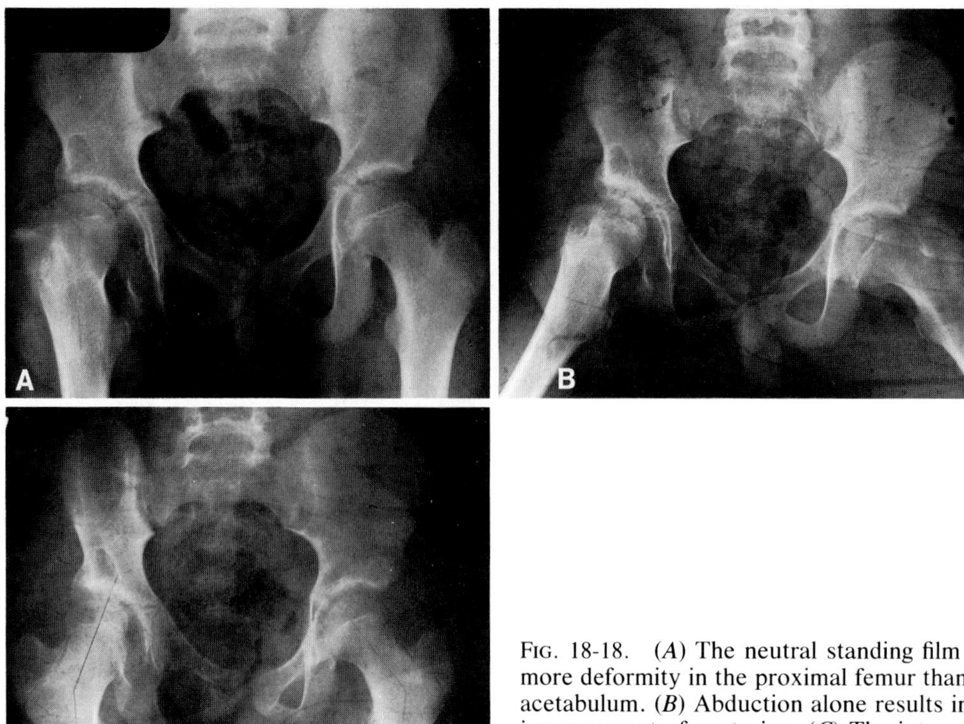

FIG. 18-18. (*A*) The neutral standing film shows more deformity in the proximal femur than in the acetabulum. (*B*) Abduction alone results in slight improvement of centering. (*C*) The internal rotation view shows further improvement. (*Continued on facing page.*)

FIG. 18-19. (*A*) This roentgenogram shows a deficient bony acetabulum. (*B*) However, arthrography shows the cartilage model to be normal. Therefore, the patient has only dysplasia of the bony acetabulum.

FIG. 18-18. (*Continued*) (*D*) Combined internal rotation and abduction results in the best centering of the hips. (*E*) A standing film after an osteotomy that combined external rotation and adduction shows that the same positioning is achieved as in *D*.

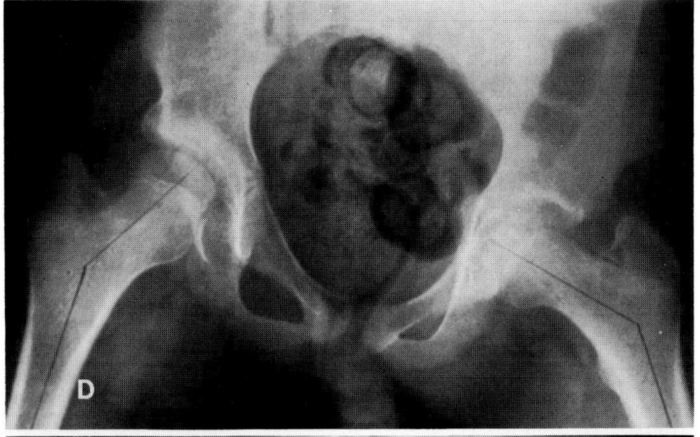

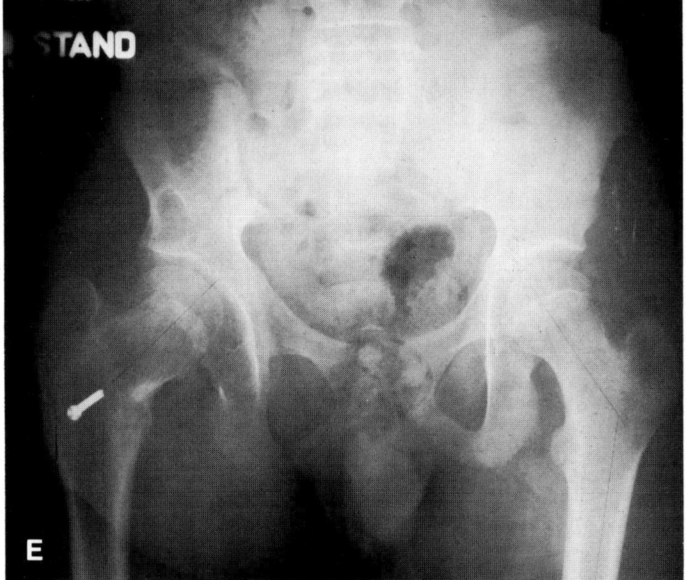

position of the head within the socket, and the femoral head must point to, or slightly below, the triradiate cartilage. A more proximal alignment of the femoral head is not compatible with a concentric reduction. Further flexion of the thigh may direct the head to the triradiate cartilage. If this is not successful, an open reduction is indicated. Following closed reduction, lateral roentgenograms yield little information other than to show a true redislocation. A plaster cast is applied with the thigh in 90° of flexion, never exceeding 60° of abduction. A modified frog-leg plaster cast is used for 6 to 9 months. An abduction brace should be used for an additional 6 months to 1 year if there are problems in maintaining the centering of the femoral head. If the hip still demonstrates subluxation with the leg in neutral position and if there is good centering with the leg in abduction, some type of extra-

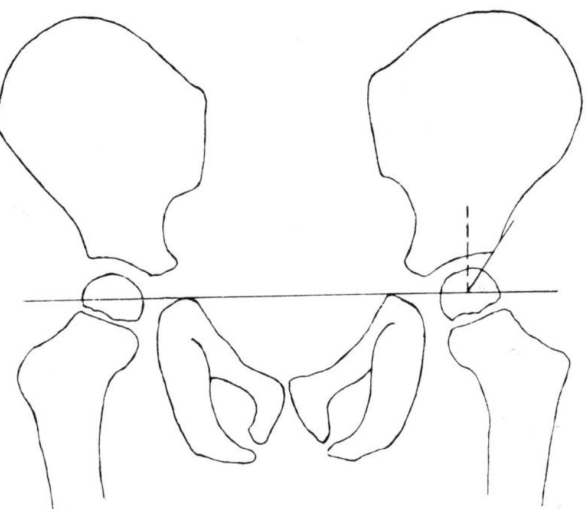

FIG. 18-20. The center-edge angle of Wiberg.

articular procedure should be considered to keep the femoral head centered.

If closed reduction proves to be unsuccessful, the surgeon should be prepared to proceed with open reduction. However, lateral displacement of the epiphysis after closed reduction is not an indication for open reduction. The clinical signs of stability are more helpful at this stage than are the results of an arthrogram. After a few days or weeks, the femoral head usually settles deeply into the acetabulum, as can be seen on follow-up roentgenograms. Persistent displacement at 6 weeks is an indication for open reduction.

Morel[55] has reintroduced and refined the technique of gradual longitudinal traction; this is followed by gradual positioning of the leg in abduction and internal rotation and the application of a spica cast, without the need for a reduction *per se*. This technique has resulted in concentric reduction in two thirds of the patients, even though many are 5 or 6 years of age, and it involves only a minimal risk of avascular necrosis. If the patient does not show full reduction 6 weeks after this maneuver, open reduction is performed. All of Morel's patients had innominate osteotomies a few weeks after stability had been obtained. This program has been highly successful in children up to approximately 6 years of age. It is based on gradual repositioning of the head of the femur in the acetabulum and the use of only extra-articular procedures, where possible. We agree with this concept.

Open Reduction

The indications for open reduction are: (1) if the femoral head persistently lies above the triradiate cartilage on roentgenographic examination, (2) if the arc of reduction and redislocation is less than 25° after an adductor tenotomy, (3) if the femoral head will not enter the acetabulum, (4) if the femoral head is still laterally placed in the acetabulum after 6 weeks of reduction, and (5) if a previous reduction has failed.

In the hands of surgeons who lack extensive experience, it is probably best to consider open reduction as the only primary procedure, reserving femoral or pelvic osteotomy as secondary measures. Too often redislocation has followed the combined procedures, and it is probably best to concentrate on performing a careful and complete open reduction. The secondary procedures can be carried out later, as after a closed reduction.

A careful open reduction should always be carried out according to an organized plan, with emphasis placed upon several important details.

The Smith-Petersen incision is most often used in children in this age group. However, the skin incision should be placed below the iliac crest, not over it. It then extends in an oblique line parallel to the inguinal ligament and should not turn distally. This allows for the same deep exposure but produces a much less noticeable scar. The psoas tendon should be sectioned if it is tight, but the iliacus muscle should always be left intact to preserve hip flexion. In the older patient, it may be necessary to peel the capsule from the articular cartilage of the femoral head. This procedure should be done with great care, and the dissection should not be carried down along the femoral neck, which would risk damage to the metaphyseal vessels and increase the risk of avascular necrosis.

If the fibrofatty tissue from the acetabulum is not thoroughly removed, it is difficult or impossible to reduce the head deeply into the socket. The use of a curette has often been suggested; however, this can result in destruction of portions of the articular cartilage. Pituitary rongeurs have been more effective in thoroughly removing the soft-tissue material, and they do not obstruct visibility during the procedure.

The inferior half of the acetabulum is one of the most important areas of the hip and is commonly overlooked. The anterolateral exposure, which is the standard approach for open reduction in the walking child, makes the distance to the inferior capsule considerable and, therefore, limits visualization in this area. The inferior capsule is usually stretched upward and across the inferior acetabulum, but is actually best pushed downward by blunt instruments, thus creating a pocket for the femoral head. The transverse acetabular ligament cannot be visualized through this approach, but, with palpation and a pair of scissors, it can be felt, outlined, transected, and opened, allowing the lower part of the acetabulum to widen. If a pocket is not developed inferiorly, the head will often not drop down into the lower part of the acetabulum, which is necessary for concentric reduction. This area is probably the most commonly overlooked in open reduction. An osteotomy is too often unwisely considered as an alternative to gaining full reduction, when in fact it should be used to develop the lower acetabular area. In such patients, to incorrectly use a pelvic osteotomy may only increase the intra-articular pressure and cause a redislocation or avascular necrosis. An accurate reduction must initially be obtained, and the lower acetabulum is the area of concern.

The infolding of the acetabular labrum (limbus) may also be an obstruction to concentric reduction. This infolding can be detected at the time of open reduction by running a curved blunt instrument about the upper half of the acetabulum. If found, it is preferable to evert the labrum and reduce the head deeply under it; this may require one or two radial cuts in the labrum before it folds outward. However, the labrum is part of the normal biologic tissue and is probably required for full acetabular development. Therefore, it should not be removed unless it is impossible to fold it outside the equator of the femoral head.

After open reduction, immobilization should not be continued past 6 to 8 weeks; otherwise, severe stiffness may result.

The older child with bilateral hip dislocation is a most difficult problem. One should strongly consider withholding treatment in a child older than 4 years of age, because the risk of stiffness in both hips is significant. This group of children has produced the greatest number of difficulties in treatment programs. Bilaterally dislocated hips, however, which are unusually mobile and in which the femoral heads pull down readily with gentle traction, may be reduced, but these are the exceptions. If roentgenograms show very high femoral heads, reduction should probably not be attempted.

The argument has been put forth that better total hip joint replacement techniques may be possible later if bilateral dislocated hips are reduced. However, we believe that it is not realistic to perform multiple surgical procedures in a patient with persistent bilateral dislocations throughout childhood and adolescence, in order to allow for better reconstructive replacement later. Most of these patients can actually get along for 25 to 40 years without treatment.[98] Although this is not an ideal situation, it is better than having repeated, unsuccessful operations. In most instances, however, the child with a unilateral dislocation is a candidate for treatment throughout childhood.

Colonna Arthroplasty

This arthroplasty is only indicated in a patient with complete dislocation of the hip. The capsule is enclosed over the femoral head and placed in an enlarged acetabulum from which the articular cartilage has been removed. Most patients treated by this procedure develop degenerative arthritis as young adults, and a significant percentage of patients will have stiff hips at an early age. The procedure has essentially been replaced by other operations and is rarely, if ever, indicated.

Complicated Reductions

If it is not possible or desirable to lower the femoral head to the level of the acetabulum with traction because of tightness in the surrounding tissues, a technique repopularized by Klisic and Jankovic[42] can be used to shorten the femur. This technique allows for the lowering of the femoral head to the acetabular level, without tension, by shortening the femur instead of elongating the muscles. However, if the surgeon is not particularly familiar with the routine methods of reduction, it is best to bring the femoral head into place with traction and concentrate all efforts on careful and complete open reduction.

If shortening of the femur is undertaken, it is important to first carry out the technique of exposing and removing the tissues that are preventing reduction before transecting the femur. This allows for better control of the fragments. The femoral osteotomy is allowed to overlap the distance previously occupied by the top of the femoral head above the roof of the acetabulum (approximately 2 cm), and some varus positioning may be desirable for stability. The anteversion may also be reduced by externally rotating the distal fragment and leaving about 10° to 15° of internal rotation. The osteotomy should be internally stabilized by pins or a plate.[18,101]

PRINCIPLES OF MAINTAINING REDUCTION BY SECONDARY PROCEDURES

The ideal goal of treatment in a child who remains untreated until after walking age is to produce a reasonably good hip joint at skeletal maturity, with no residual subluxation and only mild distortion of the acetabulum and proximal femur. Although this goal may not always be possible due to complications from the initial treatment, surgery may still be desirable. Several types of repair and reconstructive procedures must be considered. There are advantages and problems with each procedure.

As a rule, unless the hip is completely redislocated, extra-articular procedures should be performed on the proximal femur and/or pelvis, because intra-articular procedures involve an increased risk of joint stiffness in the older child.

Standing roentgenograms should always be used after a child reaches walking age. These films may help to identify leg-length discrepancy, either true or apparent, and can also establish the presence of subluxation. This subluxation may be secondary to weightbearing or to a possible malalignment of the pelvis.

If a child requires a secondary procedure, it is important to consider that both the femoral and acetabular components are abnormal to some degree. Usually, one aspect of the joint is more deformed than the other, and it becomes important to treat the more serious deformity if a good result is to be obtained. Because neither side of the joint will be fully corrected, biologic remodeling is necessary to produce the best result. Therefore, surgery should ideally be performed when there are at least 2 to 3 years of growth potential remaining—by approximately the age of 10 years in girls and 12 years in boys. Most of the procedures available may still be performed when the patient is skeletally mature, but less satisfactory results must be anticipated once the potential for remodeling with growth is gone.

The abduction test, whereby roentgenograms are obtained with the thigh abducted to varying degrees, can yield valuable information as to the extent of repositioning of the femoral head within the acetabulum. These roentgenograms can also help to determine the most desirable secondary procedure for a particular patient (Fig. 18-21). As a rule, both the pelvis and the proximal femur lose their ability to fully remodel when the child is approximately 7 to 8 years of age. After that age, in a child with a major deformity, more thought may be required in selecting a procedure to improve both the femoral and acetabular components of the deformity.

Acetabular Procedures

For a surgeon to consider performing a pelvic procedure, he should first determine (1) whether the major problem involves the acetabular component of the hip, and (2) whether the femoral head centers on the abduction test. If there is only mild to moderate deformity of the acetabulum and the affected extremity is not longer than the other, the innominate osteotomy of Salter is performed. If the acetabulum is increased in size or is more seriously deformed, as confirmed by arthrogram, the Pemberton procedure may be performed. The shelf procedure is indicated for the adolescent who needs only a stabilizing containment buttress. If the femoral head cannot be centered and the patient is having symptoms, the surgeon can resort to the reconstructive surgery of Chiari. If the femoral head can still be centered on the abduction test but the deformity is severe, the Steel or Sutherland procedures should be considered. The dial osteotomy is technically very difficult and may alter the blood supply of the acetabular roof; there are no real indications for this operation unless the surgeon has had vast experience with this type of surgery. It must, of course, be emphasized that if hip problems are recognized early, as is becoming more and more common, these latter, complex surgical procedures rarely become necessary.

Realignment Techniques. The shelf procedure was the first extra-articular acetabular containment procedure to be developed. It allows the intact acetabular cartilage to remain in contact with the femoral head. The shelf should be thought of as a stabilizer or buttress of the femoral head by the extension of the acetabulum, rather than as an additional weightbearing surface (Fig. 18-22).

It is difficult to perform the shelf procedure at exactly the correct level. It is often placed too far proximally on the side of the pelvis. (In time, the shelf will disappear if it is not giving buttress support to the femoral head). The upper portion of the capsule must be stripped down and part of it must even be split horizontally to give a smooth contour with the capsule over the femoral head. Only when dissection of the capsule is complete should a notch be created just above the acetabulum so that contoured segments of outer pelvic cortex can be placed into the notch and over the capsule and buttressed with extra bone.

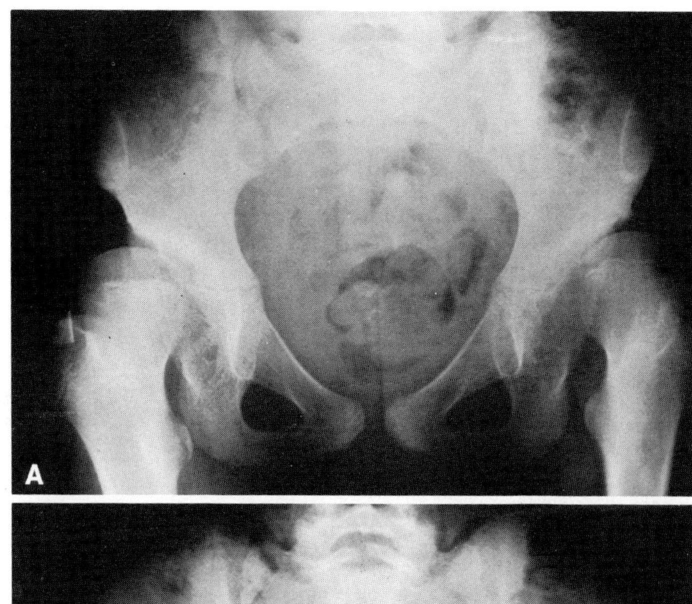

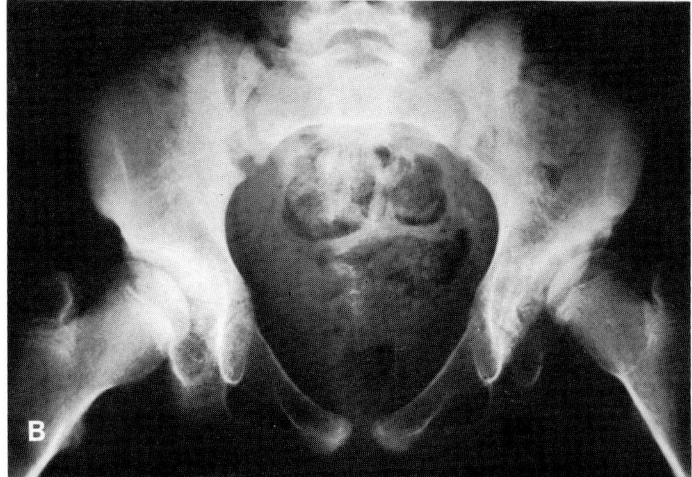

FIG. 18-21. The abduction test is performed to determine whether the femoral head will center. (*A*) The anteroposterior view shows significant subluxation of the femoral heads. (*B*) When there is abduction and internal rotation, centering results. This suggests that a technique to reposition the femoral heads is appropriate in this patient.

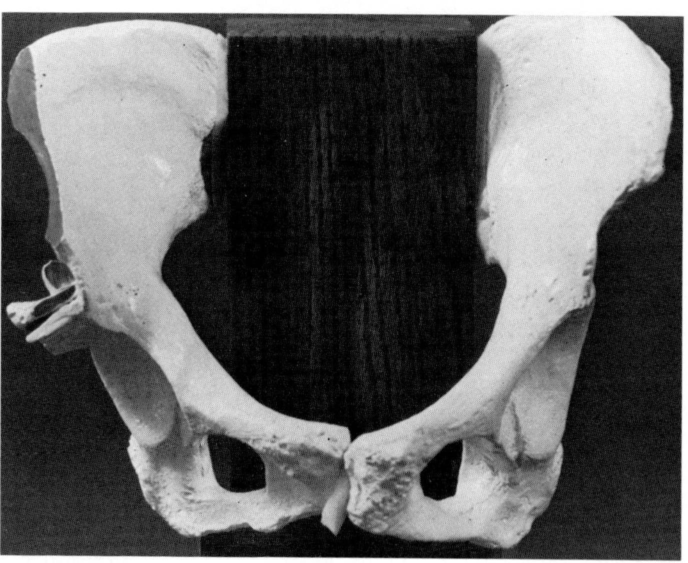

FIG. 18-22. This model shows the proper level of shelf placement for the shelf procedure.

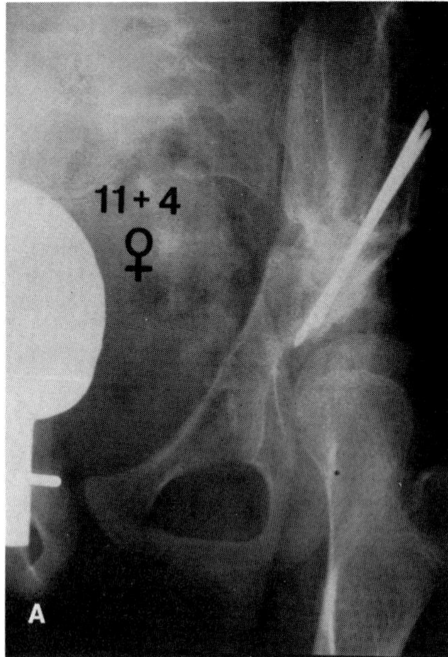

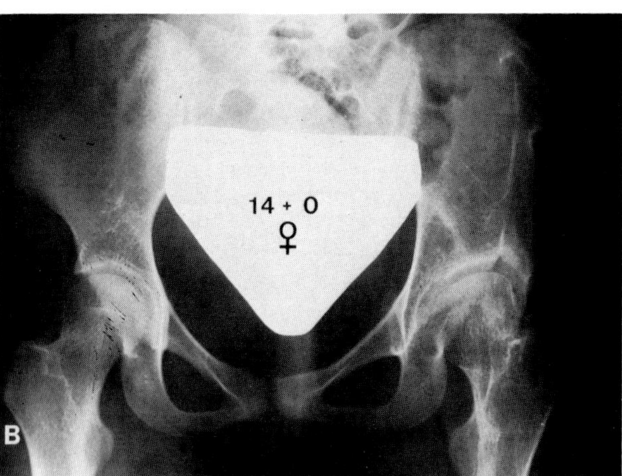

FIG. 18-23. (*A*) Immediate preoperative film of a girl 11 years and 4 months old who underwent a shelf osteotomy to salvage an inadequate Salter procedure. (*B*) Follow-up film at 14 years of age shows a contained head with the buttress effect of the shelf. One half of the femoral head must be in the acetabulum, with no gross instability, for a successful result to ensue.

Wilson[104] has reported a successful series in adolescents. Although the shelf is a reconstructive procedure, it is useful even in the older child or young adult in whom little or no biologic remodeling is to be expected when some contact exists between the femoral head and the acetabulum but when the femoral head is subluxated laterally (Fig. 18-23). An important guideline to follow is that at least half of the femoral head must be within the acetabulum with good stability for a successful result to be possible.

The innominate osteotomy of Salter is used to redirect the acetabulum in order to produce femoral head coverage laterally and anteriorly.[73,74] It is ideal for acetabular dysplasia and mild subluxation in children 3 to 10 years of age. Anterior coverage of the femoral head is accomplished by rotation of the acetabular fragment on the symphysis. The size of the patient and the resultant distance from the midline are not critical to the production of the anterior coverage (Fig. 18-24). The difficulty with this procedure arises in obtaining

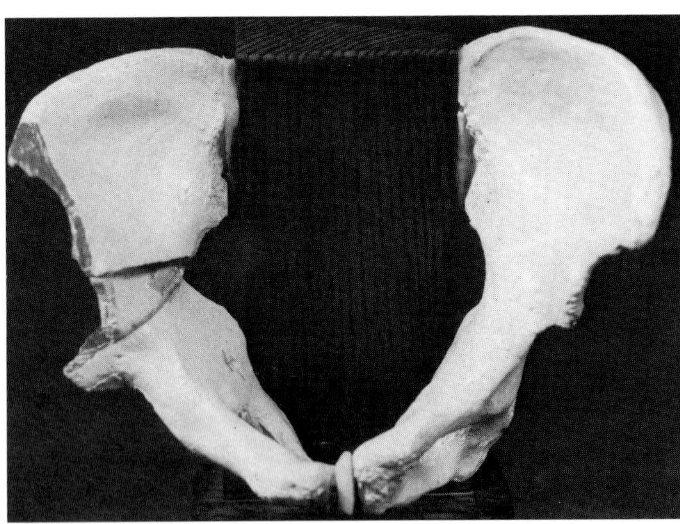

FIG. 18-24. A model of the Salter procedure, showing lateral and anterior rotation of the distal fragment and rotation at the symphysis pubis. To avoid excessive lengthening of the extremity, the graft should not separate the bony fragments posteriorly.

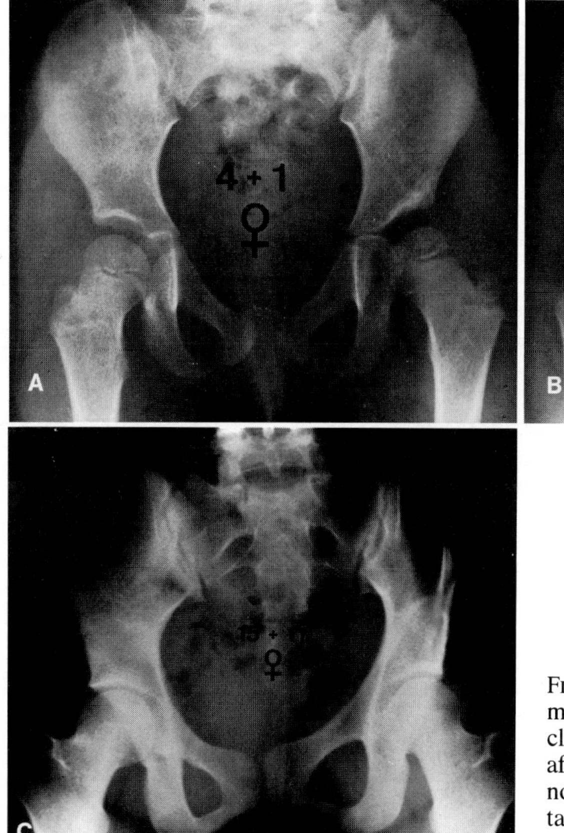

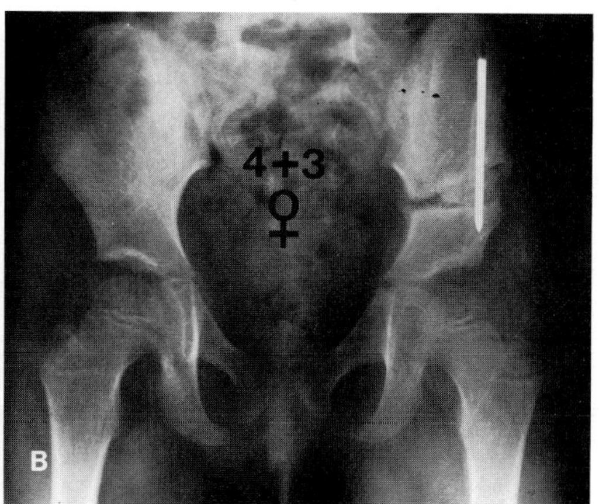

FIG. 18-25. (*A*) This female, 4 years and 1 month old, exhibits residual dysplasia following closed reduction. (*B*) A film taken immediately after Salter osteotomy shows an essentially normal acetabular roof. (*C*) The follow-up film taken at 15 years and 11 months shows an excellent result at skeletal maturity.

lateral coverage. The angulation occurs on the symphysis pubis, which is a significant distance from the acetabulum, limiting the potential for improvement. The average change in acetabular index that can be produced by the Salter technique is approximately 10°. Therefore, if the acetabulum must be changed significantly, this procedure is not technically feasible. An arthrogram is advisable before considering this osteotomy. If the cartilaginous acetabular model is normal and the hip is not subluxated, surgery can be delayed until the child is approximately 7 years of age, because there is a good possibility that the bony acetabulum may reconstitute without intervention.

If, however, there is any suggestion of subluxation, the procedure should be performed as soon as possible. In Salter's own series, the best results were obtained in the group of patients who had dysplasia without an associated dislocation. Ninety-four percent of the total series had an excellent result (Fig. 18-25). A disadvantage of the Salter innominate procedure is that it can produce a longer extremity on the involved side. Even though the osteotomy remains closed posteriorly, it tends to lengthen the extremity by approximately 1 cm. In a patient of adult size, this change is not significant, but in a child 6 years of age, the problem is magnified. All follow-up roentgenograms should be taken in the standing position rather than in the supine position to allow for better evaluation of the hips' centering and the leg lengths. If the femoral head is not fully covered after the innominate osteotomy, a heel lift on the opposite extremity may again level the pelvis. If the involved extremity is already longer, the notch technique of Kalamchi, which involves the removal of a bone wedge at the posterior section of the pelvis, may be performed with the innominate osteotomy to avoid magnifying the leg-length problem.[36]

Some innominate osteotomies are incorrectly stabilized. The pins used are often not

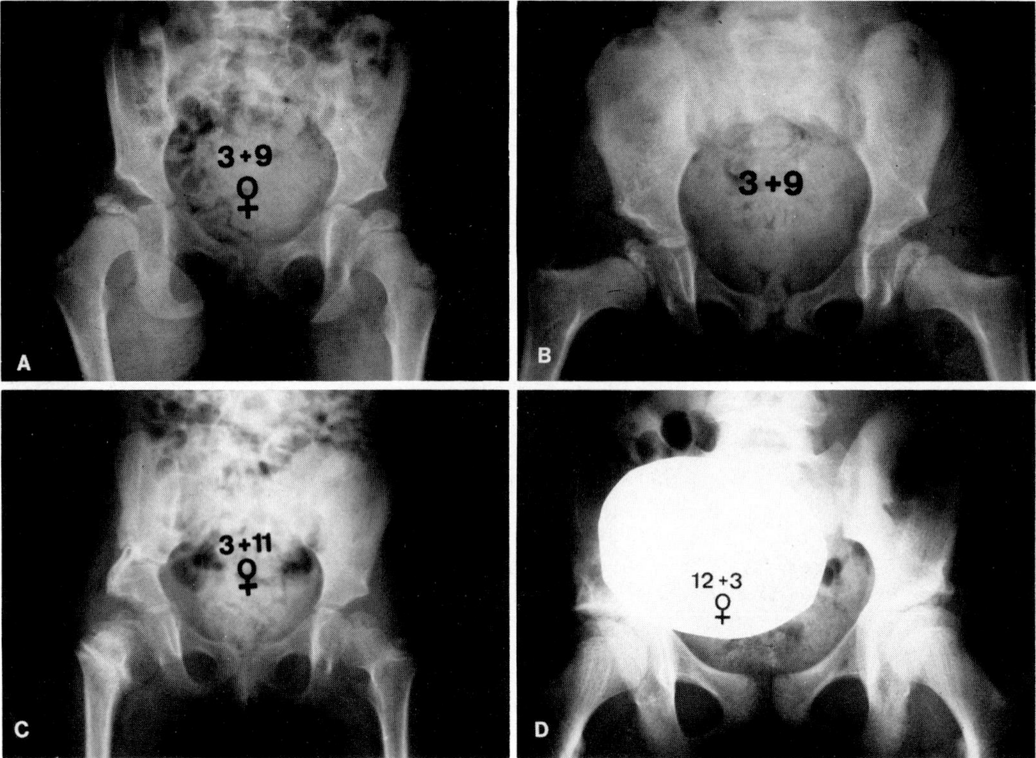

FIG. 18-26. (*A*) In this child of 3 years and 9 months, the neutral-position film shows vascular changes in the femoral head and residual acetabular dysplasia. (*B*) Significant abduction is necessary to produce centering. (*C*) Film taken 2 months later, soon after the Salter procedure and intertrochanteric varus osteotomy were performed. (*D*) At 12 years of age, there is good coverage of the femoral head.

long enough to stabilize the distal fragment, allowing the graft to dislodge and the distal fragment to slip medially. If, after this occurs, the femoral head does not subluxate, the result should be accepted. If subluxation occurs and the femoral head centers on the abduction test, a varus osteotomy is indicated rather than a second acetabular procedure (Fig. 18-26).

PEMBERTON OSTEOTOMY. In this procedure, both the direction and the shape of the acetabular roof are changed at the triradiate cartilage (Fig. 18-27).[63] The change in direction of the acetabular roof is, therefore, of much greater magnitude than in the innominate procedure of Salter, where the lateral rotation of the roof of the acetabulum is at the symphysis pubis. Both procedures, however, should be done only for a hip with a true, concentric reduction. This procedure is particularly indicated when there is a major, true deficiency in the angle of the cartilaginous acetabular roof. The actual deformity should be confirmed by an arthrogram, because the true cartilage model may be intact, even if the bone model appears grossly deficient. If the cartilage is, in fact, in good condition, the Pemberton procedure would grossly distort the hip joint and is therefore contraindicated.

The Pemberton osteotomy requires extensive surgical exposure and is technically more difficult than the Salter procedure. By altering the depth of the osteotomy medially or laterally, the distal fragment can be directed either more anteriorly or laterally, as required. Because the acetabular roof is further distorted during the procedure, there is a risk of stiffness. Therefore, as full a range of motion as possible should be obtained prior to undertaking this operation (Fig. 18-28).

Because the downward direction of the acetabular roof can be grossly altered, there is considerable risk of substantially increasing the acetabular pressure. If there has been any upward migration of the femoral head, the

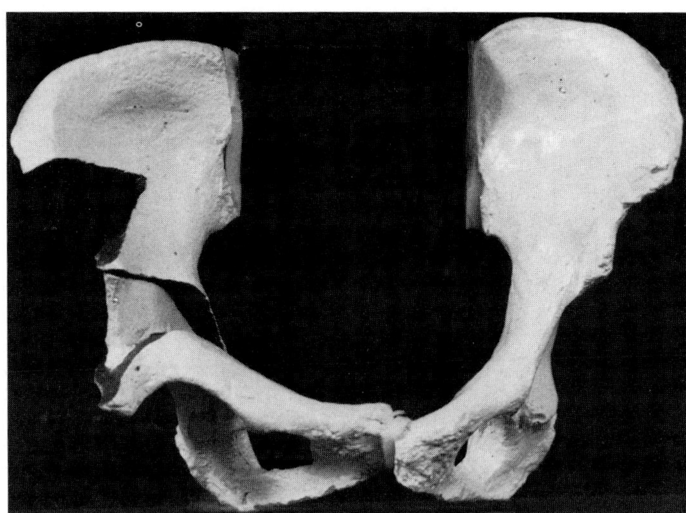

FIG. 18-27. This model of the Pemberton procedure shows the alteration in the acetabular roof achieved by angulating the hip at the triradiate cartilage.

procedure should only be performed following a period of femoral traction to bring the femoral head down to the appropriate level.

The Pemberton osteotomy necessarily deforms the acetabulum and produces an incongruity. However, this incongruity should correct itself in the growing child. The cut must not extend into the acetabulum and damage the articular cartilage. The Pemberton procedure may produce a stiff hip in the older child, because the acetabulum is deformed and incongruity is aggravated. It should, therefore,

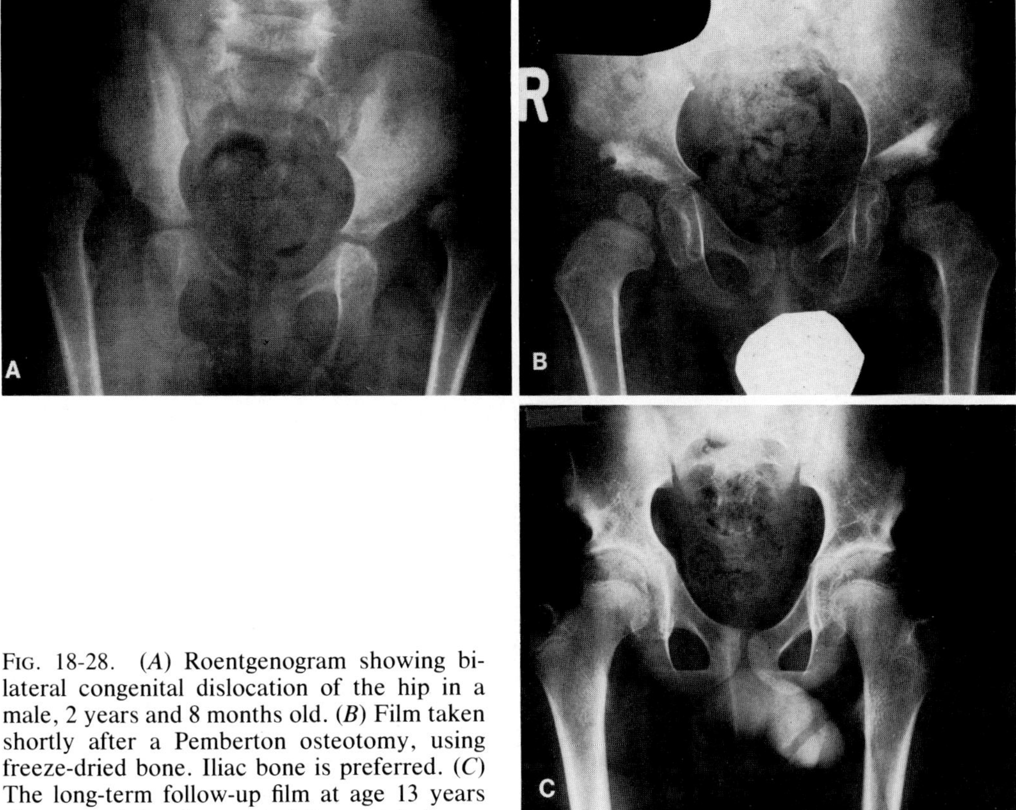

FIG. 18-28. (*A*) Roentgenogram showing bilateral congenital dislocation of the hip in a male, 2 years and 8 months old. (*B*) Film taken shortly after a Pemberton osteotomy, using freeze-dried bone. Iliac bone is preferred. (*C*) The long-term follow-up film at age 13 years shows good development of the acetabula.

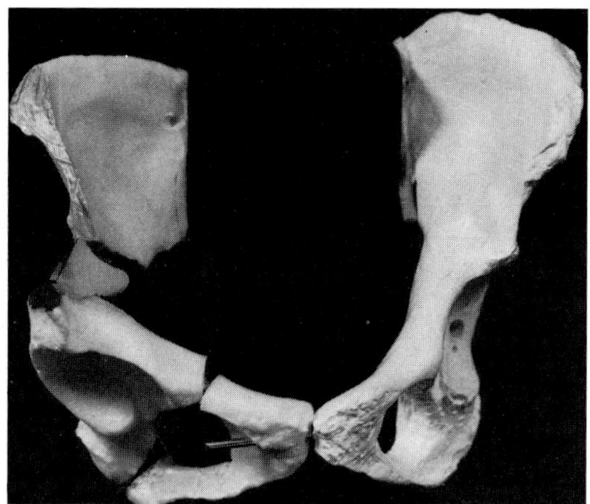

Fig. 18-29. A model of a Steel osteotomy shows cut made on the innominate bone through the three appropriate areas. (The pin across the symphysis pubis is used only to stabilize the model and is not a part of the actual procedure.)

ideally be performed several years before skeletal maturity is reached. Closure of the triradiate cartilage in the adolescent becomes an absolute contraindication for this procedure. Postoperative immobilization following a Pemberton osteotomy should not exceed 6 weeks.

Steel Procedure. This osteotomy through the innominate bone is much like Salter's procedure, but, instead of rotating at the symphysis pubis, cuts are made through both pubic rami.[80] The ischial cut is made through an incision in the buttock, and the superior ramus is sectioned from the medial aspect of the standard anterolateral Smith-Petersen approach. These extra osteotomies allow freer motion in the acetabular fragment (Fig. 18-29).

The Steel osteotomy is much more complicated than the Salter procedure. It is indicated when the femoral head still centers on the abduction test, but there is a major acetabular deformity (Fig. 18-30). The procedure is contraindicated if the femoral head cannot be reduced into the acetabulum. It is also contraindicated if the problem can be corrected by the use of simpler techniques.

Sutherland Procedure. This procedure is similar in principle and indications to the Steel osteotomy, but the osteotomy through the pubis is made from above.[84] The cut passes just medial to the obturator foramen and lateral to the symphysis pubis. A sector of bone of up to 2 cm is removed to allow medial displacement of the distal fragment (Fig. 18-31). This osteotomy allows for somewhat less rotation than does the Steel procedure but more than would be achieved with an innominate Salter procedure. It can produce more medial displacement of the distal fragment than the Steel procedure because of the removal of the bone. It does, however, require pin fixation of the medial osteotomy, which may result in complications.

Dial Osteotomy. This procedure is a periarticular acetabular osteotomy in which a cut is made around the complete acetabulum just outside the capsule. Because the osteotomy is close to the whole acetabulum, it allows the greatest potential for change in position of the acetabulum. A concentric reduction must be achieved in order to have a successful result with this osteotomy (Fig. 18-32).

Because it is technically difficult to cut out the entire acetabulum without either going medially through the pelvis or entering into

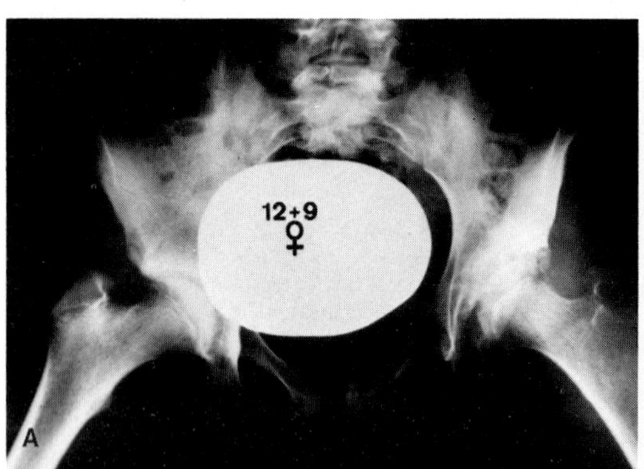

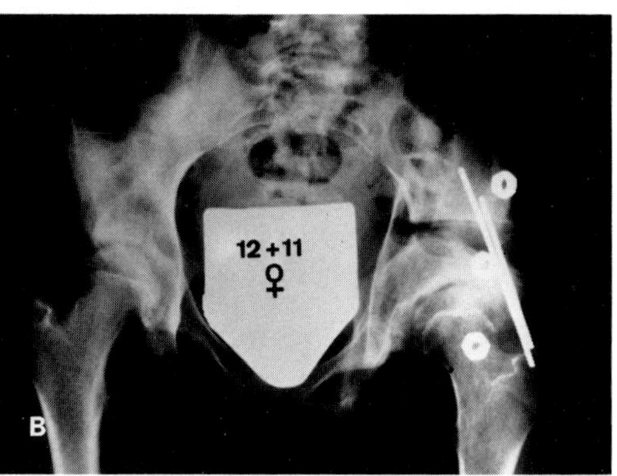

Fig. 18-30. (*A*) Preoperative film of a girl 12 years and 9 months old shows that at least 40° of abduction are required to center the femoral heads. (*B*) The roentgenogram obtained after a Steel osteotomy shows excellent coverage.

Fɪɢ. 18-31. A model of the Sutherland osteotomy. (The *arrow* indicates the midline of the pelvis.)

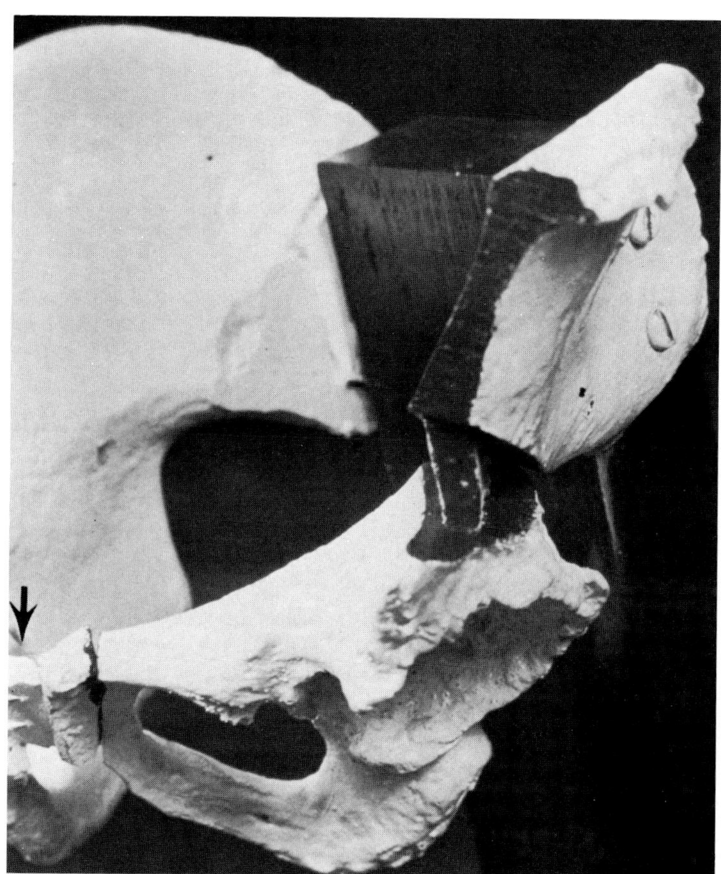

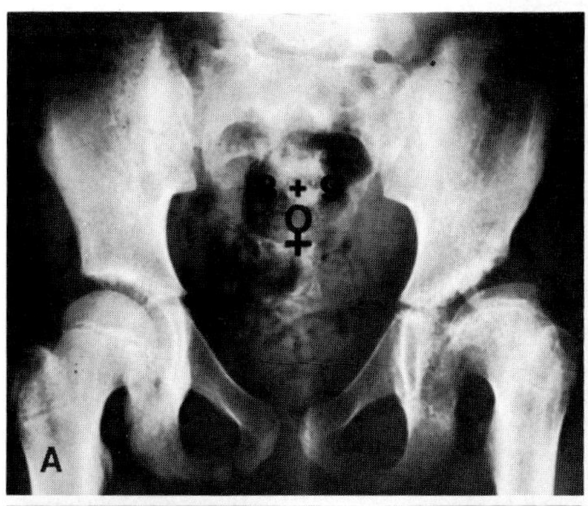

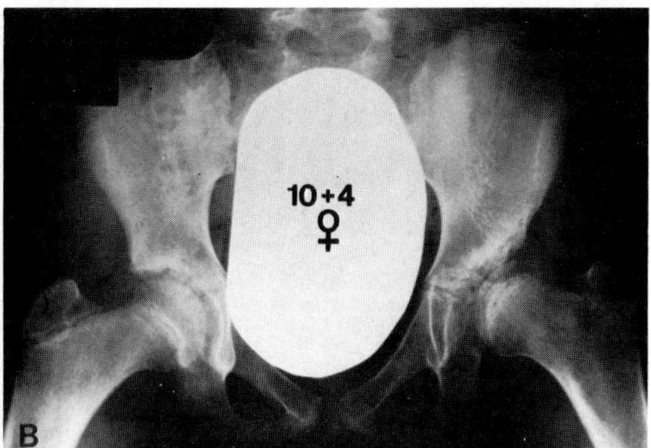

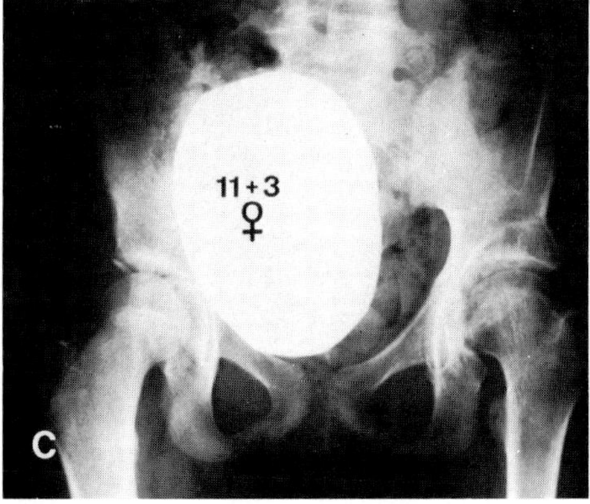

Fɪɢ. 18-32. (*A*) This film shows severe hip dysplasia in a girl 8 years and 9 months of age. (*B*) At 10 years and 4 months of age, centering is achieved on abduction. (*C*) Film taken at age 11 years and 3 months shows excellent coverage of the femoral head after a dial osteotomy.

the acetabulum, there is a relatively high risk of complication associated with the dial procedure. The sciatic nerve must be carefully avoided, and there is a risk of producing vascular changes in the acetabular fragment if the fragment is cut too thin. Although extensive experience has not been gained in the use of this operation, it would seem to be indicated in the older child or adolescent who has very severe subluxation and deformity but in whom a reduction on the abduction test is still possible. This procedure, more than all the others mentioned, is very complex and should be reserved for the patients of surgeons with vast experience in hip surgery.

Reconstructive Procedure—The Chiari Method. If the femoral head will not center on abduction because of a major abnormality of the acetabulum, the procedure developed by the late Professor Chiari may be considered.[13] This allows for good femoral coverage but also serves as an arthroplasty and a salvage procedure. It should not be considered if one of the aforementioned concentric reduction techniques is possible. However, if the femoral head has migrated laterally and proximally, it may no longer center on the abduction test. By displacing the distal fragment medially, a roof is produced for the head underneath the lateral pelvis with the capsule interposed, thus creating an arthroplasty. In theory, moving the femoral head toward the midline improves the mechanics of the joint, resulting in decreased force across the joint on weightbearing. In our experience, the femoral head actually remains displaced only minimally in the medial plane (less than 1 cm); thus, coverage of the femoral head is a more important consideration in selecting this procedure than is the medial displacement.

The osteotomy is made just above the capsule, and the capsule is pushed medially, with the distal fragment, to produce an arthroplasty above the femoral head. In other words, it

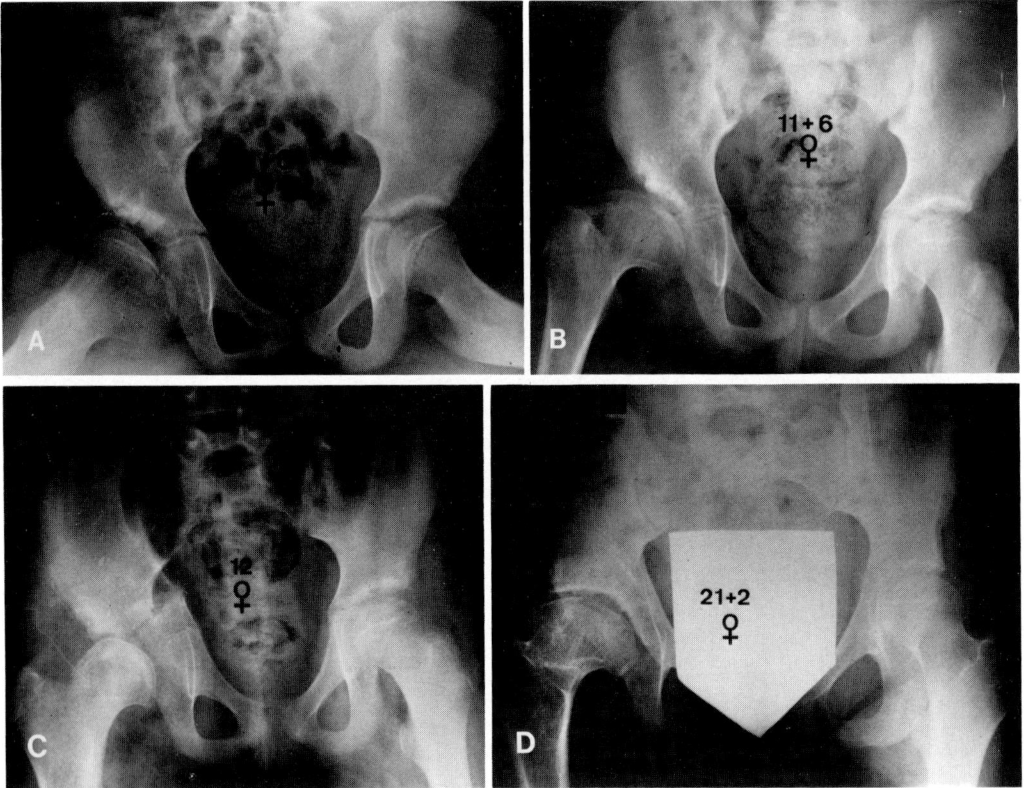

FIG. 18-33. (*A*) Lateral view shows gross deformity following avascular necrosis of the head of the femur. (*B*) Coverage of the femoral head is not achieved on abduction. (*C*) Film taken soon after the Chiari procedure shows coverage of the femoral head. (*D*) Long-term follow-up film taken at 21 years and 2 months shows good coverage of the femoral head. The patient is asymptomatic.

superimposes a Colonna arthroplasty lateral to the deficient contact of the acetabulum and femoral head. The Chiari procedure is technically exacting. The pelvic cut has to be directed medially and upward, so that the distal fragment will slide medially. This usually produces a slight shortening of the leg, which should be considered in the assessment for surgery. Ideally, the osteotomy should be domed from anterior to posterior so that the pelvic surface above the head is contoured and is as congruous as possible. Because the pelvis is essentially cancellous bone, it will contour itself with time, to some degree (Fig. 18-33). It is often of value to remove strips of bone from the outer cortex of the pelvis in order to provide extra shelf coverage both anterior and lateral to the femoral head. A relatively normal neck-shaft angle is an important consideration and, if not present, should be corrected by surgery. In most surgeons' hands, it is probably better to correct the femoral deformity and to proceed to the Chiari procedure several weeks later, after healing of the femoral osteotomy is advanced.

The displacement should be at least half the width of the pelvis (Fig. 18-34). Full displacement, with the distal fragment displaced into the pelvis, may result in nonunion. Threaded pins placed across the osteotomy site can maintain the proper amount of displacement and can avoid the need to apply a spica cast postoperatively. If stable pin fixation is obtained by placing the extremity in balanced suspension, early range-of-motion exercises are possible within days of the procedure (Fig. 18-35). This shortens the time required for rehabilitation and decreases the risk of residual stiffness.

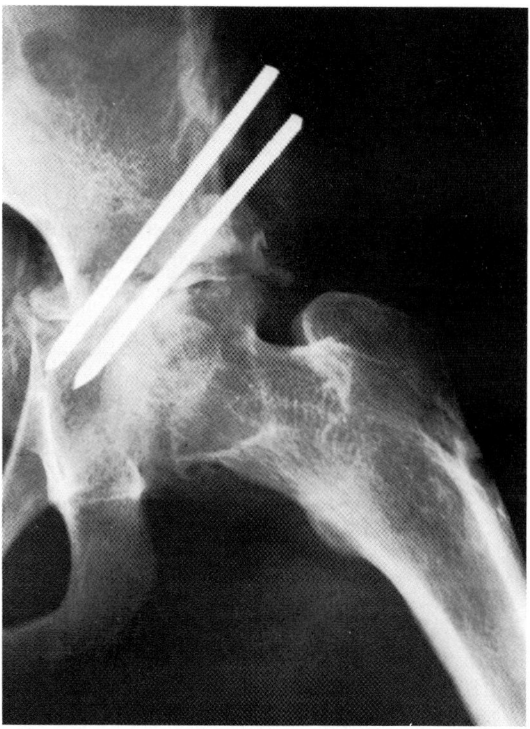

FIG. 18-35. Internal pin fixation is used to maintain the medial displacement achieved by the Chiari osteotomy.

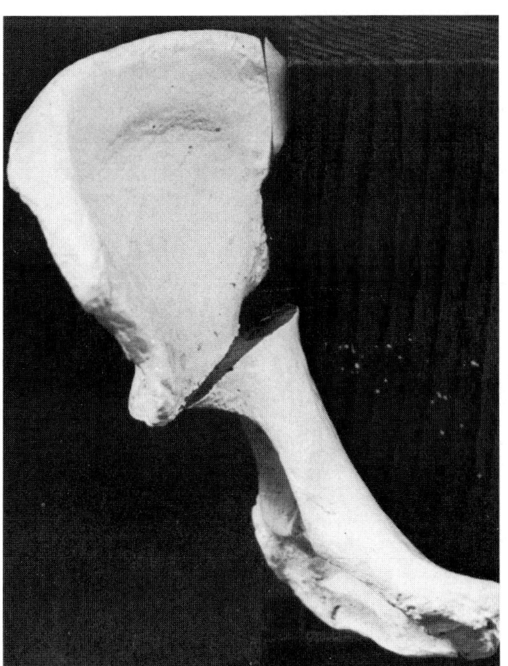

FIG. 18-34. A model of the Chiari procedure. The displacement should be at least 50% of the width of the pelvis.

Complications may result from the Chiari procedure if the cut is made below the capsule, placing the femoral head in direct contact with the bone of the pelvis and setting the stage for early degenerative changes in the femoral head. Another risk with the Chiari osteotomy is that the sciatic nerve may be injured. It is recommended that the posterior 1 cm of the notch be made with a Gigli saw, as in the Salter procedure, rather than an osteotome. The remainder of the osteotomy is then carried out with an osteotome.

Postoperatively, the interposed capsule will,

at best, develop into fibrocartilage and will never be a true articular cartilage. This type of reconstruction should result in a 15- to 25-year period of efficient joint motion. It is a worthwhile procedure in patients older than 8 to 10 years of age who have severe subluxation where there is no possibility of centering the femoral head, so that they do not have to be subjected to a more massive procedure, such as cup arthroplasty or total joint replacement.

The Chiari procedure does not preclude the use of other reconstructive procedures at a later date and also improves the acetabular space for later contact of the acetabular components.

This procedure is much more mechanical than the aforementioned procedures and is less desirable, because it uses the joint capsule as interposing substance. The articular-cartilage-to-articular-cartilage contact of the other procedures is preferred.

The Chiari procedure can be done after epiphyseal closure. Also, because it is essentially a salvage procedure, it should only be carried out in adolescents who are experiencing pain.

Femoral Procedures

A femoral deformity is associated with anteversion or true valgus of the femoral neck. The latter is rare unless previous surgery has disrupted the growth of the greater trochanteric epiphysis or there has been a previous avascular necrosis of the epiphysis, with damage to the lateral portion of the epiphyseal line of the femoral head and secondary growth into valgus. The effect of anteversion on hip stability is best determined by obtaining roentgenograms with the femur in varying degrees of internal rotation. The stabilizing effect of a varus procedure can also be similarly determined by varying the degree of abduction of the femur, as described for the evaluation of the containment potential of the acetabulum.

Rotational Osteotomy. Rarely, the acetabulum may have essentially a normal contour, and the proximal femur may have an apparent valgus, with subluxation of the femoral head. If the normal roentgenographic alignment can be restored simply by internally rotating the lower extremity, a corrective rotational osteotomy is indicated (Fig. 18-36). This procedure can be performed at either the subtrochanteric or supracondylar area. The femur should be rotated to leave approximately 15° to 25° of residual internal rotation.

The procedure is contraindicated if the hip joint is grossly unstable, because, in this situation, rotation of the femur only tends to redirect the distal fragment into external rotation, leaving the hip joint in the original pathologic position.

Varus Derotation Osteotomy. If the internal rotation test of the femur is not sufficient to stabilize the hip joint and if the thigh must be abducted to obtain the desired position of the femoral head in the acetabulum, a varus derotation osteotomy may be indicated (Fig. 18-37). The results of this procedure have been quite reliable in children less than 4 years of age.[39] However, in patients 4 to 8 years old, the results of the varus osteotomy are less certain, and it may be best to consider an innominate osteotomy. After 8 years of age, the varus derotation osteotomy has little value as an isolated procedure but may be performed in conjunction with a pelvic procedure. When the varus osteotomy is indicated, the angle should be reduced to 110° in the younger child and to no less than 125° in the child older than 7 years.

If there has been a recent avascular necrosis of the femoral head, it is better to consider the varus procedure than an acetabular procedure, because less pressure will be produced across the hip joint. However, the reduction in the angle should not be excessive because of the decreased potential of the femur (secondary to avascular necrosis) to remodel into a more valgus position. The main principle behind a femoral osteotomy is, of course, to eliminate an existing deformity; the patient will not benefit if a new significant deformity is produced.

Combined Acetabular and Femoral Procedures

Children with marked deformities on both sides of the joint cannot be expected to obtain full correction from a realignment of only one side of the joint. The abduction test roentgenograms help to determine to what degree the hip components must be realigned to achieve centering. An arthrogram may help to identify a true cartilaginous acetabular deformity and to determine the presence or absence of lateral femoral head displacement. The combined acetabular/femoral approach is more difficult, be-

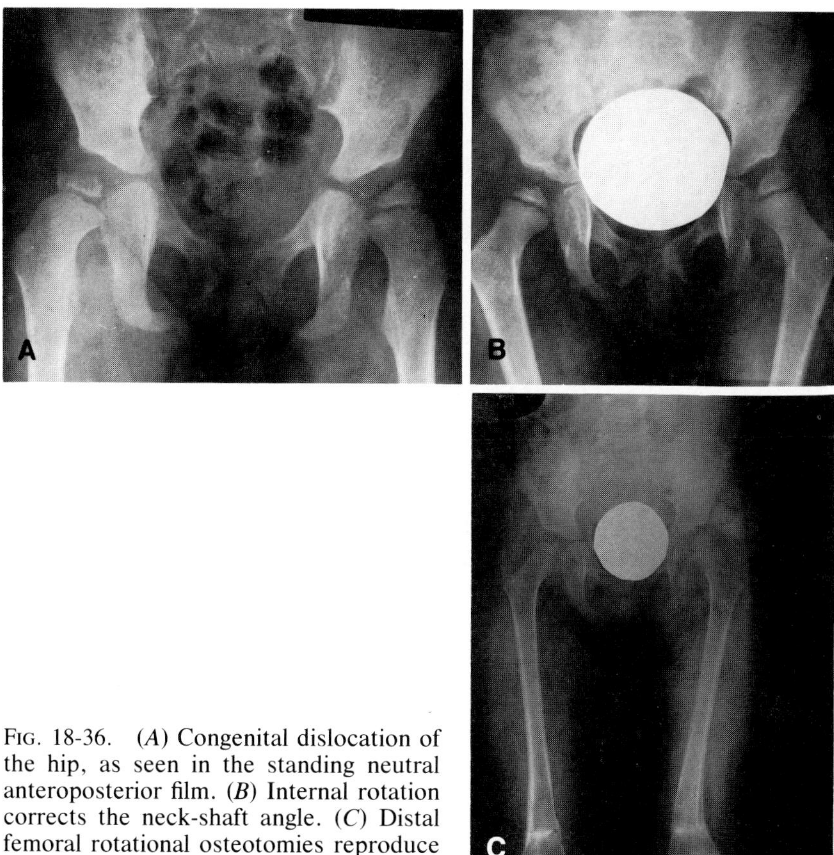

FIG. 18-36. (*A*) Congenital dislocation of the hip, as seen in the standing neutral anteroposterior film. (*B*) Internal rotation corrects the neck-shaft angle. (*C*) Distal femoral rotational osteotomies reproduce the internal rotation position, as seen in *B*.

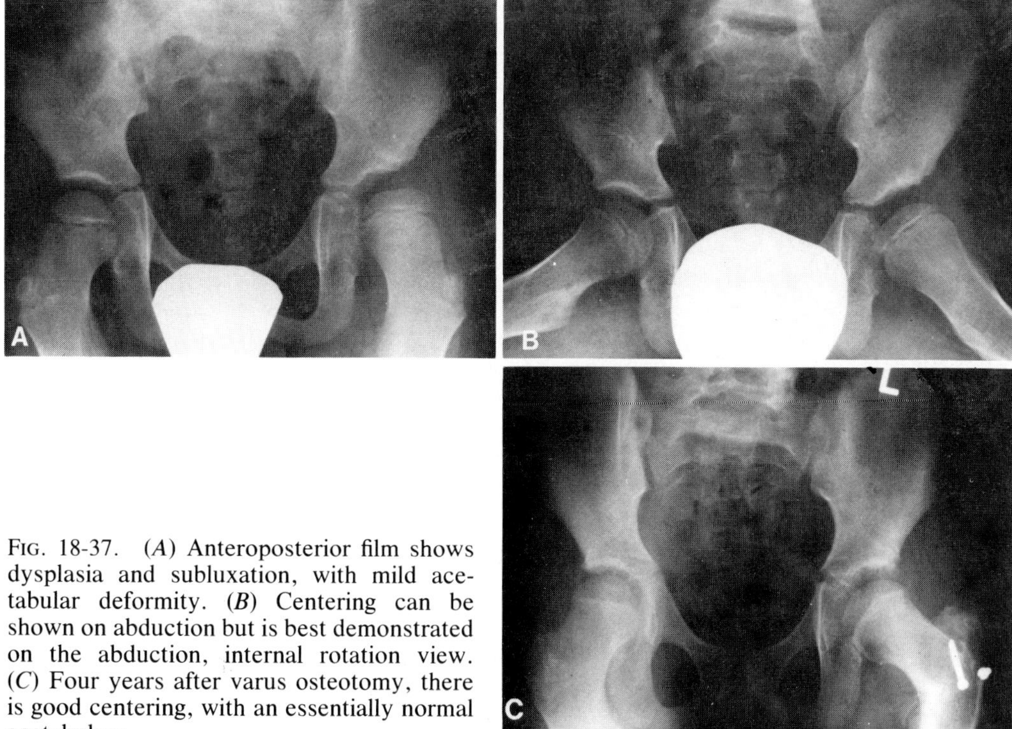

FIG. 18-37. (*A*) Anteroposterior film shows dysplasia and subluxation, with mild acetabular deformity. (*B*) Centering can be shown on abduction but is best demonstrated on the abduction, internal rotation view. (*C*) Four years after varus osteotomy, there is good centering, with an essentially normal acetabulum.

cause it requires either two standard procedures or one very difficult procedure. The question arises as to which component of the deformity should be changed first. Experience has shown us that it is probably best to change the femoral component first, especially if there has been some vascular change. The femoral osteotomy decreases joint pressure, and it can be covered above with either a Salter or a Pemberton procedure, depending on the acetabular configuration. There may be other circumstances that require an entirely different surgical approach; for example, if the hip is not centering, a Chiari procedure is preferred. The use of pins and screws for rigid fixation is also preferred when carrying out procedures on both the pelvis and the femur to maintain accurate position.

COXA VARA

Coxa vara is an abnormality of the proximal femur, characterized by a decreased neck-shaft angle and the presence of a triangular ossification defect of the femoral neck, resulting in shortening of the affected limb. Excellent reviews of the early literature on this subject have been written by several authors.[108,109,111,120,126,133]

Classifications of this abnormality have been proposed by various authors[107,129,138] and include the following groups: (1) isolated coxa vara (2) coxa vara with short or bowed femur, (3) coxa vara with congenital limb deficiency, (4) proximal femoral focal deficiency, (5) coxa vara secondary to other congenital etiology (*e.g.*, Morquio's syndrome), and (6) acquired coxa vara (*e.g.*, malunited femoral neck fracture).

ETIOLOGY

Although familial and twin occurrence of coxa vara has been reported by numerous authors,[106,114,115,121,128,130] this is rare and appears coincidental (Fig. 18-38).

It has been reported that children with a radiographically normal hip at birth can subsequently develop a classic coxa vara.[128] In light of these data, Blockey[111] has proposed the possibility of traumatic etiology. Although this theory is plausible, trauma cannot be accepted as a frequent cause of coxa vara, particularly in light of experimental work demonstrating that disordered forces of growth can also produce coxa vara.[124]

Trueta[136] has shown the delicate and changing balance in the vascular supply of the proximal femur during growth. It is reasonable to postulate that an irregularity of blood supply causes the abnormalities of growth in this condition.

There is now general agreement that the primary abnormality in coxa vara is a developmental defect in the growth of the proximal femur. Early normal growth of the proximal femur occurs from a single epiphyseal plate, which quickly differentiates into cervical and trochanteric portions. The medial portion grows most rapidly during the earliest stages, causing elongation of the femoral neck and an apparent coxa valga. Subsequent lateral growth at the area of the greater trochanter reduces the valgus angle.[125] Abnormal growth differentiation in this area may produce coxa vara or valga. Experimentally, alterations in the forces acting on this growing area produce abnormalities of the proximal femur, including coxa vara, retroversion of the femoral neck, short femoral neck, and irregularities of the femoral head.[113,124]

It has consistently been reported that the histology of the proximal femur shows disordered epiphyseal cartilage columns, disturbed cell arrangement, metaphyseal bone containing islands of cartilage, and interposed connective tissue with scanty hematopoiesis in the marrow areas.[108,118,128]

Because radiographs are normal at birth and growth disturbances have been demonstrated histologically, it seems most likely that the development of coxa vara results from abnormal growth of a radiologically normal proximal femur, resulting in weakening of the physeal plate and slipping of the capital epiphysis into the varus position when the forces of weight-bearing come into play.[128]

CLINICAL FEATURES

Coxa vara becomes evident after walking age and is most frequently diagnosed when the child is between the ages of 3 and 5 years. Males and females are affected with equal frequency, and the condition is bilateral in one third of cases.

Patients will frequently present with a painless limp or, if the deformity is bilateral, a

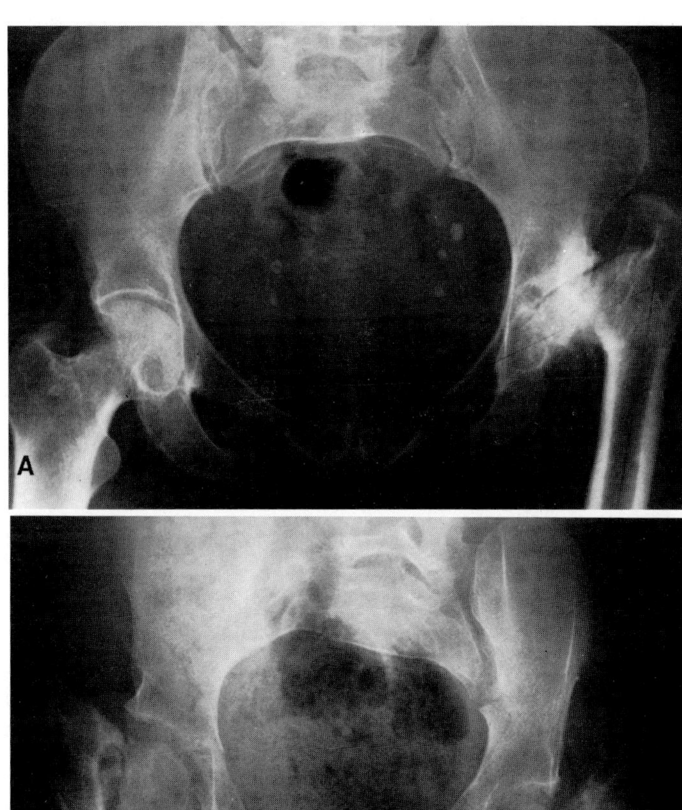

FIG. 18-38. Evidence of the familial incidence of coxa vara, as seen in (*A*) mother who presented with unilateral uncorrected coxa vara with degenerative changes, and (*B*) a son who presented with bilateral uncorrected coxa vara.

waddling gait; rarely is pain the presenting complaint. All patients have a positive Trendelenburg sign. Two thirds of patients will have decreased abduction and decreased internal rotation. All patients have a leg-length discrepancy if the condition is unilateral (always less than 2 cm if the condition is a pure coxa vara).[116,120,127,138]

RADIOGRAPHIC FINDINGS

The classic radiographic findings include a neck-shaft angle measuring less than 120°. The growth plate is rotated into a more vertical orientation than normal, and there is a triangular fragment of bone on the inferomedial aspect of the proximal femoral neck. The greater trochanter is elevated in its position relative to the femoral head, and, in advanced cases, a small notch may be noted in the ilium above the acetabulum (Fig. 18-39). At times, mild deformity of the femoral head and a shallow acetabulum may be seen.[117,123]

Measurement of the amount of rotation of the physeal plate is useful. Alsberg's angle is formed by a line parallel to the shaft of the femur and another line parallel to the growth plate. This angle should be greater than 45°.[126]

DIFFERENTIAL DIAGNOSIS

The classic findings of coxa vara with a triangular fragment in the femoral neck leave little doubt as to the diagnosis of the hip pathology. However, one must be certain to rule out other conditions with a known asso-

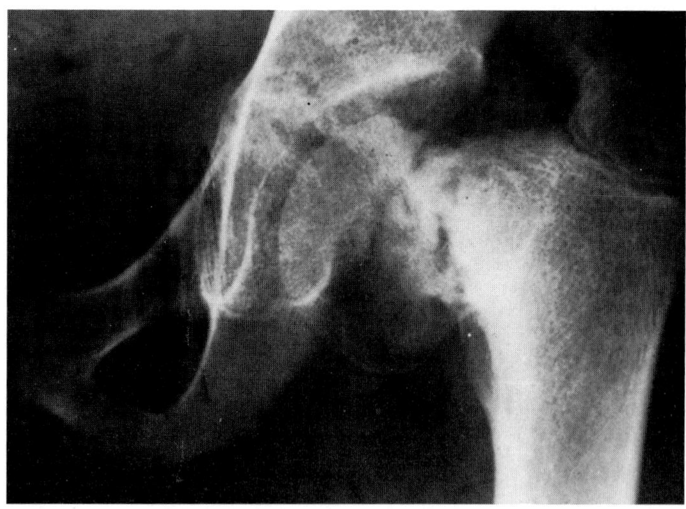

FIG. 18-39. A large triangular bone fragment is present at the inferomedial portion of the femoral neck. Because the epiphyseal line is still open, with osteotomy a good prognosis can be expected.

ciation, such as cleidocranial dysplasia, metaphyseal dysostosis, and epiphyseal dysplasias. One must also be aware of the possibility of a slipped epiphysis secondary to other generalized conditions such as endocrinopathy or renal osteodystrophy. Acquired lesions resulting in coxa vara that are less likely to be confused with developmental coxa vara include congenital dislocation of the hip with avascular necrosis, Perthes syndrome, slipped epiphysis, sepsis, or trauma.

PROGNOSIS AND NATURAL HISTORY

Untreated progressive coxa vara results in a severe hip deformity and disability in adults (Fig. 18-38).[108,118]

Weinstein and associates[138] demonstrated the value of "Hilgenreiner's epiphyseal angle" in predicting which patients will have a progressive varus deformity. This angle is formed by Hilgenreiner's line and a second line parallel with the epiphyseal plate. All patients demonstrated spontaneous correction if this angle was less than 45°. All patients in whom the angle was greater than 60° had a progressive deformity requiring surgery. The outcome of those with angles between 45° and 60° was unpredictable.

TREATMENT

The goals of treatment in this condition are (1) creation of a normal neck-shaft angle, (2) promotion of ossification of the cartilaginous femoral defect and, (3) reorientation of the growth plate into a more horizontal position (Fig. 18-40).

If the deformity is mild and nonprogressive, expectant observation is the treatment of choice. In cases of progressive deformity, nonoperative measures are completely ineffective in achieving the outlined goals.

The indications for surgical treatment of this condition include a neck-shaft angle of less than 90°, vertical physeal plate, progressive deformity, and significant limp.[127,128] If "Hilgenreiner's epiphyseal angle" is used, an angle of greater than 60° indicates surgery, whereas an angle of less than 45° indicates continued observation. Angles between 45° and 60° must be judged on individual merit.[138] Surgery should be carried out when the indications are met, regardless of the patient's age. The benefits of surgery at a younger age include a lesser degree of deformity, with fewer secondary changes in the acetabulum and abductor mechanism.

Several techniques for osteotomy have been described, most of which involve internal fixation.[110,112,122,132] There is usually no need to consider grafting in the triangular fragment.[119]

Increasing the length of the femur should not be a goal of surgery, because this places undue stress across the hip joint via the adductor mechanism. Concomitant adductor ten-

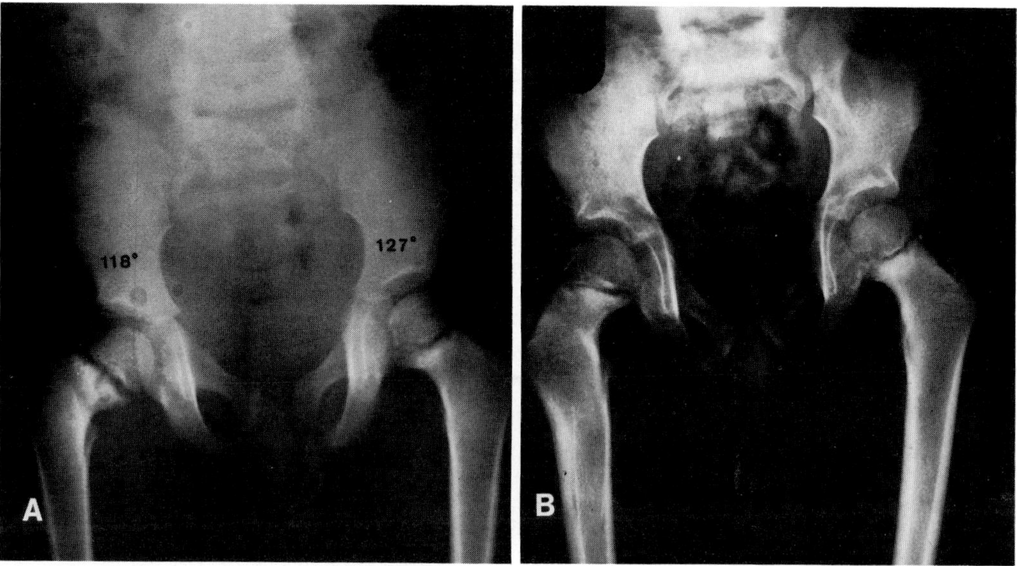

FIG. 18-40. *(A)* Congenital coxa vara seen on a standing anteroposterior film. (*B*) The neck-shaft angle is restored to normal after valgus osteotomy. The minimal defect on the right does not require surgery.

otomy may, in fact, be helpful at the time of valgus osteotomy (Fig. 18-41).[128]

A frequent complication of valgus osteotomy for coxa vara is premature closure of the femoral capital physeal plate. The explanation for this is not obvious nor can recommendations be made for ways to avoid this complication.

CONGENITAL SHORT FEMUR WITH COXA VARA

Congenital short femur may occur as an isolated anomaly or as part of a spectrum of disorders, including congenital short femur with coxa vara and dysgenesis of the proximal femur.[140–143]

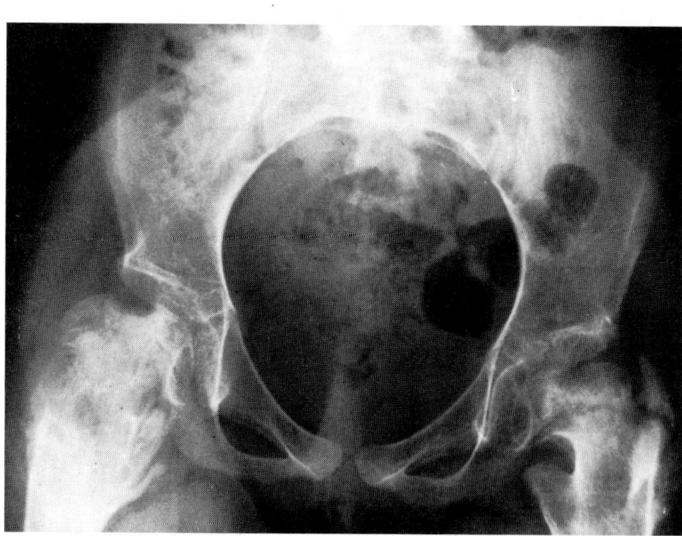

FIG. 18-41. Radiograph of a patient in whom surgical overcorrection led to avascular necrosis.

CLINICAL AND RADIOGRAPHIC FEATURES

In contrast to a pure developmental coxa vara, congenital short femur is evident at birth because of the short limb. The thigh is usually not bulky, and ranges of hip and knee motion are normal. The leg-length discrepancy is much greater than in patients with pure coxa vara, and some bowing of the leg may be evident. Frequently, genu valgum is present.

The radiographic findings frequently demonstrate completely normal architecture of the femur, with a discrepancy in length being the only difference noted between the two extremities (Fig. 18-42). There may be mild lateral bowing of the femur, with slightly increased thickness of the medial cortex. The lateral femoral condyle is frequently mildly hypoplastic, leading to the genu valgum. The growth plates at either end of the femur appear normal in the pure condition. Associated anomalies of the tibia and fibula are present in almost 30% of patients (Fig. 18-43).

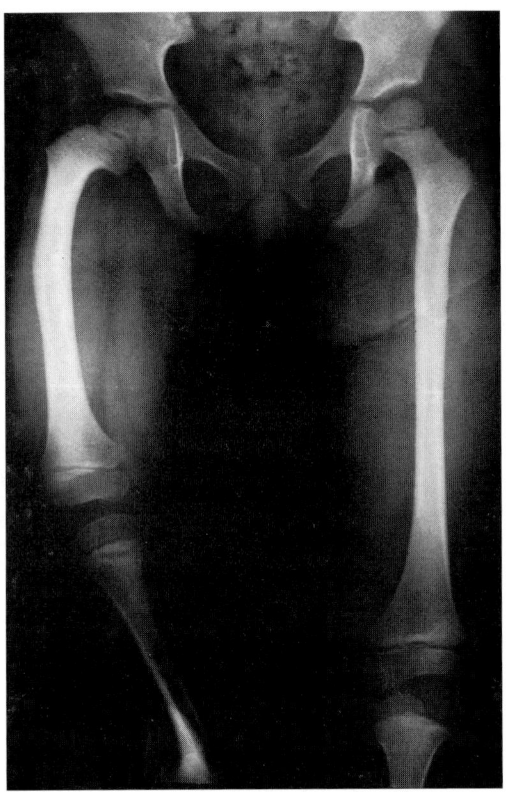

FIG. 18-43. This roentgenogram shows a congenitally short femur with coxa vara. A significant leg-length inequality is apparent.

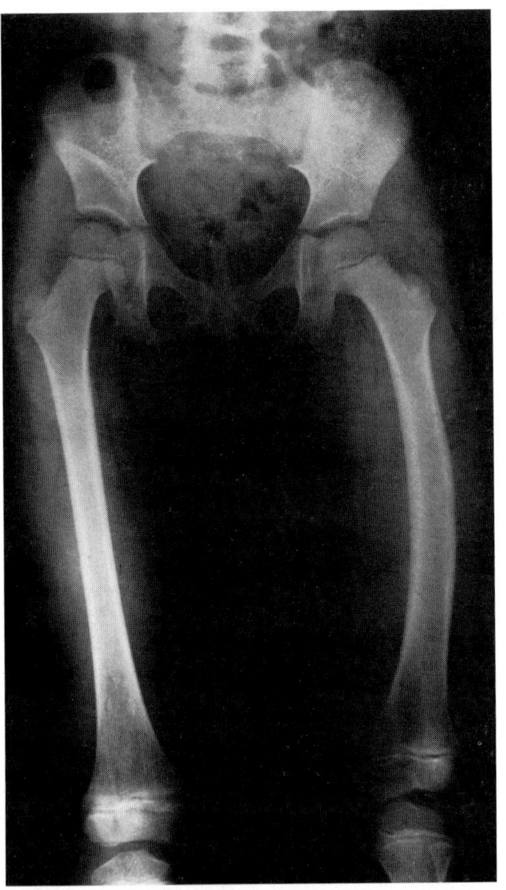

FIG. 18-42. This standing roentgenogram shows a congenitally short femur with no associated deformity. The femur is normal, but abbreviated in size, and leg-length inequality can be seen.

PROGNOSIS AND NATURAL HISTORY

Many authors have pointed out that the percentage of shortening of the femur remains constant throughout all stages of growth.[141,143,144] This serves as a valuable aid in early prediction of the ultimate leg-length discrepancy and facilitates the planning of equalization procedures.

The genu valgum that results rarely presents a major deformity and does not usually require osteotomy for realignment purposes.

TREATMENT

If the congenitally short femur is associated with a coxa vara, the treatment of coxa vara

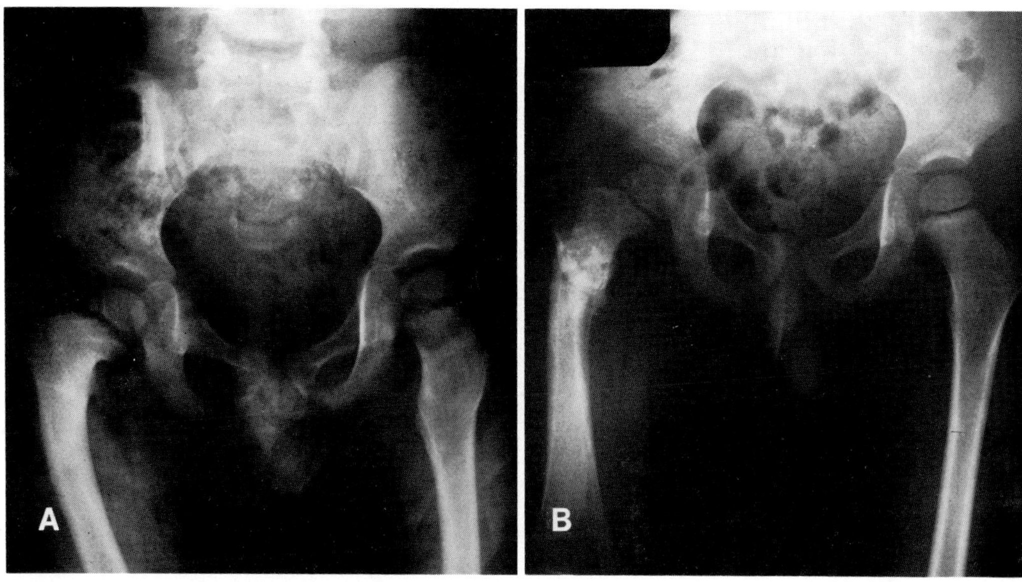

FIG. 18-44. (*A*) This preoperative roentgenogram shows a congenitally short femur with associated coxa vara. After performing a successful valgus osteotomy to correct the deformity of the proximal femur (*B*), the leg-length inequality can be treated.

should be the primary consideration. It should be emphasized that in most cases it is not feasible to attempt to lengthen the femur at the time of a valgus osteotomy of the proximal femur.

Once the problem of coxa vara has been addressed, the anticipated leg-length discrepancy should be treated according to the guidelines discussed elsewhere in this text (Fig. 18-44).

SLIPPED CAPITAL FEMORAL EPIPHYSIS

Slipped capital femoral epiphysis is the most common hip disorder occurring in adolescence. It is characterized by a growth disturbance of the capital physis, resulting in weakening of this structure and a subsequent displacement of the femoral head on the femoral neck.[152,215]

ETIOLOGY

Growth and mechanical factors appear to play an important role in the etiology of this condition. Slipping of the epiphysis always occurs during a growth spurt; it almost invariably occurs before menarche in females.[215] Patients with slips have been noted to have a significant delay in achieving final skeletal maturity.

The growth plate appears weakened in its resistance to shear stress during the adolescent growth spurt. Experimental models have demonstrated that small shear cracks develop in the cartilage plate when physiologic stresses are applied. These shear cracks may propagate, allowing displacement of the epiphysis to occur. Resistance to this shear stress is reduced by 50% if the perichondrial ring is stripped from this area.[151,155] Other evidence for mechanical factors includes a reported slip after a varus malunion of a femoral neck fracture.[204]

Most authors have reported a large number of obese patients, and Kelsey and colleagues[187] indicated that half the patients in their series were above the 95th percentile for weight. They also noted that overweight adolescents have a slower than average maturation of their epiphyseal plates, thus increasing the risk of a slip.

Genetics may be a factor in the etiology, as suggested by Rennie,[208] who reported on 14 families and suggested that the condition might be caused by an autosomal dominant trait with variable penetrance. Gorin reported the occurrence in identical twins, one with bilateral slips.[164] There also seems to be a racial predisposition, with a disproportionately high percentage of black patients.[149]

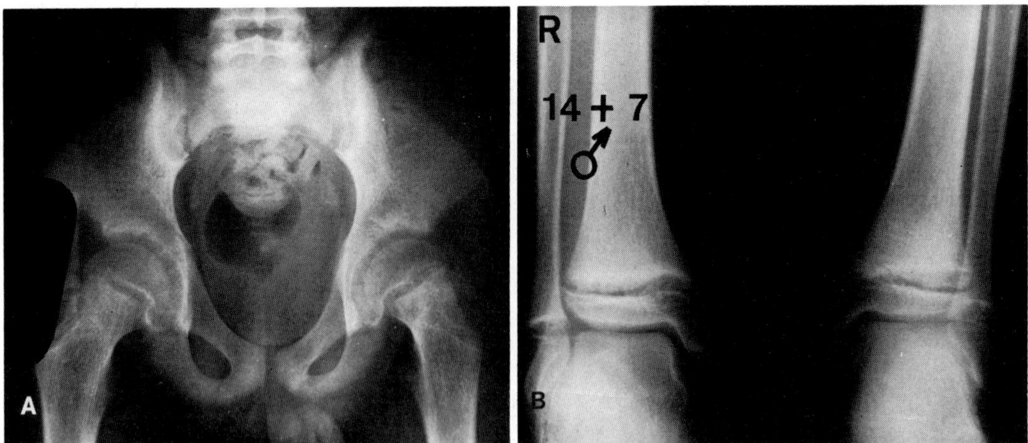

FIG. 18-45. (*A*) If slip is bilateral, as seen here, other joints should be examined roentgenographically to assist in differential diagnosis. (*B*) Note involvement of the distal fibular and tibial epiphyseal lines. This indicates the presence of a systemic condition and, in this patient, an impending renal failure.

Circumstantial evidence implicates endocrine dysfunction as a possible cause of slipping of the upper femoral epiphysis. Harris[167] has shown experimentally that growth hormone decreases the shear strength of the growth plate, whereas sex hormones increase the shear strength. Several reports associate slips with hypothyroidism[175,183,226] and treatment with chorionic gonadotropin.[176] Slipped epiphysis is frequently seen in patients with end-stage renal disease (Fig. 18-45).[162,202] Radiotherapy has also been shown to cause slipping, presumably because of an arrest of chondrogenesis.[154,220,225]

Slipped epiphysis may occur in neonates and very young children as a result of traumatic separation of the epiphysis.[198,224] This may result from birth trauma, child abuse, or conditions such as myelodysplasia.

EPIDEMIOLOGY

Kelsey[186] has written an excellent review of the epidemiology of this condition, in which he reports that the incidence is approximately 1 to 3 per 100,000 but is significantly increased in black males to approximately 8 per 100,000. Males are affected approximately twice as frequently as females. The average age at the time of slip is between 12 and 15 years for males and between 10 and 13 years for females. The left hip is affected slightly more often than the right in males but not in females. An increased incidence has been noted in lower socioeconomic classes[186] and among obese patients, as previously noted.

CLINICAL FEATURES

The most frequent presenting complaint is a painful limp. The pain and limp start simultaneously in 50% of patients, with pain preceding the limp in most of the remainder. The pain is most frequently identified at the hip but may be referred to the knee, and knee pain may be the presenting complaint. The pain is usually intermittent and gradual in onset. Half of the patients will have thigh atrophy, and half will have shortening of the extremity up to 1 inch, depending on the amount of slip.

Physical examination most frequently reveals mild pain on motion and limited motion, particularly lateral rotation and abduction (Fig. 18-46). Flexion of the hip results in an obligatory external rotation at the hip (Fig. 18-47). Stiffness is not usually apparent at the time of initial presentation.

Half of the patients will give a history of injury. Only about 14%, however, present with the acute onset of symptoms, suggesting an "acute" slipped epiphysis. These patients usually relate a sudden episode, such as a twisting or falling injury, resulting in hip pain.[152]

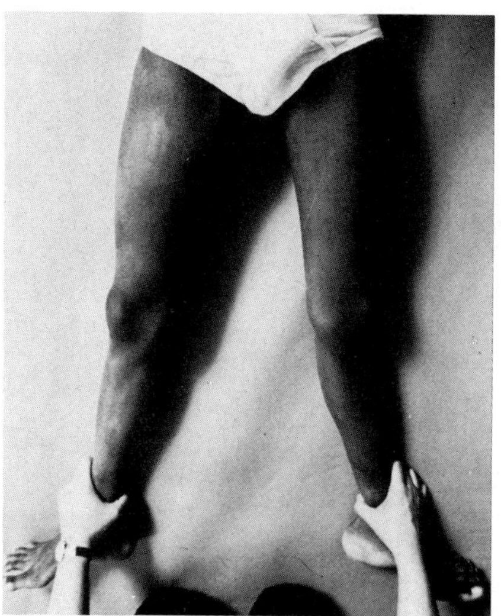

FIG. 18-46. With knees in extension, restricted abduction becomes more pronounced. This illustration shows increased external rotation of the left hip and thigh atrophy.

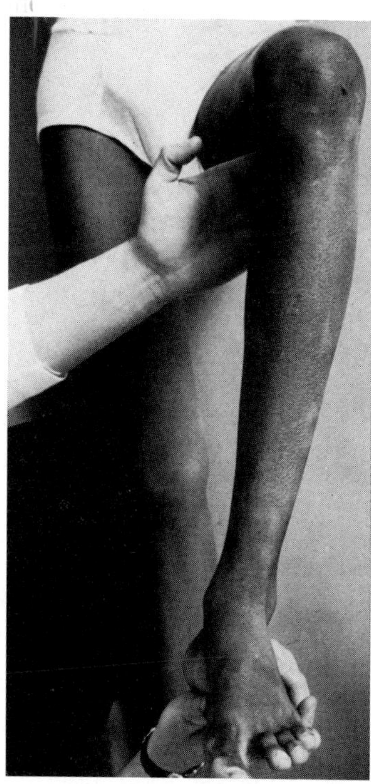

FIG. 18-47. As the thigh is flexed, it tends to roll into external rotation and abduction.

RADIOGRAPHIC FEATURES

The earliest radiographic change in slipped epiphysis is widening of the femoral capital growth plate. Minimal displacement of the epiphysis cannot usually be identified on an anteroposterior film, but a frog-leg view is mandatory in ruling out this condition. This latter view is most likely to demonstrate the displacement of the epiphysis (Fig. 18-48).

As the epiphysis displaces posteriorly and inferiorly, it drags with it the periosteum from the back of the femoral neck. This elevated periosteum then creates a "beak" of new bone formed at the posterior aspect of the neck, adjacent to the femoral head. In addition, the femoral neck becomes uncovered anteriorly, producing the characteristic "bump" of the superior femoral neck (Fig. 18-49). Rarely, displacement may occur in the opposite direction, producing a valgus slip.[213]

The severity of the condition may be determined by measuring the percentage of the slip (Fig. 18-50). If the slip is less than one third of the width of the neck, it is considered Grade I; if a slip of between 33% and 50% has occurred, it is considered Grade II; if a slip of more than 50% has occurred, it is considered Grade III. A lateral film is most likely to show the maximal slip.

The degree of slip may also be determined by measuring the head-neck angle, as described by Southwick.[216]

CLASSIFICATION

Classification may be determined based on both clinical and radiographic appearance. If the duration of symptoms is less than 3 weeks or if the clinical history indicates an acute episode, the slip may be considered acute. The condition should be considered chronic if symptoms exceed 3 weeks in duration, particularly if new bone formation is seen on the posteroinferior aspect of the metaphysis adjacent to the femoral head. An acute slip may be superimposed on an already chronically slipping epiphysis, as demonstrated by history of an acute episode and radiographic evidence of new bone formation near the posteroinferior growth plate. The slip is chronic if prolonged symptoms and new bone formation are noted.

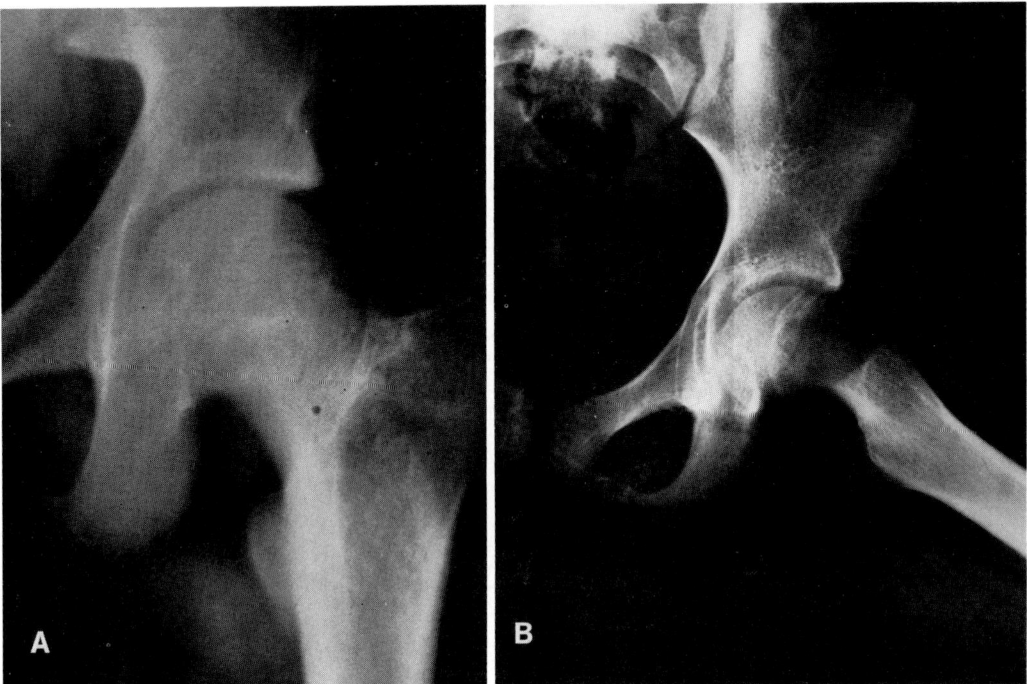

FIG. 18-48. (*A*) Slipped epiphysis can be missed on the anteroposterior projection, because it is usually posteriorly located. (*B*) Therefore, a frog-leg view should also be taken. This frog-leg view shows a Grade I slip.

PATHOLOGY

The histologic appearance of the growth plate in slipped capital femoral epiphysis is one of disorganization, particularly in its distal regions.[177,179,197] The zone of resting cartilage appears normal; the proliferative zone, however, has some early signs of disorganization, which are then greatly exaggerated in the hypertrophic zone, which is also thickened. Endochondral ossification is scanty and quite irregular. Large clusters of cartilage are seen in the metaphysis. The displacement occurs through the thickened area of the proliferative and hypertrophic zones of the growth plate.

The pathology of slipped epiphysis in real osteodystrophy is somewhat different.[195] Although the growth plate appears wide radiographically, as in a classic slip, this zone is histologically composed of a wide band of loosely woven bone that is poorly mineralized. There is also a distinct fibrous tissue layer between the cartilaginous growth plate and the metaphyseal bone.

Pathologic examination of the synovium in patients with slipped epiphysis demonstrates edema, proliferation of synovial cells, and villus formation. There is a pronounced round cell infiltration with increased vascularity and perivascular thickening and fibrosis.[200]

PROGNOSIS AND NATURAL HISTORY

Oram[205] reviewed the natural history of untreated slipped capital femoral epiphysis and reported that 51% of patients sustain significant complications, including progression of the slip, avascular necrosis, cartilage necrosis, and osteoarthritis progressing to fibrous ankylosis in some cases. Other authors have found an unexpected improvement in hip function, due primarily to resolution of the synovitis and remodeling of the upper end of the femur.[150,203]

Late radiographic findings demonstrate numerous abnormalities, including subchondral cyst formation in the femoral head, osteophytes on both the femoral head and acetabulum, subchondral bony sclerosis, and joint space narrowing. Ross and associates[209] emphasized the need for a follow-up of longer than 20 years before the final result can be

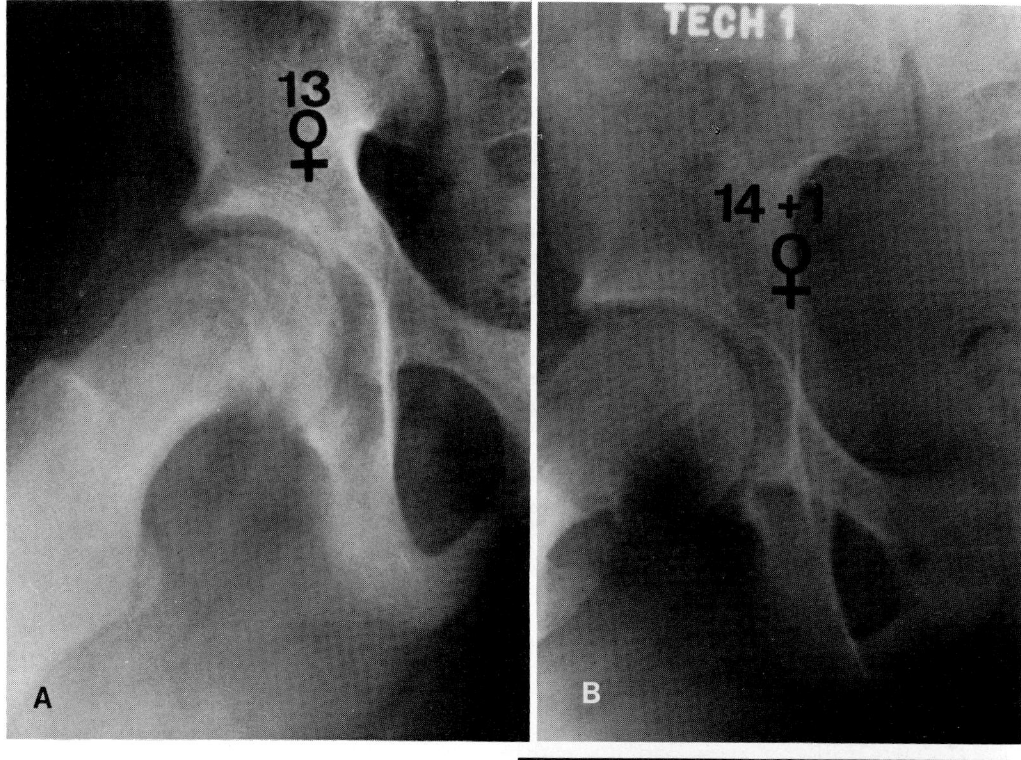

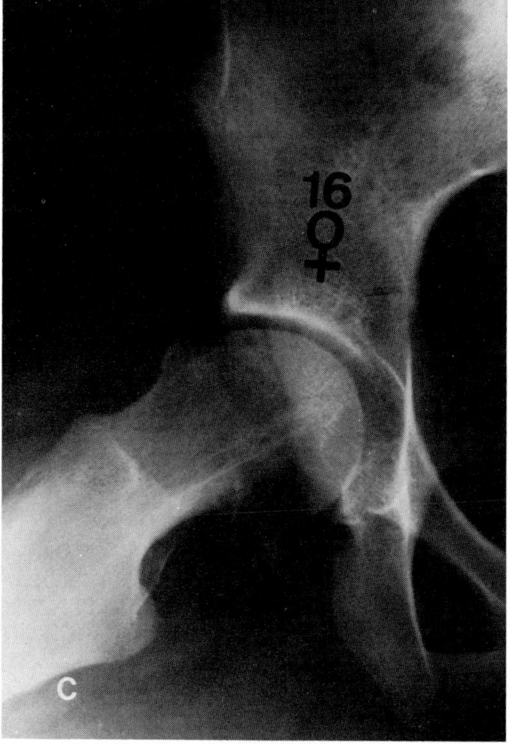

FIG. 18-49. (*A*, *B*, and *C*) These roentgenograms show the progression of calcification to ossification at the epiphyseal line, giving the impression of a moderate slip, although only a minimal slip is present. These signs are similar to those seen in adult patients with idiopathic osteoarthritis.

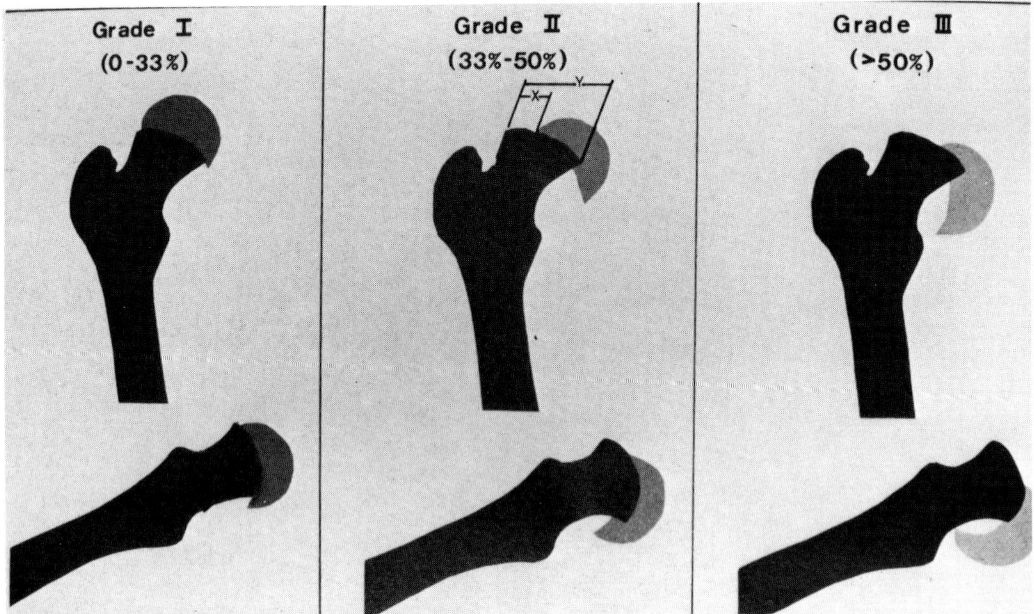

FIG. 18-50. Classification of the three grades of slip.

judged. Two thirds of their patients with a follow-up of between 10 and 20 years had a good result, whereas two thirds of those patients with a follow-up of longer than 20 years had a poor result.

The contralateral hip must be considered when making a prognosis. Approximately 20% of patients will have bilateral slips. Two thirds of these will have simultaneous slips (or a preslip) on the second side, and one third will present with a slip some months later.[150,188] Many of these are incidental findings noted on a radiograph taken because of the symptomatic hip.

Minor degrees of slipping of the femoral epiphysis as well as other minor anatomic abnormalities of the hip may cause future degenerative hip disease. Solomon[214] evaluated 327 hip specimens and noted major femoral head and neck pathology (Perthes or slipped epiphysis) in 33%. An additional 20% had minor acetabular dysplasia. He concluded that "osteoarthritis happens in joints to which other things happen first." Stulberg and associates[218] evaluated 75 patients with slipped epiphysis and 187 patients with Perthes disease and characterized the deformity of the femoral head and neck as a "pistol grip" deformity. They incidentally noted a frequent occurrence of this deformity in the contralateral "normal" hip. They then reviewed 74 patients with "idiopathic" osteoarthritis and noted the presence of the "pistol grip" deformity in 40% of these patients (66% in males). They also found a 39% incidence of mild degrees of acetabular dysplasia (68% in females). Therefore, Solomon and Stulberg and associates conclude that anatomic changes of the femoral head and neck are likely to produce osteoarthritis in later life.

TREATMENT

Several modes of treatment have been advocated, ranging from nonoperative to complex surgical methods. The choice of treatment is dictated primarily by the stage and the degree of slip.

Nonoperative Treatment

Moore[199] reported on 44 cases treated with cast immobilization; 88% of the patients with minimal slips had good or excellent final results. Other authors, however, have noted that conservative treatment is prolonged and does not produce results as good as those obtained with surgery, particularly with respect to chondrolysis.[184,210]

Fixation *In Situ*

This has been the cornerstone of treatment for slipped epiphysis of mild to moderate

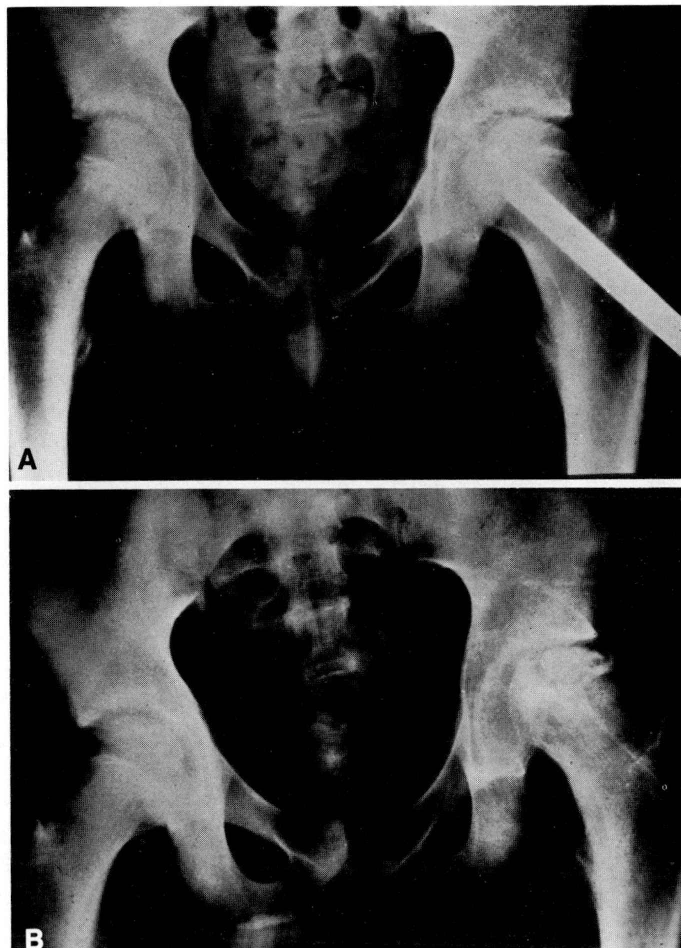

FIG. 18-51. (*A*) In this patient, a large pin separates the epiphyseal line from the metaphysis. (*B*) Radiograph demonstrating the avascular necrosis resulting from the use of the heavy nail.

degree. Early papers report on the use of a tri-fin nail (Fig. 18-51).[185,210,222] Although this provides adequate fixation, there are a number of complications associated with its use, including displacement of the epiphysis, bent guide wire, perforation of the cortex of the femoral head, migration of the nail in the postoperative period, subtrochanteric fracture, and avascular necrosis. Therefore, its use is not recommended. Fixation *in situ* with threaded Steinmann or Knowles pins remains the treatment of choice. It is essential to avoid joint penetration, and it is important to place the pins in the inferior half of the femoral head to avoid the possibility of producing segmental necrosis (Fig. 18-52).

Bone Graft and Osteoplasty

Heyman[172] and Herndon and associates[170,171] described the technique of bone graft epiphysiodesis of the capital growth plate. The advantages include quicker fusion of the growth plate, prevention of further displacement, and the elimination of the need for a second procedure to remove fixation pins. They reported 98% good and excellent results, with a very low incidence of complications. They also described an osteoplasty of the femoral neck (cheilectomy) to remove the lip of bone frequently present and blocking abduction.[172,173] Melby and colleagues[196] reviewed 252 chronic slips treated by bone graft epiphysiodesis, noting graft resorption and further slip in only 2 cases, with no reported incidence of acute cartilage necrosis or avascular necrosis. Grant[165] described a bone graft across the epiphysis, using a fibular strut graft.

McKay[194] reported a follow-up series of cheilectomy, noting that the procedure was contraindicated in patients younger than 10 years of age and in patients with a closed epiphysis, because this eliminates the possi-

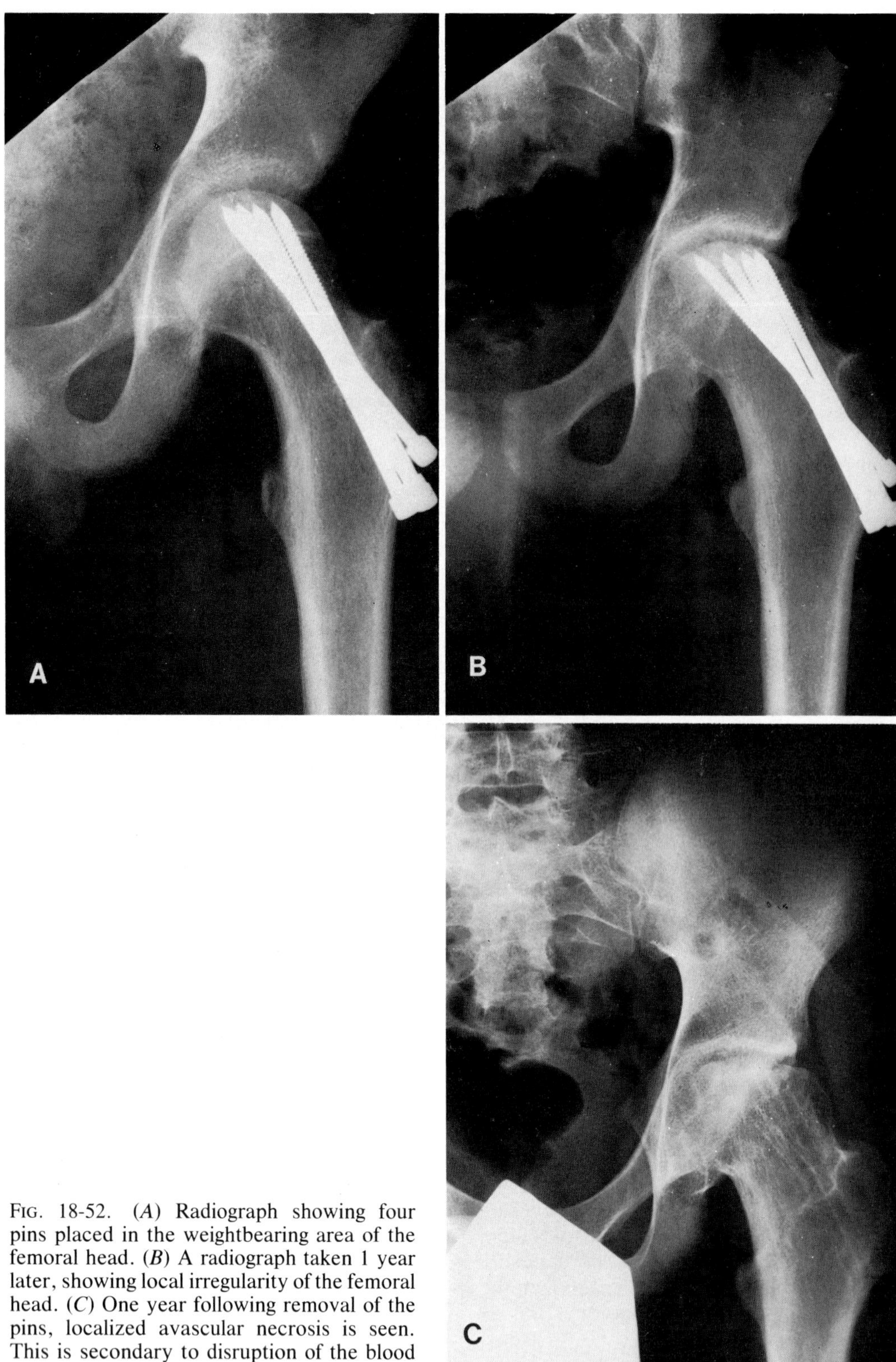

FIG. 18-52. (*A*) Radiograph showing four pins placed in the weightbearing area of the femoral head. (*B*) A radiograph taken 1 year later, showing local irregularity of the femoral head. (*C*) One year following removal of the pins, localized avascular necrosis is seen. This is secondary to disruption of the blood supply by the pins.

bility of remodeling following surgery. Avascular bone and the presence of significant osteoarthritis also contraindicate the procedure. Its primary indication is in patients with limited abduction thought to be due to the deformity of the femoral head and neck. Other procedures may be necessary in addition to the cheilectomy. Postoperative management is important, requiring motion in traction for 3 to 6 weeks and the avoidance of weight-bearing until all synovitis has subsided.

Femoral Neck Osteotomy

Osteotomies of the femoral neck are performed in an attempt to reconstruct the normal anatomic alignment of the upper end of the femur. Although several variations have been reported, they fall into two groups: those done adjacent to the growth plate, and those done at the base of the femoral neck.

The primary advantage of wedge or cuneiform osteotomy is its ability to correct the deformity at the exact location of its occurrence.[146,148,158,221] However, the high incidence of poor results of the procedure significantly outweighs this advantage. These poor results primarily involve the incidence of avascular necrosis and acute cartilage necrosis, which approaches 50% in many series.[157,161,168,174,207] The primary blood supply to the femoral head comes via the posterior and inferior periosteal vessels. Replacement of the femoral head on the femoral neck requires preservation of these vessels and, at the same time, excision of the new bone formed on the metaphyseal side posteriorly and inferiorly. This is a technically difficult procedure to perform and is clearly contraindicated if the growth plate has closed, thereby establishing a metaphyseal–epiphyseal circulation. Thus, considering the high rate of associated complications, wedge or cuneiform osteotomy cannot be the procedure of choice.

Kramer and associates[189] have recommended an osteotomy at the base of the femoral neck. Although the correction is less complete, it does satisfactorily compensate for the varus and retroversion caused by the slip and is much safer in view of the lower risk to the vascular supply. They believe that it is indicated in slips of greater than 40°, but report a 20% incidence of significant complications.

Subtrochanteric Osteotomy

A compensating osteotomy may be done at the subtrochanteric level; this has the primary advantage of avoiding the vascular complications associated with neck osteotomies. Southwick[216] described a biplane osteotomy for correction of deformity and reported 55 cases with no avascular necrosis. He later described a compression fixation device to simplify postoperative care.[217] Ireland and Newman[181] reported good results with this procedure in 35 patients, but Salvati and associates[211] noted significant complications including lost position, delayed union, avascular necrosis, and acute cartilage necrosis, in half of their patients. It must be understood that this osteotomy creates a deformity of the proximal femur, making subsequent total hip replacement difficult.

RESULTS OF TREATMENT

The results of treatment depend on the amount of slip, the method of treatment, and the occurrence of complications.

Moore[199] and Kulick and Denton[190] independently reported approximately 90% good results in Grade I slips, approximately 50% good results in Grade II slips, and only 30% good results in Grade III slips. Salenius and Kivilaakso[210] noted 80% good results if the slip was less than 50% and only 54% good results if it was greater than 50%.

Several authors have compared the results of various methods of treatment.[166,182,191,210,223] It must be recognized that the choice of treatment is influenced by the severity of the slip. However, pinning *in situ* and bone graft epiphysiodesis clearly yield superior results, with approximately 75% good-to-excellent results and 25% fair-to-poor results reported in the series cited. The need for an osteotomy clearly reflects a more severe displacement in which the overall results of treatment are much less satisfactory.

Boyer and colleagues[150] compared the long-term results in patients treated with *in situ* pinning with those who had realignment osteotomies. The long-term results, even in moderate and severe slips, were better in those patients with *in situ* pinning than in those who underwent realignment osteotomies. Ross and associates[209] noted that two thirds of patients with slipped epiphysis had a good result at 10 to 20 years but that only one third had a good result more than 20 years following their slip.

COMPLICATIONS

Avascular Necrosis

Howorth[177] reviewed 25 series reporting avascular necrosis. This complication has been noted to follow almost every method of treatment but has an especially high incidence in patients treated by closed manipulation, prolonged traction, open reduction, or osteotomy of the femoral neck.

Chondrolysis

Acute cartilage necrosis is a devastating complication of slipped capital femoral epiphysis. Maurer and Larsen[193] reviewed 17 series totaling 2044 cases of slipped epiphysis, with 135 cases of acute cartilage necrosis, an average incidence of 7%, with a range of 1 to 28%. Factors that contribute to the development of chondrolysis include increased severity of the slip and prolonged cast immobilization. Pin penetration into the joint may also be a cause.[184,192,219] The incidence in black patients is approximately three times higher than that in other racial groups.[149,206] The presence of avascular necrosis does not predispose a patient to acute cartilage necrosis.

Clinical features include pain and decreased range of motion. The time of onset of chondrolysis varies. Fifteen percent of patients exhibit chondrolysis at initial clinical presentation, whereas in almost half the patients, it will develop within 3 months of the initial presentation. A small number may develop chondrolysis more than 1 year after treatment.[169,178]

Radiographic features include persistent juxta-articular osteoporosis, a progressive narrowing of part or all of the cartilage space, and erosion of the subchondral cortices of the femoral neck and acetabulum (Fig. 18-53). Closure of the femoral capital and the greater trochanteric growth plates is frequently accelerated. The arthrographic pattern has been described as ''dappled,'' with pooling of dye in the small cartilaginous surface erosions.[163]

Microscopically, there is evidence of synovitis and an inflammatory response. The arterioles are thickened, and there is irregularity of the subchondral bone.[156,180] Some studies have demonstrated the presence of increased serum immunoglobulins and immune complexes in the synovium.[159,200]

Acute Slipped Capital Femoral Epiphysis

The diagnosis of acute slip should be made if symptoms are of less than 3 weeks duration or if there is a history of an acute episode. Approximately 5% to 25% of all cases of slipped epiphysis will be on an acute basis.[201] Fahey and O'Brien[160] reviewed the existing literature on this subject prior to 1965.

The principal decision to be made in these cases is the method of treatment. Barash and associates[147] favored manipulative reduction rather than traction in the management of acute slips. Most other authors, however, note the highest incidence of complications following this method of treatment and recommend that reduction be achieved by traction with subsequent internal fixation and no further manipulation.[145,153,201,212] The highest incidence of avascular necrosis in all of these series occurred following primary manipulation or manipulation following traction. Traction should be carried out with a pin through the tibia, and an internal rotation force must be applied to this traction. Nonweightbearing should be encouraged after fixation until closure of the growth plate is achieved. The risk of avascular necrosis approaches 50% in acute slipped capital femoral epiphysis.[201]

LEGG-CALVÉ-PERTHES SYNDROME (COXA PLANA)

In 1909, Arthur Legg,[287] from the United States, presented a paper evaluating five children who developed a limp following an injury. He believed that the injury resulted in flattening of the femoral head due to the increased pressure between the femoral head and the acetabulum. This initial description was the first attempt to differentiate this condition from tuberculosis. A French orthopaedist, Jacques Calvé,[239] published an article in 1910 about a condition he believed to be noninflammatory and self-limiting and that healed with flattening on the weightbearing surface of the femoral head. During the same year, George Perthes,[295] from Germany, described a similar condition. The similarities of these descriptions resulted in the naming of the condition *Legg-Calvé-Perthes syndrome*. Walderström[314] first wrote about the condition in 1909, and, at that time, he believed that it was a form of tuberculosis, but later he suggested the nomenclature *coxa plana,* which has also been widely accepted.

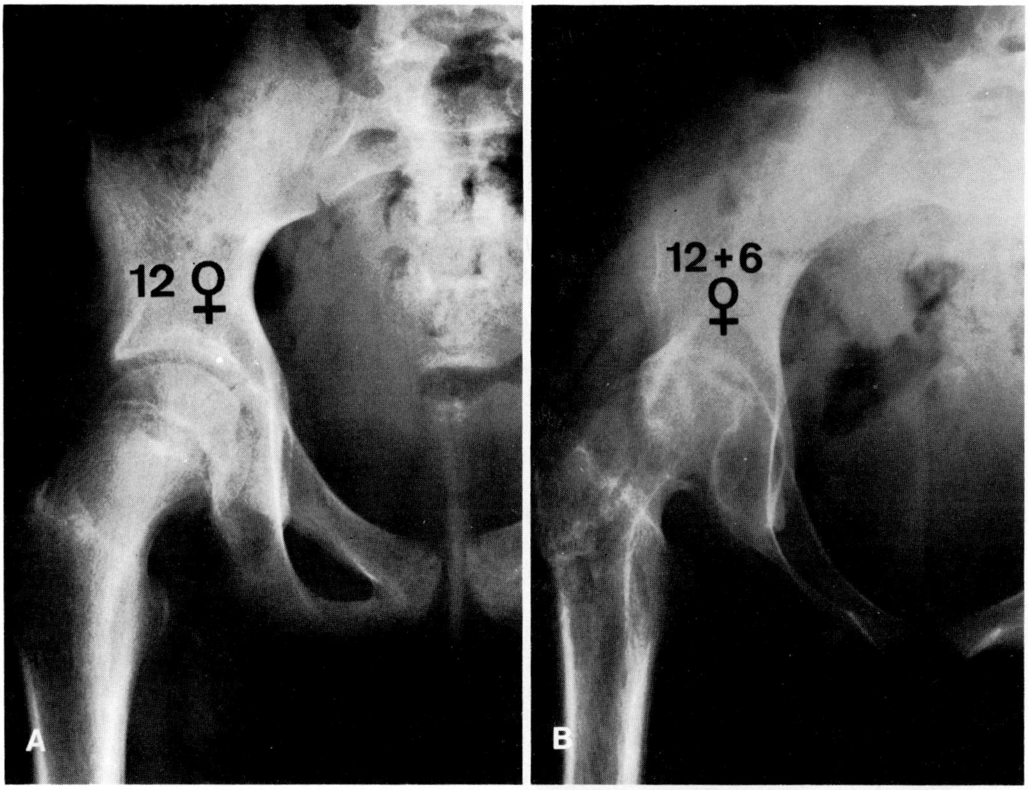

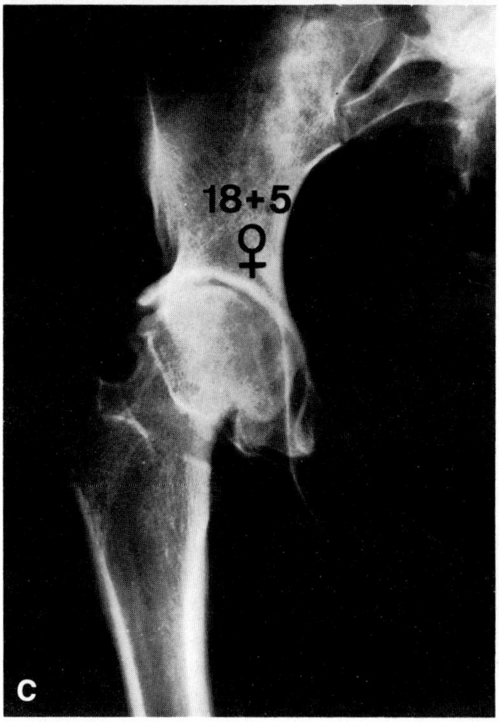

FIG. 18-53. (*A*) Roentgenogram of a hip prior to pin insertion. (*B*) Six months later chondrolysis, seen as marked narrowing of joint space with osteoporosis, is present. (*C*) A long-term follow-up film at 18 years and 5 months shows some reconstruction of the joint space.

It was Phemister,[297] in 1921, who described the pathology as necrotic bone.

INCIDENCE AND EPIDEMIOLOGY

The condition is seen in children ranging in age from 2 to 12 years, with the majority of cases reported in children between 4 and 8 years of age. Males are affected four times more frequently than are females, and the condition is bilateral in approximately 12% of the affected children. Goff [264] found that the syndrome occurred most frequently in the Japanese, Mongoloid, Eskimo, and Central European populations; the races with the fewest reported cases were native Australians, American Indians, Polynesians, and Blacks. He also found a higher incidence of the condition in first-born children.

Fisher and associates[259] conducted a study of 188 patients in which they found a 7% incidence of more than one involved family member. Only two of their patients were black, and both demonstrated atypical changes.

Molloy and MacMahon[291,292] studied single-born, white children with Legg-Calvé-Perthes syndrome. Their results showed that the birthweights were usually much lower than those of unaffected children. For example, males with a birthweight of less than 2.5 kg (5½ lb) were five times more liable to exhibit the condition than males weighing 4 kg (8½ lb). They also found that skeletal age was delayed in 89% of the involved children. Harrison and colleagues[271] confirmed that the skeletal ages of children with Perthes syndrome lagged behind their respective chronologic ages. An extension of this study in siblings of the affected children revealed that the brothers and sisters also exhibited delayed bone ages.

Cameron and Izzat compared affected children with other school-age children and found that affected males were an average of 1 inch shorter and the affected females were 3 inches shorter in height than their peers. It would therefore appear that, in addition to the localized vascular changes characteristic of Perthes syndrome,[237] there are also many unexplained constitutional factors associated with the condition.

The age at onset of Legg-Calvé-Perthes syndrome appears to be a major factor in prognosis. Children younger than 5 years of age usually do very well if they are not affected by the unusual problem of full femoral head involvement. If onset occurs in a child older than 8 years of age, the prognosis is less favorable, and a greater area of the femoral head is usually involved.

CLINICAL FEATURES

The most frequently observed symptom of this condition is a limp, which is first noted after full activity and which gradually becomes more constant. The limp is usually painless and intermittent for several weeks, often leading to a delayed visit to the family physician. The pain associated with the limp is usually in the groin and inner thigh, but it may occur only in the knee region. In our series, 15% of the patients had only knee pain. This localization of pain may direct the clinical evaluation to the incorrect joint and further delay the diagnosis. Muscle spasm usually occurs early in the course of the syndrome and limits abduction and internal rotation of the hip, producing a limp with each step. However, because aggressive treatment is not indicated during the first weeks of Legg-Calvé-Perthes syndrome, this delay in diagnosis is not as critical as in many other hip problems.

ETIOLOGY

The exact etiology of Legg-Calvé-Perthes syndrome remains unknown but is in some way related to an interruption of the blood supply, in whole or in part, to the growing femoral head. Changes in the distribution of the vessels, as shown by Trueta,[312,313] are at most only contributing factors. A direct involvement of the vessels themselves could cause the problem, although no animal model exists for this involvement, either by natural development or as a surgically induced condition. Freeman and England[261] most nearly reproduced the changes of Legg-Calvé-Perthes syndrome in the femoral heads of experimental animals by repeating vascular interruption at timed intervals.

Another investigation[274] showed a thrombus to be present in the inferior circumflex vessel in the femoral head of a child with Legg-Calvé-Perthes syndrome at postmortem examination. This thrombus was too recent in origin to produce the bone changes of Legg-Calvé-Perthes syndrome that were already present, again supporting the concept that more than one vascular interruption is necessary.

Legg considered trauma to the femoral head to be the cause of this condition, although it was in fact probably only a secondary factor. The trauma theory continues to have appeal, however, as shown by the observations of Petrie and others, who noted that in children being treated by the abduction method, the unaffected femoral head which is held deeply within the acetabulum has never developed Perthes changes; this becomes significant when one considers that approximately 12% of children with Perthes syndrome are bilaterally affected.

Synovitis with increased fluid pressure inside the joint appears to be an attractive theory as to the etiology of this syndrome; however, only rarely (1–3%) is there a history suggesting synovitis in patients who later develop Legg-Calvé-Perthes syndrome.

PATHOLOGY

Since resection of the total femoral head as a treatment method was abandoned long ago, studies of affected femoral heads are extremely rare and are based solely on accidental deaths among children with an active Legg-Calvé-Perthes condition. The pathologic process basically involves the death of part or all of the femoral head and the gradual revascularization of the area.

Jonsater,[275] using a biopsy technique, outlined the series of events during the active process of Legg-Calvé-Perthes syndrome and has linked these changes with the corresponding roentgenographic stages. These findings have been confirmed by a number of other authors who have taken biopsies, most of them by drilling through the femoral neck of an affected hip. Jonsater, in a study of 34 patients, found that during the initial stage, the epiphysis showed pronounced necrosis of bone and grossly distorted marrow trabeculae. There were no signs of an inflammatory process. At this early stage, the roentgenograms showed only an increase in density of the femoral head, but already the bone fragments were of a soft consistency. In the next stage, referred to as the *fragmentation* stage, the bone biopsy showed new bone formation. This new bone was laid down between and on the surface of the dead trabeculae. Mattner described this bone formation as "creeping apposition," even in the early stage. This observation has also been made by Larsen and Reimann.

Biopsies taken during the fragmentation stage showed that half of the bony specimens were of normal bone strength and the other half were soft. Contrary to the usual belief, the bony fragments were firmer than during the initial stage, and more normal bone marrow was also present. This finding suggests that by this stage, the femoral head is already returning to normal strength. The term *fragmentation* is actually inappropriate for this stage of Perthes syndrome, because it suggests to the clinician a fragile, defective appearance of the bone. Biopsies done later in the process show a continued gradual increase in the amount of living bone.

Investigations have consistently shown that the articular cartilage is normal or, at most, is showing faint signs of degeneration in the basilar layers.

BLOOD SUPPLY TO THE FEMORAL HEAD

The deep branch of the medial femoral circumflex artery runs behind the femoral neck, between the quadratus femoris and the external obturator muscles. It then perforates the joint capsule and runs up along the neck as retinacular vessels. These vessels penetrate the cartilage surface and, after branching, enter the femoral head.

On the anterior aspect of the femoral neck, similar branches, derived from the lateral femoral circumflex artery, course along the neck in a subsynovial level to the anterior aspect of the metaphysis and epiphysis. A small branch enters the epiphysis from the ligamentum teres. Gradually, as the epiphyseal center grows, these afferent vessels assume a more peripheral position through the epiphyseal cartilage. According to Trueta,[312,313] the blood supply to the femoral head in a child between the ages of 4 and 9 years is limited. Distribution is greater to the posterior half of the femoral head, making the anterior part of the head more susceptible to necrosis. It is this anterior part of the head that is almost always involved in the process. Trueta also found that the blood supply to the femoral head was more constant from the artery of the ligamentum teres in Black children than in Caucasian children. At the age of 4 to 6 years, first the anterior and then the distal retinacular arteries stop supplying the epiphysis. The femoral head is then dependent upon the normal function

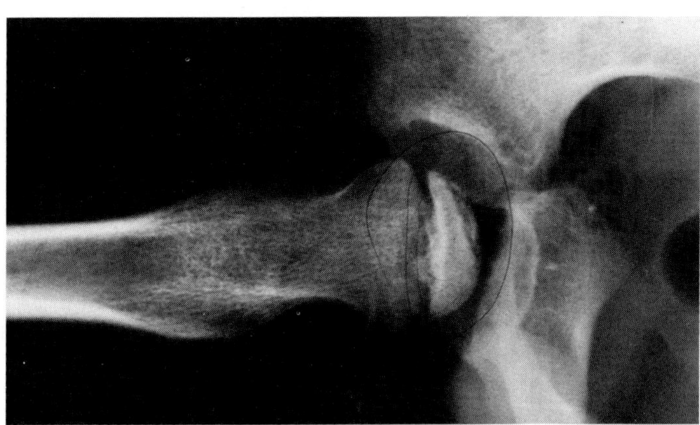

FIG. 18-54. Early segmental fracture (crescent sign), as described by Caffey.

of the deep branch of the medial circumflex femoral artery and its capillaries for blood supply. This source of blood remains until the epiphyseal line begins to close, and then it no longer forms a barrier to anastomosis between the metaphyseal and epiphyseal vascular networks. Trueta concluded that this alteration in the blood distribution may explain why the femoral head is most vulnerable to Legg-Calvé-Perthes syndrome between the ages of 4 and 8 years. This study needs to be repeated, using a much larger sample of cases, before it can be fully accepted.

ROENTGENOGRAPHIC EVALUATION

Changes in the Femoral Head

The roentgenographic appearance of the femoral head changes during the processes of necrosis and revascularization. Anteroposterior and frog-leg roentgenographic views are necessary to follow the course of the syndrome.

The earliest change in the femoral head affected by Legg-Calvé-Perthes syndrome often appears on roentgenographic study only as a slightly smaller ossific nucleus. Work by Salter[302] on 52 experimentally devascularized femoral heads in animals supported these roentgenographic findings. The change is followed by an increase in the density of part or all of the femoral epiphysis. This appearance may be caused by (1) demineralization of the adjacent femoral neck due to disuse osteoporosis, making the femoral head appear relatively dense; (2) compaction of the necrotic femoral head bone; (3) early revascularization, with new bone being laid down over the dead trabeculae, resulting in a true increase in density.[233] The soft-tissue changes at this time may include widening of the medial joint space and reactive thickening of the joint capsule.

The crescent sign of Caffey[238] may be the first bone change to appear. It is often not visible in the standard anteroposterior position. In the frog-leg position, however, the crescent sign may appear as a defined submarginal strip of decreased density on the anterolateral segment of the epiphyseal ossification center (Fig. 18-54). This radiolucent defect can cover part of the subchondral bone plate or a fragment of the superior part of the epiphysis. Caffey believed that this fragment represented a fracture. The crescent sign may help to determine the amount of avascularity, because the avascular segment almost always extends to at least the full extent of the crescent area.

The femoral head later breaks up into areas that are relatively dense, interspersed with areas of radiolucency. This change represents the resorption of the dead bone, with added areas of osteoid and new bone. At this stage, the entire femoral head may be displaced laterally in the acetabulum. Attention should also be given to the lateral half of the femoral head, which may extrude from its normal location. This extrusion is accompanied by the roentgenographic appearance of flattening of the bony portion of the femoral head, resulting from absorption of bone, but the cartilage model is usually less altered at this stage. True deformity is present in the later stages of Legg-Calvé-Perthes syndrome. Gradually, over a period of 3 to 4 years, the femoral head regains a homogeneous density. The last area to fill in is the anterior portion of the femoral head, as shown on the frog-leg view.

Roentgenographic evaluation of anteversion shows that almost all hips with the Legg-Calvé-Perthes syndrome initially have anteversion within normal limits. Therefore, anteversion cannot be implicated in the etiology of the condition. Also, follow-up studies show that patients with increased anteversion have the same results as those with no increase in anteversion. Therefore, increased anteversion *per se* does not seem to adversely affect the end result.

Arthrography

Schiller and Axer[303] found the cartilage outline of the femoral head to be enlarged in the process, as shown by arthrography. This enlargement could account for the inability of the acetabulum to contain the femoral head in some patients. Arthrography may also demonstrate changes in the spherical shape of the femoral cartilaginous surface, which occur early in the "fragmentation" phase or in the latter portion of the increased density phase if sufficient underlying bone is involved.

Arthrography in the regenerative phase can show the true joint deformity, which is helpful in outlining a treatment program. Femoral head "trenching," as described by Roberts, whereby the lateral portion of the head may be deformed by the outer corner of the acetabulum, can be seen only by arthrography during the early stages. In the residual stage, after full regeneration has occurred, arthrography is of little help, because the joint contour follows that of the regenerated subchondral bone of the femoral head.

Radioactive Isotope Studies

The use of bone-seeking isotopes can be of some value in the diagnosis and management of Perthes syndrome. It is now well recognized that isotopes can be used to identify an area of avascularity more clearly than roentgenograms. Although this is helpful in diagnosis, in most patients it will do little to alter the treatment plan, because the earliest signs and symptoms require only routine symptomatic treatment.

Reports from several centers have suggested that isotope studies may be accurate in later stages of the syndrome in determining the full extent of the avascular lesion, as well as in tailoring the treatment program. However, these techniques are not available for the majority of children with the syndrome; the treating physicians must rely, for the most part, on routine roentgenographic studies and clinical signs and symptoms.

PROGNOSIS

The great variability in the end result intrigues students of this syndrome. Several ingenious methods have been devised to assess the end result of the hip affected with Legg-Calvé-Perthes syndrome. It is generally agreed that the more spherical the femoral head at the end of treatment, the better the end result and the lower the risk that arthritis will ensue. The different quotients obtained by measuring various parameters of the femoral head are good methods of evaluation, but these are time consuming and impractical for use with the individual patient. The most practical technique seems to be the method of Goff,[264] further developed by Mose,[293] which consists of drawing concentric circles 2 mm apart on a transparent template. (Fig. 18-55). The tem-

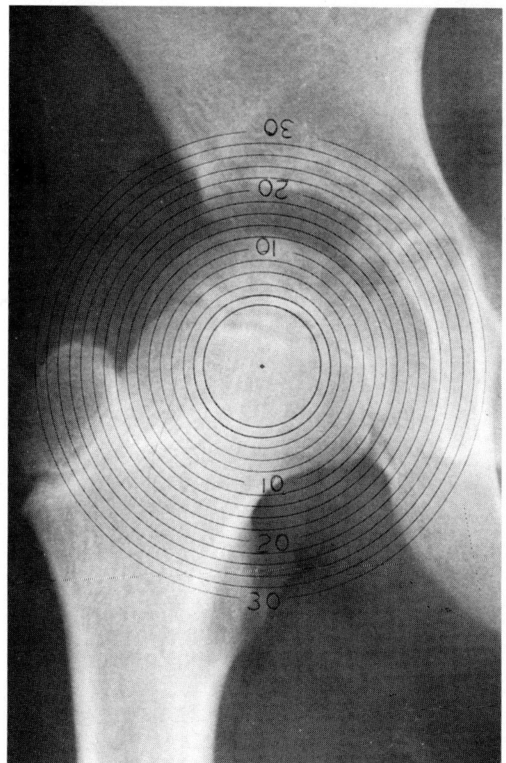

FIG. 18-55. The Mose template superimposed on a roentgenogram to evaluate sphericity of the femoral head. The template should be used to evaluate sphericity on both anteroposterior and frog-leg projections.

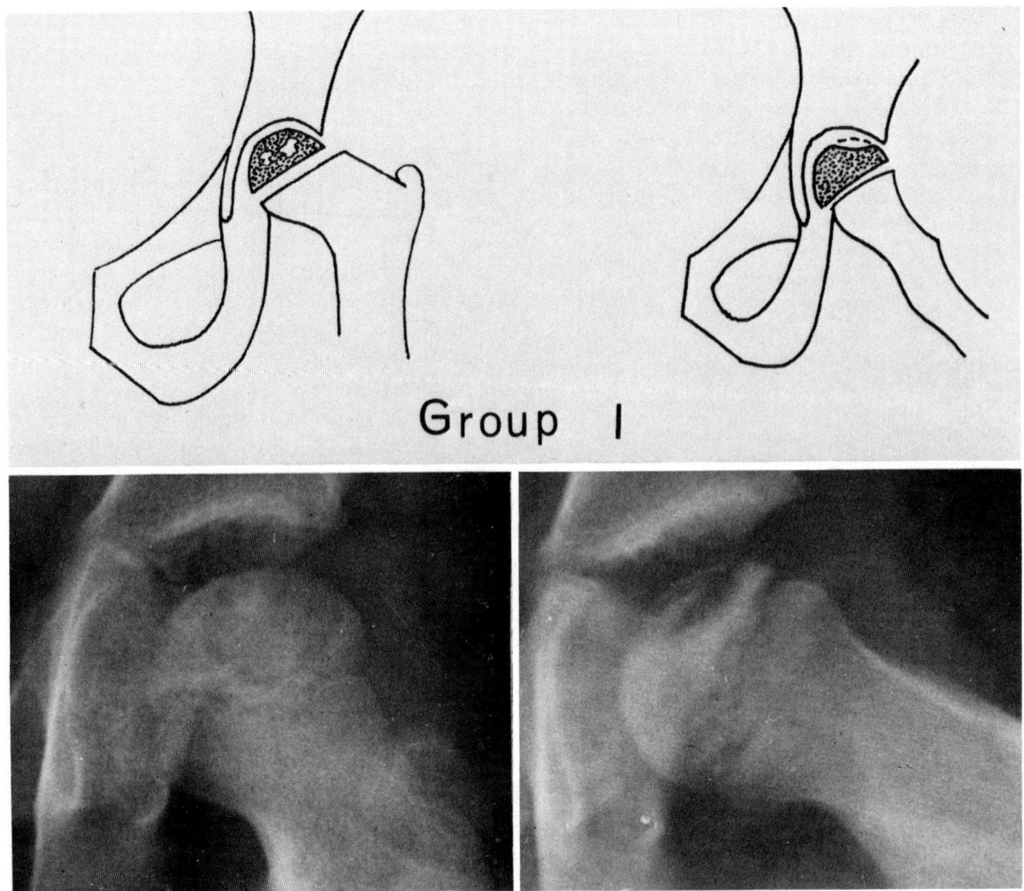

FIG. 18-56. Catterall classification, Group I. There is no significant change in density of the femoral head on the anteroposterior projection.

plate is superimposed on the anteroposterior and lateral roentgenograms and gives a satisfactory evaluation of the degree of sphericity. If the outline of the head is a perfect circle on both projections, the result is rated "good." If the outline of the head varies from a perfect circle by less than 2 mm, the result is rated "fair." If the outline of the femoral head varies from the circle by more than 2 mm in either the anteroposterior or lateral projection, the result is rated "poor." This method of measurement is rigid and quite reproducible. The CE angle of Wiberg can also be recorded to assess the acetabular coverage. However, from a practical viewpoint, the hip will be rated "poor" by the method of Mose before the CE angle will be altered to any great degree.

Catterall Classification

Catterall,[242,243] in an attempt to classify patients according to the amount of femoral epiphyseal involvement, studied the natural history of the process in a series of untreated patients and developed the following classification:

Group I. In this group of patients, the anterior part of the head is involved. There is no collapse in the involved segment. Metaphyseal changes do not occur, and the epiphyseal plate is not involved. Healing occurs without significant sequelae (Fig. 18-56).

Group II. In this group of patients, the involved segment shows increased density, as can best be recognized on the anteroposterior roentgenogram. However, the uninvolved pillars of normal bone can be seen medially and laterally, and they prevent significant collapse (Fig. 18-57). The presence of an intact lateral column in the femoral head, seen on the lateral roentgenogram, is of great prognostic significance. Metaphyseal changes may be seen, but the epiphyseal plate is usually protected by an

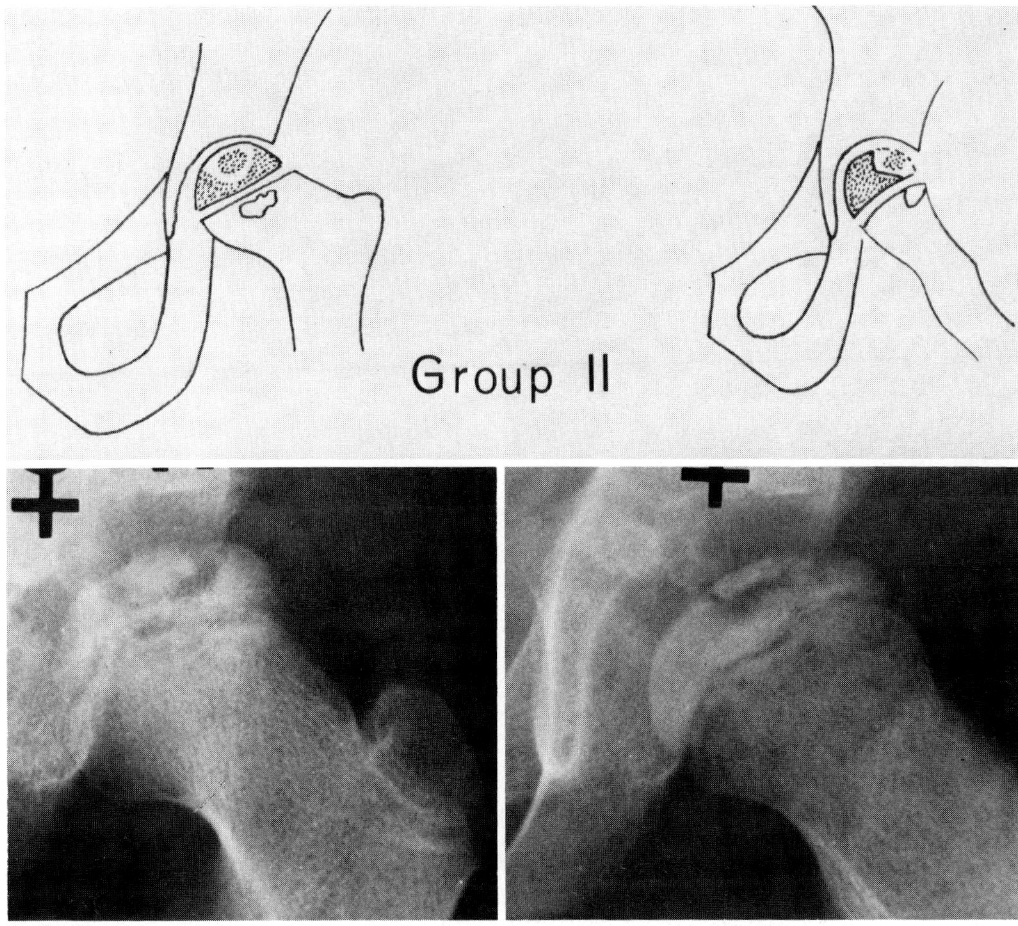

FIG. 18-57. Catterall classification, Group II. There is an intact lateral pillar on the anteroposterior projection, with minimal involvement of the epiphyseal line and metaphysis.

uninvolved tongue of epiphyseal bone that reaches anteriorly. In Group II, regeneration occurs without much loss of epiphyseal height. With an intact epiphyseal plate, the remodeling potential is not affected, and the end result is usually good, especially if several years of growth remain (Fig. 18-58).

Group III. Up to three fourths of the femoral epiphysis is affected in this group. There is no intact support laterally, and the metaphysis is usually involved. The epiphyseal plate is unprotected and is often actively involved in the process (Fig. 18-59). Collapse is more severe, and the collapsed fragment itself is larger. The process takes longer, and the results are usually poorer (Fig. 18-60).

Group IV. In this group, the entire epiphysis is affected. Collapse occurs early and is often severe (Fig. 18-61). Restoration of the femoral head is slower and is usually less complete. The epiphyseal line is most often involved directly in the process, and, if it is severely damaged and can no longer grow normally, it may greatly limit the ability of the femoral head to remodel. This sometimes contributes to a poor result, in spite of the treatment method used. However, in most of these patients, treatment does prevent a grossly deformed femoral head from occurring (Fig. 18-62).

Whereas the Catterall classification focuses on the specific degree of femoral head involvement, there are some patients who fall between the four groups. Our evaluation shows that the degree of involvement has a definite prognostic significance. For example, patients with Group III or IV involvement are more prone to poor results, and those with Group I or II involvement often require only minimal treatment. There are, however, limitations to the

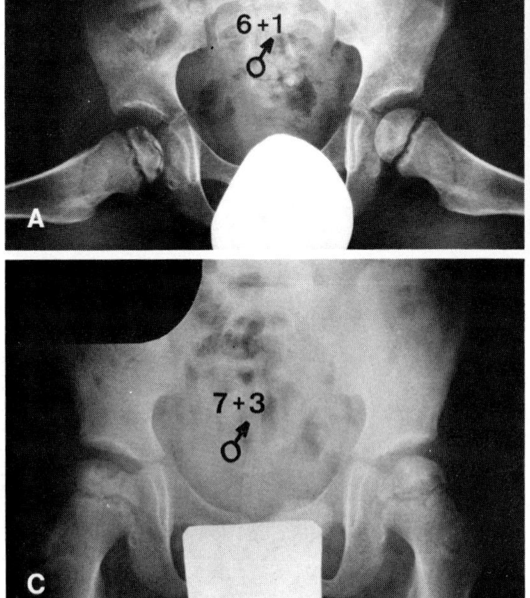

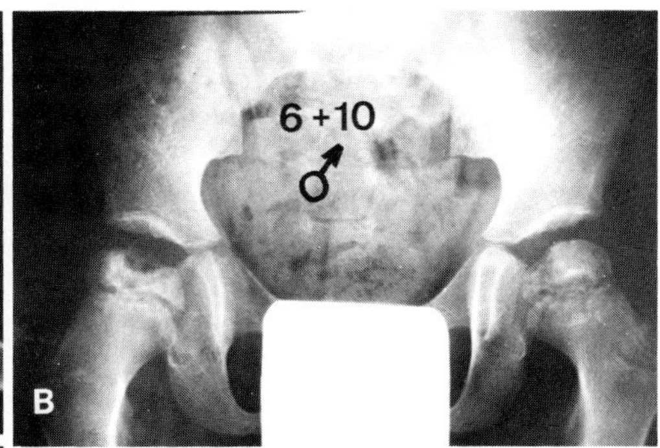

FIG. 18-58. (*A*) Catterall classification, Group II, in a child first diagnosed with Legg-Calvé-Perthes syndrome at the age of 6 years and 1 month. (*B*) The anteroposterior view 9 months later shows an intact lateral pillar. (*C*) Evaluation at age 7 years and 3 months, following early discontinuation of treatment, shows a good result.

Catterall classification in that the physician may have to wait several months to determine the true amount of involvement, and the classification may appear to change during this time (Fig. 18-63). In most patients, the simpler method of classification described by Ponseti is adequate; this method divides patients into two groups: those with less than 50% involvement of the femoral head, and those with greater than 50% involvement.

In addition to the amount of femoral head involvement, there are several other factors that influence prognosis and must also be considered.

Important Factors Influencing Prognosis

Loss of motion in the early stage of the process may be due to either soft-tissue reaction or actual contracture. Later loss of motion reflects an established bony deformity that may be irreversible. If loss of motion is allowed to persist or if it recurs after successful early treatment and is not corrected, a good result is not to be expected. The importance of obtaining and maintaining an essentially full range of motion cannot be overemphasized.

Lateral subluxation, seen as increased distance between the medial joint line and the femoral head, with an associated decrease in coverage of the femoral head, is a well-recognized feature of Legg-Calvé-Perthes syndrome. If allowed to persist, it results in abnormal stresses on a vulnerable femoral head, and a good result cannot be obtained, regardless of how small the area of involvement may be. In addition, in some patients, especially those showing Group III and IV involvement, part of the epiphysis is actually extruded laterally. This means that the amount of the proximal femur that is uncovered is greater than would be produced by an increased medial joint space alone. The changes secondary to extrusion of the lateral portion of the femoral head are usually much more significant and more common than those associated with true subluxation of the total femoral head. This extruded portion is first seen roentgenographically as a cluster of faint flecks of calcification within the cartilage model. Extrusion is the major factor in the development of an enlarged femoral head during regeneration (Fig. 18-64), and the lateral calcifications indicate that part of the femoral head will regenerate outside of the acetabulum. The head will then be larger and will be distorted unless the extruded portion can be contained within the acetabulum during the plastic stage. In an extreme case, the head can appear to be

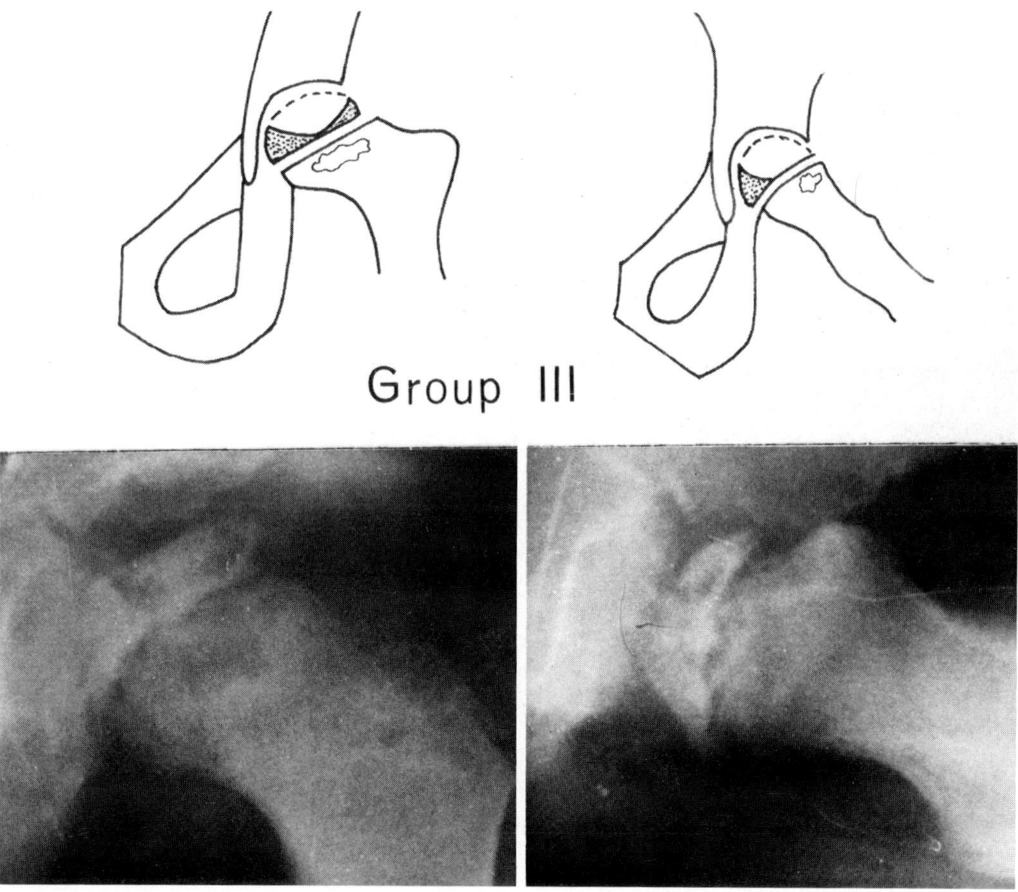

FIG. 18-59. Catterall classification, Group III. Note the loss of lateral support on the anteroposterior projection, and involvement across the epiphyseal line in the frog-leg projection. This may result in premature closure of the epiphysis and even greater distortion of the femoral head than these roentgenograms suggest.

split by the acetabular margin. Early lysis of the lateral portion of the epiphysis usually indicates loss of support laterally and vulnerability to abnormal stresses, meaning that the involved hip will fall into a Catterall Group III or IV classification.

A metaphyseal cyst may appear early in the fragmentation stage and disappear during regeneration. Biopsy of such cysts shows immature connective tissue, blood vessels, and the formation of a few giant cells (reactive-type tissue only). A biopsy is rarely, if ever, indicated. With more severe involvement, the epiphyseal line may appear to be more horizontal.

These roentgenographic changes have been described by Catterall as producing a femoral head that is "at risk" for serious deformity. However, persistent loss of motion is probably the most important early sign of impending serious problems. Again, it must be mentioned that the age at onset of Perthes syndrome significantly influences the prognosis, because increased femoral head involvement, and thus a poorer result, is usually seen in patients older than 8 years of age.

DIFFERENTIAL DIAGNOSIS

In the early stage, before roentgenographic changes may be detected in the bone, toxic synovitis, pyogenic arthritis, and osteomyelitis of the femoral neck must be considered as differential diagnoses. In Legg-Calvé-Perthes syndrome, there is little change in white blood cell count and little, if any, increase in the sedimentation rate. If true doubt exists as to the diagnosis of the syndrome, the hip should

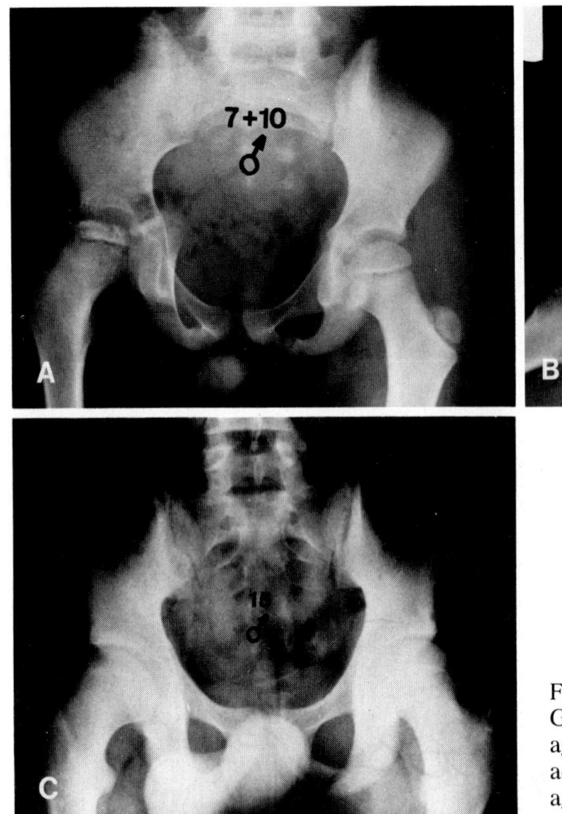

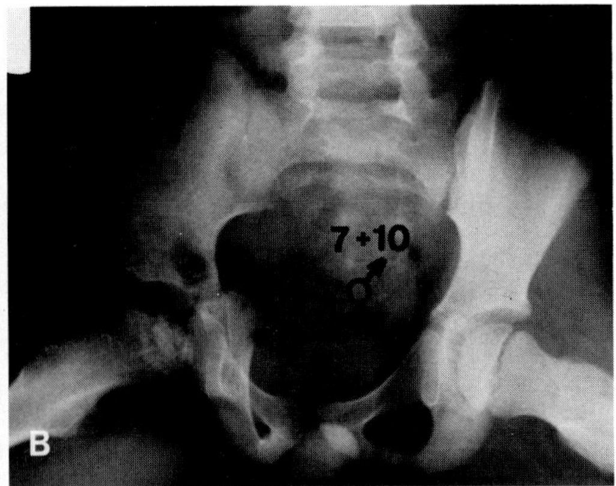

Fig. 18-60. (*A* and *B*) Catterall classification, Group III, in a child 7 years and 10 months of age. Concentric reduction was subsequently achieved. (*C*) A follow-up film at 15 years of age shows fair results according to the Mose method.

be aspirated, as should any joint suspected of harboring infection. If no fluid is recovered, a small amount of contrast fluid should be injected and a roentgenogram should be obtained to verify that the joint has been entered. If there is an unusual, fuzzy appearance of the femoral head or if the child has generalized retardation, a thyroid study may be helpful; however, this is only rarely indicated. Radioactive isotope studies may be useful in the differential diagnosis.

A major problem is differentiating Legg-Calvé-Perthes syndrome from multiple epiphyseal dysplasia. The latter should be suspected in all patients with bilateral involvement, especially when the involvement is symmetrical and the femoral heads do not have a characteristic appearance of Legg-Calvé-Perthes syndrome. Any hip joint that does not follow the classic picture of increased density and presence of the crescent sign, followed by fragmentation, should be considered suspect for multiple epiphyseal dysplasia. A family history may often be obtained. Roentgenograms of other joints, especially a tunnel view of the knee and an anteroposterior view of the ankles showing lateral tilt of the ankle mortise, help to determine the diagnosis.

TREATMENT

Principles

Treatment of Legg-Calvé-Perthes syndrome should be aimed at providing the most favorable circumstances for the disease process to run its self-limited course. All affected femoral heads eventually heal, and the main principle of treatment is to try to minimize distortion during the active stages of the process.

The most important initial treatment principle is to rapidly regain and maintain an essentially full range of motion. This is too often overlooked in the enthusiasm to proceed with a treatment program. Traction and bed rest are most helpful in regaining motion. Full abduction should be restored, and internal rotation should be regained, although the last 10° of internal rotation is not essential. Up to

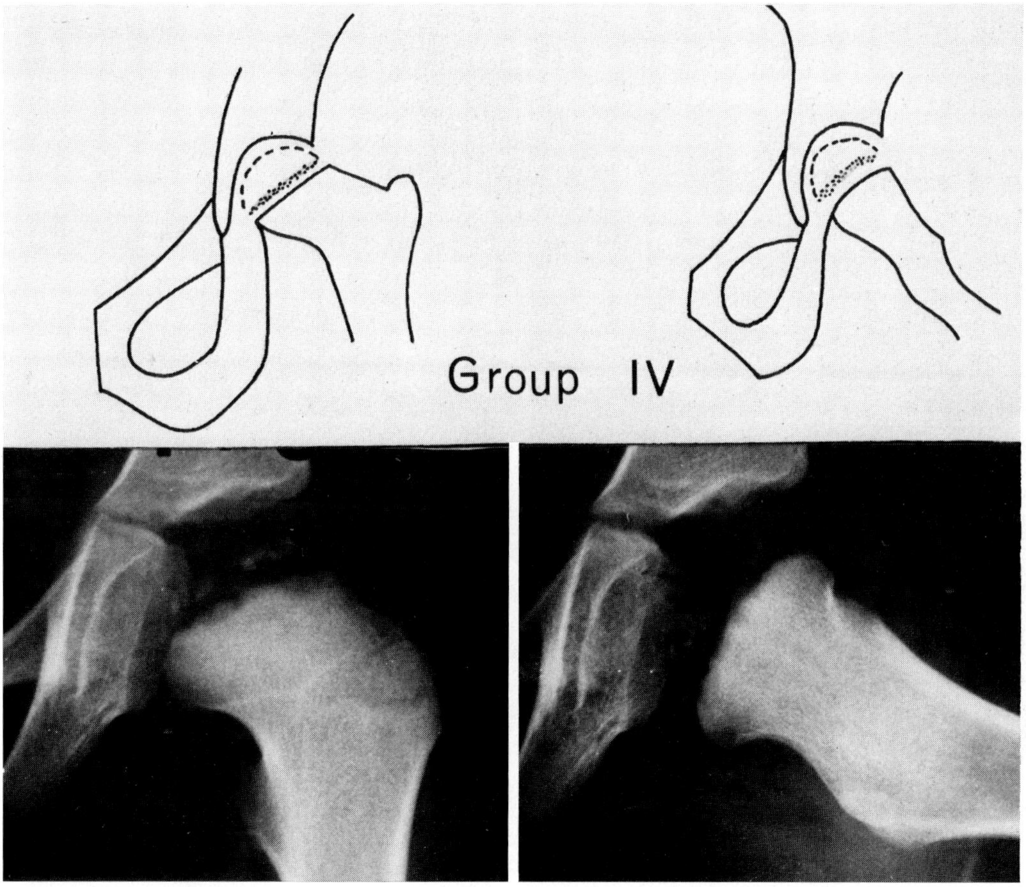

Group IV

FIG. 18-61. Catterall classification, Group IV. There is total involvement of the femoral head, with exposure of the epiphyseal line.

2 weeks of this conservative treatment may be necessary, and only after this period should an adductor release be considered. The traction program may be carried out at home if the family situation allows. In approximately 20% of the patients, an inflammatory-like reaction persists, which may be alleviated by oral salicylates. Only after motion has been restored should further treatment be considered.

In the past, most treatment efforts in Perthes syndrome were directed toward nonweightbearing. However, in recent years, it has been recognized that if the femoral head can be deeply contained within the acetabulum during the soft, vulnerable phase of the disease process, a more normal femoral head will result. It should be remembered that the acetabulum is not involved in the early phase of the disease and, therefore, can serve as an excellent mold. However, both the physician and the patient must recognize that even with a full treatment program (containment orthosis or surgery), a less-than-excellent result should be expected if the child is older than 8 years of age or has major femoral head involvement (Fig. 18-65), or if the epiphyseal line closes before skeletal maturity is reached.

Plans of Management

The following plan of management is suggested. For Group I involvement, regardless of the age of the patient, no specific treatment appears to be indicated as long as a full range of motion is maintained. A change in motion may herald a more severe form of the condition, so the patient must be watched initially for 2 to 4 months, and the program should be modified if necessary. In Group II involve-

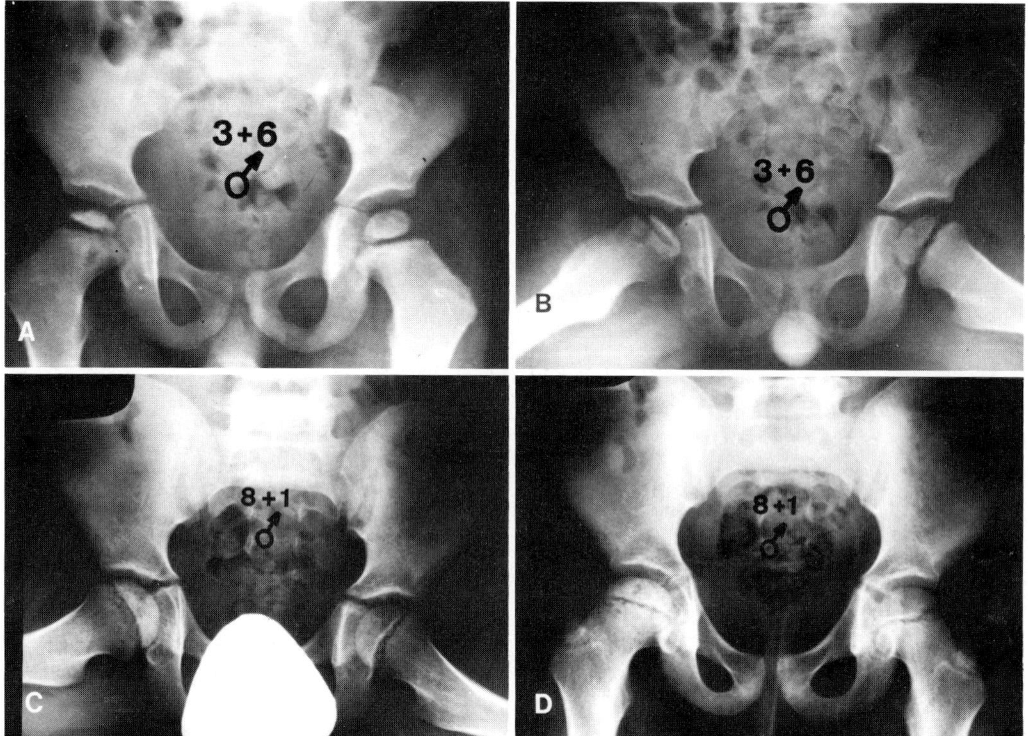

FIG. 18-62. (*A* and *B*) Catterall classification, Group IV. There is total femoral head involvement in this young child, with no resultant restriction of motion. (*C* and *D*) After treatment, minimal residual deformity is present, as seen at age 8 years and 1 month.

ment, there are rarely poor results for patients younger than 7 years of age, regardless of the type of treatment. Therefore, for the young child, containment efforts are probably not necessary with a full range of motion unless there is true subluxation. In patients 7 years of age, early containment should be achieved by an orthosis, and care should be taken to maintain motion because of the risk of more serious involvement or slight subluxation. If the hip remains in Group II, treatment can be discontinued gradually after approximately 6 months.

For Groups III and IV, regardless of patient age, emphasis should be placed on containing the femoral head within the acetabulum and maintaining a full range of motion. In very young children (3 to 4 years), if there are no signs of irritation in the joint and no evidence of subluxation, a course of observation can be carried out; however, frequent follow-up is indicated. In patients of at least 7 years of age with Group III or IV involvement, the situation may warrant surgical treatment. The work of Klisic[283] suggests that in older children with total femoral head involvement, the results are usually poor, so an active motion program without surgery is preferred. Weight-relief abduction treatment may be of help in this group of patients, but, to date, this has not been proved.

Nonweightbearing Methods

Nonweightbearing treatment may include bed rest with or without traction, an ischial weightbearing brace, or a Snyder sling. However, bed rest is only practical for as much time as is necessary to regain motion in the hip. Ischial weightbearing braces are not truly weight-relieving and may actually increase pressure across the hip joint and are therefore contraindicated. Successful use of the Snyder sling or Forte harness depends solely on the cooperation of the patient. These devices are helpful only in instances in which the diagnosis has not been confirmed and treatment is initiated only on a short-term basis.

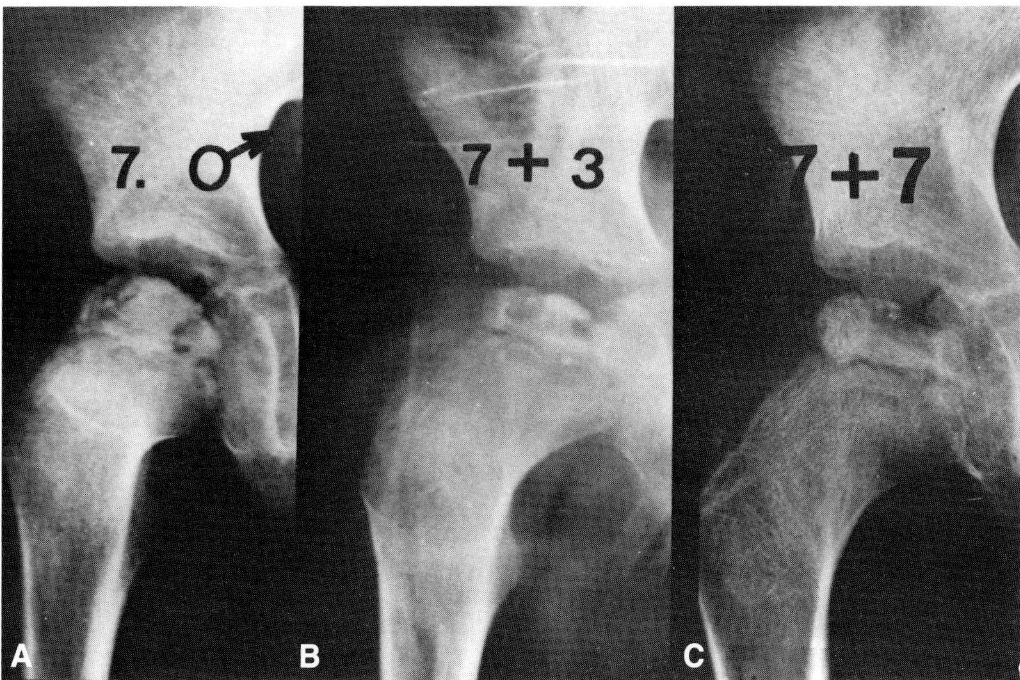

FIG. 18-63. (*A*) This roentgenogram of a 7-year-old child suggests major femoral head involvement, which is much less obvious 3 months later (*B*). (*C*) Catterall classification, Group II involvement is identifiable at the age of 7 years and 7 months, and the child was able to bear weight without a brace.

Containment Methods

The concept of containment treatment is to maintain the femoral head deeply within the acetabulum throughout its vulnerable period and to maintain a full range of hip motion. If the femoral head is placed deeply in the acetabulum, weightbearing does not seem to be an important consideration except possibly in the older child with major femoral head involvement. In abduction, the hip abductors are at a mechanical disadvantage and cannot apply strong force across the joint. Also, the soft femoral head is stabilized on all sides by the intact acetabulum.

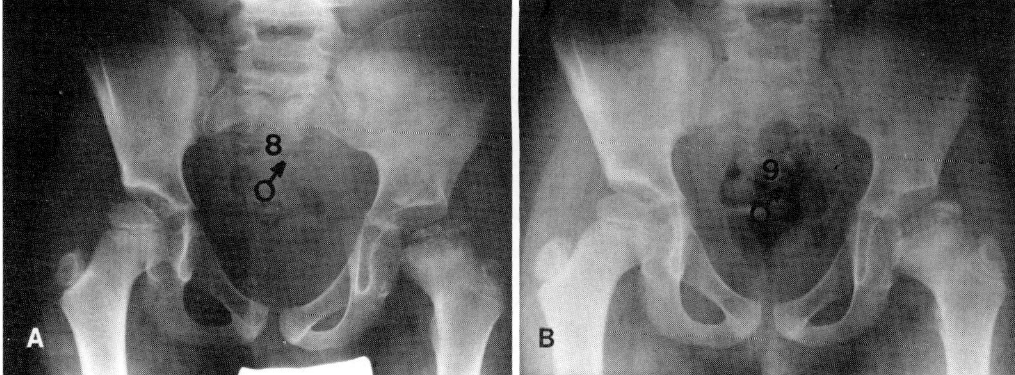

FIG. 18-64. (*A*) This male child, 8 years of age, presented with extrusion of the lateral portion of the epiphysis and lateral flecks of calcification and ossification following unsuccessful attempts at concentric reduction. (*B*) At 9 years of age, the ossification of the lateral flecks has resulted in union with and enlargement of the femoral head.

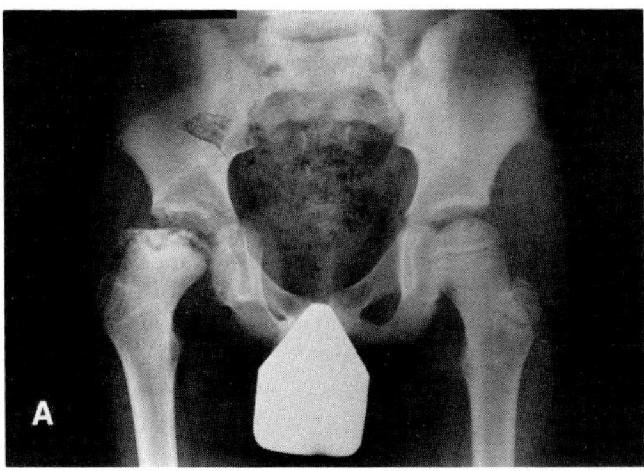

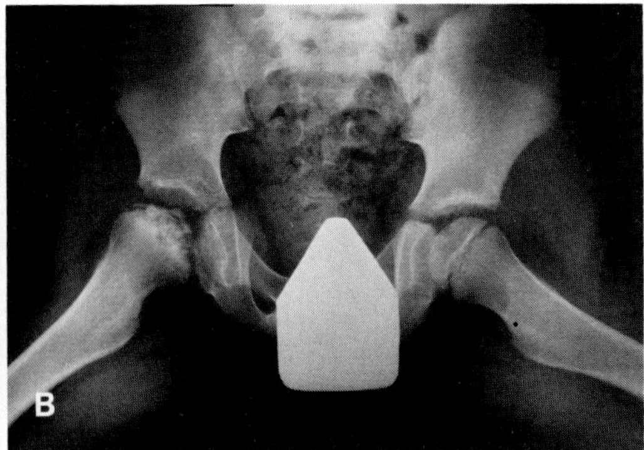

FIG. 18-65. (*A*) In this patient, a late diagnosis of Legg-Calvé-Perthes syndrome was confirmed by roentgenograms. (*B*) However, since 15° of hip abduction is possible even with the hip in full extension, surgery to remove the extruded portion of the femoral head is not necessary.

Abduction should be sufficient to allow the lateral aspect of the epiphyseal line to reach the lateral margin of the acetabulum. This lateral coverage should be confirmed by a standing roentgenogram in the holding device used for treatment (Fig. 18-66). Thirty-five to 55° leg abduction may be necessary to achieve this coverage, depending on the neck-shaft angle of the femur and the tilt of the epiphyseal line. Inadequate abduction can result in formation of a pressure point laterally and may do more harm than good. Maintaining a position with more than a few degrees of internal rotation is probably not important, because anteversion is not normally increased in the early stages of Legg-Calvé-Perthes syndrome.

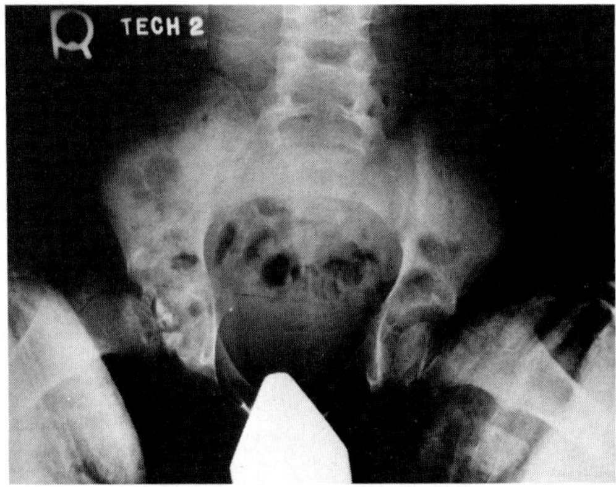

FIG. 18-66. Lateral coverage is confirmed by a standing roentgenogram in a holding device. The superior portion of the epiphyseal line is abducted to within the border of the acetabulum to prevent extrusion.

The subluxation, collapse, and extrusion that may occur in the early stages of the process can be decreased or eliminated with adequate early containment. Various methods of holding the thighs in abduction and internal rotation include nonweightbearing abduction braces, the abduction casts of Petrie and Harrison, and the abduction weightbearing orthoses of Craig, Newington, Toronto, and Atlanta (Fig. 18-67).

Plaster Method

It is important to remember that an essentially full range of motion must exist in the hip prior to placing a child in an abduction device. As soon as the child is active in any type of containment device, a standing anteroposterior roentgenogram of the pelvis is necessary to confirm that the femoral head is fully covered (see Fig 18-66).

The use of Petrie[296] abduction casts has been very helpful in short-range treatment. The casts can be applied as soon as a full range of motion is achieved, requiring no delay for fabrication of a brace. The casts also give the physician an opportunity to evaluate the total problem over a period of a few months, without the financial commitment of a brace, while the severity of the femoral head involvement is determined. A child should not remain in a cast for more than 2 to 3 months at a time. When new casts are to be applied, the child should remain out of the cast for several days in order to regain full knee motion. Except for rare situations, it is recommended that no more than two or three sets of casts be used before other containment methods are at-

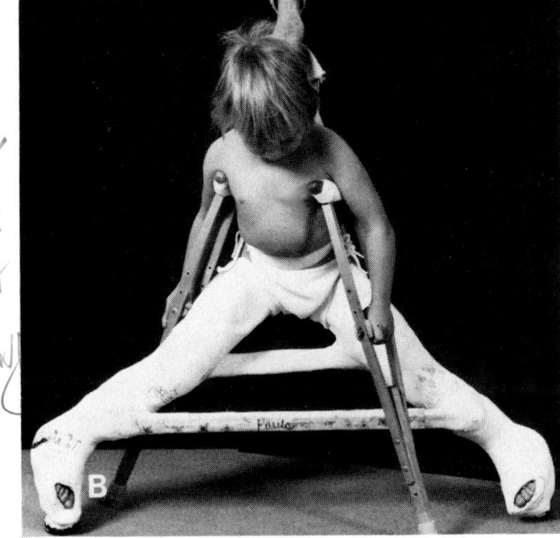

FIG. 18-67. (*A*) The Toronto brace, an abduction containment orthosis. (*B*) The Petrie cast, which achieves abduction with mild internal rotation.

tempted or treatment is discontinued because of only mild femoral head involvement. If the casts are not changed frequently, there may be damage to the articular cartilage of the knees. The casts must fit snugly about the thighs to minimize stress on the medial collateral ligament. In our patients, no late problems have resulted from this method.

Orthosis Methods

There are many types of braces and orthoses available for the treatment of patients with Perthes syndrome, all of which are designed to contain the femoral head within the acetabulum. Although there is little difference in efficiency among the methods, the local bracemaker or orthotist must be familiar with the method that is chosen and the need for repairs must be kept at a reasonable level. Any necessary repairs should be made promptly to minimize the time out of the brace. Each time that the child is re-evaluated, the device should be removed and the hip should be examined to see if a full range of motion is still present. If motion has decreased, the child should be returned to a temporary traction program. If the hip remains slightly painful or if there is only a slight decrease in motion, a nighttime home traction program may be used.

Discontinuing Treatment

In the past, most treatment programs were continued until the femoral head had filled in, as was indicated by both anteroposterior and lateral roentgenograms, or at least until the subchondral bone plate had been re-established in both views. However, this process required anywhere from 18 months to 4 years, making the program both indefinite and lengthy.

Our clinical and roentgenographic evaluations of patients who discontinued their own treatment program early have demonstrated that little, if any, distortion of the femoral head occurs if weightbearing is resumed after the increased density in the femoral head disappears (Fig. 18-68). This corresponds with observations by Ferguson and Howorth[258] and later by Thompson and Westin.[310] The increased density essentially disappears at the completion of the fragmentation stage, which is approximately 1 year after the onset of the syndrome. The studies of Jonsater[275] also demonstrated increased strength in the biopsy fragments by the time that the fragmentation stage was reached.

In most patients, once an early diagnosis has been made, a period of 6 months of observation is required to determine the full extent of femoral head involvement (using the Catterall classification). During this time, especially in the older child, there is the risk of Group II involvement changing to Group III. Studies with radioactive isotopes, when available, may allow earlier identification of the amount of involvement. If the involvement is found to be only Group II and the patient has a full range of motion, treatment can be discontinued even before the dense segment disappears. Thus, many patients can be allowed

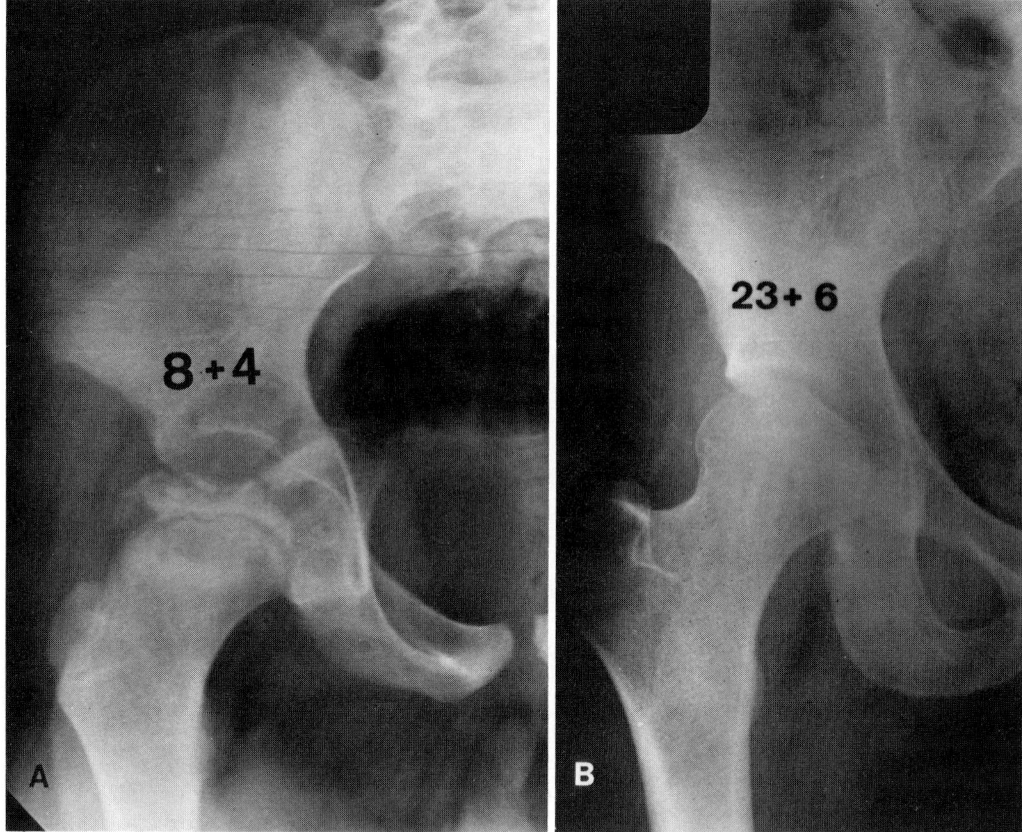

FIG. 18-68. (*A*) Treatment was discontinued at the end of the sclerotic phase for this child of 8 years and 4 months. (*B*) Long-term follow-up film taken at 23 years and 6 months shows excellent remodeling with no further collapse.

to walk unassisted by the end of the first 6 months.

If the femoral head involvement is of Group III or IV, the increased density areas usually vanish 12 to 15 months after onset, and weight-bearing can be resumed.

To wean the child from a brace program, we suggest allowing removal of the brace for only a few hours a day, starting in the house. The child should be evaluated within a week after weaning is begun in order to determine if any loss of motion has occurred. If full motion is still present, the time out of the brace can be increased and the motion can be rechecked frequently. Loss of motion is an indication that a longer period of full-time wear is necessary. It appears that at any stage in the process of Legg-Calvé-Perthes syndrome, the retention of a full range of motion is probably the most important sign that the program is under control.

Surgical Procedures

In principle, a surgical procedure should be considered for only one of two reasons: It is either done early in the process to prevent deformity and to replace a nonoperative containment method, or later in the process to improve an established, but still reversible, deformity.

The goal of surgery in the early stages of Perthes syndrome is the same as with conservative treatment: to contain the femoral head deeply within the acetabulum. This containment can be produced either by altering the acetabulum to provide further coverage (usually with the innominate osteotomy of Salter) or decreasing the angle of the proximal femur by varus osteotomy. If carried out correctly, both surgical and nonoperative containment methods should produce the same end results. Surgery is more often indicated

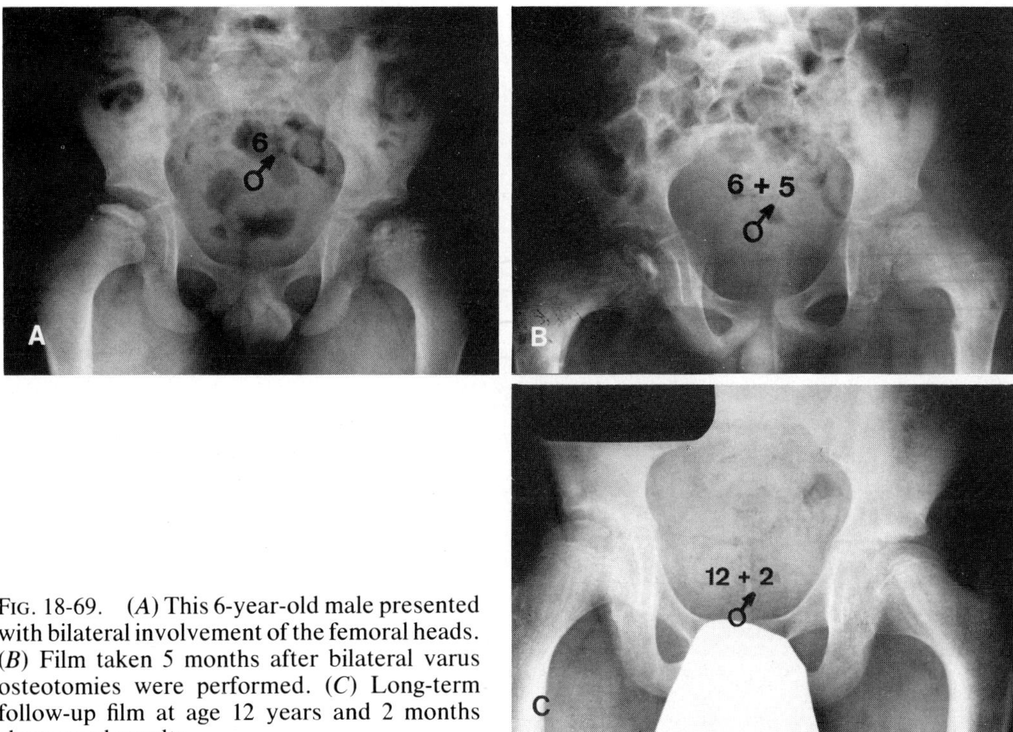

FIG. 18-69. (*A*) This 6-year-old male presented with bilateral involvement of the femoral heads. (*B*) Film taken 5 months after bilateral varus osteotomies were performed. (*C*) Long-term follow-up film at age 12 years and 2 months show good results.

when the prognosis suggests that the healing phase will be prolonged (*i.e.*, in the older child with a severely involved femoral head). Because no real deformity is expected with Group I and II involvement except for the rare hip with subluxation, surgery need only be considered for Group III or IV involvement. As mentioned earlier, this often requires a delay of up to 6 months while the extent of femoral head involvement is being determined (Fig. 18-63).

Geographic and social factors greatly influence the indications for surgery. In some areas, proper abduction braces or orthoses may not be available. Also, some children and families do not have the proper attitudes to follow a full-time bracing program. On the other hand, a surgical program should probably not be introduced unless the child can be properly followed and re-evaluated for possible complications.

It must be emphasized that the child must have an essentially full range of motion before surgery is undertaken. This motion must be maintained for several weeks prior to surgery, and, ideally, a cast or brace should be used for a few months to produce and maintain the desired motion. This also allows sufficient time for the extent of involvement to be determined, especially in the earliest stages of the process.

The varus osteotomy is usually preferred as the early surgical measure, because it allows full centering of the femoral head (Fig. 18-69). The neck-shaft angle should be reduced to no more than 115°, because a more normal angle may not be restored later if the epiphyseal line is involved (Fig. 18-70). Derotation may be carried out, but unless the child has an abnormal increase in anteversion, no more than a few degrees of correction are indicated.

The Salter osteotomy has value in the primary treatment of Legg-Calvé-Perthes syndrome, but difficulty may occur in regaining motion after this procedure, especially in the older child with total head involvement (Fig. 18-71). It is also difficult to obtain sufficient lateral coverage if the head centers fully only after 20° or more on the abduction test. The procedure should be preceded by an arthrogram, and moderate or severe distortion of the cartilage model is a contraindication. The younger child with a Group II–type uncontrolled subluxation and full range of motion can be ideally treated by this procedure.

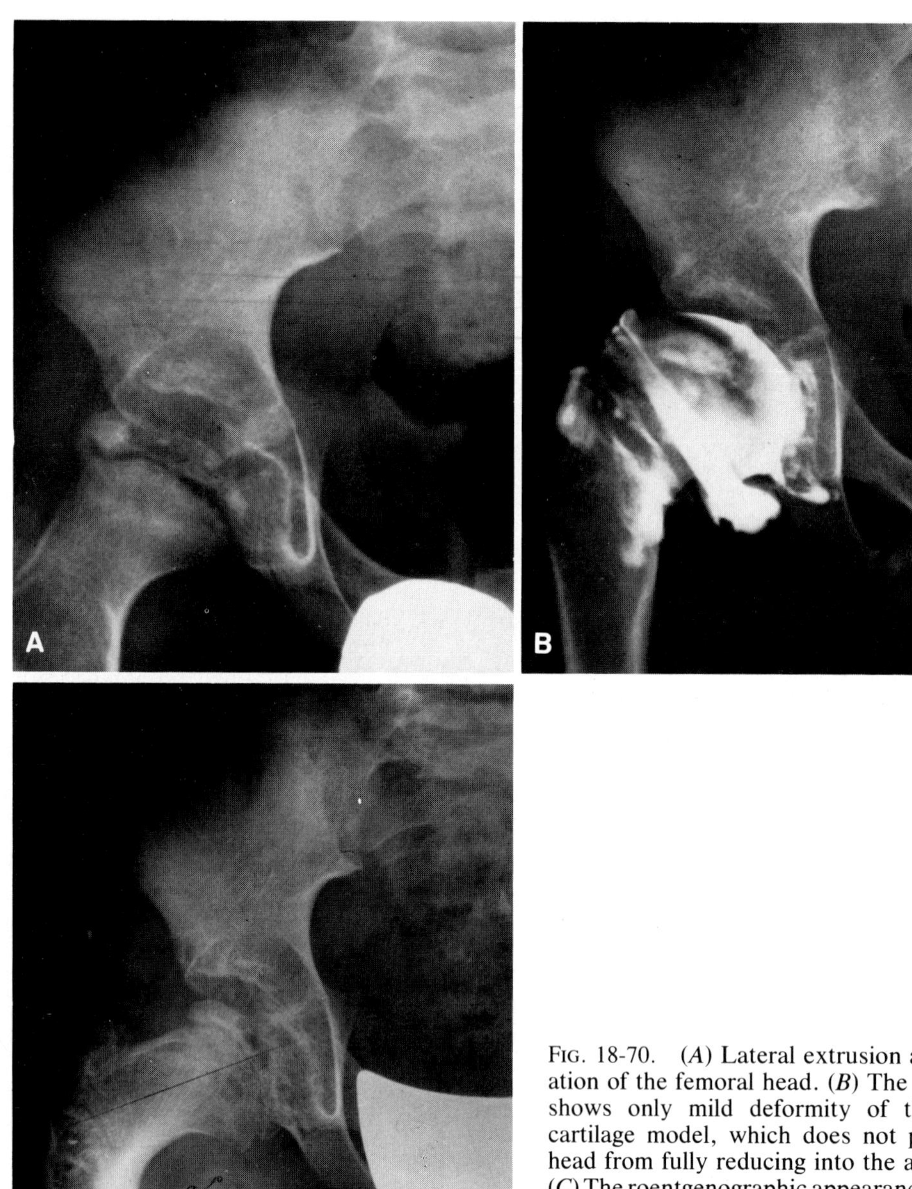

FIG. 18-70. (*A*) Lateral extrusion and subluxation of the femoral head. (*B*) The arthrogram shows only mild deformity of the femoral cartilage model, which does not prevent the head from fully reducing into the acetabulum. (*C*) The roentgenographic appearance following a varus osteotomy that was performed to re-center the femoral head, but which resulted in excessive varus.

Reconstruction

An operation performed late in Legg-Calvé-Perthes syndrome to correct an already present deformity may serve to cover the femoral head, reshape it, or translate motion into a more useful range. The improved mechanical environment will hopefully allow for further remodeling if the potential for growth still exists. If no growth potential remains, most patients are best left alone unless they have significant pain; however, such symptoms are usually rare in patients with Perthes syndrome until middle life (Fig. 18-72). If Legg-Calvé-Perthes syndrome is recognized and treated early, the need for late reconstructive procedures is lessened.

If the goal of reconstructive surgery is to re-establish containment by an indirect approach to the proximal femur or the acetabu-

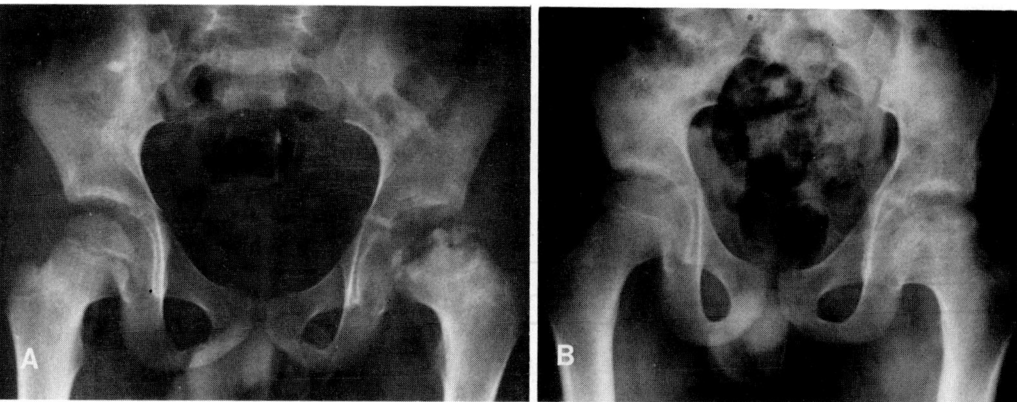

FIG. 18-71. (*A*) Preoperative roentgenogram shows total femoral head involvement. The spherical outline of the femoral head was verified by arthrogram. (*B*) Four years after Salter osteotomy was performed, a satisfactory result can be seen.

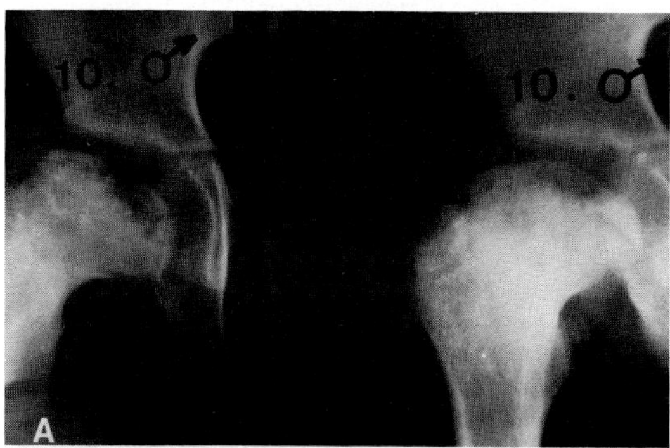

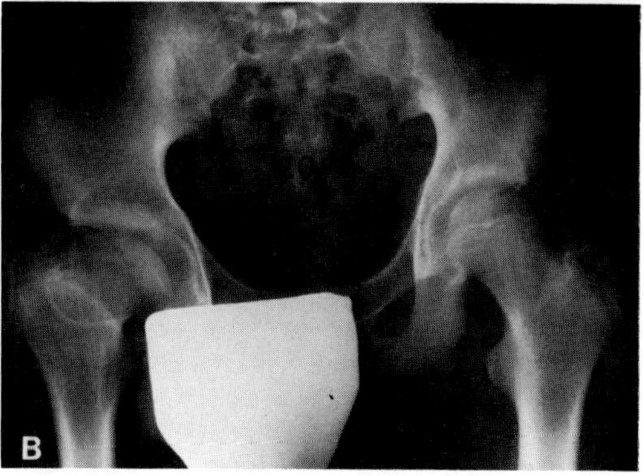

FIG. 18-72. (*A*) This film of a 10-year-old male demonstrates total femoral head involvement, extending across the epiphyseal line and to the metaphysis. (*B*) Follow-up film at 20 years shows ineffective remodeling and overgrowth of the greater trochanter due to premature closure of the epiphysis.

lum, it is mandatory that the final position be demonstrated before the surgical procedure is performed. An abduction test roentgenogram should be used to verify the position. If this is not satisfactory, a traction program is indicated to effect reduction. Unless the reduction is achieved first, the surgical procedure will fail and the malalignment may be worsened.

The Varus osteotomy may be done if the femoral head can be replaced within the acetabulum as in the primary treatment group. If, however, there has already been considerable loss in epiphyseal height, the varus procedure will exaggerate the shortening. The child may later require an epiphysiodesis of the opposite distal femur to achieve leg-length equality. The neck-shaft angle should only be reduced to 120°, because children requiring this procedure are usually older and often demonstrate involvement of the epiphyseal line; therefore, they will not regain the full normal angle.

The Salter osteotomy is seldom indicated as a reconstructive procedure in Legg-Calvé-Perthes syndrome, because there is usually already significant deformity in the femoral head. If this is to be considered, it should be preceded by an arthrogram to assess the sphericity of the head. If sphericity has been lost, the procedure should not be done.

The Chiari procedure is only rarely indicated for children with Legg-Calvé-Perthes syndrome. There is probably no indication for this procedure in an older child or adolescent who does not have pain, although it may be con-

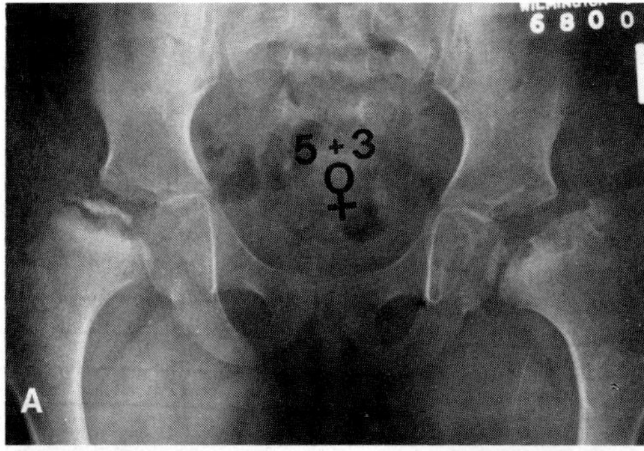

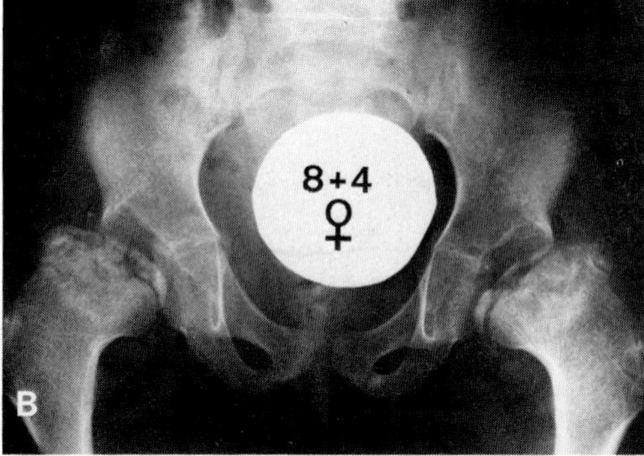

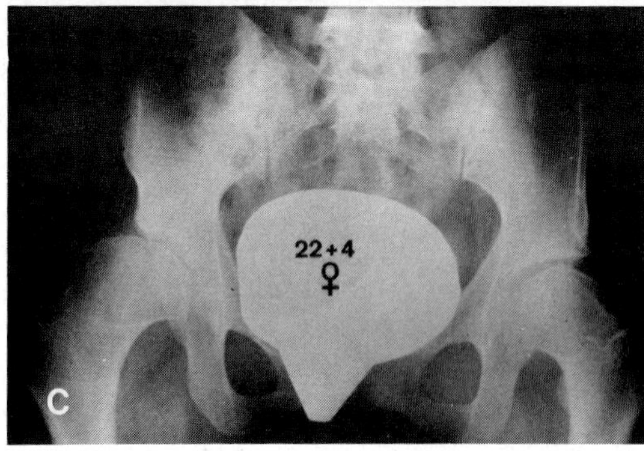

FIG. 18-73. (*A*) Roentgenogram of the hip of a child of age 5 years and 3 months, showing gross extrusion. Containment methods are not possible, and resection should not be performed at this stage. (*B*) Resection may be considered once the epiphysis is partially reconstituted, as in this film, which was obtained when the child was 8 years and 4 months of age. (*C*) This long-term follow-up film shows the improved contour of the femoral head.

sidered in the rare adolescent with coxa magna who is having considerable pain.

The Garceau procedure involves removal of the portion of the femoral head that extrudes beyond the acetabulum to such a degree that it locks the thigh in adduction or in neutral position. This procedure should not be considered until there has been adequate buildup of new bone in the weightbearing area (Fig. 18-73) and the reconstructive phase is well underway (Fig. 18-74). If treated too early, the soft weightbearing area of the femoral head may extrude again, resulting in further deformity. The Garceau procedure is only rarely indicated and should not be required if appropriate containment methods are used in the earlier phases of the process.

A valgus osteotomy may be used as an alternative to the Garceau procedure as the child approaches skeletal maturity. A roentgenogram with the hip in adduction, which may be supplemented by arthrography, should be used to define the contour of the femoral head to the acetabulum. If the congruity between the two structures is not good, the valgus osteotomy is contraindicated.

Combined Procedures

The rare patient who has had an extrusion or subluxation of the femoral head for many months may also have a true secondary dysplasia of the acetabulum. If the femoral head still centers on the abduction test, the dysplasia may be improved by combined innominate and varus osteotomies (Fig. 18-75). If this combination is considered, it should be preceded by an arthrogram to show the extent of cartilaginous changes in the acetabulum. If the cartilage model remains normal, only the femoral surgery is indicated.

TRANSIENT SYNOVITIS

Transient synovitis is the most common cause of painful hips in children. Several review articles on this subject have been published, in which synonyms such as toxic synovitis, observation hip, intermittent hydarthrosis, and coxitis serosa are used to refer to the condition.[319,322,324,329,330]

ETIOLOGY

Three major etiologies have been proposed for transient synovitis: viral infection, allergic reaction, and trauma.

Evidence for an infectious etiology is circumstantial. Spock[336] reported that 70% of his cases had a history of an upper respiratory infection within a 2-week period prior to the onset of symptoms. Of six patients tested for viral antigens, three showed an elevated titre. In addition, 30% of the patients had a positive throat culture for beta-hemolytic streptococci compared with only 10% of a control asymptomatic group. On this basis, he proposed a

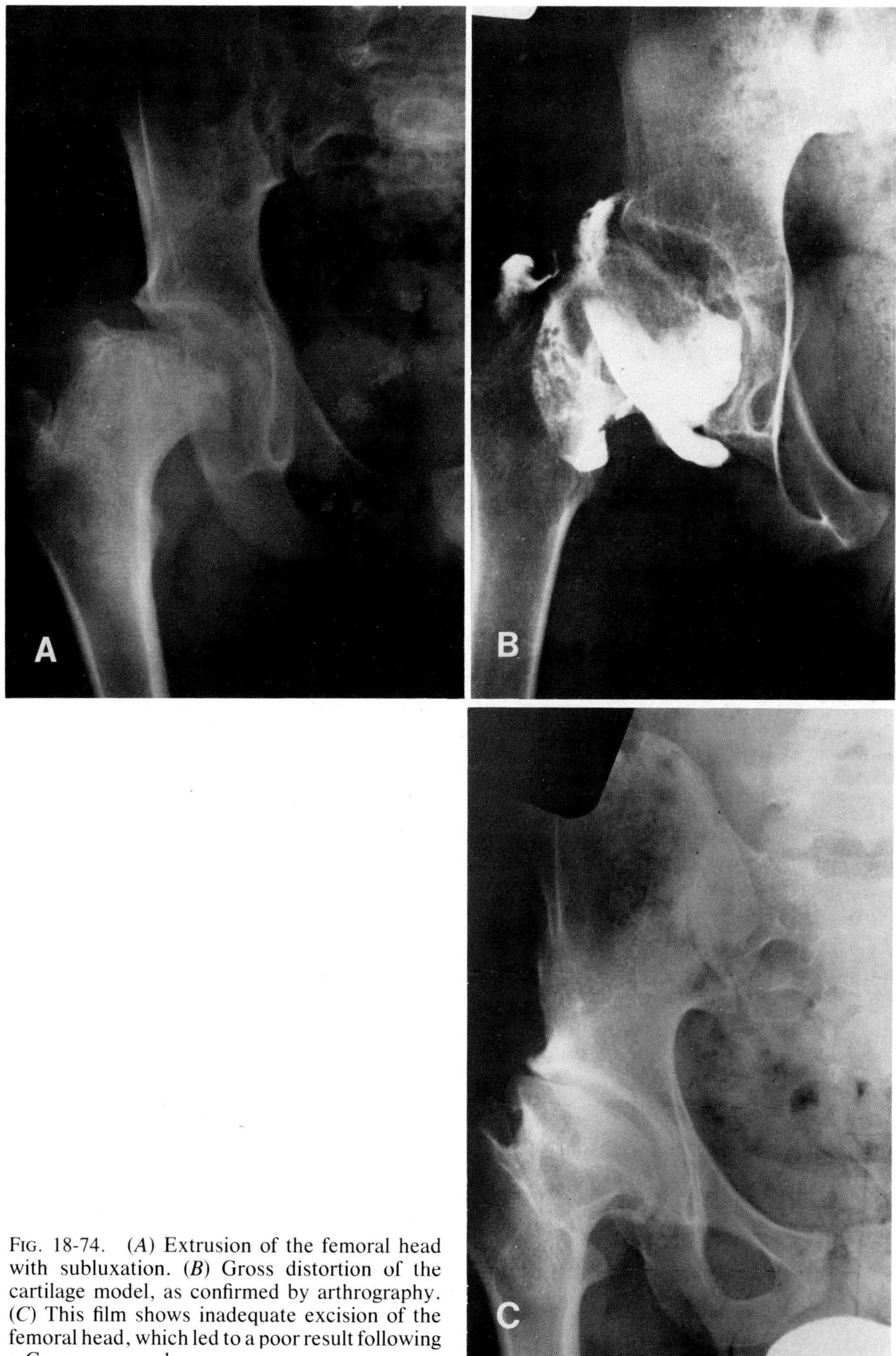

FIG. 18-74. (*A*) Extrusion of the femoral head with subluxation. (*B*) Gross distortion of the cartilage model, as confirmed by arthrography. (*C*) This film shows inadequate excision of the femoral head, which led to a poor result following a Garceau procedure.

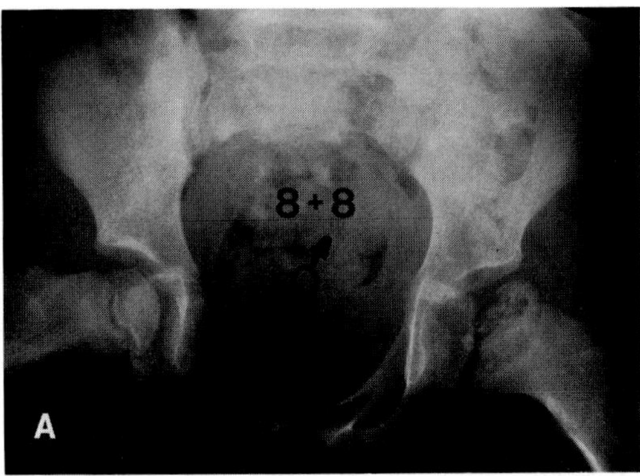

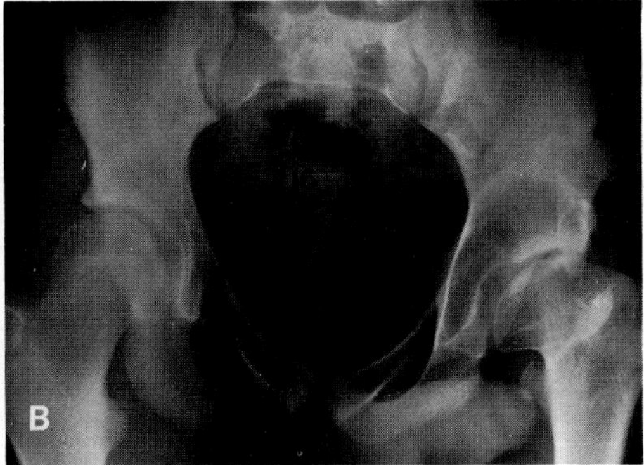

FIG. 18-75. (*A*) In this hip, the femoral head centers on abduction, despite total head involvement and secondary acetabular dysplasia. (*B*) Salter and varus osteotomies were performed; this long-term follow-up film shows improved positioning.

causal relationship between viral or bacterial infection and the presence of transient synovitis. Gledhill[328] and Donaldson[324] each report a 20% incidence of antecedent upper respiratory infection. On the other hand, Hardinge,[329] in a review of 65 patients, could establish no causal relationship between previous infection and the presence of transient synovitis. Blockey and Porter[320] reported a history of viral infection in 2 of 17 children.

Edwards[326] has suggested that synovitis may result from an allergic reaction to the presence of an infectious agent. This is supported by a rather dramatic response to antihistamines in two cases. Nachemson and Scheller,[334] on the other hand, did a careful history for allergy on patients with this condition and noted an incidence of 16%, which was identical to that for the general population, and concluded that allergy played little role in the cause of transient synovitis.

The third suspected cause of transient synovitis is minor trauma. Hardinge[329] studied the incidence of transient synovitis in patients with fracture of the tibia. Because none of these children exhibited transient synovitis, he concluded that there was no definite causal relationship between trauma and transient synovitis.

CLINICAL FEATURES

The most frequent presenting complaint is a painful limp. Approximately one half of the patients will have an acute onset, whereas the other half will have an insidious onset of the pain. The right side is affected as often as the left, and the condition is only rarely bilateral. Boys are affected twice as often as girls, and the average age at onset is 5.6 years.

The clinical findings include muscle spasm about the hip, voluntary limitation of motion, and pain on attempted motion. The child rarely appears ill and is usually afebrile.

Laboratory studies include a normal white blood count and differential and a sedimentation rate that is usually normal or minimally elevated. Fluid aspirated from the joint appears turbid but is sterile on culture in all cases.[319,322]

The characteristic radiologic appearance is normal bony architecture. Drey[325] has described edema of the muscles, causing obliteration of soft tissue and capsular shadows, including the iliopsoas, obturator internus, and gluteus minimus. Brown,[321] however, has pointed out that loss of the shadow outlining the hip capsule is a radiologic artifact related to abduction and external rotation of the hip (a position assumed by a patient with a painful hip). Demineralization of bone is not seen in acute cases; if present, it should alert one to the possibility of an alternative diagnosis.

DIFFERENTIAL DIAGNOSIS

It is of utmost importance to differentiate transient synovitis from more serious conditions involving the hip. The most urgent condition to rule out is septic arthritis of the hip joint, with or without osteomyelitis of the femoral neck. Other conditions to be ruled out include Legg-Calvé-Perthes disease, rheumatoid arthritis, and slipped capital femoral epiphysis.[322,331]

TREATMENT

The most urgent aspect of treatment is to rule out septic arthritis of the hip. Aspiration of the hip joint is mandatory if the diagnosis is in any reasonable doubt. If no fluid can be obtained, approximately 1 ml of Renografin should be injected to prove radiographically that the joint has in fact been entered.

Once the diagnosis has been confirmed, the patient should be put to rest in a position of comfort. This is most easily accomplished with light Buck's traction and a pillow under the knee to provide some hip flexion. Most patients respond promptly (within 24 to 48 hours) to rest, thus helping to verify the diagnosis. Once pain has been relieved, patients may be allowed to return gradually to normal activity. Those who resume weightbearing before complete relief of pain have a much greater risk of recurrence.[330] If a response to bed rest does not promptly occur, one must reconsider the diagnosis.

SEQUELAE

According to the literature, there is disagreement as to whether or not transient synovitis may proceed into a fully developed Legg-Calvé-Perthes disease. Adams[319] and Gledhill[328] do not think that transient synovitis is a cause of Legg-Calvé-Perthes disease. Gledhill[328] notes that 1% of patients with Legg-Calvé-Perthes disease presented with a syndrome identical to that of transient synovitis; however, none of 108 cases of transient synovitis caused Legg-Calvé-Perthes disease. Donaldson,[324] Gershuni,[327] and Jacobs[332] believe that synovitis may produce Legg-Calvé-Perthes disease and demonstrate this in their studies. Both Donaldson[324] and Gershuni[327] suggest that synovitis may represent the earliest and a potentially reversible stage of Legg-Calvé-Perthes disease.

Long-term follow-ups of patients with transient synovitis have been reported by de Valderrama,[323] Nachemson and Scheller,[334] and Sharwood,[335] whose findings in some cases included coxa magna, osteoarthritis, widening of the femoral neck, joint space narrowing, and cystic changes in the femoral neck. The incidence of these findings was low, and all agree that they most likely resulted from a prolonged nonspecific inflammatory process of the hip joint.

REFERENCES

Congenital Dislocation of the Hip

1. Andren L, Borglin ME: A disorder of estrogen metabolism as a causal factor of congenital dislocation of the hip. Acta Orthop Scand 30:169, 1960
2. Badgley CE: Correlation of clinical anatomic facts leading to a conception of the etiology of congenital hip dysplasias. J Bone Joint Surg 25:503, 1943
3. Badgley CE: Etiology of congenital dislocation of the hip. J Bone Joint Surg 31A:341, 1949
4. Barlow TG: Early diagnosis and treatment of congenital dislocation of the hip. J Bone Joint Surg 44B:292, 1962
5. Betz RR, Palmer C, MacEwen GD, Kumar SJ: Long-term follow-up of Chiari osteotomies. Presented at the 51st Annual Meeting of the American Academy of Orthopaedic Surgeons, Atlanta, GA, February 1984
6. Bjerkreim I: Congenital dislocation of the hip joint in Norway. Part III: Neonatal CDH. Acta Orthop Scand 157:47, 1974
7. Blockey NJ: Congenital dislocation of the hip (Editorial). J Bone Joint Surg, 64B:152, 1982
8. Brashear HR, Jr, Raney RB Sr: Shands' Handbook of Orthopaedic Surgery, 9th ed. St Louis, CV Mosby, 1978
9. Busanelli T, Tampieri PF: Chiari's osteotomy. Prevention and therapy of coxarthrosis secondary to hip dysplasia. Chir Organi Mov 67:281, 1981/1982
10. Caffey J, Ames R, Silverman WA, Ryder CT, Hough G: Contradiction of the congenital dysplasia-predislocation hypothesis of congenital dislocation of the hip through a study of the normal variation in acetabular angles at successive periods in infancy. Pediatrics 17:632, 1956
11. Carter C, Wilkinson J: Persistent joint laxity and congenital dislocation of the hip. J Bone Joint Surg 46B:40, 1964
12. Chapple C, Davidson D: A study of the relationship between fetal positions and certain congenital deformities. J Pediatr 18:483, 1941
13. Chiari K: Ergebnisse mit der Beckenosteotomie als Pfannendach plastik. Z Orthop 87:14, 1955
14. Chuinard EG, Logan MD: Varus-producing and derotational subtrochanteric osteotomy in the treatment of congenital dislocation of the hip. J Bone Joint Surg 45A:1397, 1963
15. Chung SM: The arterial supply of the developing proximal end of the human femur. J Bone Joint Surg 58A:961, 1976
16. Clarke NMP, Harcke HT, McHugh P, Lee MS, Borns PF, MacEwen GD: Real-time ultrasound in the diagnosis of congenital dislocation and dysplasia of the hip. J Bone Joint Surg 67B:406, 1985
17. Coleman SS, MacEwen GD: Congenital dislocation of the hip in infancy. AAOS Instruc Course Lect 21:155, 1972
18. Coleman SS: Congenital Dysplasia and Dislocation of thc Hip. St. Louis, CV Mosby, 1978
19. Colonna PC: Capsular arthroplasty for congenital dislocation of the hip; indications and technique. J Bone Joint Surg 47A:437, 1965
20. Cooperman DR, Wallensten, R, Stulberg SD: Postreduction avascular necrosis in congenital dislocation of the hip. J Bone Joint Surg 62A:247, 1980

21. Cooperman DR, Wallensten R, Stulberg SD: Acetabular dysplasia in the adult. Clin Orthop 175:79, 1983
22. Dega W: Development and clinical importance of the dysplastic acetabulum. Prog Orthop Surg 2:47, 1978
23. Dickson FD: The shelf operation in the treatment of congenital dislocation of the hip. J Bone Joint Surg 46B:198, 1964
24. Dunn P: Congenital dislocation of the hip (CDH): Necropsy studies at birth. Proc R Soc Med 62:1035, 1969
25. Edmonson AS, Crenshaw AH (eds): Campbell's Operative Orthopaedics, 6th ed. St Louis, CV Mosby, 1980
26. Eyre-Brook AL, Jones DA, Harris FC: Pemberton's acetabuloplasty for congenital dislocation or subluxation of the hip. J Bone Joint Surg 60B:18, 1978
27. Ferguson AB: Primary open reduction of congenital dislocation of the hip using a median adductor approach. J Bone Joint Surg 48B:682, 1966
28. Gage JR, Winter RB: Avascular necrosis of the capital femoral epiphysis as a complication of closed reduction of congenital dislocation of the hip: A critical review of 20 years' experience at Gillette Children's Hospital. J Bone Joint Surg 54A:373, 1972
29. Gibson PH, Benson MK: Congenital dislocation of the hip. Review at maturity of 147 hips treated by excision of the limbus and derotation osteotomy. J Bone Joint Surg 64B:169, 1982
30. Gill AB: Plastic construction of an acetabulum in congenital dislocation of the hip—the shelf operation. J Bone Joint Surg 17:48, 1935
31. Hart VL: Congenital Dysplasia of the Hip Joint and Sequelae. Springfield IL, Charles C Thomas, 1952
32. Hilgenreiner J: Zur Frühdiagnose und Frühbehandlung der angeborenen Hüftverrenkung. Med Klin 21:1385, 1425, 1925
33. Hummer CD, MacEwen GD: The coexistence of torticollis and congenital dysplasia of the hip. J Bone Joint Surg 54A:1255, 1972
34. Ilfeld FW, Makin M: Damage to the capital femoral epiphysis due to Frejka pillow treatment. J Bone Joint Surg 59A:654, 1977
35. Joseph K, MacEwen GD, Boos ML: Home traction in the management of congenital dislocation of the hip. Clin Orthop 165:83, 982
36. Kalamchi A: Modified Salter osteotomy. J Bone Joint Surg 64A:183, 1982
37. Kalamchi A, MacEwen GD: Avascular necrosis following treatment of congenital dislocation of the hip. J Bone Joint Surg 62A:876, 1980
38. Kalamchi A, Schmidt TL, MacEwen GD: Congenital dislocation of the hip: Open reduction by the medial approach. Clin Orthop 169:127, 1982
39. Kasser JR, Bowen JR, MacEwen GD: Varus derotation osteotomy in the treatment of persistent dysplasia in congenital dislocation of the hip. J Bone Joint Surg (Am) 67A:195, 1985
40. Kawamura B: Personal communication, 1976
41. Katz JF: The Chiari osteotomy in the older child with congenital hip subluxation and acetabular dysplasia. Orthopedics 1:109, 1978
42. Klisic P, Jankovic L: Combined procedure of open reduction and shortening of the femur in the treatment of congenital dislocation of the hips in older children. Clin Orthop 119:60, 1976
43. Kumar SJ: Hip spica application for the treatment of congenital dislocation of the hip. J Pediatr Orthop 1:97, 1981
44. Kumar SJ, MacEwen GD: The incidence of hip dysplasia with metatarsus adductus. Clin Orthop 164:234, 1982
45. Kumar SJ, MacEwen GD: Shelf operation. In Tachdjian MO (ed): Congenital Dislocation of the Hip, p. 695. New York, Churchill Livingstone, 1982
46. Lindstrom JR, Ponseti IV, Wenger DR: Acetabular development after reduction in congenital dislocation of the hip. J Bone Joint Surg 61A:112, 1979
47. Lloyd-Roberts GD, Harris NH, Chrispin AR: Anteversion of the acetabulum in congenital dislocation of the hip: A preliminary report. Orthop Clin North Am 9:89, 1978
48. Love BR, Stevens PM, Williams PF: A long-term review of shelf arthroplasty. J Bone Joint Surg 62B:321, 1980
49. MacEwen GD, Shands AR Jr: Oblique trochanteric osteotomy. J Bone Joint Surg 49A:345, 1967
50. Mardam-Bey TH, MacEwen GD: Congenital hip dislocation after walking age. J Pediatr Orthop 2:478, 1982
51. McKibbin B: Anatomic factors in the stability of the hip joint in the newborn. J Bone Joint Surg 52B:148, 1970
52. Michelsson JE, Langenskiold A: Dislocation or subluxation of the hip. J Bone Joint Surg 54A:6, 1177, 1972
53. Mitchell GP: Arthrography in congenital displacement of the hip. J Bone Joint Surg 45B:88, 1963
54. Mitchell GP: Problems in the early diagnosis and management of congenital dislocation of the hip. J Bone Joint Surg 54B:4, 1972
55. Morel G: The treatment of congenital dislocation and subluxation of the hip in the older child. Acta Orthop Scand 46:364, 1975
56. Morscher E: Our experience with Salter's innominate osteotomy in the treatment of hip dysplasia. Prog Orthop Surg 2:107, 1978
57. Muller GM, Seddon JJ: Late results of treatment of congenital dislocation of the hip. J Bone Joint Surg 35B:342, 1953
58. Ogden JA: Changing patterns of proximal femoral vascularity. J Bone Joint Surg 56A:941, 1974
59. Ogden JA, Moss HL: Pathologic anatomy of congenital hip disease. Prog Orthop Surg 2:3, 1978
60. Ortolani M: Un segno poco noto e sua importanza per la diagnosi précoce di prelussazione congenita dell 'anca. Pediatria 45:129, 1937
61. Ortolani M: Le diagnostic clinique fait par la recherche du signe du ressaut est la seul moyen permettant le traitement vraiment précoce et total de la luxation congénitale de la hanche. Bull Acad Natl Med 141:188, 1957
62. Pavlik A: De funktionelle Behandlungsmethode mittels Riemenbugel als Prinzip derkonservativen therapie bei angeborenen (Hüftgelenksuerren kungen) der Säuglinge. Z Orthop 89:341, 1977
63. Pemberton PA: Capsular arthroplasty for congenital dislocation of the hip: Indications and techniques. Some long-term results. J Bone Joint Surg 47A:437, 1965
64. Peterson HA, Klassen RA, McLeod RA, Hoffman AD: The use of computerized tomography in dislocation of the hip and femoral neck anteversion in children. J Bone Joint Surg 63B:198, 1981

65. Plattou E: Rotation osteotomy in the treatment of congenital dislocation of the hip. J Bone Joint Surg 35A:48, 1953
66. Pogrund H, Finsterbush A: Hip dysplasia associated with abduction contracture of the contralateral hip. J Bone Joint Surg (letter) 65A:1029, 1983
67. Ponseti IV: Nonsurgical treatment of congenital dislocation of the hip. J Bone Joint Surg 48A:1392, 1966
68. Ponseti IV: Morphology of the acetabulum in congenital dislocation of the hip. Gross, histologic, and roentgenographic studies. J Bone Joint Surg 60A:586, 1978
69. Pous JG, Dimeglio A, Daoud A: Is treatment of CDH by progressive reduction by traction still advisable? (author's translation) Rev Chir Orthop 65:327, 1979
70. Race C, Herring JA: Congenital dislocation of the hip: An evaluation of closed reduction. J Pediatr Orthop 3:166, 1983
71. Ramsey PL: Congenital hip dislocation before and after walking age. Postgrad Med 6:114, 1976
72. Ramsey PL, Lasser S, MacEwen GD: Congenital dislocation of the hip: Use of the Pavlik harness in the child during the first 6 months of life. J Bone Joint Surg 58A:1000, 1976
73. Salter RB: Role of innominate osteotomy in the treatment of congenital dislocation and subluxation of the hip in the older child. J Bone Joint Surg 48A:1413, 1966
74. Salter RB, Dubos J: The first 15 years' personal experience with innominate osteotomy in the treatment of congenital dislocation and subluxation of the hip. Clin Orthop 98:72, 1974
75. Schuster W: Radiologic interpretation of dysplasia of the acetabulum. Prog Orthop Surg 2:73, 1978
76. Somerville EW: A long-term follow-up of congenital dislocation of the hip. J Bone Joint Surg 60B:25, 1978
77. Somerville EW: Displacement of the Hip in Childhood. New York, Springer-Verlag, 1982
78. Staheli LT, Dion M, Tuell JI: The effect of the inverted limbus on closed management of congenital hip dislocation. Clin Orthop 137:163, 1978.
79. Staheli LT: Slotted acetabular augmentation. J Pediatr Orthop 1:321, 1981
80. Steel HH: Triple osteotomy of the innominate bone. J Bone Joint Surg 55A:343, 1973
81. Stephens DC, MacEwen GD: Comparison of pelvic osteotomies in the treatment of congenital hip dislocation. Prog Orthop Surg 2:147, 1978
82. Strauss, J.: Chiari pelvic osteotomy for hip dysplasia in patients below the age of twenty. Prog. Orthop. Surg., 2:121, 1978.
83. Strayer, L.M.: Embryology of the human hip joint. Yale J. Biol. Med., 16:13, 1943.
84. Sutherland DH: Personal communication, 1975
85. Tachdjian MO: Pediatric Orthopedics. Philadelphia, WB Saunders, 1972
86. Thieme WT, Wynne-Davies R, Blair HAF, Loraine JA: Clinical examination and urinary estrogen assays in newborn children with congenital dislocation of the hip. J Bone Joint Surg 50B:546, 1968
87. Thomas, CL, Gage JR, Ogden JA: Treatment concepts for proximal femoral ischemic necrosis complicating congenital hip disease. J Bone Joint Surg, 64A:817, 1982
88. Tönnis D: An evaluation of conservative and operative methods in the treatment of congenital hip dislocation. Clin Orthop 119:76, 1976
89. Tönnis D (Ed): Congenital Hip Dislocation: Avascular Necrosis. New York, Thieme-Stratton, 1982
90. Tönnis D, Behrens K, Tscharani F: A modified technique of the triple pelvic osteotomy: Early results. J Pediatr Orthop 1:241, 1981
91. Tronzo, RG: Surgery of the Hip Joint. Philadelphia, Lea & Febiger, 1973
92. Utterback TD, MacEwen GD: Comparison of pelvic osteotomies for the surgical correction of the congenital hip. Am Orthop 98:104, 1974
93. von Rosen S: Early diagnosis and treatment of congenital dislocation of the hip joint. Acta Orthop Scand 26:136, 1957
94. Voutsinas SA, MacEwen GD, Boos ML: Home traction in the management of congenital dislocation of the hip. Arch Orthop Trauma Surg. 102:135, 1984
95. Wagner H: Experiences with spherical acetabular osteotomy for the correction of the dysplastic acetabulum. Prog Orthop Surg 2:131, 1978
96. Wagner H: Femoral osteotomies for congenital hip dislocation. Prog Orthop Surg 2:85, 1978
97. Watanabe RS: Embryology of the human hip. Clin Orthop 98:8, 1974
98. Wedge HJ, Wasylenko MJ: The natural history of congenital disease of the hip. J Bone Joint Surg 61B:334, 1979
99. Weiner DS, Hoyt WA Jr, O'Dell HW: Congenital dislocation of the hip. The relationship of premanipulation traction and age to avascular necrosis of the femoral head. J Bone Joint Surg 59A:306, 1977
100. Weinstein SL, Ponseti IV: Congenital dislocation of the hip. J Bone Joint Surg 61A:119, 1979
101. Westin GW, Dallas TG, Watanabe BM, Ilfeld FW: Skeletal traction vs. femoral shortening in treatment of older children with congenital hip dislocation. Isr J Med Sci 16:318, 1980
102. Wilkinson JA: Prime factors in the etiology of congenital dislocation of the hip. J Bone Joint Surg 45B:268, 1963
103. Wilkinson JA: Post-natal survey for congenital displacement of the hip. J Bone Joint Surg 54B:40, 1972
104. Wilson JC Jr: Surgical treatment of the dysplastic acetabulum in adolescence. Clin Orthop 98:137, 1974
105. Yamamuro T, Hama J, Shilcato J, Sanada H, Takeda T: Connective tissue of the joint capsule and sex hormones. Conn Tissue (Tokyo) 6:151, 1974

Coxa Vara

106. Almond HG: Familial infantile coxa vara. J Bone Joint Surg 38B:539, 1956
107. Amstutz HC, Freiberger RH: Coxa vara in children. Clin Orthop 22:73, 1962
108. Babb FS, Ghormley RK, Chatterton CC: Congenital coxa vara. J Bone Joint Surg 31A:115, 1949
109. Barr, JS: Congenital coxa vara. Arch Surg 18:1909, 1929
110. Becton JL, Diamond LS: Persistent limp in congenital coxa vara. South Med J 60:921, 1967
111. Blockey NJ: Observations on infantile coxa vara. J Bone Joint Surg 51B:106, 1969
112. Blount WP: Blade-plate internal fixation for high femoral osteotomies. J Bone Joint Surg 25:319, 1943
113. Calhoun JD, Pierret F: Infantile coxa vara. Am J Roentgenol Radium Ther Nucl Med 115:561, 1972
114. Compere EL, Garrison M, Fahey, JJ: Deformities

of the femur resulting from arrestment of growth of the capital and greater trochanteric epiphyses. J Bone Joint Surg 22:909, 1940
115. Duncan GA: Congenital coxa vara occurring in identical twins. Am J Surg 37:112, 1937
116. Fisher RL, Waskowitz WJ: Familial developmental coxa vara. Clin Orthop 86:2, 1972
117. Golding FC: Congenital coxa vara. J Bone Joint Surg 30B:160, 1948
118. Hark FW: Congenital coxa vara. Am J Surg 80:305, 1950
119. Hasue M, Kimura F, Funayama M, Ito R: An unusual case of coxa vara, characterized by varying degrees of metaphyseal changes and multiple slipped epiphyses. J Bone Joint Surg 50A:373, 1968
120. Johanning K: Coxa vara infantum. I. Clinical appearance and aetiologic problems. Acta Orthop Scand 21:273, 1951
121. Johanning K: Coxa vara infantum. II. Treatment and results of treatment. Acta Orthop Scand 22:100, 1952
122. Knowles KG: Congenital coxa vara: Presentation of a case. RI Med J 46:594, 1963
123. Langenskiöld F: On pseudarthrosis of the femoral neck in congenital coxa vara. Acta Chir Scand 98:568, 1949
124. LeMesurier AB: Developmental coxa vara. J Bone Joint Surg 30B:595, 1948
125. Letts RM, Shokeir MHK: Mirror-image coxa vara in identical twins. J Bone Joint Surg 57A:117, 1975
126. MacEwen GD, Shands AR Jr: Oblique trochanteric osteotomy. J Bone Joint Surg 49A:345, 1967
127. Magnusson R: Coxa vara infantum. Acta Orthop Scand 23:284, 1954
128. Michelsson JE, Langenskiöld A: Coxa vara following immobilization of the knee in extension in young rabbits. Acta Orthop Scand 45:399, 1974
129. Morgan JD, Somerville EW: Normal and abnormal growth at the upper end of the femur. J Bone Joint Surg 42B:264, 1960
130. Noble TP, Hauser EDW: Coxa vara. Arch Surg 12:501, 1926
131. Pavlov H, Goldman AB, Freiberger RH: Infantile coxa vara. Radiology 135:631, 1980
132. Pylkkanen PV: Coxa vara infantum. Acta Orthop Scand (Suppl) 48:1, 1960
133. Ring PA: Congenital abnormalities of the femur. Arch Dis Child 36:410, 1961
134. Rubin A, et al: Adolescent's coxa vara—an attempt toward an etiologic view and the possible explanation of endocrine effects (author's transl). Acta Chir Orthop Traumatol Cech 48(6):496, 1981 (Engl abstract)
135. Say B, Taysi K, Pirnar T, Tokgozoglu N, Inan E: Dominant congenital coxa vara. J Bone Joint Surg 56B:78, 1974
136. Trueta J: The normal vascular anatomy of the human femoral head during growth. J Bone Joint Surg 39B:358, 1957
137. Weighill FJ: The treatment of developmental coxa vara by abduction subtrochanteric and intertrochanteric femoral osteotomy with special reference to the role of adductor tenotomy. Clin Orthop 116:116, 1976
138. Weinstein JN, Kuo KN, Millar EA: Congenital coxa vara. A retrospective review. J Pediatr Orthop 4:70, 1984
139. Zadek I: Congenital coxa vara. Arch Surg 30:62, 1935

Congenital Short Femur With Coxa Vara

140. Aitkin GT: Amputation as a treatment for certain lower-extremity congenital abnormalities. J Bone Joint Surg 41A:1267, 1959
141. Fock G, Sulamaa M: Congenital short femur. Acta Orthop Scand 36:294, 1965
142. Frantz CH, O'Rahilly R: Congenital skeletal limb deficiencies. J Bone Joint Surg 43A:1202, 1961
143. Hamanishi C: Congenital short femur. Clinical, genetic, and epidemiologic comparison of the naturally occurring condition with that caused by Thalidomide. J Bone Joint Surg 62B:307, 1980
144. Ring PA: Congenital short femur. Simple femoral hypoplasia. J Bone Joint Surg 41B:73, 1959

Slipped Capital Femoral Epiphysis

145. Aadalen RJ et al: Acute slipped capital femoral epiphysis. J Bone Joint Surg 56A:1473, 1974
146. Badgley CE, et al: Operative therapy for slipped upper femoral epiphysis. An end-result study. J Bone Joint Surg 30A:19, 1948
147. Barash HL, et al: Acute slipped capital femoral epiphysis. A report of nine cases. Clin Orthop 79:96, 1971
148. Barmada R, et al: Base of the neck extracapsular osteotomy for correction of deformity in slipped capital femoral epiphysis. Clin Orthop 132:98, 1978
149. Bishop JO, et al: Slipped capital femoral epiphysis. A study of 50 cases in black children. Clin Orthop 135:93, 1978
150. Boyer DW, et al: Slipped capital femoral epiphysis. Long-term follow-up study of 121 patients. J Bone Joint Surg 63A:85, 1981
151. Bright RW, et al: Epiphyseal-plate cartilage. A biomechanical and histologic analysis of failure modes. J Bone Joint Surg 56A:688, 1974
152. Burrows HJ: Slipped upper femoral epiphysis. Characteristics of one hundred cases. J Bone Joint Surg 39B:641, 1957
153. Casey BH, et al: Reduction of acutely slipped upper femoral epiphysis. J Bone Joint Surg 54B:607, 1972
154. Chapman JA, et al: Slipped upper femoral epiphysis after radiotherapy. J Bone Joint Surg 62B:337, Aug. 1980
155. Chung SMK, et al: Shear strength of the human femoral capital epiphyseal plate. J Bone Joint Surg 58A:94, 1976
156. Cruess RI: The pathology of acute necrosis of cartilage in slipping of the capital femoral epiphysis. A report of two cases with pathologic sections. J Bone Joint Surg 45A:1013, 1963
157. Dunn DM, Angel JC: Replacement of the femoral head by open operation in severe adolescent slipping of the upper femoral epiphysis. J Bone Joint Surg 60B:394, 1978
158. Dunn DM: The treatment of adolescent slipping of the upper femoral epiphysis. J Bone Joint Surg 46B:621, 1964
159. Eisenstein A, Rothschild S: Biochemical abnormalities in patients with slipped capital femoral epiphysis and chondrolysis. J Bone Joint Surg 58A:459, 1976
160. Fahey JJ, O'Brien ET: Acute slipped capital femoral epiphysis. Review of the literature and report of 10 cases. J Bone Joint Surg 47A:1105, 1965
161. Gage JR et al: Complications after cuneiform osteotomy for moderately or severely slipped capital femoral epiphysis. J Bone Joint Surg 60A:157, 1978

162. Goldman AB, et al: Slipped capital femoral epiphyses complicating renal osteodystrophy: A report of three cases. Radiology 126:333, 1978
163. Goldman AB, et al: Acute chondrolysis complicating slipped capital femoral epiphysis. Am J Roentgenol 130:945, 1978
164. Gorin RL: Slipped capital femoral epiphyses in identical twins: Report of case. J Am Osteopath Assoc 77:124, 1977
165. Grant IR: The treatment of slipped upper femoral epiphysis by fibular grafting. Clin Orthop 114:270, 1976
166. Hall JE: The results of treatment of slipped femoral epiphysis. J Bone Joint Surg 39B:659, 1957
167. Harris WR: The endocrine basis for slipping of the upper femoral epiphysis. An experimental study. J Bone Joint Surg 32B:5, 1950
168. Hauge MF: Wedge osteotomy in slipped femoral epiphysis. With special reference to technique. Acta Orthop Scand 28:51, 1959
169. Heppenstall RB, et al: Chondrolysis of the hip. Clin Orthop 103:136, 1974
170. Herndon CH: Treatment of minimally slipped upper femoral epiphysis. AAOS Instr Course Lect 21:188, 1972
171. Herndon CH, et al: Treatment of slipped capital femoral epiphysis by epiphysiodesis and osteoplasty of the femoral neck: A report of further experiences. J Bone Joint Surg 45A:999, 1963
172. Heyman CH, Herndon CH: Epiphysiodesis for early slipping of the upper femoral epiphysis. J Bone Joint Surg 36A:539, 1954
173. Heyman CH, et al: Slipped femoral epiphysis with severe displacement. A conservative operative treatment. J Bone Joint Surg 39A:293, 1957
174. Hiertonn T: Wedge osteotomy in advanced femoral epiphysiolysis. Acta Orthop Scand 25:44, 1956
175. Hirano T, et al: Association of primary hypothyroidism and slipped capital femoral epiphysis. J Pediatr 93:262, 1978
176. Hirsch PJ, Hirsch SA: Slipped capital femoral epiphysis. Occurrence after treatment with chorionic gonadotropin. JAMA 235:751, 1976
177. Howorth MB: Pathology: Slipping of the capital femoral epiphysis. Clin Orthop 48:33, 1966
178. Ingram AJ, et al: Chondrolysis complicating slipped capital femoral epiphysis. Clin Orthop 165:99, 1982
179. Ippolito E, et al: A histochemical study of slipped capital femoral epiphysis. J Bone Joint Surg 63A(7):1109, 1981
180. Ippolito E, Ricciardi-Pollini PT: Chondrolysis of the hip (idiopathic and secondary forms). Ital J Orthop Traumatol 7(3):335, 1981
181. Ireland J, Newman PH: Triplane osteotomy for severely slipped upper femoral epiphysis. J Bone Joint Surg 60B:390, 1978
182. Jacobs B, Wilson PD: The treatment of slipping of the upper femoral epiphysis. A follow-up study of 300 cases. Arch Orthop Unfallchir 56:349, 1964
183. Jayakumar S: Slipped capital femoral epiphysis with hypothyroidism treated by nonoperative method. Clin Orthop 151:179, 1980
184. Jerre T: A study in slipped upper femoral epiphysis. With special reference to the late functional and roentgenologic results and to the value of closed reduction. Acta Orthop Scand (Suppl) 6, 1950
185. Jerre T: Early complications after osteosynthesis with a three-flanged nail *in situ* for slipped epiphysis. Acta Orthop Scand 27:126, 1958
186. Kelsey JL: Epidemiology of slipped capital femoral epiphysis: A review of the literature. Pediatrics 51:1042, 1973
187. Kelsey JL, Acheson DM, Keggi KJ: The body build of patients with slipped capital femoral epiphysis. Am J Dis Child 124:276, 1972
188. Klein A, et al: Management of the contralateral hip in slipped capital femoral epiphysis. J Bone Joint Surg 35A:81, 1953
189. Kramer WG, et al: Compensating osteotomy at the base of the femoral neck for slipped capital femoral epiphysis. J Bone Joint Surg 58A:796, 1976
190. Kulick RG, Denton JR: A retrospective study of 125 cases of slipped capital femoral epiphysis. Clin Orthop 162:87, 1982
191. Lindstrom N: Surgical treatment of epiphysiolysis capitis femoris. Acta Orthop Scand 28:131, 1959
192. Lowe HG: Avascular necrosis after slipping of the upper femoral epiphysis. J Bone Joint Surg 43B:688, 1961
193. Maurer RC, Larsen IJ: Acute necrosis of cartilage in slipped capital femoral epiphysis. J Bone Joint Surg 52A:39, 1970
194. McKay DW: Cheilectomy of the hip. Orthop Clin North Am 11(1):141, 1980
195. Mehls O, et al: Slipped epiphyses in renal osteodystrophy. Arch Dis Child 50(7):545, 1975
196. Melby A, et al: Treatment of chronic slipped capital femoral epiphysis by bone-graft epiphysiodesis. J Bone Joint Surg 62A:119, 1980
197. Mickelson MR, et al: The ultrastructure of the growth plate in slipped capital femoral epiphysis. J Bone Joint Surg 59A:1076, 1977
198. Milgram JW, Lynn ED: Epiphysiolysis of the proximal femur in very young children. Clin Orthop 110:146, 1975
199. Moore RD: Conservative management of adolescent slipping of the capital femoral epiphysis. Surg Gynecol Obset 80:324, 1945
200. Morrissy RT, et al: Synovial immunofluorescence in patients with slipped capital femoral epiphysis. J Pediatr Orthop 1:55, 1981
201. Nielson HO: Acute slipped capital femoral epiphysis. Treatment in 8 cases. Acta Orthop Scand 46:987, 1975
202. Nixon JR, Douglas JF: Bilateral slipping of the upper femoral epiphysis in end-stage renal failure. A report of two cases. J Bone Joint Surg 62B:18, 1980
203. O'Brien ET, Fahey JJ: Remodeling of the femoral neck after *in situ* pinning for slipped capital femoral epiphysis. J Bone Joint Surg 59A:62, 1977
204. Ogden JA, et al: Slipped capital femoral epiphysis following ipsilateral femoral fracture. Clin Orthop 110:167, 1975
205. Oram V: Epiphysiolysis of the head of the femur. A follow-up examination with special reference to end results and the social prognosis. Acta Orthop Scand 23:100, 1953
206. Orofino C, et al: Slipped capital femoral epiphysis in Negroes. A study of 95 cases. J Bone Joint Surg 42A:1079, 1960
207. Pearl AJ, et al: Cuneiform osteotomy in the treatment of slipped capital femoral epiphysis. J Bone Joint Surg 43A:947, 1961
208. Rennie AM: The inheritance of slipped upper femoral epiphysis. J Bone Joint Surg 64B:180, 1982

209. Ross PM, et al: Slipped capital femoral epiphysis long-term results after 10 to 38 years. Clin Orthop 141:176, 1979
210. Salenius P, Kivilaakso R: Results of treatment of slipped upper femoral epiphysis. Acta Orthop Scand (Suppl.) 114, 1968
211. Salvati EA, et al: Southwick osteotomy for severe chronic slipped capital femoral epiphysis: Results and complications. J Bone Joint Surg 62A:561, 1980
212. Schein AJ: Acute severe slipped capital femoral epiphysis. Clin Orthop 51:151, 1967
213. Skinner SR, Berkheimer GA: Valgus slip of the capital femoral epiphysis. Clin Orthop 135:90, 1978
214. Solomon L: Patterns of osteoarthritis of the hip. J Bone Joint Surg 58B:176, 1976
215. Sorenson KH: Slipped upper femoral epiphysis. Acta Orthop Scand 39:499, 1968
216. Southwick WO: Osteotomy through the lesser trochanter for slipped capital femoral epiphysis. J Bone Joint Surg 49A:807, 1967
217. Southwick WO: Compression fixation after biplane intertrochanteric osteotomy for slipped capital epiphysis. A technical improvement. J Bone Joint Surg 55A:1218, 1973
218. Stulberg SD, Cordell LD, Harris WH, Ramsey PL, MacEwen GD: Unrecognized childhood hip disease: A major cause of idiopathic osteoarthritis of the hip. In The Hip Society: The Hip. St Louis, CV Mosby, 1975
219. Tillema DA, Golding JSR: Chondrolysis following slipped capital femoral epiphysis in Jamaica. J Bone Joint Surg 53A:1528, 1971
220. Walker SJ, et al: Slipped capital femoral epiphysis following radiation and chemotherapy. Clin Orthop 159:186, 1981
221. Whiteside LA, Schoenecker PL: Combined valgus derotation osteotomy and cervical osteoplasty for severely slipped capital femoral epiphysis: Mechanical analysis and report of preliminary results using compression screw fixation and early weightbearing. Clin Orthop 132:88, 1978
222. Wiberg G: Considerations on the surgical treatment of slipped epiphysis with special reference to nail fixation. J Bone Joint Surg 41A:253, 1959
223. Wilson PD, et al: Slipped capital femoral epiphysis. An end-result study. J Bone Joint Surg 47A:1128, 1965
224. Wojtowycz M, et al: Neonatal proximal femoral epiphysiolysis. Radiology 136:647, 1980
225. Wolf EL, et al: Slipped femoral capital epiphysis as a sequela to childhood irradiation for malignant tumors. Radiology 125:781, 1977
226. Zubrow AB, et al: Slipped capital femoral epiphysis occurring during treatment for hypothyroidism. J Bone Joint Surg 60A:256, 1978

Legg-Calvé-Perthes Syndrome

227. Apley AG, Wientroub S: The sagging rope sign in Perthes' disease and allied disorders. J Bone Joint Surg 63B:43, 1981
228. Axer A, Gershuni DH, Hendel D, Mirovski Y: Indications for femoral osteotomy in Legg-Calvé-Perthes disease. Clin Orthop 150:78, 1980
229. Axer A, Schiller MG: The pathogenesis of the early deformity of the capital femoral epiphysis in Legg-Calvé-Perthes syndrome (LCPS). Clin Orthop 84:106, 1972
230. Barnes JM: Premature epiphyseal closure in Perthes' disease. J Bone Joint Surg 62B:432, 1980
231. Bensahel H, Bok B, Cavailloles F, Csukonyi Z: Bone scintigraphy in Perthes disease. J Pediatr Orthop 3:302, 1983
232. Bobechko WP: The Toronto brace for Legg-Perthes disease. Clin Orthop 102:115, 1974
233. Bobechko WP, Harris WR: The radiographic density of avascular bone. J Bone Joint Surg 42B:626, 1960
234. Bowen JR, Foster BK, Hartzell CR: Legg-Calvé-Perthes disease. Clin Orthop 185:97, 1984
235. Bowen JR, Schreiber FC, Foster BK, Wein BK: Premature femoral neck physeal closure in Perthes' disease. Clin Orthop 171:24, 1982
236. Brotherton BJ, McKibbin B: Perthes' disease treated by prolonged recumbency and femoral head containment: A long-term appraisal. J Bone Joint Surg 59B:8, 1977
237. Burwell RG, Dangerfield PH, Hall DJ, Vernon CL, Harrison MHM: Perthes' disease: An anthropometric study revealing impaired and disproportionate growth. J Bone Joint Surg 60B:461, 1978
238. Caffey J: The early roentgenographic changes in essential coxa plana; their significance in pathogenesis. Am J Roentgenol Radium Ther Nucl Med 103:620, 634, 1968
239. Calvé J: Sur une forme particuliere de cosalgie greffee sur des déformations caractéristiques de l'extremité supérieure du fémur. Rev Chir 42:54, 1910
240. Calver R, Venugopal V, Dorgan J, Bentley G, Gimlette T: Radionuclide scanning in the early diagnosis of Perthes' disease. J Bone Joint Surg 63B:379, 1981
241. Canario AT, Williams L, Wientroub S, Catterall A, Lloyd-Roberts GC: A controlled study of the results of femoral osteotomy in severe Perthes' disease. J Bone Joint Surg 62B:438, 1980
242. Catterall A: The natural history of Perthes' disease. J Bone Joint Surg 53B:37, 1971
243. Catterall A: Legg-Calvé-Perthes Disease. New York, Churchill Livingstone, 1982
244. Chuinard EG: Femoral osteotomy in treatment of Legg-Calvé-Perthes syndrome. Orthop Rev 8:113, 1979
245. Chung SMK: The arterial supply of the developing proximal end of the human femur. J Bone Joint Surg 58A:961, 1976
246. Clarke NMP, Harrison MHM: Painful sequelae of coxa plana. J Bone Joint Surg 65A:13, 1983
247. Clarke TE, Finnegan TL, Fisher RL, Bunch WH, Gossling HR: Legg-Perthes disease in children less than 4 years old. J Bone Joint Surg 60A:166, 1978
248. Coleman SS: Observations on proximal femoral osteotomy and pelvic osteotomy. Orthop Rev 8:139, 1979
249. Coleman SS, Kehl D: An evaluation of Perthes' disease: Comparison of nonsurgical and surgical means. American Academy of Orthopaedic Surgeons meeting. Las Vegas, 1981
250. Danielsson LG, Hernborg J: Late results of Perthes' disease. Acta Orthop Scand 36:70, 1965
251. DeCamargo FP: Revascularization of the neck of the femur in Legg-Calvé-Perthes syndrome. Clin Orthop 10:79, 1957
252. Dickens DRV, Menelaus MB: The assessment of the prognosis of Perthes' disease. J Bone Joint Surg 60B:189, 1978

253. Dolman CL, Bell, HM: The pathology of Legg-Calvé-Perthes disease; a case report. J Bone Joint Surg 55A:184, 1973
254. Eaton GO: Long-term results of treatment in coxa plana. J Bone Joint Surg 48A:1031, 1967
255. Edgren W: Coxa plana. Acta Orthop Scand (Suppl):84, 1965
256. Edvardsen P, Slrdahl J, Svenningsen S: Operative versus conservative treatment of Legg-Calvé-Perthes disease. Acta Orthop Scand 52:553, 1981
257. Fasting OJ, Bjerkreim I, Langeland N, Hertzenberg L, Nakken K: Scintigraphic evaluation of the severity of Perthes' disease in the initial stage. Acta Orthop Scand 51:655, 1980
258. Ferguson AB, Howorth B: Coxa plana and related conditions at the hip. J Bone Joint Surg 16:781, 1934
259. Fisher RL, Roderique JW, Brown DC, Danigelis, JA, Ozonoff MB, Sziklas JJ: The relationship of isotopic bone imaging findings to prognosis in Legg-Perthes disease. Clin Orthop 150:23, 1980
260. Fotter R, Lammer J, Ritter G: [5-year scintigraphic study of children with Perthes' disease. Diagnostic evaluation and therapeutic consequences] ROFO 137:141, 1982
261. Freeman MAR, England JPS: Experimental infarction of the immature canine femoral head. Proc R Soc Med 62:431, 1969
262. Gaucher A, Colomb JN, Naoun A, Pourel J, Robert J, Faure G, Netter P: Radionuclide imaging in hip abnormalities. Clin Nucl Med 5:214, 1980
263. Glimcher MJ: Legg-Calvé-Perthes syndrome: Biological and mechanical considerations in the genesis of clinical abnormalities. Orthop Rev 8:33, 1979
264. Goff CW: Legg-Calvé-Perthes syndrome (LCPS). Clin Orthop 22:93, 1962
265. Gower WE, Johnston RC: Legg-Perthes disease: Long-term follow-up of 36 patients. J Bone Joint Surg 53A:759, 1971
266. Green NE, Beauchamp RD, Griffin PP: Epiphyseal extrusion as a prognostic index in Legg-Calvé-Perthes disease. J Bone Joint Surg 63A:900, 1981
267. Green NE, Griffin PP: Intraosseous venous pressure in Legg-Perthes disease. J Bone Joint Surg 64A:666, 1982
268. Hall D, Harrison MHM: An association between congenital abnormalities and Perthes disease of the hip. J Bone Joint Surg 60B:138, 1978
269. Hardcastle PH, Ross R, Hamalainen M, Mata A: Catterall grouping of Perthes' disease: An assessment of observer error and prognosis using the Catterall classification. J Bone Joint Surg 62B:428, 1980
270. Harrison MHM, Burwell RG: Perthes' disease: A concept of pathogenesis. Clin Orthop 156:115, 1981
271. Harrison MHM, Turner MH, Jacobs P: Skeletal immaturity in Perthes disease. J Bone Joint Surg 58B:37, 1976
272. Ingman AM, Paterson DC, Sutherland AD: A comparison between innominate osteotomy and hip spica in the treatment of Legg-Perthes disease. Clin Orthop 163:141, 1982
273. Inoue A, Freeman MAR, Vernon-Roberts B, Mizuno S: The pathogenesis of Perthes' disease. J Bone Joint Surg 58B:453, 1976
274. Jensen OM, Lauritzen J: Legg-Calvé-Perthes disease: Morphological studies in two cases examined at necropsy. J Bone Joint Surg 58B:332, 1976
275. Jonsater S: Coxa plana; a histopathologic and arthrographic study. Acta Orthop Scand (Suppl):12, 1953
276. Kamhi E, MacEwen GD: Osteochondritis dissecans in Legg-Calvé-Perthes disease. J Bone Joint Surg 57A:506, 1975
277. Kamhi E, MacEwen GD: Treatment of Legg-Calvé-Perthes disease: Prognostic value of Catterall's classification. J Bone Joint Surg 57A:651, 1975
278. Katz JF: Conservative treatment of Legg-Calvé-Perthes disease. J Bone Joint Surg 49A:1043, 1970
279. Katz JF: Nonoperative therapy in Legg-Calvé-Perthes disease. Orthop Rev 8:69, 1979
280. Kenzora JE, Steele RE, Yosipovitch ZH, Glimcher MJ: Experimental osteotomies of the femoral head in adult rabbits. Clin Orthop 130:8, 1978
281. King EW, Fisher RL, Gage JR, Gossling HR: Ambulation-abduction treatment in Legg-Calvé-Perthes disease (LCPD). Clin Orthop 150:43, 1980
282. Klisic PJ, Blazevic U, Seferovic O: Approach to treatment of Legg-Calvé-Perthes disease. Clin Orthop 150:54, 1980
283. Klisic PJ: Treatment of Perthes' disease in older children. J Bone Joint Surg 65B:419, 1983
284. Lamont RL, Muz J, Heilbronner D, Bonwhuis JA: Quantitative assessment of femoral head involvement in Legg-Calvé-Perthes disease. J Bone Joint Surg 63A:746, 1981
285. Laurent LE, Poussa M: Intertrochanteric varus osteotomy in the treatment of Perthes' disease. Clin Orthop 150:73, 1980
286. Lauritzen J: Legg-Calvé-Perthes disease: A comparative study. Acta Orthop Scand (Suppl):159, 1975
287. Legg AT: An obscure affection of the hip joint. Boston Med Surg J 162:202, 1910
288. Lloyd-Roberts GC, Catterall A, Salamon PB: A controlled study of the indications for and the results of femoral osteotomy in Perthes' disease. J Bone Joint Surg 58B:31, 1976
289. MacEwen GD: Treatment of Legg-Calvé-Perthes disease. AAOS Instruc Course Lect 30:75, 1981
290. Marklund T, Tillberg B: Coxa plana: A radiological comparison of the rate of healing with conservative measures and after osteotomy. J Bone Joint Surg 58B:25, 1976
291. Molloy MK, MacMahon B: Birthweight and Legg-Perthes disease. J Bone Joint Surg 49A:498, 1967
292. Molloy MK, MacMahon B: Incidence of Legg-Perthes disease (osteochondritis deformans). N Engl J Med 275:988, 1966
293. Mose K: Legg-Calvé-Perthes disease: A comparison among three methods of conservative treatment. Arhus, Universitets Fortuget, 1964
294. Muirhead-Allwood W, Catterall A: The treatment of Perthes' disease: The results of a trial of management. J Bone Joint Surg 64B:282, 1982
295. Perthes G: Uber osteochondritis deformans juvenilis. Dtsch Z Chir 10:111, 1910
296. Petrie JG, Bitenc I: The abduction weightbearing treatment in Legg-Perthes disease. J Bone Joint Surg 53B:54, 1971
297. Phemister DB: Perthes' disease. Surg Gynecol Obstet 33:87,1921
298. Ponseti IV: Legg-Perthes disease. J Bone Joint Surg 38A:739, 1956
299. Ponseti IV, Cotton RL: Legg-Calvé-Perthes disease; pathogenesis and evolution. J Bone Joint Surg 43A:261, 1961
300. Purvis JM, Dimon JH III, Meehan PL, Lovell WW:

Preliminary experience with the Scottish Rite Hospital abduction orthosis for Legg-Perthes disease. Clin Orthop 150:49, 1980
301. Ratliff AHC: Perthes' disease. J Bone Joint Surg 49B:102, 1967
302. Salter RB: Legg-Perthes disease: The scientific basis for the methods of treatment and their indications. Clin Orthop 150:8, 1980.
303. Schiller MG, Axer A: Hypertrophy of the femoral head in Legg-Calvé-Perthes syndrome (LCPS). Acta Orthop Scand 43:45, 1972
304. Schiller MG, Axer A: Legg-Calvé-Perthes syndrome (LCPS): A critical analysis of roentgenographic measurements. Clin Orthop 86:34, 1972
305. Somerville EW: Perthes' disease of the hip. J Bone Joint Surg 53B:639, 1971
306. Somerville EW: Osteotomy in treatment of Perthes' disease of the hip. Orthop Rev 8:61, 1979
307. Stevens P, Williams P, Menelaus M: Innominate osteotomy for Perthes' disease. J Pediatr Orthop 1:47, 1981
308. Stulberg SD, Cooperman DR, Wallensten R: The natural history of Legg-Calvé-Perthes disease. J Bone Joint Surg 63A:1095, 1981
309. Sutherland AD, Savage JP, Paterson DC, Foster BK: The nuclide bone scan in the diagnosis and management of Perthes' disease. J Bone Joint Surg 62B:300, 1980
310. Thompson GH, Westin GW: Legg-Calvé-Perthes disease: Results of discontinuing treatment in the early reossification phase. Clin Orthop 139:70, 1979
311. Trias A: Femoral osteotomy in Perthes' disease. Clin Orthop 137:195, 1978
312. Trueta J: The normal vascular anatomy of the human femoral head during growth. J Bone Joint Surg 39B:358, 1957
313. Trueta J, Amato VP: The vascular contribution to osteogenesis. III. Changes in the growth cartilage caused by experimentally induced ischaemia. J Bone Joint Surg 42B:571, 1960
314. Walderström J: Der obere tuberkulöse cullumherd. Z Orthop Chir 24:487, 1909
315. Weinstein SL: Legg-Calvé-Perthes disease. AAOS Instruc Course Lect XXXIII:272, 1983
316. Wenger DR: Selective containment for Legg-Perthes disease: Recognition and management of complications. J Pediatr Orthop 1:153, 1981
317. Wolcott WE: The evolution of the circulation in the developing femoral head and neck; an anatomic study. Surg Gynecol Obstet 77:61, 1943
318. Wynne-Davies R: Some etiologic factors in Perthes' disease. Clin Orthop 150:12, 1980

Transient Synovitis

319. Adams JA: Transient synovitis of the hip joint in children. J Bone Joint Surg 45B:471, 1963
320. Blockey NJ, Porter BB: Transient synovitis of hip. A virological investigation. Br Med J 4:557, 1968
321. Brown I: A study of the "capsular" shadow in disorders of the hip in children. J Bone Joint Surg 57B:175, 1975
322. Caravias DE: The significance of the so-called irritable hips in children. Arch Dis Child 31:415, 1956
323. de Valderrama JAF: The "observation hip" syndrome and its late sequelae. J Bone Joint Surg 45B:462, 1963
324. Donaldson WF: Symposium on pediatric orthopedics. Transient synovitis of the hip joint. Pediatr Clin North Am 2:1073, 1955
325. Drey L: A roentgenographic study of transitory synovitis of the hip joint. Radiology 60:588, 1953
326. Edwards EG: Transient synovitis of the hip joint in children; report of 13 cases. JAMA 148:30, 1952
327. Gershuni DH, et al: Arthrographic findings in Legg-Calvé-Perthes disease and transient synovitis of the hip. J Bone Joint Surg 60A:457, 1978
328. Gledhill RB: Transient synovitis and Legg-Calvé-Perthes disease; a comparative study. Can Med Assoc J 100:311, 1969
329. Hardinge K: The etiology of transient synovitis of the hip in childhood. J Bone Joint Surg 52B:101, 1970
330. Hermel MB, Albert SM: Transient synovitis of the hip. Clin Orthop 22:21, 1962
331. Illingworth CM: One hundred twenty-eight limping children with no fracture, sprain, or obvious cause. Clin Pediatr 17:139, 1978
332. Jacobs BW: Synovitis of the hip in children and its significance. Pediatrics 47:558, 1971
333. Lucas, L.S.: Painful hips in children. AAOS Instructional Course Lectures, 5:144, 1948.
334. Nachemson A, Scheller S: A clinical and radiological follow-up study of transient synovitis of the hip. Acta Orthop Scand 40:479, 1969
335. Sharwood PF: The irritable hip syndrome in children. A long-term follow-up. Acta Orthop Scand 52:633, 1981
336. Spock A: Transient synovitis of the hip joint in children. Pediatrics 24:1042, 1959
337. Tudor RB: Hip synovitis in children. Lancet, 80:51, 1960.

19

Lower Limb Length Discrepancy

Sherman S. Coleman

In this chapter on the management of inequalities in length of the lower limb, the term *limb length discrepancy* will be used, rather than the term "leg length inequality" because of its greater accuracy and specificity. Because the leg is, by definition, only that part of the lower limb extending from the knee to the ankle and because lower limb inequality may be manifest in any segment from the pelvis to and including the foot, it seems more appropriate to refer to the "lower limb" rather than to the "leg."

Proper management of the problem of limb length inequality is mainly contingent upon three factors. First, all the available data surrounding and having bearing on the case must be examined and cross-evaluated in order to arrive at a competent decision of whether or not the inequality warrants some form of surgical correction. Second, the various methods of surgical equalization must be understood, and it must be decided which method or combination of methods would be most desirable for the case in question. Finally, a comprehensive understanding of all the technical aspects of surgical equalization must be mastered.

The problem of limb length discrepancy is common, and its importance will likely not diminish, despite the fact that the etiologic factors have changed considerably during the past 15 years. Prior to the advent of the poliomyelitis vaccine, lower limb length discrepancies due to muscle paralysis of poliomyelitis were the most common. However, in the United States and in those countries where the poliomyelitis vaccine has been effectively used, the problem of limb length inequality due to poliomyelitis has almost vanished, and other causes of discrepancy have assumed greater importance (see below).

Minor discrepancies in limb length are often seen, and many can be either ignored or treated with a small shoe lift. Yet, when the discrepancy approaches 2 cm, some form of surgical equalization should be considered.

NORMAL GROWTH AND BEHAVIOR OF A LONG BONE

It is essential that one understand the normal process of longitudinal growth of the long bones of the lower limb in order to appreciate not only the mechanisms by which limb length inequality can be produced but also the current methods of treatment. The appendicular skeleton is preformed in cartilage and longitudinal growth of a bone takes place by interstitial cartilage proliferation, both at the physeal plate and at the articular cartilage, followed by gradual and orderly replacement of the cartilage by bone. This has been called *endochondral ossification*. In the femur and tibia, each has a primary center of ossification (diaphysis) and two secondary ossification centers, one at each end (epiphyses). The physeal plate makes a much greater contribution to the length of any long bone than does its companion arti-

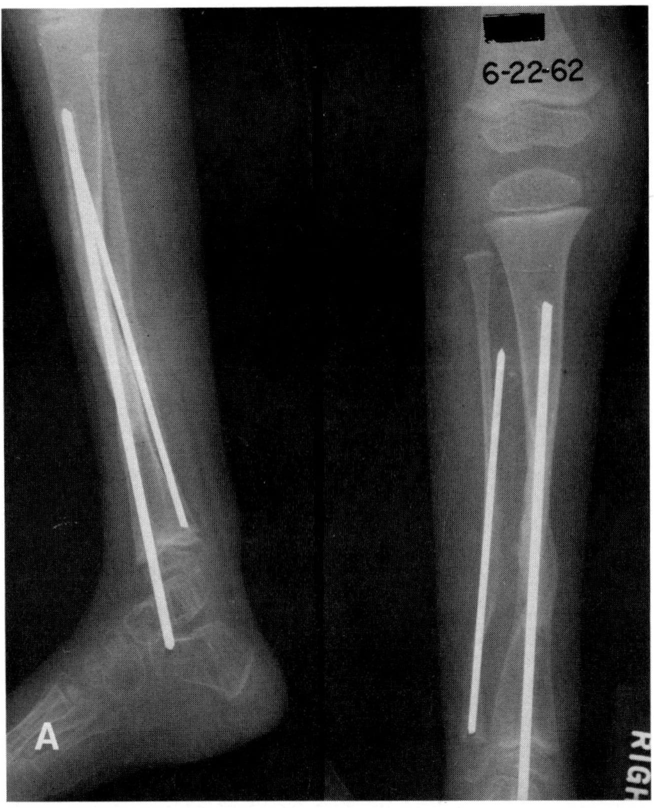

FIG. 19-1. A patient with congenital pseudarthrosis of the tibia who was treated with intramedullary rodding and autogenous bone grafting. *(A)* Early postoperative film, taken 1 year following surgery. The smooth rod is passing through the epiphyseal plate, as well as the articular surfaces of the talocalcaneal and talotibial joints. *(Legend continued on facing page.)*

cular cartilage. Yet, chondrogenesis and chondral ossification of the proliferating articular cartilage are essential for normal epiphyseal growth, both longitudinal and peripheral. Studies have shown that the femur contributes 54% of the total length of the lower limb and the tibia contributes 46%. Furthermore, the distal femoral and proximal tibial physeal plates provide a greater length increment to their respective bones than do the proximal femoral or distal tibial growth centers. In the femur, the distal end provides approximately 70% of the ultimate total length of that bone, and the proximal end of the tibia contributes about 60% of the total longitudinal growth of that bone. Therefore, injuries and diseases affecting the growth centers about the knee result in much greater alteration in growth than do similar insults occurring elsewhere in the lower limb.

The portion of these physeal growth cartilages that is most sensitive to insult is the germinal layer, because irreparable damage to this layer of cartilage cells, either from trauma or infection, can lead to complete growth arrest. Different kinds and degrees of injury are tolerated differently. For example, a smooth metal device of considerable size can be passed through the center of a physeal plate and remain there indefinitely without significant or irreparable influence upon growth (Fig. 19-1). However, a similar sized threaded device may interrupt growth permanently if it is left for several weeks or months. Furthermore, damage to the peripheral (perichondral and periosteal) areas of the growth plate are poorly tolerated, whereas small areas of the central portion may be traumatized without significant alteration in growth. The exception is a crushing injury to the physeal plate, which may totally destroy its growth potential, leading to early epiphyseal-metaphyseal closure. Significantly displaced epiphyseal fractures that affect the germinal and proliferating layers of the cartilage can also cause growth arrest unless appropriately treated. This is because the physeal plate becomes effectively bridged by the bone of either the metaphysis or the

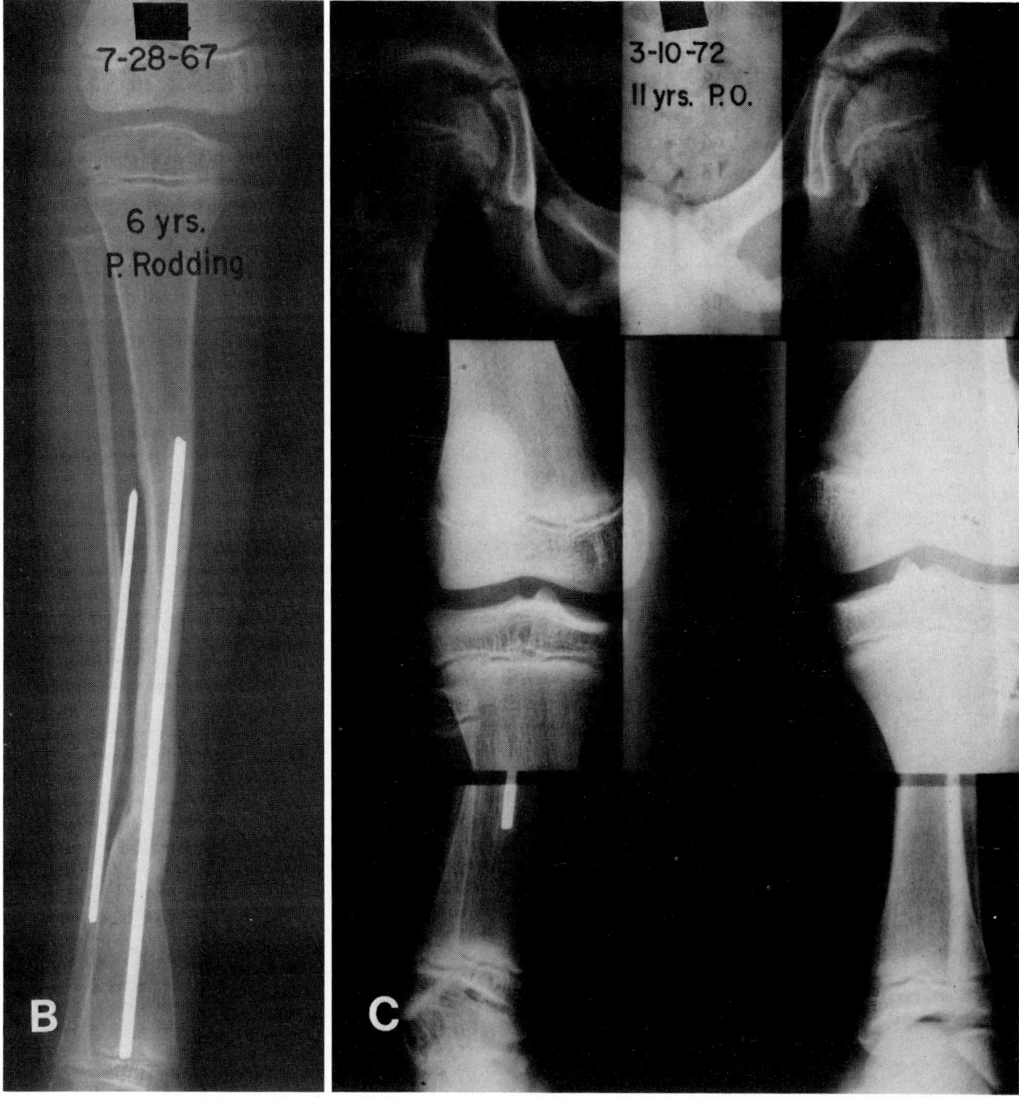

FIG. 19-1 *(Continued). (B)* Six years after surgery, the smooth Steinmann pin has now gradually migrated into the tibia by virtue of continued growth of the distal and proximal physeal plates. *(C)* Eleven years postoperatively, the tibia remains solidly united, and limb lengths are equal, indicating that there has been no interference with epiphyseal growth, despite the fact that a smooth rod passed through the physeal plate for several years.

epiphysis. Limb length discrepancies can also be produced by any chronic process that stimulates excessive chondrogenesis in these growth centers. Any condition that produces hyperemia of the entire limb or of even a single bone can cause overgrowth to such a degree that a treatable limb length discrepancy results. The amount of additional skeletal growth expected at the time of injury or affliction also has great influence on the amount of discrepancy to be expected. It is, therefore, apparent that the cartilaginous growth centers play a vital role in the problem of limb length inequality, and the degree of discrepancy and the nature of the discrepancy (shortening or angulation) are a reflection not only of the type of injury or noxious influence but also of the skeletal age at which such insult occurs.

FACTORS GOVERNING THE DECISION FOR EQUALIZATION

There are many factors that govern the need for equalization of a limb length discrepancy, especially when surgical equalization is being considered. Because each case must be considered on an individual basis, it is essential that all the circumstances be evaluated, both singly and in conjunction with the other factors involved, when any method or combination of methods for correction of any inequality is being considered.

The factors include the following:

- Cause of the discrepancy (etiology)
- Degree of discrepancy
- Skeletal age
- Progression of the discrepancy
- Anticipated adult height
- Strength and balance of the musculature
- Status of the foot and ankle
- Localization or predominant site of the inequality (thigh or leg)
- Sex of the patient
- General or extenuating health factors
- Needs and desires of the patient and the parents

CAUSE OF THE DISCREPANCY

There are five broad etiologic categories that embrace the majority of instances of limb length discrepancy. These can be listed as follows:

Etiologies of Limb Length Discrepancy

- Congenital and Developmental
  - Terminal limb deficiencies
    - Paraxial hemimelias
    - Proximal femoral focal deficiencies
  - Congenitally short femur
  - Hemiatrophy or hemihypertrophy
  - Posterior bow of tibia
  - Ollier's disease
  - Congenital dislocation of the hip
- Paralytic
  - Poliomyelitis
  - Encephalopathy (cerebral palsy)
  - Myelopathy
  - Miscellaneous other causes of flaccid paralysis
- Infections of Bone and Joint
  - Causing growth retardation or arrest
    - Osteomyelitis; acute
    - Pyarthrosis
  - Causing growth acceleration
    - Osteomyelitis, chronic
- Trauma of Bones and Joints
  - Causing growth retardation or arrest
    - Injuries to physeal plate
  - Causing growth acceleration
    - Fractures of metaphysis and diaphysis
  - Resulting in shortening
    - Malunion (excessive overriding) of fractures
- Miscellaneous
  - Tumors and tumorous conditions producing "overgrowth"
    - Fibrous dysplasia
    - Osteoid osteoma
    - Hemangiomatosis
    - Neurofibromatosis
  - Tumor or tumorous conditions producing growth retardation
    - Solitary enchondroma
    - Solitary bone cyst
    - Neurofibromatosis

The cause of the limb length discrepancy is extremely important when contemplating surgical corrections of that discrepancy. Each etiologic type can accomplish shortening or lengthening in a different manner and to a different degree. There also exists a broad spectrum with respect to the type and significance of other limb abnormalities associated with each cause. These factors carry much of the weight in evaluating the indications for or against surgical equalization. Subsequently, and as will be discussed in more depth later in this chapter, the type of corrective measure used will depend on the cause of the shortening.

Congenital and Developmental Causes

As noted above, *congenital and developmental* causes of limb length discrepancy include a wide variety of conditions. Almost all terminal limb deficiencies, whether unilateral or bilateral, result in some discrepancy of limb length. Paraxial hemimelia of the fibula, either partial or complete, is the most common cause of excessive congenital shortening. Often the shortening is severe and the foot and ankle are deformed. Therefore, most often, ablation of the foot is required, and equalization of the length discrepancy is achieved by means of an orthosis or a prosthesis (Fig. 19-2). However, some select patients, wherein the shortening is not severe and the foot and ankle are in good condition, can be treated by equalization procedures that preserve the foot (Fig. 19-3).

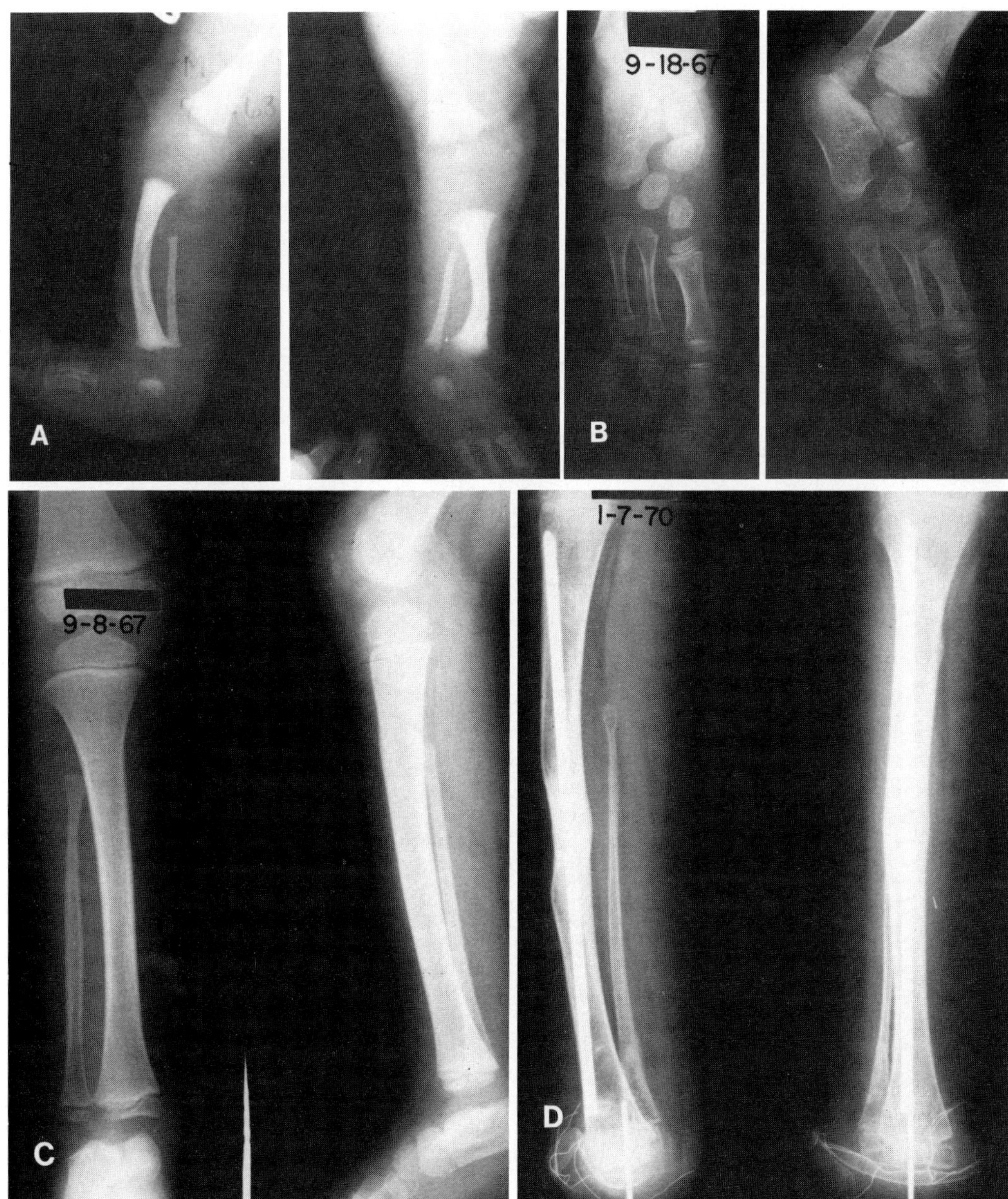

FIG. 19-2. *(A)* A patient with a partial hemimelia of the fibula with significant shortening, presenting shortly after birth. *(B)* Gross abnormality of the foot, with only three rays and tarsal coalition. *(C)* Preoperatively the tibia is foreshortened, with some 6 cm of discrepancy in limb lengths. The foot, however, is still not plantigrade. *(D)* The success of tibial lengthening following bone grafting is evident; however, a disarticulation of the ankle was accomplished. Thus, in this case, even though equalization was achieved, the foot was so deformed that the results of the surgery were negated. It would have been better to disarticulate this foot in the beginning, rather than to subject the patient to the multiple lengthening procedures. The importance of the need for a plantigrade foot prior to lengthening is evident in this patient.

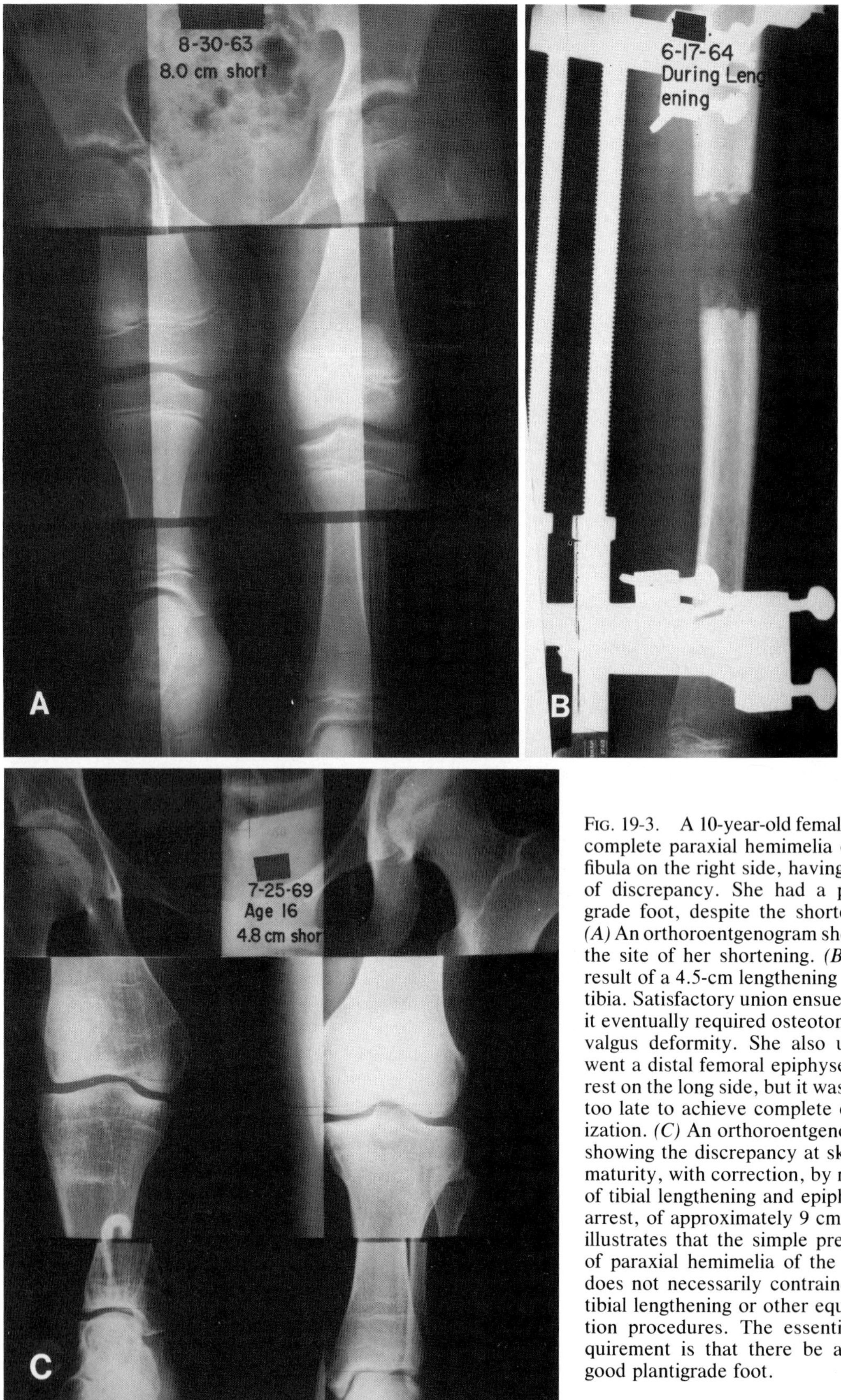

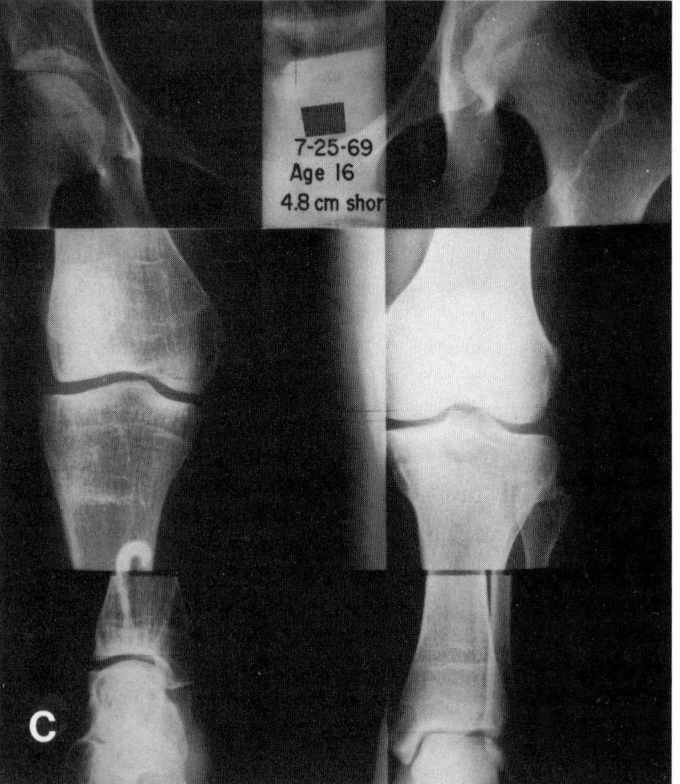

Fig. 19-3. A 10-year-old female with complete paraxial hemimelia of the fibula on the right side, having 8 cm of discrepancy. She had a plantigrade foot, despite the shortening. *(A)* An orthoroentgenogram showing the site of her shortening. *(B)* The result of a 4.5-cm lengthening in the tibia. Satisfactory union ensued, but it eventually required osteotomy for valgus deformity. She also underwent a distal femoral epiphyseal arrest on the long side, but it was done too late to achieve complete equalization. *(C)* An orthoroentgenogram showing the discrepancy at skeletal maturity, with correction, by means of tibial lengthening and epiphyseal arrest, of approximately 9 cm. This illustrates that the simple presence of paraxial hemimelia of the fibula does not necessarily contraindicate tibial lengthening or other equalization procedures. The essential requirement is that there be a very good plantigrade foot.

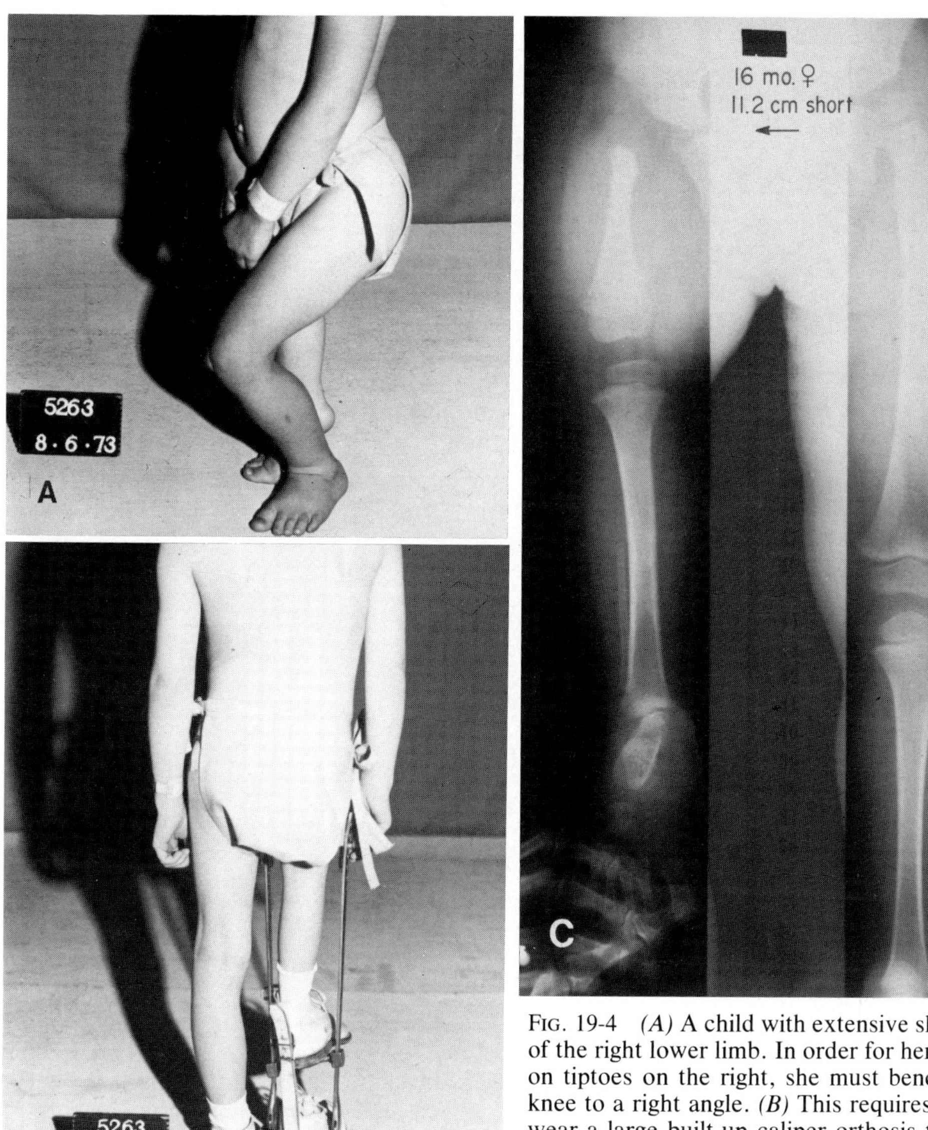

FIG. 19-4 *(A)* A child with extensive shortening of the right lower limb. In order for her to stand on tiptoes on the right, she must bend the left knee to a right angle. *(B)* This requires that she wear a large built-up caliper orthosis to permit more effective ambulation. *(C)* The discrepancy, as seen on scanogram. In such a case, ablation of the foot and use of a prosthesis are indicated.

Proximal femoral focal deficiency is less common but far more dramatic in its manifestations. It is a very challenging and unique condition, which, in unilateral cases, virtually always requires ablation of the foot. Limb length equalization is then achieved by use of a prosthesis (Fig. 19-4). Monographs have been written about this subject, emphasizing the many complicated problems that this abnormality poses and underscoring the need for individualized treatment.

Instances of the congenitally short femur are often accompanied by an anterolateral bow of the femur, which is usually located at the subtrochanteric level or in the region of the proximal third of the femur. Such instances are also frequently accompanied by shortening of the tibia and fibula. Usually, there is a normal foot and ankle, and the degree of shortening is quite variable. The solution must, therefore, be approached individually.

Discrepancies due to hemiatrophy or hemi-

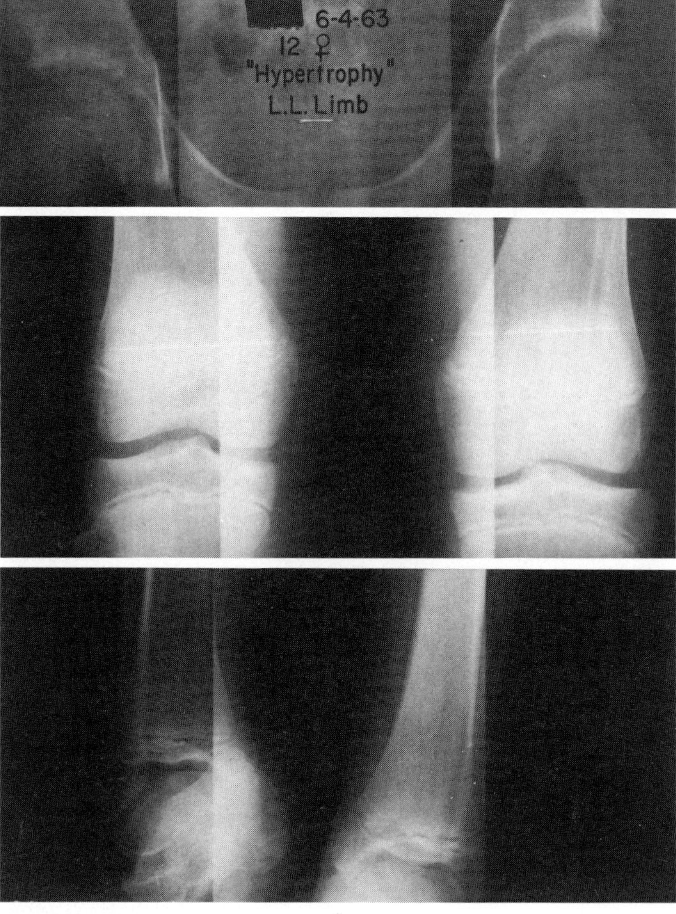

FIG. 19-5. This orthoroentgenogram shows approximately a 4-cm difference in limb length due to simple hemihypertrophy or hemiatrophy. The musculature and the bones and joints are all normal, but they simply differ in size from one side to the other.

hypertrophy (Fig. 19-5) are uncommon, but they are significant in that they may be due to some other underlying cause. For example, in the case of hemiatrophy, associated factors may exist, such as neurofibromatosis, an obscure neurologic disorder, or even a Wilms' tumor. In hemihypertrophy, localized neurofibromatosis or excessive proliferation of subcutaneous fat are frequently encountered.

Ollier's disease (enchondromatosis of bone) is very rare, but it almost always results in some degree of limb length discrepancy because of its variable, but predominantly unilateral, manifestation (Fig. 19-6). Likewise, hemangiomata, lymphangiomatosis, and hemangiomatosis can produce limb length discrepancies by hyperemia and resultant overgrowth or rarely, by progressive bone dissolution, which produces shortening (Fig. 19-7).

Congenital dislocation of the hip causes an unusual type of shortening. It is unique in that its treatment is largely directed toward reducing the dislocation. Only when reduction is contraindicated or impossible or when complications of treatment such as epiphyseal necrosis or physeal arrest become evident, do methods of correction other than reduction of the dislocation become serious considerations.

PARALYTIC CAUSES

These causes of limb length discrepancy include poliomyelitis, unilateral flaccid paralysis due to other causes, and hemiplegia due to spastic paralysis. As noted earlier, poliomyelitis, though rare in the United States, will continue to occasionally offer the problem of shortening (Fig. 19-8). The cause of the shortening is twofold: the first and most significant factor is the muscle atrophy, the accepted belief being that this results in reduced stimulation of normal skeletal growth. On the other hand, there are studies, such as those by Haas,

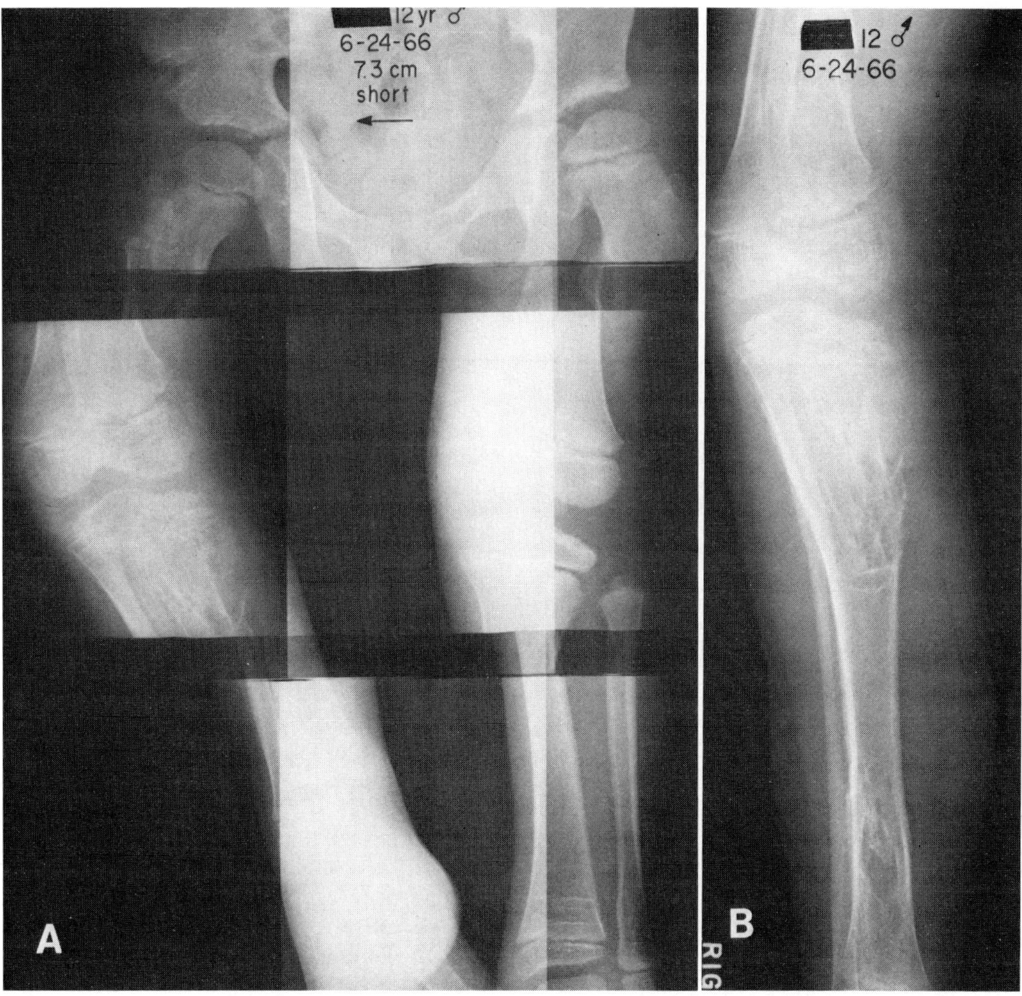

FIG. 19-6. A 12-year-old male with a 7.3-cm shortening of the right lower limb, secondary to multiple enchondromatosis. *(A)* The orthoroentgenogram. *(B)* A more detailed view of the tibia, with its multiple cartilaginous lesions.

that suggest that growth is not necessarily dependent upon muscle function. The second factor is a peculiar coldness of the limb, which in some instances seems to produce even further atrophy or lack of growth. The latter is a highly variable manifestation due to some poorly understood disturbance in vasomotor control. This peculiar vascular manifestation seems to be the best explanation for the unpredictable degree of shortening seen in various patients with poliomyelitis who have similar degrees of muscle weakness or paralysis. Encephalopathy (cerebral palsy) or myelopathy with spastic paralysis, on the other hand, rarely produces a degree of discrepancy that requires an equalization procedure. In the past 25 years at the Intermountain Unit of the Shriners Hospital, only four surgical equalization procedures have been performed upon children having a limb length discrepancy due to cerebral palsy. This indicates that a degree of discrepancy requiring surgical equalization is seldom encountered in cerebral palsy. The explanation for this is that, first, the paralysis is often rather symmetrical, and, second, there is usually an intact reflex motor arc with preserved functioning anterior horn cells innervating muscles that continue to function, even though at a spastic, somewhat reflex level. Thus, a degree of muscle atrophy comparable to that seen in poliomyelitis is much less likely to occur.

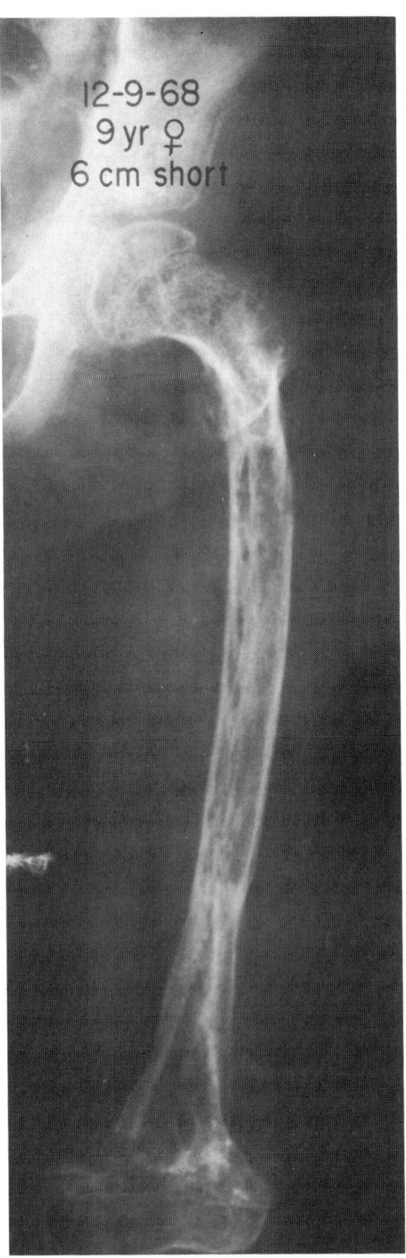

FIG. 19-7. Extensive hemangiomatosis of the femur may produce significant shortening.

INFECTIOUS CAUSES

It is very likely that pyogenic disease of the skeleton will continue to occur, despite the fact that prudently prescribed and effective antibiotic therapy is available. Depending upon the location, degree, and duration of a bone or joint infection, a limb can become either shortened or lengthened. Epiphyseal arrest due to bone infection may occur as the result of pyogenic disruption of the physeal plate (Fig. 19-9). Similarly, destruction of part or all of the epiphysis due to pyarthrosis is not rare, especially in the hips of infants and young children (Fig. 19-10). Destruction or premature closure of normal growth centers in this age group can produce impressive and challenging limb length discrepancies. On the other hand, stimulation of longitudinal limb growth can be produced by chronic osteomyelitis, wherein the long-standing hyperemia of chronic infection serves to stimulate epiphyseal growth (Fig. 19-11). Discrepancies resulting from overgrowth due to chronic infection, however, rarely are of significant magnitude to justify or require surgical equalization.

TRAUMATIC CAUSES

Trauma can produce three different types of discrepancies. First, overgrowth may occur due to stimulation of bone growth following fracture of the femur or tibia. This seems to be the result of the hyperemia invoked by the trauma and the resultant healing process. Overgrowth is commonly seen in children younger than 10 or 12 years of age who have fractures, even though a slight amount of overriding usually follows most fractures of the lower limb. Longitudinal overgrowth of bone following trauma, especially in fractures of the femur, has always been of interest and importance to orthopaedic surgeons. David[35] and Gatewood and Mullen[39] were among early observers. Cole,[29] Phemister,[73] and Barford and Christensen[8] maintained that overgrowth resulting from fracture was a natural compensatory phenomenon. Those believing that overgrowth was secondary to hyperemia were Aitken, Blackett, Ciacotti,[2] and Speed.[84] Compere and Adams[34] agreed and also believed that the increased length was possibly the result of medullary blood supply interruption. Furthermore, on the basis of experimental studies on rabbits, they found that the period of overgrowth lasts only as long as the healing period. Bisgard's[13] animal experiments supported those of Compere and Adams. Trueta[91] was among those to note that the greater the extent of overriding of the fracture fragments, the greater the subsequent overgrowth. Recently, Staheli[85] showed in his clinical observations that greater stimulation of overgrowth occurs in fractures of the proximal third of the

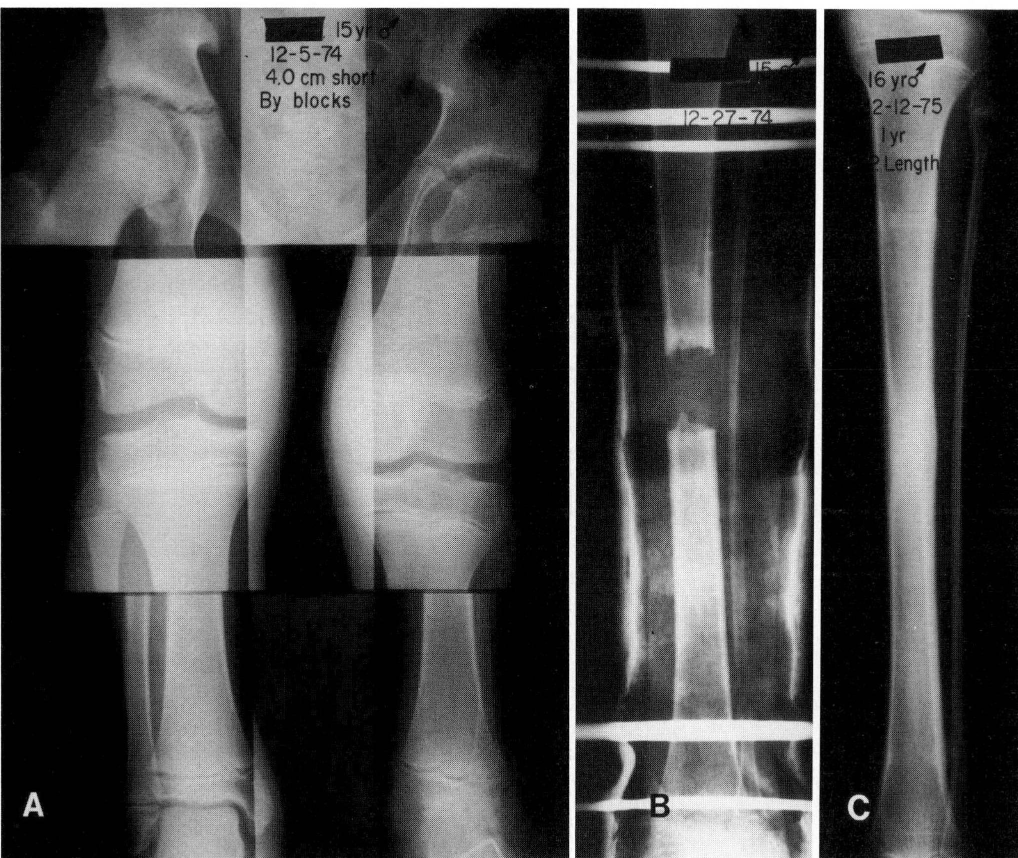

FIG. 19-8. *(A)* Orthoroentgenogram of a 15-year-old male with 4 cm of shortening as the result of poliomyelitis acquired when he was a young child. A pantalar arthrodesis had been done because of the completely flail foot and ankle. *(B)* The results of a tibial lengthening. *(C)* One year following the tibial lengthening, the tibia is solidly united, and the patient has been bearing full weight for 6 months.

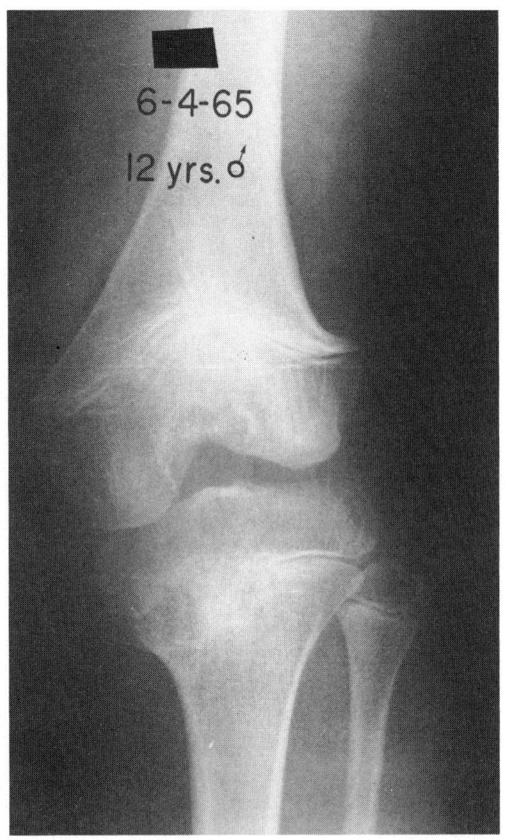

Fig. 19-9. Partial distal femoral and proximal tibial growth arrests have been produced by acute osteomyelitis in this 12-year-old male. He has had osteotomies of the distal femur and the proximal tibia to maintain alignment.

femur, with the least amount of stimulation being found in the distal third.

Shortening, on the other hand, may be produced as the result of significant angulation or excessive overriding following fracture. Also, excessive growth retardation can occur as the result of irreversible damage to the physeal plate, producing premature epiphyseal-diaphyseal fusion.

It is very important to distinguish between different types of limb length discrepancy following infection or trauma, because treatment may vary significantly from one type to another. For example, in cases of shortening due to fracture with overriding or malunion of the fragments, the degree of shortening will likely remain static due to the fact that the epiphyses on the short side can be expected to grow at the normal and equal rate of the opposite member. Discrepancy in these situations can be corrected by epiphyseal arrest on the long side, accomplished during the time of skeletal development when continued growth of the short side corrects the discrepancy. Conversely, and correspondingly, when shortening is the result of epiphyseal arrest due to trauma or bone infection, the shortening will not be static but, rather, will be progressive as long as the patient continues to grow. Surgical arrest of the opposite companion physeal plate under these circumstances will *not* effect any correction, but rather only stops the inevitable progression of the discrepancy. Any correction must, therefore, be accompanied by arrest of additional growth centers or by some other means of equalization. The above circumstances underscore and emphasize the most important basic principle involved in correcting limb length discrepancy by growth arrest, namely, that any correction of the discrepancy is predicated upon continued normal longitudinal limb growth on the shortened side.

Shortening due to traumatic growth arrest is the result of irreversible damage to a growing physeal plate in the lower limb following fracture. The type of epiphyseal injury has a direct realtionship to the possibility of epiphyseal-metaphyseal fusion (growth arrest). Salter and Harris[80] have developed an anatomic classification of these injuries, which enables the surgeon not only to define the nature of the injury but also, more importantly, to have some idea of the prognosis following injury (Fig. 19-12). Five different anatomic types have been outlined, but, from a practical clinical standpoint, only two major clinical types are useful. Functionally and clinically, Types 1 through 3 can be grouped together, because, if appropriate treatment is administered, growth arrest is very unlikely to occur. Conversely, Types 4 and 5 can be similarly grouped because growth arrest is very likely to develop, either symmetrically or asymmetrically (shortening or angulation), regardless of the treatment instituted.

In the majority of patients, the anatomic nature of the injuries can be readily ascertained by means of roentgenographic examination. In some situations, however, more than one anatomic type may occur in the same injury (Fig. 19-13). These episodes of multiple epiphyseal injuries require that several months be allowed to pass before a prognosis is made, in order to observe the functional behavior of

(*Text continues on p. 797*)

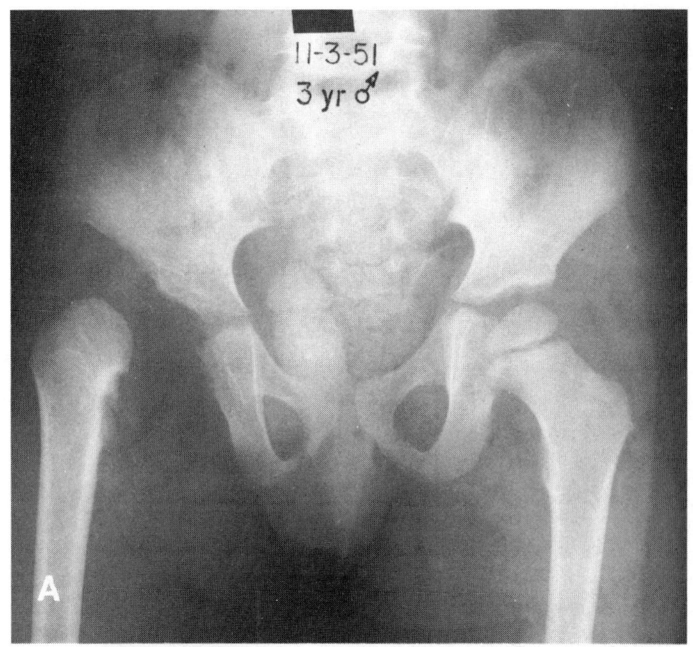

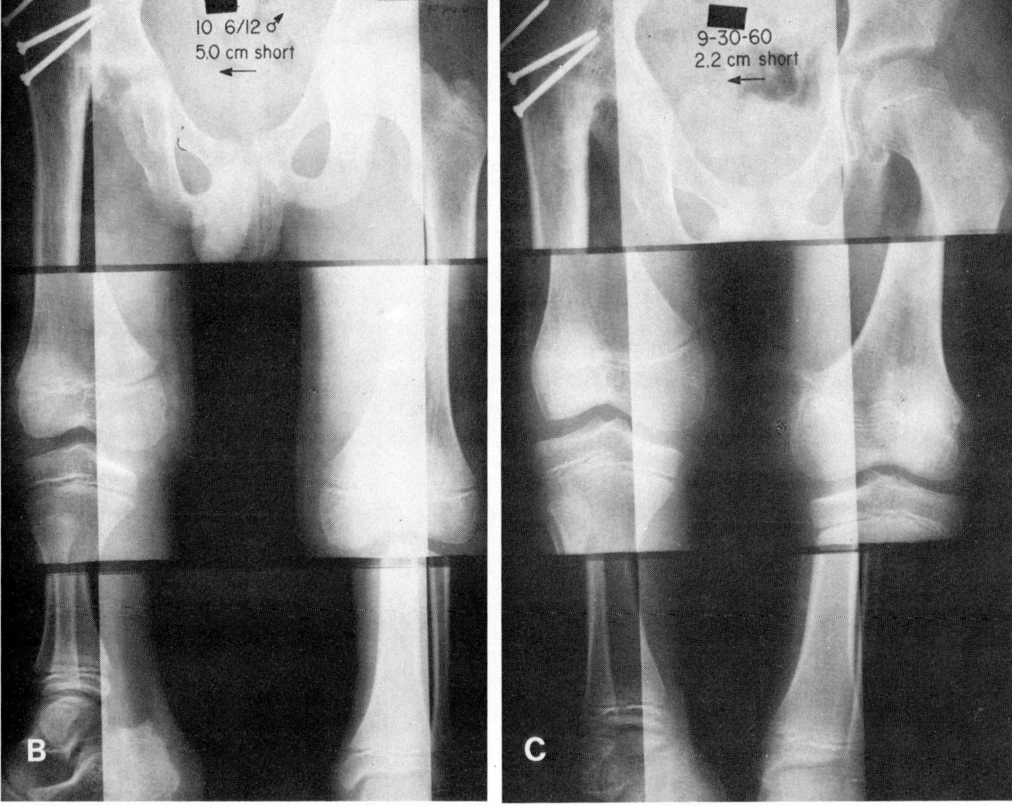

FIG. 19-10 *(A)* Results of pyogenic arthritis of the right hip with complete loss of the femoral head and complete hip dislocation. *(B)* The limb is 5 cm short, and a hip fusion has been accomplished. *(C)* A distal femoral epiphyseal arrest was performed. At skeletal maturity, limb lengths were within 1 cm.

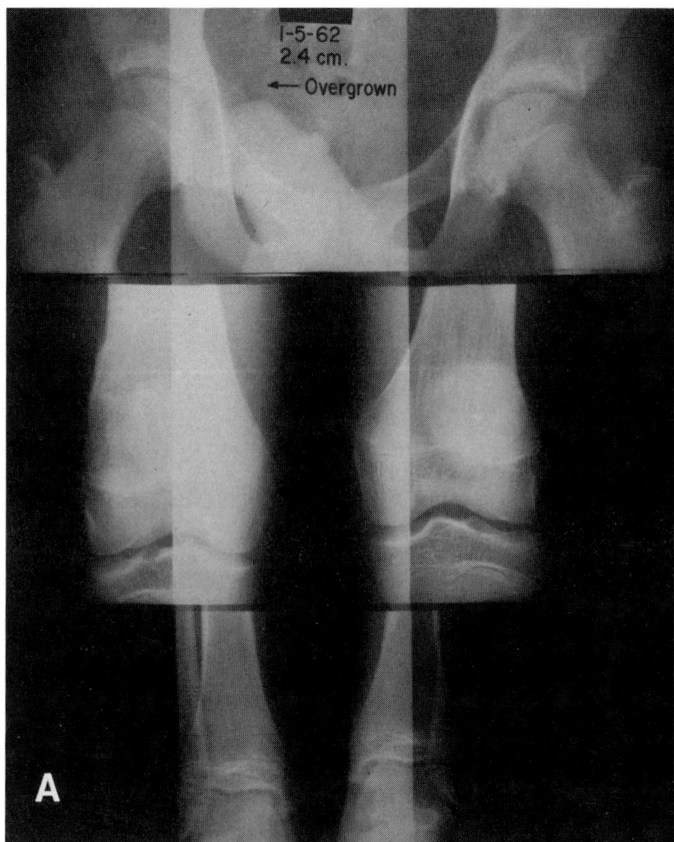

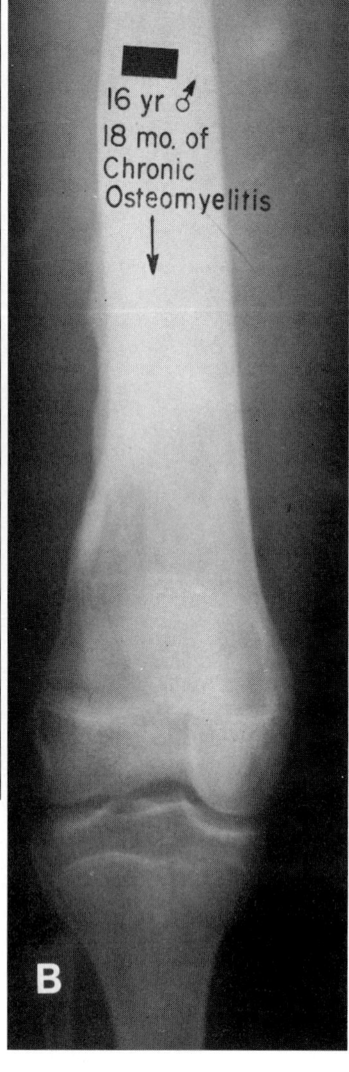

FIG. 19-11. A 13-year-old male with 2.4 cm of limb length discrepancy as the result of chronic osteomyelitis of the right distal femur. *(A)* An orthoroentgenogram, showing that the discrepancy is located exclusively in the femur. *(B)* A better view of the chronic inflammatory process can be seen. Unfortunately, this young man was seen too late to achieve equalization by simple epiphyseal arrest.

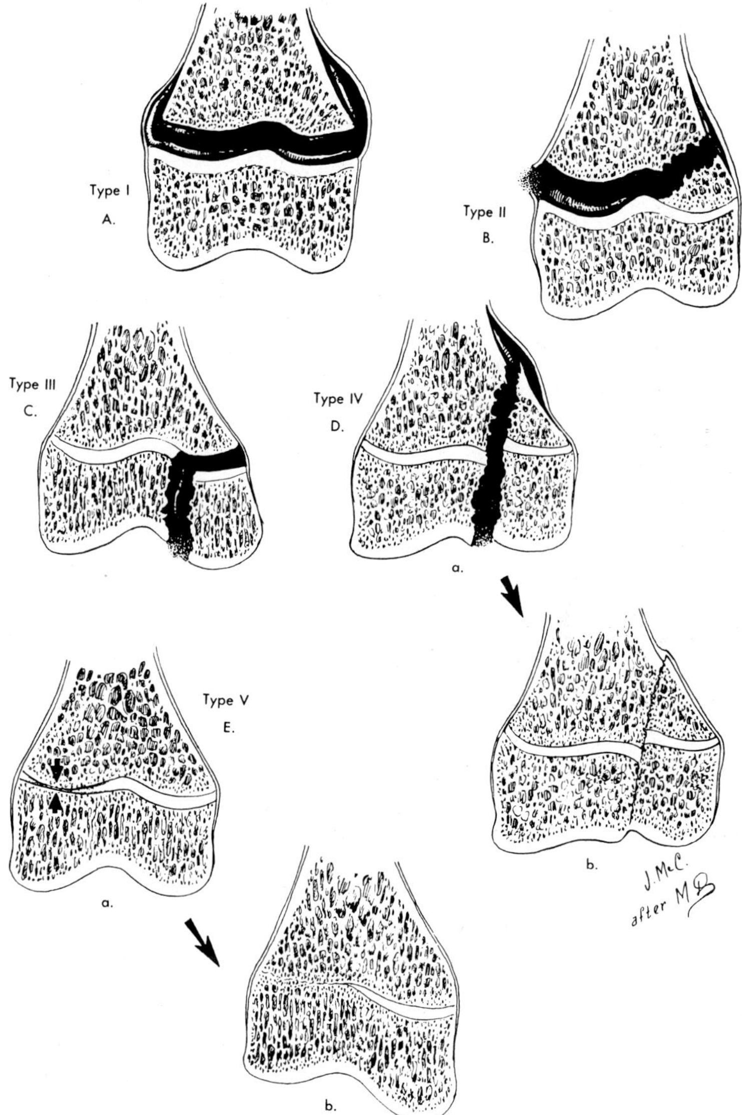

FIG. 19-12. Salter-Harris classification of epiphyseal injuries. (Redrawn after Salter RB, and Harris WR: Injuries involving the epiphyseal plate. J Bone Joint Surg 45A:587, 1963)

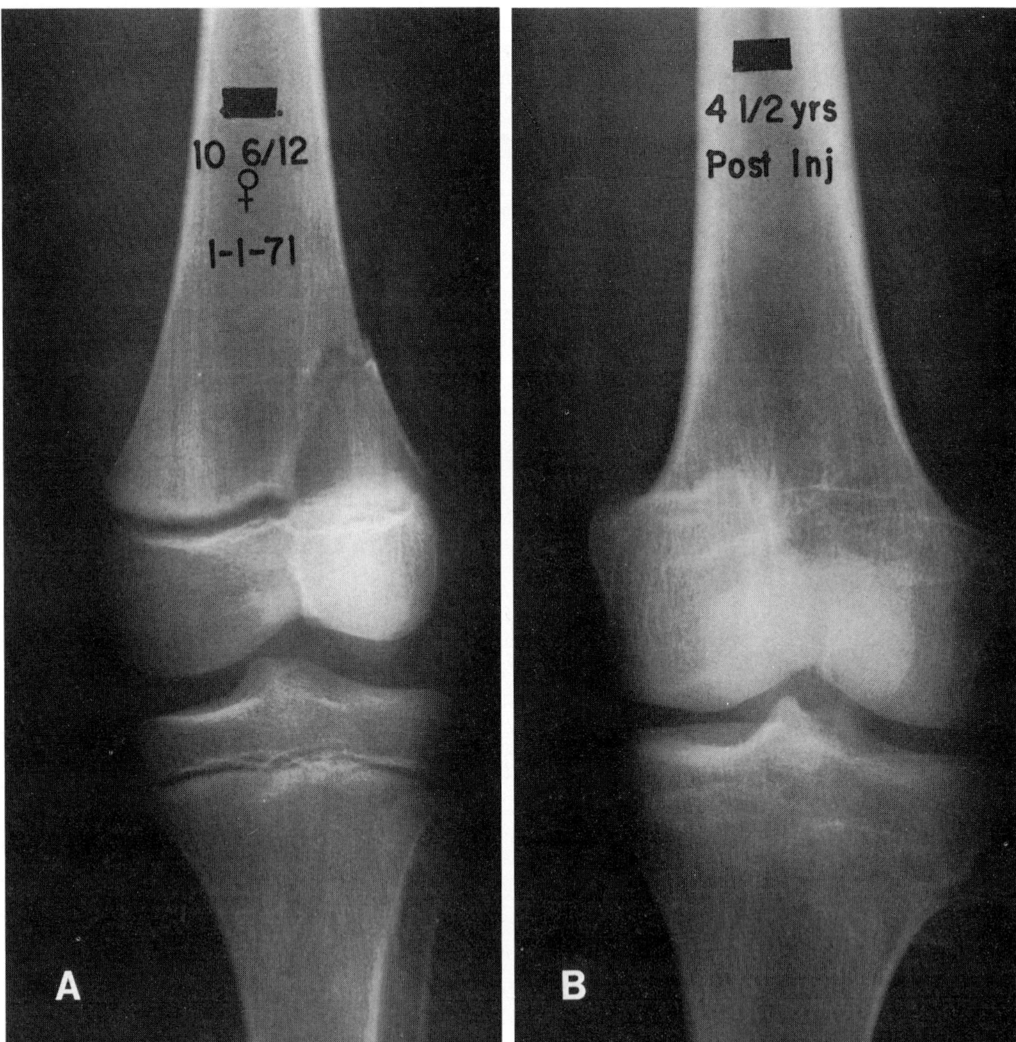

FIG. 19-13. A 15-year-old female who, 4½ years previously, sustained a complex epiphyseal fracture in the left distal femur. *(A)* The combination of a Type 2 and a Type 4 epiphyseal injury. Complete arrest of the epiphyseal plate occurred, resulting in a 4.2-cm shortening at skeletal maturity. *(B)* The x-ray film of the distal femur at maturity. This case demonstrates how a combination of epiphyseal injuries can occur, and, in such situations, predictions with respect to future behavior of a growth plate must be guarded. It would have been better if the arrest had been recognized early so that the opposite companion epiphysis could be arrested. At skeletal maturity, a femoral shortening by resection had to be accomplished.

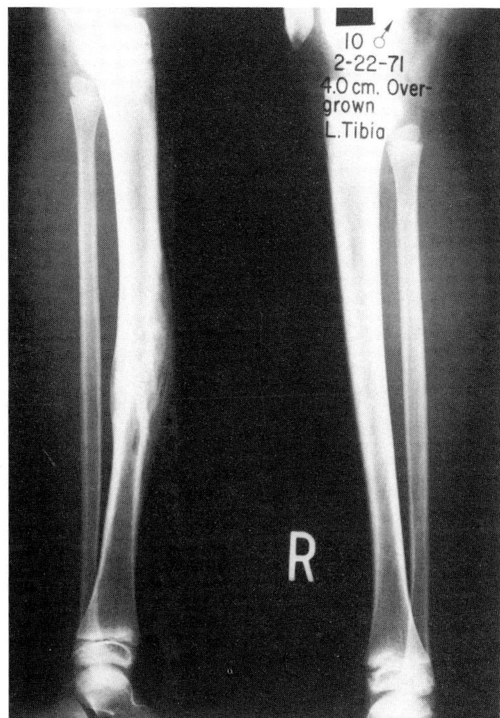

FIG. 19-14. A case of fibrous dysplasia of the tibia known to be present for 8 years. The resulting 4 cm of overgrowth of the tibia is evident.

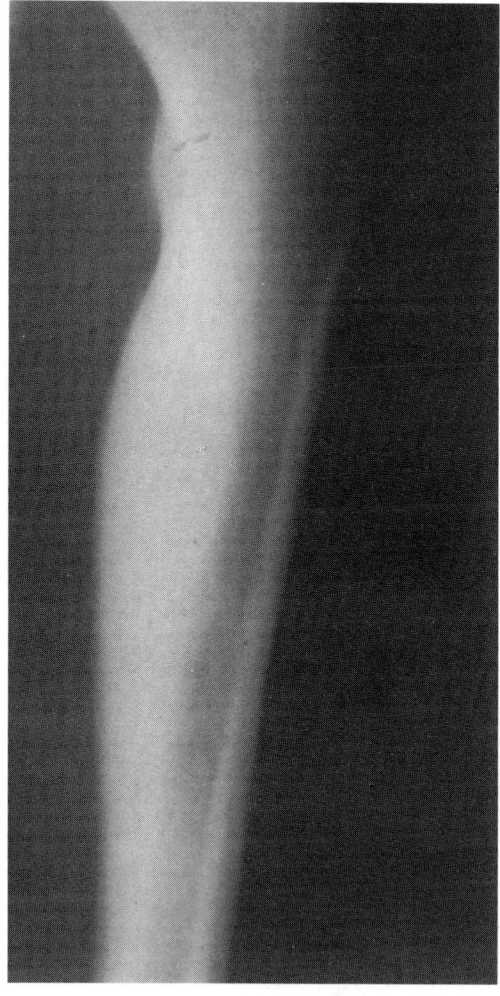

FIG. 19-15. Osteoid osteoma of the proximal femur, with symptoms of at least 2 years' duration. The chronic hyperemia produced a 2.5-cm increased length of this involved left femur.

the physeal plate. Unfortunately, Type 5 cannot often be detected by roentgenographic examination in the early post-traumatic period, and Type 4 may not respond favorably to conscientious efforts at closed or open reduction. It is also suggested by Speed[84] and others that traumatic epiphyseal displacement may incur overgrowth in some cases, just as it occurs in shaft fractures.

MISCELLANEOUS CAUSES

Miscellaneous causes of limb length discrepancy include a variety of unusual conditions that may stimulate or retard bone growth. Any tumor or tumorous condition that invokes a chronic increase in vascularity of the limb or a major bone can produce a limb length discrepancy requiring consideration of correction.

Examples of conditions that may stimulate bone growth include fibrous dysplasia (Fig. 19-14), osteoid osteoma (Fig. 19-15) and soft-tissue hemangiomatosis and neurofibromatosis. Conversely, conditions resulting in retardation or shortening of the limb include solitary bone cyst, enchondroma, hemangiomatosis of bone (see Fig. 19-7) and neurofibromatosis (Fig. 19-16). Most often, discrepancies produced by such lesions are not great, and, because of their rarity, they are not particularly important.

Thus, the importance of the etiology of any limb length discrepancy is evident, and it must be a major consideration when contemplating surgical correction. Whether the inequality is due to growth retardation, growth acceleration, growth arrest, fracture with overriding and malunion, or cogenital dislocation of the hip has a significant influence on what form of

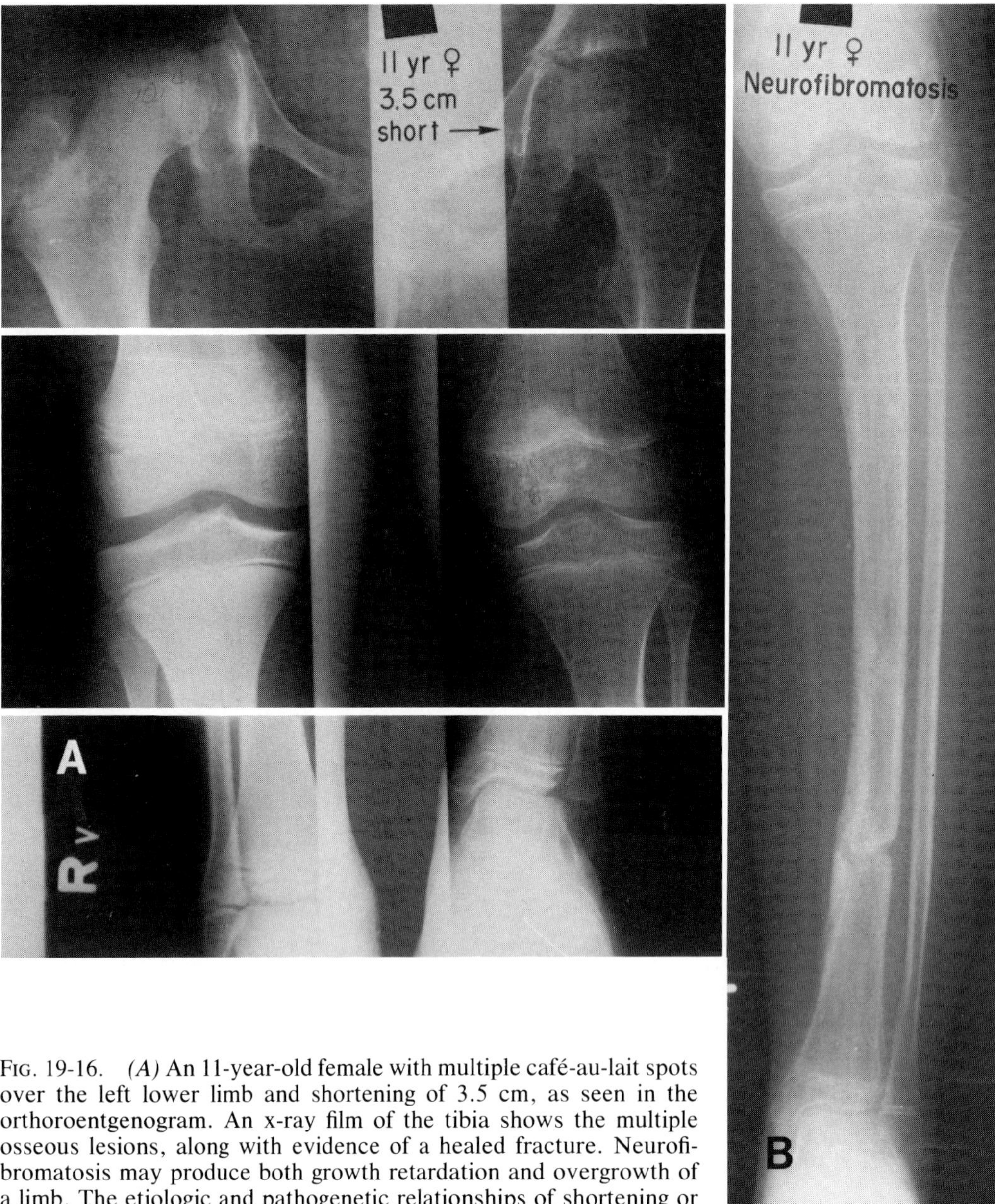

FIG. 19-16. *(A)* An 11-year-old female with multiple café-au-lait spots over the left lower limb and shortening of 3.5 cm, as seen in the orthoroentgenogram. An x-ray film of the tibia shows the multiple osseous lesions, along with evidence of a healed fracture. Neurofibromatosis may produce both growth retardation and overgrowth of a limb. The etiologic and pathogenetic relationships of shortening or lengthening in neurofibromatosis are not well understood.

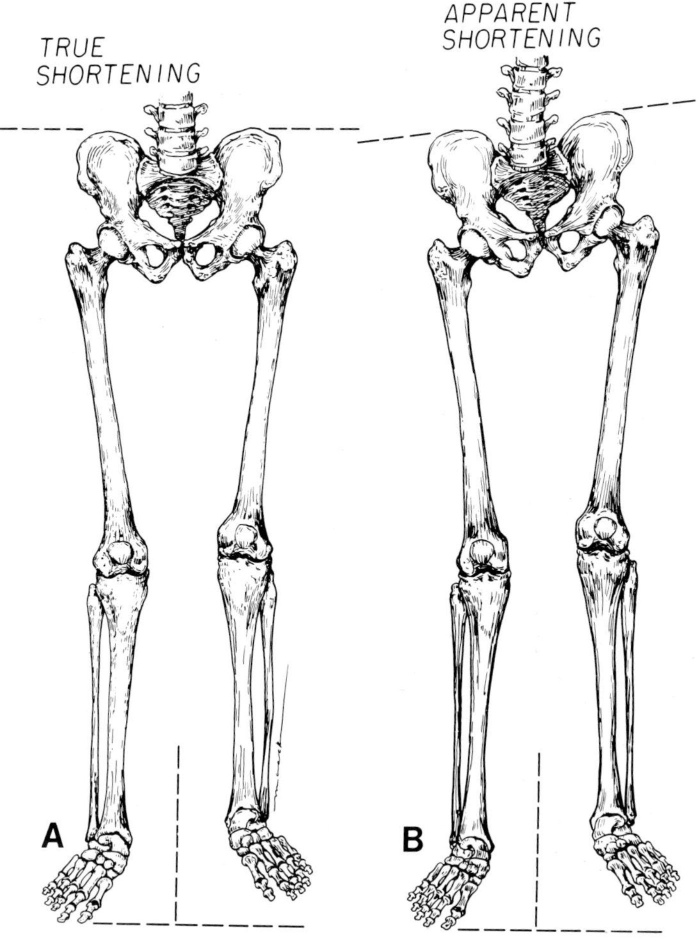

FIG. 19-17. The difference between true shortening *(A)* and apparent shortening *(B)*. In the case of true shortening, the limb from the hip joint to the ankle is truly short by actual measurement. In *(B)*, as a result of pelvic obliquity, adduction contracture of the apparent short side or abduction contracture of the apparent long side, the side on which the pelvis is elevated, appears shorter than its opposite member. The limb lengths, however, are actually the same.

equalization program might be required. As a specific example, highly divergent therapeutic considerations would be exercised when dealing with a limb length discrepancy due to poliomyelitis and an inequality resulting from a traumatic epiphyseal arrest.

THE DEGREE OF DISCREPANCY

This is a most significant factor in deciding the appropriate management of limb length discrepancy. Differences of less than 2.0 cm (under 0.75 inches) are customarily accepted and can be treated by nonsurgical methods, such as a shoelift or no treatment at all. At the other end of the scale, any projected inequality exceeding 18 cm (over 7.0 inches) is usually in excess of the amount that any combination of procedures can be effectively or predictably used to equalize the discrepancy. The only exception is when surgical conversion (amputation or disarticulation) and application of a prosthesis are used. For the most part, therefore, only a limb length inequality between 2.0 and 18 cms warrants serious consideration toward surgical correction. These are not rigid figures, and they represent only practical guidelines, which may be modified by the many other factors involved in the deliberation.

It is critically important to distinguish between a relative (apparent) and an absolute (true) limb length discrepancy. An absolute limb length discrepancy is defined between the iliac crest and the foot. Relative (apparent) shortening or lengthening can be produced by an abduction contracture of the apparently long limb or an adduction contracture of the apparently short limb (Fig. 19-17). This situation is commonly seen in neurologic disorders, such as poliomyelitis and cerebral palsy. The apparent shortening or lengthening is basically the result of pelvic obliquity, which can sometimes cause a significant functional lower limb length discrepancy. In such instances, all efforts at treatment should be directed toward correcting the pelvic obliquity and its cause by whatever means is necessary. Correspondingly, implementation of limb shortening or lengthening procedures in relative disorders of limb length is almost always contraindicated, because the real problem, the pelvic obliquity, will remain uncorrected.

After identifying the nature of the discrepancy, the next step is to document accurately the amount of discrepancy by means of photographs and roentgenograms. To ascertain the amount of discrepancy, three techniques should be used: (1) leveling the pelvis with an appropriate elevation under the shoe, (2) measuring the limbs by tape measure, and (3) measuring the limbs by roentgenographic examination (scanogram or orthoroentgenogram).

The first and most practical procedure is that of placing elevations of variable thickness under the short limb in order to level the pelvis when the patient is standing in bare feet. The amount of elevation required to level the pelvis is easily determined. This is the most reliable method, because it accomplishes the ultimate goal of equalization—a level pelvis. It readily accounts for any variation in bony landmarks and differences in pelvic size and shape, as well as foot size and shape. A photograph should be made of the patient, showing that the pelvis is level and recording the precise amount of lift required to achieve this (Fig. 19-18). The best roentgenographic technique for determining limb length discrepancy is the

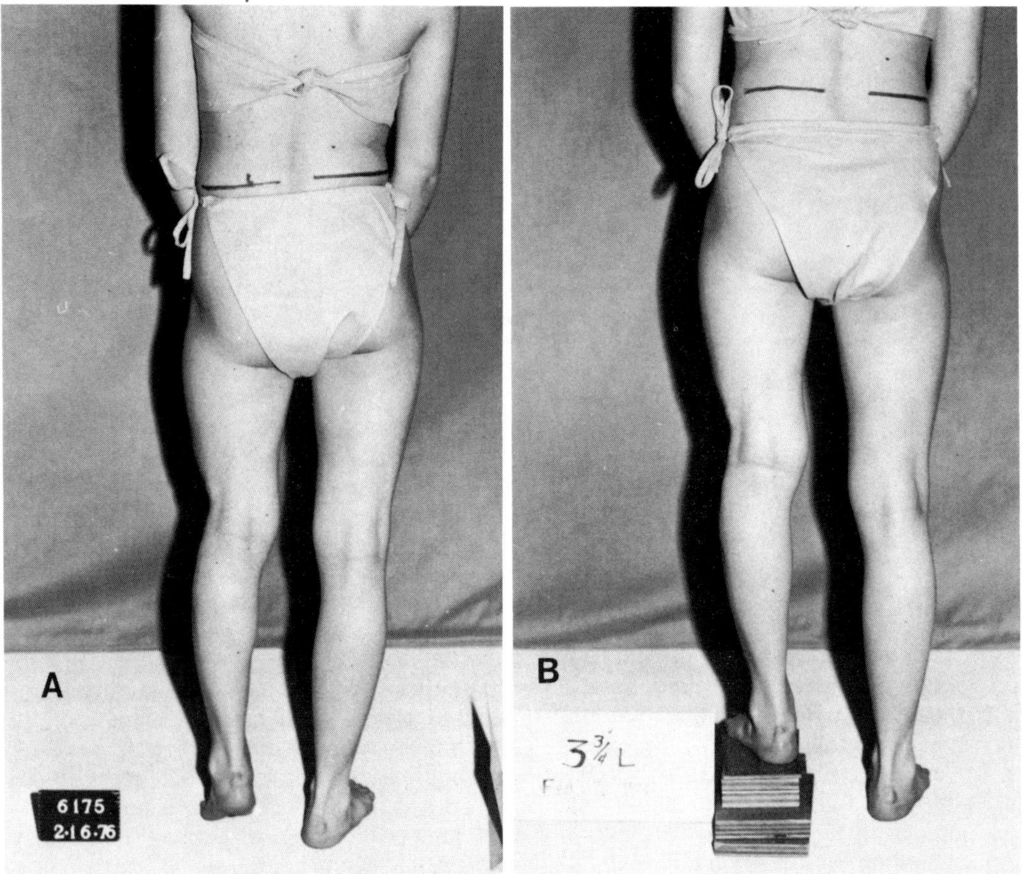

FIG. 19-18. *(A)* A child with almost 4 inches of shortening, due to traumatic distal femoral and proximal tibial epiphyseal arrests. *(B)* The amount of lift needed under the heel to achieve a level pelvis. The exact height of the blocks necessary to achieve equalization is included in the photograph.

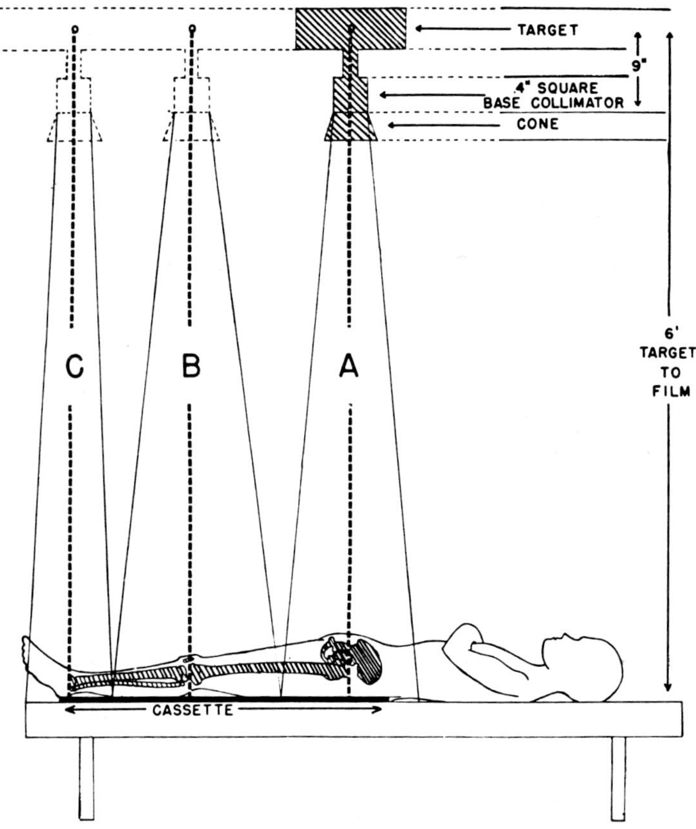

FIG. 19-19. Method of making an orthoroentgenogram. (Tachdjian MO: Pediatric Orthopedics. Philadelphia, WB Saunders, 1972)

orthoroentgenogram. This procedure uses three separate roentgen exposures, with the beam sequentially centered directly over the hip, the knee, and the ankle joints (Fig. 19-19). The distances between the major joint surfaces are calibrated by means of a centimeter rule placed at the same level as that upon which the patient lies. The resultant film can be used to establish with reasonable accuracy not only the total amount of discrepancy between the hip and ankle joints but also the location of the discrepancy, that is, whether it is in the femur, the tibia, or both. There are two deficiencies of orthoroentgenography that offer potential errors in measurement. First the technique ordinarily does not take into account any variation in size of the pelvis or the foot, and these must be calculated into the final determination of discrepancy. Second, if the patient's position is altered between any of the roentgen exposures, the examination is invalidated. Thus, the need to double check the orthoroentgenogram by other methods of measurement is evident.

The tape measure should be used to provide corroborative measurements of various bony prominences, measured from the pelvis to the lower limb. Conventionally, the anterosuperior iliac spine is used on the pelvis, and the medial malleolus is the standard prominence used in the lower limb. Measurements from the umbilicus to the malleolus and to the heel are frequently used, because this latter measurement takes into account any variation in size of the foot and pelvis and any abnormalities or variations in the bony prominences. This technique also assists in determining whether the discrepancy is true or apparent. Care must be taken to ascertain that the pelvis is level. Even though it is the determination most subject to error and it is the one that lends itself least well to documentation, one of the most important values of the tape measurement is that of confirming and double checking the values derived from the other examinations. Ideally, all three should validate and complement each other. In this way, any errors can be detected, and accurate determination of the discrepancy is virtually ensured. It is essential to remember that any flexion contracture of the hip or knee and any equinus contracture of the ankle may seriously influence any of these determinations. A careful and comprehensive effort must be made to measure and record the exact amount of discrepancy. Without this measurement, a responsible approach to the problem of limb length inequality is impossible.

SKELETAL AGE

Once the degree of discrepancy has been established accurately, it is necessary to determine the skeletal age of the patient, especially if correction by growth arrest is being contemplated.

The skeletal age of the patient is important for several reasons. First, if skeletal maturity has been reached (or nearly so), correction by growth arrest is impossible. Furthermore, if skeletal age is grossly different from chronologic age or if the patient is skeletally very immature, correction of limb length discrepancy by growth arrest may be unpredictable or impractical. In order to achieve equalization safely and effectively in patients having limb length inequality who are approaching skeletal maturity, one must resort to either shortening of the long limb by bone resection or using some selective lengthening process. In cases in which unpredictability of correction by epiphyseal arrest exists or when the patient is very young, equalization can be accomplished by mechanical lengthening, application of a shoe lift, amputation and prosthesis or, in rare cases, temporary growth arrest (stapling), depending on the degree of discrepancy and the cause of the discrepancy. In some cases, a combination of lengthening and shortening may be used. It is obvious that there are a challenging number of variables that must be dealt with in assessing the factor of skeletal age.

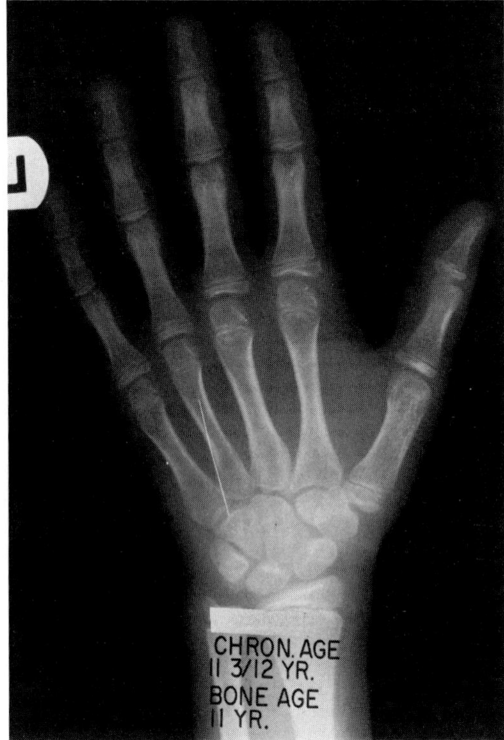

FIG. 19-20. An x-ray film of the wrist and hand in a young female whose chronologic age is 11 3/12 years and whose skeletal age is 11 years. This determination is essential when contemplating any form of equalization by growth arrest.

There are several ways in which skeletal age can be assessed, none of which is critically accurate. In all the methods, there is a relatively wide standard of deviation (12 months). The most popular method of determining skeletal age is the use of a single anteroposterior roentgenogram of the wrist and hand (Fig. 19-20). By comparing the patient's wrist and hand film with a known standard, a reasonably accurate determination of skeletal age can be achieved. The Greulich and Pyle Atlas[44] is the most highly accepted documentation of skeletal age. Standards of skeletal age for both males and females are based on the stage of development of various primary and secondary ossification centers in the wrist and hand. There are other methods of determining skeletal age, an example being interpretation of the state of epiphyseal development of the long bones of the lower limbs. None of these methods, however, has been as well accepted or universally used as evaluating the roentgenogram of the wrist and hand.

By using these data appropriately, a sufficiently accurate assessment of skeletal age can be made, and, from a clinical standpoint, a soundly based therapeutic program can be devised. When wide and erratic variations are encountered between chronologic and skeletal age, greater care must be exercised in formulating a therapeutic program, especially when permanent epiphyseal arrest is being contemplated as a method of equalization. This is because epiphyseal arrest relies upon critical calculations of skeletal age and relatively predictable growth patterns in order to obtain appropriate correction and to avoid over- or undercorrection.

Studies such as as those by Green and Anderson[41] and Bayley[11] agree that skeletal age is a far more accurate measurement than chronologic age in evaluating and predicting the status of a discrepancy. In addition, they cite a very close correlation between skeletal age and sexual maturity.

PROGRESSION OF THE DISCREPANCY

Once the discrepancy has been documented and the patient's skeletal age has been identified as well as it can be, this knowledge can be effectively applied in reaching some understanding as to the progressional qualities of the discrepancy.

Progression of the discrepancy is important for several reasons. On one hand, if a difference in limb length is static or relatively so, the best form of equalization treatment can be planned more accurately and more specifically. On the other hand, if the discrepancy is progressive, it is extremely important that it be accurately documented and that its progression be plotted. By this means, it can be ascertained whether the shortening is along a linear, rather predictable course or whether it is following a more erratic and unpredictable course. It should be recognized that on rare occasions, minor limb length discrepancies may stabilize or largely correct themselves spontaneously, and, in such rare situations it is probable that no treatment will be needed.

Throughout the literature, many methods of plotting the factors surrounding a limb length discrepancy have been described. They represent efforts to correlate the relative rates of growth of the long and short limb, the sex variables, the degree of skeletal maturity, the chronologic age, and the degree of limb length discrepancy. From these data, one attempts to determine what types of equalization procedures would best suit the individual case and when the procedures should be performed. At present, one of the most widely used growth prediction methods is that which was published (as revised from an earlier study) by Green and Anderson.[43] The *growth remaining* methods, as it is called, uses a chart depicting the amount of additional growth to be expected from a normal proximal tibia and distal femur in different sexes and at different skeletal ages (Fig. 19-21).

In addition, the percentage of growth inhi-

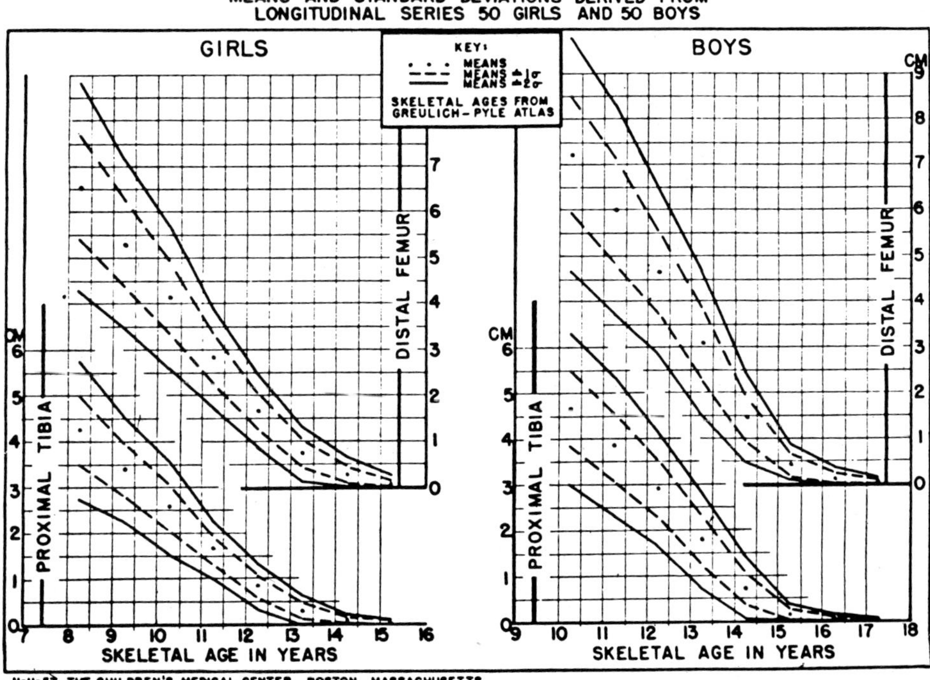

FIG. 19-21. The Green-Anderson growth-remaining chart. (Anderson M, Green WT, Messner MB: Growth and predictions of growth in the lower extremities. J Bone Joint Surg 45A:10, 1963)

bition of the shorter limb is determined over a given time interval (suggested as at least 3 months) by subtracting the amount of growth in the short limb from the amount of growth in the normal limb, dividing the remainder by the amount of growth in the normal limb, and then multiplying by 100:

$$\frac{\text{growth normal} - \text{growth involved} \times 100}{\text{growth normal}}$$

This ratio, used in conjunction with the growth remaining chart, is evaluated, and the patient's growth curves are manipulated in an effort to decide upon a course of action and the optimal time to pursue that course.

The second method of evaluating a limb length inequality has been developed by Moseley.[68] It is referred to as the "straight line" graph for limb length discrepancies. Although the author has not yet felt the need to use it, the method appears to have significant advantages over other methods. This is an ingenious and very graphic method of plotting the progession of a lower limb length discrepancy. The parameters for its use are essentially the same as those for the "growth remaining" method. Skeletal age is determined by the Gruelich and Pyle method[44] as the corresponding limb lengths (of both short and long limbs) are recorded. It is recommended that several determinations be made, as in the Anderson-Green method. The advantages of the "straight line" method are the following: no mathematical calculations are necessary; the growth rates of short and long sides can be easily compared at a glance; the patient's height, relative to his or her skeletal age group, is quickly determined, as are lengths of the limbs at maturity. One can also see graphically exactly when and where the best equalization procedure should be accomplished. In addition to the simplicity of the method, it appears that it is significantly more accurate than the alternative methods. An example of the "straight line" graph is seen in Figure 19-22.

Shapiro[81] studied 803 patients with lower

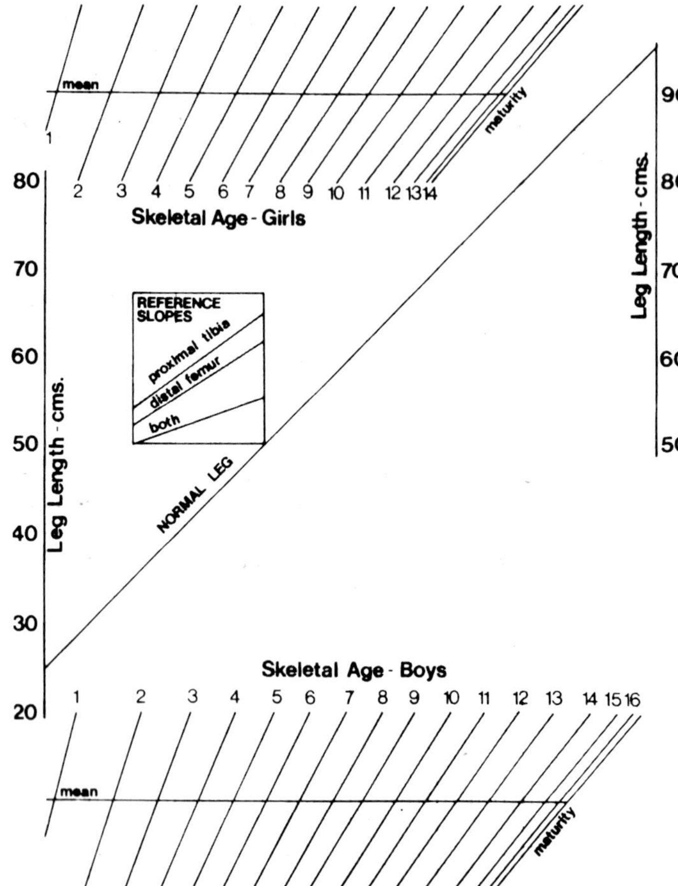

FIG. 19-22. The Mosely "straight-line" graph is educationally a very attractive technique of documenting the progression of a lower limb length inequality. It requires several serial scanographic and bone age measurements to be accurate. (Mosely CF: J Bone Joint Surg 59A:176, 1977)

limb length inequality and found a substantial difference in the progression of the discrepancy, depending largely on the cause of the length difference and the place and time of its occurrence. He identified at least five different patterns of progression. These are illustrated graphically in Fig. 19-23. These observations clearly have a direct influence on the decision-making process as it relates to the ultimate discrepancy, and, when they are coupled with the growth-remaining tables, a more accurate determination can be made regarding a program of equalization.

ANTICIPATED ADULT HEIGHT

Anticipated adult height is one of the most elusive factors to determine accurately. This also requires a periodic skeletal age determination, provided that the patient's growth is plotted against normal height and growth patterns, and this information is compared with genetic data. Even when parental stature is known, ultimate stature is difficult to predict with a high degree of confidence. All determinations must be considered estimates, as evidenced by earlier studies. For example, in a study by Bayley[11] in 1946, it was noted that skeletal age is much more highly correlated with relative size than is chronologic age. She presented a series of tables for use in approximating expected adult heights from skeletal age and relative heights. Some general relationships with respect to relative maturity and adult height were outlined, including: (1) Early-maturing girls are usually large when young, their growth slows down to about an average rate at 13 years, and they complete growth rapidly, becoming smaller adults. (2) Late-maturing girls are more often small when young, catching up to the average at about age 13, and becoming tall adults. (3) Early maturing boys do not exhibit the abrupt curtailment of growth as in girls (this is attributed to the action of sex hormones), but the rate of growth slows down more gradually. They seem to have an equal likelihood of becoming tall, medium, or short; however, they tend to be of a larger, broader, or heavier build at all ages than do late-maturing boys. (4) Late-maturing boys continue to grow, some even into their early 20s, and more often than not they become tall adults. They are usually slender and long-legged, their greater adult height being due primarily to continued growth of the lower limbs.

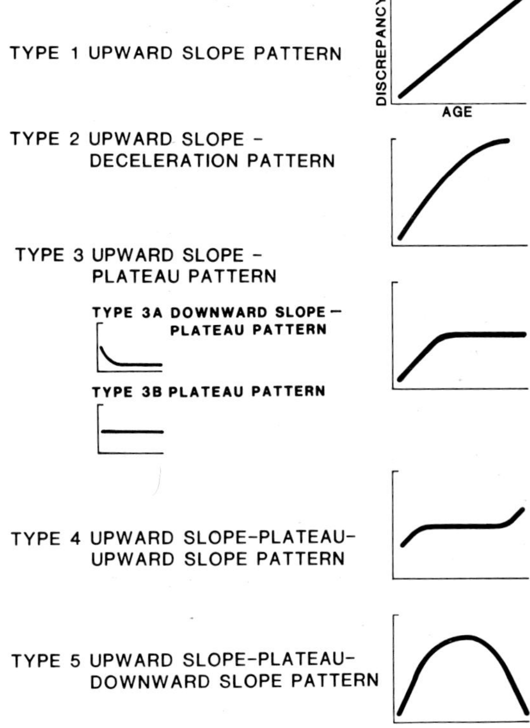

FIG. 19-23. Developmental patterns of lower limb length discrepancies are shown in these five types. Each of these is directly related to the etiologic factors responsible for the discrepancy. For details, the reader is urged to consult Shapiro's original article. (Shapiro F: Development patterns in lower extremity length discrepancies. J Bone Joint Surg 64A:639, 1982)

In any event, the importance of this factor is related not only to its consideration in accurate plotting of the progression of an inequality but also to the assumption that a patient of anticipated significantly short stature will more likely desire some form of lengthening rather than shortening procedure. Conversely, a patient with a predictable ultimate stature of normal or taller-than-average proportions will be more amenable to, and probably more appropriately treated by some form of shortening procedure, if the discrepancy does not exceed 4 or 5 cm.

STRENGTH AND BALANCE OF THE MUSCULATURE

The strength and balance of the musculature in the shortened limb is important for two reasons. First, it is a questionable practice to lengthen a short limb where an above-knee brace is already required for independent ambulation. Second, to elongate a very weak, shortened limb may possibly create a situation in which an above-knee brace may be required for independent ambulation, whereas prior to lengthening, a brace was not necessary. This unfortunate circumstance may result from one of two mechanisms: (1) weakening existing musculature by elongation, or (2) producing a longer lever arm with a resultant mechanical disadvantage. Alternatively, there is some valid concern that lengthening of a limb that has completely normal musculature may result in some degree of paresis of muscles due to neuropraxia (temporary), muscle stretch (probably temporary), or ischemic necrosis (permanent). Finally, by virtue of a combination of the above circumstances, any previously existing imbalance of muscle strength may be accentuated by lengthening. Thus, an accurate knowledge of the strength and balance of the musculature of the limb must be ascertained prior to considering any form of equalization procedure that requires elongation of the shorter limb.

STATUS OF THE FOOT AND ANKLE

The status of the foot and ankle becomes of major importance when discrepancies exist that may require tibial lengthening for equalization. Foot and ankle deformities existing prior to lengthening are almost invariably accentuated by the elongation process, and any uncorrected pre-existing ankle equinus is almost always made worse by lengthening. Therefore, in contemplating a lengthening procedure in the tibia, the patient should have a plantigrade foot and a stable ankle, and there must be no fixed or uncorrectable ankle equinus.

Conversely, when the shorter side has a foot that is neither plantigrade nor capable of being made plantigrade or when there is an unstable ankle, tibial lengthening is contraindicated. Therefore, when discrepancies exist that are correctable only by a combination of epiphyseal arrest and some form of lengthening, it is essential that the status of the foot and ankle be carefully appraised.

LOCALIZATION OF PREDOMINANT SITE OF THE INEQUALITY (THIGH OR LEG)

The principal site of the shortening (or lengthening) is important for the simple reason that it is desirable to keep the segments of the lower limb as equal as possible. Thus, any discrepancy in the thigh or leg portion would be most appropriately corrected by equalizing the corresponding segment of the opposite member. This is not always possible, nor necessarily desirable, but it is a factor that must be taken into account.

SEX OF THE PATIENT

The sex of the patient is significantly less important than skeletal age when considering equalization. However, in some instances, it can be a very substantial factor. Generally speaking, a girl will accept a shorter ultimate anticipated stature than a boy. Correspondingly, a boy would likely prefer lengthening to shortening, when confronted with the alternative of being significantly shorter than his peers. This factor is subtle, but one that cannot be ignored, and it must be weighed carefully in all instances of inequality.

GENERAL OR EXTENUATING HEALTH FACTORS

Evaluation of general or extenuating health factors for each patient, with respect to the indications and the techniques for correcting limb length inequality, is frequently not given appropriate attention. However, if this issue is given proper consideration from the first evaluation, a significant number of physical and psychological complications can be prevented, or at least anticipated. The ultimate goal in the treatment of unequal limb lengths is to give the patient as great a degree of normality of function as is possible. When the welfare of the patient as a whole is not taken into account, complications worse than the limb length discrepancy may be encountered.

Physiologic Factors

The organic problems of the patient who is being considered for limb length equalization are usually easier to evaluate than are those stemming from psychological problems, which may be covert. In an effort to uncover and define such problems, it is, of course, essential that a complete history be taken and a comprehensive physical examination be done. It should be ascertained that the patient is in the best possible physical and psychological condition prior to any attempt at major methods of equalization. This is especially true in situations that involve extensive surgery or prolonged hospitalization. Certain physical and medical factors may even be considered as possible contraindications to the use of a particular procedure. Some of the more obvious examples are hypertension, heart disease, any previous osteomyelitis of the limb, angular or flexion deformities, muscle weakness in borderline cases, extensive scarring of soft tissues, and neurologic or vascular abnormalities. These and other disturbances must be evaluated whenever considering any major equalization procedure. Furthermore, if it is elected to undertake correction, all these factors must be monitored carefully throughout the treatment program.

Psychological Factors

Whenever contemplating a major equalization procedure, the psychological condition of the patient is a subject of considerable importance. Even to a patient who is psychologically healthy, the ordeal of long-term treatment and a convalescence that may involve prolonged immobilization can be an emotionally draining experience. When either the parent or patients suffer from psychological problems, as may often be the case in children having a deformity, major surgery and prolonged convalescence may be less well tolerated. Little satisfaction can be gained by improving the patient's physical condition while his emotional condition deteriorates. A patient who is very frightened, poorly prepared, or undergoing great psychological stress often experiences more pain during treatment and may often exhibit many psychosomatic manifestations, such as depression, irritability, anorexia, and weight loss. On the other hand, patients filled with abnormally strong feelings of inadequacy and insecurity that they attribute to the deformity often view surgery as the answer to their problems, and they may be overzealous, almost desperate, for treatment. Any complications encountered during treatment of this type of patient could be disastrous. Also, they are more likely to find fault with the operative procedure or result. This type of problem may manifest in a patient who has a minor discrepancy but who is highly conscious of the discrepancy and is convinced that it is conspicuous to others. Therefore, the patient may insist that treatment be effected for its correction. Naturally, medical care should not be withheld from these patients, but the many factors involved must be given serious consideration. In an instance in which the patient is not strong enough emotionally to endure an extended ordeal, perhaps the lengthening procedure should not be used, even at the expense of losing some height by means of the alternate method of limb shortening. Furthermore, it may be desirable that, in some cases, the patient, as well as the parents, undergo professional counseling, both initially and throughout the convalescent period.

In any problem as complex as the treatment of limb length inequality, early and careful attention to all the general and extenuating health factors of the patient can very possibly lessen or prevent many potential problems, not only for the patient but also for the surgeon.

NEEDS AND DESIRES OF THE PATIENT AND PARENTS

The final and very important factor that must be evaluated in arriving at a satisfactory approach to treatment of limb length discrepancy is the issue of the personal needs and desires of the patient and parents. Most often, the patient is not mature or knowledgeable enough to weigh all facets of the problem to the extent that an informed opinion can be expressed. However, this does not mean that a full explanation of all the ramifications of the problem and its treatment should not be given. The parents must be informed as to all of the advantages, disadvantages, and potential complications of all appropriate and feasible techniques of equalization. Once the many factors and subleties of each procedure have been thoroughly discussed, the decision often becomes apparent. It is not uncommon to have several evaluation and discussion periods before a satisfactory conclusion is reached by the three parties concerned (patient, parents, and physican). Therefore, in formulating a therapeutic program, the needs and desires of the patient and parents must be given strong consideration, provided that they have been fully informed and that they understand the advantages and disadvantages of the treatment modalities.

The treatment of limb length inequality has traditionally involved a multiplicity of approaches that are enormously dissimilar and, in many instances, are controversial in principle, technique, and result. It is essential that the surgeon be as well informed and as objective as possible so that all methods for equalization may be evaluated according to their relative merit. Only in this way can the surgeon choose the method most appropriate for the patient while also considering the other factors surrounding the discrepancy and the decision to correct it.

METHODS OF EQUALIZATION OF LIMB LENGTHS

Equalization of limb lengths can be achieved by several techniques, either nonsurgically or surgically. Nonsurgical methods include shoe lifts and a variety of braces and prosthetic devices. Surgical modalities can be grouped into five broad categories and are those that (1) convert a limb with a terminal deficiency, by ablation of a portion of a limb, to a limb that will facilitate use of an artificial limb; (2) shorten the long side; (3) lengthen the short side; (4) use a combination of lengthening and shortening; and (5) restore growth by means of surgical epiphyseolysis. As mentioned earlier, any solution to a problem of limb length inequality requires a sound knowledge of all these technical procedures in order to arrive at the best possible therapeutic program.

NONSURGICAL METHODS

A shoe lift is a simple method of equalizing limb lengths, but children often refuse to wear it or are unhappy if forced to do so. Furthermore, the indications for a shoe lift prescription are difficult to define accurately. Large discrepancies, those in excess of 5 or 10 cm, require cumbersome and unattractive shoe alterations in order to equalize a limb length discrepancy, but such lifts are often accepted because, by their use, ambulation is made easier. On the other hand, smaller lifts of 2.0 cm or less are usually refused. A shoe elevation of 2.0 cm or less exerts its effect only during the act of walking or standing with the knees extended. Once the knee on the long side is flexed, the effect of the lift is lost. Correspondingly, when the patient sits or lies down, a shoe lift obviously exerts no effect. The ultimate need for the lift must then be based either on the effect of the shortening on gait or on any symptoms that might possibly result from a discrepancy. These may include low back discomfort and lumbosacral and lower lumbar scoliosis. Low back pain during childhood is rarely caused only by a limb length discrepancy. Whether limb discrepancies by themselves cause significant structural scoliosis is controversial. As a matter of fact, the best available evidence reveals the contrary. Nickel and associates [69] studied two hundred patients having a combination of limb length inequality and structural scoliosis. In 51%, the convexity of the scoliotic curve was directed toward the short limb as one might expect. However, in 49%, the curve convexity went in the opposite direction. Thus, a causal relationship between the two is highly conjectural. Assuming that a shortened limb can produce structural scoliosis, the duration and amount of limb length discrepancy necessary to produce a structural scoliotic curve of significance is not accurately known, but it is reasonable to assume that the greater the discrepancy and the earlier it occurs during the period of a child's growth, the more likely it is that a structural curve may result. Still, it is not known whether such a curve is clinically significant. Therefore, whether to equalize limb lengths by shoe lifts in order to forestall the onset of the development of scoliosis is a moot issue, and specific guidelines are impossible to contrive. It largely becomes a matter of philosophy. I am not convinced that the presence of a limb length discrepancy necessarily means that a shoe lift should be prescribed. Furthermore, it is extremely difficult to establish how much of a lift to prescribe, although some elaborate and detailed tables have been devised as guidelines for shoe lifts.[36] In some cases, complete equalization is undesirable, such as in cases of muscle weakness about the hips, knees, or ankles, because equalization may make the limb so long that foot clearance is made difficult. Thus, it becomes difficult to outline any specific solution to such a highly individualized problem. On the other hand, if ambulation is prevented or compromised because of shortening, an elevation of some sort is undoubtedly required and indicated. Also, if the patient has significant symptoms of limb length inequality, if he or she needs or wants the lift, and if his or her symptoms are relieved by the lift, there is a positive indication for it. These are obviously situations that may vary greatly from one patient to another.

SURGICAL METHODS

SURGICAL CONVERSION TO AN ARTIFICIAL LIMB

Very large shoe lifts, orthoses, and caliper extensions may provide a practical aid to ambulation in cases of extreme limb length discrepancy, deformity, or terminal deficiency. However, a child or parent rarely desires permanent use of an orthosis such as that shown in Figure 19-4. Almost always, a more definitive equalization procedure is desired. Cosmetically, as well as functionally, the most satisfactory solution is frequently ablation of the foot or a portion of the limb in order to facilitate the use of an artificial limb. From a practical point of view, the earlier this decision can be confidently reached, the sooner one can enable the patient to accept the conversion to a prosthesis. As emphasized by Aitken,[3] conversion to a prosthesis is indicated and is most appropriately accomplished when the natural history of the deformity is sufficiently well known that the surgeon is confident of the need for ablation and is convinced that the other methods of equalization of limb lengths are either impossible or impractical.

Shortening of the Long Side

Shortening of a limb can be accomplished in three ways: (1) The physeal growth centers of the distal femur or the proximal tibia and fibula can be arrested prematurely by epiphysiodesis; (2) the same centers can be arrested temporarily or permanently by epiphyseal stapling; or (3) the femur and/or the tibia can be shortened by resection of bone. As with all surgical procedures, each has its advantages and disadvantages, and each has its prerequisites, indications, and contraindications.

Epiphysiodesis

The primary goal of epiphysiodesis is to achieve surgical epiphyseal growth arrest in the distal femur or the proximal tibia and fibula, or both. If physeal closure is successfully accomplished and if the short limb continues to grow, gradual correction of the inequality takes places according to the amount of growth remaining in the short limb.

History. Early studies, such as those by Gatewood and Mullen[39] showed that the cartilaginous epiphyseal lines were responsible for almost all the longitudinal growth in bones of the lower limbs and that their fusion, even if premature, is sufficient to stop any subsequent growth except for that small portion contributed by the articular cartilages. Prompted by such studies, Phemister[73] developed a simple technique for epiphyseal-diaphyseal fusion. In his procedure, fusion is accomplished by excising a block of the cortex on both sides of the physeal plate and reinserting it with the ends reversed (Fig. 19-24). Except for minor modifications such as those suggested by Green and Anderson[42] and Eyre-Brook,[37] who recommend removal of a block of bone containing much more than just the cortex (which thus

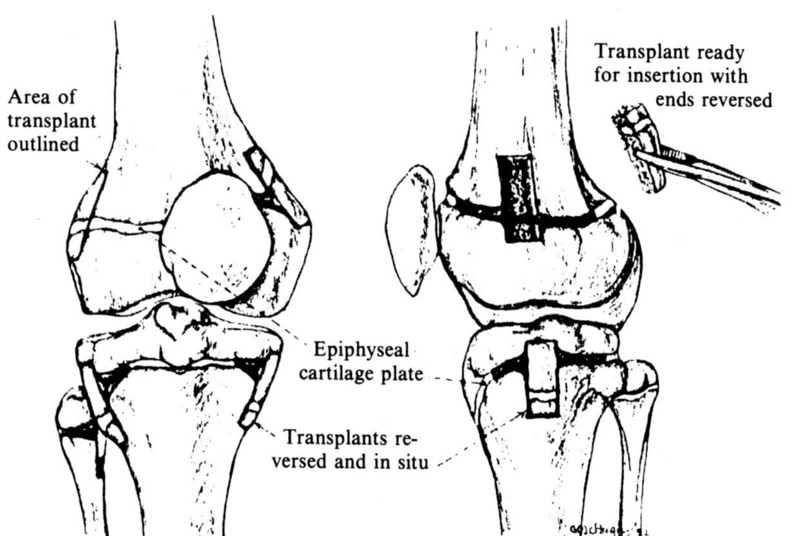

Fig. 19-24. Epiphyseal arrest by epiphysiodesis, according to Phemister. (Courtesy C. Howard Hatcher, M.D. From Phemister DB: Operative arrestment of longitudinal growth in bones in the treatment of deformities. J Bone Joint Surg 15:1, 1933)

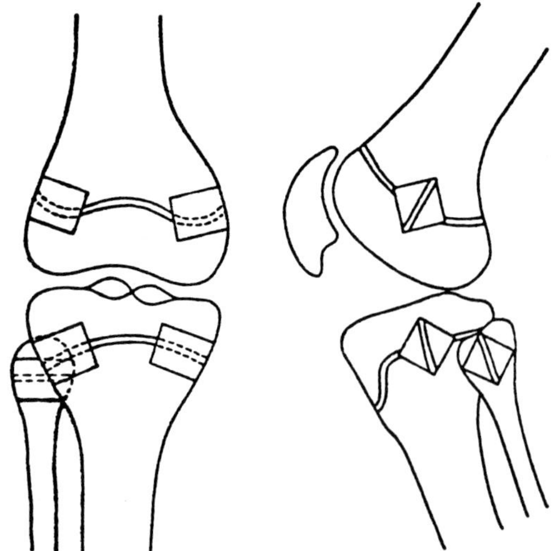

FIG. 19-25. The White modification of the Phemister epiphysiodesis. (White JW, Stubbins SG Jr: Growth arrest for equalizing leg lengths. JAMA 126:1146. Copyright 1944, American Medical Association)

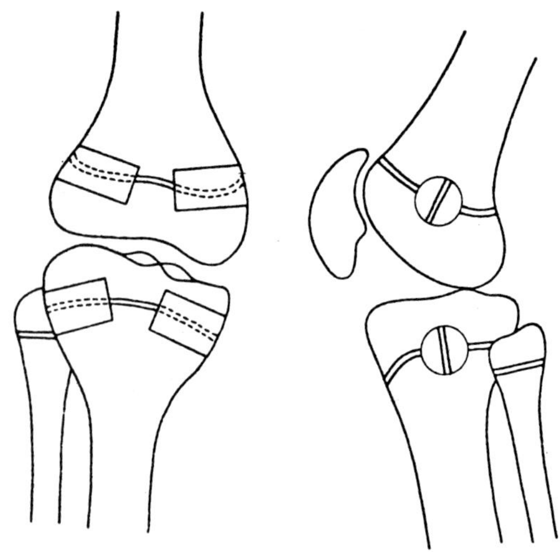

FIG. 19-26. A modification of White's technique of epiphysiodesis. (Blount WP: Trauma and growing bones. Septième Contrès de la Société Internationale de Chirugie Orthopédique et de Traumatologie. Barcelona, 1957)

accomplishes a wider, longer, and thicker fusion), the Phemister technique has survived with very little alteration. Other variations from the Phemister technique include the White modification (Fig. 19-25)[103] and the modifications of the White and Stubbins technique (Fig. 19-26)[104] as cited by Blount,[17] both of which strive to achieve a greater degree of operative simplicity.

Other early literature dealt mainly with various aspects of epiphysiodesis. Green and Anderson[43] stress the importance of accurate assessment of skeletal maturity and expected growth, with respect to the time at which the procedure is accomplished. Straub, Thompson, and Wilson,[88] who carefully documented their cases, signified that "a good result" could be claimed if final length differed by less than ¾ inch or if there was 75% or better correction of the total discrepancy. They found that 10% of their cases developed angular deformities, ultimately requiring surgical correction. This closely paralleled other early results, such as those by Regan and Chatterton,[78] who found that 11% of their cases developed significant deformities. Since that time, more exact operative technique and improved, more knowledgeable planning of the cases have greatly decreased the incidence of deformities resulting from this procedure. Thus, Phemister's simple yet ingenious method of equalizing limb lengths by permanently arresting growth of the appropriate physeal center on the long side in growing patients persists as one of the most effective means of equalizing modest discrepancies in limb lengths.

Indications. Generally speaking, equalization of lower limb length inequality by permanent epiphysiodesis is the most commonly accepted method of equalizing moderate limb length inequalities in North America. This procedure is indicated when the limb length discrepancy is not great and when there is sufficient anticipated growth of the opposite long limb, so that correction of the inequality can be reasonably expected. If expected growth on the long side is insufficient to produce adequate correction, this procedure is obviously not indicated.

Prerequisites. To qualify for this operation, the patient should have a discrepancy not exceeding 5 cm. However, in patients whose anticipated ultimate stature may be greater than normal, limb length inequalities in excess of 5 cm may still be appropriately treated by epiphysiodesis. On the other hand, when the expected adult height is less than normal, or when there is significant discrepancy between chronologic age and skeletal age, correction by epiphysiodesis may be inappropriate or unacceptable. Thus, even though certain broad and general guidelines can be recognized, latitude of interpretation must be exercised when considering equalization by epiphyseal arrest. It must be remembered also that epiphysiodesis is permanent and irreversible, and its purpose is to produce a calculated, premature physeal plate closure. It is necessary that the growth potential of the short side, the skeletal age of the patient, and the anticipated adult height be predicted with a high degree of certainty in order to achieve a good result.

Technique. As noted earlier, arresting growth of a major physis requires that a symmetrical bony bridge be created between the epiphysis and the metaphysis. It must be strong enough to produce a permanent and ultimately complete bony fusion. This is not difficult to accomplish, provided that certain basic orthopaedic surgical principles are followed. The medial and lateral aspects of the distal femur or proximal tibia and fibula (or all three, if indicated) are exposed through a 2-inch vertical, transverse, or oblique incision placed over the center of the physeal plate. The physis is identified by passing a Keith needle through the overlying periosteum and perichondrium into the plate. A flap of periosteum and perichondrium is elevated, exposing at least 1 square inch of the femur, including equal portions of the metaphysis and epiphysis on either side of the epiphyseal plate. A generous-sized square plug of bone (approximately ¾ inch square and ¼ inch thick) which contains the physis and adjacent portions of the epiphysis and metaphysis, is removed. The plate is then thoroughly curetted and drilled, leaving only the peripheral portions intact. The defect is packed with bone taken from the adjacent metaphysis, and the bone plug is replaced after rotating it 90°, thus bridging the plate with solid bone. The periosteum and perichondrium are then closed snugly to help hold the plug in place. The same procedure is accomplished on the opposite side of the bone.

The fibular epiphysiodesis is done by a radical curettage. The bone is so small that removing a plug of bone is more difficult and is usually not necessary, provided that the curettage is thorough.

Appropriately and thoroughly accomplished, epiphyseal-diaphyseal fusion ordinarily occurs within 3 months. There is some evidence to show that a brief period of growth stimulation occurs immediately after this procedure, but from a practical standpoint, it has not been of significance in the ultimate clinical result.

Advantages and Disadvantages. The advantages of this procedure include the following: (1) It is technically relatively simple and has a low morbidity; (2) the correction of the inequality is accomplished by normal growth of the short side; (3) the rate of acceptable corrections is attractively high (more than 90%); and (4) significant complications are rare.

The disadvantages are the following: (1) The patient's ultimate stature is shortened; (2) often the unaffected (longer) limb is operated on; and (3) the operation is virtually irreversible.

Complications. Aside from the usual complications of any major surgery on bone, there are specific potential complications inherent in this procedure, including (1) failure to calculate bone age accurately, resulting in over- or undercorrection; (2) asymmetrical growth arrest, producing valgus or varus deformity; and (3) failure to effect an epiphysiodesis. Most of these complications are rare or their effect is insignificant with respect to the end result.

Epiphyseal Plate Stapling

Haas[47] showed that by encircling the epiphyseal plate of the femurs of growing dogs with wire loops, retardation of longitudinal growth of the involved limb was effected. When the loops were untied, growth resumed. Staples were then used in a similar study in 1948.[48] Stimulated by this work, Blount and Clark[18] published a paper outlining the use of stainless steel staples to correct limb length inequalities and angular deformities such as knock knees (Fig. 19-27). Green and Anderson[43] observed that inhibition of growth with staples is less rapidly facilitated than when epiphysiodesis is used. They also noted the potential complications related to stapling, especially the danger of premature epiphyseal fusion. They suggested that stapling be regarded as simply another method of complete growth arrest. Most of the remaining pertinent literature, such as works by Poirier,[75] May and Clemens,[63] and Brockway, Craig, and Cockrell,[22] deals with the numerous complications that can arise from the stapling procedure. In his review of the number of complications reported in the literature, Tachdjian[89] recom-

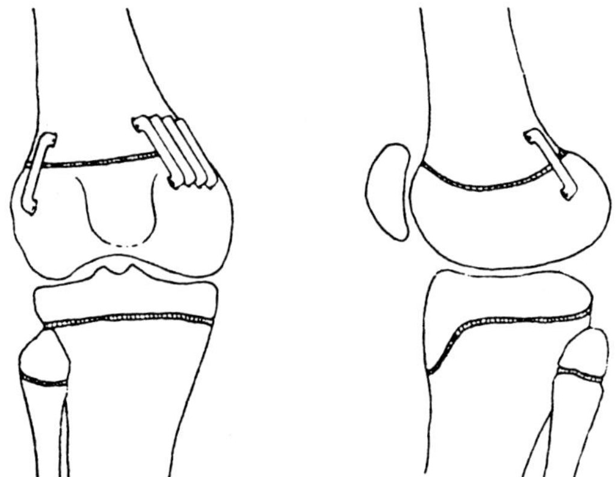

FIG. 19-27. The stapling procedure for angular deformity at the knee. (Blount WP, Zeier F: Control of bone length. JAMA 148:451. Copyright 1952, American Medical Association)

mended that stapling be discarded in favor of epiphysiodesis for growth arrest.

Thus, Blount's procedure of correcting limb length inequality by stapling the physeal plate has achieved dubious acceptance. It was developed with the concept that correction could be accomplished in a younger patient with limb length inequalities expecting a permanent growth arrest. The staples placed across the physeal plate are of sufficient strength that they are able to interrupt growth of the growth center. If equalization takes place prior to skeletal maturity, the staples are removed, and normal growth is then expected to resume. Conceptually, therefore, the stapling procedure is a method of temporarily interrupting growth, which can be applied to younger children who have a significant limb length discrepancy on whom a shortening procedure is considered acceptable.

Indications. According to Blount and others, the best indication for the use of staples to correct a limb length inequality is a situation in which the discrepancy, preferably one that is not progressive, occurs in a child who is skeletally immature, so that sufficient additional growth will take place in the short limb to correct the discrepancy after stapling is accomplished.

It might be noted that the ideal indication for the use of staples in the growing skeleton is for the correction of developmental angular deformities about the knee (Fig. 19-27). However, the author prefers to delay use of the staples until the patient is almost skeletally mature, so that the staples will not have to be removed prior to cessation of growth. This avoids the possibility of overcorrection, in the event that permanent growth arrest occurs.

Because there is some potential latitude in the age at which stapling can be done and because stapling may be safe to accomplish in children who have not yet reached the skeletal age for permanent epiphysiodesis, the operation *may* be indicated in other circumstances, such as: (1) children with limb length discrepancies in whom there is difference between skeletal and chronologic age of more than 18 months, and (2) children with proven static limb length discrepancies who are too young for permanent epiphysiodesis. In light of these indications, the need for physeal stapling is obviously rare, but, in these occasional instances, the procedure may offer a valuable method of temporarily interrupting longitudinal growth.

It is extremely important to recognize, however, that any stapling procedure involving the physis of children older than 12 years of age very often and almost predictably results in a permanent, premature fusion of the physis, and removal of the staples does not restore growth. From a practical point of view, therefore, I agree with Tachdjian that in this age group, physeal plate stapling is an alternative to epiphysiodesis as described previously.

Advantages of Stapling. When properly executed, according to the strict procedural techniques outlined and emphasized by Blount[18] this operation is relatively simple, though technically demanding. Because the subperiosteal and interior portions of the bone are not openly violated, the morbidity is less than in epiphysiodesis. Convalescence is much more rapid because there is less surgical trauma and the bone is not temporarily weakened, as with epiphysiodesis. The patient may resume full activities as soon as the wound is healed and full range of motion of the knee has returned.

Theoretically, the principal advantage that the operation offers over permanent epiphysiodesis is the latitude that it permits for errors in calculations of skeletal age or limb length discrepancy. If it appears that overcorrection might occur, the staples may be removed in anticipation that normal growth will resume on the operative side. Blount has shown that this can occur, but whether resumption of growth consistently occurs following staple removal has not been proved in a statistically useful series of patients, and, in fact, much evidence points to the contrary. Thus, although this procedure possesses a distinct potential advantage over epiphysiodesis because of its proposed safety factor, the reliability of this procedure has not been proved.

Disadvantages of Stapling. As implied above, there are some uncertainties about this procedure that represent potentially serious disadvantages. Whether or not resumption of growth occurs following staple removal can pose a serious problem. However, this applies only if stapling has been done in a younger child, wherein resumption of growth is critical to maintenance of limb length equality. If the physeal plate closes prior to normal skeletal maturity, an obvious overcorrection may occur, resulting in excessive shortening. Conversely, if compensatory acceleration of growth takes place upon removal of the staples, the procedure will not have achieved its purpose. The occurrence of these adverse situations is unpredictable, and the possibility of their occurrence may reflect the *technique* by which the procedure is done more than the procedure itself. If the staples do not have to be removed prior to skeletal maturity, this disadvantage is largely vitiated.

Another disadvantage has to do with the operative procedure required to remove the staples. Even though it appears minor, this operation is essentially of the same extent as the procedure used to insert the staples. Often the devices must be removed, even after skeletal maturity has been achieved, because they frequently are the source of discomfort due to the formation of overlying bursae or simply the palpable presence of metallic structures under the subcutaneous tissues. Sometimes the removal can be difficult, especially if the cross-member of the staple is initially sunk into the bone, resulting in its subsequent burial. However, if they have been properly inserted outside the periosteum, this is usually not a problem.

This operation is demanding on the technical skills of the surgeon, because the staples must be precisely inserted under roentgenographic control. It requires much more meticulous attention to detail than epiphysiodesis, because any significant injury to the physeal plate must be assiduously avoided in the stapling procedure in order to avoid permanent growth arrest. There is also the possible consequence, as stated by Tachdjian, of damaging the periosteum and the epiphyseal vessels during stapling. Therefore, because of the greater technical demand placed upon the surgeon in the stapling procedure, a relative disadvantage exists, when compared with the operation for permanent physeal arrest, as described earlier.

Complications. Because this procedure carries with it some uncertainties, the number of possible complications is somewhat greater than those encountered in epiphysiodesis. The most significant are those that are clearly related to the technical aspects of the procedure. These include: (1) premature growth arrest resulting in excessive shortening; (2) asymmetrical growth arrest, either temporary or permanent, producing valgus or varus deformity (Fig. 19-28); and (3) failure of the devices, or the techniques by which they are inserted, resulting in no growth retardation or correction.

Bone Shortening (Resection)

This method of equalization is reserved for those patients who have a significant limb length inequality but who are not candidates for lengthening or who are skeletally too old to qualify for equalization by growth arrest. This is a much more formidable method of equalization compared with simple growth arrest, because it requires resection of a generous portion of the shaft of either the femur or tibia and fibula, coupled with appropriate rigid internal fixation and local autogenous bone grafting. Nevertheless, it represents a valuable and practical method of equalization in skeletally mature patients whose needs justify its execution.

History. As cited by Goff,[40] the first recorded case of bone shortening was accomplished by Rizzoli in 1846, when he allowed the fractured fragments of a femur to override. The patient was a woman whose unfractured limb was more than 10 cm shorter than the other. The results of Rizzoli's procedure were such that they seemed to justify the use of this method in achieving correction of limb length inequality, in some cases. Throughout the history of bone shortening procedures, a multitude of different approaches are cited (mainly with respect to femoral shortening), which differ more in technical details than in philosophy. Calvé and Galland[25] described an oblique osteotomy with overriding. White[103] proposed

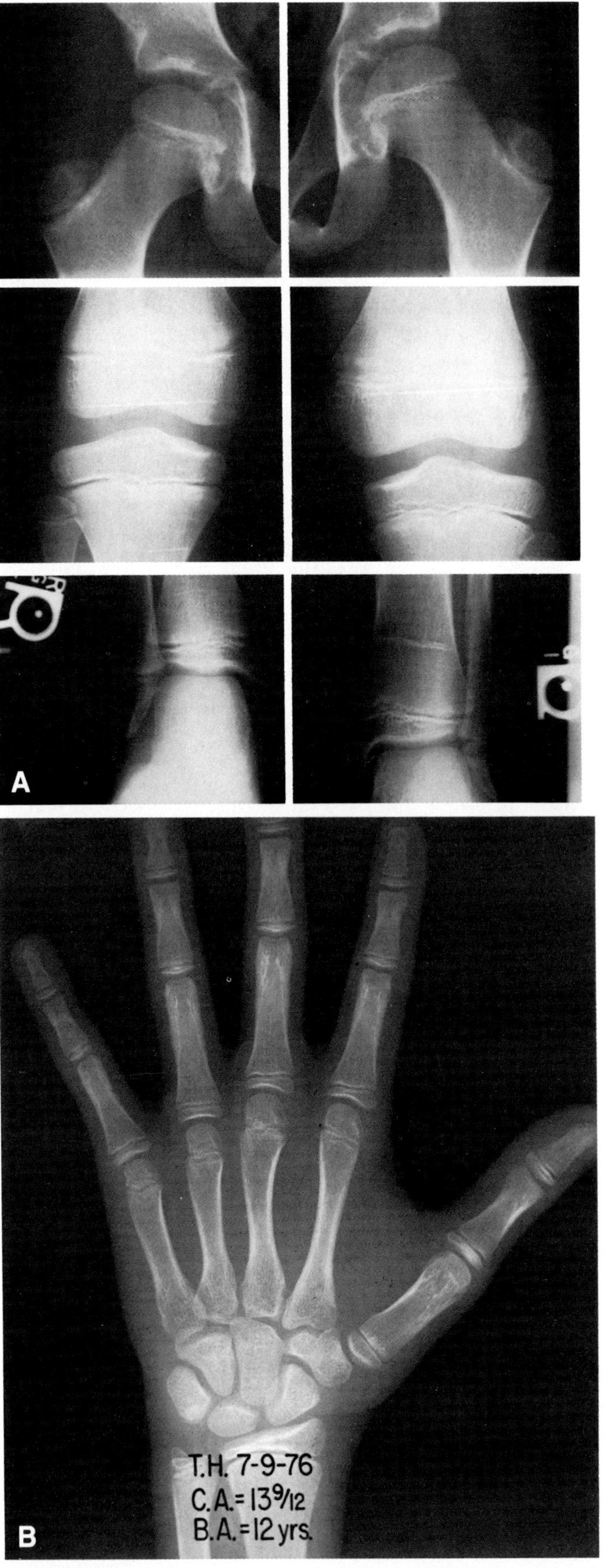

FIG. 19-28. Scanogram in this boy aged 12 years 4 months showed 4 cm of limb length discrepancy *(A)*. A film of the left wrist and hand taken a year later revealed almost a 2-year difference between chronologic and bone ages *(B)*. Therefore, a stapling procedure was accomplished on the distal femoral physis of the long side *(C)*. Almost 4 years later, the femoral physis has fused with almost 4° of varus due to the spreading of the staple tines on the lateral side *(D)*. The physis has fused (as expected), but a small amount of growth remains in the proximal tibia.

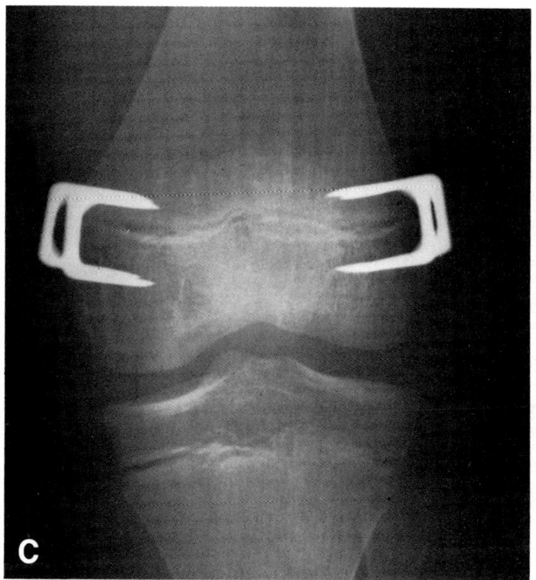

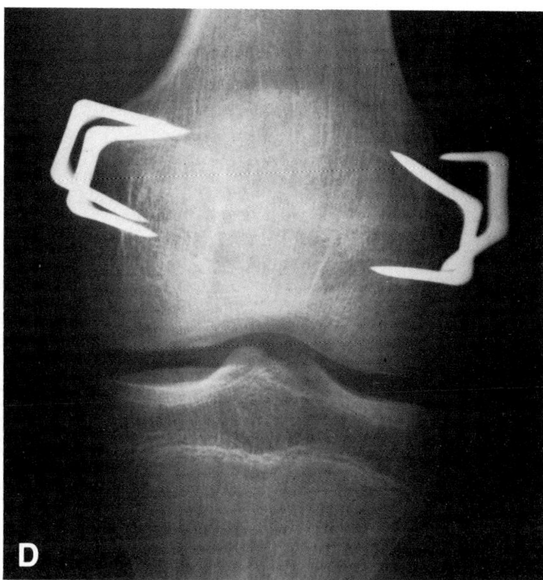

a femoral shortening by simple overlap of a transverse osteotomy and internal fixation with screws. The use of tibial onlay graft following resection of a step-cut osteotomy of the femur was favored by J.R. Moore[66] and Phalen and Chatterton.[72] Harmon and Krigsten[51] also suggested that the excised bone portion be used in creating an onlay bone graft, when performing tibial and femoral resection. Howorth[53] used an end-to-end or step-cut resection, with the internal fixation being accomplished by use of a metal plate. Blount[14] recommended that the shortening be done in the subtrochanteric region, whereas R.D. Moore[67] suggested a method of supracondylar shortening of the femur. Thompson, Straub, and Campbell[90] and Stirling[87] summarized their preference for an oblique osteotomy with multiple screw fixation. Cameron[26] dealt with resection by parallel V-shaped osteotomies, followed by screw fixation. Although not original with them, Merle D'Aubigne and Dubousset[64] preferred using a step-cut osteotomy, with resection of both ends and internal fixation with an intramedullary rod and screws.

During the past decade, a very ingenious and technically demanding method of femoral shortening has been developed by Winquist, Hansen, and Pearson.[106] It consists of midshaft shortening of the femur, using closed resection and intramedullary rodding of the femur. It requires substantial technical expertise, in addition to special devices that can cut the femur by means of an expanding saw, break the resected fragments into pieces, and then permit the shortening to occur over the intramedullary rod. Clearly, this should be done only by those surgeons who have had considerable experience with such a procedure. It does have the advantages of being relatively bloodless and also avoids a scar on the thigh. Its disadvantages lie in its technical difficulty and the fact that the femur must be shortened in the midshaft. This does result in some temporary quadriceps weakness, but, with a proper rehabilitation program, this weakness apparently can be largely reversed.

Indications. As noted above, only those patients who are nearing skeletal maturity or those who are skeletally mature should be subjected to this procedure. Prior to skeletal maturity, the previously described growth arrest procedures performed alone, or in combination with some form of lengthening (when excessive discrepancy exists), are usually more appropriate than bone resection.

As a general rule, such a major procedure as this is not justified unless the discrepancy exceeds 2.5 or 3 cm. On the other hand, no rigid minimal figure should cause a patient to be denied the operation if the discrepancy is less than that, provided that the patient strongly desires it and fully understands all of the potential complications of the operation. I personally have never performed resection of bone for lower limb length equalization unless the discrepancy exceeded 2.5 cm.

Clearly, shortening by resection alone is

indicated only when the procedure can effect equal or almost equal limb lengths through resection of less than 5 or 6 cm, which is about the maximum amount of shortening tolerated in the femur. Therefore, any discrepancy greater than 5 or 6 cm probably should not be corrected by resection alone, but rather in combination with a lengthening procedure. In the case of the tibia, the maximum amount of shortening safely tolerated is about 3.0 cm. In my opinion, the ideal indication for equalization by resection of bone is a skeletally mature patient who is of acceptable height and whose discrepancy can be fully corrected by femoral rather than tibial resection.

Femoral Versus Tibial Resection. Other things being equal, it is much easier and safer to shorten the femur rather than the tibia and fibula. Femoral resection, recommended to be performed at the subtrochanteric level, has the following advantages over tibial resection: (1) There is relative ease of accomplishment; (2) it lends itself well to internal fixation; (3) it requires no external fixation; (4) union is usually rapid; (5) there is little weakening of the thigh or hip musculature, and any resultant weakness rapidly disappears, and (6) correction up to 6.0 cm is technically possible and safe.

In the tibia, on the other hand, one has to deal with two bones. There are complicated fascial planes and muscle compartments, which render the neurovascular bundle more susceptible to injury during sudden shortening of any significant degree. The level of shortening must be accomplished in the middle or upper shaft, which is below the major areas of origin of the leg musculature. This makes at least temporary weakness of the musculature almost inevitable; and recovery of strength takes much longer, if it ever recovers completely. A cast is usually necessary, which temporarily compromises ankle and knee motion. Furthermore, the limb is usually restricted to a maximum of about 3 cm of correction.

From my experience, it is evident that femoral resection is preferable to tibial-fibular shortening, and I have done this procedure almost exclusively, regardless of the portion of the lower limb having the maximum discrepancy (Fig. 19-29). Nevertheless, occasionally an instance may arise in which the discrepancy is exclusively in the leg segment (below the knee) and in which equalization of knee levels is highly desirable. Ordinarily, this is in an adolescent girl or young woman whose circumstances may justify the increased risks attendant upon tibial shortening. When it is done, I strongly recommend that a radical fasciotomy be performed in the anterior compartment, and even possibly in the posterior compartment, in anticipation of potential neurovascular complications.

Technique. For equalization of limb length discrepancy by femoral resection, the author prefers the technique illustrated in Figure 19-30. The shortening is accomplished at the subtrochanteric level, and a compression nail plate or screw plate combination is used for internal fixation. It embraces all the advantages of the various methods of femoral shortening and capitalizes on the advantages outlined further on in this discussion.

With the patient supine on the operating table, an appropriate lateral incision is made over the proximal thigh, with the upper limb of the incision extending to a level 1 inch below the greater trochanter. The fascia lata is split longitudinally, and the vastus lateralis and underlying periosteum is elevated from the base of the trochanter, distally, for about 3½ inches. A drill hole is made for passage of a guide pin into the femoral head and neck, just as in the nailing of a femoral neck or an intertrochanteric fracture. The placement of this guide pin is checked roentgenographically for position. A small trough or "score" about 2½ inches long is made parallel to the long axis of the femur, which is used as reference for control of rotation after the femur is sectioned. The "score" must extend at least ½ inch proximal to the site of initial osteotomy and well below the lowest point of resection. The periosteum is elevated completely around that portion of the femur to be excised. The compression screw is placed into the head and neck, and its length and position are verified by roentgenogram. The primary osteotomy is accomplished, and the appropriate length of femur is resected. The distal end of the femur is brought proximally and clamped to the barrel and sideplate of the compression device. Accuracy of rotation is verified by aligning it with the "score" previously made on the femur, and the sideplate is screwed to the distal fragment. Using compression screw technique, the fragments are then impacted firmly.

After verifying the position of the compression screw plate device by roentgenographic examination, the segment of bone removed is

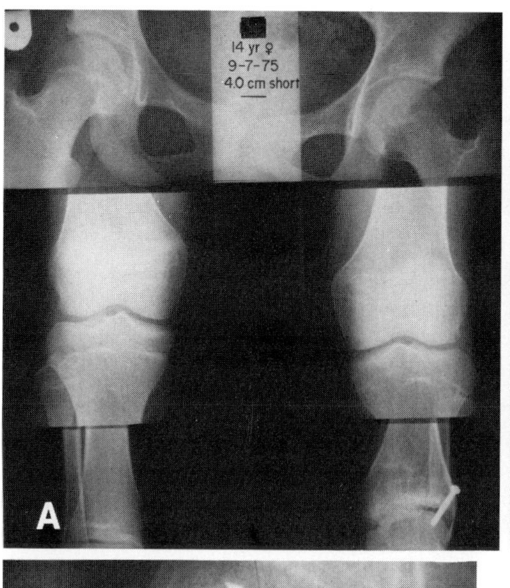

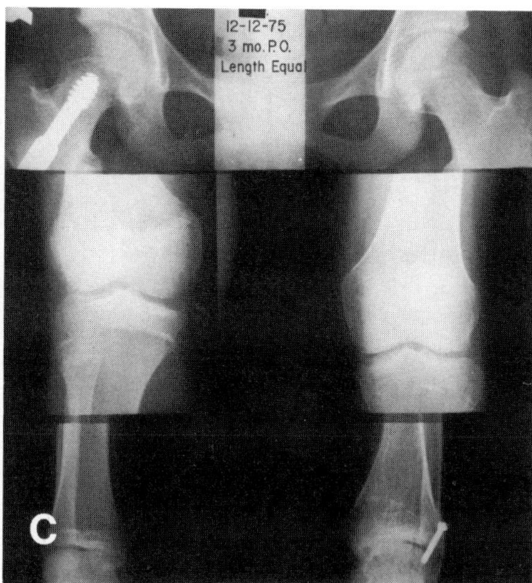

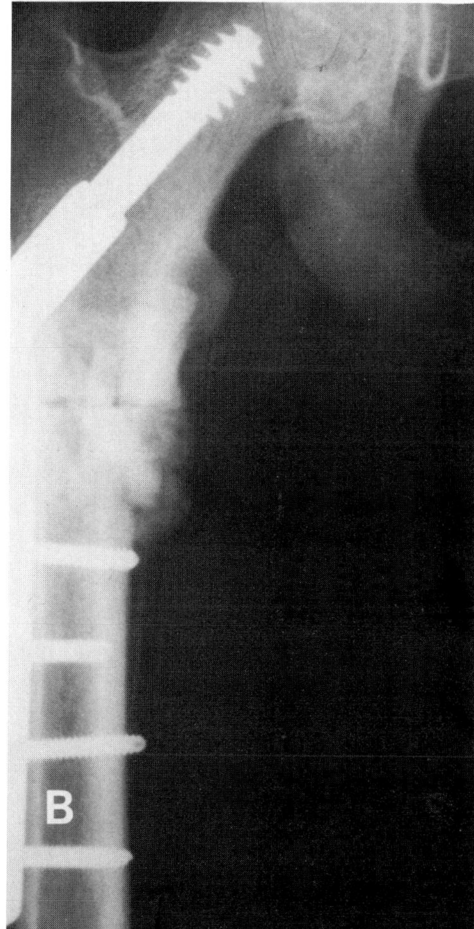

FIG. 19-29. *(A)* The orthoroentgenogram of a 14-year-old female whose limb length difference is 4 cm as a result of a traumatic distal tibial epiphyseal arrest. Correction of the angular deformity in the ankle has been achieved. *(B)* Three months following femoral shortening to achieve equalization, the osteotomy has healed. *(C)* The orthoroentgenogram shows the limb lengths to be exactly equal.

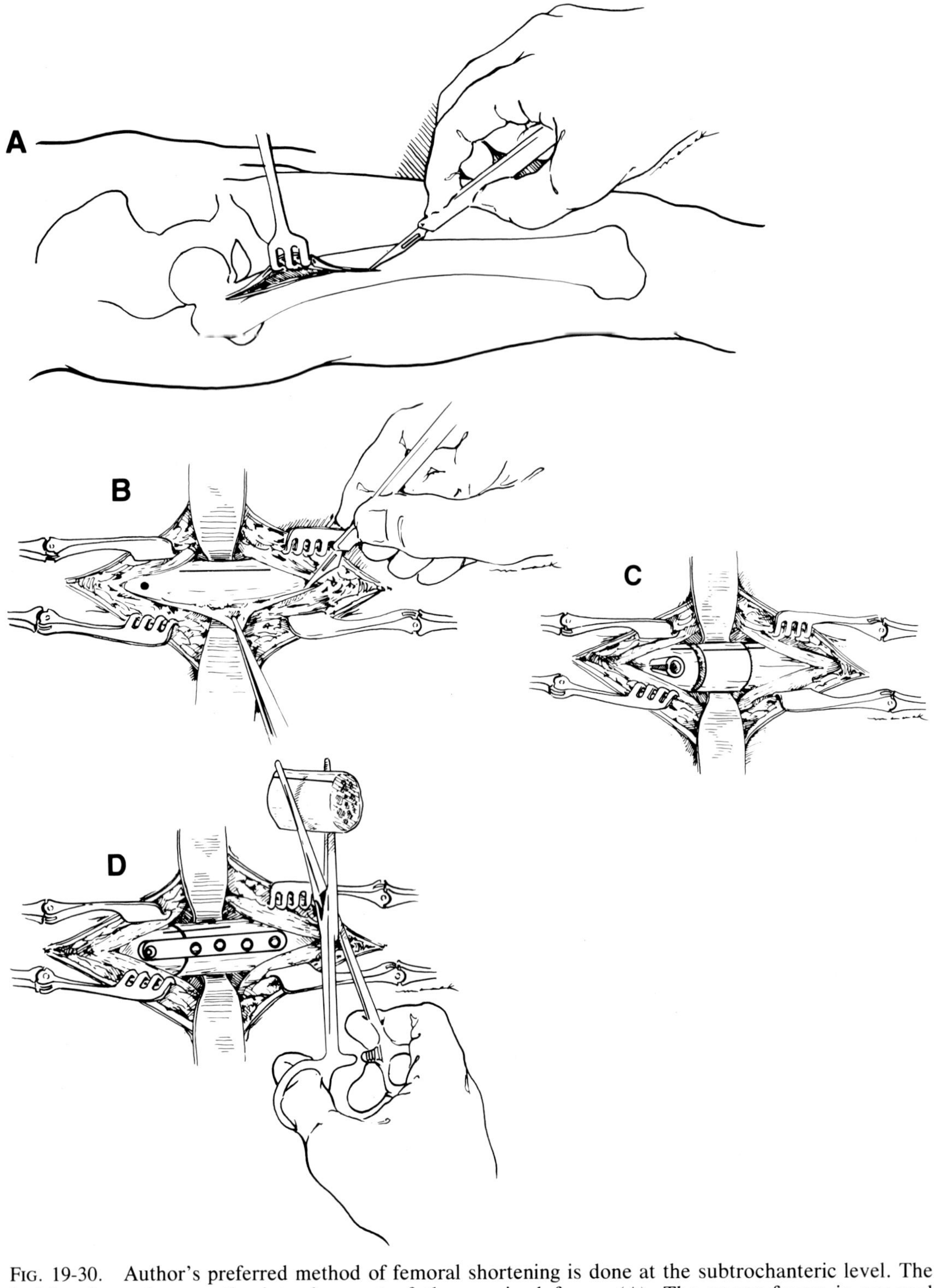

FIG. 19-30. Author's preferred method of femoral shortening is done at the subtrochanteric level. The incision is made over the lateral aspect of the proximal femur *(A)*. The upper femur is exposed subperiosteally and a longitudinal "score" is made on the anterior aspect of the femur. This is done in order to establish rotational orientation *(B)*. The compression (sliding) screw is placed in the proximal fragment, and the appropriate length of femur is resected *(C)*. The side plate is applied with compression, and the excised fragment of bone is cut into grafts that are placed about the osteotomy site *(D)*.

cut into small grafts, which are placed about the osteotomy site. The wound is then closed in layers. At this point, the thigh appears more bulky than it did previously. This is due to the increased muscle mass over the area of resection. This bulkiness gradually recedes as the muscles adapt to their new length.

No cast is necessary, and the patient can be ambulatory with crutches and nonweightbearing on the operated side as soon as comfort permits. Graduated weightbearing is begun in about 3 months or when early union of the osteotomy is evident on roentgenograms.

Advantages. Despite the fact that this procedure is much more formidable than growth arrest operations, there are certain distinct advantages to equalization by bone resection, even in this comparison. First, it can be done at any time after skeletal maturity, and, therefore, there are no time constraints for accomplishing the procedure. Second, a highly accurate equalization can be accomplished, without having to calculate or be concerned about the patient's exact skeletal age. Finally, if properly done in the skeletally mature patient, overcorrection cannot occur.

Disadvantages. The major disadvantages to the operation are (1) the fact that a major resection of bone is required along with a large metal implant or internal fixation device, and (2) the attendant potential complications. Therefore, the preoperative evaluation must be very thorough in order to ensure that the indications and the needs of the patient justify undertaking this major procedure.

Correction of Lower Limb Length Inequality By Lengthening

Conceptually, lengthening of the short side in treatment of limb length inequality is, in most instances, the most attractive approach to this problem. Unfortunately, because of the many problems and uncertainties inherent in lengthening, this method of equalization has justifiably become relegated to a position in which it is only occasionally indicated. At the present time, lengthening by any technique is indicated *only* when the simpler methods of shortening are, by themselves, either unacceptable or inappropriate. However, because there is always the occasional patient who requires both lengthening of the short side and shortening of the long side, or lengthening of the short side alone, this method of equalization will always occupy a small but important sector of our therapeutic armamentarium in the treatment of limb length inequality.

There are two conceptually different methods of lengthening a limb: (1) lengthening by stimulation of growth, and (2) mechanical lengthening. They are widely divergent approaches to the problem, both as to concept as well as to technique, and are outlined as follows:

Lengthening by Stimulation of Growth

Stimulation by creation of arteriovenous fistula
Stimulation by subepiphyseal implantation of dissimilar foreign materials
Periosteal stripping
Stimulation by multiple surgical insult
Stimulation by ganglionectomy (sympathectomy)

Lengthening by Mechanical Means

Lengthening by osteotomy and gradual distraction
Femoral lengthening and tibial lengthening
Lengthening by osteotomy, sudden distraction, and implantation of bone or foreign materials, such as a "spacer"
Iliac osteotomy (modified Salter osteotomy)

Lengthening by Stimulation of Growth

Prior to having developed our currently more acceptable methods of mechanical lengthening of long bones, a variety of methods were used, designed to stimulate growth of the short lower limb. These unpredictable and sometimes risky procedures have now been abandoned for more conventional means, but because of their historical interest, they are discussed briefly.

Arteriovenous Fistula. It has long been known that children with congenital or acquired arteriovenous fistulae or hemangiomata of a limb often develop increased growth in the involved limb. In some situations, the vascular lesions have produced lower limb length discrepancies requiring surgical correction. It is, of course, also well established that disease conditions that produce increased vascularity by means of hyperemia also may produce overgrowth of the limb. On the strength of these observations, it was thought that a surgically created arteriovenous fistula in the superficial femoral vessels could result in stimulation of growth in the shorter limb, with resultant gradual "physiological" correction of the discrepancy.[46,54–56,93,94] In concept, this seems logical, but, from a practical standpoint, the long-term results have not stood up to critical analysis. In general, the disadvantages and complications have outweighed the value of any correction achieved.

Metaphyseal Stimulation of Subepiphyseal Implantation of Foreign Material. Based on the observation that hyperemia and other irritative metaphyseal lesions can produce increased physeal growth, Pease[71] believed that a shortened lower limb could be stimulated to grow faster than the opposite limb by means of implanting dissimilar metals (the battery effect) and other foreign materials in the metaphyseal region of the distal femur or the proximal tibia. In a follow-up review of the patients operated on, the following observations are significant: He found that ivory was the most suitable material for implantation. However, his results were extremely variable. In one case, he achieved 3 cm of correction, but for most of his patients, insignificant or nonexistent correction was obtained. Pease concluded that no valid predictions could be drawn from his endeavors. In addition, Haas,[49] Bohlman,[19] Carpenter and Dalton,[27] and Tupman[92] all experienced disappointments in use of this technique because of its lack of reliability. In many cases, there was actually a loss of growth in the treated limb. The possibility of infection also posed a threat, and, in some cases, foreign body reactions produced such ill effects as flexion contractures of the knee.

It is clear that the complications and unpredictability of results obtained render the Pease procedure obsolete, and it is being mentioned here only for historic interest and to emphasize that it should not be done.

Periosteal Stripping. In 1867, Ollier[70] showed that periosteal stripping of the tibia stimulated growth. Since that time, there has been periodic interest in the procedure as a possible mode of treating limb length inequality.[59] Despite multiple experimental and clinical trials in the past,[107] it appears that the merit of the procedure is negligible, because the effect of the stripping lasts only a few weeks following the operation and the most length that can be gained is a few millimeters.

Multiple Surgical Insults. It is a well-known fact that "overgrowth" of the limb often follows fracture repair in the long bones of young children. This can be observed clinically, especially in patients with femoral fractures who are younger than 12 years of age.[8,15,16] If the fractured ends are anatomically reduced, a limb length discrepancy may result due to overgrowth, presumably as the result of hyperemia of the reparative process. Such overgrowth is not uniformly predictable, even though a rather consistent pattern is identified following certain fractures of the femur. Although overgrowth following a variety of limb fractures has been reported, it would appear that the greatest incidence of overgrowth follows fractures of the proximal diaphysis. Most records show an average of about 1 cm of overgrowth occurring in the first year following the fracture.[83] However, more extensive lengthening has been reported in cases in which the fracture initially resulted in shortening of 1 cm or greater. Most investigators believe that accelerated growth lasts only as long as the healing process, usually about 1 year.

Despite a substantial number of investigative efforts to explore the practicality of this mode of lengthening, there is little statistically valid evidence to support a program that is designed to stimulate bone growth by surgical trauma alone.

Ganglionectomy or Sympathectomy. Due to the frequent "coldness" associated with the polio limb, wherein frequently there is shortening, and in view of the contrary observation that lesions associated with increased vascularity sometimes produce overgrowth of an involved limb, it has been proposed that sympathectomy might enhance growth of shortened limbs. The literature on treatment of the limb length inequalities associated with poliomyelitis by means of sympathetic ganglionectomy is controversial. Harris and McDonald[52] failed to effect growth stimulation by this means in animals, but they observed favorable results in children under highly controlled conditions. Barr and associates[10] also reported some degree of success but advocated that the procedure be used only in conjunction with other equalization procedures. Opponents to the use of sympathetic ganglionectomy for limb growth stimulation include Bisgard,[12] Fahey,[38] and Green.[42] I believe that the procedure is unreliable in producing limb growth stimulation and should be used only when it is otherwise desirable to stimulate circulation to the limb.

Lengthening by Electrical Stimulation. Wagner[100] stated that he used electrical stimulation of the bones of a shortened lower limb on several patients. He reported no success with this method of stimulation. I have had no experience with this technique, and I know of no reports in the literature dealing with electrical stimulation of growth that demonstrated proven and predictable results.

Mechanical Lengthening

It is my opinion that this method of lower limb elongation is the most proven and reliable method, despite the many controversies surrounding the indications and potential complications of the procedure. Historically, lower limb lengthening by osteotomy and distraction has been highlighted by alternating periods of enthusiasm and almost total rejection. In order to understand and appreciate the qualified acceptance of mechanical limb lengthening, it is essential to review the historic features surrounding its evolution, with respect to both tibial lengthening and femoral lengthening.

History. Codivilla[28] introduced the concept of femoral lengthening in 1905. His technique included an oblique osteotomy, with skeletal traction applied to the calcaneus. Others who used Codivilla's method modified the traction device, such as Magnuson[62] who facilitated traction in femoral lengthening by use of a Hawley table. Putti[76,77] accomplished limb lengthening by initially placing the patient in traction on a Braun frame, passing Kirschner wires through the proximal and distal ends of the bones to be lengthened, and applying traction to opposite ends of an oblique osteotomy. He then used his special "osteotone," which consisted of two pins connected with a telescoping tube and a spring extension device. Abbott and Crego,[1] finding that Putti's device was unstable and offered no control of bone fragments, devised an apparatus consisting of four stainless steel drill pins (two above and two below), a pin guide, and a device that combined traction with a supporting splint. They also suggested a method of tibial and fibular lengthening using a similar device while emphasizing the need for release of soft tissue prior to lengthening. Both Putti and Abbott stressed the importance of directly applying both traction and countertraction to the bone to be lengthened. Despite further improvements made on the lengthening device, Compere[33] in 1936, dissatisfied not only with the length of convalescence following lengthenings but also with the high incidence of delayed or non-union recommended bone grafting at the time of femoral lengthening. This consisted of an onlay graft of cortical tibial bone applied on the proximal fragments of the femur. He also outlined the complications of limb lengthening. Harmon and Krigsten[51] and Phalen and Chatterton[72] believed that bone shortening should be used in place of lengthening because of the many poor results following lengthening. Bost[20] like Abbott, stressed the need for release of soft tissues prior to femoral lengthening. Later, in 1956, he and Larsen[21] proposed a technique of femoral lengthening using an intramedullary rod. Brockway and Fowler's[23] review in 1942 of 105 limb lengthening operations showed that they were in favor of tibial lengthening (Abbott method) and that femoral lengthenings were much too dangerous. McCarroll[61] wrote that the Phemister technique of epiphyseal arrest had essentially made limb lengthening, especially femoral lengthenings, obsolete. He recommended that when indicated, femoral lengthening should be done using a slotted blade and a subtrochanteric Z-type osteotomy. Crego, in 1957, as cited by Goff,[40] thought that tibial lengthening, because of the frequent necessity of secondary heel cord lengthenings and because of muscle weakness resulting from the lengthenings, should be completely discarded in deference to bone shortening or femoral lengthening. Sofield[82] also cited numerous cases of subsequent muscle weakness and believed that limb lengthening was too hazardous to continue. Goff[40] also had given up the procedure almost entirely in favor of other simple modes of equalization. Allan[4] discussed simultaneous lengthening of the tibia and femur but emphasized that knee stiffness often ensues. He also dealt extensively with the complications of lengthening.[5,6]

Despite the fear and unacceptance shown by many surgeons with respect to mechanical limb lengthening, much has been accomplished in the last 30 years to greatly improve the techniques, results, and acceptance of the procedure. In 1952, Anderson[7] published a paper that rekindled much of the lost enthusiasm for tibial lengthening. His procedure consisted of distal fibular osteotomy, a distal tibiofibular synostosis, division of the tibia by percutaneous drilling and osteoclasis, and slow lengthening by means of transfixion pins held in a distraction device. Currently, the most popular method in mechanical limb lengthening is that described by Wagner. His apparatus and the technical details of the operation can be applied equally to the femur and the tibia. It is the technique that I prefer at this time. Westin[102] described a method of femoral lengthening using a periosteal sleeve to bridge the gap in the bone fragments. His findings indicated that the sleeve was at least partly responsible for increased rapidity of bridging the distraction gap with new bone during and immediately following lengthening. Gross[45] and Kawamura and colleagues[58] both recommended bone grafting as early as 8 weeks in the event of delayed union or non-union. On the other hand, Wagner[98] almost routinely planned to plate and graft (if necessary) the femur as well as the tibia once the desired length had been achieved. This was done in order to ensure healing of the distracted fragments and to hasten rehabilitation. Kawamura[57,58] further broadened our understanding of the complications in his studies of 1968 and 1969. It is reasonable to assume that the improvements in our knowledge and technical expertise make this procedure increasingly more useful and practical, as long as the indications and prerequisites are clearly defined and strictly followed.

Osteotomy and Gradual Distraction. Throughout the evolution of lengthening procedures, the method that has remained most consistently acceptable is osteotomy followed by gradual distraction. A variety of techniques has been used, but the fundamental principles have remained more or less constant in all. These technical principles include (1) a semi-open or open transverse, oblique or step-cut osteotomy in the femur or tibia, (2) application of a mechanical distraction device, and (3) gradual (usually daily) distraction of approximately 1 to 2 mm per day. Variations in these basic issues result largely from minor differences in concepts regarding the physiology of bone repair and differences in approaches to the biomechanics of the hardware used. It is reasonable to predict that as our technical knowledge and skills become further refined, current methods may soon become outmoded. However, the basic mechanical approach to the solution of this problem will likely be unchanged for some time to come. Because almost all the principles apply equally to operations done on the femur and the tibia, the discussion of those principles can, therefore, encompass procedures done on either bone.

THE OSTEOTOMY. For many years, the technique of osteotomy involved subperiosteal exposure of the shaft of the tibia or femur, followed by either a step-cut or an oblique osteotomy. This technique is still preferred in some modern lengthening procedures. By serendipity, Anderson[7] developed a method of percutaneous osteoclasis when one of his patients scheduled for a tibial lengthening sustained a closed, transverse fracture of the tibia of the short limb. He applied the distraction device and proceeded to lengthen the tibia without open surgery. Rapid union ensued, and, since that time, the technique of percutaneous drilling and "semi-closed" osteoclasis has become a well-established method of osteotomy. The potential advantages of this technique over the open method are theoretical and can be listed as follows: (1) The magnitude of the surgery is lessened, (2) wide exposure of bone is avoided, and (3) the environment of a closed fracture is simulated. The obvious disadvantage is that the ends of the bone become much more widely spaced during the distraction process than in the step-cut or the open, oblique osteotomy. Wagner[95] prefers to make an open transverse osteotomy at which time the periosteum and the intermuscular septa and interosseous membrane (in tibial lengthening) are sectioned completely. This makes it an easier and, in my experience, a less painful elongation. Despite the arguments that may support one method over the other, it has not been unequivocally proved that the union is more rapid or more certain with anyone of these techniques of osteotomy, and there is evidence to support either of the techniques. Therefore, as far as can be determined at present, the surgeon may confidently choose the type of osteotomy that lends itself best to the specific aspects of a particular lengthening technique or device.

THE DISTRACTION DEVICE. Many distraction devices have been developed over the years in an effort to provide a reliable, simple, and uncomplicated means of separating the bones. All the devices currently being used have several features in common: (1) two skeletal transfixion pins above and below the osteotomy; (2) some mechanism for controlling angulation, rotation, and displacement during distraction; and (3) parallel longitudinal threaded rods for systematic and controlled separation of the transfixed bony fragments (Fig. 19-31).

THE PROGRAM OF DISTRACTION. There are two well-accepted axioms regarding the distraction

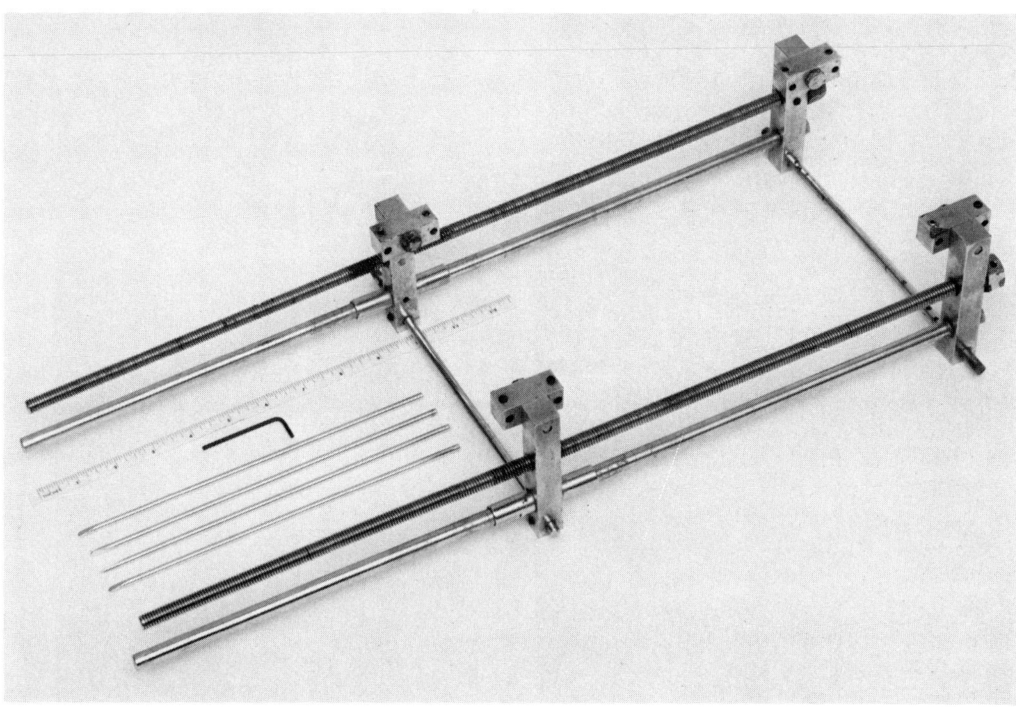

FIG. 19-31. The tibial lengthening device that we used prior to adopting the Wagner technique. The two uprights are held by two longitudinal steel rods, one smooth and one threaded. The uprights are then connected by two transverse steel rods, which maintain the uprights perpendicular to each other. Also illustrated are the 5/32-inch smooth Steinmann pins and the Allen wrench.

process. One has to do with the rate of lengthening and the other has to do with the ultimate limits of distraction (or lengthening). The guidelines regarding rapidity of lengthening are less well established, and there is a fairly wide degree of latitude governing this parameter. For example, the difficulty of achieving the desired amount of length is much greater and the problem and complication rate much higher in discrepancies of *congenital* or *developmental* etiology than in those resulting from *acquired* cause. This is a well-known and now well-established observation that reinforces the concept that each case must be individualized with respect to the rapidity and magnitude of elongation.

LIMITS OF DISTRACTION. In 1968, Kawamura and associates[58] published their findings from extensive research in the field of limb lengthening. Their experiments, which involved blood chemical, histologic, and electromyographic studies, put forth suggestions governing technique, rate, and limits of lengthening. The recommended technique was tibial lengthening, using a small incision, a tube-like elevation of periosteum, and an oblique "subcutaneous" osteotomy. Electromyography of the lengthened muscles indicated that a 10% lengthening of the bone's initial total length was a safe limit, with 15% being the absolute maximum. Beyond this, any increased length resulted in a significantly increased number of complications.

Until Kawamura's study, which established some defensible guidelines, the amount of ultimate length to be gained by lengthening had been arbitrarily set at 5.0 cm, or 2 inches, in either the femur or the tibia. Unfortunately, this figure was used regardless of the age of the patient or the initial length of the bone. Consequently, many complications were encountered that might otherwise not have occurred. My personal experience holds that the maximum amount of total distraction usually should not exceed 15% of the original length of the bone. This applies equally well to the femur and to the tibia. However,in some shortenings of substantial degree, *resulting from acquired causes*, I have occasionally exceeded 30 to 35% of the original length of the bone

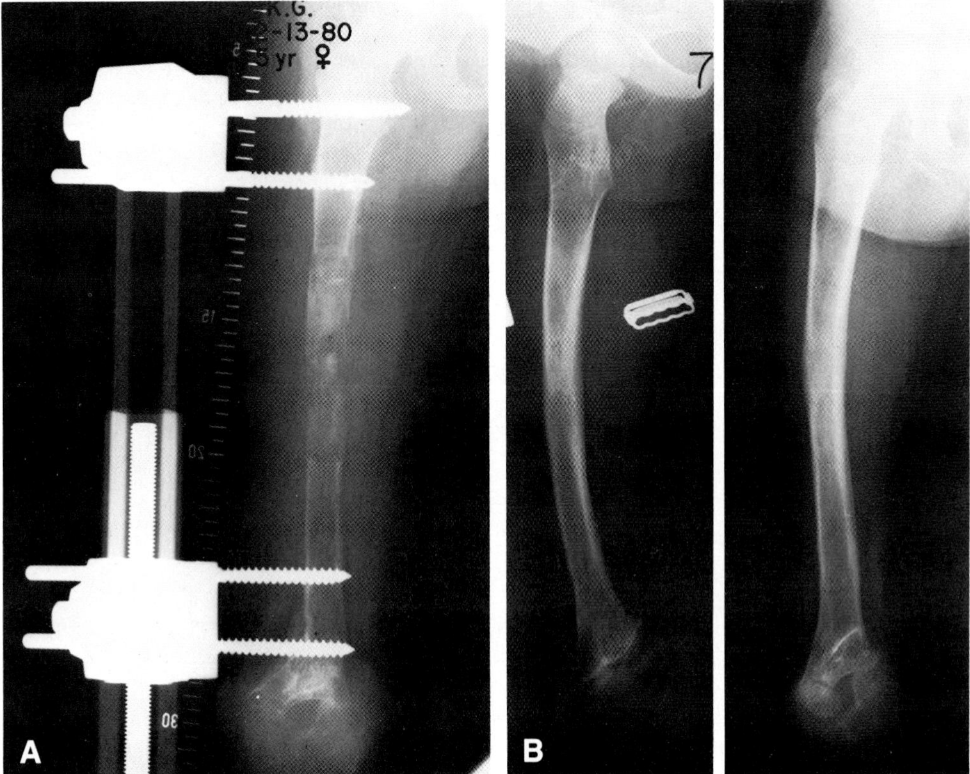

FIG. 19-32. An illustration of the degree of lengthening that can be achieved in an instance of acquired shortening caused by septic destruction of the distal femoral physis. Almost 8.0 cm of distraction was safely achieved *(A)* in this 5-year-old girl who had undergone a below-knee amputation for septic gangrene. The femur united without bone grafting, and the final result more than 2 years later is seen in *B*. A second lengthening was planned to be done in 1984.

without serious problems or complications (Fig. 19-32).

RATE OF LENGTHENING. Kawamura's findings (using biomechanical studies of enzymes of the elongated muscles) concluded that slow lengthening should be done in several stages, with the first lengthening being limited to 3% of the total bone length. This should be done during the first 2 weeks or more. He thought that this was the best compromise between the need for rapid lengthening, which theoretically ensures against nonunion, and the need for slower lengthening, which protects soft tissues.

Some children tolerate a more rapid rate of lengthening than do others. Also, some types of discrepancies, such as that due to poliomyelitis, lend themselves to more rapid lengthening than do discrepancies from congenital causes. These are individual circumstances that must be treated accordingly. As a general rule, however, in considering all the factors outlined below, the standard accepted rate of lengthening is 1/16 inch or about 1.6 mm per day. As noted earlier, this may be exceeded in some situations, or, in other instances, this rate of distraction may not be tolerated. Each patient must be managed individually, using certain subjective and objective observations.

The following clinical guidelines are available, which are especially helpful in governing the rate of distraction: (1) the development of muscle paresis, (2) the degree of pain, (3) the development of a sensory or motor neurologic deficit, (4) any alterations in local circulation, and (5) any significant elevation of diastolic blood pressure (above 95 mm). These facts must be monitored at regular intervals throughout each day of lengthening, and, if adverse signs appear, the distraction must cease or be reversed, if necessary. The reason for most of the local alterations appear rather obvious;

however, an exact explanation of any alterations in the muscles to lengthening has until just recently been somewhat vague.

In a very sophisticated study using electromicroscopy, Calandriello[24] has shown that in order for muscles to be elongated, the fibrils actually have to rupture and then become restored by regeneration. This phenomenon occurs readily under circumstances of slow lengthening, but if rapid lengthening is accomplished, there may be failure of the muscle fibrils to repair themselves, and hemorrhage will occur, followed by cicatrix formation. Therefore, care must be taken in the rapidity with which lengthening is accomplished. Conceptually, because of the greater length and excursion of thigh musculature, it would appear that more rapid lengthening could be tolerated in the femur than in the tibia, wherein the muscles are shorter and have less excursion.

Femoral Lengthening by Osteotomy and Gradual Distraction

This surgical procedure is more formidable than tibial lengthening, has more potential complications, and usually has a higher morbidity rate. Consequently, I believe that femoral lengthening, as herein described, should be reserved for only those patients whose limb length inequality cannot be corrected by any other currently acceptable means. Using this rather rigid criterion, the indications for the femoral lengthening operation will be extremely uncommon. Nevertheless, there will undoubtedly always be a few instances in which the procedure is justified and desirable. Before this procedure is seriously considered, however, all prerequisites must be satisfied and all the technical aspects must be thoroughly understood. In addition, the indications and contraindications, the advantages and disadvantages, as well as all the potential complications must be thoroughly known by the surgeon and the patient.

Indications. As noted above, correction of limb length inequality by lengthening of the femur is indicated when no other method or combination of methods of equalization are acceptable or appropriate. If one reviews the many considerations that are operative in a case of limb length inequality, it appears impossible to provide a concise list of indications with any practical value. Nevertheless, some broad guidelines can be set down that may be of assistance in determining whether femoral lengthening is feasible. These should not be viewed as restrictive considerations, because each patient will present different problems, both physical and psychological, all of which must be put into proper perspective.

It is convenient to group the guidelines under four broad categories having to do with: (1) degree of discrepancy, (2) etiology of the discrepancy, (3) location of the discrepancy, and (4) established or anticipated height of patient.

Degree of Discrepancy. When inequalities of length exceed 10.0 cm, it becomes very difficult to achieve equalization by epiphyseal arrest alone, or even in combination with tibial lengthening. In such instances, femoral lengthening is indicated. If a discrepancy approximates 15.0 cm, the only way in which surgical equalization can possibly be achieved is with a combination of epiphyseal arrest, tibial lengthening, and femoral lengthening. Thus, if one uses the degree of discrepancy as a major parameter, femoral lengthening is often indicated in individuals having 10.0 cm or more of limb length discrepancy; femoral lengthening is *necessary* in those patients with 15.0 cm of length discrepancy if surgical equalization is to be accomplished without ablation.

Etiology of Discrepancy. As mentioned earlier, there are some instances of limb length inequality that lend themselves well to femoral lengthening on the basis of their underlying cause, such as in adolescents and young adults whose shortening is the result of poliomyelitis, fracture with overriding of the fragments (malunion), and premature epiphyseal arrest due to trauma or infection.[74,96] The reasons why these patients tolerate femoral lengthening so well may be due to the fact that the soft tissues and neurovascular elements were at one time longer (in overriding fragments) or were destined to be longer (in retarded or arrested growth). On the other hand, femoral shortening of congenital or developmental origin responds less well to lengthening. In these instances, there may be a more difficult lengthening process and a greater likelihood of the need for bone grafting and subsequent operative procedures.

Location of Discrepancy. Clearly, it is desirable to have equal thigh and leg segments. Thus, if the discrepancy is largely in the femur, it can be argued that the equalization procedure should take place in the femur. Conceptually

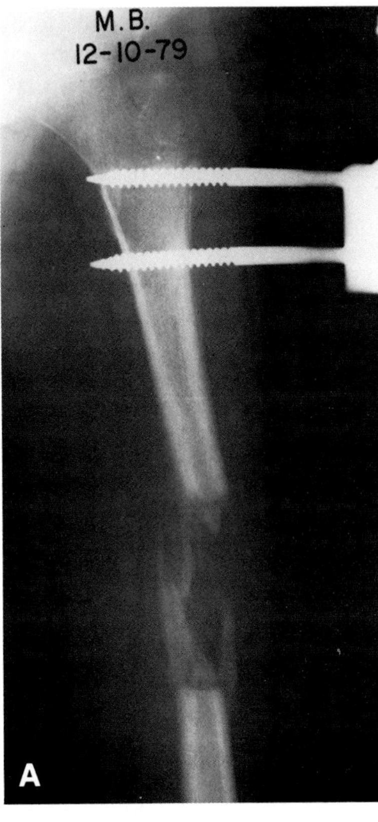

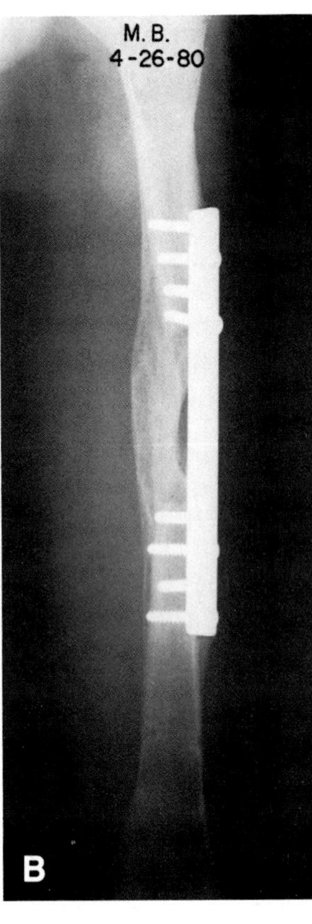

FIG. 19-33. This case illustrates how an unstable hip can tend to subluxate during and following femoral lengthening. The intitial lengthening process in this 12-year-old boy is seen in *A*. After a gain of 6.0 cm, the femur was plated and grafted *(B)*. Because of left hip discomfort that developed during vigorous range-of-motion exercises, a pelvic film was taken, which revealed a subluxated hip *(C)*. An innominate osteotomy was accomplished to achieve a painless and stable hip *(D)*.

this is fundamental, but, practically, the problems of femoral lengthening must be weighed against the desirability of equal knee heights. When all the factors support the need or desirability of equalizing the femoral lengths, lengthening of the femur may be indicated.

ESTABLISHED OR ANTICIPATED ADULT HEIGHT. In patients who have completed growth, this factor can be accurately established. In growing patients, some latitude with respect to the final determinations must be exercised. The principal issue has to do with whether it is more appropriate to lengthen or shorten the limb by surgery on the femur. Faced with comparable degrees of discrepancy, it is clear that in any male patient having 5.0 cm of femoral shortening and in one who is or can plan to be 72 inches tall, shortening of the femur by 4 or 5 cm is preferable to a lengthening procedure. Correspondingly, if the patient is a female and less than 62 inches tall or a male and shorter than 68 inches tall, femoral lengthening may be the more desirable therapeutic program.

Prerequisites. If it is determined that femoral lengthening is indicated, it is necessary that all prerequisites be met before the procedure is undertaken, in order to avoid catastrophic and disabling complications. First, it is essential that there be a stable, preferably normal hip joint. If this does not exist, the possibility of dislocating the femoral head during distraction is a serious concern (Fig. 19-33). Second, the knee joint must have a normal range of motion, or nearly so. Mechanical lengthening of the femur exerts a tremendous force across the knee joint by means of the stretch on the quadriceps and hamstring muscles. Therefore, any prior compromise of motion of function of the knee will undoubtedly be accentuated by femoral lengthening. Third, the musculature and soft tissues of the thigh must be pliable and distensible in order to permit lengthening. Severe scar or cicatrix formation in the skin, subcutaneous tissues, or muscles renders effective lengthening difficult or impossible. Finally, the patient must be normotensive and must have no vascular compromise in the limb to be lengthened. As noted earlier, hypertension may be a serious complication during femoral lengthening. If the patient has an elevated blood pressure prior to lengthening,

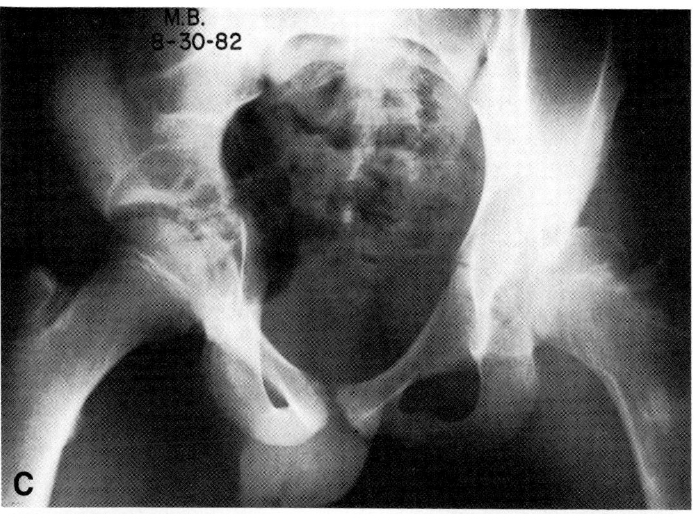

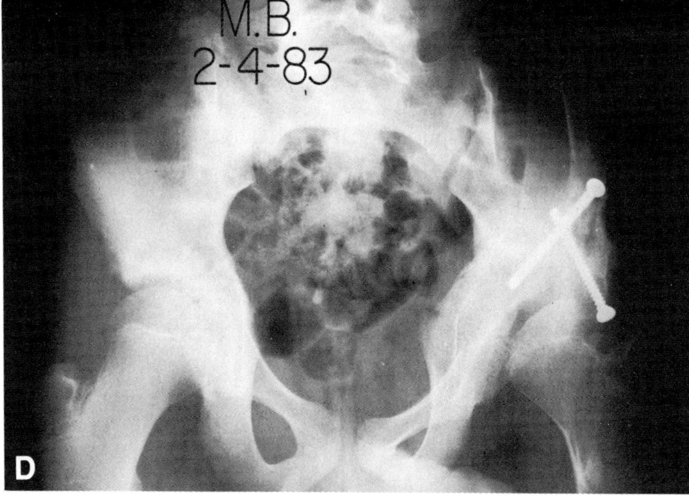

the possibility that further elevation might occur must weigh heavily against lengthening.

Contraindications. It is clear that in any patient whose clinical situation does not meet the indications and the prerequisites for lengthening, as outlined above, lengthening is contraindicated. Also, any aspect of the patient's general health, either psychological or physiologic, that might seriously compromise the femoral lengthening procedure must be considered a contraindication to the technique.

Advantages. There are two circumstances in which femoral lengthening has an advantage over other methods of surgical equalization. These include those situations in which (1) the major or entire amount of shortening is in the femur, and (2) the discrepancy is so great that any other method or combination of other methods cannot effectively or acceptably accomplish equalization. In the former case, its advantage applies to those instances in which it is important to achieve equalization in that particular portion of the limb that is short; in the latter case, the procedure has an advantage because it can possibly provide additional length unobtainable by any other means. Equalizing discrepancies that reside primarily in the femur by femoral lengthening has more than just a philosophical advantage. The alternative is shortening, and shortening the femur in a child who is already short has serious cosmetic and psychological drawbacks. Shortening of the long femur in an effort to equalize a discrepancy in the thigh in a short person may impart a simian appearance to the patient. This is because the upper limbs and the leg segment of the lower limb may thereafter appear disproportionately long when compared with the entire lower limb.

Disadvantages. The disadvantages of gaining lower limb length equalization by femoral lengthening are the complications of the procedure. It is the threat of complications and the seriousness of them when they occur that argue against doing the procedure. These complications are multiple and are probably reflective of the fact that such an operation, generally speaking, is unphysiologic. Because of the importance of these complications, it is essential that they be thoroughly discussed.

One of the major disadvantages of femoral lengthening is inherent in the fact that the technical aspects of the operation are still undergoing refinement. Until the procedure can be made technically simpler and until greater agreement can be reached regarding the best surgical approach, this disadvantage will continue to remain a serious drawback.

One of the major complications includes the effect femoral lengthening has upon the knee joint. Prolonged and occasionally permanent restriction of knee motion is a major concern following this procedure. Knee motion is always seriously restricted during the lengthening process, and, in some cases, it has required as long as 12 months or more for motion to return to preoperative levels. To what extent articular cartilage necrosis is produced by the pressure exerted across the knee joint and whether it is reversible are unknown factors. If one insists upon a daily range of knee motion of at least 60° (−10° to 70°), the likelihood of any permanent restriction of knee motion or damage to the articular cartilage of the knee joint is greatly vitiated or even obviated.

A second complication is delayed union or non-union of the lengthened area. Although such an occurrence may be considered an expected development of the lengthening procedure, it usually requires a second operation, consisting of bone grafting and internal fixation. If this becomes necessary, it represents a technical challenge, due to the fact that it is preferable to do the grafting operation with the distraction device in place. This requires great care, not only in preparation of the operative field but also in clinical judgment to avoid another dreaded complication, namely, a deep wound infection.

Hypertension not infrequently develops during the lengthening process, and it represents one of the most worrisome problems. The cause of the elevated blood pressure is not well established, but it has been the subject of several studies. The elevation is seen in both the diastolic and systolic levels.

Wilk and Badgley[105] were among the first to report an increase in blood pressure during bone lengthening, especially in the femur. They noted increases from normal to 185 mm Hg systolic pressure and to 140 mm Hg diastolic pressure. In 1967, Yosipovitch and Palti[108] studied the phenomenon by experiments with dogs, and they examined records of patients undergoing limb lengthening. Their results suggested that the more immediate rise in blood pressure was probably the result of a reflex response to the rapid tension developed in the sciatic nerve in the upper portion of the thigh during lengthening. The condition was aggravated by the common sitting posture in bed assumed by patients during lengthening. A later manifestation of hypertension has also been suggested as being due to ischemia of the kidney caused by an increased afferent activity in the sciatic nerve, a condition long known to cause reflex spasms in renal blood vessels. Recently, Harandi and Zahir[50] reported development of hypertension in two patients following correction of severe hip and knee flexion contractures due to polio. They concluded that the elevation of blood pressure was mediated by the sympathetic nerves accompanying the femoral and popliteal arteries. Therefore, it is still uncertain as to whether the cause of the hypertension is mediated through the large nerve trunks or the sympathetic nerves that accompany the major vessels. In any event, upon the development of hypertension, specific treatment is indicated. Treatment consists primarily of one thing, namely, cessation of the lengthening process. Occasionally, antihypertensives may be indicated. Most often, the pressure elevation is transient, and, usually when lengthening is interrupted, the pressure returns to normal levels within a 24- to 48-hour period, at which time lengthening may safely be resumed. Although no permanent, irreversible, catastrophic changes have been reported as a result of lengthening-induced hypertension, it nevertheless represents a serious and treacherous complication.

Pin tract infections of significance are rare, but serous drainage about the pins is common.

Unless a deep infection occurs, the only unattractive aspect of the transfixion pins is the subsequent scarring, which is almost always unavoidable. Because of the large muscle mass through which the pins pass in the thigh, pin tract problems and resultant scarring can be somewhat troublesome. This potential complication of pin tract infections can likely be avoided if the incision made for introduction of the pins or screws is generous, especially if these incisions are periodically elongated under local anesthesia if any tension about the skin develops. The elongation of the incisions must be generous and must extend through the deep fascia. Once a deep pin tract infection occurs, removal of the pin or pins may be required. Obviously, if union has not occurred at the time that the pin tract problem is recognized and treatment is aggressively instituted, a major problem exists with respect to maintaining increased length of the femur. Furthermore, such an infection temporarily contraindicates any bone grafting procedure that is designed to gain union. Treatment of deep pin tract infections, which force premature removal of the pins, requires massive antibiotic therapy and skeletal traction to maintain length while awaiting a surgical environment receptive to a delayed surgical approach to grafting and internal fixation. This potential complication has encouraged me to do early bone grafting and plating of the distracted fragments just as soon as the desired amount of length is achieved. In some instances, plating and grafting will not be necessary because of unusually rapid union that may take place, especially in children with acquired femoral shortening (Fig. 19-32). My technique of bone grafting and plating using the Wagner method of femoral lengthening is discussed further on.

There is a miscellaneous group of complications that can be very troublesome, but, because of their singular nature, they must be handled on an individual basis. These include (1) fracture of the lengthened area, (2) angulation with malunion, (3) temporary neurovascular disturbances during the lengthening process, and (4) the occurrence of some degree of knee instability. All these adverse situations must be recognized as early as possible and be thoroughly defined in order to provide appropriate treatment.

Methods. Many techniques of femoral lengthening have been used for the past 75 years, ever since Codivilla of Italy performed a femoral lengthening in 1905.[28] Most of these earlier methods have been abandoned because of serious technical problems and serious complications. In recent years, the technical aspects of the procedure have become more refined, but the operation still offers a serious challenge to anyone desirous of undergoing mechanical elongation of a short femur. The fact that newer and more innovative techniques are being developed simply re-emphasizes the persistent need for a safer, more effective and more proven technique for femoral lengthening. Currently, the most well accepted and proven method of femoral lengthening is that of Wagner, which is my preference. The technique of Bost and associates has largely, if not entirely, been supplanted by the Wagner method, and the technique of Walter Barnes[9] is not yet well established.

BOST-LARSEN TECHNIQUE.[21] This procedure was introduced in 1955, and it has been one of the most popular techniques used during the past 25 years. A vertical through-and-through pin is placed in the proximal femur near the femoral neck, and a transverse pin is placed through the supracondylar region. These skeletal fixation devices are attached to a spring-loaded distraction mechanism designed for gradual lengthening (Fig. 19-34). An open, transverse osteotomy is made at the subtrochanteric level of the femur, and alignment, angulation, and displacement are controlled by means of an intramedullary rod placed downward from the greater trochanter. A periosteal "sleeve" is created at the level of the osteotomy, through which the distal fragment is distracted (Fig. 19-35). Conceptually, this preserves an intact periosteum in the area of distraction, therefore promoting more rapid bone deposition. A pin is also placed in the proximal tibia in order to maintain a fixed position of the femur and tibia across the knee joint. This is done with the intent of reducing the pressure on the articular surfaces of the distal femur and proximal tibia during lengthening. An illustration of a patient who has undergone femoral lengthening conducted by this method is seen in Figure 19-36.

Despite the time-proven value of this technique, there are two specific disadvantages to the operation: (1) the problems encountered in nursing care of a patient with a vertical proximal pin and the large circular device to which the pin is attached, and (2) the difficulty in placing internal fixation across the osteot-

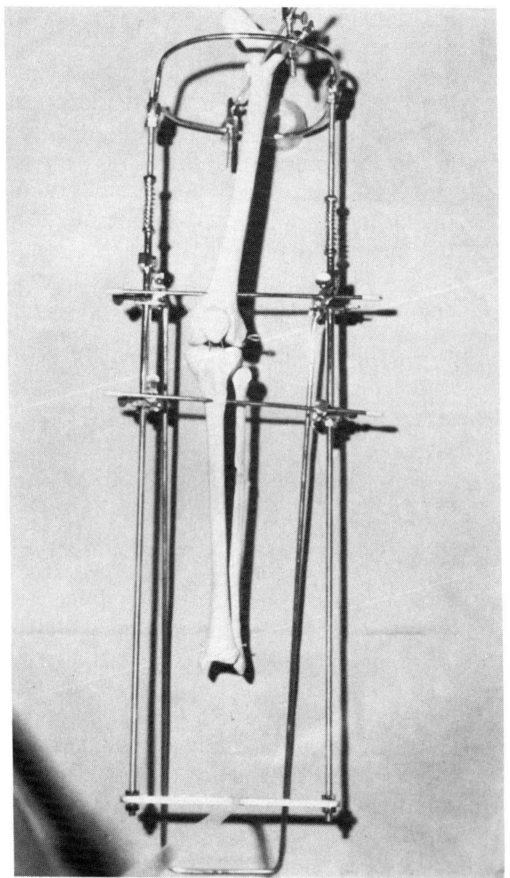

FIG. 19-34. The Bost device for femoral lengthening.

omy site if delayed or non-union ensues or if the pins have to be removed prematurely because of loosening or infection.

BARNES' TECHNIQUE. With this procedure, an internal fixation device (plate) is used that can not only lengthen the femur but also maintain the distracted fragments in excellent position and alignment. The apparatus consists of two plates joined together with one longitudinal telescoping rod. The device is placed in the midshaft of the femur, following a midshaft osteotomy. Primary bone grafting is accomplished using fibular isografts. Distraction of the fragments is achieved by means of a "driving screw" that is turned by a ratchet wrench. At the initial operation, about 1.25 cm (½ inch) can be gained. Rarely, the femur can be lengthened 2.0 cm. At 2- to 4-week intervals, subsequent successive lengthening is achieved by operations in which the proximal femoral wound is opened and the driving screw is turned until 1.2- to 2.0-cm lengthening is again accomplished. The operated limb is maintained in an above-knee brace with pelvic band, and the patient is ambulatory on crutches throughout the entire procedure. Ranges of joint motion and muscle strengthening are encouraged during the lengthening process.

Barnes claims few complications and now has had experience with more than 40 femoral lengthening operations. The maximum gain in length in his series was 2½ inches.

THE WAGNER TECHNIQUE. The limb to be lengthened is approached from the lateral side (Fig. 19-37). A sandbag is placed under the buttock of the limb to be operated on. The greater trochanter is identified, and a generous stab wound is made through the skin at about the level of the lesser trochanter, or slightly above. A template is placed over the stab wound, and a drill guide is inserted through the proximal hole of the template. The guide is placed against the outer cortex of the femur as close as possible to the center of the anteroposterior diameter of the femur. A long 4.5-mm drill is then placed through the guide, and the femur is drilled transversely through both cortices. It is extremely important that the direction of the drill hole be perpendicular to the long axis of the femur. A 6.0-mm Schanz screw of appropriate length is then inserted into the drill hole until it firmly engages both cortices of the femur. Verification of its depth and location should be made by roentgenograms. Using the template, a second stab wound is made at a proper distance from the first so as to receive the proximal portion of the distraction device. A second Schanz screw is placed into the femur, exactly parallel to and in the same manner as the first screw. Its depth can be verified by comparing it to the first screw.

The template is then used in the same manner over the distal femur, or, alternatively, the distraction device may be used if desired. I find it easier to insert the drill guide through the template. Exercising care to avoid the distal femoral physis, if it is still open, two Schanz screws are inserted into the distal femur parallel to the previous two screws. Depth can usually be verified by palpation over the medial aspect of the distal femur. However, the placement and depth of the screws should be verified by radiographs prior to performing the osteotomy. After all four screws are appropriately inserted, the distrac-

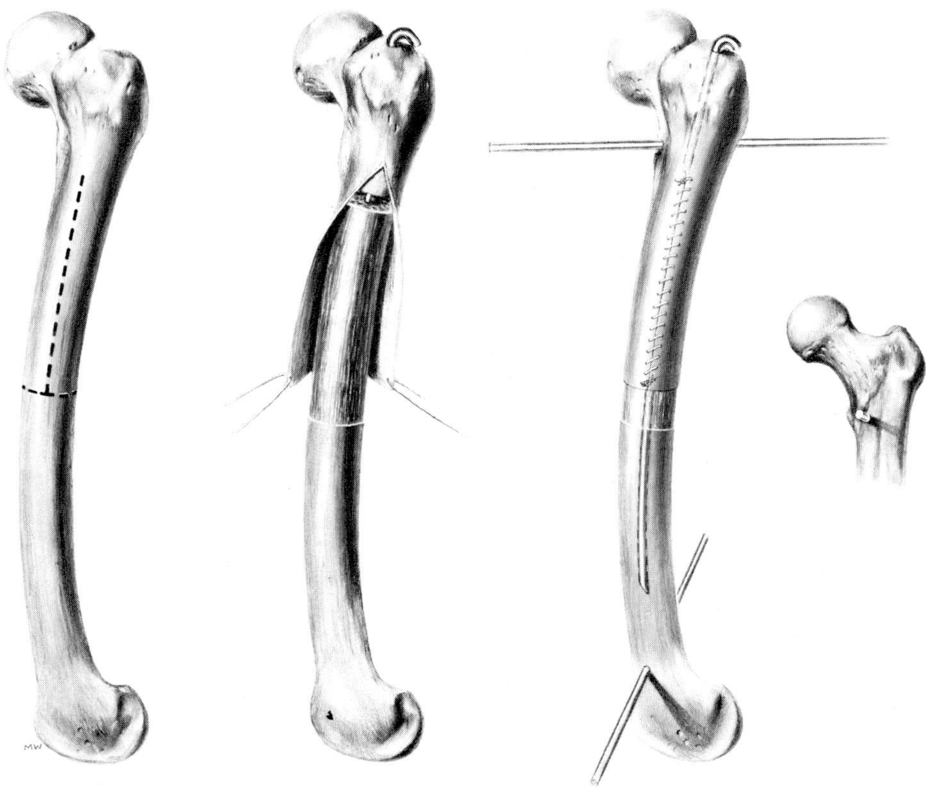

FIG. 19-35. The Bost technique for femoral lengthening, as modified by Westin. (Westin GW: Femoral lengthening using a periosteal sleeve. Report of 26 cases. J Bone Joint Surg 49A:83, 1967)

tion device is applied, and all lock nuts are secured. This is necessary so that after the femur is osteotomized, proper orientation of the fragments will be achieved upon replacement of the distraction device. The device is then removed in order to facilitate the exposure of the femur for the osteotomy.

The knee and hip are then flexed, and a *posterolateral* incision of appropriate length is made parallel to the long axis of the femur, centering over the midpoint between the two sets of screws. The incision should be at least 4 to 5 cm *posterior* to the level of the site of insertion of the screws. This is necessary in order to facilitate later exposure of the femur for plating and bone grafting if they become necessary. The fascia lata is exposed, and it is incised completely and thoroughly both anteriorly over the quadriceps and posteriorly as far as the hamstring muscles. The lateral intermuscular septum is also incised down to the periosteum of the femur. The vastus lateralis is then elevated subperiosteally, over a distance of at least 5 cm. With the femur exposed, the lengthening device is then reapplied, and several turns are made with the knob in order to put the screws on tension. Then a transverse osteotomy is made exactly midway between the two sets of screws. The reason why the osteotomy is best made transversely at this location is because of the possible need for subsequent bone grafting and plating. The latter procedure is greatly assisted by having comparable lengths of the full thickness of the femur on both sides of the distraction defect. Clearly, a step-cut osteotomy would grossly complicate the subsequent use of a plate, if needed.

At this point, I turn the distraction knob another series of full turns, which distracts the fragments about ½ inch (1.25 cm) with the knee flexed 45°. The peripheral pulses are palpated, and the blood pressure is checked. If these are normal, the osteotomy site is again exposed to ensure that the alignment is satisfactory. At this point, it is essential that any remaining portions of the intermuscular septum and periosteum be transected. This re-

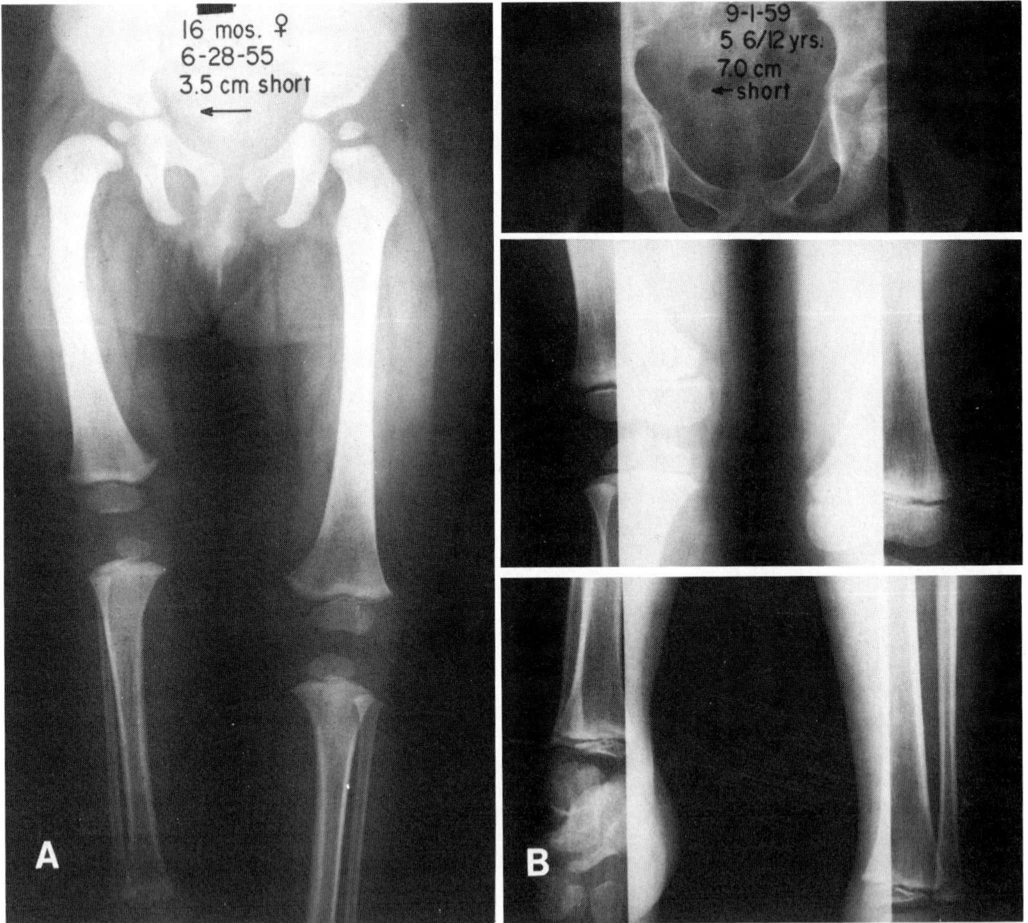

FIG. 19-36. *(A)* This 16-month-old female was initially measured to have 3.5 cm of shortening, due to a congenital short femur on the right, as seen in the scanogram. *(B)* At age 5½ years, the orthoroentgenogram shows 7 cm of shortening. *(Legend continued on facing page.)*

quires great care because of the close proximity of a very large perforating vessel that is commonly found in this location. The wound is closed, but the fascia lata cannot and should not be closed. Wagner recommends flexing the knee fully at the close of the operative procedure in order to loosen any fibers of the quadriceps that might be pierced by the distal screws. At this time, the lateral retinaculum should be *completely incised* at the level of the distal screw with a set of heavy scissors. This is done in order to free up any adherence between the screw and the retinaculum that might hinder knee motion. Whether an adductor tenotomy is done at this time is optional.

Postoperatively, no lengthening is performed until the second postoperative day. Thereafter, the distraction knob is turned one full turn daily (1/16 inch or 1.6 mm). The peripheral pulses, motor and sensory functions, and blood pressure must be monitored at least four times daily. Any compromise of the neurovascular status or any elevation of the diastolic pressure over 105 mm Hg requires immediate temporary cessation of the lengthening and may even require reversing the mechanism by one or two turns. A graph of the daily and the total lengthening that has been accomplished and the neurovascular and blood pressure status should be at the patient's bedside at all times. Also, it is best if only one person accomplishes the lengthening in order to avoid failure to lengthen or overlengthening.

Acute and active assistive knee motion and quadriceps setting should be carried out daily, as soon as symptoms permit. Most often, the

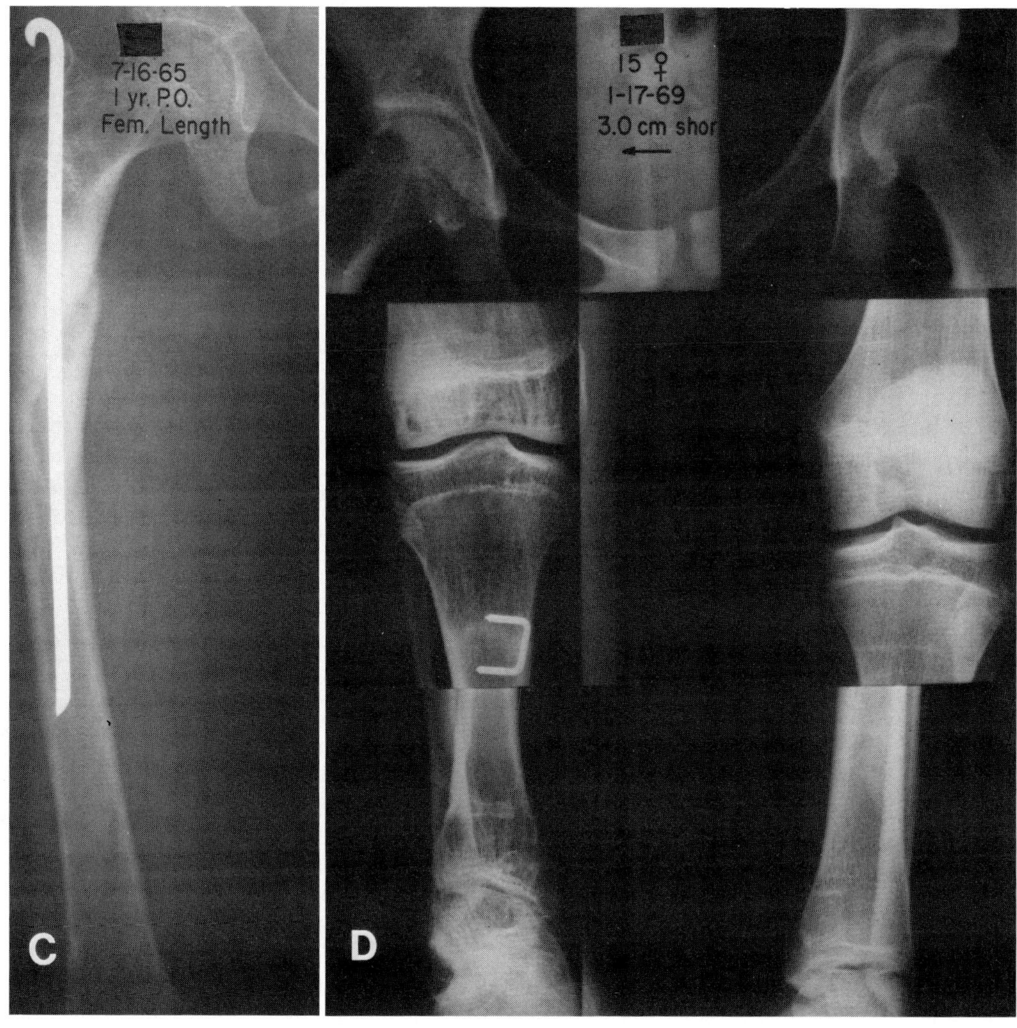

FIG. 19-36. *(Continued). (C)* Due to increasing discrepancy, a femoral lengthening was accomplished by the Bost technique at age 12. *(D)* The final orthoroentgenogram, taken at skeletal maturity. In the interim, a right tibial lengthening had been accomplished, in addition to a left distal femoral arrest.

knee motion is reduced immediately preoperatively and during the period of distraction. This underscores the critical importance of maintaining knee motion during the lengthening process. At least 60° of knee motion (−10° to 70°) should be required daily before lengthening is carried out.[101] Usually, the daily services of a qualified therapist are essential. It may take as long as 1 hour to achieve this motion. However, this range of motion is essential in order to avoid pressure necrosis of cartilage, to provide nourishment to the articular cartilage, and to ensure full return of preoperative knee function. If this motion cannot be achieved, the lengthening process must cease until it can bc accomplished.

Throughout the elongation process, a weekly roentgenogram should be taken to verify the position of the fragments and to confirm the amount of distraction achieved. As long as the screws are in place, daily attention is essential. I prefer a daily alcohol wash, followed by application of Neosporin ointment.

I believe that hospitalization for the duration of the distraction process is essential. Once the desired length has been achieved, however, and the neurovascular and blood pressure status is stabilized and normal, the patient may

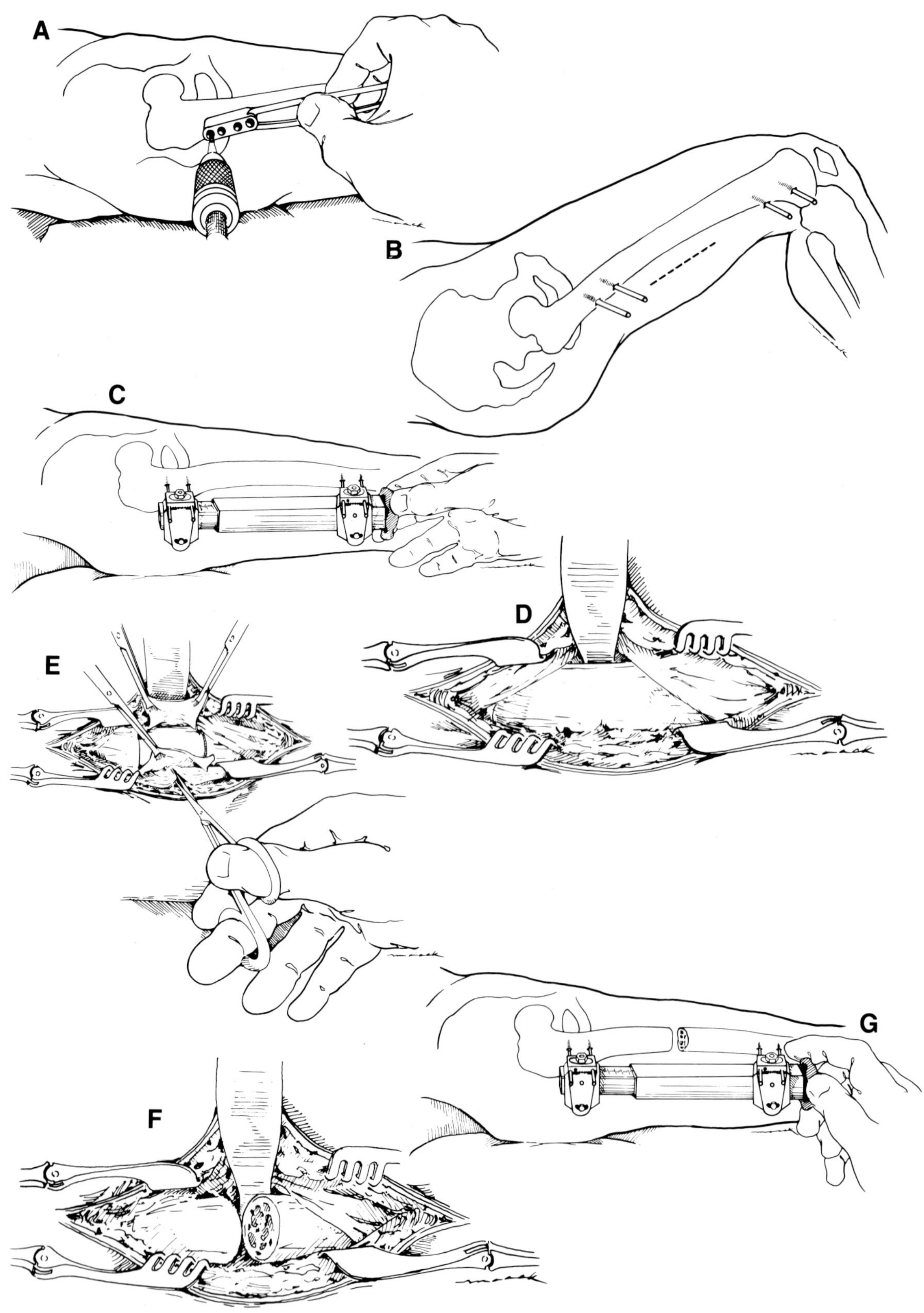
A
B
C
D
E
F
G

be discharged to a responsible home. Ambulation with crutches is optional, but I discourage any activities other than ambulation within the home. Active knee motion is encouraged and should be done as often as possible. At least 60° of knee motion must be maintained daily, as mentioned earlier.

Once the desired distraction has been accomplished, a determination must be made regarding the need for bone grafting and plating. If there is failure of early bridging callus to appear, I favor immediate bone grafting and plating. This permits removal of the distraction device, enhances bony union, and gives greater ensurance of solid, strong union. It also makes increased knee motion possible, because the pins are removed from their location in the distal portion of the vastus lateralis muscle. Furthermore, the limb can be used more functionally, although *no* weightbearing is permissible at this point.

BONE GRAFTING AND PLATING OF WAGNER. If it is elected to graft and plate the distraction defect, it is essential to accomplish it with the distraction device in place. This can only be done safely, however, if the pin tracts are clean and there is no sign of a pin tract infection. This is another reason why an early decision is helpful when contemplating grafting. The longer the pins remain in, the greater the likelihood of pin tract problems.

The patient is placed prone on the operating table, and the iliac crest and the entire length of the posterior aspect of the thigh are surgically prepared (Fig. 19-38). The distraction device is carefully sealed out of the field by sterile adhesive drapes prior to the surgical preparation. This renders the field clean over the posterior aspect of the femur. Prior to making the thigh incision, a generous quantity of iliac bone is obtained through an incision over the posterior iliac crest. This wound is then closed, and the same incision on the posterolateral thigh that was used for the osteotomy is again opened and extended in length. The remaining and regrown fascia lata is incised, and the interval between vastus lateralis and hamstrings is developed. The proximal and distal fragments are exposed subperiosteally for a distance long enough to receive the specially designed 8- or 10-hole plate. The defect between the bone is cleaned of any soft tissue, and the ends of the bone are appropriately denuded, so as to receive the bone graft. The plate is applied, using 4.5-mm hex-head screws, and the defect is filled with the iliac bone. The wound is closed routinely, and the distraction device is removed. Usually no cast is necessary (Fig. 19-39).

Postoperatively, active knee motion is begun. Complete knee motion may not be achieved for several months. In the meantime, solid strong union of the lengthened femur should have occurred. Weightbearing is permitted, according to the judgment of the surgeon. Because of the rigidity and strength of the plate, its removal is advisable at a time when its need has been exceeded.

TECHNIQUE OF PLATE REMOVAL. The timing and technique of plate removal are very important. First of all, the plate should never be removed until a good solid femoral cortex has developed and some degree of medullary cavity has formed. This often requires 1 to 2 years, depending on the age of the patient, the cause of the discrepancy, and the distance that the fragments were distracted.

Because the 4.5-mm screws are of substantial size and because the plate is so rigid, I have made it a policy to remove the plate and screws in two stages. The first is done when the femoral cortex has been formed. One half of the screws are removed, and the other half are loosened by one or two turns. This leaves the plate in as an "internal splint" but removes a considerable amount of the stress-shielding effect of the plate and screws. Six months to

---

◀ FIG. 19-37. The Wagner method of femoral lengthening consists of placing two 6.0-mm Schanz pins in the distal fragment. A template is used, and, with the patient supine, a 3.2-mm drill hole is made at the level of the lesser trochanter *(A)*. The Schanz screws are placed in the femur as illustrated in *B*. They are placed well anterior to the incision for osteotomy indicated in *B*. The lengthening device is applied, but the device should be reversed to that shown in *C*. That is, the distraction bar should be anterior. Through the posterolateral incision, the femur is exposed, just anterior to the lateral intermuscular septum *(D)*. The periosteum is elevated, and the intermuscular septum is carefully severed transversely *(E)*. This maneuver is facilitated by distraction of the fragments following osteotomy *(F)*. The fragments are distracted at least 1.0 cm, and the wound is closed *(G)*.

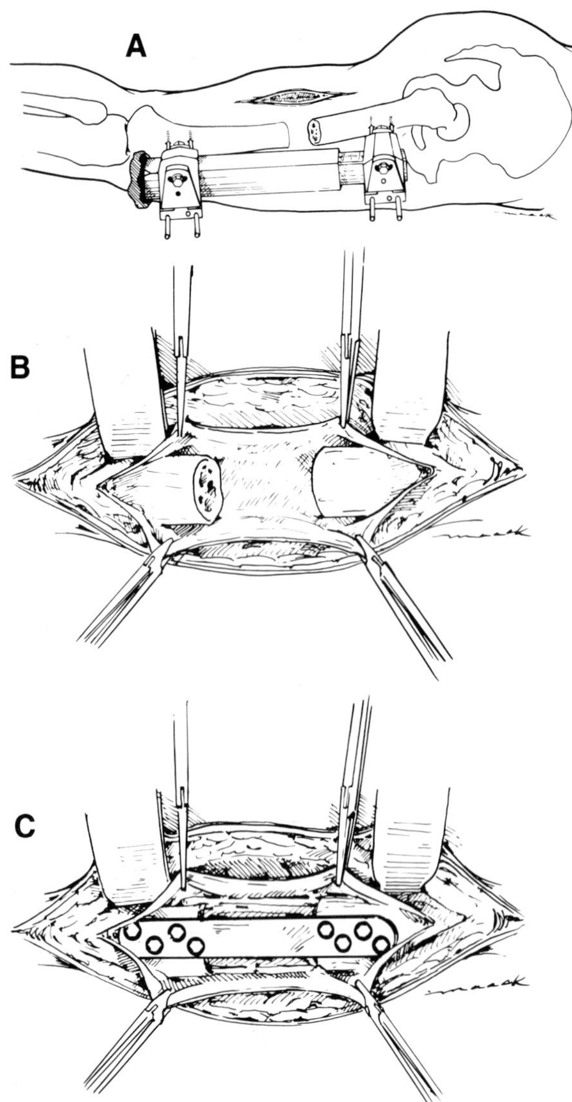

FIG. 19-38. Method of plating and bone grafting the femur following achievement of desired lengthening. The patient is placed prone, and the previous incision for osteotomy is opened *(A)*. The soft tissue about the lengthened area is opened up as an envelope as shown in *B*. The bone ends are freshened, the specially designed eight- or ten-hole plate is applied, and autogenous iliac bone grafts are placed in the defect *(C)*.

1 year later, the remainder of the screws and the plate are removed.

Having followed this program for the past 4 years, there have been no pathologic femoral fractures in my patients, whereas prior to that time, three chldren in whom the plate and screws were removed in one procedure sustained fractures, either through a screw hole or through the lengthened area. It seems that this one extra relatively uncomplicated procedure is justified in view of the increased security that it conveys. It is important to emphasize that following each procedure to remove the screws and ultimately the plate and screws, that the patient should exercise protected and gradually increasing weight-bearing for at least 6 weeks.

OSTEOTOMY AND SUDDEN DISTRACTION. Codivilla's[28] initial effort to increase the limb length by femoral elongation involved a principle of sudden or rapid distraction. This was accompanied by a significant number and variety of complications. Since then, several techniques have been practiced, which conceptually have been designed to achieve lengthening without the prolonged morbidity and technical challenge of gradual distraction. As far as popularity and acceptance are concerned, however, no technique has achieved or maintained the level of acceptance of the

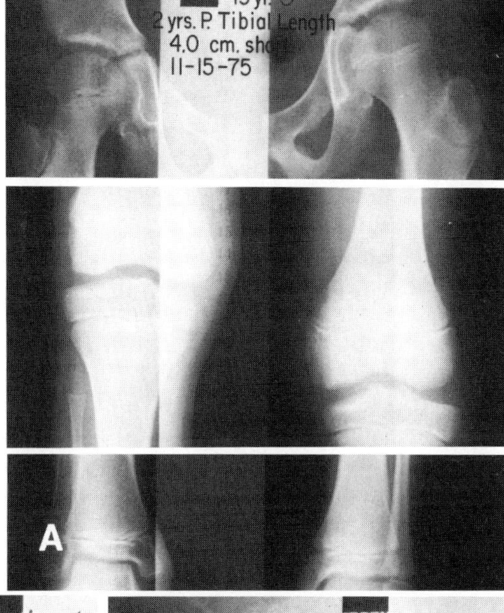

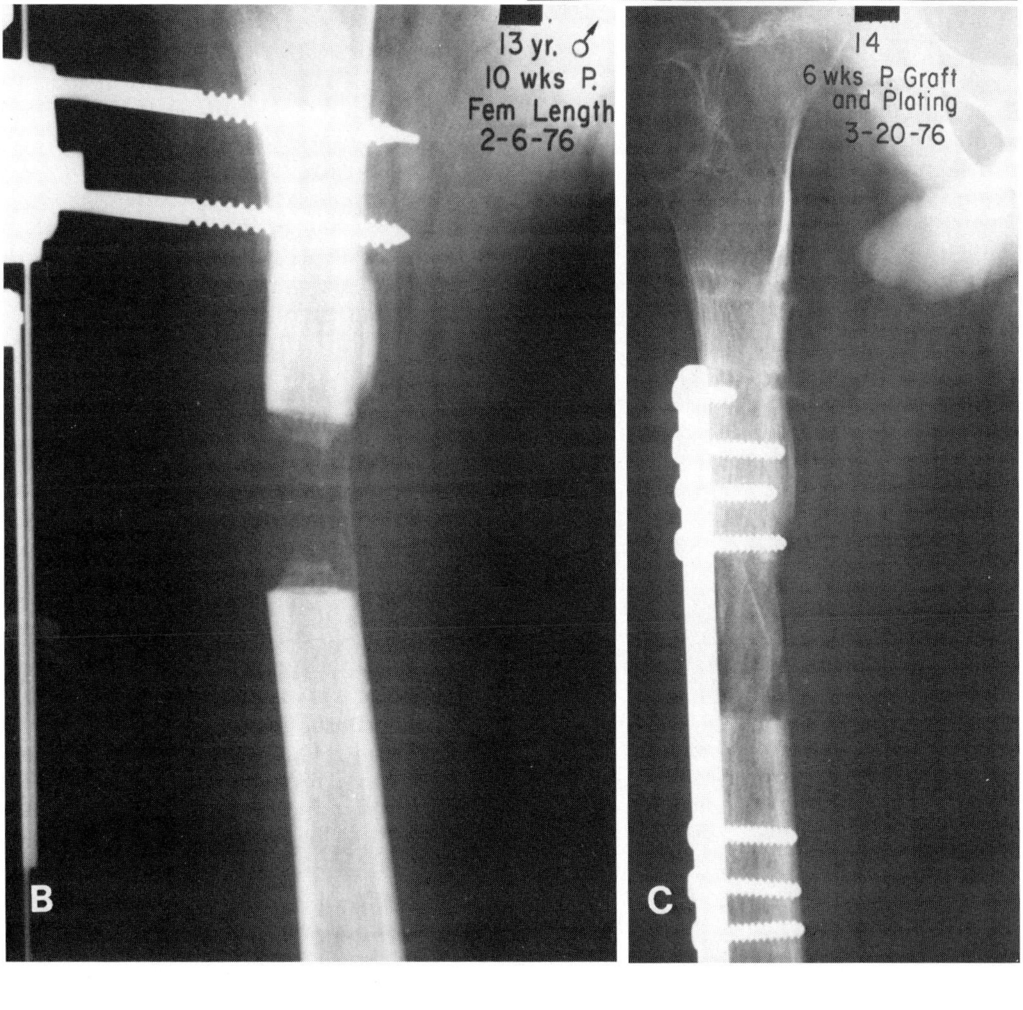

FIG. 19-39. A 13-year-old male with a congenital shortening of the right lower limb who had previously undergone tibial lengthening for a shortening of 8 cm. *(A)* The orthoroentgenogram shows that the lower limb is still 4 cm short. *(B)* Ten weeks after Wagner femoral lengthening, the amount of bone bridging the distracted fragments is obviously inadequate; therefore, an autogenous bone grafting and plating of the femur were accomplished. *(C)* The results of the plating and grafting procedure.

technique outlined above. It is appropriate, however, that each be mentioned with reference to the original source.

Sudden, immediate lengthening of the femur on the short side, along with simultaneous shortening of the contralateral femur has been suggested by Merle d'Aubigne and Dubousset.[64] The technique involves removal of a 1- or 2-inch long full segment of femur on the long side, with insertion of this autograft into a similar distraction defect on the short side. The osteotomized fragments are internally fixed by an intramedullary rod in both femora. It was thought that this procedure could accomplish 2 inches of correction in a single operative exercise. The two negative features that have vitiated the value of this operation are (1) both limbs had to undergo simultaneous major surgery, and (2) the bone graft placed in the lengthened side frequently underwent some degree of resorption. The increased morbidity caused by the bilateral surgical procedure and the lack of predictable equalization are self-evident; this operation has, therefore, largely been abandoned.

In 1912, Magnuson[62] attempted a femoral lengthening on a Hawley table by distracting the bone fragments suddenly at one time. He experienced disastrous results, and one patient actually died of shock. Since that time, no convincingly favorable results have been reported with the sudden distraction technique. Furthermore, as shown by Calandriello,[24] sudden stretch of muscles may produce extensive scarring and ultimate compromise of muscle function. The methods using sudden elongation of the femur, therefore, have not been well accepted, not only because of the uncertainty with respect to the degree of lengthening that can be expected but also because of the serious potential complications inherent in the techniques. I have had no personal experience with any of the foregoing technical procedures involving sudden lengthening, and I recommend that they not be used.

Pelvic Osteotomy. Although uncommonly practiced, and the indication for its use being rare, pelvic osteotomy can be used to gain up to 1 inch of length by sudden separation of the distal fragment of a complete innominate osteotomy. With downward and outward displacement of an appropriately executed osteotomy, little resistance to the lengthening is encountered. The tendinous portion of the iliopsoas muscle must be released, and the abductors must be recessed downward from the iliac crest. All else then moves distally with the inferior fragment. A trapezoid- rather than a triangular-shaped graft is removed from the iliac crest and is placed in the osteotomy defect in the same manner as described by Salter.[79] Two or three large 4.5-mm hex-head screws must be used to hold the fragments in the corrected position while union occurs. In young children, a one and one half hip spica cast is usually used for at least 6 weeks, followed by nonweightbearing and crutch walking until firm union and maturation of the bridged defect has occurred. (Fig. 19-40). The same technical pitfalls exist as for Salter's innominate osteotomy.

When the acetabulum is normal, this procedure should probably be used only in instances of severe shortening as an adjunct to other equalization procedures. The uncertainty inherent in altering the relationships of a normal acetabulum does not warrant its routine use; however, for obvious reasons, the procedure may be indicated in the rare case exhibiting a dysplastic acetabulum. As an extension of this concept, the innominate osteotomy is *always* required before femoral lengthening whenever a dysplastic acetabulum exists. This is done in order that a stable hip can be achieved (Fig. 19-41). It is clear that the need for such a procedure is rare indeed if the above indications are followed.

Tibial Lengthening by Osteotomy and Gradual Distraction

Historically, this is the most time-proven and consistently reliable method of elongating the lower limb. As noted earlier, Abbott and Crego[1] are given credit for developing the basic concepts of tibial lengthening and demonstrating that it is a feasible procedure. It has survived the many controversies surrounding lengthening procedures in general, and currently it remains a very valuable procedure when properly done under the right circumstances. In 1952, Anderson[7] introduced a novel variation in the technique whereby the osteotomy is accomplished through a percutaneous drilling operation. This simplified the procedure and minimized some of the complications that were so feared when the open osteotomy was done. However, for the past several years, the technique of Wagner has been my preference. It involves an open osteotomy just as is

Fig. 19-40. An anteroposterior view of the pelvis, showing a 1-inch gain in elongation of the left lower limb by means of a modified Salter osteotomy. A large trapezoid-shaped graft was used, with no specific effort made toward rotation of the distal fragment. The gain in length from the iliac crest to the floor was 1 inch.

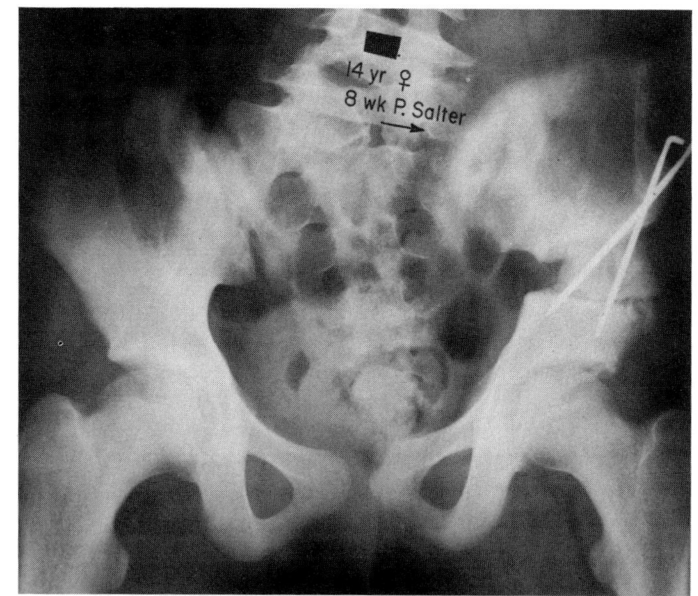

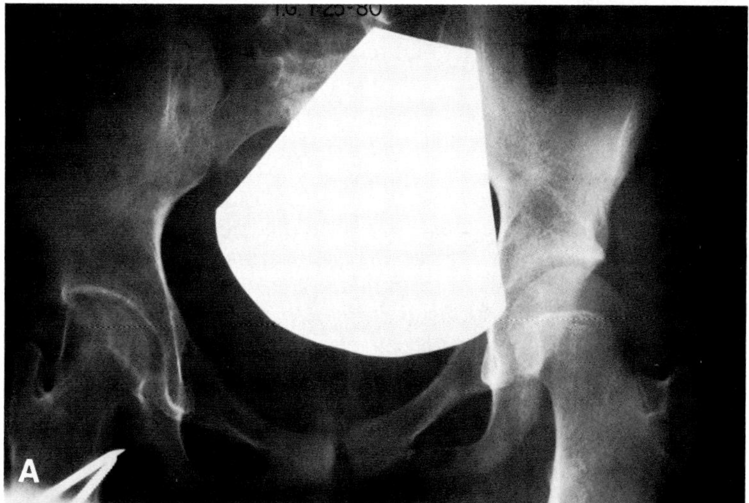

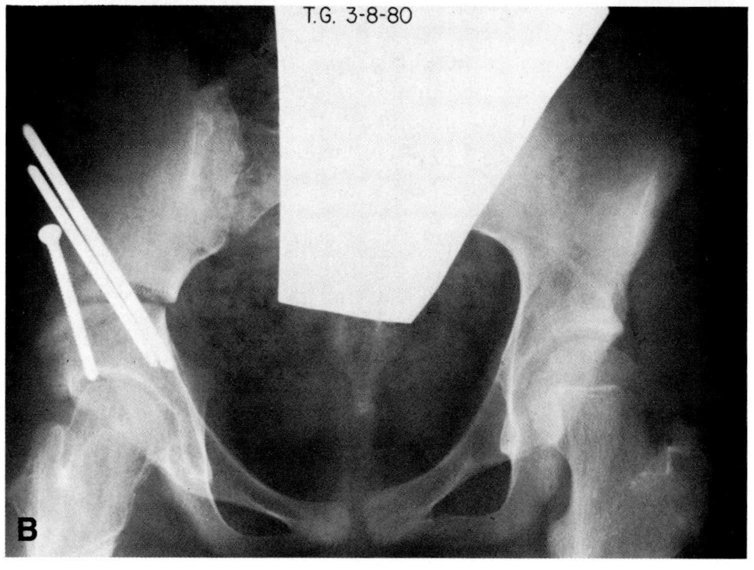

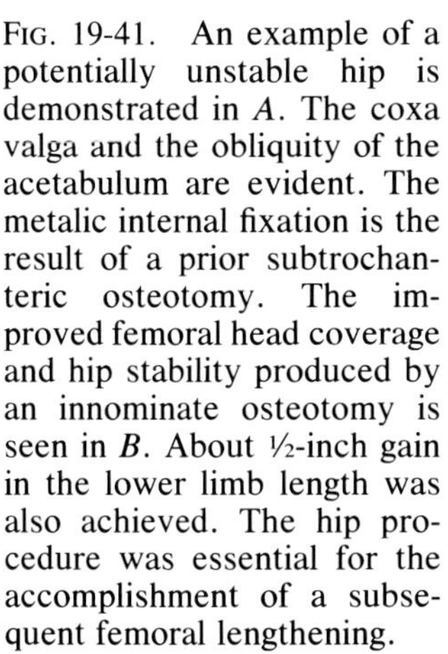

Fig. 19-41. An example of a potentially unstable hip is demonstrated in *A*. The coxa valga and the obliquity of the acetabulum are evident. The metalic internal fixation is the result of a prior subtrochanteric osteotomy. The improved femoral head coverage and hip stability produced by an innominate osteotomy is seen in *B*. About ½-inch gain in the lower limb length was also achieved. The hip procedure was essential for the accomplishment of a subsequent femoral lengthening.

done in femoral lengthening. In fact, many of the technical details for tibial lengthening are very similar to those described in femoral lengthening.

Indications. This procedure may be indicated in one of the situations listed below. It is essential, however, that all the factors mentioned earlier be reviewed prior to reaching a decision to perform this operation. The possible indications are as follows: (1) in a patient with shortening in excess of 4.0 cm, preferably with the majority of the discrepancy being located in the tibia; (2) in a patient whose discrepancy justifies surgical equalization but who is skeletally too old for epiphyseal arrest; (3) in a patient who has a major discrepancy exceeding that which can be acceptably corrected by epiphyseal arrest or shortening alone; and (4) in patients in whom amputation (and prosthetic prescription) is a likely alternative. In evaluating the indications, it is essential that the prerequisites for tibial lengthening be identified.

Prerequisites. Several criteria must be met before tibial lengthening can be seriously considered. The prerequisites can be listed as follows: (1) a plantigrade foot or one that can be made so; (2) a stable ankle; (3) good muscle balance in the foot and ankle; (4) normal vasculature of the limb; (5) a stable knee with a normal range of motion; and (6) a patient who is normotensive, with no serious and evident extenuating physical or emotional problems.

Contraindications. Clearly, this procedure is contraindicated in anyone not meeting the indications or the prerequisites for tibial lengthening. In addition, severe soft-tissue scarring, poor skin condition, sclerotic bone, and instances in which there is a prior history of bone infection or non-union or pseudarthrosis may represent contraindications. However, even these must be viewed with circumspection, since Stelling[86] and I have safely and effectively performed tibial lengthening in cases of shortening due to congenital pseudarthrosis once union has been achieved. However, this is not recommended except for the surgeon who is conversant with all the problems inherent in tibial lengthening, as well as with those accompanying the treatment of congenital pseudarthrosis. The need for concern regarding the other soft tissues and bones is self-evident.

Advantages. Because of the subcutaneous location of the tibia and because of the usual presence of the fibula, certain advantages are present in tibial lengthening compared with femoral lengthening. First, the procedure is technically less complicated; second, the hardware used is much simpler to use; and third, the procedure has fewer major complications, and treatment of them is rendered simpler by the unique anatomy the leg.

Disadvantages and Complications. Lengthening is an unphysiologic operation, and it results in a variety of complications, which must be anticipated whenever this procedure is done. These complications represent the disadvantage of this procedure, as opposed to simpler forms of equalization, such as shortening by resection or growth arrest. The complications and their treatment may represent a very important feature of this section, because it is with these issues that the surgeon and the patient must contend when considering tibial lengthening. In the skeletally mature patient, the complication rate from tibial lengthening is substantially greater than in the skeletally immature patient. Also, as noted earlier, patients whose shortening is the result of congenital or developmental problems have a higher incidence of complications than those whose discrepancy is due to paralysis or the complications of skeletal infection or trauma. It is convenient to group the complications of lengthening as follows: (1) systemic; (2) local, at the tibial osteotomy site or in the pin tracts; (3) local, at the fibular osteotomy site; (4) regional, in the adjacent bones or joint; (5) neuromuscular; and (6) vascular (compartment syndromes).[30–32]

Systemic complications include emotional lability, mental depression, hypertension, anorexia, and weight loss. These are temporary conditions and respond dramatically to cessation of lengthening. In rare instances, weight loss and anorexia persist for several months, but once normal activity is resumed, these symptoms gradually subside. Hypertension does not seem to be as much of a problem in tibial lengthening as in femoral elongation.

Local complications most frequently consist of inadequate union, delayed union, and non-union of the tibial osteotomy site. Judgment is required to determine the indications for bone grafting. In cases of "inadequate union," the distracted area requires grafting when the bridging bone fails to hypertrophy over a period of 8 to 12 weeks (Fig. 19-42). In cases

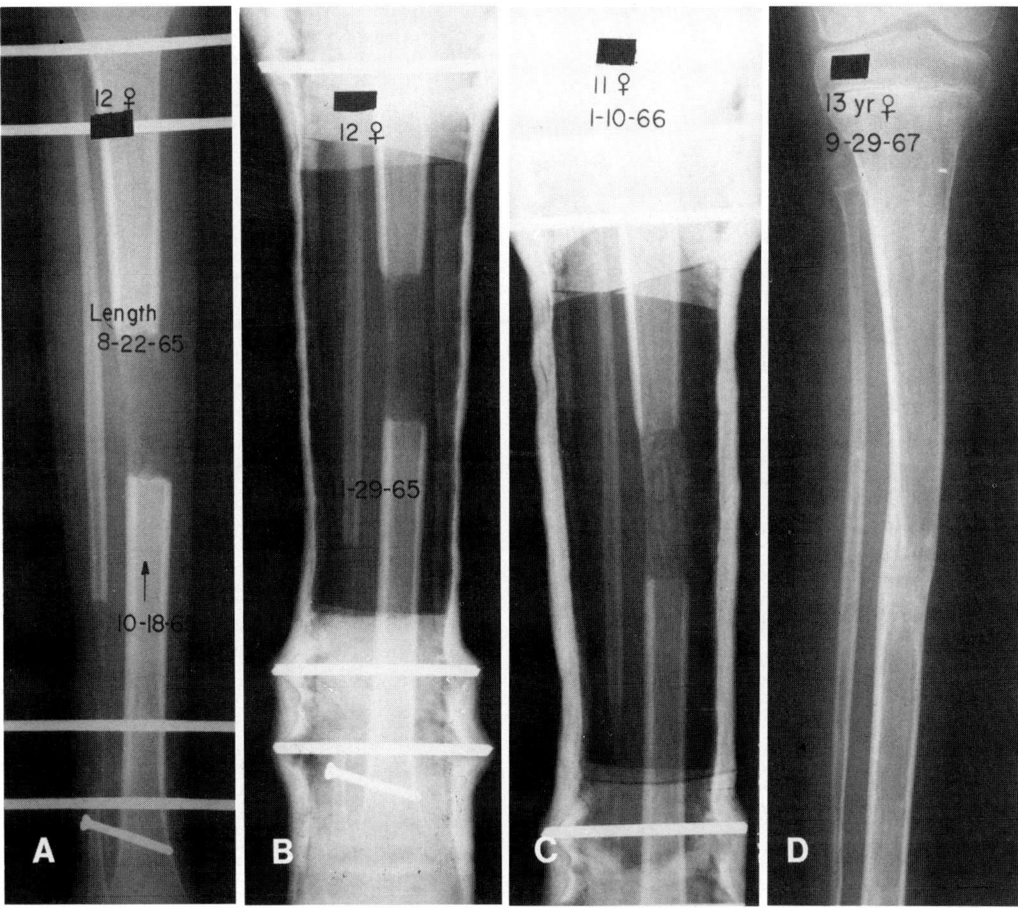

FIG. 19-42. *(A)* Tibial lengthening, approximately 10 weeks following the initial lengthening procedure. Note that there is little bone evident in the lengthened area. *(B)* Six weeks later, there is little increase in bridging of the lengthened area. *(C)* The iliac bone grafts placed between the bone ends in the defect are seen. *(D)* Solid union is seen not only in the tibia but also in the fibula 9 months after the grafting procedure.

of delayed union, usually the bridged area strengthens with judicious use of weightbearing casts (Fig. 19-43). When non-union exists, there is no evidence of bridging bone 6 to 8 weeks following cessation of lengthening, and grafting is mandatory (Fig. 19-44). Other complications include seepage about the pin tracts, which is very common, but a true pin tract infection is rare if appropriate care is given to the pins during and immediately following lengthening. Infection of the tibial osteotomy site occurred only once in our series. When it occurs, treatment must be given according to the usual principles of bone infection. Local complications may also occur in the area of the fibular osteotomy or resection. If the osteotomy fails to unite and if there is remaining skeletal growth, the transfixion screw between the tibia and the fibula must not be removed unless union of the fibula is achieved by bone grafting or unless the distal fibula is fused to the distal tibia. Because the fibula does not grow normally unless solidly united, failure of fibular union in this area results in progressive valgus deformity of the ankle as a result of continued tibial growth and reduced growth of the distal fibula. Correction of this complication requires distal tibial osteotomy and creation of a tibiofibular synostosis (Fig. 19-45).

Regional complications include knee flexion contracture, equinus of the ankle, accentuated valgus of the subtalar joint, and valgus deformity of the tibia. Most of these are revers-

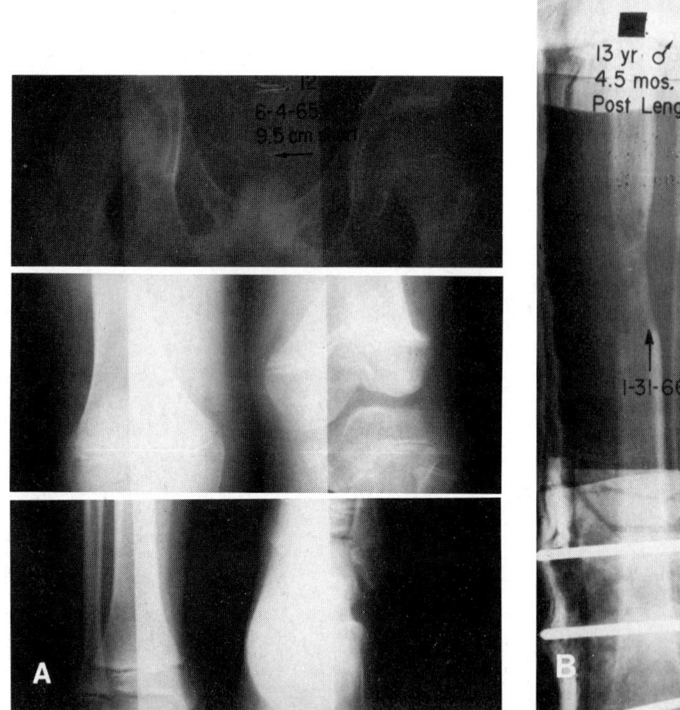

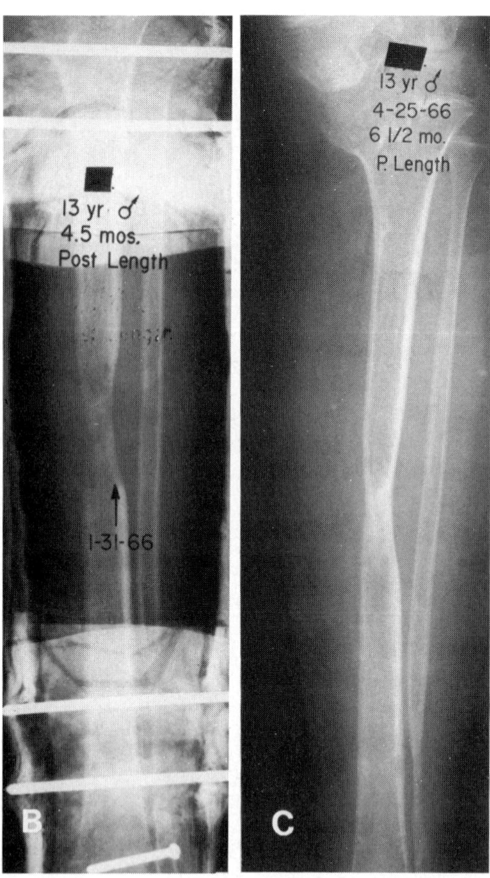

FIG. 19-43. *(A)* The orthoroentgenogram of a 12-year-old male with excessive shortening as the result of pyogenic osteomyelitis and arrest of the proximal tibial and distal femoral epiphyses on the left. *(B)* A tibial lengthening was accomplished, and in 4½ months following lengthening, the fragments had united but were not quite solid enough for weightbearing. *(C)* Six and one-half months after lengthening, with no intervention by bone grafting, solid union ensued, with sufficient strength to permit protected weightbearing. If progressively increasing strength of the bone bridging the defects is evident, bone grafting probably is not necessary.

ible and respond well to an exercise program. Occasionally, triple arthrodesis is necessary to correct the subtalar valgus of the foot.

Neuromuscular complications of any significance have been rare in our experience. Occasionally, temporary interruption of lengthening has been necessitated because of the development of transient sensory changes in the foot and leg. None has persisted. Significant motor loss occurred in one of our patients who sustained an anterior compartment syndrome and lost function of all her dorsiflexors. This is discussed below under vascular complications.

Vascular complications of significance are exceedingly uncommon. One patient in our series developed an anterior compartment syndrome and lost her entire anterior compartment as a result of muscle ischemic necrosis. The diagnosis was delayed and clouded by the relative absence of pain and the presence of a palpable dorsalis pedis pulse. We have had several instances of cavus feet develop following lengthening, and this seemingly is the result of unrecognized ischemia occurring in the intrinsic musculature of the foot. Because of this experience, as noted earlier, I now routinely perform an anterior compartment fasciotomy at the time of the initial lengthening procedure. It may be that fasciotomy of the posterior compartment is also indicated. Wagner[98] has made a unique and extremely valuable observation with respect to the neurovascular response of the limb to lengthening.

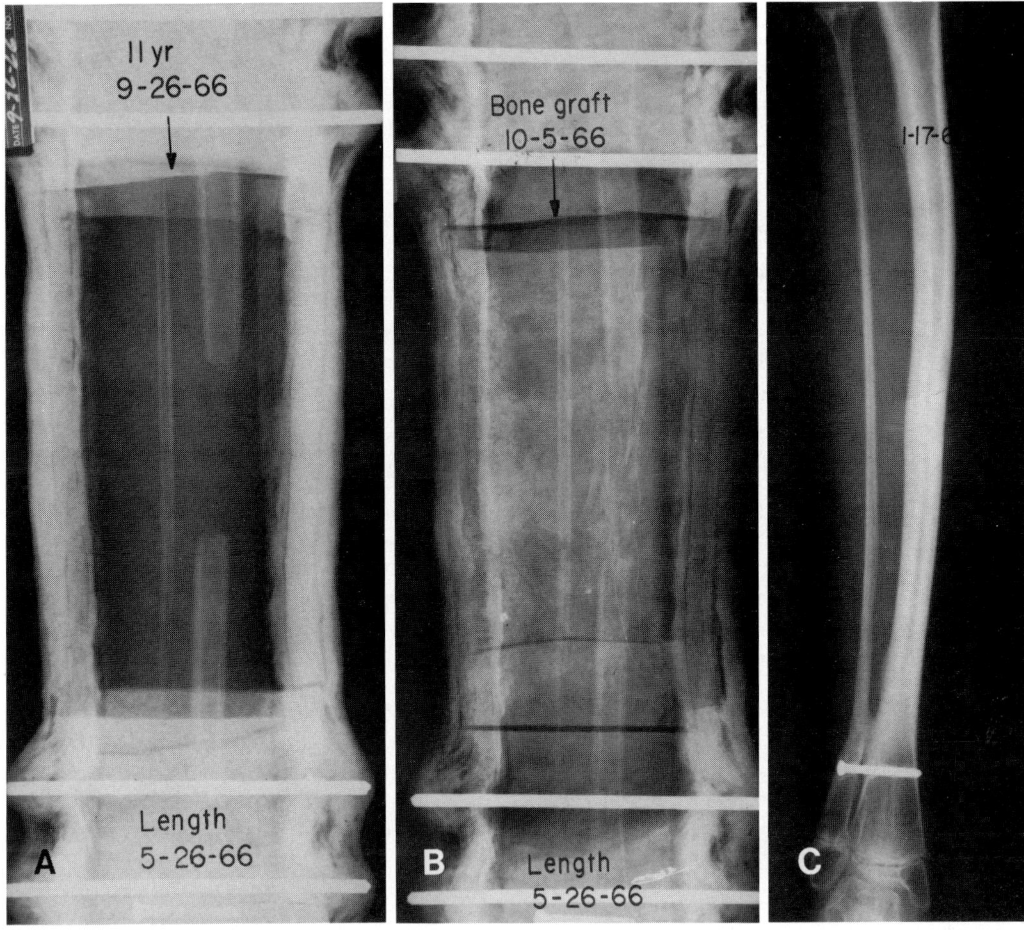

FIG. 19-44. *(A)* Four months after lengthening, there is no evidence of bone formed between the two distracted fragments. *(B)* The immediate postoperative film through the cast shows the bone grafts in place. *(C)* The final result demonstrates solid bony union and the reformed medullary cavity.

Although neuropraxia with resulting neurologic deficit may definitely occur with elongation of the limb, he has concluded that *compression* of the nerves by the enveloping fascia is a much more likely cause of compromise of nerve function. During tibial lengthening, the fascia about the fibular neck and the shelving edge of the biceps femoris tendon can restrict the excursion and freedom of movement and thereby produce compression of the common peroneal nerve. Thus, whenever paresthesias develop over the peroneal nerve distribution, or if paresis of the muscles innervated by this nerve develops, decompression of the nerve is accomplished immediately around the neck of the fibula and underneath the distal insertion of the biceps femoris. During the past 4 years, I have routinely done a decompression of the common peroneal nerve as described above at the initial surgical procedure whenever I perform lengthening of a tibia that is of congenital or developmental cause. In those shortenings due to acquired causes, I have waited for the possible development of some evidence of neural deficit before doing the decompression. Since this program has been instituted, no cases of paresis have developed, and only occasionally has transient hypesthesia of the first web space occurred. Furthermore, since doing both the routine fasciotomy and the nerve decompression, I have not observed any evidence of compartment syndromes or the sequelae of these syndromes.

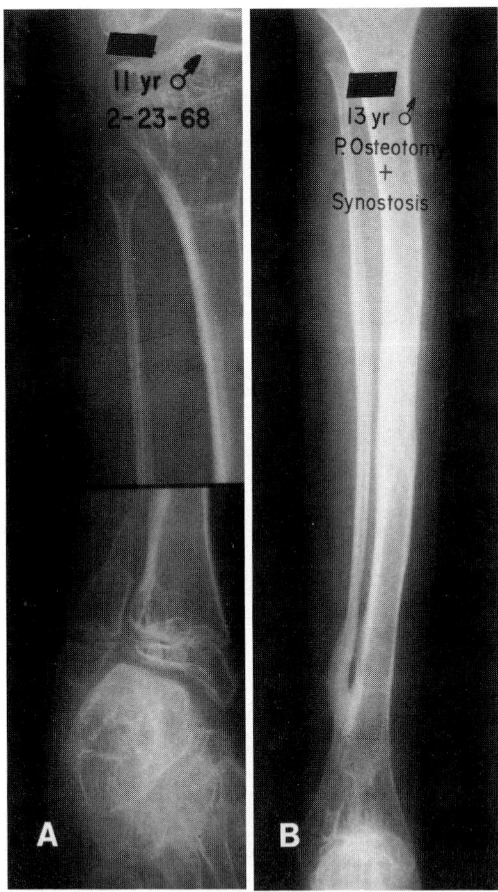

FIG. 19-45. *(A)* A valgus deformity of the ankle and deformation of the distal tibial epiphysis secondary to failure of union of the fibula. *(B)* Osteotomy of the distal tibia and synostosis of the fibula to the tibia resulted in correction of the deformity.

Technical Aspects. The surgical technique involved in tibial lengthening has been recorded in detail below, but I believe that some innovations and qualifications in the technical details deserve special mention, as illustrated in Figure 19-46. In recent years, I have modified the procedure of tibial lengthening in several ways. First, I use the Wagner device (see Fig. 19-38). Second, I no longer resect the fibula, as described earlier; rather, a long, oblique osteotomy is performed just above the tibiofibular transfixion. This is done in order to reduce the amount of separation of the fibula required during lengthening; it is believed that this discourages delayed union and non-union of the fibula. Third, I routinely perform anterior compartment fasciotomy. As noted above, since doing this, I have had no cases of early or late sequelae traceable to neurovascular compromise of this compartment. As mentioned previously, possibly even a posterior compartment fasciotomy may be indicated in some cases, but I have not yet performed it. Fourth, I perform a transverse open osteotomy and cut the periosteum and interosseous membrane circumferentially. Finally, in cases of congenital and development tibial shortening, I decompress the common peroneal nerve routinely as described in the previous section. It is also very important to monitor the blood pressure during tibial lengthening just as in femoral lengthening. Occasionally, it will be necessary to cease lengthening due to transient hypertension, but in more than 150 tibial lengthening procedures that I have performed, permanent cessation of the elongation procedure due to this circumstance has not been required.

Technique (Anderson Principle). A 1½-inch incision is made over the lateral aspect of the distal fibula, just above the level of the distal tibia physis (Fig. 19-46). The fibula is exposed subperiosteally and a 7/64-inch screw is placed across the fibula into the tibia at least ¼ to ½ inch above the distal tibial physis. This stabilizes the mortise of the ankle joint and protects the fibular physis during lengthening. A long, oblique fibular osteotomy is then made just above the screw. This is necessary to allow fibular distraction during the tibial lengthening process. The wound is closed. Next, a vertical incision about 2 inches in length is made over the anterior aspect of the leg, being centered over the anterior tibial muscle. The fascia of the calf is exposed and split longitudinally as far proximally and distally as possible in order to accomplish a decompression of the anterior compartment. Then, only the skin and subcutaneous tissues are closed. The purpose of this is to anticipate and possibly avoid the development of an anterior compartment syndrome during lengthening.

With the distraction device in place, a generous stab wound is made over the medial aspect of the proximal tibia, just below the tibial tubercle. Through the proximal hole of the distraction device, a smooth 5/32-inch Steinmann pin is placed transversely through the long axis of the tibia in such a way that it passes through the companion hole of the distraction device on the lateral side. It is very important to place this pin properly, because

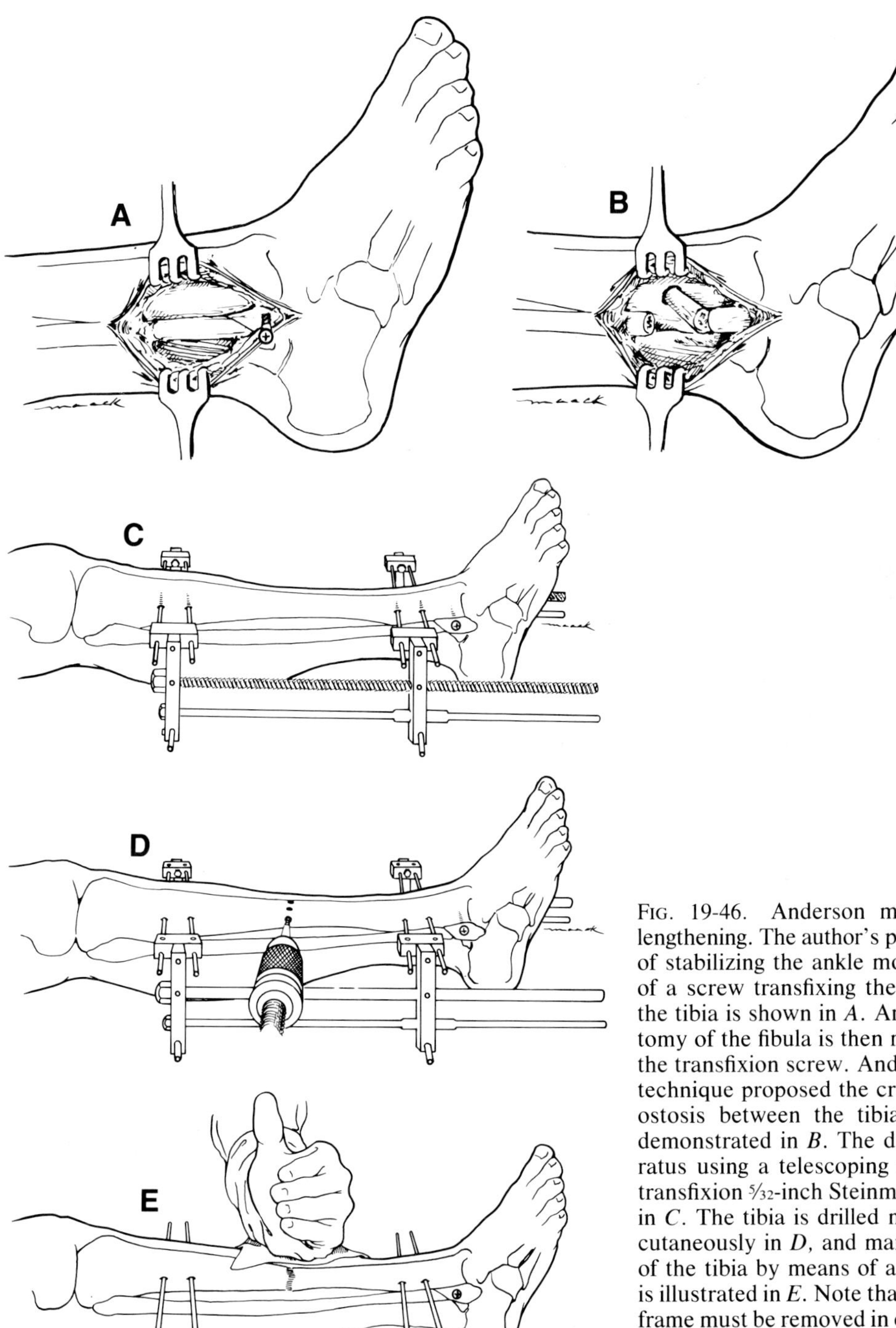

FIG. 19-46. Anderson method of tibial lengthening. The author's preferred method of stabilizing the ankle mortise by means of a screw transfixing the distal fibula to the tibia is shown in *A*. An oblique osteotomy of the fibula is then made just above the transfixion screw. Anderson's original technique proposed the creation of a synostosis between the tibia and fibula as demonstrated in *B*. The distraction apparatus using a telescoping frame and four transfixion 5⁄32-inch Steinmann pins is seen in *C*. The tibia is drilled many times percutaneously in *D*, and manual osteoclasis of the tibia by means of a "karate" blow is illustrated in *E*. Note that the distraction frame must be removed in order to achieve the "closed" fracture of the tibia. The frame is then reapplied in the precise manner that existed when placed into the intact tibia.

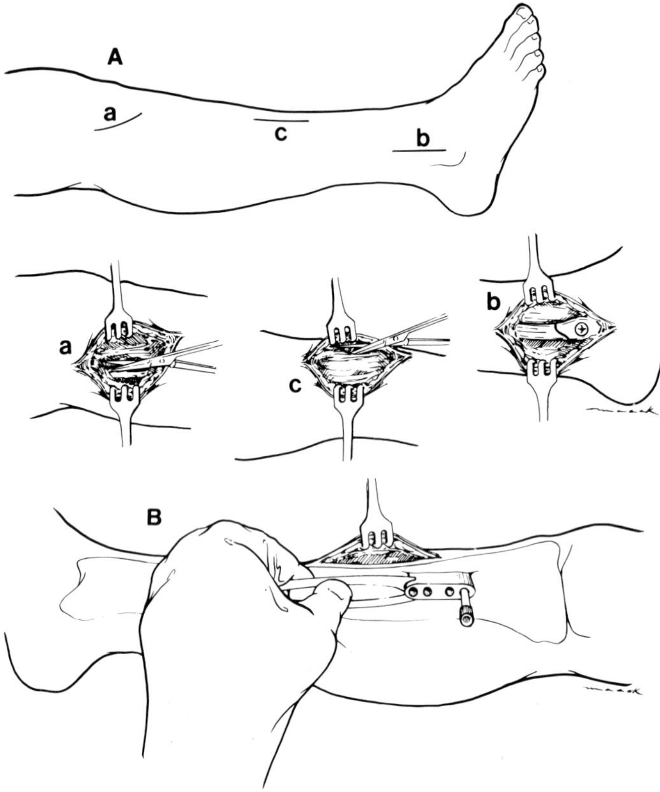

FIG. 19-47. Three incisions are essential in order to accomplish my modification of the Wagner tibial lengthening *(A)*. An incision over the fibular neck is made in order to decompress the peroneal nerve *(a)*. A transfixion screw between the tibia and fibula and an oblique osteotomy of the fibula is accomplished through incision *b*. A fasciotomy and a transverse osteotomy of the tibia are made through incision *c*. The placement of the 6.0-mm Schanz screws is accomplished in the proximal and distal portions of the tibia on the medial side. The same technique as that used in femoral lengthening is used *(B)*.

all other pins have to align with this pin. Care must be taken so that the pin pierces both cortices of the tibia. The second pin is then placed in the lower hole of the distal portion of the distraction device. At this point, it is wise to pull the skin toward the midpoint of the tibia to reduce the stretch on the skin about the pin tracts during lengthening. This pin should be exactly parallel to the first pin in all directions. Similarly, the other two pins are placed so that the tibia is firmly transfixed above and below. The device is then removed, leaving the pins in place.

A stab wound is made over the anterior crest of the tibia in its midportion. Using a 7/64-inch drill, the tibia is drilled transversely percutaneously many times so as to weaken the bone. The leg is then suspended between two elevations of sterile surgical drapes, and the tibia is broken by means of a sharp, direct blow over the drilled portion. The pretibial skin should be well padded to protect not only the skin of the tibia but also the surgeon's hand. If excessive difficulty is encountered in fracturing the tibia, a small 1/4-inch osteotome can be inserted to complete the osteotomy.

After the percutaneous osteotomy has been accomplished, the lengthening device is reapplied exactly as it has been placed in the intact tibia. Palpation of the subcutaneous crest of the tibia usually verifies the absence of any offset or angulation. An x-ray film should be taken to verify proper alignment of the fragments. The device is secured to the pins, and six turns of the lengthening screw are made. This accomplishes two things: it separates the fragments, which may reduce the immediate postoperative pain, and it reduces the duration of subsequent elongation. If the heel cord is tight, a percutaneous lengthening may be done if it had not been done earlier in the surgery. The pins are sealed with collodion over sterile sheet wadding. A below-knee cast is applied, which extends up to *but not including* the proximal pins. The ankle and foot should be held in a neutral position. If there is any tendency to valgus or varus angulation, a transverse pin may be placed through the calcaneus, and this is incorporated in the cast. When the cast is dry, that portion of the cast over the dorsum of the foot and ankle is removed to enable the surgeon to keep close

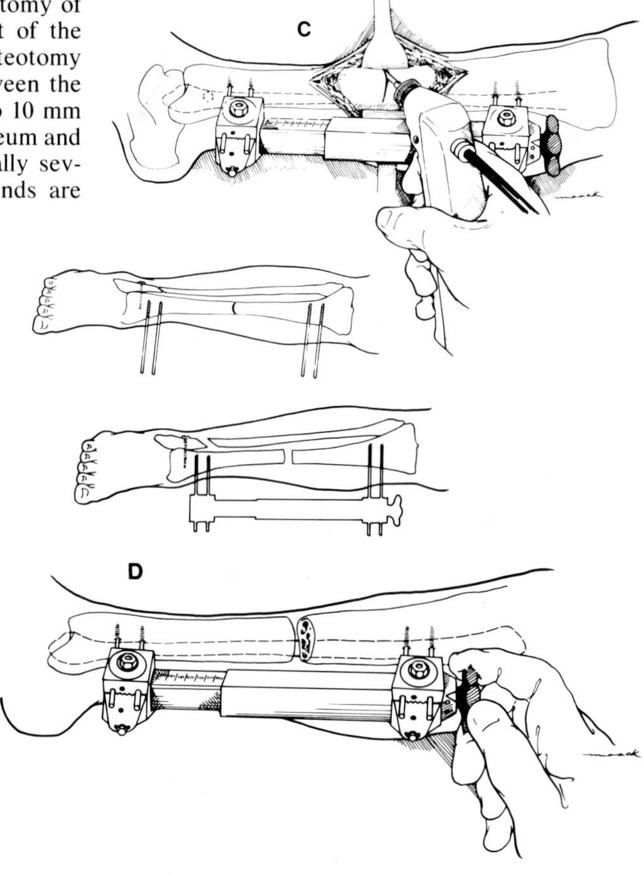

FIG. 19-47. (*Continued*). Following fasciotomy of the anterior compartment and attachment of the lengthening device, an open transverse osteotomy is made in the tibia, exactly midway between the two sets of Schanz screws *(C)*. About 8 to 10 mm of lengthening is then achieved, the periosteum and interosseous membrane are circumferentially severed at the osteotomy site, and the wounds are closed *(D)*.

watch over the neurovascular status of the foot and limb.

Technique (Wagner Principle). Since 1978, I have preferred the technique of tibial lengthening using slight personal modifications of the Wagner method (Fig. 19-47). With the patient supine and a tourniquet on the thigh, the distal fibula is managed in the same manner as described in the previous section. The wound is closed, and, if the shortening is the result of congenital causes, the common peroneal nerve is decompressed. This wound is closed, and four 6.0-mm Schanz screws are inserted into the medial aspect of the tibia, two proximal and two distal. The same guides and templates are used as those used in femoral lengthening. The screws are placed as far proximal and as far distal as possible, care being taken to avoid the physeal plate. They are placed at right angles to the long axis of the tibia. Generous incisions are made for the insertion of the screws, and they should securely engage both cortices of the tibia. A roentgenogram is taken to verify the position and depth of the screws. The lengthening device is then applied, all nuts are tightened securely, and about six or eight turns of the lengthening knob are accomplished. This puts the screws on tension. Then a 5- to 7-cm incision is made over the anterolateral aspect of the leg, centering exactly over the midpoint between the two sets of Schanz screws. The tibia is exposed, and a complete fasciotomy of the anterior compartment is done using a long Metzenbaum scissors. The tibia is then subperiosteally exposed and sectioned transversely with a saw. The fragments will immediately spring apart a few millimeters; this facilitates circumferential sectioning of the periosteum and the interosseous membrane. As these tight structures are cut, the fragments usually distract another few millimeters. Finally, the ankle and foot are checked to see that there is at least 20° to 30° of motion permissible, a range that must be maintained throughout lengthening. One or two more turns

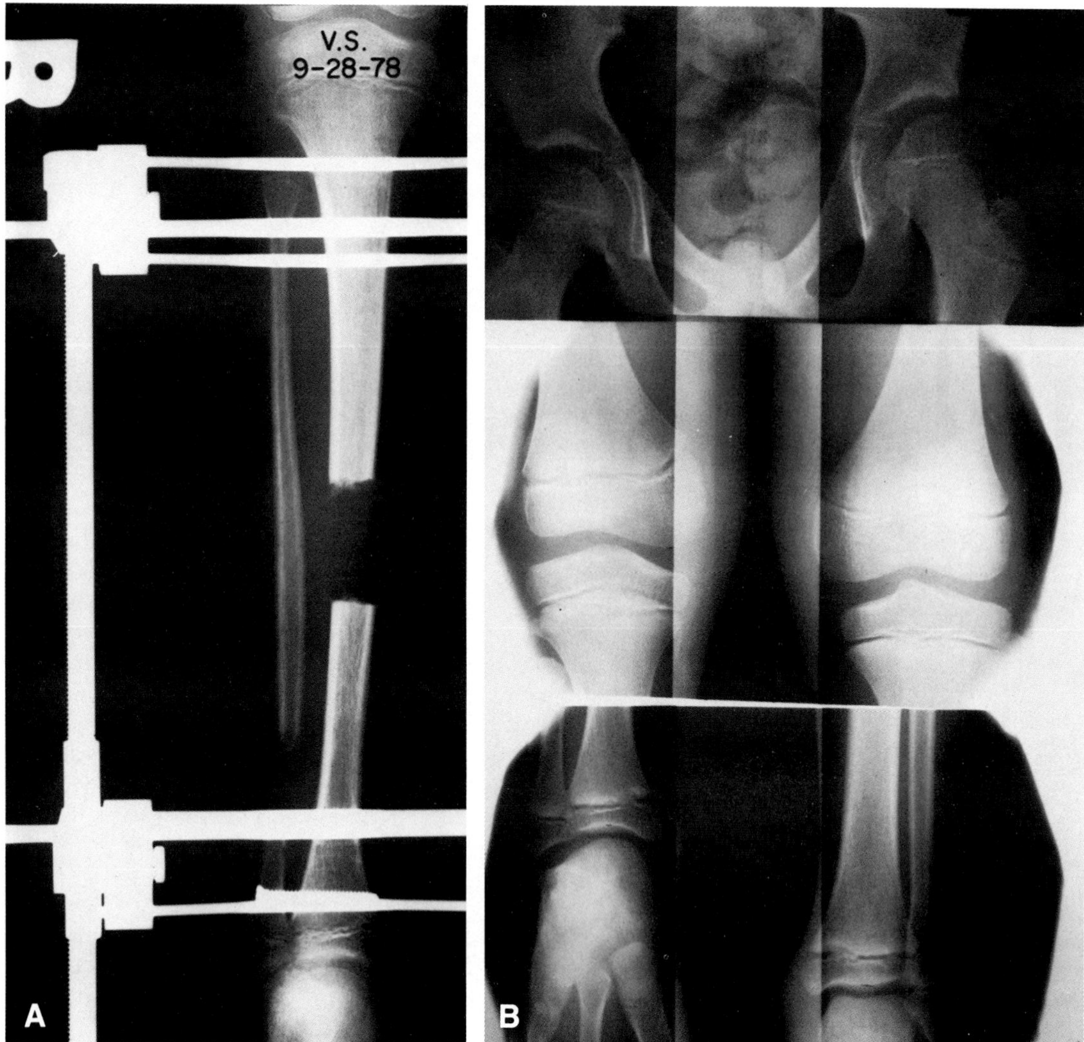

FIG. 19-48. Orthoroentgenogram of a 9-year-old boy with developmental (congenital) shortening of the femur and tibia *(A)*. The "ball and socket" ankle joint on the short side is readily apparent. Tibial lengthening using the Wagner apparatus achieved 5.0 cm of length, but, at the conclusion of lengthening, there was no evidence of union *(B)*. Plating and bone grafting were accomplished, and the result 1 year later is seen in *C*.

of the knob can now be readily achieved and the wound is closed. No cast is necessary; in fact it is considered inappropriate, because it is essential that ankle ranges of motion be maintained during the lengthening process.

Postoperatively, the lengthening is begun on the second day, and the same postoperative routine is exercised here as with femoral lengthening. It is extremely important that the ankle be taken through the range of motion of at least 20° daily through the duration of the lengthening process and thereafter. Just as with femoral lengthening, to maintain this range requires the skilled daily assistance of a qualified therapist. Weekly roentgenograms should be taken to verify that elongation is occurring properly and to assess the integrity and security of the screws and lengthening device.

When the desired length has been achieved, most patients will not show sufficient bridging callus between the fragments to avoid plating and grafting. Therefore, just as in the case of femoral lengthening, plating and bone grafting are accomplished as shown in Figure 19-48.

The lengthening device is assiduously ex-

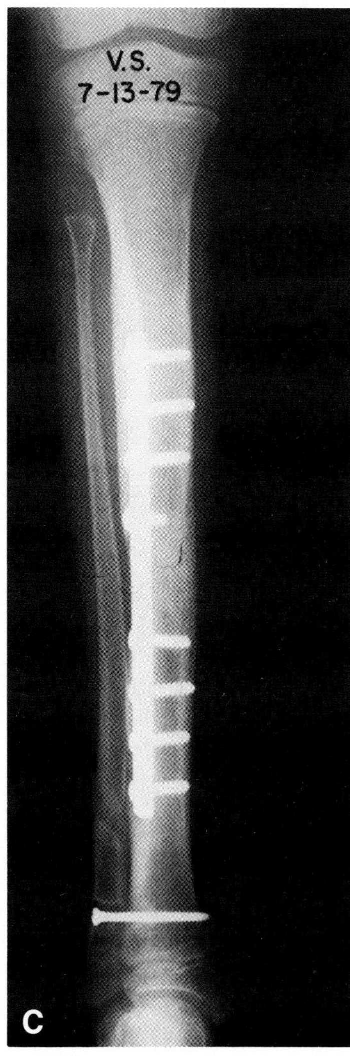

cluded from the surgical prep and drape. The same incision that was used for the osteotomy is opened and enlarged. The distracted fragments are exposed, and the same method of plating and bone grafting is accomplished as was done for the femoral plating procedure. The wound is closed, and the distraction device and Schanz screws are removed. At this point, it is advisable to assess any degree of equinus that may exist resulting from tightness of the heel cord. Clinical judgment and experience are required to decide whether a percutaneous heelcord lengthening is appropriate at this time while the patient is under anesthesia. I do not hesitate to accomplish this simple procedure following removal of the distraction device. If it is done, however, a cast is necessary in order to maintain the correction achieved. Ankle capsulotomy is not necessary, because the lengthening has not affected the joint capsule itself. The cast is usually left on for 4 to 6 weeks, and then a removable ankle-foot orthosis is applied in order to protect the tendon lengthening. Range-of-motion exercises are resumed as soon as the cast is removed.

Nonweightbearing with crutches is permitted, and progressive weightbearing can be permitted according to the degree and rapidity of healing of the distracted fragments. The same principles apply here as in the femoral lengthening procedure. Also, the same approach to removal of the plate is used as for femoral lengthening.

Simultaneous Femoral and Tibial Lengthening

Wagner[99] has shown that the main deterrents to lengthening of the long bones of the lower limb are not the neurovascular structures, but rather the musculotendinous units. Thus, he has concluded and demonstrated that to lengthen the femur and the tibia simultaneously is a practical and safe operation, provided that all indications and prerequisites are met with respect to lengthening of either bone. Clearly, this is an ambitious undertaking and requires considerable experience in lengthening of either bone before simultaneous lengthening is attempted.

The projected discrepancy should exceed 10 to 12 cm, and all other prerequisites should be carefully assessed. When the decision is reached to perform this combined procedure, the tibia should be done first so that a sterile tourniquet can be used. When plating is required, however, it is more appropriate to approach the femur first with the patient prone. Following plating and grafting, the device is removed and the patient is turned to the supine position. A tourniquet is applied to the thigh, the calf and foot are reprepped and redraped, and the tibia is plated and grafted. Heelcord lengthening can be accomplished just as described in the previous section.

The advantages of such an ambitious procedure are obvious. There is only one hospitalization, the length of hospitalization rarely exceeds 5 to 7 days more than with lengthening, plating, and grafting of a single bone. Furthermore, total morbidity and disability are cut essentially in half because the healing of both bones occurs with the same predictability and rapidity as with the procedure on only one bone. Meticulous attention to detail is *especially* important in this operative program. Again, only those surgeons who have substantial experience in bone lengthening should venture into this ambitious and aggressive exercise.

Lengthening by Physeal Distraction

Recently, Monticelli and Spinelli[65] have had experience with a new and novel method of lower limb lengthening. After a series of operations on young goats showed this to be feasible, they carried out a number of tibial and femoral lengthening procedures in which the intact physis (distal femur and proximal tibia) is gradually pulled apart. Two pins must be placed in the epiphysis, and two pins in the metaphysis or diaphysis. Then, a distraction force is exerted across the physis, which essentially produces a longitudinal epiphyseal separation. The physeal cartilage continues to proliferate into the distracted area and is slowly replaced by bone. As much as 5 cm of lengthening has been achieved in one bone (Fig. 19-49).

The advantages are: (1) The distracted area almost always heals, and (2) no internal fixation or bone grafting is required. *The disadvantages* are: (1) This can only be done in a bone with an intact physis; thus, bones suffering from an epiphyseal arrest due to trauma or infection cannot be lengthened in this manner; (2) the physis usually fuses once the desired length is achieved; therefore, it can only be effectively accomplished in patients toward the end of skeletal growth; (3) lengthening can only be accomplished once in the same bone; and (4) knee motion is difficult to maintain with the pins so close to the joint.

I have had no experience with this technique, and because of the above listed disadvantages and despite its conceptual advantages, I have no intention at this time of attempting this procedure.

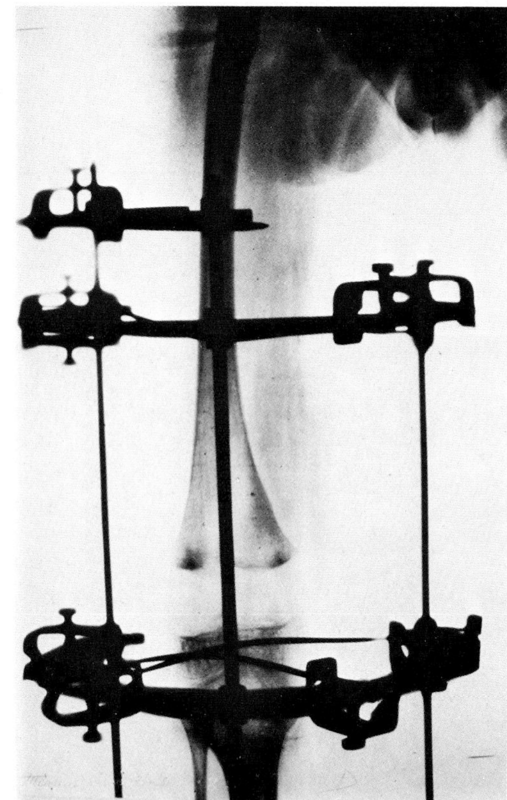

FIG. 19-49. X-ray films of a lengthening through the physis as described by Monticelli and Spinelli. The two distal distraction pins are in the distal femoral epiphysis, and the proximal pins traverse the femoral diaphysis. The device separates the epiphysis from the metaphysis by distraction through the proliferating and maturation zones of the physis. The cartilage then ossifies, and the physis fuses.

Limb Length Inequality Due to Angular Deformity

Angular deformities can produce alterations in limb lengths in three ways: (1) shortening as a result of an asymmetrical growth arrest due to trauma or infection (2) elongation as a result of asymmetrical stimulation of growth following malunion of a fracture, or (3) angulation following malunion of a fracture. The most significant problem in limb length discrepancy is that associated with asymmetrical growth arrest, because this may, depending on the age at which it occurs, result in a very challenging therapeutic problem. Shortening of a lower limb due to an asymmetrical growth arrest means that a significant portion of the epiphyseal plate has been closed as a result of trauma or infection. The most common etiologic factor is trauma, which may be either surgical or nonsurgical (Fig. 19-50). The problem differs from symmetrical growth arrest in that there is not only a true limb length discrepancy but also an angular deformity. The solution to the problem, therefore, must take into account both abnormalities.

The degree of limb length discrepancy and, to a comparable extent, the degree of angu-

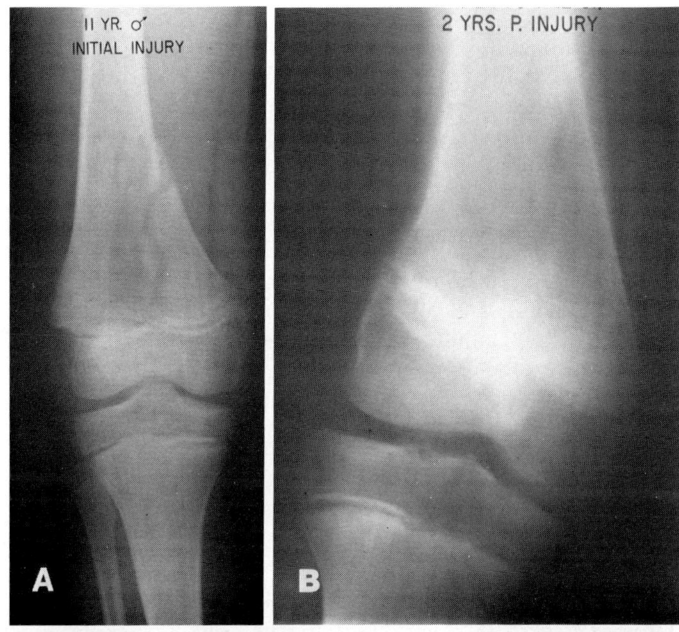

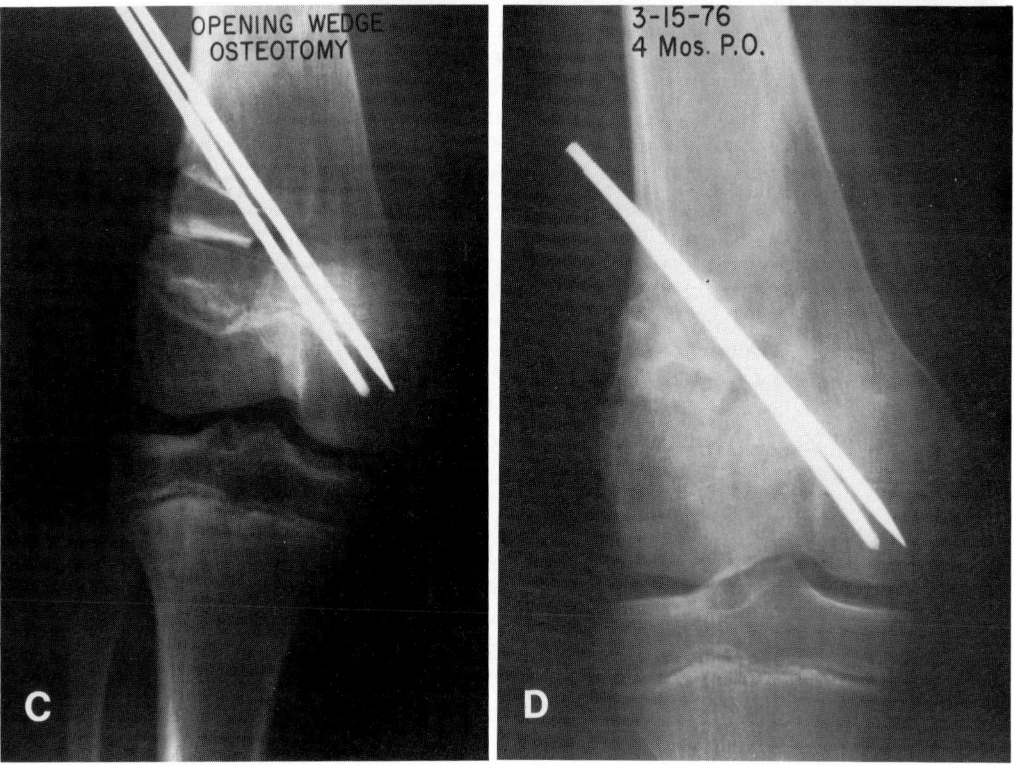

FIG. 19-50. *(A)* Roentgenogram of the distal femur and proximal tibia of a 10-year-old male who sustained a Type 2 epiphyseal injury. *(B)* Two years following injury, the lateral aspect of the distal femoral epiphyseal plate is obviously fused, and there is an angular deformity of 30°. There is also a 2-cm shortening of the same limb. *(C)* The results of an opening wedge osteotomy. The angular deformity is corrected and there is a 2-cm gain in length. *(D)* Four months postoperatively, the healed osteotomy is evident.

lation not only depends on the age at which the insult occurs, but also depends on the particular growth centers involved. Thus, damage to the growth centers about the knee, at comparable skeletal ages, produces greater degrees of limb length discrepancy and angular deformity than comparable injuries occurring at the hip or ankle, simply because of the difference in their contribution toward longitudinal growth of the limbs. In principle, however, the length and angular alterations must be approached similarly, regardless of their skeletal location.

In treating conditions involving limb shortening due to asymmetrical growth arrest, therefore, two fundamental problems surface: (1) correction of the angular deformity, and (2) correction of the limb length discrepancy. The solution to the length discrepancy embodies all the fundamental issues that were discussed earlier. The problem of the angular deformity, on the other hand, poses several different philosophical, biological, and technical questions. Philosophically, the issue centers around the factors of ultimate height, the need or tolerance for repeated operations such as osteotomies, and the willingness to accept an operation in which the results cannot be accurately predicted. Biologically, the question involves such issues as the reversibility of an asymmetrical skeletal growth arrest and the ability of a surgeon to alter a growth aberration in the bone after it has undergone such an arrest. Technically, of course, the issues focus on the various procedures available for correcting limb length inequalities and angular deformities. Acquired deformities are almost always possible to correct from a technical standpoint, but deciding upon the procedure or procedures best suited to accomplish correction can tax the ingenuity of the most experienced surgeon. All factors mentioned in the earlier section on limb length inequality must be taken into account and, in addition, the technical problem of correcting angulation must be considered.

The special philosophical issues principally concern the willingness of the patient (and the parents) to undergo multiple operative procedures in order to correct angulation and shortening. In turn, this has a direct relationship to the problem of the ultimate length of the limb, as well as limb-trunk proportions. On the other hand, some degree of increased length can be achieved by multiple corrective angulation (opening wedge) osteotomies. By this means, the degree of discrepancy can be minimized but probably never completely corrected unless the child sustained the growth arrest toward the end of skeletal maturity. Conversely, by arresting growth completely by means of an angulation osteotomy through the physeal plate, prevention of the recurrence of deformity can be ensured. However, ultimate total height will automatically be reduced on that side, and, almost surely, some form of major shortening or lengthening procedure will become necessary to achieve correction, especially if the initial asymmetrical arrest occurred when the possibility of significant skeletal growth remained. In summary, therefore, the complexity of the problem is even greater than in cases of pure limb length inequality, because decisions occasionally have to be made, which, by virtue of unique growth and skeletal age characteristics, may create new and different problems.

Clinically and biologically, there is good evidence to show that an asymmetrical bony bridge across the growth plate can be excised, and the deforming and shortening process can be reversed. Langenskiold[60] reported instances wherein resection of the osseous bridge, accompanied by replacement of the resected defect by fat, resulted in resumption of normal longitudinal growth. In Langenskiold's series, even some degree of correction of the angular deformity occasionally occurred. Peterson has had an extensive experience with surgical epiphysiolysis, and this subject is covered in detail in Chapter 25.

Technically, all the various procedures discussed under correction of limb length inequality may be used at one time or another in different circumstances to correct the limb length discrepancy. In addition, the use of angulation osteotomy (both opening and closing wedge) or asymmetrical epiphyseal plate stapling (temporary growth arrest) is almost always required for correction of the angular component of the problem. These procedures have been proved and are predictable as well as versatile.

Treatment

In approaching the problems of limb length inequality and angular deformity due to malunion or fracture or asymmetrical growth arrest, each patient presents with a singular set of anatomic facts, variables, and circumstances. The solutions to the problem are equally variable and versatile. It is impossible to design a specific program of treatment that will satisfactorily solve all problems. One must take all factors into account, weigh the importance of each facet of the problem, and fabricate a solution that best meets the needs and desires of the patient and parents. The analysis of the problem and the synthesis of the solution clearly require, in each instance, knowledge and compassionate consideration of philosophical issues, thorough understanding of the biology of the physeal plate, and well-founded technical expertise and experience in performing the various operative procedures.

Implementation of Equalization Procedures

It is impossible to provide explicit guidelines for any given method of equalization. This becomes particularly obvious when the wide variety of techniques are reviewed and the many factors influencing the decision for or against equalization are considered. However, in addition to those situations described earlier, a few examples of how certain specific procedures and combinations of equalization procedures may be used are illustrated below.

CASE HISTORIES

Tibial Lengthening Only

Tibial lengthening for congenital shortening of the tibia was accomplished in a skeletally mature 14-year-old girl. She was born with a posterior bow of the tibia and fibula, and, at skeletal maturity, the bones had straightened spontaneously, but there was 4.0 cm of limb shortening, all in the tibia. Because her height was only 59 inches and because she did not want to be further shortened, it was elected to accomplish a tibial lengthening, as described in the text. She required a bone graft for ultimate union, but bone grafting is not unusual following lengthening of any congenitally short bone.

The salient point to emphasize in this patient is that tibial lengthening alone is suitable for a patient of unusually short stature, especially when the shortening is predominantly in the tibia (Fig. 19-51).

Tibial Lengthening, Contralateral Distal Femoral Epiphysiodesis and Ipsilateral Medial Femoral Stapling

Tibial lengthening was thought to be indicated in a 9-year-old girl whose congenital lower limb shortening of 6.0 cm was located predominantly in the tibia. The lengthening procedure was successful, and this was followed by epiphysiodesis of the distal femur on the long side. Because of an angular deformity at the knee on the congenitally short side, a stapling of that distal femoral physeal plate was accomplished, as described in the text (Fig. 19-27). At skeletal maturity, her limb lengths were equal, despite a slight discrepancy in the knee heights.

This patient demonstrates the occasional need for a combination of equalization procedures that are appropriately timed (Fig. 19-52).

Femoral Lengthening Only

A femoral lengthening alone was accomplished in a 14-year-old boy whose 5.0-cm limb length discrepancy was confined to the femur. The shortening was due to traumatic premature physeal plate arrest in the distal femur. His anticipated adult height was 67 inches, and the patient preferred lengthening to shortening. This etiologic type of acquired shortening is most appropriately suited to a lengthening procedure, if indicated. Union rapidly occurred in this patient, whose femur was lengthened by a modified Wagner technique.

When the shortening is located predominantly in the femur and is acquired rather than congenital in etiology, femoral lengthening is preferred over tibial lengthening (Fig. 19-53).

Femoral and Ipsilateral Tibial Lengthening and Contralateral Distal Femoral Epiphysodesis

Femoral lengthening (Bost type), tibial lengthening (Anderson type), and distal femoral physeal arrest on the long side were necessary in a 12-year-old boy to achieve satisfactory equalization. The shortening was due to partial physeal plate arrest secondary to osteomyelitis, and the projected discrepancy was in excess of 16.0 cm. He previously had distal femoral and proximal tibial osteotomies in order to correct angular deformities.

This patient illustrates how multiple equalization procedures may occasionally be justified, even when the projected discrepancy exceeds 18.0 cm (Fig. 19-54).

(Text continues on p. 859.)

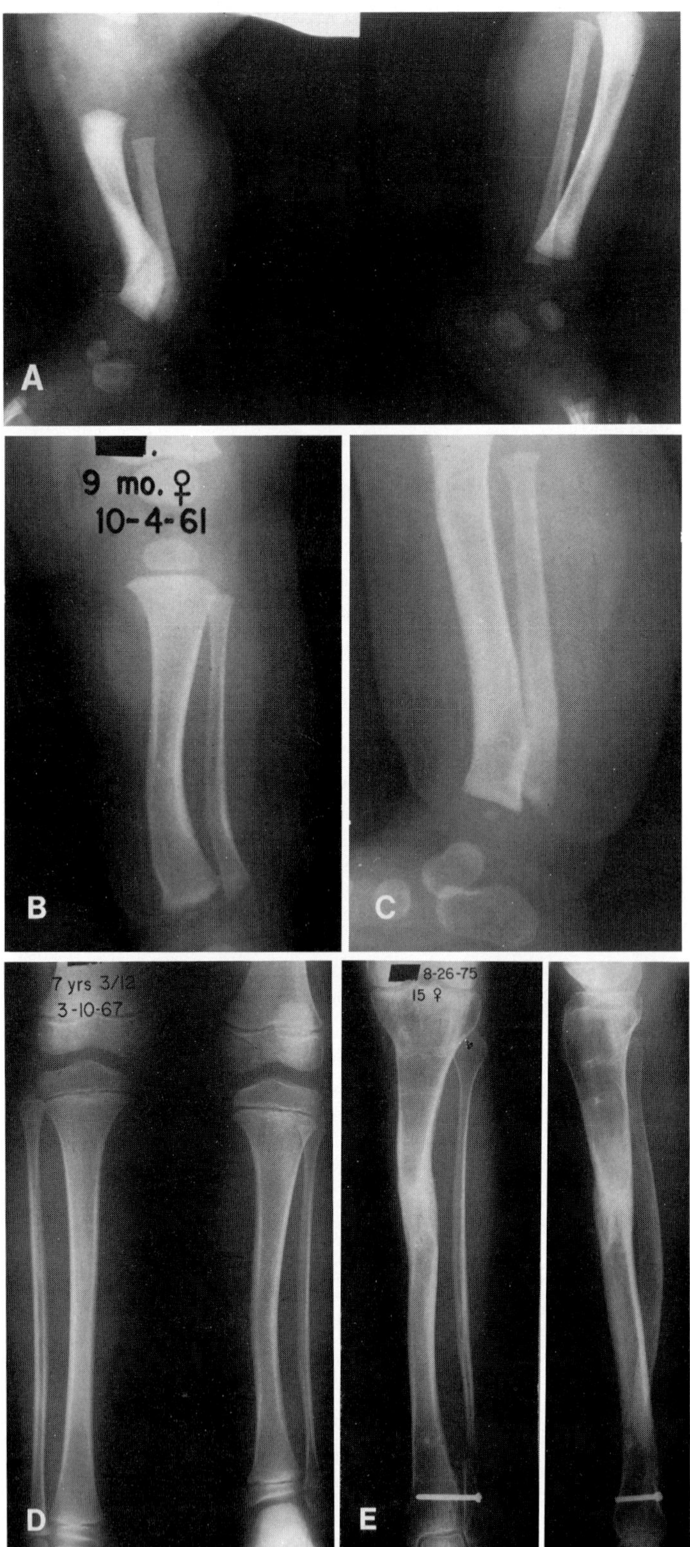

FIG. 19-51. *(A)* Roentgenogram of a child born with a congenital posterior bow of the left lower limb. *(B and C)* Ten months later, much of the deformity had corrected. *(D)* By the age of 7 years, almost complete correction had taken place, but there was 4.5 cm of shortening of the left lower limb, predominantly in the tibia. This young girl was 59 inches tall at age 14, and because of the discrepancy being located predominatly in the tibia, a tibial lengthening was accomplished. *(E)* Bone grafting was required for union, but a satisfactory union with equal limb lengths is evident.

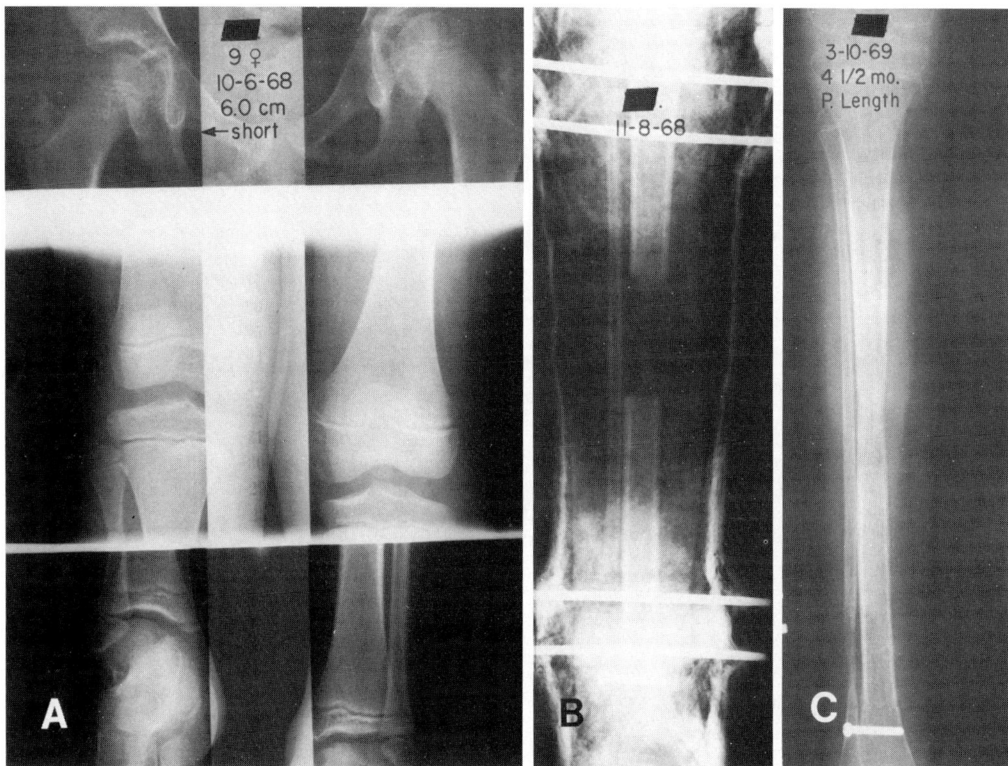

FIG. 19-52. A 9-year-old female with 6 cm of shortening as the result of congenital shortening of the right lower limb. *(A)* Approximately equal shortening exists in both the femur and the tibia, as seen in the orthoroentgenogram. *(B)* The results of a 5.0-cm tibial lengthening. *(C)* Four and one-half months after lengthening, the tibia is solidly united, and the patient is fully ambulatory without protection. (*Continued overleaf.*)

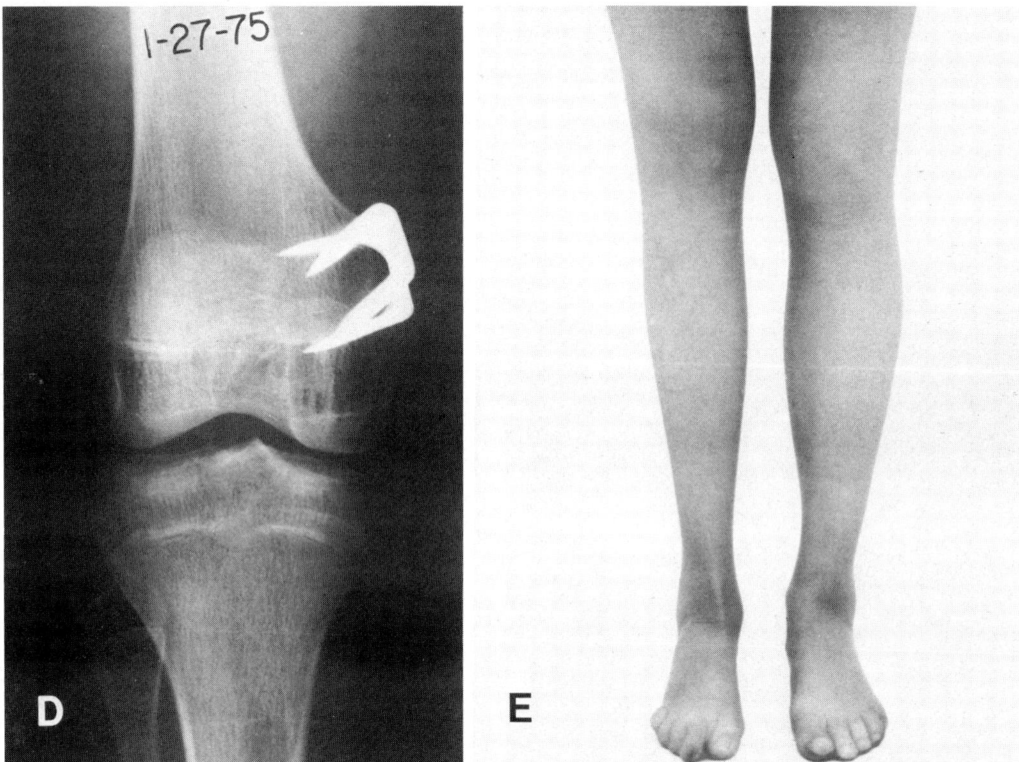

FIG. 19-52. *(Continued). (D)* Because of an angular deformity of the knee and the residual shortening, a simultaneous medial femoral stapling on the short side and an arrest of the longer distal femoral epiphysis was accomplished. *(E)* A standing photograph shows equal limb lengths. It demonstrates that a slight difference in knee levels is not cosmetically significant. This illustrates the value of using bone lengthening procedures, shortening procedures (epiphyseal arrest), and epiphyseal stapling for correction of angular deformities.

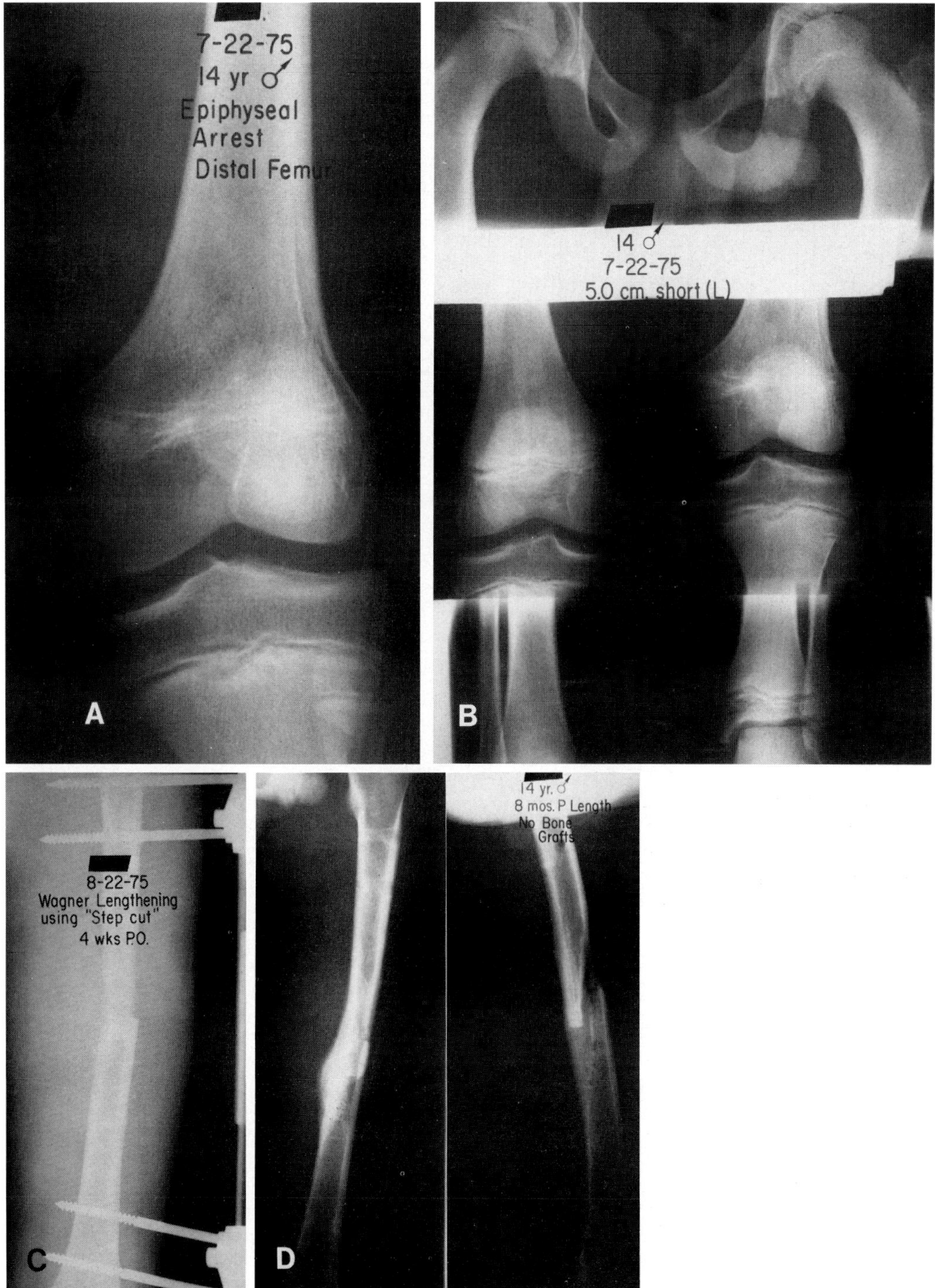

FIG. 19-53. *(A)* A 14-year-old male presenting with a 5 cm-shortening due to arrest of the distal femoral epiphysis following trauma. *(B)* The scanogram reveals the amount of discrepancy and shows that it is entirely in the femur. This patient was only 66 inches tall, with an anticipated adult height of 68 inches. It was his desire that his femur be lengthened on the short side, rather than shortened on the long side. *(C)* Four weeks postoperatively, the distraction device can be seen in place, with lengthening of 5 cm. *(D)* Eight months postoperatively, solid union of the femur has been achieved. This step-cut lengthening is not recommended for the Wagner technique, because it compromises the technique of plating and bone-grafting, if it is necessary.

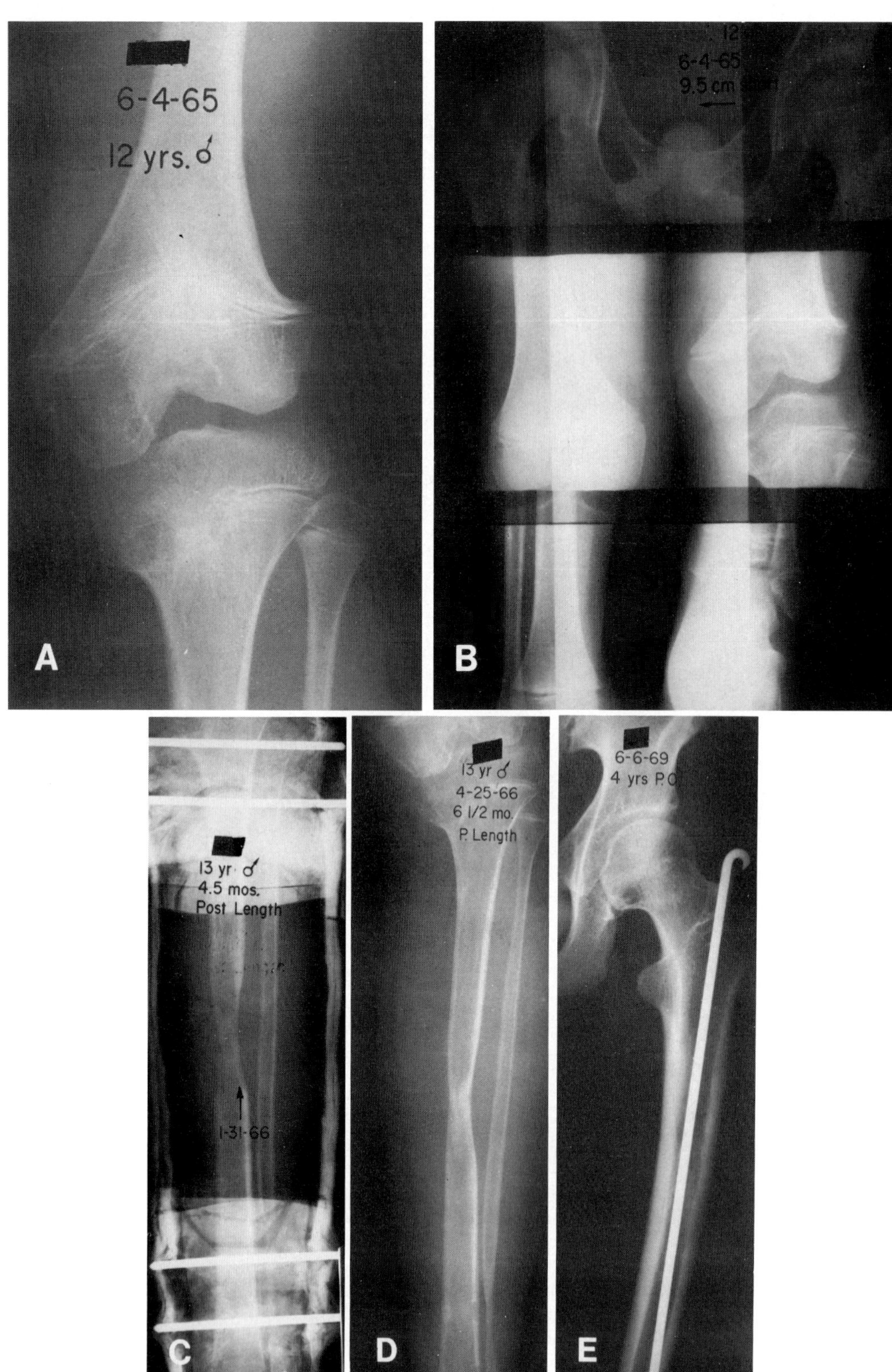
6-4-65
12 yrs. ♂
A
6-4-65
9.5 cm
B
13 yr ♂
4.5 mos.
Post Length
1-31-66
C
13 yr ♂
4-25-66
6 1/2 mo.
P. Length
D
6-6-69
4 yrs P.O.
E

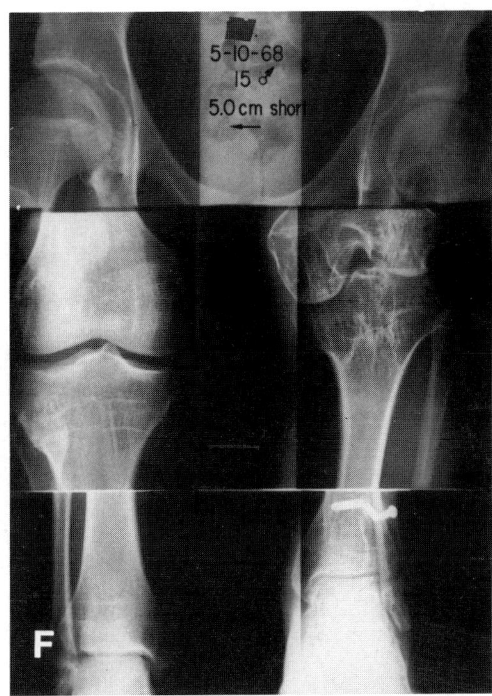

FIG. 19-54. A 12-year-old male was seen initially for lower limb shortening secondary to pyogenic osteomyelitis of the distal femur and proximal tibia, resulting in arrest of the distal femoral epiphysis and partial arrest of the proximal tibial epiphysis. Osteotomies of the distal femur and proximal tibia had been done to correct angular deformities. *(A)* The deformity of both physeal plates and the angular deformity of the knee joint. *(B)* The limb length inequality by orthoroentgenogram measures 9.5 cm. *(C)* The results of tibial lengthening. *(D)* The appearance some 6½ months postoperatively. *(E)* A Bost-type femoral lengthening was accomplished, and the results of that procedure are shown. *(F)* An orthoroentgenogram shows the discrepancy at skeletal maturity. In the interim, a distal femoral epiphyseal arrest had been accomplished, and the combined procedures, therefore resulted in equalization of some 14 cm, with 5 cm of correction in the tibia and 5 cm in the femur by lengthening, and a 4-cm correction was achieved by distal femoral arrest. This illustrates how a variety of equalization procedures may be used to achieve satisfactory correction.

SIMULTANEOUS FEMORAL AND TIBIAL LENGTHENING

C.K. This child was first observed at 3 to 5 years of age to walk with a limp. A diagnosis of Ollier's enchondromatosis was established, with predominant involvement of the right lower limb. At the time she was first seen by me, at age 8 years, she had a lower limb length inequality of 9 cm. It was projected that her discrepancy would ultimately reach 15 cm or more at maturity. After due deliberation, it was agreed that she would have a simultaneous lengthening of the femur and the tibia on the short side, followed at the appropriate time by an epiphyseal arrest of the distal femur and possibly the proximal tibia of the short side.

On April 6, 1981, she simultaneously underwent a Wagner-type lengthening of the right tibia and right femur. At the time of surgery, 5 mm of length was gained in both the femur and the tibia.

Postoperatively, both bones underwent gradual daily distraction of 1.6 mm each until 5.0 cm of length was gained in both the femur and tibia, resulting in a total gain of 10 cm. During the process, the patient received daily intensive physical therapy in order to maintain both ankle and knee motion. On two or three occasions, a delay of 1 or 2 days was necessitated because of lack of motion of the ankle; however, by May 11th, 5 weeks after the initial surgery, the planned degree of lengthening of both bones had been achieved and both underwent plating and grafting. Grafts were obtained from the posterior portion of the ilium during the prone position used for plating and grafting of the femur and from the anterior crest of the ilium during the supine position used for plating and grafting of the tibia. Each of these operations was performed under the same anesthesia, but under separate preps and drapes.

She continued with the program of physical therapy directed toward getting greater ranges of motion in the knee and ankle, but because she retained a 20° to 30° plantar flexion equinus deformity, a heelcord lengthening was accomplished in September of 1981.

The tibia and femur rapidly consolidated and, therefore, she began partial weightbearing. She was able to demonstrate active dorsiflexion of the ankle above a right angle and had normal knee motion. On December 10, 1982, at which time she was fully ambulatory without aids, every other screw in the plates of her femur and tibia was removed and the alternate screws were loosened.

She was last seen on June 6, 1983, just over 2 years following the initial lengthening. She had a bone age of 11 years 6 months and was scheduled to undergo final plate and screw removal and an arrest of her distal femoral and proximal tibial and fibular physes on the long side. At skeletal maturity, considering her growth inhibition of 18%, she should be equalized to within 5 mm.

This case demonstrates the ability to achieve simultaneous lengthening of both femur and tibia and, along with appropriately timed growth arrests, to correct discrepancies exceeding

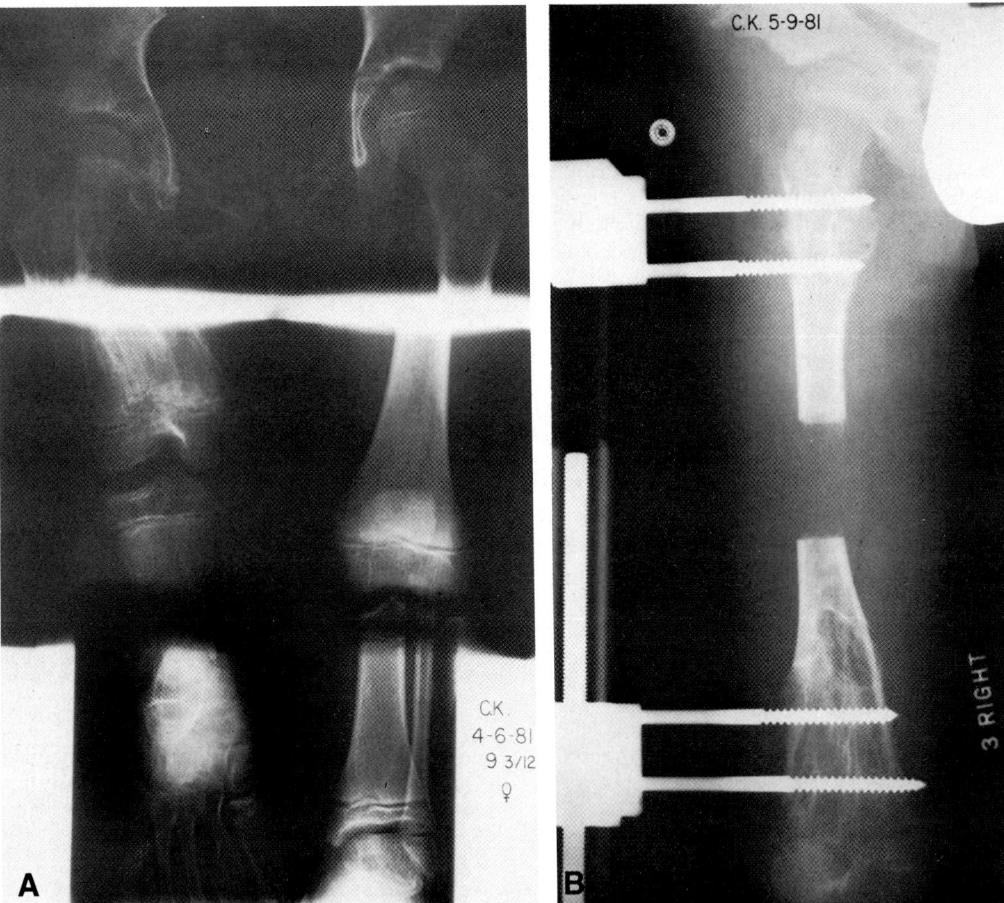

FIG. 19-55. A 9-year-old girl with Ollier's disease had 10.0 cm of shortening of the right lower limb, equally distributed between the femur and the tibia *(A)*. A simultaneous femoral and tibial lengthening was accomplished, and 5.0 cm were gained in the femur *(B)* as well as in the tibia *(C)*. The appearance 1 year later is seen in *D, E,* and *F*.

15.0 cm. The major advantage in this patient is that both femur and tibia were lengthened simultaneously, thus reducing the morbidity to approximately one half of what it would have been if the lengthenings had been done separately (Fig. 19-55).

These cases demonstrate how the various equalization procedures can be used under a variety of circumstances. In each instance, all factors influencing the choice of equalization procedures were evaluated in depth. In addition to these deliberations, all indications and prerequisites of each procedure had to be met, and the patient and parents were sufficiently well informed so that they could intelligently participate in the decision to proceed with the operative program. It is sometimes extremely difficult to arrive at these decisions, and, often, repeated discussions are required to clarify the various aspects of the problem. It is impossible to devise a "cookbook" equalization program on the basis of x-ray films and physical examination alone. The need for individualization and selective evaluation of an equalization program cannot be overemphasized, because only by carefully weighing all the facets of a problem of limb length inequality is it possible to arrive at the appropriate solution.

REFERENCES

1. Abbott LC, Crego CH: Operative lengthening of the femur. South Med J 21:823, 1928
2. Aitken AP, Blackett CW, Ciacotti JJ: Overgrowth of the femoral shaft following fractures in childhood. J Bone Joint Surg 21:334, 1939

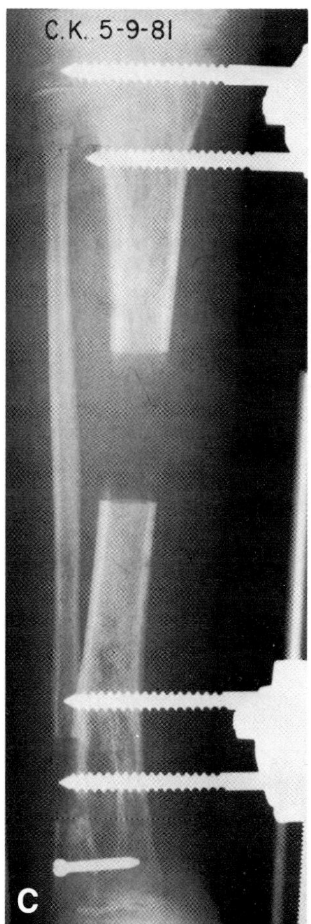

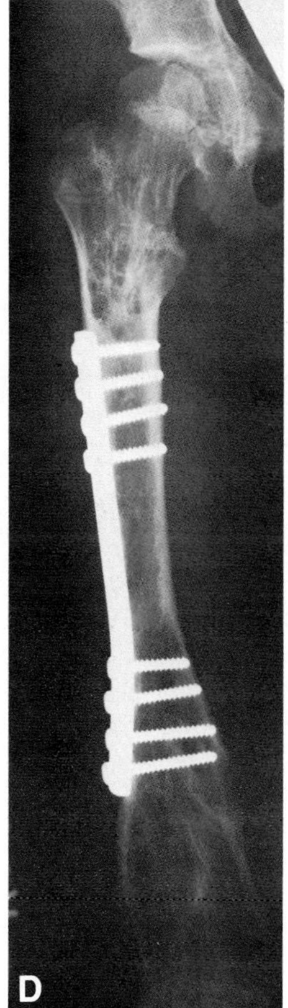

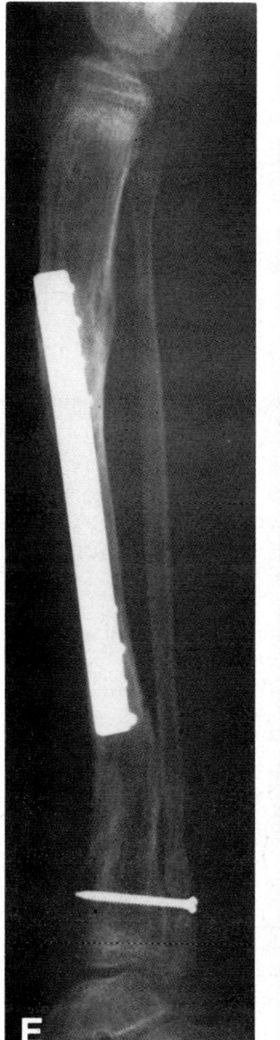

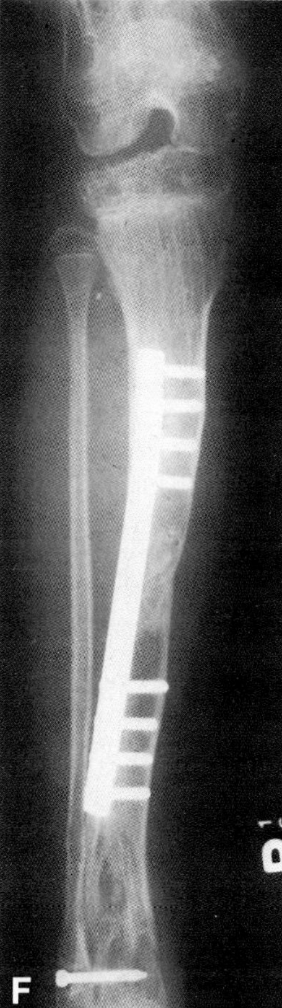

3. Aitken GT: Personal communication, 1976
4. Allan PG: Bone lengthening. J Bone Joint Surg 30B:490, 1948
5. Allan PG: Leg lengthening. Br Med J 1:218, 1951
6. Allan PG: Simultaneous femoral and tibial lengthening. J Bone Joint Surg 45B:206, 1963
7. Anderson WV: Leg lengthening. J Bone Joint Surg 34B:150, 1952
8. Barford B, Christensen J: Fractures of the femoral shaft in children with special reference to subsequent overgrowth. Acta Chir Scand 116:235, 1958–1959
9. Barnes W: Personal communication, 1983
10. Barr JS, Stinchfield AG, Reidy JA: Sympathetic ganglionectomy and limb length in poliomyelitis. J Bone Joint Surg 32A:793, 1950
11. Bayley N: Tables for predicting adult height and skeletal age and present height. J Pediatr 28:49, 1946
12. Bisgard JD: Longitudinal bone growth, the influence of sympathetic deinnervation. Ann Surg 97:374, 1933
13. Bisgard JD: Longitudinal overgrowth of long bones with special reference to fractures. Surg Gynecol Obstet 62:823, 1936
14. Blount WP: Blade-plate internal fixation for high femoral osteotomies. J Bone Joint Surg 25:319, 1943
15. Blount WP: Fractures in Children. Baltimore, Williams & Wilkins, 1954
16. Blount WP: Trauma and Growing Bones. Septiéme Congres de la Société Internationale de Chirurgie Orthopédique et de Traumatologie, Barcelona, 1957
17. Blount WP: Unequal leg length in children. Surg Clin North Am 38:1107, 1958
18. Blount WP, Clark GR: Control of bone growth by epiphyseal stapling. Preliminary report. J Bone Joint Surg 31A:464, 1949
19. Bohlman HR: Experiments with foreign materials in the region of the epiphyseal cartilage plate of growing bones to increase their longitudinal growth. J Bone Joint Surg 11:365, 1929
20. Bost FC: Operative lengthening of the bones of the lower extremity. AAOS Instruc Course Lect 1, 1944
21. Bost FC, Larsen LJ: Experiences with lengthening of the femur over an intramedullary rod. J Bone Joint Surg 38A:567, 1956
22. Brockway A, Craig WA, Cockrell BR Jr: End result of 62 stapling operations. J Bone Joint Surg 36A:1063, 1954
23. Brockway A, Fowler SB: Experiences with 105 leg-lengthening operations. Surg Gynecol Obstet 72:252, 1942
24. Calandriello B: The behavior of muscle fibres during surgical lengthening of a limb. Ital J Orthop Traumatol 1:231, 1975

25. Calvé J, Galland M: A new procedure for compensatory shortening of the unaffected femur in cases of considerable asymmetry of the lower limbs (fractures of the femur, coxalgia, etc.). Am J Orthop Surg 16:211, 1918
26. Cameron BM: A technique for femoral shaft shortening. A preliminary report. J Bone Joint Surg 39A:1309, 1957
27. Carpenter EB, Dalton JB Jr: A critical evaluation of a method of epiphyseal stimulation. Follow-up notes on article previously published. J Bone Joint Surg 45A:642, 1963
28. Codivilla A: On the means of lengthening in the lower limbs, the muscles, and tissues which are shortened through deformity. Am J Orthop Surg 2:353, 1905
29. Cole WH: Results of treatment of fractured femurs. Arch Surg 5:702, 1922
30. Coleman SS: Management of Complications of Tibial Lengthening. Proc of the 11th Congress, Soc Internat de Chirgurgie Ortopedique et de Traumatologie, Mexico City, 1969
31. Coleman SS: Current concepts of tibial lengthening. Orthop Clin North Am 3:201, 1972
32. Coleman SS, Noonan TD: Anderson's method of tibial lengthening by percutaneous osteotomy and gradual distraction. Experiences with 31 cases. J Bone Joint Surg 49A:263, 1967
33. Compere EL: Indications for and against the leg lengthening operation. J Bone Joint Surg 18:692, 1936
34. Compere EL, Adams CO: Studies of the longitudinal growth of long bones, the influence of trauma to the diaphysis. J Bone Joint Surg 19:922, 1937
35. David VC: Shortening and compensatory overgrowth following fractures of the femur in children. Arch Surg 9:438, 1924
36. Diveley RL: Foot appliances and shoe alterations. Orthopedic Appliances Atlas 1:471, 1952
37. Eyre-Brook AL: Bone shortening for inequality of leg lengths. Br Med J 1:222, 1951
38. Fahey JJ: The effect of lumbar sympathetic ganglionectomy on longitudinal bone growth as determined by the teleroentgenographic method. J Bone Joint Surg 18:1042, 1936
39. Gatewood, Mullen BP: Experimental observations on the growth of long bones. Arch Surg 15:215, 1927
40. Goff CW: Surgical Treatment of Unequal Extremities. Springfield, Illinois, Charles C Thomas, 1960
41. Green WT, Anderson M: Experiences with epiphyseal arrest in correcting discrepancies in length of the lower extremities in infantile paralysis. J Bone Joint Surg 29:659, 1947
42. Green WT, Anderson M: The problem of unequal leg lengths. Pediatr Clin North Am 2:1137, 1955
43. Green WT, Anderson M: Skeletal Age and Control of Bone Growth. AAOS Instruc Course Lect 17:199, 1960
44. Greulich WW, Pyle SI: Radiographic Atlas of Skeletal Development of the Hand and Wrist, 2nd ed. Stanford, California, Stanford University Press, 1959
45. Gross RH: An evaluation of tibial lengthening procedures. J Bone Joint Surg 53A:693, 1971
46. Haas SL: The relation of the blood supply to the longitudinal growth of bone. Am J Orthop Surg 15:157, 305, 1917
47. Haas SL: Retardation of bone growth by a wire loop. J Bone Joint Surg 27:25, 1945
48. Haas SL: Mechanical retardation of bone growth. J Bone Joint Surg 30A:506, 1948
49. Haas SL: Stimulation of bone growth. Am J Surg 95:125, 1958
50. Harandi BA, Zahir A: Severe hypertension following correction of flexion contractures of the knee. A report of 2 cases. J Bone Joint Surg 56A:1733, 1974
51. Harmon PH, Krigsten WM: The surgical treatment of unequal leg length. Surg Gynecol Obstet 71:482, 1940
52. Harris RI, McDonald JL: The effect of lumbar sympathectomy upon the growth of legs paralyzed by anterior poliomyelitis. J Bone Joint Surg 18:35, 1936
53. Howorth MB: Leg-shortening operation for equalizing leg length. Arch Surg 44:543, 1942
54. Janes JM, Jennings WK: Effect of induced arteriovenous fistula on leg length. Ten-year observations. Proc Mayo Clinic 36:1, 1961
55. Janes JM, Musgrove JE: Effect of arteriovenous fistula on growth of bone. Preliminary report. Proc Mayo Clinic 24:405, 1949
56. Janes JM, Musgrove JE: Effect of arteriovenous fistula growth on bone. Surg Clin North Am 30:1191, 1950
57. Kawamura B: Leg Lengthening, Principles Involved and the Limiting Factors. Proc. of the 11th Cong., Soc. Internat. de Chirgurie et de Traumatologie. Mexico City, 1969
58. Kawamura B, Hosono S, Takshaski T, Yano T, Kobayashi Y, et al: Limb lengthening by means of subcutaneous osteotomy. J Bone Joint Surg 50A:851, 1968
59. Khoury SC, Silberman FS, Cabrine RL: Stimulation of the longitudinal growth of long bones by periosteal stripping. J Bone Joint Surg 45A:1679, 1963
60. Langenskiold A: Personal communication, 1975
61. McCarroll HR: Trials and tribulations in attempted femoral lengthening. J Bone Joint Surg 32A:132, 1950
62. Magnuson PB: Lengthening of shortened bones of the leg by operation. Surg Gynecol Obstet 17:63, 1913
63. May VR Jr, Clemens EL: Epiphyseal stapling with special reference to complications. South Med J 58:1203, 1965
64. Merle D'Aubigne R, Dubousset J: Surgical correction of large length discrepancies in the lower extremities of children and adults. J Bone Joint Surg 53A:411, 1971
65. Monticelli G, Spinelli R: Distraction epiphysiolysis as a method of limb lengthening; I. Experimental study. II. Morphologic investigation. III. Clinical applications. Clin Orthop Rel Res 154:254, 1981
66. Moore JR: Tibial lengthening and femoral shortening. Pa Med J 36:751, 1933
67. Moore RD: Supracondylar shortening of the femur for leg length inequality. Surg Gynecol Obstet 84:1087, 1947
68. Moseley CF: A straight line graph for leg length discrepancies. J Bone Joint Surg 59A:174, 1977
69. Nickel V: Personal communication, 1980
70. Ollier L: Traite experimental et clinique de la regen-

eration des os et de la production artificielle du tissu asseux. Paris, Masson, 1867
71. Pease CN: Local stimulation of growth of long bones, a preliminary report. J Bone Joint Surg 34A:1, 1952
72. Phalen GS, Chatterton CC: Equalizing the lower extremities: A clinical consideration of leg lengthening versus leg shortening. Surgery 12:678, 1942
73. Phemister DB: Operative arrestment of longitudinal growth of bones in the treatment of deformities. J Bone Joint Surg 15:1, 1933
74. Phemister DB: Bone growth and repair. Ann Surg 102:261, 1935
75. Poirier H: Epiphyseal stapling and leg equalization. J Bone Joint Surg 50B:61, 1968
76. Putti V: The operative lengthening of the femur. JAMA 77:934, 1921
77. Putti V: Operative lengthening of the femur. Surg Gynecol Obstet 58:318, 1934
78. Regan JM, Chatterton CC: Deformities following surgical epiphyseal arrest. J Bone Joint Surg 28:165, 1946
79. Salter RB: Innominate osteotomy in the treatment of congenital dislocation and subluxation of the hip. J Bone Joint Surg 43B:518, 1961
80. Salter RB, Harris WR: Injuries involving the epiphyseal plate. J Bone Joint Surg 45A:587, 1963
81. Shapiro F: Developmental patterns in lower extremity length discrepancies, J Bone Joint Surg 64A:639, 1982
82. Sofield HA: Leg lengthening. Surg Clin North Am 19:69, 1939
83. Sofield HA: Personal communication, 1965
84. Speed K: Longitudinal overgrowth of long bones. Surg Gynecol Obstet 37:787, 1923
85. Staheli LT: Late femoral and tibial length inequality following femoral shaft fractures in childhood. J Bone Joint Surg 43A:1224, 1966
86. Stelling FH: Personal communication, 1975
87. Stirling RI: Equalization of limb length. J Bone Joint Surg 37B:511, 1955
88. Straub LR, Thompson TC, Wilson PD: The results of epiphysiodesis and femoral shortening in relation to equalization of leg length. J Bone Joint Surg 27:254, 1945
89. Tachdjian MO: Pediatric Orthopedics, Vol 2, p 1469. Philadelphia, WB Saunders, 1972
90. Thompson TC, Straub LR, Campbell RD: An evaluation of femoral shortening with intramedullary nailing. J Bone Joint Surg 36A:43, 1954
91. Trueta J: The influence of the blood supply in controlling bone growth. Bull Hosp Joint Dis 14:147, 1953
92. Tupman GS: Treatment of inequality of the lower limbs. The results of operations for stimulation of growth. J Bone Joint Surg 42B:489, 1960
93. Vanderhoeft PJ, Kelly PJ, Janes JM, Peterson LFA: Growth and structure of bone distal to an arteriovenous fistula: Quantitative analysis of the tetracycline-induced transverse growth patterns. J Bone Joint Surg 45B:582, 1963
94. Vesely DG, Mears TM: Surgically induced arteriovenous fistula. Its effect upon inequality of leg length. South Med J 57:129, 1964
95. Wagner H: Operative Beinverlängerung. Der Chirurg 42(6):260, 1971
96. Wagner H: Personal communication, 1977
97. Wagner H: Personal communication, 1978
98. Wagner H: Pediatric Orthopedic International Seminar, San Francisco, 1978
99. Wagner H: Pediatric Orthopedic International Seminar, Chicago, 1979
100. Wagner H: Personal communication, 1979
101. Wagner H: Pediatric Orthopedic International Seminar, Chicago, 1980
102 Westin GW: Femoral lengthening using a periosteal sleeve. Report of 26 cases. J Bone Joint Surg 49A:83, 1967
103. White JW: Overlapping procedure for shortening bone defects. AAOS Instruc Course Lect 2:201, 1949
104. White JW, Stubbins SG Jr: Growth arrest for equalizing leg lengths. JAMA 126:1146, 1944
105. Wilk LH, Badgley CE: Hypertension, another complication of leg lengthening procedure. Report of a case. J Bone Joint Surg 45A:1263, 1963
106. Winquist RA, Hansen ST Jr, Pearson RE: Closed femoral shortening. J Bone Joint Surg 57A:135, 1975
107. Yabsley RH, Harris WR: The effect of shaft fractures and periosteal stripping on the vascular supply to epiphyseal plates. J Bone Joint Surg 47A:551, 1965
108. Yosipovitch ZH, Palti Y: Alterations in blood pressure during leg lengthening. A clinical and experimental investigation. J Bone Joint Surg 49A:1352, 1967

20

The Lower Limb

Paul P. Griffin

TIBIAL TORSION

Torsion in the tibia may be directed either internally or externally. Its significance as a psychological or an anatomic problem is controversial, as are the methods of measurements and the effectiveness of treatment. Such controversy is brought about by the lack of a scientifically sound study that demonstrates the effectiveness of treatment, as well as the well-known fact that torsion of the tibia is seldom a problem in the adult.

Internal tibial torsion may be measured roentgenographically[35,40] or by a tropometric method.[35,66] These methods, although more accurate than clinical measurements, are still inaccurate to a certain degree. If the angle between the transmalleolar and transcondylar axis of the tibia is used to measure torsion, there is a progressive external rotation from birth to maturity, so that in the adult, there is 20° of external torsion.[35,40]

The patient with internal torsion is usually brought for evaluation because of toeing-in or because of a bowleg appearance. Many babies with internal tibial torsion have an external rotation "deformity" of the femur, in that the hip has excessive external rotation with internal rotation limited to 10° to 20°. This combination of external rotation of the thigh and internal torsion of the lower leg gives an appearance of bowing whether or not there is true tibia vara or genu varum.

In my experience, there has seldom been a need for orthopaedic devices in treating internal torsion. From the number of children that I have seen who have worn various orthoses for months or years and who still have tibial torsion, I am inclined to believe that those patients in whom internal torsion does not spontaneously correct are not likely to improve with the devices presently used.

I have seen the appearance of medial torsion in young infants changed within 6 to 8 weeks by the use of a Denis Browne brace attached to shoes. In spite of the improved appearance, the relationship of the transcondylar to the transmalleolar axis was altered very little, and the correction obtained was through the ankle and knee joints where I think many infants have a medial rotation from their position in utero. Most toddlers who appear to have medial torsion below the knee have excessive medial rotation of the tibia on the femur. In these children, the tibia can frequently be internally rotated on the femur to where the foot may point 90° to the sagittal plane, but external rotation is limited so the foot points only 10° to 15° outwardly. This relaxation of the ligaments of the knee is most likely related to *in utero* position. Correction of the medial torsion at the knee responds rapidly to the Denis Browne bar, but treatment is not necessary because this positional deformity spontaneously corrects. The spontaneous correction of this torsion is delayed by sleeping and sitting and kneeling postures that hold the feet and knees in an internally rotated position.

In line with the present limited data that support the need for treatment, splinting should be reserved for the 18- or 24-month-old child who has severe intoeing from internal tibial torsion but who does not have excessive external rotation of the hip. If a Denis Browne bar is used, its width should not exceed the width of the pelvis. A wider bar puts a valgus stress on the foot and knee. Tibial torsion may be familial,[8] and, where there is a familial pattern, it is not likely to correct with or without an external rotation brace, but, in this group of patients, I do treat the child when first evaluated, but with little evidence that it changes the torsion deformity.

Whereas internal torsion is more bothersome to parents, excessive external torsion is probably mechanically less desirable. External torsion gives an out-toe gait that increases stress on the feet and later may have some influence on running. Certainly, boys and girls with external torsion who participate in sports have more difficulty with shin splints than those with normal torsion or internal torsion.

GENU VALGUM

Physiologic Genu Valgum

Clinical Features. It is common for children between the ages of 2 and 6 years to have up to 15° of valgus deformity at the knee. This is usually but not always symmetrical. Children with as much as 15° of valgus deformity may complain of leg or foot pain and may fatigue easily. They seldom run well, and they are likely to be less active than their peers who have less valgus deformity. When the amount of valgus exceeds 15°, when it is asymmetric, or if the child is unusually short of stature, a growth abnormality should be suspected as a possible cause of the valgus and appropriate roentgenograms made of the knee.

Treatment. The natural history of physiologic genu valgum is one of progressive improvement, beginning around 30 months of age, and most are corrected by 5 years of age, although a few go on until 7 or 8 years of age. Those children who have valgus deformity at 8 years of age seldom spontaneously correct. The valgus knee puts unusual stress on the medial side of the foot and may cause foot strain. In children with 15° of genu valgum I use a ⅛- to 3/16-inch medial heel wedge and occasionally an arch pad.

In a child with excessive genu valgum, that of 20° or so, particularly if the father or mother has genu valgum, I use a night brace to attempt to correct the deformity. The brace is a lateral straight single upright, without a knee joint, which is attached to a shoe. It has a thigh and calf band and a large knee pad that is used to pull the knee toward the upright. This is worn only at night.

The adolescent with genu valgum presents a special problem. Genu valgum is a functional as well as a cosmetic disability. It is rare to find an adolescent with genu valgum who can run well; therefore, most of these patients are not active in sports and do poorly in physical activities. A valgus knee also places stress on the patellofemoral joint and possibly contributes to patellofemoral instability.

When the genu valgum is great enough to produce approximately 10 cm of space between the malleoli with the knees together or if it measures more than 15° to 20° when the child is 10 years old, surgical correction should be considered. There are several important observations to make before attempting to correct the deformity. One must be sure that the distance between the malleoli is due to valgus deformity at the knee and not to fat thighs. The latter is a common finding in adolescent girls and must not be overlooked. By losing weight, improvement in the appearance is gained. A valgus deformity may be secondary to elongation of the distal medial condyle of the femur or to more rapid growth of the medial part of the proximal epiphysis of the tibia.

The correction should take place at the proper level, that is, at the site of deformity. If the deformity is in the tibia and correction is through the femur, the knee joint will be tilted laterally when the feet are together. The opposite is true when the deformity is in the femur and correction is obtained through the tibia. There is normally a slight valgus angulation between the shaft of the femur and the distal articular surface, which is necessary to keep the knee joint horizontal when the thighs are together, because the upper ends of the femora are separated by the pelvis. This necessary valgus angulation is greater in girls than boys and must be considered when looking at roentgenograms of the knees. On an average, girls have about 9° to 10° of valgus angulation of the distal femur, boys have slightly less.

In most patients with genu valgum, the deformity is in the distal femur and therefore should be corrected through the femur. If the epiphyseal plate has sufficient growth potential, stapling of the medial part of the epiphysis with three staples gradually corrects the deformity (Fig. 20-1).[59] Once correction is ob-

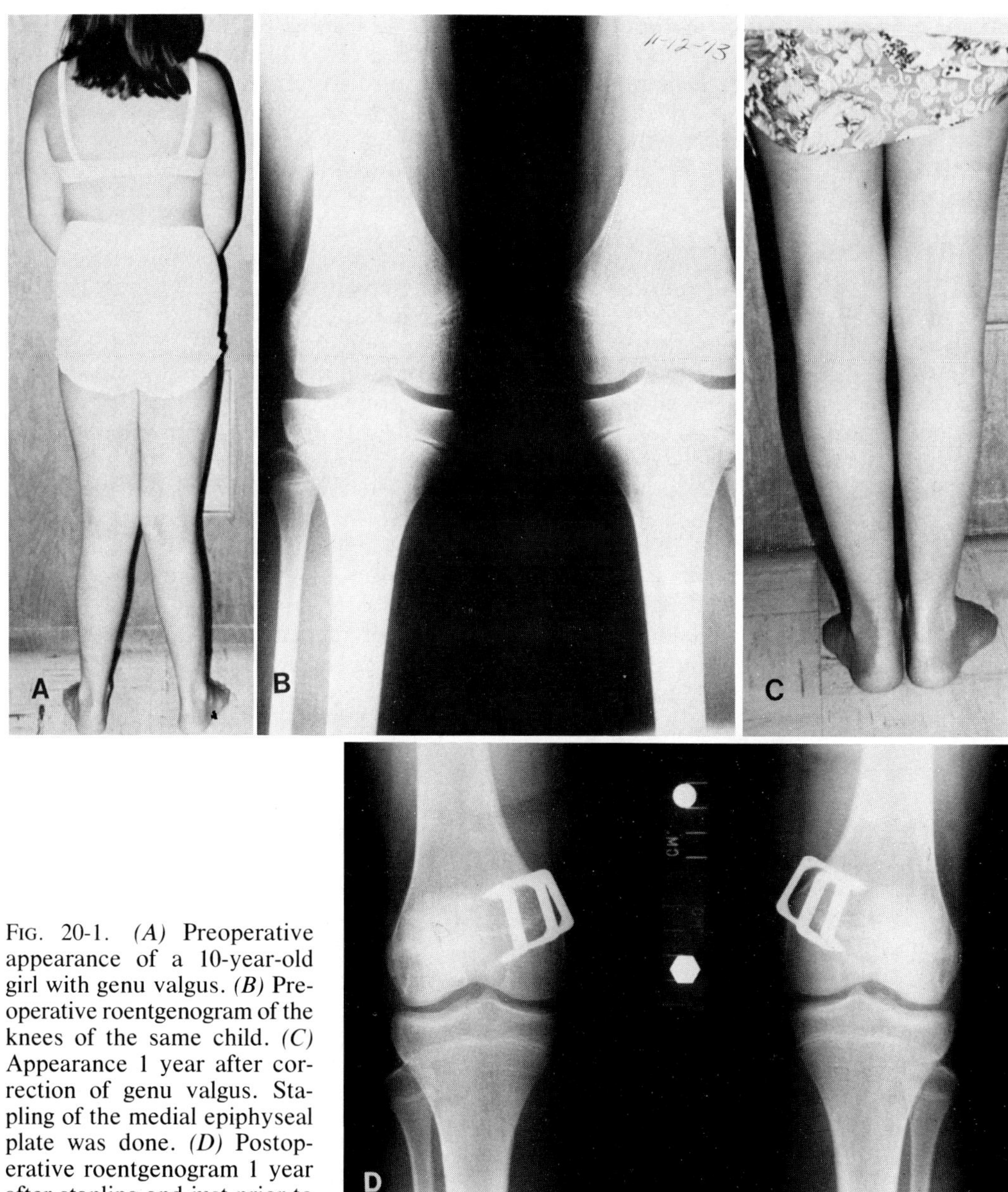

FIG. 20-1. *(A)* Preoperative appearance of a 10-year-old girl with genu valgus. *(B)* Preoperative roentgenogram of the knees of the same child. *(C)* Appearance 1 year after correction of genu valgus. Stapling of the medial epiphyseal plate was done. *(D)* Postoperative roentgenogram 1 year after stapling and just prior to staple removal.

tained, the staples should be removed. Timing is important. If done too late, correction will be inadequate. As a rule, surgery on girls should be done at a skeletal age of 10 years and on boys at a skeletal age of 11 years. The amount of correction that is obtained by stapling is mathematically related to the transverse width of the plate, the length of the leg distal to the plate, and the growth that occurs on the unstapled side of the plate. A simple way to decide whether there is sufficient growth remaining to obtain correction is to trace the legs on a long, clear, x-ray film, divide the femur at the level of the femoral epiphysis, and visualize the distance of medial elongation necessary to straighten the extremity. An osteotomy of the distal femur can be done to correct the deformity when remaining growth potential is not sufficient.

When the deformity is in the tibia, the same

principles apply. Stapling of the medial part of the proximal tibial epiphysis, if growth is sufficient to correct the deformity, is an effective method of treatment. If the remaining growth is insufficient to correct the deformity, an osteotomy of the tibia should be done after the epiphysis is closed.

Post–Traumatic Genu Valgum

An injury to the distal femoral physis or proximal tibial physis may cause a valgus or varus deformity if growth of the epiphyseal plate is disturbed. Management of this is discussed under leg length inequality. However, there is a special situation that results in valgus deformity of the tibia after a fracture of the proximal metaphysis of the tibia. Valgus deformity may follow an undisplaced fracture or a displaced fracture that is well reduced. (Fig. 20-2). Most fractures of the proximal tibial metaphysis open on the medial side, and great care should be taken to completely reduce the fragments and close any separation on the medial side. At times, even maximum effort may be insufficient to completely reduce the fracture by manipulation. However, open reduction and anatomic reduction are likely to be followed by valgus deformity. The family should always be told of the possibility that a valgus deformity may develop following this fracture.

The cause of this valgus growth pattern is uncertain. It is seen in children between 2 and 7 years of age who usually have genu valgum. The natural growth pattern toward valgus may have some influence. After a fracture occurs, there is an increase in blood flow to the area. This stimulates growth that is greater on the medial side than the lateral. The fibula possibly tethers the growth from the lateral side. Incomplete reduction may contribute to the valgus. Soft-tissue interposition may prevent adequate reduction of the fracture.[71] If the reduction is not anatomic, one should give serious consideration to open reduction. However, after open reduction, the growth differential may still cause the valgus deformity to develop.

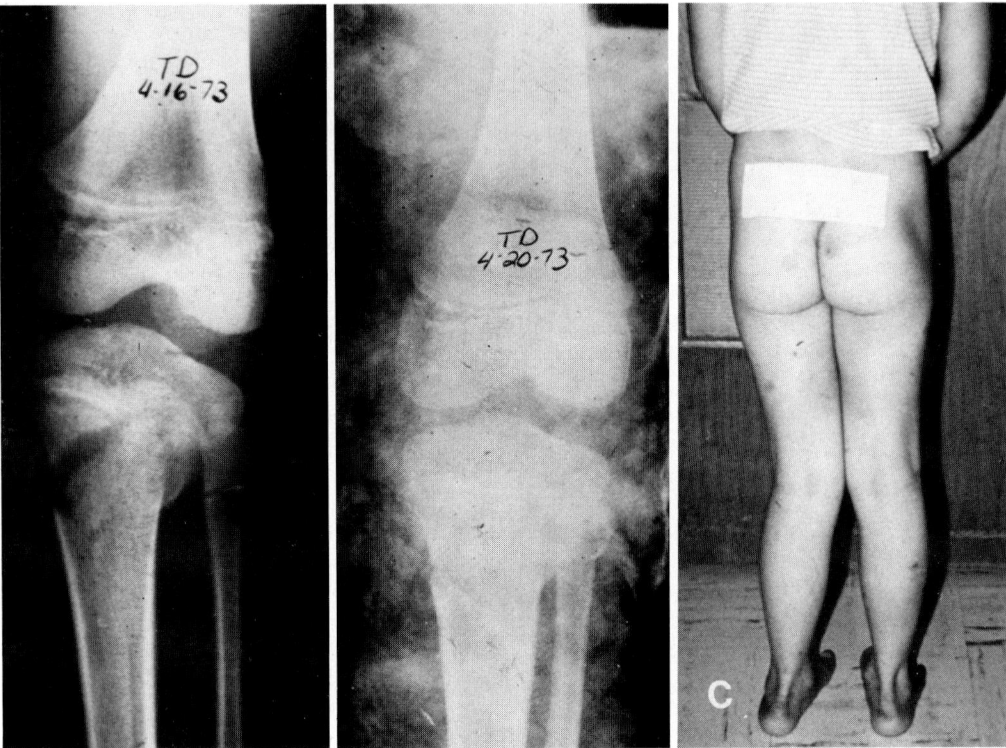

FIG. 20-2. *(A)* Fracture of the proximal tibia and fibula. *(B)* After reduction, the medial side remains slightly open, in spite of manipulation. Note that the lateral joint space has opened. *(C)* Two years later, genu valgum is evident.

Management of the valgus is difficult. To immediately correct the valgus by osteotomy of the tibia usually results in recurrence of the valgus. The medial side of the tibial epiphyseal plate may be stapled and correction obtained gradually, but, in young children, stapling of the medial epiphysis is technically difficult and must be done with great care. The staple is removed after correction has been obtained. I prefer to wait until the child is 8 or 9 years old and correct the deformity by a closing wedge osteotomy of the tibia through the proximal metaphysis, with an oblique osteotomy of the fibula. When the valgus deformity is too severe to postpone correction until the child is 8 or 9 years of age, the osteotomy must overcorrect the valgus to allow for the tendency of the deformity to recur.

PHYSIOLOGIC GENU VARUM

In the infant and young child, mild medial bowing of the lower extremities is normal. The bowing involves both the femur and the tibia. Gradual spontaneous correction is the natural course of genu varum, and the great majority are straight at 2 to 2½ years. Some of these children later develop genu valgum, which is also a temporary condition that begins to straighten at 4 years. Most are straight somewhere between 5 and 8 years of age. The presence of medial torsion exaggerates the bowed appearance.

Most parents seek medical help for their children with bowlegs after walking begins. Important in the history of the child is whether the deformity increased after walking began. If so, roentgenographic examination is probably warranted. The roentgenographic characteristics of physiologic genu varum are: (1) medial angulation of the upper one third of the tibia and lower end of the femur; (2) a thickened medial cortex of the tibia and, to a lesser degree, the femur; (3) prominence of the medial metaphysis of the tibia and femur; (4) normal-appearing epiphyseal plate, and (5) usually symmetric involvement (Fig. 20-3). The differential diagnosis includes rickets, metaphyseal dysplasia, and Blount's disease.

Levine and Drennan showed that by measuring the metaphyseal-diaphyseal angle on an anteroposterior roentgenogram, physiologic bowlegs can be distinguished from Blount's disease (tibia vara) before the characteristic radiographic changes of Blount's disease appear. The angle created by the intersection of a line through the transverse plane of the proximal tibial metaphysis and a line perpendicular to the long axis of the tibia is greater in those patients who develop Blount's disease. When this angle is less than 11°, the development of Blount's disease is very unlikely, but, over 11° most patients subsequently have the classic changes of Blount's disease.[46]

Treatment for physiologic bowlegs is not necessary, because the deformity improves spontaneously. Use of a Denis Browne bar may exaggerate the subsequent genu valgum that follows the correction of the bowleg. It is the responsibility of the orthopaedist to rule out other causes of genu varum that need specific treatment.

TIBIA VARA (BLOUNT'S DISEASE)

In 1937, Dr. Walter Blount reported on a series of 13 patients with bowed tibiae secondary to a growth disturbance of the medial portion of the proximal epiphysis of the tibia, and he reviewed 15 additional cases from the literature.[7] His excellent description of the tibia vara has resulted in its being commonly called "Blount's disease," even though the condition was reported in 1922 by Erlacher.[17]

Blount described an infantile type of tibia vara that begins between the first and third years of life and an adolescent type that has its onset after 9 years of age. The infantile type is the more common of the two. Both males and females are affected. Golding and co-workers[24] reported a male-to-female ratio of 17 to 11, whereas both Langenskiold[43] and Blount reported a predominance of females.

Infantile-type tibia vara usually occurs in obese children who have short stature and walk early. The course of the disease is usually progressive, with increasing varus of the proximal tibia, secondary joint changes that include ligamentous laxity, hypoplasia of the posterior medial plateau, which results in a flexion of the diaphysis on the proximal epiphyseal, and lateral shift of the tibia on the femur. There is, in addition, a medial torsion of the tibia. Rarely does mild Blount's disease remain static for some time and then progressively improve. Generally, the deformity is progressive.

There are characteristic histologic findings in the resting layer of epiphyseal cartilage in tibia vara.[43] These are (1) islands of densely packed cells showing a greater degree of hy-

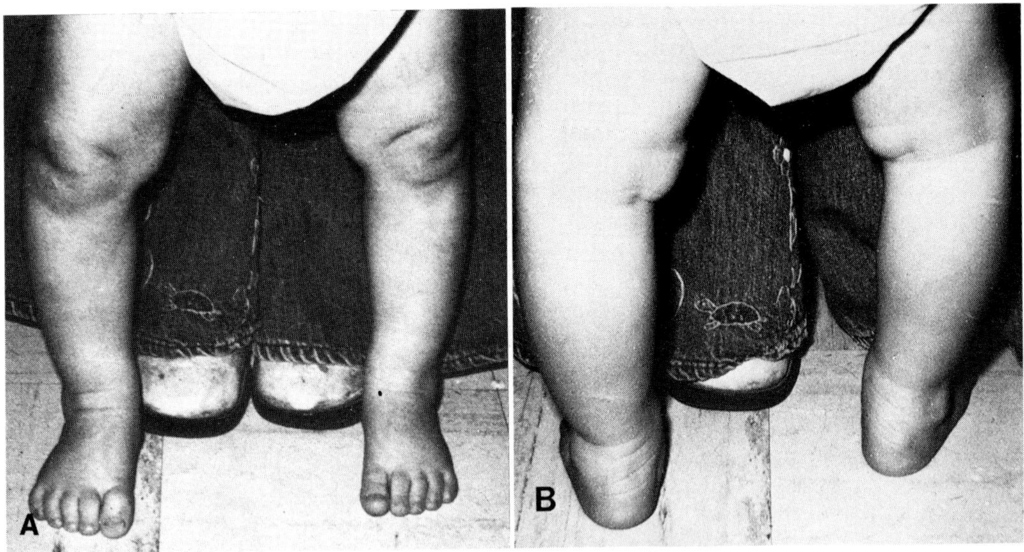

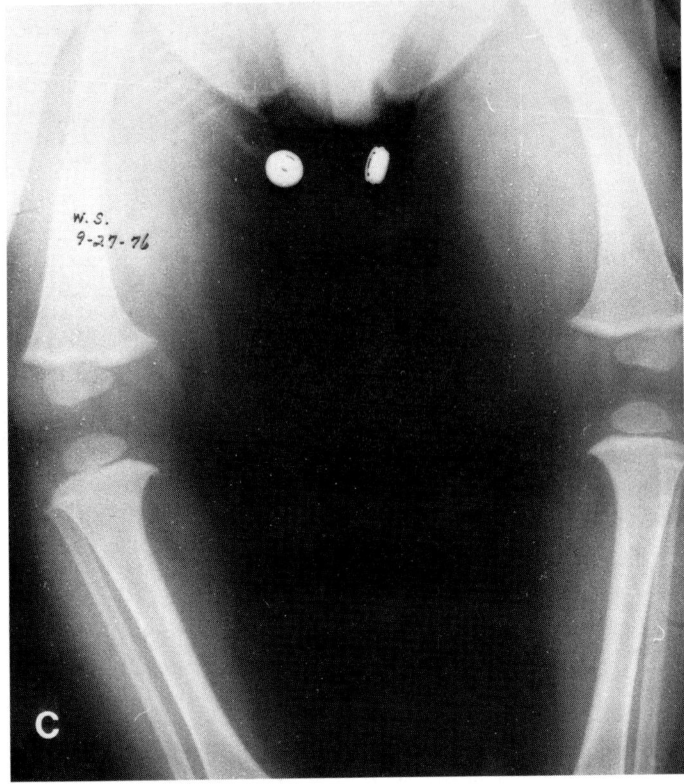

FIG. 20-3. *(A and B)* Physiologic genu varum. *(C)* Roentgenographic view of physiologic genu varum.

pertrophy than could be expected from their topographical position, (2) islands of almost cellular fibrous cartilage, and (3) abnormal groups of capillary vessels.

Etiology

The infantile type of tibia vara is caused by a disturbance in growth and ossification of the posterior medial part of the proximal epiphysis of the tibia. It has not been clearly delineated as to why the growth disturbance occurs. There is no evidence that infection, trauma, or ischemia are contributing factors. It may be a response to abnormal stress from weight-bearing on an already bowed leg. This is difficult to prove, but it is typically the case that heavy children whose legs are already bowed and who walk early are those most likely to develop Blount's disease.

"Necroses of epiphyseal cartilage both in the growth plate and in the cartilage of the epiphysis is the chief cause of the growth disturbance in tibia vara."[45] Langenskiold writes that "The histological picture at the borderline between the cartilage and metaphyseal bone reveals areas of dead cartilage or severely damaged cartilage intermingled with an area showing reparative changes."[45] These changes are possibly secondary to pressure. This concept is supported by the fact that relief of the pressure in the medial side of the proximal tibia by valgus osteotomy is followed by healing of the damaged growth plate and metaphysis. Bathfield and Beighton,[5] however, did not find that their patients were unusual in size or height or that pressure on the medial side of the proximal tibia was not a significant force in the pathologic changes seen in Blount's disease.

Clinical Features

Clinically there is difficulty in differentiating the severe physiologic bowleg from Blount's disease. The diagnosis is made by the roentgenographic picture. Until there are definite changes in the medial metaphysis, the physician cannot be certain whether the patient has Blount's disease. However, recently, Levine and Drennan[46] demonstrated that by measurement of the metaphyseal-diaphyseal angle of the tibia, physiologic bowlegs can be distinguished from Blount's disease before the characteristic roentgenographic changes appear.[46] Usually by the age of 2 years, physiologic bowlegs will have shown improvement, whereas the deformity in Blount's disease will have increased and roentgenographic changes in the proximal tibia will be well developed.

On physical examination, there is a sharp bowing just below the knee. A prominence is palpable on the medial tibial metaphysis. With the knee flexed 10° to 15°, there may be significant instability of the tibia on the femur. The child walks with the knee flexed, and the varus may increase during the single support phase of gait.

Rickets, radiation change, multiple chondromatoses, traumatic epiphyseal disturbance, congenital bowing, in addition to the physiologic bowlegs, must be differentiated.

The clinical course varies from population to population. Langenskiold had two patients who improved, but the remainder of his patients progressed. Golding found in his Jamaican population that the deformity always progressed.[24] I have had several patients who improved after Stage I. Bathfield found that in the Witwatersrand region of South Africa, patients with tibia vara progressed until age 3 years, after which the deformity became static or improved. He found that residual deformity of the tibia in the adult population was very rare.[5]

The diagnosis of tibia vara is a roentgenographic one. Langenskiold[44] has separated the roentgenographic changes into six stages that are related to age. It is important that the orthopaedist treating tibia vara recognize these stages (Fig. 20-4).

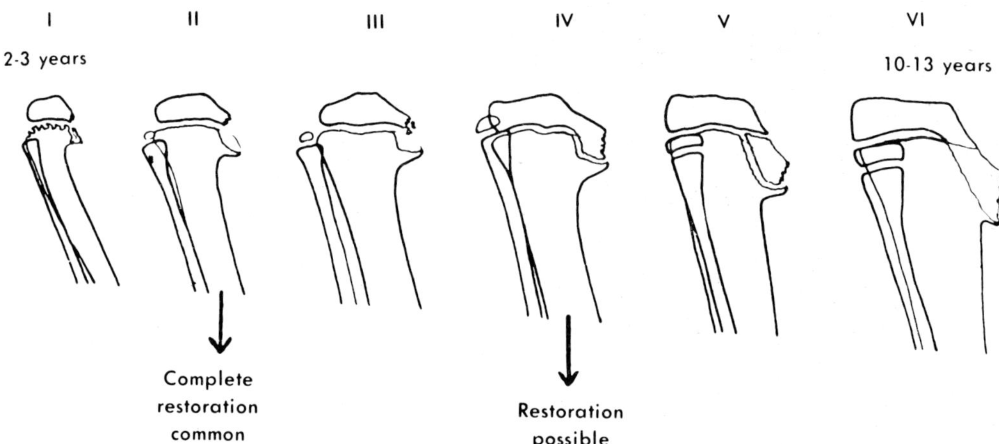

FIG. 20-4. The six stages of tibia vara, as related to age. (Langenskiold A: Tibia vara. Acta Chir Scand 103:9, 1952)

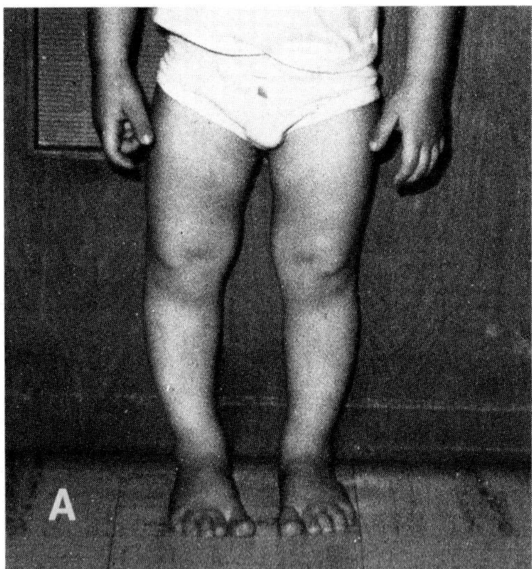

FIG. 20-5. *(A)* A 2-year-old with varus on weightbearing. *(B)* Roentgenogram of same patient at age 2 years, showing early Blount's disease. *(C)* At age 2½ years, the changes of Blount's disease have progressed. *(Legend continued on facing page.)*

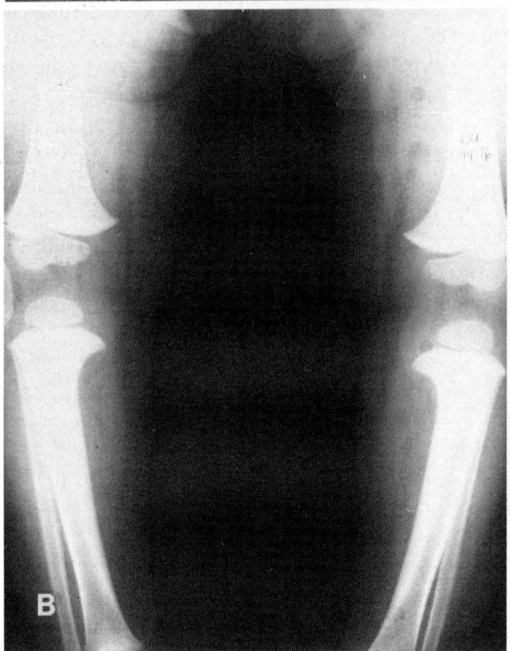

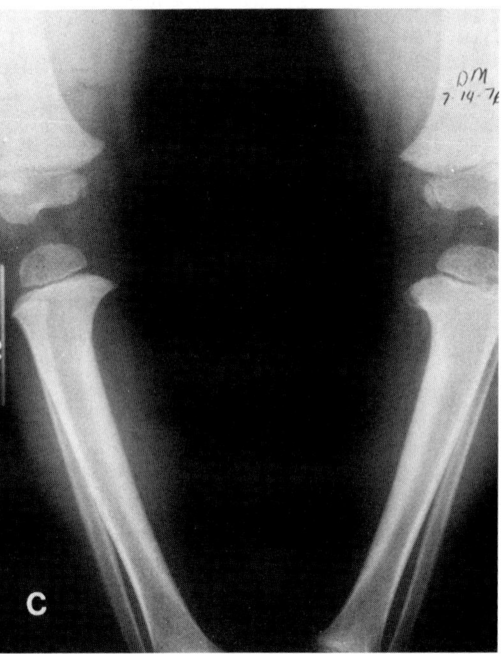

Stage I. This stage is seen in children up to 3 years of age. There is an irregularity of the entire ossification of the metaphyses, with radiolucent zones separating islands of calcified tissue from the bony metaphysis. The medial part of the metaphysis protrudes and is beaked medially and distally.

Stage II. This is seen in children between 2½ and 4 years of age. There is a sharp lateromedial depression in the ossification line of the medial one third of the metaphysis that forms the characteristic beak. The upper portion of the beak is more radiolucent than the other parts of the metaphysis. The medial part of the bony epiphysis becomes more wedge shaped and still is less developed than its lateral part.

Stage III. This occurs in children in the 4- to 6-year age group and is characterized by deepening of the depression filled by cartilage in the metaphyseal beak, with the radiolucent area giving the appearance of a step in the metaphysis. The medial part of the bony epiphysis is still wedge shaped and is less distinct,

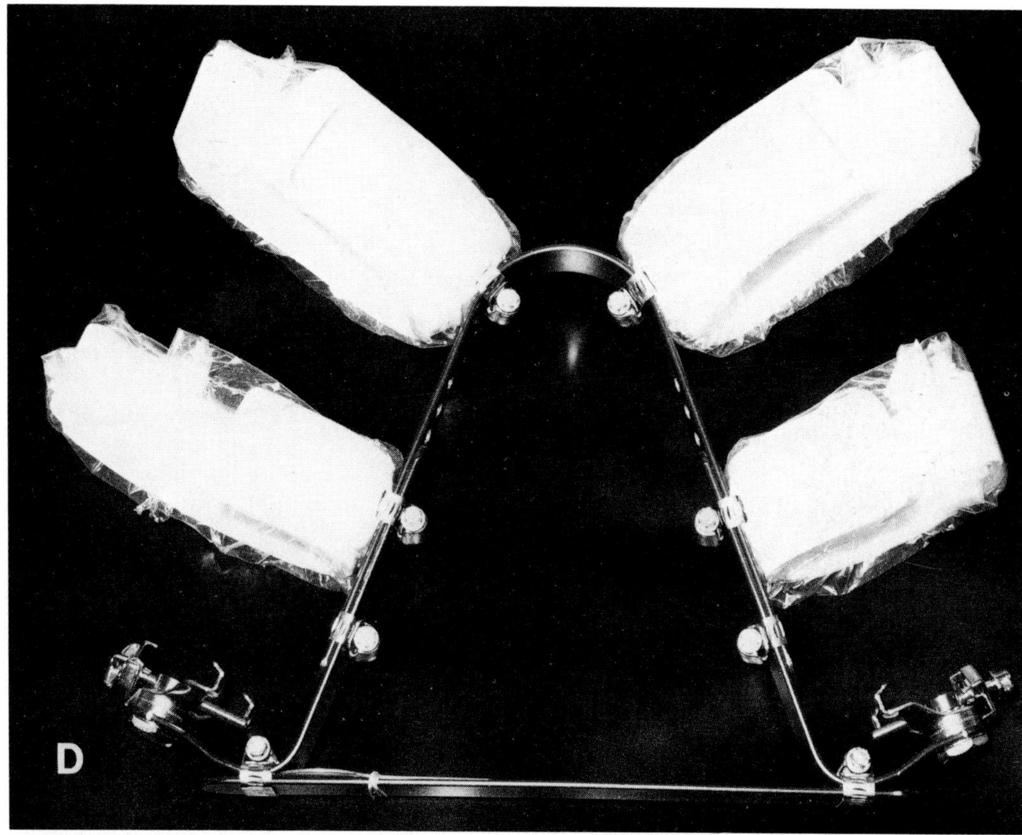

FIG. 20-5. *(Continued). (D)* The patient now wears this orthosis at night.

and small areas of calcification may be present beneath the medial border.

Stage IV. This may be seen in children between 5 and 10 years of age. The epiphyseal growth plate narrows, and the bony epiphysis enlarges. Consequently, the step in the metaphysis increases in depth, and the bony epiphysis occupies the depression in the medial part of the metaphysis. There is a marked irregularity of the medial border of the bony epiphysis.

Stage V. This occurs in children between 9 and 11 years of age. A clear band traverses medially the lateral portion of the epiphyseal plate to the articular cartilage, separating the bony epiphysis into two portions and giving the appearance of a partial double epiphyseal plate. There is some irregularity of the triangular area of the bony epiphysis against the joint cartilage and the cartilage that covers the medial aspect. The articular surface of the medial part of the tibia is deformed, sloping medially and distally from the center condyle notch. As pointed out by Golding, the slope is posteriorly as well as medially directed.[24]

Stage VI. This is seen in children between 10 and 13 years of age. The branches of the medial part of the epiphyseal plate ossify and growth continues in its normal lateral part.

Treatment

In the 2- to 3-year-old child with Stage I or Stage II changes, specific treatment is not necessarily needed. These may be watched and periodically evaluated, or the physician may choose to prescribe a corrective orthosis for nighttime use. If the deformity has caused sufficient changes in the knee so that on weightbearing there is a definite increase in the varus of the knee but the roentgenographic changes are not severe enough to warrant surgical correction, an orthosis that exerts a corrective force on the knee should be used at night (Fig. 20-5). The varus and the medial torsion in patients who have shown progressive roentgenographic changes to Stage III or

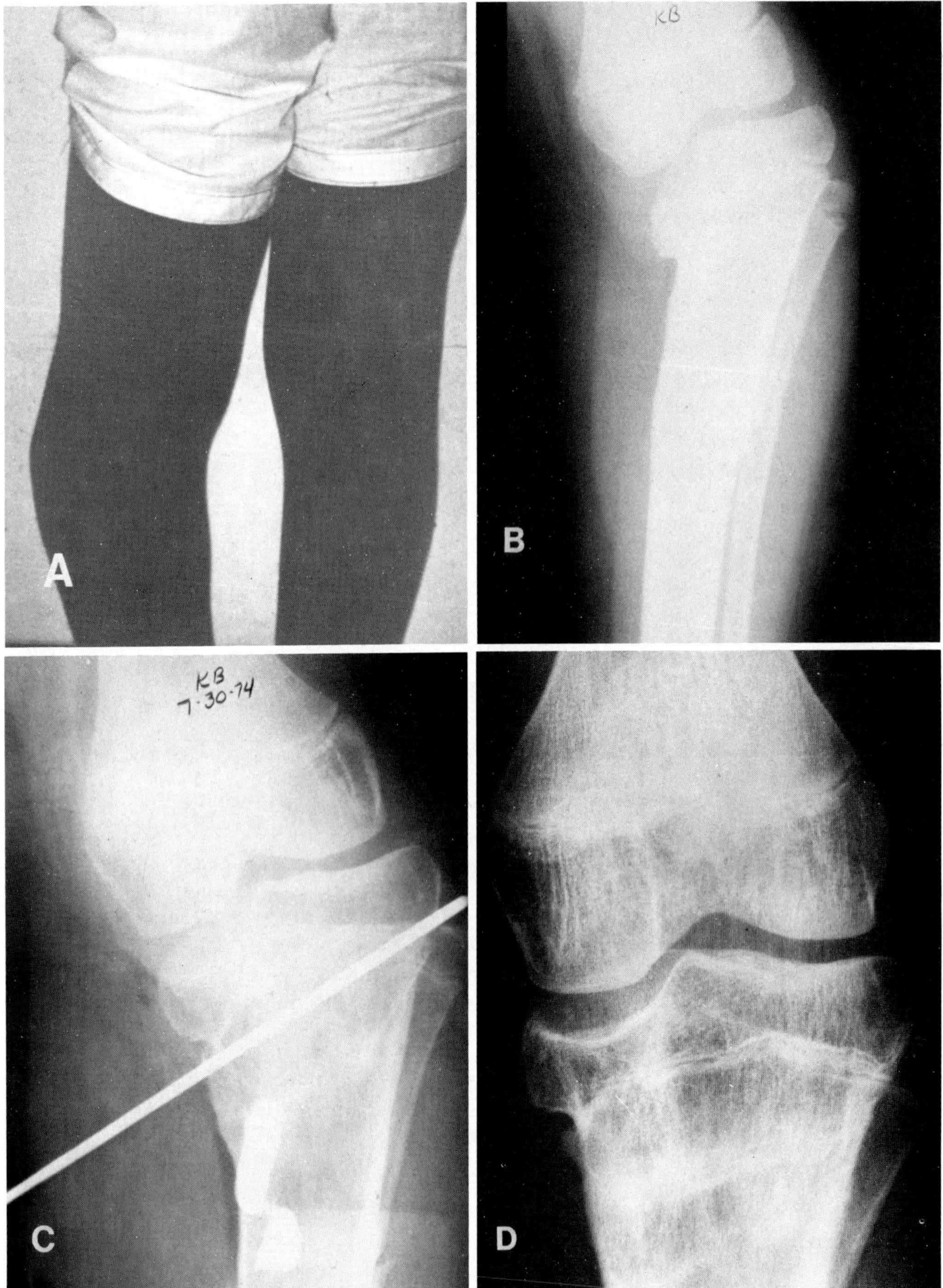

FIG. 20-6. *(A)* A 10-year-old girl with unilateral Blount's disease. *(B)* Two previous osteotomies were too far distal to the tubercle. The deformity is still severe (Stage IV). *(C)* A guide drill is placed parallel to the articular surface and as close as possible to the tubercle. *(D)* Roentgenogram taken after open-wedge osteotomy was performed. No further surgery was required.

Stage IV can usually be corrected and the progressive course of the disease controlled by a reversed dome osteotomy at the level of the distal tip of the tibial tubercle. The fibula should be osteotomized at a lower level but in the upper third of the diaphysis. Excessive overcorrection should be avoided, because the valgus obtained may remain. However, the osteotomy should produce sufficient valgus to shift the stress of weightbearing onto the lateral plateau. In children over 9 years of age, the medial epiphysis may be closed (Stage VI), and, if so, an epiphysiodesis of the lateral part of the proximal epiphysis of the tibia and the proximal epiphysis of the fibula should be done at the time of the osteotomy. Most patients younger than 8 years of age can be corrected, and recurrence is not a problem. However, after 8 years of age, recurrence requiring a second osteotomy is not uncommon.

Up to and including Stage IV disease in children younger than 8 years of age, an adequate reversed dome-shaped osteotomy of the proximal tibia is usually very effective. In patients with the changes of Stage V and over, a repeat osteotomy is likely to be needed if the child is 8 years old. Langenskiold has found that the neglected Stage VI patient older than 8 years of age with excessive deformity of the medial plateau may need to have the medial plateau elevated and an epiphysiodesis of the tibia and fibula performed.[44] After this is healed, a dome osteotomy of the tibia, or an open-wedge osteotomy and an oblique osteotomy of the fibula are needed to complete the correction. A common error in the management of the tibia vara is to make the osteotomy of the tibia too low. It must be made as close to the tubercle as possible to obtain adequate correction without excessive distortion of the contour of the tibia (Fig. 20-6). In older children, the osteotomy may be made closer to the epiphyseal plate and a better correction may be obtained.

Adolescent Tibia Vara

The adolescent type of Blount's disease usually has its start when the child is older than 9 years. The roentgenographic appearance in the adolescent type is quite different. There is no steplike deformity of the epiphyseal plate, and the ossified portion of the epiphysis appears to be relatively normal. The overall appearance is of a prematurely closed medial portion of the growth plate. With tomograms, there can be seen a line of bone that crosses the epiphyseal plate in some patients.

In the adolescent tibia vara, the changes on the medial side of the growth plate are suggestive of a response to trauma as a bridge of bone develops from the epiphysis to the metaphysis. Langenskiold has suggested that it is effective to excise the bridge and replace it with fat.[45] There must be sufficient growth remaining in the remainder of the plate for correction of the deformity to take place. If the patient does not have at least 2 years of growth remaining, osteotomy and epiphysiodesis of the tibia and fibula should be done.

Treatment by dome osteotomy high on the tibia with an oblique osteotomy of the fibula can correct the varus. However, the surgical correction should wait until the child is grown, because some of these correct spontaneously.

CONGENITAL ANGULAR DEFORMITIES OF THE TIBIA

Posterior Bowing

Congenital posterior bowing of the tibia occurs at the junction of the lower and middle thirds of the tibia. The bow is primarily posteriorly directed, but it may be posteromedial. The fibula has a similar bow. Because the distal tibia is directed somewhat anteriorly in comparison to normal, the foot is in a calcaneous position. Plantar flexion is limited, and the anterior muscles of the ankle and foot are shortened. This may be due to the foot and ankle resting in a dorsiflexed position *in utero*.

No treatment except passive stretching of the tight anterior musculature is required. The natural course is a progressive straightening of the tibia, and usually by 4 years of age, the tibia appears normal. Osteotomy is not indicated and should not be done. If the linear growth of the tibia or fibula shows inhibition, appropriate correction may be required later (Fig. 20-7).

Most of these patients develop a leg length discrepancy from inhibition of growth in the tibia. Epiphysiodesis to correct the discrepancy is indicated if the estimated discrepancy will exceed 2.0 cm. The discrepancy may become as great as 5 cm or more, but this degree of discrepancy is unusual.[32] Tibial lengthening to achieve equal leg lengths may be considered in those patients with 5 cm of discrepancy, but I would be hesitant to rec-

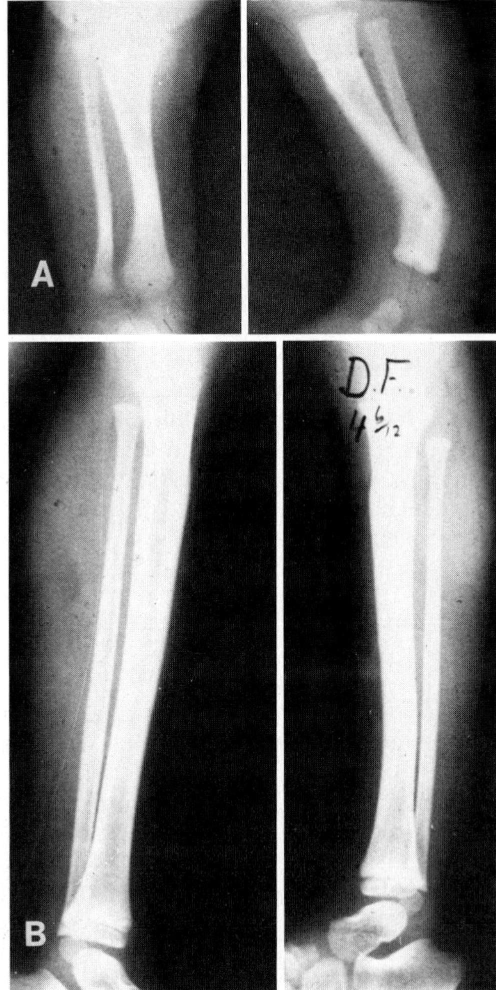

FIG. 20-7. *(A)* Posterior bowing of the tibia in a 3-month-old child. *(B)* The same child at age 4½ years. No treatment was given. Both tibiae are shown for comparison. Note that the fibula on the affected side is slightly shorter.

ommend lengthening except when the difference in length cannot be satisfactorily corrected by epiphysiodesis.

Anterior Bowing

The congenital anteriorly bowed tibia occurs more frequently, is more serious, and has more variations in pathology at the area of bowing than does the posteriorly bowed tibia. The bowing is in the middle and lower thirds of the tibia, and almost always the fibula is similarly bowed and may have the same pathology.

Clinical Features

There are several types of anteriorly bowed tibiae. The first type occurs in association with a congenital absent fibula. In these patients, the tibia is short, bowed, and has a thick sclerotic cortex. The primary problem in these children is the leg length inequality, and these are not considered further in this section.

Congenital pseudarthrosis of the tibia may generally describe the second and third types of anterior bowing. These two types are different in many ways, but both have the serious problem of pathologic fracture and pseudarthrosis at the apex of the bow. The fibula is similarly involved and may also fracture and develop non-union alone or in combination with the tibia.

The second type of anterior bow presents as a narrowing of the tibia with sclerosis and partial or complete obliteration of the intramedullary canal. Surrounding the narrowed area of tibia is a thick fibrous tissue, which Aegerter[1] described as a hamartomatous proliferation of fibrous tissue. After the narrow segment fractures, the ends of the fragments become tapered.

The anterior bow with narrowing of the tibia (the second type) is associated with neurofibromatosis, although some authors have not described neurogenic material in the microscopic examination of specimens removed from the area of pseudarthrosis (Fig. 20-8). Green[28] did describe such changes. Others have reported a high incidence of associated neurofibromatosis in patients who developed pseudarthrosis of the tibia.[3,16] Neurofibromatosis is seen less frequently in the third type.

In the third type of bowing, there is a cystic lesion of the apex of the bow. The tibia may be slightly narrow in the area of the lesion, but usually there is no narrowing, and occasionally, the width may be greater than normal. In the third type, the bow is generally not as severe as it is in the tibia with the narrowed sclerotic segment. The lytic lesion contains material that has the appearance of fibrous dysplasia, not neurogenic material.

Treatment

In all anteriorly bowed tibiae, the treatment is directed toward prevention of fracture. The leg should be protected. A long-leg brace with a molded cuff for the tibia can be used to protect the tibia when the child begins to stand.

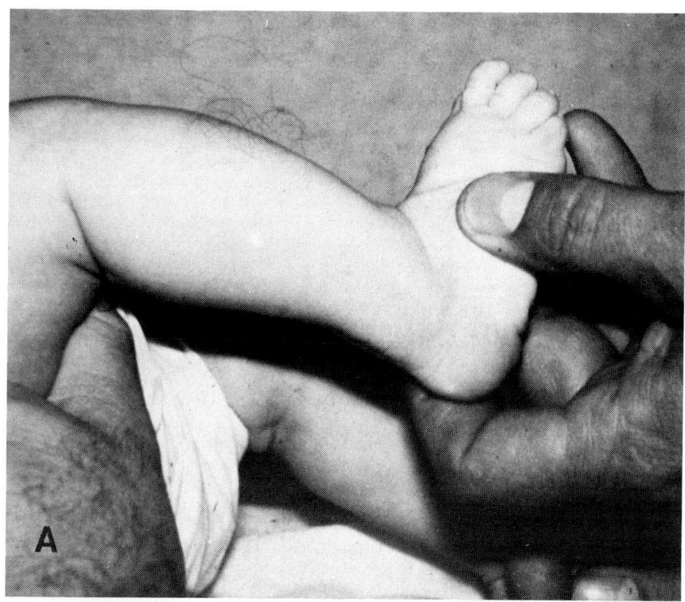

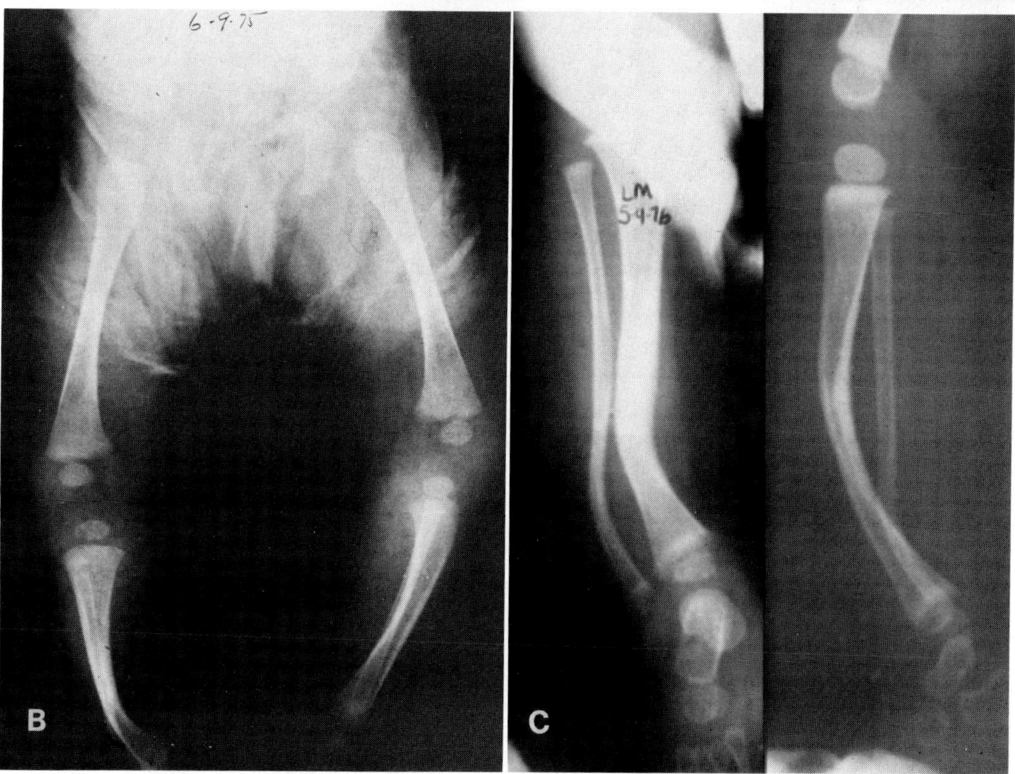

FIG. 20-8. *(A)* Anterior bow in a child with neurofibromatosis. The child's father also has neurofibromatosis. *(B)* Roentgenogram of the same child at age 2 months. Note the narrow sclerotic segment of the tibia with the lateral anterior bow. *(C)* One year later. The tibia was protected first with a plaster cast and later with a foot-ankle-knee orthosis. Note the continued anterolateral bow and the narrow sclerotic segment, as seen on the lateral film. Simlar changes are present in the fibula. The foot-ankle-knee orthosis protects the ankle joint from mediolateral stress, as well as giving protection to the tibia.

Excision of the thick hamartomatous fibrous tissue from around the narrowed area of the tibia and bone grafting posteriorly along the concave side of the bow before the tibia fractures, in Morrissy's[51] experience, has not been beneficial.

After a fracture has occurred, there are many methods used in attempting to obtain union. In fact, there are so many techniques described, it is clear that none are highly successful. One of the basic procedures used in most techniques is excision of the relatively avascular, thick, hamartomatous fibrous tissue from around the bone fragment, excision of the sclerotic bone ends, and bone grafting (autogenous, if possible). Double onlay bone grafts with screw fixation; bypass bone grafts; intramedullary rods, and additional bone grafts; or compression clamps and bone grafts are some of the more frequently used techniques of treatment.[10,49,70]

The success rate of the many types of grafting and the different fixation devices is not sufficiently different to strongly recommend one over the other, but I prefer the intramedullary rod fixation plus grafting.

It is apparent, as suggested by Morrissy,[51] that the severity of the biologic disorder is the most significant factor in the prognosis. The prognosis for healing of a pseudarthrosis is not significantly different in those patients with neurofibromatosis than in those without. Children who are born with a pseudarthrosis have a poorer prognosis than others. Except for this newborn group, the average age of fracture is not significantly different in those patients who achieve an acceptable result from those who are either unacceptable or who have amputations.

The technique I prefer is to excise the fibrous hamartoma from about the pseudarthrosis and obtain fixation by inserting an intramedullary Steinmann pin through the calcaneus and talus and into the distal tibia across the pseudarthrosis and high into the proximal tibia; bone grafts are placed around the pseudarthrosis. Postoperatively, the leg is immobilized in a plaster cast. After 12 to 14 weeks in plaster, the cast is replaced by a long-leg brace with a gauntlet about the tibia. Patersen has added electrical stimulation with implanted cathode at the pseudarthrosis and reported healing in 9 of 11 patients.[57] Electrical stimulation, through electromagnetic fields, has been reported to improve the success rate of healing.[6] The 71% success rate reported by Bassett is higher than I have seen at other institutions that use the electromagnetic field technique.

Regardless of the technique used, the prognosis for healing is guarded. Even if union is obtained, leg length discrepancy is likely to be present. The earlier the fracture occurs and the more distal the pseudarthrosis, the poorer the prognosis. Although primary amputation has been advised as the treatment of choice, I believe a reasonable attempt at obtaining union should be used in all cases, with even up to three or four attempts at bone grafting. Once it is obvious that even if union were to be obtained, the leg would be unacceptably short and small, amputation is advised.

The future may bring a more biologic approach in the management of the congenital pseudarthrosis. Early reports suggest that vascularized fibular grafts are encouraging.[72] Gilbert[23] reported a large series of vascularized fibular grafts with very encouraging results. This approach appears so promising that it will very likely become the procedure of choice in the near future. Only time is needed to prove that the early success in union develops into satisfactory survival and growth of the graft.

RECURRENT SUBLUXATION AND DISLOCATION OF THE PATELLA

Recurrent subluxation and dislocation are a spectrum of multiple anatomic and biomechanical variations of degrees of severity. Before the great athletic and physical exercise boom of the 1970s, the majority of patients with these problems were girls. However, today there is a majority of male patients with patella problems of instability.

However, the frequency of complete recurrent dislocation is far greater in girls than in boys.[9,25,48]

Etiology

There are multiple abnormal anatomic relationships that contribute to the development of recurrent dislocation of the patella.

Most patients have generalized relaxation of joint ligaments. Laxity of the medial capsule has to be a factor, because unless it is lax, the patella cannot dislocate. Whether the medial capsule is lax as part of the elastic nature of the patient's ligaments or is lax because of repeated stress from the patella being pulled laterally by other forces is unclear, but both aspects are probably important.

The iliotibial band may be contracted or may have an abnormal attachment to the patella. A contracted iliotibial band or abnormal patellar attachment may play a role in displacing the patella laterally as the knee is flexed.

Both genu valgum and external torsion of the tibia encourage lateral dislocation of the patella.

A high-lying patella can more easily be displaced lateral to the lateral condyle when the tibia is externally rotated on the femur while slightly flexed and abducted and tension is produced by contracting the quadriceps muscle. These are the conditions that prevail when the patella dislocates in a patient who turns while dancing or twists while standing, and during running and changing direction. This is more likely to occur if the lateral condyle is small, the femoral groove shallow, and the "q" angle is increased.

All these anatomic variations may play a role in the recurrent dislocation or subluxation of the patella. There are, however, instances when none of these can be identified with certainty, yet the patient has a history of dislocation or symptoms suggesting subluxation.

The normal excursion of the patella as the knee goes from full extension to flexion is first to strike the lateral condyle and then to move medially into the femoral sulcus. The medial facet of the patella does not contact the femoral surface until the knee is well flexed. If the lateral condyle is insufficient or the resultant dynamic force between the quadriceps and the patellar tendon insertion is directed too far laterally, the patella initially moves lateral to the lateral condyle and then moves medially back into the sulcus with further flexion of the knee. The medial return to the sulcus causes abnormal wear on the medial facet, which is the location of chondromalacia in most patellae.

The abnormality of patellar movement may be so slight that the lateral excursion of the patella is too limited for the patient to appreciate a displacement, or it may be such that it allows the patella to migrate laterally on flexion and then jump back medially over the condyle, or it may be severe enough for the patella to stay laterally displaced until the knee is again passively extended under the appropriate circumstances.

Clinical Features and Diagnosis

Recurrent dislocation may begin in the child as young as 5 or 6 years but usually does not manifest itself until adolescence, and, indeed, at times it is not manifested until the third decade of life. In many patients with recurrent dislocation, the history is usually relatively simple. The patella frankly dislocates and may spontaneously reduce when the knee is extended either passively or actively.

With such a history, diagnosis is no problem. There are, however, patients who complain that they feel the patella (or feel something) move laterally with certain motions of the knee. This is associated with pain and rarely is followed by effusion in the joint. A more subtle patellofemoral abnormality may be present, in which the patella is pulled laterally by pathologic forces but does not displace enough for the patient to appreciate any patellar displacement. Diagnosis is difficult in this type of patient. The symptoms may be confined to sudden pain while running or "giving way" of the knee when changing directions during walking or running.

In the patient whose patella frankly dislocates, physical examination usually shows a hypermobile patella that can be or can almost be dislocated by pushing it laterally. The patella is frequently higher than normal, and the patient is likely to have, in general, loose ligaments. The vastus medialis is flat and small and does not extend as far distally as normal. Varying degrees of genu valgum may be present.

The patient without a history of complete dislocation may have essentially the same physical findings except that the patella is not quite as mobile. Patients with either type frequently have a positive so-called apprehension test. That test is done with the patient sitting on a table, the leg resting at 45° of flexion, and the quadriceps relaxed. A lateral-directed force is put on the patella. The fear of the pain that will result from displacement causes the patient to contract the quadriceps and to assume a facial expression showing apprehension of pain, with or without verbal comment.

Patients who present with the complaint of peripatellar pain when running, cutting, or going up and down stairs are difficult to diagnose. These patients fall into that group of patients that Ficat[19] has called Excessive Lateral Pressure syndrome (ELPS). In addition to pain on activity, there may be complaints of locking, giving way, crepitus, and intermittent swelling. Ficat describes ELPS as a loss of dynamic equilibrium of the patella in the trochlea. It is this lateral pressure and loss of dynamic equilibrium that leads to narrowing of the joint space with subsequent fragmentation of the cartilage.[19] Patients with ELPS are likely to have a lateral tilt to the patella, a tight retinaculum may or may not be present, and the iliotibial band is usually contracted as shown by the Ober test. The Q angle may be normal, as may routine x-rays. However, axial views of the patella taken at 30°, 60°, and 90° of flexion will, with time, show narrowing of the lateral patellofemoral joint. If neglected, the changes of fissuring of the cartilage and sclerosis of the subchondral bone can be seen on axial arthrography of the patellofemoral joint.

Green and others demonstrated the lateral position of the patella in the femoral sulcus by an axial view of the patella with the knee flexed 45°, the x-ray beam tilted 30° off the horizontal, and the cassette held resting on the tibia with the x-ray beam perpendicular to the cassette.

Merchant and associates[50] analyzed and redefined and measured a large population of patients to make this technique more meaningful. They measured the sulcus and the position of the patella in the sulcus and called the relationship the *patellofemoral congruence angle*.

The sulcus of the femur is bisected with a line that extends through the patella. The lowest point in the posterior surface of the patella is marked, and a line is drawn through it from the point where the sulcus is bisected. The angle between the two lines is called the *congruence angle*. (Fig. 20-9). Angles that are medial to the line of bisection are negative and those lateral to it are positive. The average angle is −6°, with an 11° standard deviation. An angle less than +16° is within the 95th percentile. In spite of carefully taken roentgenograms and measurement, there will be patients whose history and physical findings are sufficient to make the diagnosis of subluxation or dislocation when the roentgenogram is normal.

Treatment

More than 100 operative procedures for the treatment of congenital dislocation of the patella have been described. This alone attests to the complexity of the problem and to the ineffectiveness of the operative procedures.

The problems faced in treating subluxation and dislocation of the patella are directed at prevention of recurrence without creating either a destructive force against the patellofemoral articulation or a growth disturbance of the proximal tibia that would cause recurvation.

Patients with the diagnosis of recurrent subluxation should initially perform isometric exercises to strengthen the quadriceps.

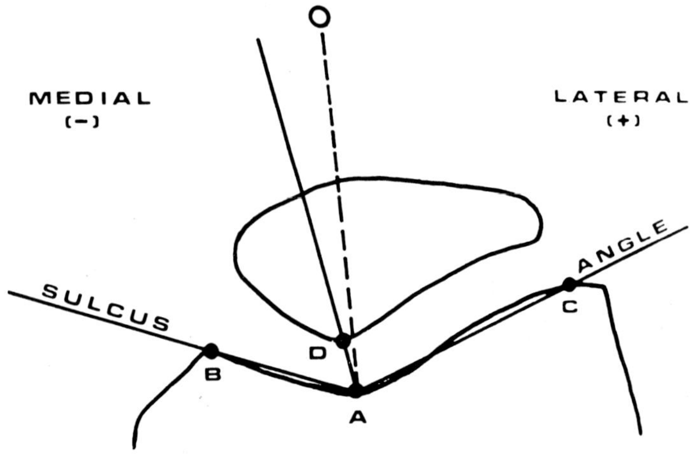

FIG. 20-9. Diagram showing plotting of the congruence angle. (Merchant CC *et al*. Roentgenographic analysis of patellofemoral congruence. J Bone Joint Surg 56A:1391, 1974)

The first incident of dislocation of the patella should be treated by immobilization of the knee in extension for 4 weeks, followed by a program of isometric exercises. This may be successful in preventing recurrent dislocations. If conservative treatment does not relieve symptoms or prevent recurrent dislocations, surgical correction should be undertaken.

There are many recorded surgical approaches to the treatment of this problem. The most popular over the years has been the transfer of the insertion of the patellar tendon. If the tendon insertion is moved, it should not be moved distally. It should be moved medially only enough to have the patella articulate with the center of the femoral sulcus when the knee goes from extension to flexion. Excessive medial displacement can cause the patella to articulate too forcefully and too early in the flexion motion, so that there is a clicking sensation as the patella slides over the superior lip of the medial condyle when the knee flexes. This appears to be harmful to the medial facet of the patella. If, in addition, the insertion is transferred distally, the interarticular force between the femur and patella is increased, which may also cause further wear on the patellar articular surface.

In my opinion, transfer of the patellar tendon alone is not sufficient treatment for recurrent subluxation or dislocation, and the location of the patellar tendon insertion is not the primary factor in subluxation and dislocation of the patella. I believe that the essential dynamic force in subluxation and dislocation of the patella is the action of the quadriceps muscle and the iliotibial band. If the quadriceps mechanism is properly aligned surgically, and if the lateral reticulum is released, there is seldom a need to transfer the patellar tendon.

When the treatment has been delayed and the articular surface has sustained extensive chondromalacia, patellectomy must be considered. If possible, it seems preferable to shave and drill the patella rather than to do a patellectomy, but excision is at times necessary.

The operative technique I prefer is the one described and used by Green.[26,68] In this procedure, the lateral influence of the iliotibial band on the patella is negated by dividing the lateral retinaculum and iliotibial band on the flat, completely freeing all fibers that seem to pull on the patella. By lengthening on the flat, two layers are identified that can be closed loosely to prevent herniation of the synovium. This technique of release is not essential, but the iliotibial band must be completely released from any attachment on the patella and the patellar ligament. The medial retinaculum capsule is opened, the joint is inspected, and the medial capsule and retinaculum are reefed "pants over vest." The vastus medialis is advanced distally and laterally so that the distal lateral edge of the muscle is advanced to the distal lateral edge of the patella. The medial fibers should be left attached medially so that the dynamic force of the vastus medialis pulls the patella medially as the knee is extended and prevents lateral displacement. In older teenagers and young adults whose quadriceps patellar tendon angle is more than 25°, the insertion of the tendon may need to be moved medially, but only enough to decrease this angle to about 10°. In young children, this should be avoided, because it may interfere with growth and may cause genu recurvatum.[30,48] When the patella tendon insertion needs to be moved medially to improve the patella alignment, I prefer the Elmslie-Trillat technique. In this procedure, the lateral tightness is released, the medial structures are tightened, and the patellar tendon insertion is moved medially to decrease the Q angle without posteriorly displacing the insertion. The Hauser procedure displaces the insertion posteriorly, which decreases the momentum and causes greater patellofemoral pressure.

If the patellar tendon is not transferred, flexion and extension of the knee in the side-lying position and with assistance is started 5 to 6 days postoperatively. A bivalved cast is used for 6 weeks, and crutches are used for an additional 6 weeks, with partial weight-bearing being allowed. In those patients who have the tendon transferred medially, the beginning of the exercise program is delayed until 4 weeks after surgery.

Where other procedures of realignment have failed, the use of the semitendonesis as a tether into the patella may be effective. I have not used this technique for preventing recurrent dislocation and prefer the realignment techniques mentioned, but, where this fails, the semitendonesis transfer may be effective in the child who is too young for the Elmslie-Trillat procedure.

The subluxating patella is treated the same as the dislocating patella. However, major emphasis is on releasing the lateral structures and transferring the vastus medialis laterally and distally. Occasionally in a teenage athlete with pain about the patella that occurs only when changing direction while running, but who has essentially normal appearing quadriceps, patellar, femoral, and tibial relationships, I have limited the surgery to a release of the iliotibial band and lateral retinaculum from the patella, with relief of symptoms in most patients.

ELPS, recurrent subluxation, and recurrent dislocation are probably a continuum of the abnormality of different severity. The approach to treatment should be with this concept in mind.

The initial treatment of ELPS is nonoperative. An exercise program to stretch the iliotibial band and to strengthen the quadriceps and hamstrings should be started. The tight iliotibial is demonstrated by the Ober test. In my experience, if it is tight, the symptoms in ELPS will not respond to strengthening exercises until the iliotibial band is stretched. The quadriceps and hamstrings exercises should be isometric with progressively increasing resistance. If after 10 to 12 weeks of exercises the symptoms persist, release of the iliotibial band should be considered. The customary way of lengthening the band has been to release the lateral retinaculum. Because the problem is a dynamic one and the tightness is in the iliotibial band, I have divided the iliotibial band transversely two fingers' breadths above the lateral condyle of the femur. It should be divided anteriorly until there is no tightness with the knee flexed and posteriorly to where the intermuscular septum is attached to the femur. Postoperative exercise in order to rapidly get full flexion of the knee is important.

CONGENITAL AND HABITUAL DISLOCATION OF THE PATELLA

Congential dislocation of the patella is less common than the ordinary recurrent dislocation. Most of my patients have had associated anomalies of the musculoskeletal system or other systems.

The extent of the patellar dislocation may be such that the patella dislocates with each flexion of the knee and reduces with extension (habitual dislocation), or the patella may be so laterally displaced that it remains dislocated at all times. In the congenitally dislocated patella, the primary anomaly is in the vastus lateralis and its fascia, the vastus intermedius, and the iliotibial band. The tightness in these structures prevents the patella from staying in the femoral sulcus during flexion of the knee.

In the patient with a patella that dislocates each time the knee is flexed, the complaint may be the recognition by the parent of a clicking sensation on flexion and extension of the knee. After a period of time, this becomes painful and the child keeps the knee flexed so that the patella is perpetually dislocated, because it is the relocation motion that is painful. By keeping the knee flexed, a flexion contracture develops and the child walks with an unusual gait where the knee does not extend during weightbearing. Finding a laterally displaced patella upon palpation makes the diagnosis, which may be confirmed by a roentgenogram of the knee if the patella has ossified. As seen in Figure 20-10, the tibia may be subluxed laterally on the femur as a result of the lateral tightness.

The contracture of the vastus lateralis may be so great that the patella is perpetually dislocated. When the patella stays dislocated in the newborn, the knee does not extend. Attempts at correcting the persistent flexion contracture by traction or casting will be unsuccessful. The small unossified patella is difficult to palpate, but when there is a high level of suspicion and a careful examination, it can be palpated in a lateral position. The treatment is surgical release of the lateral retinaculum and the iliotibial band, excision of any fibrotic bands found in the vastus lateralis or vastus intermedius, extensive mobilization of the vastus lateralis from the lateral intermuscular septum, recession of the vastus lateralis from the patella, and central slip of the quadriceps mechanism, and transfer of the vastus medialis distally and laterally, as described above. In older children, in addition, the patellar tendon may require medial transfer if, after the releases are performed, the patella rides laterally on flexion. Occasionally the patella is adherent to the periosteum and perichondrium over the lateral condyle. Great care is needed to free the patella without injury to its articular surface.

CONGENITAL DISLOCATION AND SUBLUXATION OF THE KNEE

Congenital dislocation of the knee is an uncommon anomaly seen with equal frequency in both sexes.[60] The dislocation may be either unilateral or bilateral. In the congenitally dislocated knee, the tibia is displaced anteriorly. It is usually rotated in relation to the femur and may also have lateral displacement. There are associated congenital anomalies in 60% of patients born with a congenital dislocation of the knee.

The diagnosis is made by the physical finding of anterior displacement of the tibia, with or without lateral displacement. Roentgenograms of the knee confirm the diagnosis. The condyles of the femur are prominent posteriorly and help to orient the rotation of the tibia to the femur. Usually the tibia is internally rotated, and the femur is frequently capable of only limited internal rotation, making it difficult to correctly align the tibia and femur. The collateral ligaments of the knee are stretched, and it is difficult to know the appropriate plane for flexion-extension, because the mediolateral range of motion of the knee is usually as great or greater than the anteroposterior range. The finding may be present even after the dislocation is reduced.

Hyperextension is always present in the congenitally dislocated knee. However, hyperextension is frequently present in normal knees of a breech baby, as well as in those knees that are subluxated but not completely dislocated. It is important that these latter entities be differentiated from the dislocated knee, because the treatment and results vary significantly.

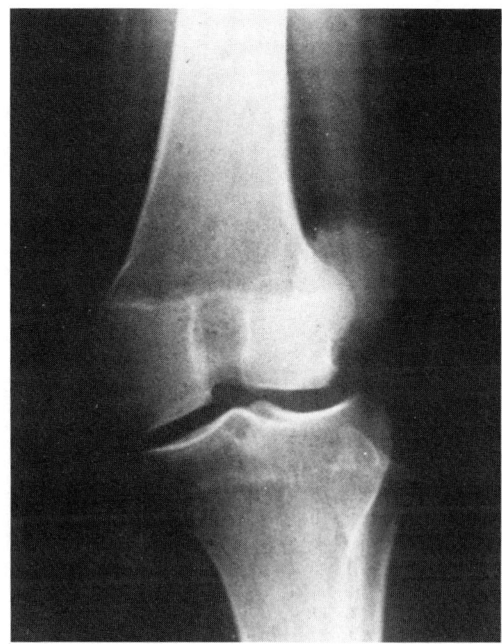

FIG. 20-10. Congenitally dislocated patella, moderately displaced. This could be reduced with full extension. The patient walked with the knee in flexion.

Etiology

Both congenital and environmental causes have been postulated.[39] There are cases in which there is a familial history, but the majority of patients have no positive family history. The position *in utero* may influence the development of a dislocated knee when the fetus is in the breech position with the feet under the mandible, but the majority of the patients are not breech births. Fibrosis of the vastus lateralis or vastus intermedius is present in some cases. Those patients with fibrosis in the quadriceps muscle are likely to have lateral displacement of the patella in addition to dislocation of the knee.

For the knee to dislocate, the posterior capsule has to be very loose and the cruciate ligaments either stretched, hypoplastic, or absent. These changes are possibly secondary to the dislocation, but they could be primary factors. Dislocation of the knee is a frequent finding in children with arthrogryposis multiplex congenita. In these children the muscle abnormality certainly must be an important factor in producing the dislocation.

Congenital *subluxation* of the knee is more common than dislocation. The difference can best be seen by roentgenographic examination, because the appearance of the subluxated knee on inspection is similar to that of the dislocated knee. The subluxated knee usually has up to 25° to 40° of flexion. The tibia may be moved manually, anteriorly, and posteriorly, which easily causes subluxation and reduction of the knee (Fig. 20-11). The same etiologic factor that causes dislocation may also cause subluxation of the knee. It is important to make the correct diagnosis, because the treatment is different.

Treatment

Treatment should begin immediately after birth. If the roentgenogram shows subluxation, the affected knee is treated by passively flexing the knee as far as it will easily go. After manual

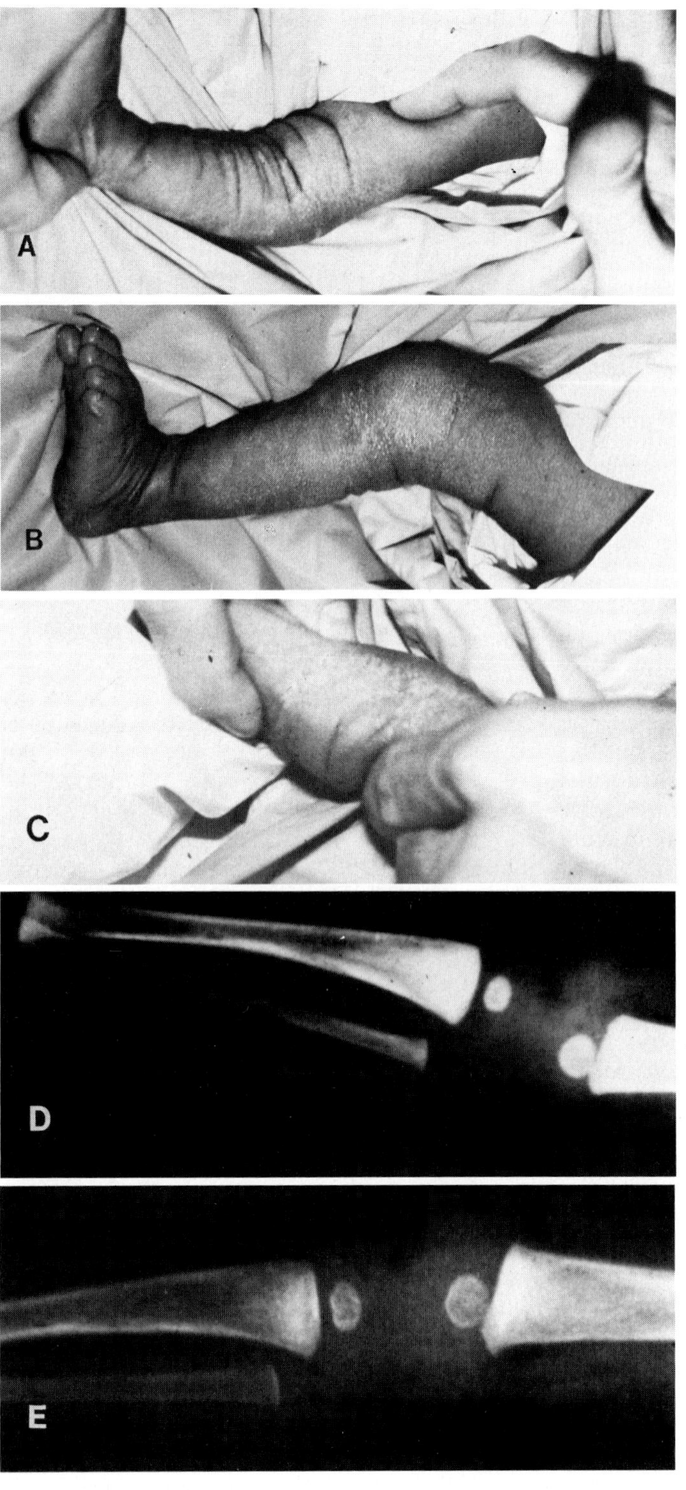

FIG. 20-11. Subluxation of the knee. *(A)* The knee in hyperextension. *(B)* The knee in flexion. *(C)* The tibia could be moved manually, anteriorly to the subluxed position and posteriorly to a position of reduction. *(D)* A lateral roentgenogram taken before traction was applied. *(E)* Lateral roentgenogram taken after treatment with traction followed by plaster immobilization flexion.

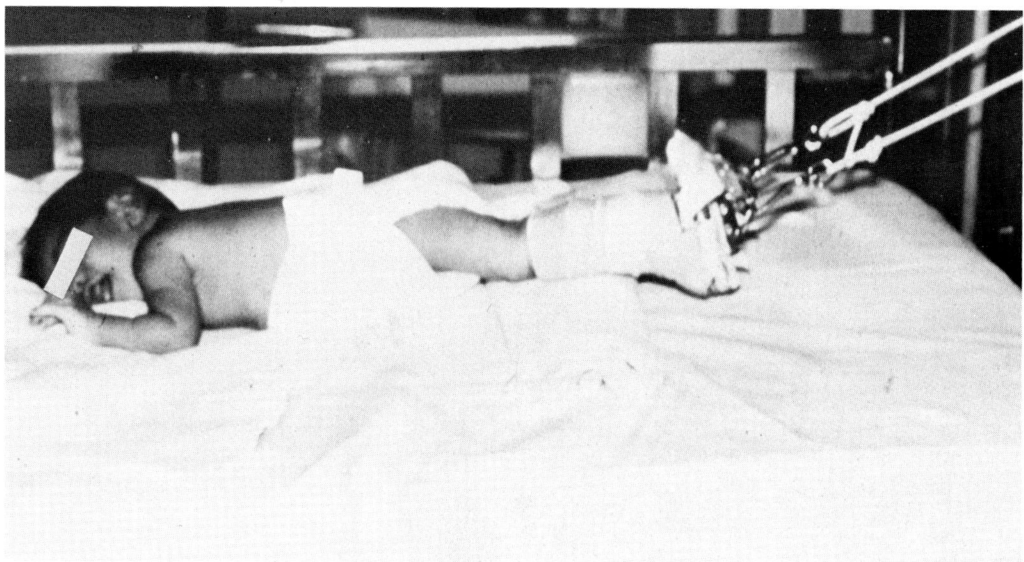

FIG. 20-12. This child has been placed in skin traction for reduction of subluxation.

pressure has been applied for 2 or 3 minutes, the knee is held in this position by a plaster cast. The cast is changed at weekly intervals, and further flexion is obtained with each cast change until 90° of flexion is present. Further immobilization for 4 to 6 weeks, with the knee held in flexion with a bivalved cast or an orthosis that is removed several times each day, is usually sufficient to prevent recurrence of the subluxation. Great care must be taken to avoid the use of excessive force, because the distal femoral epiphysis can be displaced by this technique.

If there is uncertainty as to whether the knee is subluxated or dislocated, skin traction with the baby in the prone position and the traction directed so as to flex the knees may be used as the initial treatment (Fig. 20-12). Daily knee-flexion exercises can be performed on the baby by the therapist. These should be continued until the knees flex to 90°, after which a bivalved cast or orthosis is applied and the exercises are continued for 4 to 6 more weeks. I prefer to use skin traction initially on my patients before putting the leg in plaster in managing congenital subluxation.

The dislocated knee should *not* be manipulated but should be treated initially with skeletal traction. The technique used by Green[26] is to place a Kirschner wire in the distal femoral metaphysis, one through the distal tibia and one through the proximal tibia (Fig. 20-13). A weight placed on the femoral wire is directed forward and cephalad to counteract the distal force on the tibia. The proper rotational position is maintained by proper placing of the wires. After the tibia is pulled distally to clear the end of the femur, the direction of the forces is changed to allow gradual flexion of the knee. If the rotational position is not corrected, the flexion obtained may be tangential or even perpendicular to the correct flexion-extension axis. It is necessary to have an infant on a Bradford frame or some similar device to obtain appropriate traction.

When it is apparent that traction is not sufficient to correct the deformity, open reduction is required. The operative procedure may vary in each patient, but certain basic features should be mentioned. The approach is best done through a long, anterior incision. After exposing the quadriceps, patella, anterior capsule, patellar tendon, and collateral ligaments, the quadriceps is the first structure that is corrected. If there is a discrete fibrous mass in the vastus lateralis or the vastus intermedius, it should be excised. If the vastus lateralis and vastus intermedius form a fibrous mass that is adherent to the femur and that obliterates the suprapatellar pouch, the quadriceps should be lengthened by a V incision, with approximation of the V cephalad with a Y closure. The anterior capsule is then transversely divided. If the knee flexes to 80° or

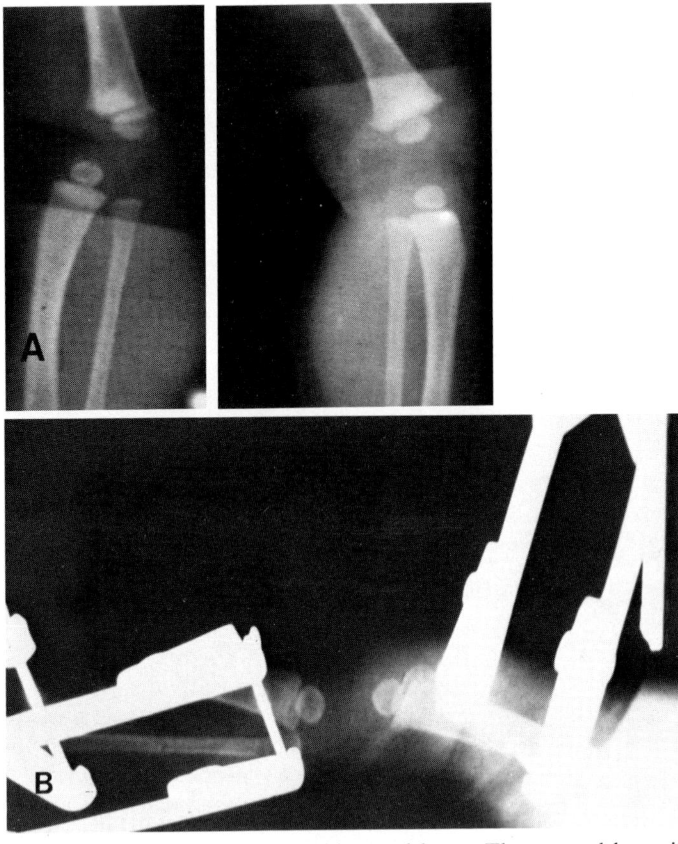

FIG. 20-13. *(A)* A severely subluxated knee. The normal knee is shown on the right for comparison. *(B)* The three-pin technique for reducing the severely subluxated or the truly dislocated knee.

90°, no further dissection is needed. However, if flexion is still limited, the collateral ligaments should be freed so that they will slide posteriorly. The posterior capsule may need to be bluntly dissected from the femoral condyles and the iliotibial band divided. If, after the knee is reduced and flexed to 90°, there is anterior instability, the anterior cruciate may be moved forward on the tibia, but if the anterior cruciate is absent, I would not reconstruct it at this time, because with time, the instability may improve. If it does not improve, repair of the posterior capsule may be preferable to an attempt at cruciate reconstruction.

Prognosis

Almost all those patients with knees that are subluxed and reduced by simple traction or cast do well. Those that have knees that are completely dislocated and need skeletal traction or open reduction do less well. It is uncommon to obtain more than 90° of motion, but the patient can usually expect sufficient function to live at least a sedentary life.

BIPARTITE PATELLA

The bipartite patella is a congenital anomaly with little clinical significance except that frequently it must be differentiated from a fracture.

The patella usually arises from one center of ossification, but, at times, there are two or more centers. These centers usually fuse to form one bone but may remain separate, creating a bipartite or multiple-partite patella. The second or smaller ossified section of the patella is almost always in the upper outer section of the patella.

The diagnosis is made by roentgenographic examination, and, unfortunately, the roentgenogram is usually made following an injury.

However, the distinguishing features of the congenital anomaly should separate it from an acute fracture. In the bipartite patella, the margins between the fragments are smooth and the edge is cortical bone, whereas in an acute fracture, the edges are irregular and are cortical cancellous bone. Often the anomaly is bilateral, and, when there is doubt, the opposite patella should also be examined.

DISCOID MENISCUS

A discoid meniscus is a condition in which the fibrocartilage structure of the knee is discoid in shape rather than semilunar. It usually occurs in the lateral compartment of the knee, but it may occur in the medial compartment.[14,52] Generally it is unilateral, but it may be bilateral, and it occurs with equal frequency in males and females.

Etiology

The etiology of discoid meniscus is controversial. Ross, Tough, and English thought it to be a congenital lesion resulting from arrest of the development of the meniscus in the embryo.[63] Kaplan was unable to find any evidence that the meniscus was ever discoid in shape during its development.[38] Since no one had ever described a discoid-shaped meniscus in an embryo, he believed there must be another explanation. His studies led him to believe the discoid-shaped meniscus was an acquired lesion resulting from the lateral femoral condyle repeatedly riding over the lateral meniscus during flexion and extension of the knee. According to Kaplan, in the discoid meniscus there is no attachment of the meniscus posteriorly to the tibia, and the ligament of Wrisberg is short. Whereas the normal lateral meniscus moves posteriorly with flexion and anteriorly with extension, the discoid meniscus is displaced posteriorly and medially by the short thick ligament of Wrisberg as the knee extends. The short ligament of Wrisberg does not allow the meniscus to move forward with the lateral condyle as the knee extends. On flexion of the knee, the popliteal and coronary ligament pull the meniscus laterally. This medial and lateral movement of the meniscus beneath the pressure of the lateral condyle gradually deforms the cartilage into its discoid shape.

Clinical Features

The child with a discoid meniscus may present with the complaint of a "clunk" or "click" in the knee or may have pain as the major complaint or both. There may be a snapping in the knee that on observation gives the appearance of the tibia subluxating during flexion-extension, or the knee may give way while walking or running. Other patients have a dull ache that is intermittent, that is aggravated by activity, but that also is present at night and during inactive periods.

The physical findings are usually limited. Often the snap can be reproduced by flexing and extending the knee. If the meniscus is torn, pressure over the lateral compartment at the joint line may cause pain. A discoid meniscus may undergo cystic degeneration. The cyst is palpable along the joint line, usually just anterior to the lateral collateral ligament. If pain has been present for some time, there should be atrophy of the thigh muscle. Arthroscopy and arthrography are both helpful in confirming the diagnosis.

Treatment

No treatment is indicated in the nonpainful discoid meniscus. However, if the symptoms of a torn meniscus are present or if a cyst is palpable over the lateral joint space, the meniscus should be removed. Meniscectomy of a discoid meniscus is more difficult to perform than removal of a torn semilunar meniscus. The meniscus is difficult to see because it displaces medially and posteriorly on extension and lateroposteriorly on flexion. A transverse incision over the lateral joint line is used to remove the meniscus. Care must be taken to protect both the popliteal artery, which lies close to the ligament of Wrisberg that connects the discoid meniscus to the medial femoral condyle and the lateral inferior genicular artery that lies between the fibular collateral ligament and the synovium over the posterior lateral aspect of the meniscus. Postoperative care is the same as that for any other meniscectomy.

OSTEOCHONDRITIS DISSECANS

Osteochondritis is a lesion that affects the subchondral bone and articular surface of a joint. It is generally thought of as a disease of young adults but occurs not infrequently in children between 10 and 15 years of age. The youngest reported patient was 4 years old.[27] The distal femur is the most common site of involvement, but it may also occur in the dome of the talus, the patella, the capitellum of the humerus, and in the femoral head. About 10% of the patients have more than one lesion, with the involvement being usually symmetrical, but multiple lesions may be present without being symmetrical in distribution.

Alexander Pare described the removal of a loose body from a joint in 1558. In 1870, James Paget described this lesion and called it *joint necrosis*, but Konig in 1887 gave the lesion the name by which it is now known. He believed that the lesion was due to trauma that resulted in "dissecting inflammation."

Etiology

Trauma, either directly or indirectly, with occlusion of the subchondral blood supply, is generally thought to be the cause of osteochondritis dissecans.[12,18,65] Lesions similar to osteochondritis dissecans have been produced experimentally by Rehbein, both by repeated hyperextension of the knee and by a direct force on the patella.[61]

Smillie separates this condition into juvenile and adult types. According to Smillie, the adult type is attributed to trauma brought about by a displacement of a meniscus or by instability of the joint. In the child, irregular ossification with isolation of a nidus of bone in the subchondral area creates the environment in which minimal trauma causes the blood supply to the nidus to be interrupted.[65]

There is a hereditary or constitutional predisposition for development of osteochondritis dissecans. I have treated several patients and their cousins. Others have had similar experiences.[21,54,67] About 10% of the patients have more than one lesion, which suggests a constitutional factor. Furthermore, the patients are more likely to have osteochondrosis of other areas, such as Osgood-Schlatter disease, osteochondrosis of the lower pole of the patella, and vertebral osteochondrosis. Six of 27 children in Green's series showed other osteochondritic lesions.[27]

I have observed an asymptomatic irregular ossification defect in the distal end of the femur in a 10-year-old boy progress to a symptomatic typical osteochondritis dissecans by the time he was 13 years old. It is my belief that in the child, the isolation of a nidus of ossified bone surrounded by cartilage in the subchondral area sets the stage for a fracture to occur at the interface between the bone and the nonossified cartilage. The cartilage may ossify, and the necrotic nidus may be gradually incorporated. However, if the articular cartilage fractures, joint fluid will circulate into the fracture, preventing healing, and a loose body develops, which eventually drops out of its bed.

Necroses of the subchondral bone have been reported as the primary pathology.[1] I believe that it is only after the articular surface fractures that the nidus of bone becomes necrotic. When the osteochondritic lesion is examined microscopically before the articular cartilage has a fracture, the bone is not necrotic.

Clinical Features

The major symptom in the child is pain, which is intermittent early in the course but later becomes constant. Strenuous activities increase the discomfort, not so much during the action, but rather after resting from vigorous activity. Mild swelling may be observed intermittently, and the child may have an antalgic gait. Occasionally the joint is asymptomatic, or the symptoms may be too mild for the patient to seek help until the fragment separates, the loose body causes locking of the joint and swelling, and other signs of synovitis become more prominent.

The physical findings are usually minimal and depend on the duration of symptoms and the joint affected. In the knee, it is usually the case to find a full range of motion, no synovial thickening, and minimal thigh atrophy. When a loose body is present, there may be a synovitis with effusion, and, occasionally, the loose body can be palpated. Pressure by palpation over the involved surface usually causes pain. The test described by Wilson is particularly helpful when the knee is affected. In this test, the tibia is internally rotated on the femur with the knee flexed 90°. As the knee is extended, internal rotation is maintained and pain is experienced at about 30° of flexion if the lesion is on the medial condyle. The pain is relieved by externally rotating the tibia.

The diagnosis is made by roentgenogram. Early, there is a radiolucent area with a small spicule of bone (Fig. 20-14 *A*, *B*). Later the picture is one of a subchondral fragment of bone demarcated by a radiolucent line. The lesion in the knee may be seen on the routine anteroposterior roentgenogram in some pa-

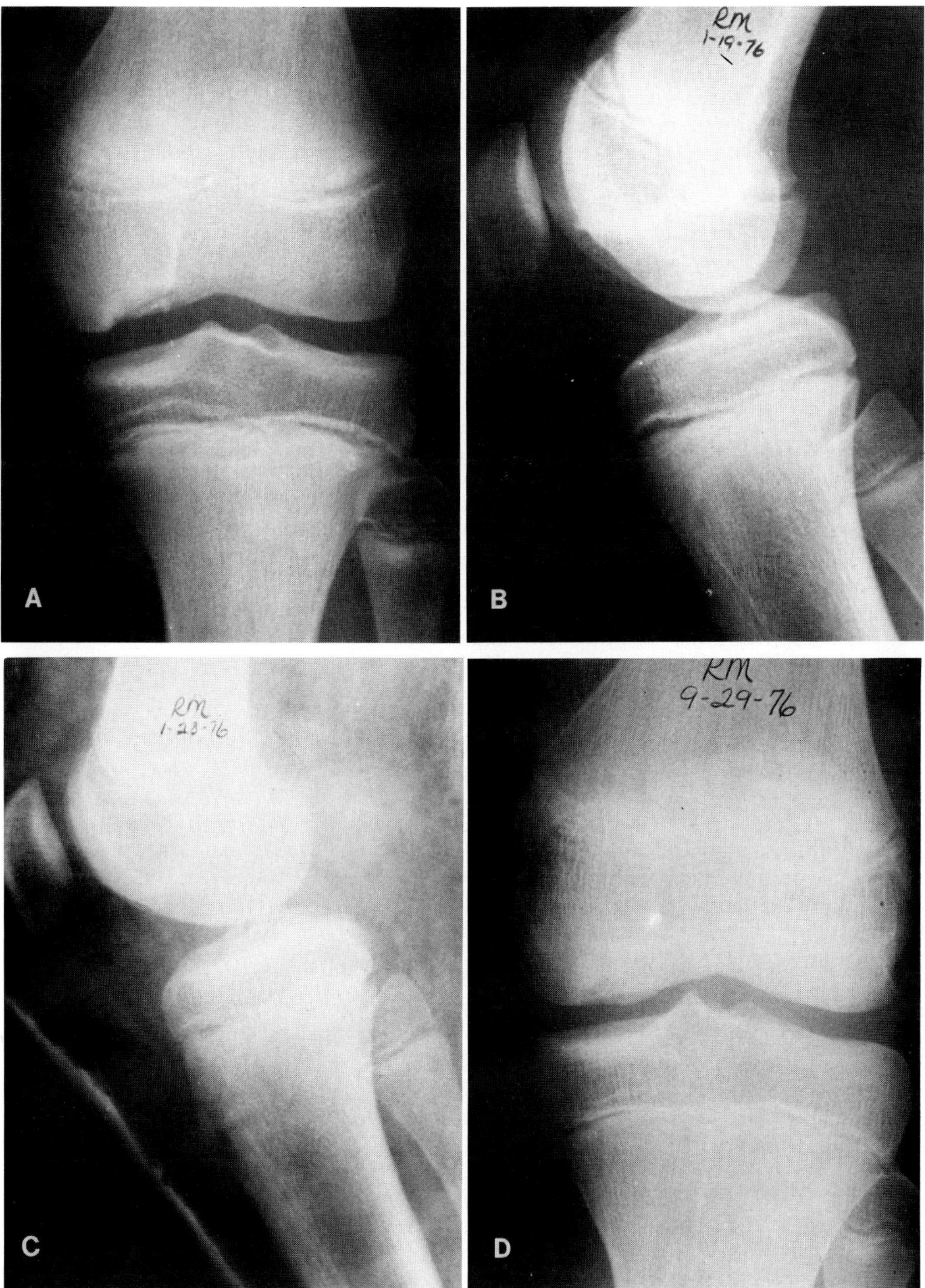

FIG. 20-14. *(A* and *B)* Anteroposterior and lateral views of the knee showing a typical osteochondritic lesion in a young adolescent. *(C)* This film, taken through the cast, shows the position of immobilization that removes weightbearing stress from the lesion. *(D)* After 18 weeks of immobilization, the lesion is healing.

tients. However, if it is located posterior to the most distal projection of the femur, a tunnel view is needed for it to be seen. The usual position of the lesion is on the lateral portion of the medial condyle, but it also occurs on the lateral condyle.

Treatment

Green and Banks[27] showed that, in children, conservative treatment gave an excellent prognosis for healing without residual deformity. In children, when the diagnosis is made before the articular cartilage fractures, immobilization of the knee almost always leads to healing of the lesion in 16 to 20 weeks and in some patients even at 12 weeks. The immobilization is effected by means of a cylinder cast that extends from the upper thigh to just above the ankle (Fig. 20-14 *C*, *D*). The position in which the knee is immobilized is of utmost importance, because weightbearing between the tibia and femur should not exert pressure in the area of the lesion. Using a lateral roentgenogram of the knee, the position of flexion necessary to relieve the pressure exerted by the tibia on the lesion is determined and the plaster is applied with the knee held in that position. A follow-up roentgenogram is made after the cast is applied to be certain that the lesion is free of pressure. The lesion is usually located so that the knee has to be either in full extension to clear the posteriorly located lesion or in 40° to 45° of flexion to avoid the lesions that are more anteriorly located. There is no evidence that healing of the intact lesion is hastened by drilling. If the knee has to be flexed, the patient walks more comfortably with the heels of the shoes raised by adding appropriate lifts.

Almost without exception, the knees of patients younger than 15 years of age heal if appropriate treatment is started before the defect separates. If the patient is skeletally mature or near maturity, healing after conservative treatment is unlikely. When the lesion has separated, I prefer to remove the loose body and drill the bone in the base of the defect for medial condylar defects. However, when the fragment is large or is on the lateral condyle, the fragment should be replaced. Removal of a large posterior area of the lateral condyle causes instability of the knee and interferes with participation in sports. Smillie advocates replacement of the fragment and grafting of the bone, if necessary, to level the articular surface on both the medial and lateral defects. He uses small Smillie nails to hold the fragment in place. These need to be removed later. Kirschner wires, inserted so that they can be removed anteriorly without an incision, are preferable to Smillie nails. Fixation of the loose fragment may be done with bone pegs 2 mm in diameter instead of Kirschner wires.

After the fragment is removed and the base of the defect drilled, motion with minimal stress is started on the first or second postoperative day. The leg is suspended in a Thomas splint with a Pearson attachment so that the patient can passively flex and extend the knee. This is done every 30 minutes for 2 to 3 minutes during the day for about 7 to 10 days. Ambulation can begin on the seventh to tenth postoperative day with crutches and minimal weightbearing. Flexion and extension exercises are done from the side-lying position six to eight times a day for several minutes. This regimen is continued for about 10 to 12 weeks. Motion without stress is important for rapid healing of the defect. The results of surgical excision of the defect and drilling of the base are not as satisfactory as when healing of the lesion takes place with conservative treatment.

OSGOOD–SCHLATTER DISEASE

This syndrome, described first by Osgood in 1903, presents during adolescence as a swelling around the tibial tubercle and patellar tendon.[53]

Etiology

The etiology is controversial. Both Osgood and Schlatter, who described the entity a few months after Osgood, thought that the cause was trauma with partial avulsion of the tibial tubercle.[53] Woolfrey[73] and Hughes,[33] however, presented evidence that the lesion is a result of traumatic tendonitis of the patellar tendon resulting in heterotopic bone formation in the tendon.

Neither of these concepts can be confirmed or denied by present information. Codman, in his discussion of Osgood's paper, stated that he thought the cause was periostitis or new-bone formation from injury to the patellar tendon. The idea of traction on the tibial tubercle appeals to me as a reasonable etiologic factor, resulting in a traumatic epiphysitis.

Certainly the mechanics of the quadriceps pull during the age at which there is rapid growth and widening of the epiphyses and apophyses support this view. If trauma to the patellar tendon was the cause, why does the age of these patients fall within such a limited range? The tendonitis that is present is secondary to the epiphysitis. Further evaluation is needed to elucidate the exact etiology.

Clinical Features and Diagnosis

The typical patient is an 11- to 15-year-old child, usually a boy, who is active in sports. Pain is the presenting complaint. The pain occurs over the tibial tubercle when pressure is exerted and also when the quadriceps is stressed, as in ascending and descending stairs, running and jumping. There is soft-tissue swelling over the tibial tubercle. The remainder of the joint examination is negative.

The roentgenogram of the knee shows soft-tissue swelling anterior to the tubercle and thickening of the patellar tendon. In older patients, there are bony changes in and around the patellar tendon insertion that have been divided into three types by Woolfrey.[73] In Type I, the tibial tuberosity is prominent and irregular; in Type II, the tibial tubercle is irregular, and there is a small free fragment of bone anterior and superior to the tubercle; and, in Type III, there is a small regular tubercle with a small fragment of bone anterior and superior to the tubercle. These free fragments of bone are the result of heterotopic bone formation and are not fragments off the tubercle.

Treatment

This is a self-limiting disease that spontaneously subsides with fusion of the tubercle about 15 years of age. The longer the symptoms are present and the more severe the swelling, the more likely it is that there will be residual enlargement of the tubercle and heterotopic bone in the patellar tendon. When symptoms are severe enough to interfere with the patient's activities, I have recommended immobilization in a cylinder cast for 6 to 8 weeks. After removal of the cast, activity is limited to walking for another 2 to 3 weeks, and then full activity is resumed. Most patients are able to return to full activity without further difficulty.

Operative treatment has been recommended for those patients with recurring symptoms following conservative therapy. I have had no occasion to use surgical therapy, because immobilization has been an effective treatment.

POPLITEAL CYST

The popliteal cyst in children is a synovial cyst that arises from the semimembranous bursa, from beneath the medial head of the gastrocnemius, or from the joint capsule. Baker described a popliteal cyst arising as a herniation from the joint. This is a frequent finding in adults with rheumatoid or osteoarthritic arthritis, but it is not common in children.[4] Burleson and co-workers[11] reported on 83 cysts occurring in the popliteal area of children of all age groups, which were treated by excision. Of these, 46 arose from the semimembranous bursa, 26 from herniations of the joint, and 11 could not be accurately classified. The cyst is always found between the semimembranous bursa and the medial head of the gastrocnemius.

The typical popliteal cyst in the child, in my experience, arises from the semimembranous bursa. It is filled with a gelatinous fluid, and the lining of the cyst may be either fibrous tissue, synovial cells, inflammatory cells, or a mixture of the fibrous and synovial cell lining.

The popliteal cyst of childhood presents as a swelling of the medial side of the popliteal space just lateral to the semitendinosus. Tumors that are not located just lateral to the semitendinosus and between it and the medial head of the gastrocnemius should be looked upon as being something other than a typical Baker's cyst, because they are usually lesions of another type, such as fibroma, sarcoma, or a vascular anomaly. The cyst is usually asymptomatic, but it can cause discomfort if it enlarges excessively. In my experience, the massive cyst seen in adults that dissects downward and spreads beneath the posterior muscle does not occur in children except in a rare rheumatoid arthritic joint. The cyst transilluminates, and this diagnostic test should always be done to prevent confusing it with a fibrous or vascular anomaly.

Observation of the asymptomatic nonenlarging cyst is appropriate in the child, because some cysts may regress and others may remain asymptomatic. In those that cause symptoms or that continue to enlarge, surgical excision should be done.

REFERENCES

1. Aegerter EE: The possible relationship of neurofibromatosis, congenital pseudarthrosis, and fibrous dysplasia. J Bone Joint Surg 32A:618, 1950
2. Aegerter EE, Kirkpatrick JA: Orthopedic Diseases, 4th ed. Philadelphia, WB Saunders, 1975
3. Andersen KS: Congenital pseudarthrosis of tibia and neurofibromatosis. Acta Orthop Scand 47:108,1976
4. Baker WM: On the formation of synovial cysts in the leg in connection with disease of the knee joint. St Bart Hosp Rep 13:245, 1877
5. Bathfield CA, Beighton PH: Blount's disease: A review of etiologic factors in 110 patients. Clin Orthop 135:29, 1978
6. Bassett CA, et al: Congenital pseudarthrosis of the tibia. Treatment with pulsing electromagnetic field. Clin Orthop 154:136, 1981
7. Blount WP: Tibia vara: Osteochondrosis: Deforman's tibiae. J Bone Joint Surg 19:1, 1937
8. Blumel J, Eggers GWN, Evans B: Eight cases of hereditary bilateral medial tibial torsion in four generations. J Bone Joint Surg 39A:1198, 1957
9. Bowker HH, Thompson EB: Surgical treatment of recurrent dislocation of the patella. A study of 48 cases. J Bone Joint Surg 46A:1451, 1964
10. Boyd HB, Sage FP: Congenital pseudarthrosis of the tibia. J Bone Joint Surg 40A:1245, 1958
11. Burleson RJ, Bickel WH, Dahlin D: Popliteal cyst: a clinicopathologial survey. J Bone Joint Surg 38A:1265, 1956
12. Burrows HJ: Osteochondritis juvenilis. J Bone Joint Surg 41B:455, 1958
13. Campbell WC, Crenshaw AH (eds): Campbell's Orthopaedics, 5th ed. St Louis, CV Mosby, 1971
14. Cave EF, Staples OS: Congenital discoid meniscus: A cause of internal derangement of the knee. Am J Surg 54:371, 1941
15. Cheu C, Yu Z, Waus Y: A new method of treatment of congenital tibial pseudarthrosis using free vascularized fibular graft. Ann Acad Med 8:465, 1979
16. Ducroquet R, Cottard A: Pseudarthrosis congenitale de jambe deformation osstua de la neurofibromatoses. J Chir 53:483, 1939
17. Erlacher P: Deformerierende prozesse der epiphysengegend bei kindern. Arch Op Unfallchir 20:81, 1922
18. Fairbank HAT: Osteochondritis dissecans. Br J Surg 21:67, 1933
19. Ficat RP, Hungerford DS: Disorders of the patellofemoral joint. Baltimore, Williams & Wilkins, 1977
20. Fienman NL, Yakovac WC: Neurofibromatosis in childhood. J Pediatr 76:339, 1970
21. Gardiner TB: Osteochondritis dissecans in three members of one family. J Bone Joint Surg 37B:139, 1955
22. Gillespie HS: Bone peg fixation in the treatment of osteochondritis dessicans of the knee joint. Clin Orthop 143:125, 1979
23. Gilbert A: AAOS Annual Meeting, 1983
24. Golding JSR, McNeil-Smith JDG: Observations on the etiology of tibia vara. J Bone Joint Surg 45B:320, 1963
25. Goldthwait JE: Dislocation of the patella. Trans Am Orthop Assoc 8:327, 1897
26. Green WT Sr: Personal communication, 1965
27. Green WT, Banks HB: Osteochondritis dissecans in children. J Bone Joint Surg 35A:26, 1953
28. Green WT, Rudo N: Pseudarthrosis and neurofibromatosis. Arch Surg 46:61, 1943
29. Harrison MHM: The results of realignment operation on recurrent dislocation of the patella. Clin Orthop 18:96, 1960
30. Heywood AWB: Recurrent dislocation of the patella. A study of its pathology and treatment of 106 knees. J Bone Joint Surg 43B:508, 1961
31. Heyman CH, Herndon CH, Kingsbury KG: Congenital posterior angulation of the tibia with talipes calcaneus. J Bone Joint Surg 41A:476, 1959
32. Hofmann A, Wenger DR: Posteromedial bowing of the tibia. Progression of discrepancy in leg length. J Bone Joint Surg 63A:384, 1981
33. Hughes ESR: Osgod Schlatter's disease. Surg Gynecol Obstet 86:323, 1948
34. Hughston JC: Subluxation of the patella. J Bone Joint Surg 50A:1003, 1968
35. Hutter CG Jr, Scott W: Tibial torsion. J Bone Joint Surg 31A:511, 1949
36. Jakob RP, et al: Tibial torsion calculated by computerized tomography and compared to other methods of measurement. J Bone Joint Surg 62B: 238, 1980
37. Jones JB, Francis KC, Mahoney JR: Recurrent dislocating patella—a long-term followup study. Clin Orthop 20:230, 1961
38. Kaplan EB: Discoid lateral meniscus of the knee joint: nature, mechanism, and operative treatment. J Bone Joint Surg 39A:77, 1957
39. Katz MP, Grogone BJJ, Sope KC: The etiology and treatment of congenital dislocation of the knee. J Bone Joint Surg 49B:112, 1967
40. Khermosh O, Lior G, Weissman SL: Tibial torsion in children. Clin Orthop 79:26, 1971
41. Konig F: Ueber frei körper in den gelenken. Deutsche Zertschrift für Chir 27:90, 1887
42. Lancourt JE, Christini JA: Patella alta and patella infera—their etiological role in patellar dislocation, chondromalacia and apophysitis of the tibial tubercle. J Bone Joint Surg 57A:1112, 1975
43. Langenskiold A: Tibia vara. Acta Chir Scand 103:9, 1952
44. Langenskiold A, Riska EB: Tibia vara. J Bone Joint Surg 46A:1405, 1964
45. Langenskiold A: Tibia vara: Osteochondrosis deformans tibial. Blount's disease. Clin Orthop 158:77, 1981
46. Levine AM, Drennan JC: Physiological bowing and tibia vara. The metaphyseal-diaphyseal angle in the measurement of bowleg deformities. J Bone Joint Surg 64a:1158, 1982
47. Malekafzali S, et al: Tibial torsion—A simple clinical apparatus for its measurement and its application to a normal adult population. Clin Orthop 145:154, 1979
48. Macnab I: Recurrent dislocation of the patella. J Bone Joint Surg 34A:957, 1952
49. Masserman RL, Peterson HA, Bianco AJ: Congenital pseudarthrosis of the tibia. Clin Orthop 99:140, 1974
50. Merchant AC, Mercer RL, Jacobsen RH, Cool CR: Roentgenographic analysis of patellofemoral congruence. J Bone Joint Surg 56A:1391, 1974
51. Morrissy RT: Congenital pseudarthrosis of the tibia. J Bone Joint Surg 63B:367, 1981
52. Murdock G: Congenital discoid medial semilunar cartilage. J Bone Joint Surg 38B:564, 1956
53. Osgood RB: Lesions of the tibial tubercle occurring during adolescence. Boston Med Surg J 148:114, 1903
54. Nielsen NA: Osteochondritis dissecans, capituli humeri. Acta Orthop Scand 4:307, 1933

55. Paget J: On the production of some loose bodies in joints. St. Bartholomew Hosp Rep 6:1, 1870
56. Pare A: Oeuvres Completes, Vol. 3. Paris, JB Balliere, 1841
57. Patersen D: Successful treatment of congenital pseudarthrosis of the tibia using electrical stimulation. J Bone Joint Surg 64B:632, 1982
58. Phemister DB: The causes of and the changes in loose bodies arising from articular surface of the joint. J Bone Joint Surg 61:278, 1924
59. Pistevos G, et al: The correction of genu valgum by epiphyseal stapling. J Bone Joint Surg 59B:72, 1977
60. Provenzano KW: Congenital dislocation of the knee. N Engl J Med 236:360, 1947
61. Rehbein F: Die entstehung der osteochondritis dissecans. Arch Klin Chir 265:69, 1950
62. Rosen H, Sandlick H: Measurement of tibiofibular torsion. J Bone Joint Surg 37A:847, 1955
63. Ross JA, Tough ICK, English IA: Congenital discoid meniscus. J Bone Joint Surg 40B:262, 1958
64. Salter RB et al: The biologic effect of continuous passive motion on the healing of full-thickness defects in articular cartilage. An experimental investigation in the rabbit. J Bone Joint Surg 62A:1232, 1980
65. Smillie IS: Osteochondritis dissecans. Baltimore, Williams & Wilkins, 1960
66. Staheli LT, Engel GM: Tibial torsion: A method of assessment and a survey of normal children. Clin Orthop 86:183, 1972
67. Stougaard J: Familial occurrence of osteochondritis dissecans. J Bone Joint Surg 46B:542, 1964
68. Tachdjian M: Pediatric Orthopaedics, p 723. Philadelphia. WB Saunders, 1972
69. Tolon S: Torsion of the lower extremity. Proc 12th Cong of Int Soc Orthop Surg Traumatol Amsterdam, Excerpta Medica, 1972
70. Van Nes CP: Congenital pseudarthrosis of the leg. J Bone Joint Surg 48A:1467, 1966
71. Weber BG: Fibrous interposition causing valgus deformity after fracture of the upper tibial epiphysis in children. J Bone Joint Surg 59B:290, 1977
72. Weiland AJ, Daniel RK, Congenital pseudarthrosis of tibia treated with vascularized autogenous fibular graft. A preliminary report. Johns Hopkins Med 147:89, 1980
73. Woolfrey BF, Chandler EF: Manifestation of Osgood-Schlatter's diease in late teenage and early adulthood. J Bone Joint Surg 42A:327, 1960

21

The Foot

Wood W. Lovell
Charles T. Price
Peter L. Meehan

STRUCTURE AND FUNCTION

The foot is in constant contact with the environment. It serves to propel the body and give information regarding our surroundings. Since we bear four times our body weight on each extremity at rest, the feet must be strong. The surfaces that we walk on vary, so the foot must be able to accommodate to these changes.

EMBRYOLOGY

Willis[22] points out that the human foot and leg are adaptations of the pelvic fin of an aquatic animal to terrestrial locomotion. The evolution from fin to foot is reviewed briefly in the embryology of the human fetus. For the first 6 months of intrauterine life, the feet are inverted, the soles directed toward the abdomen. A more rapid growth of the scaphoid and cuneiform bones then occurs. The neck of the talus, which has been directed downward, has relatively delayed growth and turns inward and upward. The inner border of the talus grows upward. Lack of this change in growth rate leaves the foot in the equinovarus position.

Willis[22] further states that in the primitive foot, there are five tarsal bones, plus an os tibiale and an os fibulare. Between the last two are the os intermedium proximally and the os centrale distally. Tarsals one, two, and three become the cuneiforms. Tarsals four and five unite to form the cuboid. This occurs in the feet of all mammals. The os intermedium fuses with the posterior tubercule of the os tibiale to form the posterior process of the astragalus or, failing to fuse, persists as the anomalous os trigonum.

The os fibulare undergoes great posterior development to form the human heel. The os centrale becomes the scaphoid. The extension of the heel interrupts the tendons of the gastrocnemius and plantaris.

White[21] called attention to the torsion in the Achilles tendon and its surgical significance. Prior to this, Hoke used this in developing his method of heelcord lengthening. Those fibers of the Achilles tendon that occupy a medial portion proximally twist laterally as they approach the calcaneus, so that they are then posterior to those fibers that originally occupied the lateral position. These are the fibers that originally inserted on the os tibiale.

ANATOMY

INTEGUMENT

The skin of the sole of the foot at the heel and over the metatarsal heads is equipped with special tissue. In running and jumping, the feet must bear up to 10 times the body weight. Kuhns[14] emphasized that the elastic adipose tissue in these locations serves to cushion the stresses of weightbearing on the underlying bone and soft tissue. It is believed that part of the prolonged disability after os calcis fracture is related to rupture of the septae in the elastic adipose tissue.

Bony Architecture

The bony architecture of the foot must accommodate the great variability in terrain over which we course throughout our lives. In contradistinction to the hand, the foot must be stable. The wedge-shaped mortise and tenon articulation between the talus and the tibia exemplifies this fact.

There are two arches in the foot. The longitudinal arch is keystoned medially by the neck of the talus. This is reinforced by the spring ligament between the sustentaculum tali and the navicular. The Y ligament of Bigelow between the calcaneus, navicular, and cuboid supports it as well. The posterior tibial tendon and, indirectly, the flexor hallucis longus support the medial arch. The lateral longitudinal arch is keystoned by the cuboid. The transverse arc of the foot exists only at the level of the metatarsal bases. At the level of the metatarsal heads, there is no arch.

Acton[1] states that the weight borne by various positions of the foot varies according to the phase of gait and the position of the foot. In normal standing, weight is borne equally on the forefoot and hindfoot. The first metatarsal bears more weight than the lesser rays. If total weight is 24 units in normal stance, each foot would bear 12 units. The hindfoot of each would bear 6 units, and the forefoot would bear 6 units. In the forefoot, the weight would be borne in a ratio of 2:1:1:1:1 from the first to the fifth metatarsal.

According to Jones,[11] with the triceps surae relaxed, four fifths of the load is borne by the hindfoot.

The slings affected by the tibial muscles and the peroneus longus tendon would seem to provide dynamic support for the longititudinal arch. They are, however, silent during the stance phase of gait.[2] Dynamic support is provided more indirectly through the reflex contraction and shift of body weight. The plantar aponeurosis and short muscles act as tie rods for the longitudinal arch.

Ligamentous support for the ankle is symmetrical. There are discrete structures laterally, but medially they blend into a fan-shaped ligament. Laterally the three components, anterior and posterior, talofibular and calcanofibular, are under equal tension throughout a full range of motion. They radiate from the approximate axis of motion of the ankle. Medially, the axis of motion is 1 cm distal to the medial malleolus. For this reason, the posterior talotibial ligament is a check rein to plantar flexion. Beneath the calcaneotibial ligament is the middle portion of the tibiotalar ligament—a most important structure for stability of the ankle. Smith[19] has evaluated the subtalar region of the foot. He credits Jones[11] with redefining the area between the talocalcaneonavicular joint in front and the talocalcaneal joint behind into two parts. The sinus tarsi is the wide lateral part of this region. Jones refers to the narrower medial part as the canalis tarsi. This was the terminology used in older writings. Smith[19] found these ligaments in this area: (1) The inferior extensor retinaculum is a continuation of a retinaculum that lies in front of the ankle. This was fully described by Frazer[6] in 1920. Traced laterally, the retinaculum turns downward around the lateral aspect of the neck of the talus, to which it is sometimes attached, and enters the sinus tarsi. Within the sinus, it divides into well-defined lateral, intermediate, and medial roots. The lateral root becomes incorporated into the deep fascia on the lateral aspect of the foot. The larger intermediate root descends vertically into the calcaneus. The slender medial root inclines into the canalis tarsi before being attached to the sulcus calcanei. (2) The cervical liagment lies in the anterior part of the sinus tarsi. Jones[11] used this term, and it is now accepted terminology. It is a broad flattened band that lies anterior to the intermediate route of the retinaculum. It is attached below to the dorsal surface of the calcaneus, medial to the extensor digitorum brevis, and extends medially and upward to a tubercle on the inferolateral aspect of the neck of the talus. (3) The ligament of the canalis tarsi extends between the talus and the calcaneus. Other authors refer to this as the interosseous ligament. It is a broad band, flattened in the coronal plane, in which the fibers extend downward and laterally from the sulcus tali to the sulcus calcanei, crossing in its course either anterior or posterior to the medial route of the inferior extensor retinaculum.

The cervical ligament limits inversion; the ligament of the canalis tarsi limits eversion.

Muscles

There are ten tendons that span the ankle joint when considering the plantaris and triceps surae as one. In order to prevent bowstringing of the tendons on the anterior aspect of the ankle, the thin crural fascia of the lower leg is reinforced by transverse bundles. This comprises the extensor retinaculum or the anterior annular ligament. Distally, there is a Y-shaped reinforcement. It attaches to the anterolateral surface of the calcaneus where it has three divisions, as previously noted. It spreads medially as two limbs blending into the medial malleolus of the tibia and into the plantar aponeurosis.

Because the triceps surae inserts into the tuberosity of the calcaneus 2 inches posterior to the axis of motion of the ankle, it is a powerful plantar flexor. The anterior tibial tendon is 2 inches from the axis of motion while the toe extensors are 1½ inches from that point. Thus, they have ample leverage to act as ankle dorsiflexor muscles.

The muscles of the foot can be divided into extrinsic and intrinsic groups. There are similarities to the hand. The leg may be divided into four compartments. The anterior compartment containing the extensor digitorum longus, the extensor hallucis longus, and the anterior tibial muscle are supplied by the deep portion of the peroneal nerve. They receive their vascularity from muscular branches of the tibial or anterior tibial artery. The lateral compartment of the leg contains the peroneus longus and peroneus brevis muscles. They are supplied by the superficial portion of the peroneal nerve and muscular branches of the peroneal artery. The superficial posterior compartment of the leg contains the gastrocnemius, the soleus, and the popliteus muscles. They are innervated by the tibial nerve and receive their blood supply from sural branches of the popliteal artery. The deep posterior compartment contains the flexor hallucis longus, the flexor digitorum longus and the posterior tibial muscle. They, as well, are supplied by the tibial nerve and receive muscular branches from either the posterior tibial artery or the peroneal artery.

Anterior Compartment

The extensor digitorum longus passes along a straight line from its origin on the proximal three fourths of the anterior surface of the fibular shaft and the interosseous membrane as well as along the lateral tibial condyle. The peroneus tertius is actually a part of the extensor digitorum longus. All tendons pass beneath the extensor retinaculum in the same canal. The peroneus tertius inserts on the dorsum of the base of the fourth or fifth metatarsals or on both sites. The extensor digitorum longus inserts onto the dorsal surface of the middle and distal phalanges of the lateral four toes. It functions to extend the phalanges of the lateral four toes and acts as a secondary dorsiflexor of the foot. The peroneus tertius acts to dorsiflex the foot while everting it. The tibialis anterior arises from the proximal two thirds of the lateral aspect of the tibia and interosseous membrane. As in the proximal muscles of the forearm, it also arises from investing fascia and adjoining planes. It inserts onto the medial and plantar surfacc of the first cuneiform and base of the first metatarsal. It dorsiflexes the foot and inverts it.

The extensor hallucis longus arises from the middle one half of the anterior surface of the fibula crossing the anterior tibial artery proximal to the ankle and passes distally to insert into the base of the distal phalanx. It functions to extend the great toe and acts secondarily to dorsiflex the ankle.

The extensor digitorum brevis has no counterpart in the hand. It is an intrinsic muscle of the foot. It arises from the dorsal lateral surface of the calcaneus. It has three tendons that insert into the fibular borders of the extensor digitorum longus tendons to the second, third, and fourth toes. The most medial belly of the extensor digitorum brevis is actually a separate muscle of the extensor hallucis brevis, which inserts into the dorsum of the base of the proximal phalanx of the great toe.

The lateral compartment contains the peroneus longus and peroneus brevis muscles. The peroneus longus arises from the lateral condyle of the tibia, the head and upper two thirds of the lateral surface of the fibula, adjacent fascia, and intermuscular septae. It inserts into the lateral side of the first cuneiform and the base of the first metatarsal. It functions to plantar flex the foot while everting it.

The peroneus brevis arises from the lower two thirds of the lateral surface of the fibula and the adjacent intermuscular septae. It inserts into the lateral side of the base of the fifth metatarsal. It functions to plantar flex and evert the foot.

As stated before, the posterior compartment of the leg is divided into deep and superficial compartments by the deep transverse fascia. This is a distinct sheet stretching from the tibia to the fibula. Each compartment has three extrinsic muscles to the foot. Those in the superficial compartment act as one.

The gastrocnemius arises from two heads: The medial head arises from the medial condyle, the adjacent part of the femur, and the capsule of the knee joint. The lateral head arises from the lateral condyle, the adjacent part of the femur, and the capsule of the knee joint. They insert into the calcaneus by means of a common tendon with the soleus. It functions to plantar flex the foot while secondarily flexing the knee and inverting the foot.

The soleus originates from the posterior surface of the head and upper one third of the shaft of the fibula, the middle third of the medial border of the tibia, and the tendinous arch between the tibia and fibula. It inserts into the calcaneus by means of a common tendon with the gastrocnemius. It functions to plantar flex the foot and secondarily to invert the foot.

The plantaris crosses over from its origin on the lateral prolongation of the linea aspera of the femur and crosses distally between the gastrocnemius and the soleus to the medial side of the tendo Achilles, then inserts into the calcaneus. It is absent in 6% to 8% of normal individuals. It functions to flex the leg and to rotate the tibia medially at the beginning of flexion. It serves as a secondary flexor of the ankle and invertor of the foot. The deep posterior compartment is comprised of the flexor hallucis longus, the flexor digitorum longus, and the posterior tibial muscles.

The flexor hallucis longus arises from the inferior two thirds of the fibula and passes distally on the lower end of the tibia into a definite groove in the posterior aspect of the talus. It passes forward, turning around another pulley, the sustentaculum tali, to contribute a strong slip to the flexor digitorum longus before running between the two heads of the short flexor to insert into the base of the great toe. Its primary function is that of flexion of the great toe, while secondarily it aids in plantar flexion and inversion of the foot.

The flexor digitorum longus arises from the posterior aspect of the tibia between the popliteal line and the lower 3 inches of the tibia. Its primary function is that of flexion of the lateral four toes. Its secondary function is that of plantar flexion of the ankle and inversion of the foot. The flexor digitorum longus receives the total insertion of the quadratus plantae muscle. The point of attachment covers all but the medial side of the tendon.

The posterior tibial muscle arises from the entire posterior surface of the interosseous membrane except its lower portion and from the adjacent surfaces of the tibia and fibula. It inserts into the tuberosity of the navicular, the plantar surfaces of all cuneiform bones; the plantar surfaces of the base of the second, third, and fourth metatarsal bones; the cuboid; as well as the sustentaculum tali. It functions to plantar flex and invert the foot.

The relationship of the tendons and neurovascular bundle with the medial malleolus is well known. It was pointed out by Ben-Menachem and Butler[3] that the blood supply to the foot in congenital anomalies is not constant. He demonstrated absence of either the dorsalis pedis or posterior tibial arteries in association with congenital abnormalities.

Acton[1] has written a comprehensive article on the surgical anatomy of the foot. The reader is encouraged to review this article.

After removing the skin and subcutaneous tissue from the sole of the foot, the plantar aponeurosis is visible. It arises from the medial process of the tuberosity of the calcaneus and sends forward strong longitudinal fibers that terminate in five bands, one on each toe. These five bands send a superficial slip to the skin crease at the base of each toe and a deep slip that splits to embrace each toe flexor tendon. The two halves of this deep slip attach to and contribute to the fibrous digital sheath and the transverse metatarsal ligaments. In addition to the central portion of the plantar aponeurosis, a medial portion invests the abductor hallucis and a lateral portion invests the abductor digiti quinti. A strong cord of the lateral portion acts as a tie rod from the lateral process of the calcaneus to the tuberosity of the fifth metatarsal.

The muscles of the sole of the foot can be considered four layers of intrinsics, with extrinsics added to the second and fourth layers.[10] The first layer includes the two abductors and a short flexor; the second, an accessory flexor and the lumbricals; the third, two short flexors and an adductor; and the fourth, the interossei.

The first layer of muscles includes the abductor hallucis, the flexor digitorum brevis, and the abductor digiti quinti. Both abductors insert, by a conjoined tendon shared by the respective short flexor, into the base of the proximal phalanx of the first and fifth digits. The flexor brevis arises from the medial tuberosity of the calcaneus, passes forward and divides into four tendons—exactly analogous to the tendons of the flexor sublimis in the hand.

The second layer is composed of the flexor digitorum longus, the flexor hallucis longus, the quadratus plantae, and the lumbricals. The quadratus plantae arises from two pointed heads from the calcaneus and inserts on all but the medial side of the flexor digitorum longus. The lumbricals arise from the long flexor tendons and pass around the medial or hallux side of each lesser ray. Each lumbrical has a bipenniform origin from the two flexor tendons. The exception to this is the first lumbrical, which supplies the second toe. It arises only from the flexor tendon to the second toe.

The third layer consists of the flexor hallucis brevis, the flexor digiti quinti brevis, and the adductor brevis. The flexor of the great toe arises from the cuboid and third cuneiform. The fifth toe flexor arises from the base of the fifth metatarsal. The flexor hallucis brevis inserts through a conjoined tendon shared with the abductor and the adductor hallucis. The flexor of the fifth toe inserts into the fifth digit by a conjoined tendon shared by the abductor.

The fourth layer consists of the interossei. They differ from those of the hand in that the second instead of the third ray is the axis about which abduction and adduction take place in the foot. The four dorsal interossei are bipenniform, filling the four intermetatarsal spaces. The three plantar ones are unipenniform, with their origins and insertions on the same ray. Mann and Inman[17] studied the phasic activity of the intrinsics of the foot by implanting electrodes in six intrinsics of the foot, including the short extensors, the three muscles of the first layer, the flexor hallucis brevis, and one interosseous. They concluded that the intrinsic acts as a functional unit and plays an important role in the stabilization of the foot for propulsion.

Opinions vary as to the function of the interossei and lumbricals. Spalteholz[20] believes that they only flex the proximal phalanges of the lesser toes without extending the second and third phalanges, as in the hand. From this and the evidence presented by Forster,[5] Manter,[18] and Kelekian[12] concluded that the long extensors of the toes and the surface walked upon are the two factors that maintain extension of the interphalangeal joints of the toes. Acton's[1] dissections did not bear this out. He noted that in specimens from younger individuals, it was possible to demonstrate extension of both interphalangeal joints by placing tension on either the interosseous or lumbrical muscles if gentle tension on the long flexor and extensor was maintained. He was also able to trace fibers from the lumbrical and interosseous tendons to the extensor hood.

The deep transverse metatarsal ligament in the foot joins the plantar plate of the metatarsophalangeal joints of all five rays. This description is at variance with the description in *Gray's Anatomy*[8] but corresponds to Cunningham's[4] description. The plantar plates are attached in a similar manner to the palmar plates in the hand.

The glenoid ligament of Cruveilhier is a term synonymous with plantar plate. The glenoid ligament of Cruveilhier corresponds to the volar, palmar, or vaginal ligaments in the hand. These are pivotal to understanding the anatomy of this portion of the foot. With an understanding of all the structures that attach to the glenoid ligaments and their relationships, much of the anatomy will become clearer.

The following structures attach directly to the glenoid ligaments: (1) the deep transverse ligament of the sole (also called the transverse metatarsal ligament); (2) the extensor hood; (3) the plantar aponeurosis through its divergent bands; (4) the flexor tendon sheath; (5) the fanlike portions of the collateral ligaments of the metatarsophalangeal joints; and (6) the capsule of the metatarsophalangeal joints.

The distal two thirds of the glenoid ligament is a dense, thick fibrocartilaginous structure forming a broad rectangular plate. In its proximal one third, it is composed of a more pliable tissue, which is continuous with the capsule of the metatarsophalangeal joint and attaches relatively loosely to the metatarsal neck. This latter portion begins to fold upon itself when the joint is flexed to a position midway between the extremes of flexion and extension. It is elongated when the joint is in extension.

The glenoid ligament of the metatarsophalangeal joint of the great toe differs from that of the corresponding joint in the thumb. In the great toe, this ligament contains two sesmoid bones, whereas in the thumb, the sesmoids are within the substance of the conjoined tendons related to the respective sides of the joint.

These ligaments form the volar portion of the metatarsophalangeal capsular ligaments. Their grooved volar surfaces form the dorsal wall of the flexor tendon sheath. This permits the profundus tendon to glide on the plantar aspect of the metatarsophalangeal joint regardless of the degree of flexion. The extensor hood girdles the metatarsophalangeal joint (more properly, the proximal phalanx just distal to it) and is anchored into the glenoid ligament.

BIOMECHANICS

In evaluating the biomechanical aspects of the foot, definitions are essential to proper discussion. Rotation about a transverse axis will be termed *flexion* and *extension*. Rotation about a vertical axis when the foot is moving is termed *abduction-adduction* and when the leg is moving is termed *medial rotation-lateral rotation*. Rotation about an anteroposterior axis is *pronation* and *supination*. *Inversion* and *eversion* are used differently by various authors. We use it to refer to rotation about an anteroposterior axis of the talocalcaneonavicular joint.

Hicks[9] has demonstrated in studies of normal cadaver feet that all movements in the foot are rotations. Hinged joints have their motion predetermined. A ball and socket joint has its plane of movement determined by the direction of forces acting upon it. Different tendons, though they may run in oblique directions, always produce one of two movements—clockwise or counterclockwise rotation about an axis. Due to this, motion in the foot is of a compound nature. This holds true for other forces such as body weight. For example, a force that tends to produce abduction at the talocalcaneonavicular joint only succeeds in producing pronation—abduction and extension because this (or its opposite) is the only movement of which this joint is capable. This occurs because the axis of motion only permits this complex movement.

The talonavicular articulation, being of a ball and socket shape, might be expected to show a greater degree of freedom of movement. This may seem incompatible with the assertion that all joints are hinged joints. Hicks[9] explains that this joint is peculiar in being one half of two different joint complexes. In conjunction with the talocalcaneal articulation, it forms the talocalcaneonavicular joint complex. In conjunction with the calcaneocuboid articular, it forms the midtarsal joint complex. The navicular, therefore, rotates on the talus about three different axes—about the talocalcaneonavicular axis when the talocalcaneonavicular complex is in action and about one or the other of the midtarsal axes when the midtarsal complex is in action. The motion remains a simple hinge movement in each case. He does state that action at all these complexes may occur simultaneously.

During normal gait, internal rotation of the limb progressively develops until ground contact and foot flat. External rotation begins and progresses until toe-off, when the cycle repeats. Rotation about the foot occurs largely in the subtalar joint complex.

The surgical implications of these and other biomechanical principles have been outlined by Mann.[16] An ankle arthrodesis should be placed in slight valgus, neutral dorsiplantar flexion and in the same degree of external rotation as the opposite leg. A subtalar arthrodesis should be aligned in 5° of valgus.

The effect of forefoot twist in standing is interesting to analyze. Table 21-1 may be helpful in enabling one to understand the interrelationships.

Talocalcaneonavicular movement provides for rotation between the foot and leg, whereas the midtarsal joint provides for rotation between the anterior and posterior parts of the foot.

Lateral rotation of the leg results in supination of the foot.[15] This apparent double movement is nothing more than a simple hinge movement at the talocalcaneonavicular joint. It is difficult to visualize because the hinge is oblique. Thus, supination of the hindfoot in response to pronation of the forefoot results in raising of the medial arch. Kite[13] has called attention to the association of lateral torsion of the leg and flatfeet.

Several authors have called attention to the fact that the arrangement of axes of motion of the subtalar joint and a transverse tarsal joint

Table 21-1. Interrelationships of Joint Motion in Standing

Foot standing:				
Arch high	Supination-adduction-flexion	Supination	Flexion–pronation	Extension-pronation
			(*i.e.*, pronation twist of forefoot)	
Arch low	Pronation–abduction-extension	Pronation	Extension–supination	Flexion-supination
			(*i.e.*, supination twist of forefoot)	

play a role in increasing the stability of the foot when it is in supination. The axes of motion of the component joints of the transverse tarsal joint are divergent in the normal supinated foot but coincide in a pronated foot. This permits an unstable hingelike action in the midtarsal region of the pronated foot. Support of the longitudinal arch is not accomplished by muscle pull,[2] but by maintaining the tarsal bones in positions of overlapping girders of the arch. Pes planus develops through medial rotation of the bones, not by direct downward collapse.

EQUINOVARUS DEFORMITIES

CONGENITAL TALIPES EQUINOVARUS

Introduction

Congenital talipes equinovarus is a complex deformity involving all the bones of the foot. The incidence in the United States and England is said to be one per one thousand live births. The sex ratio is approximately two males to one female. Wynne-Davies[103–105] reports that the incidence of the same deformity among first-degree relatives is between 20 and 30 times higher than the normal incidence in Caucasians. The authors are not aware of any studies relating to the incidence of congenital talipes equinovarus in blacks. It is more often unilateral than bilateral.

Genetic Implications

The genetics of congenital idiopathic talipes equinovarus is not yet well defined. According to Wynne-Davies,[103–105] the inheritance pattern is multifactorial, the manifestation of which is dependent upon predisposing environmental influences as well as a genetic background for the anomaly. Under these circumstances, the predictability of occurrence within a family is less straightforward than a simple gene defect. Family studies have shown the incidence of congenital idiopathic talipes equinovarus is 20 to 30 times higher in first-degree relatives than in the general population, illustrating the genetic tendency. Such studies have also been helpful in counseling the parents of an affected child. For example, the risk to a future sibling of a child with congenital club foot and the normal parents is about 3%, whereas if the parents are also affected, the risk may be as high as 25%. Further studies are needed, however, to more clearly define the probability of recurrence within a family.

Cowell and Wein[39] concluded in an excellent review that congenital clubfoot is the result of a multifactorial inheritance system modified by environmental factors.

Etiology

The etiology of congenital talipes equinovarus remains an enigma, although many theories have been advanced. Scarpa believed that the deformity was related to medial twisting of the navicular, cuboid, and calcaneus bones in their relation to the talus. Adams[24] investigated a number of fetal and adult specimens and found that all soft-tissue abnormalities were secondary. He stated that the principal deformity was in the talus. The head and neck of the talus in his dissections were found to be attenuated and directed toward the plantar and medial aspects of the foot. Böhm[34,35] believed that the congenital clubfoot was due to an arrest in development. He postulated that the foot in a normal embryo at the 5-week stage was in a position of equinovarus and that an arrest in development was responsible for persistance of the deformity at birth. Other theories that have been suggested include abnormal tendon insertions and dysplasia of peroneal muscles.[22,73]

Settle,[93] in his study to determine the gross anatomic abnormalities in congenital clubfoot, found in 16 dissected infantile clubfeet that the tibiae were essentially normal except for a slight degree of internal torsion in four specimens. All the tali were found to be severely distorted. The talus was reduced in size by approximately one fourth and was plantar flexed at the ankle joint. The neck of the talus presented the most significant changes and was deviated medially and plantarward on the body. The navicular was dislocated medially and plantarward also in its relation to the head of the talus. The subtalar articular facet was also severely distorted. Only one articular surface was noted, and its axis was slanted medially.

The calcaneus was of normal shape but appeared slightly smaller than normal and was displaced into varus, equinus, and internal rotation.

Settle[93] concluded by saying that congenital clubfoot appears to be a primary developmental deformity of the hind part of the foot and is present as early as the twelfth gestational week.

Irani and Sherman[59] dissected 11 extremities with equinovarus in stillborns and found no primary abnormalities of nerves, vessels, muscles, or tendon insertions. In every specimen, the neck of the talus was found to be short and distorted and the anterior portion of the talus was found to rotate in a medial and plantar direction. The deviation of the anterior end of the talus was thought to be the primary fault. The deviations were attributed to a defective cartilaginous anlage that was dependent upon a primary germ-plasm defect. Environmental factors very likely contribute to the deformity as well.

Gray and Katz,[51] in 1981, found in a histochemical study of muscles in clubfeet that the muscle structure was normal except for a reduction in muscle fiber numbers in the calf and an increase in type 1 fiber in the soleus.

Ninety muscle biopsies were taken from 13 clubfoot patients during surgical correction by Handelsman and Badalamente.[52] The age range was from 3 months to 12 years. In most instances, the tibialis posterior, soleus, flexor hallucis longus, and flexor digitorium longus muscles were biopsied. In some instances, the intrinsic muscles were also examined. All were studied electron microscopically. In all muscle samples examined, consistent ultrastructural abnormalities were found that were compatible with a neurogenic etiology. The findings suggested that an underlying neurogenic disorder is significant in the pathogenesis of clubfoot. The bony deformity present in this disorder follows the persistent muscle imbalance. They caution that because of the muscle imbalance forces, the tendency to relapse is everpresent; therefore, following correction, prolonged night splint usage is necessary to negate the muscular imbalance.

Ippolito and Ponseti,[58] in 1980, reviewed the pathologic anatomy in five clubfeet comparing it with three normals. Soft-tissue alterations located posterior and medial were noted. These changes consisted of ligament thickening and shortening, muscle atrophy, and increased fibrous connective tissue. The tarsal bones were altered in size, shape, and anatomic relationship.

Bell and Versfeld,[31] in 1982, studied 22 patients with congenital idiopathic clubfoot electromyographically. The age of the patients varied from 1 day to 22 months. They concluded that conventional electromyographic techniques were unable to demonstrate abnormalities suggesting neuropathic or myopathic changes in idiopathic clubfoot.

Simon and Sarrafian[95] presented the results of a microsurgical dissection of a severe teratologic fetal club foot of a 7-month stillborn fetus with camptomelic dysplasia. The most striking anatomic alteration was marked rotation of the calcaneous beneath the talus with the rotation in a vertical axis. A complete subtalar release as well as a posteromedial and plantar release was necessary to reposition the bones of the hindfoot.

Pathology

The deformity in congenital idiopathic clubfoot is that of forefoot adduction combined with inversion and supination, as well as varus of the hindfoot with the calcaneus inverted under the talus. The talus is found to be in equinus. These changes, although present at birth, become pronounced with the passage of time due to soft-tissue contracture. The head of the talus is prominent at the dorsal lateral aspect of the foot. The navicular is medial to the head of the talus and may lie adjacent to the medial malleolus. The cuboid is also displaced medially in front of the calcaneus. The cuneiforms as well as the metatarsals contribute to the deformity as a result of the adduction deformity. The cavus deformity is related to contracture of the plantar aponeurosis as well as the abductor hallicus, the short toe flexors, and the abductor digiti quinti. The plantar flexed position of the first metatarsal also aggravates the cavus deformity.

In unilateral congenital clubfoot, there is usually minimal shortening of the involved foot and extremity as well as a slight discrepancy in the calf. The shortening of the extremity may involve the femur, the tibia, or the foot, and, in some instances, all the bones of the extremity are involved. This discrepancy in the involved extremity and foot may be more noticeable in females.

McKay[83] has emphasized that the major deformity in congenital clubfoot is the medial rotation of the entire foot on the talus. This inward rotation takes place primarily at the midtarsal and subtalar joints. The navicular moves around the head of the talus anterior to the ankle joint. He does not feel that there is internal rotation of the talus in the ankle joint or an abnormal plane of motion of the talus relative to the bimalleolar plane of the tibiotalar articulation.

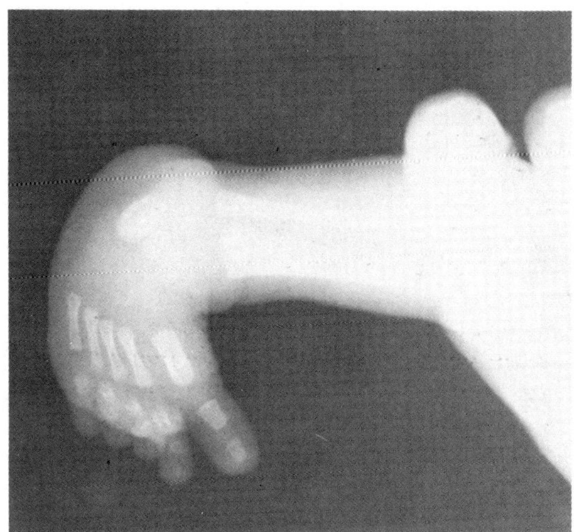

FIG. 21-1. Congenital clubfoot showing forefoot adduction and varus of the hindfoot. The foot is positioned at a right angle to the long axis of the tibia.

Clinical Findings

Generally, congenital clubfoot may be classified into two distinct groups.[26,75] In the first group, commonly referred to as a normal or conventional congenital clubfoot, the foot presents the usual deformities. The foot is, however, much more supple than the second type. The second group, by contrast, is characterized as having a greater degree of stiffness, and the foot is very likely to show considerable difference in size. In our experience, the first type accounts for approximately 70% to 75% of cases. In the second type, the calcaneus is smaller than normal, and, because of the overlying adipose tissue, it is difficult to palpate. There is often a transverse crease present in the region of the midfoot. This can be attributed to contracture of the plantar aponeurosis and the first layer of plantar muscles. The second type constitutes the recalcitrant type of deformity and is extremely difficult to correct by nonoperative means. The reduction in circumference of the calf is probably secondary to reduction in total muscle bulk.

Clinically, the foot in both types is held at a right angle to the ankle and long axis of the tibia. There is often very little prominence at the upper border of the heel. The talus is usually palpable at the dorsal lateral aspect of the foot and fills the sinus tarsi. The tubercule of the navicular is palpable medially. If an attempt is made to abduct the forefoot, resistance is encountered and the soft-tissue contractures are palpable on the medial aspect of the foot. Attempts at dorsiflexion of the foot demonstrate the marked contracture of the posterior soft tissues, including the Achilles tendon and posterior capsule of the ankle. Finally, if the infant is supported and held erect, weight is borne on the dorsal lateral aspect of the foot rather than on the plantar aspect.

Roentgenographic Examination

At birth, the primary centers of ossification include the talus and calcaneus and, in some instances, the cuboid. These structures can be demonstrated roentgenographically. The ossifiation center for the navicular appears at age 3 years in females and usually 1 year later in males. At the forefoot, the phalanges and metatarsals are ossified at birth (Fig. 21-1).

The technique of obtaining appropriate roentgenograms is of importance if the foot is to be assessed accurately. Beatson and Pearson[28] have described a method of obtaining anteroposterior and lateral roentgenograms that is simple and easily adapted to use. The child's hips are flexed 90° and the knees are flexed approximately 45° to 60°. The feet for the anteroposterior view are then held closely together and placed in 30° of plantar flexion on the cassette. The x-ray tube is then directed cranially from the vertical. The lateral view of the foot should be made with the foot plantar flexed 35° and the x-ray tube centered over the ankle and hindfoot. A stress lateral film following correction is also made, with the foot and ankle in extreme dorsiflexion. Lines drawn through the long axis of the talus as well as the inferior margin of the calcaneus should subtend an angle of 35° or greater if the deformity is corrected. Turco[98,99] has emphasized the importance of the stress lateral roentgenogram in determining that the foot is satisfactorily corrected. The stress lateral view will also demonstrate overlap of the talus and calcaneus at their anterior ends.

In the anteroposterior view, similar lines are drawn through the long axes of the calcaneus and the talus, and the resulting angle represents the talocalcaneal angle or Kite angle. The line through the talus should coincide with the first metatarsal and the line drawn through the calcaneus should coincide with the fifth metatarsal. The normal angle in the anteroposterior view varies between 20° and 35°. An angle greater than 35° indicates valgus and an angle less than 20° indicates varus of the hindfoot.

Simon[94] has developed the concept of analytical roentgenography of congenital clubfeet. He defines this term as an analytical method for roentgenographic evaluation of the four major deformities of clubfeet in whatever combination they may exist. The technique is based on positioning the foot as close to the plantar grade or maximally corrected position as possible. If the foot is positioned properly, the degree of residual deformity following conservative treatment can be determined. In addition to the anteroposterior and lateral views of the foot, Simon[94] has suggested that the talo-first metatarsal angle (TMT angle) be determined. The normal TMT angle is zero to −20°. Measurements in a positive direction are abnormal. This angle is indicative of medial deviation of the foot at either the distal or proximal row of tarsal bones or both. It is not helpful unless used in conjunction with the hindfoot talocalcaneal angle.

Weinstein and associates[100] evaluated the abnormalities in 32 patients with unilateral clubfoot and correlated the roentgenographic findings with the functional results. The average follow-up averaged 20 years. Notching of the anterior distal tibia, diminished anteroposterior and lateral talocalcaneal angle, flattening and wedging and medial displacement of the navicular, lateral displacement of the cuneiforms, decreased posterior tibial calcaneal distance, and decreased talocalcaneal index were noted. Other roentgenographic abnormalities included small flattened talar heads and misshapen facets of the subtalar joints.

Classification of Idiopathic Congenital Talipes Equinovarus

Congenital clubfeet do vary in severity.[26,75] All such deformities have in common forefoot adduction, varus of the hindfoot, and equinus of the ankle and subtalar joint, as well as subluxation of the talonavicular joint.

We believe that aside from the congenital clubfoot that results from positional deformity, there are two major types of deformity. The most frequent type is the usual or conventional type. This accounts, as previously mentioned, for approximately 75% of the congenital clubfeet seen, and this group fortunately is much easier to correct by nonoperative means than the second type. The second type is extremely resistant to conservative measures and is characterized by a transverse crease (Fig. 21-2). The foot is short and rather stiff and seems to have a small calcaneus with associated contracture of the plantar structures. It has been our experience that this type of deformity virtually always requires surgical correction.

Treatment

Conservative Management

It should be possible to correct congenital clubfeet in a very significant number of children by conservative measures.[30] Success requires that the foot shows correction both clinically and roentgenographically. It would also imply that the foot is fully flexible, normal in appearance, and painless and accepts conventional shoes.

A retrospective review was conducted in all patients treated at the Scottish Rite Hospital for idiopathic congenital clubfoot from 1950 to 1956 by Price and Lovell.[90] This time period was selected to allow at least a 20-year follow-up. During this period, 85 consecutive patients younger than 4 months of age were treated. Of this group, 63 patients were male and 22

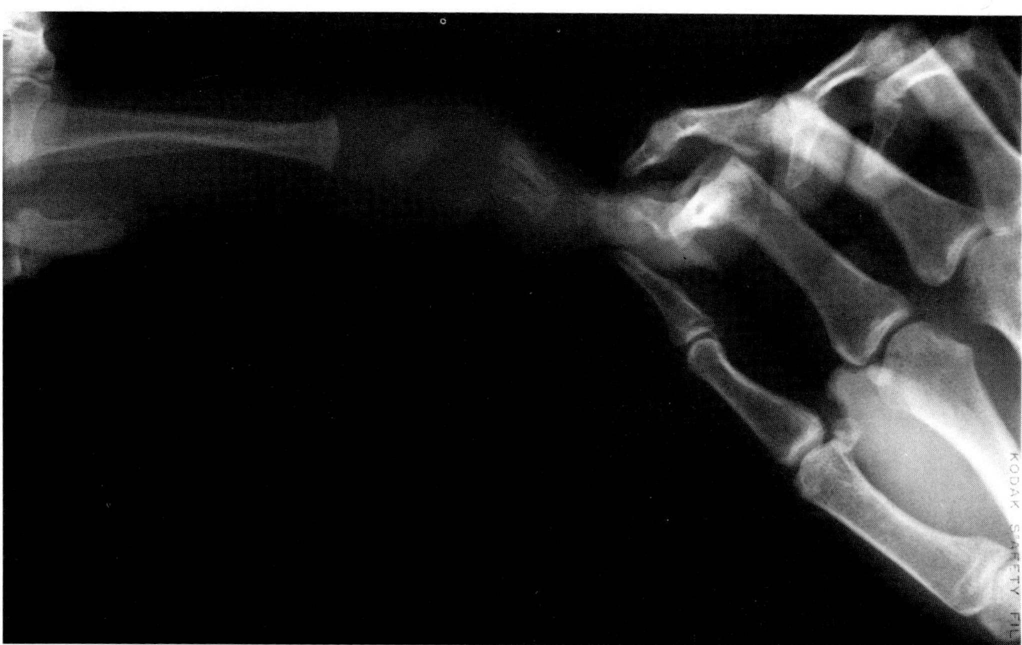

FIG. 21-2. Lateral roentogenogram of congenital clubfoot. Note the marked equinus of both the forefoot and the hindfoot. There is a transverse crease at the plantar aspect of the foot.

patients were female; all were Caucasian. Forty-nine patients had unilateral and 36 patients had bilateral clubfoot involvement, thus giving a total of 121 feet. The average age at initiation of treatment was 6 weeks. Thirty-eight patients with 54 clubfeet were lost to follow-up before the age of 10 years. Forty-seven patients with 67 affected feet were followed 10 years or longer. The average follow-up for this group was 17.8 years. Treatment consisted of weekly cast changes for 3 to 4 months and then biweekly changes. Recurrences were treated with further manipulations and cast application. The average total length of time in plaster casts was 20.4 months. Only 3 of the 67 clubfeet followed had operative procedures before the age of 10 years.

Results were classified as good, fair, or poor by chart review. Approximately two thirds qualified as a good result. Twelve feet were rated fair with slight residual deformity, slight overcorrection, slight forefoot adduction, or normal with tight heelcord. Twelve feet were poor with rocker-bottom deformity, residual clubfoot, or required triple arthrodesis.

In this series, there was a striking difference in results according to sex. Only 31% of females with clubfeet had a good result, whereas 76% of males with clubfeet had a good result.

As a part of the study, an attempt was made to recall patients for clinical and roentgenographic examination. Twenty-two patients returned for follow-up at an average age of 23.6 years. There were 32 affected feet in this group. Sex, ratio, bilaterality, age at initial treatment, length of time in plaster, number of recurrences, and percentage of good results were found to be similar in all respects to the overall series. Using very strict criteria, 21 of 32 feet or approximately two thirds had a good result by nonoperative means alone. An additional five patients or one sixth had fair results and one sixth had poor results.

We prefer the Kite method of nonoperative correction, although this method has now been modified.[61,63,66–68,70,71,73,89]

Treatment with serial casting should be initiated as early as possible. Early treatment suggests that treatment begin within the first few days of life, prior to development of secondary contractures. The earlier treatment is initiated, the greater the likelihood of success by nonoperative means.[74] The converse is also true. An effort should be made to achieve correction of the deformity within the first 3 months of life.[88]

Criteria for Correction. A corrected congenital clubfoot is one that is fully mobile with

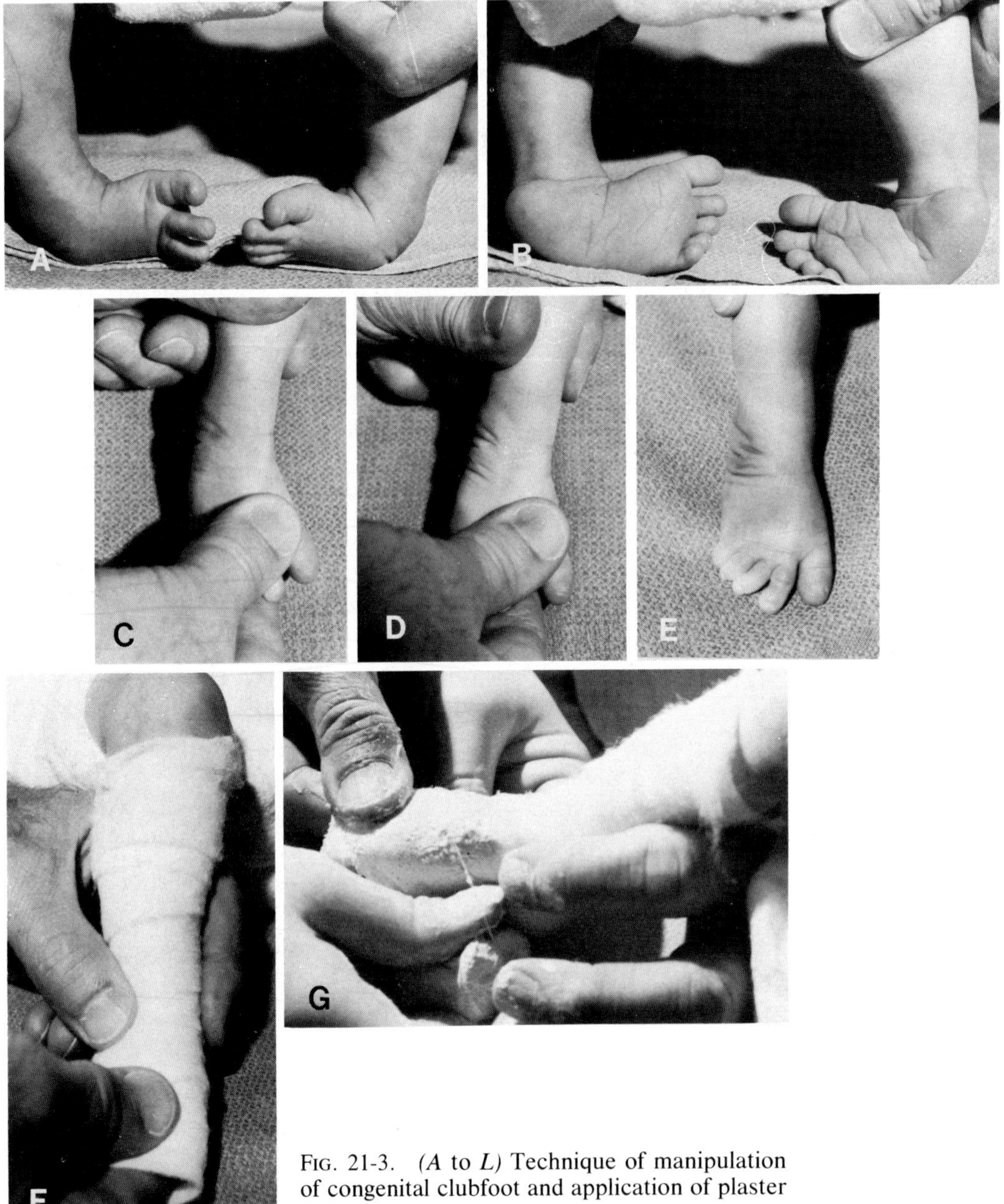

FIG. 21-3. *(A to L)* Technique of manipulation of congenital clubfoot and application of plaster casts.

no restriction of motion at the subtalar joint with dorsiflexion of 15° to 20° and with the heel in slight valgus. The forefoot can also be abducted slightly beyond the midline and is quite supple. If there is unilateral involvement, its appearance should be similar to the contralateral foot.

Manipulation of Foot. The foot is manipulated prior to each change of cast.[72,75] This is a very important procedure and should be done extremely carefully as well as gently in order not to injure the hyaline cartilage. It is this procedure that actually corrects the foot, and the plaster cast maintains the correction that follows each manipulation.

The technique of manipulation that we use consists of grasping the forefoot between the thumb and index finger (Fig. 21-3). The leg is stabilized with the opposite hand. A distracting force is applied with elongation of the foot.

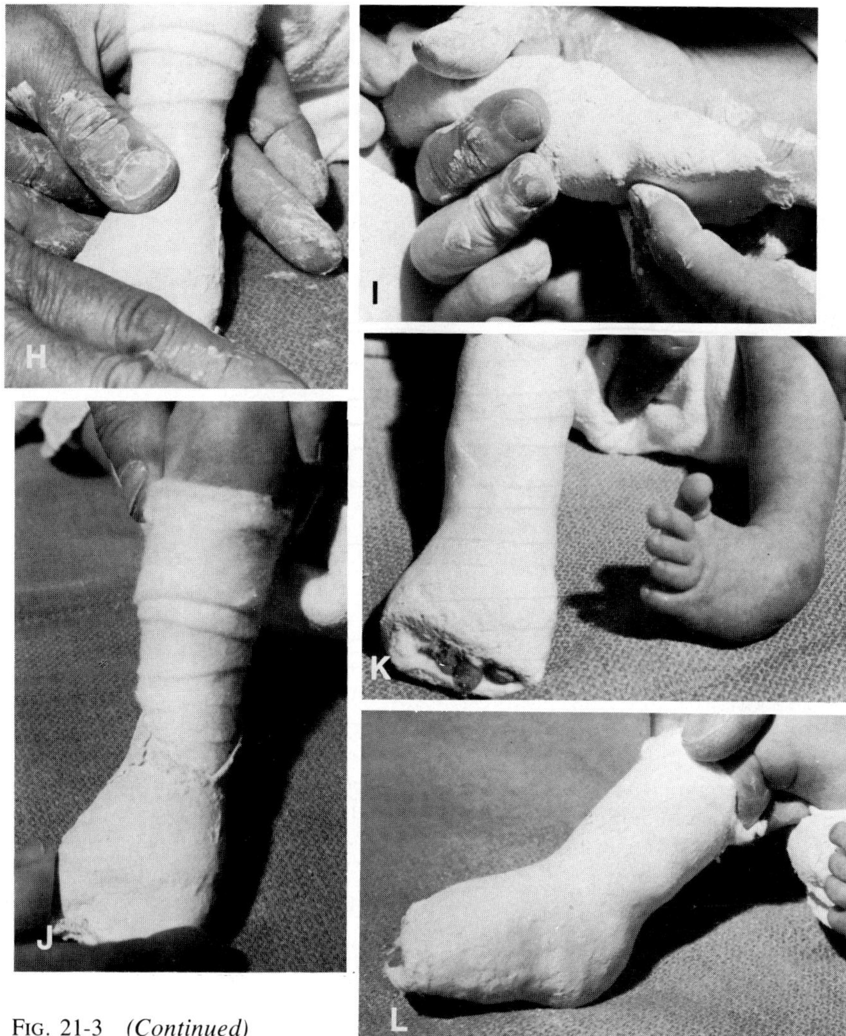

FIG. 21-3 *(Continued)*

This maneuver permits unlocking of the subtalar joint and eversion of the calcaneus. As the tarsus elongates due to the distraction force, slight pressure is applied at the sinus tarsi, and the head of the talus is displaced medially. The navicular is then gently displaced laterally to correct the talonavicular subluxation. This permits abduction of the forefoot in preparation for cast application.

Technique of Cast Application. In the newborn, a single 3-inch roll of plaster is adequate. The plaster is divided with a sharp knife and one half of the roll is used for the foot in order to prepare a plaster slipper, and the remainder of the roll of plaster serves to attach a slipper to the leg portion of the cast. The cast extends only to the knee and is changed weekly. Following manipulation in the manner described with the foot held in maximum correction, a single layer of sheet cotton is applied, extending from toes to the knee. The plaster is then applied in a circular manner about the forefoot and hindfoot by an assistant. A piece of plexiglass or some similar substance should be used to stabilize the foot during molding of the cast. Very careful molding of the cast follows in order that the correction that has resulted from manipulation be maintained. In order to correct the forefoot adduction deformity, it is particularly important to abduct the forefoot at the calcaneocuboid joint. A rocker-bottom deformity (Fig. 21-4) can be

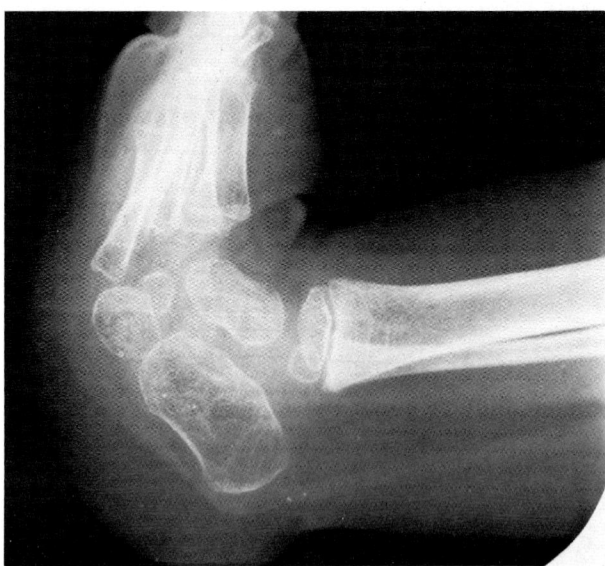

FIG. 21-4. Rocker-bottom deformity.

avoided if the forefoot is plantar flexed and the cast molded under the midtarsal joint. The foot is then everted, displaced posteriorly, and dorsiflexed slightly. No attempt should be made to dorsiflex the foot above a right angle until the forefoot adduction and varus of the hindfoot is corrected. Following correction of these deformities clinically and with verification of position by appropriate roentgenograms (Fig. 21-5), the foot is manipulated gently in dorsiflexion to correct the equinus deformity. This is done with the knee extended and with uniform pressure applied by the cupped hand at the plantar aspect of the foot.

Following correction of all deformities, a series of holding casts are necessary to permit the foot to accommodate to its newly corrected position. Generally, this requires a minimum of 2 or 3 months.

A recent review of the results of Ghali and associates[50] of 125 patients with 194 congenital club feet is of interest. Of the 70 patients representing 68 affected feet seen within 4 weeks of birth, it was thought that excellent or good results were achieved in 94% of feet treated conservatively and in 82% of feet that required a plantar release. Of the 55 patients seen after 4 weeks of age, satisfactory results were achieved in 75%.

In reviewing 338 patients with congenital club foot deformity over a 5-year period, Yip and colleagues[106] noted that talipes equinovarus was present in 229 patients; 130 patients had bilateral deformity, and, of the 99 patients with unilateral deformity, the right side was involved in 51 cases and the left side in 48 cases. The initial treatment was conservative with manipulation, strapping, and splinting on a daily outpatient basis. Of the 368 feet with talipes equinovarus deformity, 291 feet responded to conservative treatment. The duration of treatment varied from 3 months to 3 years, with an average of 8 months. Fifty-seven patients with 77 feet required surgical correction.

In reviewing 123 unselected treated congenital clubfeet, Harrold and Walker[53] found that those feet classified as severe did the worst. Of the 48 feet seen in this group, 1 in 10 responded to serial casting. Surgical correction succeeded in 2 of 3 of the resistant feet but had to be repeated in others.

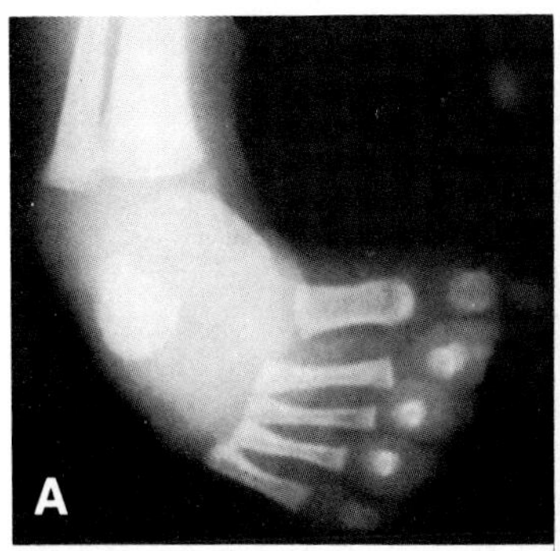

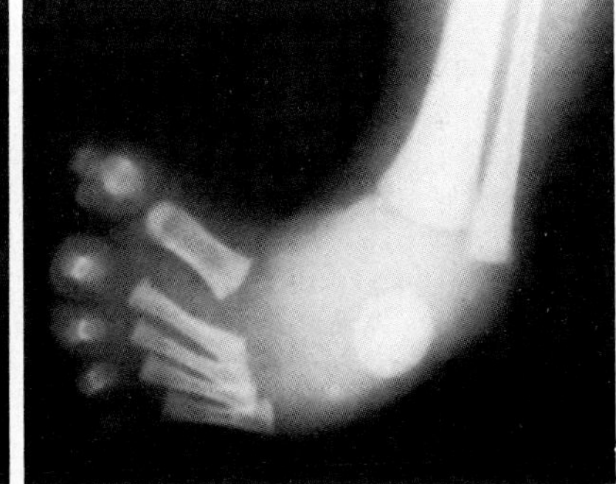

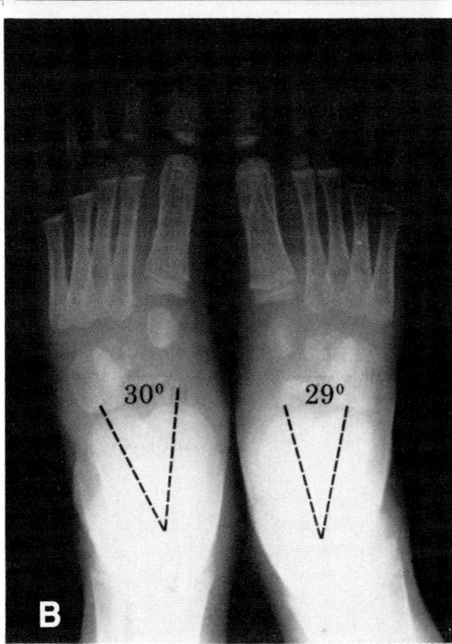

FIG. 21-5. Typical congenital clubfoot deformity showing forefoot adduction and varus of hindfoot bilaterally. *(A)* Before treatment. *(B)* After closed treatment. Note the restoration of the talocalcaneal angle and correction of the forefoot varus. *(C* and *D)* Clinical photographs after correction of deformity on both sides.

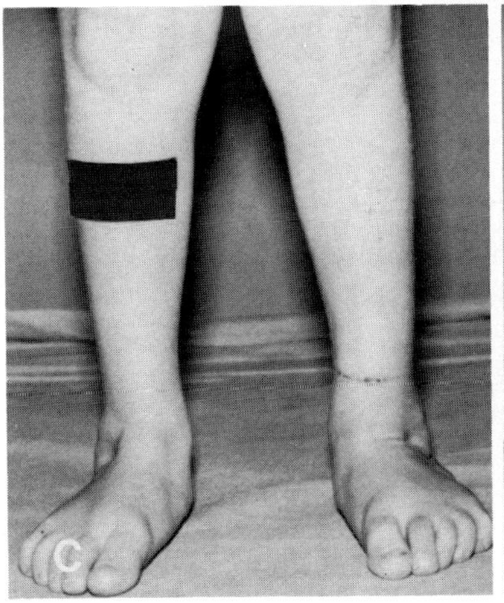

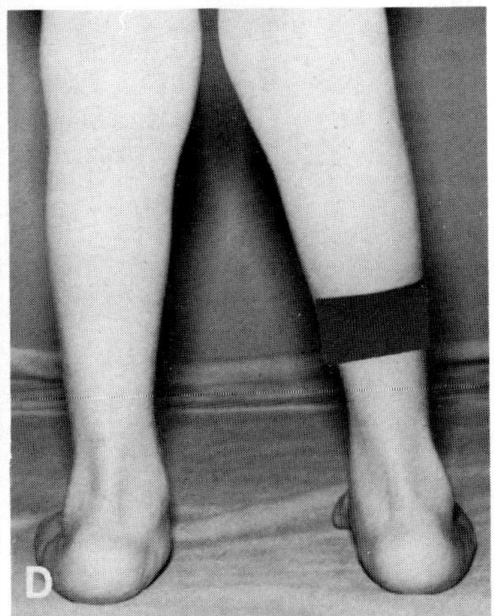

Retentive Splints. Retentive splints aid in maintenance of correction. Splintage should be combined with dedicated passive stretching of the foot by the parents. Straight last shoes are attached to a Denis Browne split, turning the involved foot outward 10°. Splintage may be discontinued when the child is walking well, but passive stretching of the feet should be continued until the child is approximately 2 or 3 years of age and shows no tendency toward recurrence.

If there is recurrence of the deformity, the physician must make the decision as to whether additional casting or surgical correction is appropriate.

Operative Management

The attending physician, upon reaching an impasse in the nonoperative management, must make a decision as to what surgical procedure or procedures are indicated in order to correct the existing deformities. Often a combination of procedures may be necessary. Each foot must be evaluated carefully and dealt with in the appropriate manner. Many operative procedures have been described and all have merit.[26,36,38,55,62,77,78,86] It is a mistake for the surgeon to attempt to adapt all feet to a particular operation. Bony procedures must not be done in the infant and young child, because damage to bone and articular cartilage will ensue. After analyzing the foot carefully in determining the extent of involvement of the various deformities, the appropriate surgical procedure must then be chosen.[62]

Forefoot Adduction. If the deformity is confined to the forefoot only, a Heyman, Herndon, and Strong[54] procedure should be considered. Although the bases of the metatarsals may be exposed by vertical incisions, a curved incision extending from the base of the first metatarsal to the cuboid bone is preferred. The neurovascular structures are protected, and the intermetatarsal joints are released by capsulotomy and division of the ligaments. Injury to the articular cartilage and the growth plates must be avoided. Heyman, Herndon, and Strong[54] have recommended that this procedure be limited to children younger than 7 years of age.

Tendon Transfer. Transfer of the anterior tibial tendon to the dorsum of the foot in the region of the fifth metatarsal base has been advocated by Garceau.[46–48] This procedure should not be done until correction of fixed structural deformity of the forefoot has been done. This can usually be accomplished with serial plaster casts with wedging of the forefoot in abduction. In our experience, there is an occasional instance when this procedure is indicated. If the forefoot is flexible and tends to supinate during the swing phase of the gait, we have used the split anterior tibial transfer, moving the detached lateral one half of the tendon to the second or third cuneiform. If the tendon is transferred too far laterally, overcorrection is possible. The second possible disadvantage of transferring the entire tendon is plantar flexion of the first metatarsal and clawing of the first toe due to the unopposed action of the peroneus longus muscle.

Transfer of the Posterior Tibial Tendon. Gartland advocated transplantation of the posterior tibial tendon through the interosseous membrane anteriorly to the third cuneiform in the relapsed clubfoot.

Fried[45] dissected the insertion of the tendon of the tibialis posterior in 56 recurrent clubfeet. The insertion was found to be abnormal in all instances. He believed that the abnormal contracture of this muscle contributed to the development of clubfoot. In view of this, the tendon was transferred after excision of the abnormal insertion to the third cuneiform. A posterior release consisting of lengthening of the Achilles tendon and posterior capsulotomy were performed at the same time to correct the equinus deformity.

We have not found it necessary to use the posterior tibial tendon transplant for recurrent clubfoot. It is difficult to accept the hypothesis that release and forward transplantation of this tendon will result in correction of the residual deformities.

Posterior Release. A posterior release alone is indicated in congenital clubfoot only after there has been complete correction of forefoot adduction and hindfoot varus both clinically and roentgenographically. If dorsiflexion is attempted before these deformities are corrected, a rocker-bottom deformity will follow.

All too often, a posterior release is done when an impasse is reached, with persistence of forefoot adduction and hindfoot varus. A simple posterior release alone will not result in correction of these residual deformities. This is a very common error and will very likely result in increased stiffness in the foot because of adhesions secondary to lengthening of the Achilles tendon and posterior capsulotomy of the ankle and subtalar joints.

Posterior release consists of lengthening of the Achilles tendon by the Z-plasty method. It is necessary to lengthen the tendon in this manner in order to do an adequate posterior capsulotomy at the ankle and subtalar joints. The posterior deltoid ligament should be sectioned, as well as the posterior talofibular ligament and the calcaneofibular ligament. Sectioning of these structures enables correction of the equinus deformity of the talus and also permits the anterior end of the calcaneus and talus to ascend, with restoration of the normal talocalcaneal angle.

A long-leg plaster cast is applied, with the foot at a right angle, for 6 weeks. Upon removal of the cast, passive stretching of the foot is indicated, as well as application of a night splint.

Soft-Tissue Release. Numerous authors have advocated a one-stage surgical release for correction of all residual elements of congenital talipes equinovarus.

Turco[98,99] popularized this procedure, stating that in his experience, a significant number of all clubfeet treated from birth had incomplete corrections and recurrent deformities requiring repeated manipulations and casts and finally one or more surgical procedures. He expressed disenchantment with the results of nonoperative treatment, saying that the one-stage posterior medial release corrects all existing deformities and results in a flexible plantargrade foot.

Turco[98,99] described three groups of contractures in the congenital clubfoot, namely, posterior, medial, and subtalar. In the recalcitrant clubfoot, all the contractures must be released surgically. The posterior contractures involve the posterior capsule of the ankle and subtalar joints, the Achilles tendon, the posterior talofibular, and the calcaneofibular ligaments. The medial contractures involve the deltoid and calcaneonavicular ligaments, the talonavicular joint capsule, and the sheaths of the posterior tibial, flexor digitorum longus, and flexor hallicus longus tendons. The subtalar contractures involve the anterior talocalcaneal interosseous ligament and the bifurcated ligament.

All contractures must be released by meticulous dissection, avoiding injury to the articular cartilage of the joints as well as injury to the neurovascular structures. Anomalies of the blood supply to the foot may exist with absence of the anterior vessels. Absence of the anterior vessels has been reported by Ben-Menachem and Butler[32] following selective arteriography. If the posterior tibial artery is compromised in the dissection, a catastrophic result may occur.

We have found the posteromedial release as described by Turco[98,99] to be satisfactory (Fig. 21-6). In most instances, the interosseous talocalcaneal ligament is not sectioned, because it is thought that this may result in excessive valgus deformity at the hindfoot. The posterior tibial tendon is not sacrificed but is lengthened in a Z-plasty manner above the medial malleolus. The circumferential soft tissue release utilizing the Cincinnati incision and following the surgical technique as advocated by McKay is the author's current choice. It permits adequate utilization of the anatomical structures and excellent correction of the residual deformity.

In many instances, the complete plantar release as described by Lucas[76] is also done. This procedure has been popularized by Westin[101] and consists of release of the abductor hallicus, the plantar aponeurosis, the short toe flexors, and the abductor digiti quinti at their attachment to the calcaneus. These structures are released medially through the same incision. It appears that the addition of the plantar release aids in elongation of the foot and correction of the forefoot adduction deformity.

Turco[98,99] assessed 31 feet having the one-stage posteromedial release and followed the patients for 2 years or more. He found 27 feet to be excellent or good, 3 were considered to be fair results, and 1 was considered a failure, requiring additional surgery.

Barrett and Lovell,[27] in an unpublished review, studied 83 one-stage posteromedial releases performed at the Scottish Rite Hospital from 1975 to 1977. Thirty-two feet involving 22 patients with a diagnosis of idiopathic congenital talipes equinovarus were evaluated. Using very strict criteria, 11 feet in eight patients were graded excellent, 13 feet in nine patients were graded good, 5 feet in four patients were graded fair, and 3 feet in two patients were graded poor.

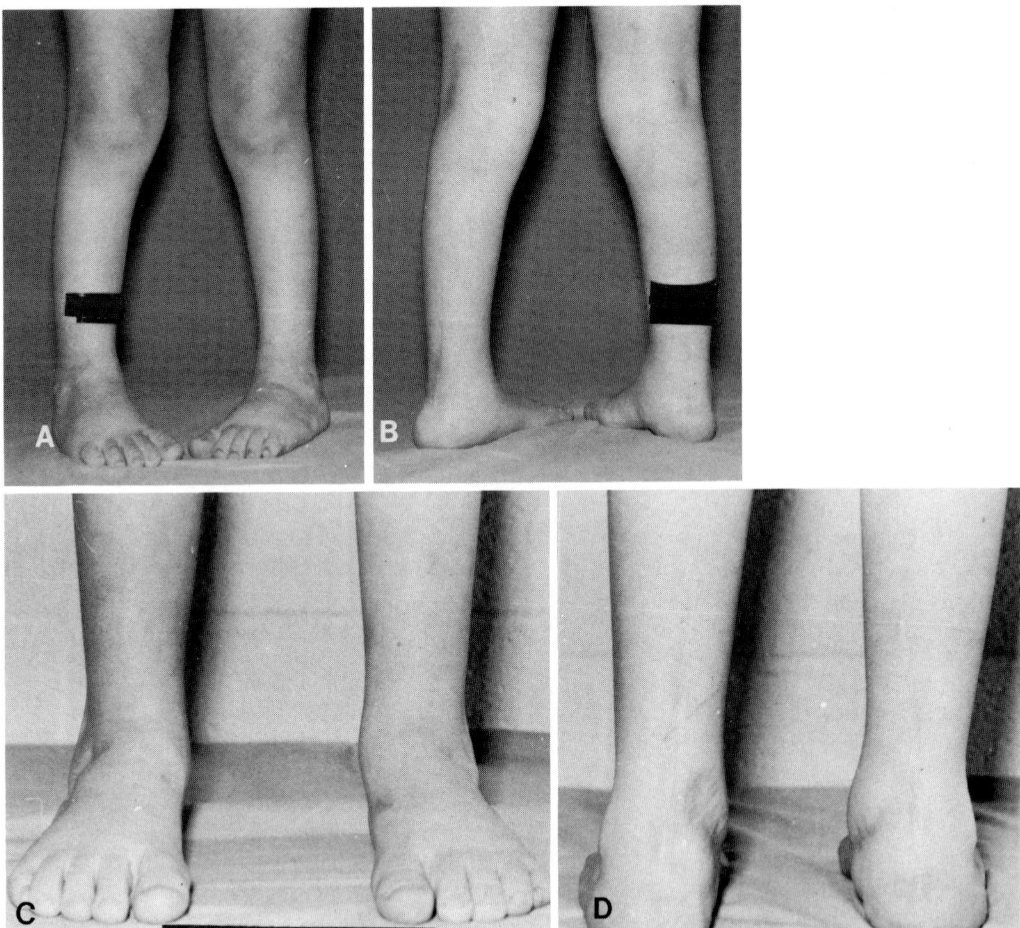

FIG. 21-6. *(A and B)* graphs showing deformity of forefoot and hindfoot. *(C and D)* Postoperative clinical photographs following posteromedial release. Note correction of forefoot as well as hindfoot deformities.

The age at the time of surgery varied from 6 months to 7 years. The average age at time of surgery was 3 years. The average time of follow-up was 20.3 months. Ten patients had bilateral congenital clubfeet requiring bilateral posteromedial releases. Five patients had bilateral clubfeet and responded to cast correction on one side, and unilateral posteromedial release was necessary on the opposite side. Seven patients had unilateral clubfeet and posteromedial releases.

The one-stage posteromedial release combined with the plantar release has not been done at the Scottish Rite Hospital in patients younger than 4 months of age. Ideally, the procedure should be done after the age of 6 to 12 months. The use of magnification glasses and small instruments is a necessity when the procedure is done in a small foot.

The upper limit for age for the posteromedial release has been 7 years, with the best results in children younger than 3 years of age.

Ryöppy and Sairanen[91] in a preliminary report described their results following soft-tissue release in 94 resistant clubfeet involving 67 patients. The mean age of the patients was 12 days, with the range of 2 to 41 days. No treatment was attempted before the operation, which was done as soon as all other postnatal problems were under control. These authors stated that the aim of early surgery was to obtain total correction of the foot with minimal surgical release. Seventy percent were graded as excellent, 29% were considered good, and only one foot was graded poor. They concluded that although neonatal surgery in their hands has proved satisfactory in correcting the resistant club foot, it cannot be recommended for general use without reservations.

Smith, Campbell, and Bonnett[96] advocated splitting the interosseous tibiofibular ligament to allow the mortise to accommodate the wider anterior third of the talus if equinus could not be corrected at operation.

In a recent review, Scott, Hosking, and Catterall[92] studied dorsiflexion in three normal feet and three feet with talipes equinovarus to determine the anatomic factors that might contribute to the failure of operative treatment to correct the deformity. In the normal feet, dorsiflexion movement was noted to be essentially rotary, whereas in the clubfeet, a posterolateral tether was found, which prevented forward movement of the fibula, thus blocking dorsiflexion. Dorsiflexion cannot occur in a normal manner if movement of the lateral malleolus is restricted. Shortening of the structures attached to the posterior and lateral aspect of the fibula prevented its normal excursion. It was the recommendation of these doctors that a posterior and lateral release be done for the operative correction of the hindfoot in a child with clubfoot deformity, especially if he is younger than 1 year of age.

Operations on Bone. OSTEOTOMY OF THE METATARSALS. Berman and Gartland[33] suggested osteotomy of the bases of the metatarsals for structural adduction deformity of the forefoot. This procedure should be reserved for children older than 6 or 7 years of age. After exposure of the bases of the metatarsals, using a transverse slightly curved incision or three longitudinal incisions between the metatarsals, a dome-shaped osteotomy is done. The osteotomy of the first metatarsal is done just distal to the growth plate in order to avoid injury. Stout Kirschner wires are then used to transfix the first and fifth metatarsal bases. These may be cut subcutaneously and are removed 6 weeks later. The short-leg cast can usually be discontinued 6 weeks following surgery. Berman and Gartland[33] performed metatarsal osteotomy for the correction of rigid adduction of the forepart of the foot in 115 feet. Forty-four of the operations were done to correct resistant adduction of the forefoot associated with congenital clubfoot. In evaluating the end results, 84% were classified as good and excellent, and 16% were classified as fair and poor.

OSTEOTOMY OF THE CALCANEUS. Dwyer[41,42] noted that conservative measures often fail in a high number of children with talipes equinovarus. He expressed belief that the persistence of an inverted heel is the most important factor in preventing complete correction, in that relapse is encouraged by its presence.

In describing the deforming forces, Dwyer[41,42] stated that in a clubfoot, the heel is inverted and elevated so that the outer border of the foot receives most of the weight. As a result, the plantar fascia becomes contracted.

The operation advocated by Dwyer[41,42] aims at correction of the varus of the heel, increasing its height and placing it directly under the line of weightbearing. Although the ideal age for this procedure is said to be 3 to 4 years, it can be done in older children.

Through a posterior incision, the Achilles tendon is exposed and divided in a sagittal plane, with the medial half dissected from its insertion at the calcaneus. The calcaneus is then divided with a broad osteotome more or less in the line of the flexor hallucis tendon. The distal fragment is tilted laterally, and a bone graft taken from the proximal tibia is inserted in the interval, thus creating an opening wedge osteotomy.

Immobilization is recommended for 10 weeks, and normal activity returns rapidly with an improved gait.

In assessing his results in 56 feet in 48 patients, Dwyer[41,42] stated that emphasis was placed on function rather than appearance. Twenty-seven of the 56 feet were regarded as a good result, and 29 were considered to be a fair result.

The authors prefer a closing wedge laterally at the calcaneus, as described by Dwyer[41,42] for pes cavus. This is a much simpler procedure and appears to correct the varus deformity of the hindfoot satisfactorily.

WEDGE RESECTION OF THE CALCANEOCUBOID JOINT. Evans[43] described an operation for the relapsed clubfoot. He stated that the essential deformity in clubfoot is in the midtarsal joint and that all other deformities are secondary. It would, therefore, appear that the essential lesion in a clubfoot is a congenital dislocation of the navicular on the talus, that the cuboid bone as well as the calcaneus is included with the dislocation, and that changes in the skeleton and soft tissue are secondary and adapted. Finally, the manipulative reduction must achieve replacement of the navicular on the talus. In doing so, the medial column of the foot is restored. Manipulation of a clubfoot invariably encounters resistance; the older the child, the greater the resistance. The resistance, as previously mentioned, is secondary to contracted soft tissues and joint surfaces that are very likely incongruous. The elongated lateral column of the foot as well as the shape of the calcaneocuboid joint contributes to the resistance, according to Evans.[43] The aim of the operation is to secure a significant lateral rotation of the navicular to bring the first metatarsal into line with the talus and to correct equinus. Evans[43] correctly makes a strong point of applying serial plaster casts to correct the deformity as much as possible and to increase the suppleness of the foot prior to operation.

The operation consists of Z-plasty lengthening of the posterior tibial tendon and the tendo Achilles. A posterior capsulotomy at the ankle is also usually necessary, thus permitting correction of the equinus to a right angle or greater. The calcaneocuboid joint is then exposed through a lateral incision and an appropriate wedge or bone is excised at this joint. Evans[43] advises the use of two staples to hold the calcaneus and cuboid and to maintain apposition of their surfaces. Immobilization in a short cast is recommended for 5 months, with walking permitted after 6 weeks.

In discussing the results, Evans[43] operated on 30 feet between 1953 and 1956. The ages of the children ranged from 3 years to 14 years, with the majority being between 4 and 8 years. He was impressed with the permanent correction of the deformity, finding that if the shape of the foot is satisfactory following removal of the plaster, it is likely to retain its correction. A second advantage according to Evans is that the operation can correct all elements of the deformity. Finally, the operation preserves the foot that is of good shape, accepts normal shoes, and is plantargrade.

Abrams,[23] in 1969, concluded, in reviewing the early results of the Evans operation in 31 feet, that 23 were good, 7 were fair, and 1 was poor. His results, he thought, were comparable to the results of Evans.[43] He also agreed with Evans in that following fusion at the calcaneocuboid joint, no subsequent loss of correction will occur. Abrams advised that the operation not be done before the age of 4 years or after the age of 9 years. It would seem that the ideal age is 6 years. If the procedure is done too early, overcorrection of the hindfoot may ensue, because wedge resection of the calcaneocuboid joint may remove too much cartilage.

Addison and colleagues[25] reported on their experiences with a modified form of the collateral operation described by Dillwyn Evans used in severe relapsed clubfeet. Forty-five feet in 37 patients were reviewed. Of this group, 35 were considered satisfactory. Although the majority of the feet were stiff, they were relatively free of pain. It was noted that 42 of the 45 feet had previous surgery. Most of the feet fit into normal shoes, and 34 patients were able to participate in essentially normal activities. A pronated forefoot was a common residual deformity, but this did not prevent a satisfactory functional outcome.

Osteotomy of the Medial Cuneiform. Hofmann and co-workers[56] performed a biplane osteotomy of the first cuneiform on 18 feet in 14 patients with residual deformity of congenital clubfoot. The procedure consisted of doing an opening-wedge biplane osteotomy of the first cuneiform, accompanied by a radical plantar release. The average correction was 72% for the adduction of the fore part of the foot and 47% for the equinus deformity of the fore part of the foot. The indication for the operation was that preoperative radiographs demonstrated an adduction deformity of the fore part of the foot with an abnormal angle of the first metatarsocuneiform joint.

Derotational Osteotomy of the Tibia and Fibula. Internal tibial torsion is extremely uncommon in congenital talipes equinovarus, in our experience. Occasionally, derotational osteotomy of the proximal tibia and fibula may be indicated. It is important in the child who has corrected clubfeet and who toes inward to determine whether the toeing inward is related to uncorrected forefoot adduction or to increased femoral anteversion. The intoeing is more likely to be the result of abnormal sitting, with a resultant increase in femoral anteversion. Many children with congenital clubfeet that have been corrected tend to sit with feet tucked under their buttocks or in the reverse tailor position. In this instance, it is possible that a derotational osteotomy of the distal femur may occasionally be indicated in children older than 8 or 10 years of age.

Triple Arthrodesis. We have used the Hoke[57]

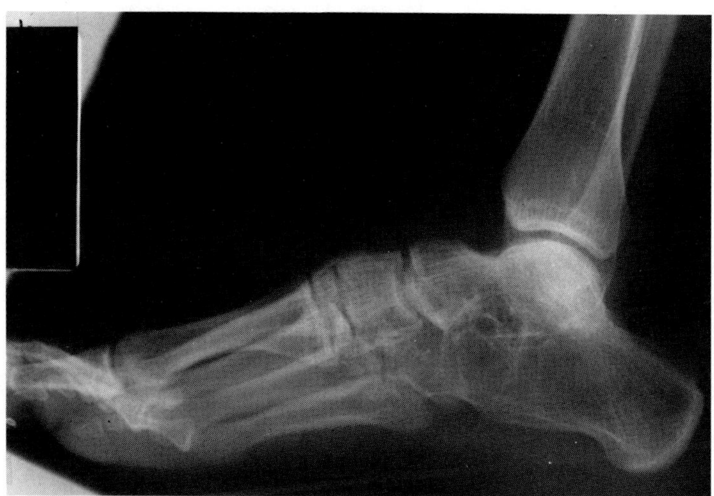

FIG. 21-7. Postoperative triple arthrodesis.

or Dunn[40] triple arthrodesis as a salvage procedure (Fig. 21-7). It should only be done in children with a skeletal age of 12 years or older. This procedure is primarily indicated in the stiff, rigid, and often painful foot that has not responded to serial casting or to other operative procedures. Often, such children have been subjected to multiple soft-tissue as well as other operative procedures.

In the Hoke triple arthrodesis, an oblique incision 7 cm in length is made overlying the midportion of the sinus tarsi. This incision is deepened to the floor of the sinus tarsi, and the areolar tissue is excised. The skin flaps must not be undermined in order to avoid skin loss. After exposure of the calcaneocuboid, subtalar, and talonavicular joints, appropriate wedges are excised with correction of the deformities.

The joint surfaces are fish scaled, and a long-leg plaster cast is applied, with the foot held in the corrected position. Staples or strong Kirschner wires may also be used to maintain fixation of the involved joints in their properly corrected position. There should be total immobilization for a period of 3 months, with a short-leg walking cast being applied at 6 weeks.

CONGENITAL METATARSUS VARUS

Congenital metatarsus varus is a relatively common condition, and it appears to occur with increasing frequency. The deformity, although present at birth, may not be recognized until several months later or possibly after the child begins to walk.

A significant number of deformities related to congenital metatarsus varus, if untreated, will improve or correct completely. If the deformity persists or worsens, the child may be clumsy and may exhibit a toe-in gait. The adolescent and adult with this condition may complain of pain at the lateral border of the foot near the tarsometatarsal area. The shoe often irritates the prominence at the midportion of the foot laterally. It is possible that this deformity, if uncorrected, may also contribute to bunion formation with hallux valgus.

The incidence of congenital metatarsus varus is said to be one per one thousand live births.[124] If one child in a family has the deformity, the chances of a second having a similar deformity is 1 in 20.

Colonna[109] and Jacobs[112] noted the association of congenital hip dysplasia and congenital metatarsus varus. Jacobs[112] reviewed 300 consecutive cases of metatarsus varus and found 30 cases of dysplasia of the hip—an incidence of 10%. A child with metatarsus varus deformity should, therefore, have a careful evaluation of the hips.

CLINICAL APPEARANCE

Kite has suggested that congenital metatarsus varus, for descriptive purposes, represents one third of a congenital clubfoot.[114–116] McCormick and Blount[118] introduced the term *skewfoot* (Fig. 21-8).

The forefoot is adducted and supinated and

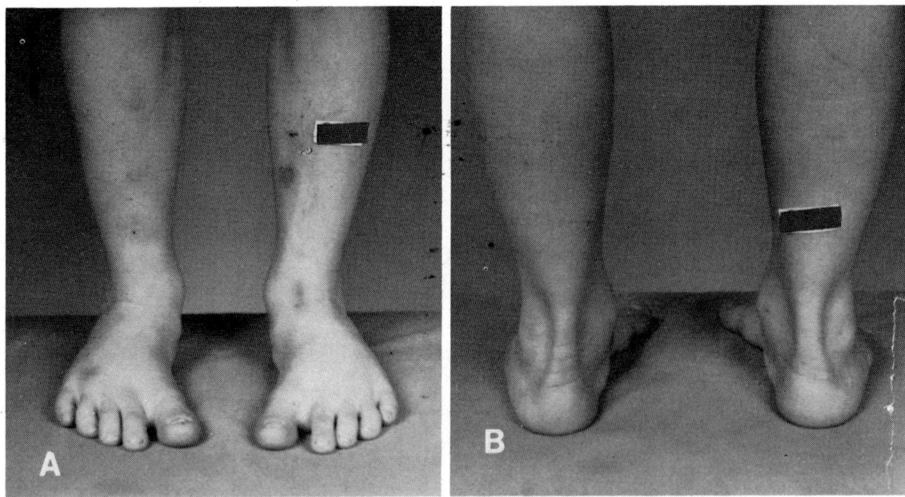

FIG. 21-8. *(A)* Congenital metatarsus varus showing forefoot adduction and hallux varus. Note the convex appearance of the lateral border. *(B)* The heels are in valgus.

the hindfoot is usually in a neutral position, although, in a significant number of instances a valgus heel may be present.[118] The lateral border of the foot is convex, and a prominence is noted at the tarsometatarsal area. The medial border of the foot is concave. There is an increased interval between the first and second toes, with the great toe held in slight varus. Dorsiflexion of the foot and ankle is normal. If the forefoot is abducted passively and released, it returns to its original adducted and inverted position. An increase in the normal internal tibial torsion is also commonly seen in this condition.

The serpentine type of deformity as described by Peabody and Muro[121] is rare but has been reported by Kite. Such feet are difficult to correct conservatively because of a tendency to recur. They very often require surgical correction.

In the walking child with uncorrected metatarsus varus, a toe-in gait is noted. This may result in clumsiness with frequent falls. Abnormal shoe wear may be present, with the lateral portion of the shoe showing greater wear.

Roentgenographic Findings

Anteroposterior roentgenograms confirm the clinical findings, as outlined above, with forefoot adduction and apparent closeness and overlap of the lateral four metatarsals (Fig. 21-9). The talocalcaneal angle is increased if the heel is in a valgus position. The navicular, if ossified, is, in such an instance, subluxated laterally at the head of the talus. No abnormalities are usually present in the lateral film.

Incidence

It would appear that congenital metatarsus varus is occurring with increasing frequency.[115,122] At the Scottish Rite Hospital, Kite noted an average of one case per year from 1924 to 1938. For the following 5 years, the average number of cases was four each year. Since then, the incidence has gradually increased, with the average for the past few years being 200 cases. A slightly greater preponderance has been noted in males.

Treatment

Conservative Treatment

Whereas correction of the congenital idiopathic clubfoot by serial plaster casts is not always successful, the converse is usually true, in our experience, with respect to congenital metatarsus varus. Treatment should be initiated as soon as possible. The foot is quite supple, and secondary contracture of the forefoot can be avoided. If the deformity is a mild one, simple observation is in order or perhaps straight-last shoes may be used. Almost one fourth of children seen with this deformity do not require treatment. McCauley, Lusskin, and Bromley[117] expressed the belief

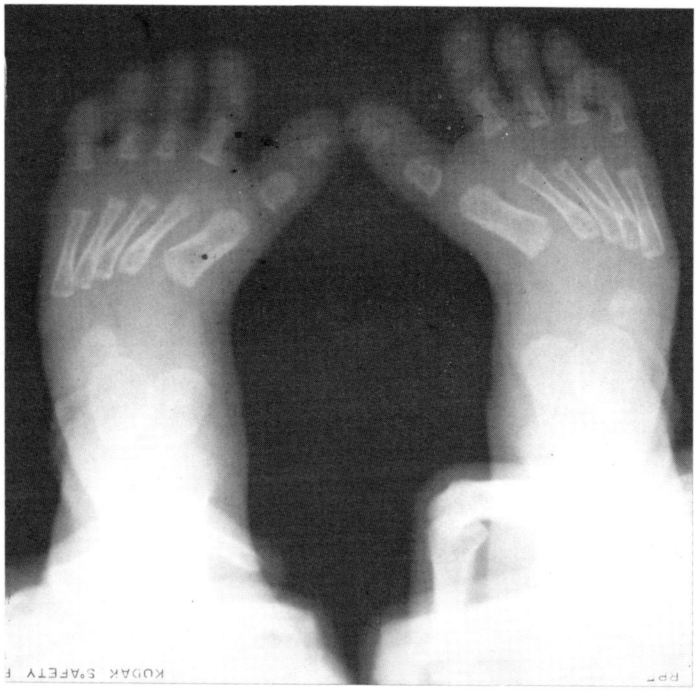

FIG. 21-9. Anteroposterior roentgenogram of the feet in congenital metatarsus varus showing an increased talocalcaneal angle with supination and adduction of the forefoot. The increased space between the first and second toes can be seen.

that there is a significant tendency toward recurrence of the deformity following conservative management.

We have not found manipulation of the foot necessary prior to application of a plaster cast, although Kite,[114] McCormick and Blount,[118] as well as Ponseti and Becker,[122] have advocated manipulation in conjunction with serial plaster casts.

The technique of plaster of Paris cast application is similar to that used for congenital clubfoot. The plaster slipper is fashioned, abducting the forefoot with the point of fulcrum at the tarsometatarsal joint. The plaster slipper is then joined to the leg component of the cast. If the heel is in valgus, the foot should be inverted slightly as the cast is continued to below the knee. The cast is changed weekly until the deformity is corrected. A holding cast should then be used for approximately 2 to 4 weeks. The period for correction varies from 4 to 10 or 12 weeks, depending on the severity of the deformity. Wedging of the cast in abduction is not advocated in the young infant. It may be advantageous in the older child.

Full correction implies that there is no deformity and the forefoot can be abducted fully both actively and passively. The convex appearance of the lateral border of the foot must be corrected, and the prominence at the tarsometatarsal junction must be absent. It is not necessary to use retentive splints following correction. The abnormal internal tibial torsion associated with congenital metatarsus varus usually corrects spontaneously. A mild hallux varus deformity may persist for several years following cast correction and may be of concern to the parents. This deformity will eventually disappear with the wearing of shoes.

Forty-three patients with 69 feet affected by metatarsus adductus were reviewed by Ghali and associates.[110] Twenty of the patients with involvement of 31 feet corrected without treatment. The remaining 23 patients with 38 feet involved required surgical correction. Two indications for operative intervention were suggested: (1) persistent adduction of the forefoot, which is not passively correctible into axial alignment with the heel; and (2) supination of the forefoot, which is present during walking. Surgical release is advised only if both elements of the deformity are present. Surgery is designed to realign the metatarsus at the level of the tarsometatarsal joint and to control the supinating action of the tibialis anterior muscle. The surgical procedure proposed by these authors consists of dividing that portion of the tibialis anterior tendon that attaches to the plantar and medial surfaces of the medial cuneiform. The medial metatarsocuneiform and the naviculocuneiform joints are opened by dividing their capsular ligaments on the medial, dorsal, and plantar aspects. The foot is then immobilized in an above-knee plaster cast in the corrected position for a period of 3 months.

Bleck[108] in reviewing results of treatment in 160 children involving 265 feet with metatarsus adductus noted that in 147 patients treated with plaster casts or casts followed by derotation splints, a good result was related to the age of the patient. Results were statistically significantly better when treatment was begun from ages 1 day to 8 months. Additionally, he concluded that it appears reasonable not to treat the mild cases, because such feet do not progress to a more serious involvement.

Mitchell[120] concluded that contracture of the abductor hallucis is the major deforming factor in resistant congenital metatarsus varus. It is therefore necessary in some instances to release this structure.

Surgical Treatment

In the child with congenital metatarsus varus who is older than 4 years of age, surgical correction may be indicated. Serial plaster casts with wedging in abduction should first be used. If this fails, a tarsometatarsal and intermetatarsal release is an effective procedure for correction of the forefoot deformity.[111,113] This operation should not be done in children who are older than 7 years of age. For the older child, osteotomy at the base of the metatarsals, as advocated by Berman and Gartland,[107] is occasionally necessary.

Thompson[123] concluded that the abductor hallucis muscle may contribute to a persistent hallux varus following correction of the metatarsus varus deformity. This muscle originates from the medial process of the tuberosity of the calcaneus, the plantar aponeurosis, and the intermuscular septum. It inserts by a tendon, with the medial head of the flexor hallucis brevis to the medial side of the base of the first phalanx of the great toe. Thompson[123] advised resection of the entire abductor hallucis muscle to correct the hallux varus and also to reduce the metatarsus varus. He resected the abductor hallucis in 40 children with recurrent metatarsus varus.

Mitchell[119] has also suggested release of the abductor hallucis and advises that the procedure be restricted to the severe deformity that resists correction by serial plaster casts. He cautions that the child should be at least 1 year of age. The operation as practiced by Mitchell consists of release of the abductor hallucis at its origin at the calcaneus. The foot should be held in plaster for 8 weeks following release with the forefoot abducted.

If the great toe exhibits an adducted position in the stance phase, division of the abductor hallucis tendon at its insertion is indicated, according to Mitchell.

HABITUAL TOE WALKERS (CONGENITAL SHORT TENDO CALCANEUS)

This entity was first described by Hall, Salter, and Bhalla[126] in 1967 (Fig. 21-10). It is not uncommon and predominates in boys. At the beginning of independent walking, toddlers may walk with the foot in equinus. By 2 years of age, children normally develop walking patterns similar to adults, and by the age of 3 years, a mature gait pattern should be well established.[127] Most children who present as persistent toe walkers are able to lower the heels to the ground when standing. Heel-toe gait is possible but is usually awkward.

Examination reveals limited dorsiflexion, ranging from mild restriction of motion to severe fixed equinus. Careful neurologic examination is entirely normal. Differential diagnosis includes cerebral palsy, diastematomyelia, spinal dysraphism, muscular dystrophy, spinal cord tumor, acute toe walking syndrome, functional toe walking in a hyperactive child, and delayed maturation of the corticospinal tract.

Griffin and co-workers[125] performed electromyographic gait analysis on a group of six children who were habitual toe walkers. Electromyographic analysis demonstrated swing-phase activities of the gastrocnemius and soleus muscles during toe-toe gait in both toe walkers and normal children. However, on attempted heel-toe gait, prolonged and increased activity of the tibialis anterior muscle was necessary in toe walkers to overcome the force of the shortened tendo Achilles. Following treatment, electromyographic studies returned to normal and no longer reflected the contracture of the triceps surae muscles.

Initial management should be nonoperative. Stretching exercises and manipulations have generally been unsuccessful. Serial stretching

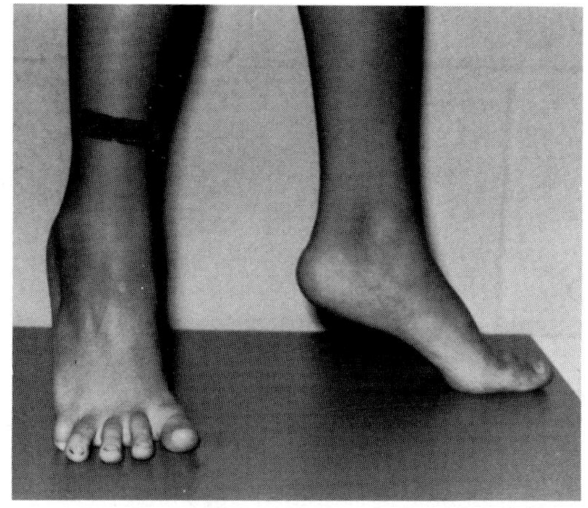

FIG. 21-10. A 5-year-old female with congenital contracture of the Achilles tendon, showing the weight borne on the forefeet during erect stance.

casts should be applied every 2 weeks for 6 to 8 weeks. Generally, casts alone restore a normal range of motion and gait pattern. However, if the ankle does not dorsiflex to neutral position despite a trial of nonoperative management, cautious sliding lengthening of the heel cord is indicated. We confirm Hall, Salter, and Bhalla's observations that tendo Achilles lengthening alone will restore dorsiflexion. In severe deformity, posterior capsulotomy has occasionally been performed, but with little additional gain in range of motion. The results of surgery were generally rewarding. The postoperative regimen consists of long-leg casts for 6 weeks, followed by night splinting for several months.

FLATFOOT DEFORMITIES

CONGENITAL VERTICAL TALUS

Congenital vertical talus is uncommon. The first clinical, anatomic, pathologic, and roentgenographic study of this condition was published in 1914 by Henken.[137] Osmond-Clark,[146] in emphasizing its comparative rarity, stated that he had encountered the deformity in young children only on four occasions.

It is known by a variety of names including "congenital convex pes planus," "congenital rigid rocker-bottom foot," and "congenital flatfoot with talonavicular dislocation." Lamy and Weismann[143] as well as Heyman and Herndon[138,139] prefer the term *congenital vertical talus* because of its simplicity and its usefulness as a descriptive term that is easily recognized.

Although congenital vertical talus may occur as an isolated entity, in the experience of Coleman, Stelling, and Jarrett,[129] it is very often seen in association with arthrogryposis multiplex congenita, myelodysplasia, mental retardation, or other congenital anomalies. We have seen it associated with Turner's syndrome and also in one instance with a congenital idiopathic clubfoot. Drennan and Sharrard[130] emphasized its frequent association with central nervous system abnormalities. Lamy and Weismann[143] also noted the high incidence of neurologic abnormalities in children with congenital vertical talus. Lloyd-Roberts and Spence[144] as well as Hark[135] found in their patients a preponderance of associated neurologic abnormalities, particularly arthrogryposis.

The etiology of congenital vertical talus is unknown. Familial incidence involving mother and child has been observed by the authors. It is more common in males and very often is bilateral.

Silk and Wainwright[150] believe that this condition is due to disparity in growth between the muscles and bones of the leg.

PATHOLOGIC ANATOMY

The pathologic abnormalities in congenital vertical talus are well known and have been described by several writers, including Hughes,[141] Hark,[135] Coleman, Stelling, and Jarrett.[129] The sustentaculum tali is hypoplastic and does not provide adequate support to the head of the talus.[148] Patterson, Fitz, and Smith[149] were the first to report the histologic and anatomic findings in a 6-week-old white female infant who had bilateral congenital vertical talus and who succumbed to congenital heart disease. In the description of the dissection of the feet, they found abnormal tightness in the anterior tibial, extensor hallucis longus, extensor digitorum longus, and peroneus longus muscle–tendon units. The muscles were grossly and histologically normal. The posterior tibial tendon and the peroneal tendons were anteriorly displaced and lying in grooves on the medial and lateral malleolus, respectively. The vertical position of the talus was described as one of equinus, and the head of the talus was noted to be oval rather than spherical. Only two of the three normally present articulating facets on the superior surface of the calcaneus were present, and these were found to be abnormal. The talonavicular and subtalar joints showed subluxation, and the calcaneus occupied a position of equinus due to the contracture of the Achilles tendon.

Drennan and Sharrard[130] described the pathologic anatomy in a white female with myelomeningocele who died shortly after birth following closure of the myelomeningocele and spinal osteotomy. Their observations suggested that an imbalance between a weak tibialis posterior and strong dorsiflexors and evertors is the underlying cause of the deformity.

Clinical Findings

There is no mistaking the clinical appearance of a newborn infant with this condition. The plantar aspect of the foot is convex, thus giving it a rocker-bottom appearance. The head of the talus is palpable medially and at the sole. The talus is likely to be parallel to the long axis of the tibia and in marked equinus. The hindfoot is in valgus and equinus, and the forefoot is abducted and dorsiflexed at the midtarsal joint. The foot is exceedingly rigid, and wearing of shoes may be difficult. In an older child who is walking, the shoes become misshapen and callosities develop under the head of the talus. The gait is usually clumsy and quite awkward, and there is very little push-off with the forefoot. The posterior aspect of the heel does not touch the ground. Pain usually develops at adolescence or soon thereafter.

Of 16 children with congenital vertical talus reviewed at the Scottish Rite Hospital, 5 had bilateral involvement, giving a total of 21 feet. Eight of the patients were male, and eight were female. The age when seen varied from 4 weeks to 7 years.

Roentgenographic Features

The roentgenographic appearance of congenital vertical talus has been described by numerous authors.[128,131,135,136,138–140,143,147,152] The talus occupies a vertical position and is often parallel with the long axis of the tibia (Fig. 21-11). The head of the talus lies medially and is palpable in the sole of the foot. The forefoot is dorsiflexed, and the navicular, if ossified, is seen to lie on the neck of the talus. A marked lateral deviation of the calcaneus results in an

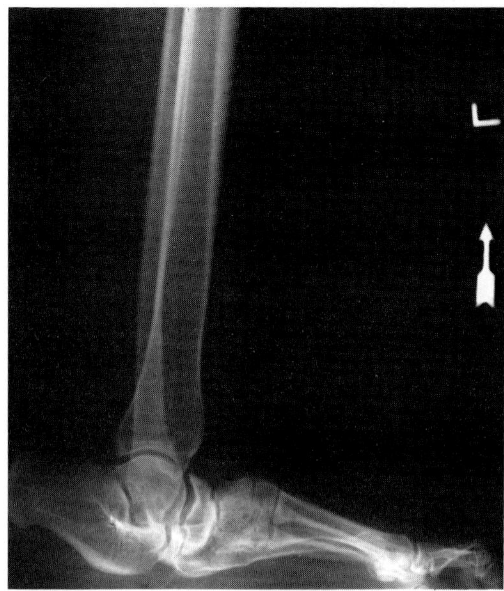

Fig. 21-11. Note the vertical position of the talus, the equinus position of calcaneus and the convexity of the plantar aspect of the foot.

increased talocalcaneal angle in the anteroposterior view. In the lateral view, notching of the neck of the talus results from the abnormal position of the navicular.

Differential Diagnosis

A severe flexible flatfoot may be confused with a vertical talus. It lacks the rigidity that is always present in congenital vertical talus. The rocker-bottom deformity is also absent in the flexible flatfoot, and the hindfoot can be passively corrected. Furthermore, the Achilles tendon does not show the severe degree of contracture that is seen in the congenital vertical talus.

A paralytic flatfoot may be associated with cerebral palsy, myelomeningocele, and anterior poliomyelitis. No difficulty should be experienced in differentiating these conditions from a congenital vertical talus. Tarsal coalition usually results in a rigid flatfoot.

Treatment

Nonoperative Treatment

We believe that it is of utmost importance to initiate treatment as early as possible for congenital vertical talus. Soft-tissue contractures occur rapidly, and delay in diagnosis and treatment results in increased rigidity and greater resistance to correction.

If the infant is seen within the first few days of life, it is possible by manipulation and corrective casts that an acceptable result may be obtained.

Manipulation of the foot is important in order to stretch the contracted soft tissues. The forefoot is placed in extreme equinus, thus aligning it with the hindfoot, and a distraction force is applied by grasping the foot between the thumb and the index finger. As the tarsus elongates, the forefoot is adducted and supinated. The hindfoot is inverted, and an upward pressure is made under the head of the talus at the plantar aspect of the foot. The foot is held in this position as a plaster cast is applied. Careful molding of the cast is necessary, particularly at the midtarsal area, in order to correct the rocker-bottom deformity and to elevate the talus. The plaster slipper is then joined to the leg portion of the cast, which is extended to the knee with the foot maintained in a position of equinus and inversion.

The cast should be changed twice weekly until satisfactory correction of the deformity, both clinically and roentgenographically, is accomplished. If the foot cannot be corrected by conservative means, it is then necessary to proceed to surgical correction.

Tachdjian,[153] in discussing treatment, states that this should begin at birth. If closed reduction fails, he advises open reduction at 3 months of age. He emphasizes that if reduction is to be maintained, it is necessary to repair the capsule of the talonavicular joint inferiorly and medially, as well as to tighten the posterior tibial tendon and the calcaneonavicular ligament.

Surgical Treatment

It is generally accepted that conservative measures, particularly in the older child, are usually not successful in the treatment of congenital vertical talus. In order to achieve lasting correction, the talonavicular dislocation must be reduced and maintained. Additionally, the talus must be elevated and the normal talocalcaneal relationship restored and held for an adequate period if recurrence is to be prevented.

Many different surgical techniques have been used by various authors to achieve correction.[129] Osmond-Clark[146] advocated the reduction of the talonavicular and subtalar joints and maintenance of elevation of the talus by transplanting the distal end of the peroneus brevis tendon through the neck of the talus. A vertical tunnel is made in the neck of the talus, and the tendon of the peroneus brevis, after detaching it from the base of the fifth metatarsal, is passed through the tunnel and sutured back on to itself. He reported success in two children with bilateral deformity.

Grice[132,133] reported use of the anterior tibial tendon to the neck of the talus for support and advised that this procedure be combined with the extra-articular subtalar fusion.

Outland and Sherk[147] described a 3-year-old boy with congenital vertical talus who had been unsuccessfully treated with conservative measures for 2 years. Operative correction was achieved by lengthening the anterior structures, reducing the talonavicular joint, followed by fixing with Kirschner wire to maintain reduction. Six weeks later, the pin was removed and the plaster immobilization continued for an additional 6 weeks. An extra-articular subtalar arthrodesis was then done, and this was followed by an Achilles tendon lengthening 3 months later.

Lamy and Weismann[143] advocated partial or total talectomy combined with lengthening of the tight peroneal and the extensor tendons.

Lloyd-Roberts and Spence,[144] in assessing results in 28 feet in 22 patients treated at the Hospital for Sick Children by several nonoperative methods, concluded that the deformity was neither corrected nor significantly improved in any instance.

Eyre-Brook[131] devised an operation consisting of lengthening of the extensor digitorum longus, the tibialis anterior, and extensor hallucis longus tendons. The navicular is then reduced opposite the head of the talus. A wedge, based dorsally, is removed from the proximal part of the navicular and placed below the head of the talus to maintain the head in its proper position. Additionally, the spring ligament is reefed, and the posterior tibial tendon is shortened. The extremity is immobilized with the foot in full plantar flexion and slight inversion. The cast is removed after 4 to 8 weeks, depending on the age of the child.

Eyre-Brook[131] used this procedure in four cases, and the results 5 to 10 years after the operation disclosed that the stable reduction at the talonavicular joint was maintained.

Herndon and Heyman[138] reported open reduction of the deformity in six feet. The procedure consisted of division of the ligaments and capsular attachments of the subtalar and talonavicular joints. The navicular is then reduced after elevating the head of the talus. Lengthening of the peroneals and common toe extensors is advisable in older children. The forefoot is placed in marked equinus in order to align it with the calcaneus and to reduce the deformity at the midtarsal region. Two transfixing Kirschner wires have aided in maintaining reduction, with one driven through the base of the first metatarsal and the navicular into the body of the talus, and the second passing from the plantar aspect of the foot through the calcaneus into the talus. Six weeks later, a heel-cord lengthening and posterior capsulotomy are done. Plaster immobilization is advised for 4 months.

Coleman, Stelling, and Jarrett[129] emphasized that from a pathologic and therapeutic standpoint, it appears that two major types of congenital vertical talus exist—namely, Type I, in which the calcaneocuboid relationship is normal, and Type II, which is associated with a calcaneocuboid dislocation or subluxation.

These authors express disappointment with nonoperative treatment, and in their series none of the feet could be corrected by wedging casts or manipulation. They suggested preliminary casting of the foot into equinus, with stretching of the extensor tendons as well as the skin on the dorsum of the foot.

Coleman, Stelling, and Jarrett[129] advise that operative correction be performed in two stages following 4 to 6 weeks of plantar flexion wedging casts (Fig. 21-12). A dorsolateral incision centered over the sinus tarsus is made, and the extensor digitorum longus, extensor hallucis longus, and anterior tibial tendons are lengthened. A complete capsulotomy is done at the talonavicular and calcaneocuboid joints, permitting reduction of the talonavicular joint. Release of the talocalcaneal interosseous ligament aids in reducing the talonavicular joint. The forefoot is placed in plantar flexion, and the talonavicular joint is transfixed with a percutaneous Kirschner wire. Plantar flexion of the forefoot aids in aligning the foot properly because of the hindfoot being in a fixed equinus position. This also permits the posterior tibial and peroneus longus tendons to return to their normal position with improvement in the mechanics of the foot. In the child between 2½ and 3 years of age, a talocalcaneal extra-articular bone block is done to provide stability to the subtalar joint and to maintain reduction and elevation of the talus. The procedure as described results in four accomplishments: (1) The talonavicular dislocation has been reduced and stabilized; (2) the talocalcaneal subluxation has been reduced and stabilized; (3) foot alignment has been corrected; and (4) muscle balance of the foot has been restored.

Following suturing of the lengthened tendons, the wound is closed and a long-leg cast is applied with the knee in comfortable flexion and the foot and ankle in equinus. In 6 or 8 weeks, the Kirschner wires are removed and the second stage follows. This consists of Achilles tendon lengthening, posterior capsulotomy, and the advancement of the posterior tibial tendon to the plantar surface of the navicular. The cast is removed 6 weeks later, and a spring-loaded dropfoot brace is used for approximately 2 months.

These authors also recommend that in the child younger than 1 year of age, satisfactory reduction of the deformity and maintenance of the correction can be achieved in most instances without the use of the subtalar bone block.

In the Type II form, lesions with an abnormal calcaneocuboid joint require exposure of the calcaneocuboid joint and maintenance of the reduction with transfixion wire if some degree of recurrence of the deformity is to be prevented.

Jacobsen and Crawford,[142] in an excellent review, described their experience with the Coleman-Stelling two-stage realignment procedure in 11 patients with 17 involved feet. Eleven of the feet were operated upon. All the feet had initial manipulation with serial casting. Those feet that did not respond to nonoperative treatment were operated upon. The Coleman-Stelling two-stage procedure was used in 9 feet, and 2 feet were treated with soft-tissue release without lengthening the dorsal tendons. Three feet were treated with manipulation and casting alone. Three patients were not treated because of their poor general condition. The 9 feet that underwent the Coleman-Stelling procedure obtained a satisfactory result. One patient in this group required a subsequent Grice subtalar arthrodesis.

Forty-four cases of idiopathic vertical talus were reviewed by Hamanishi.[134] The male to female ratio was found to be 1.2:1. Six cases

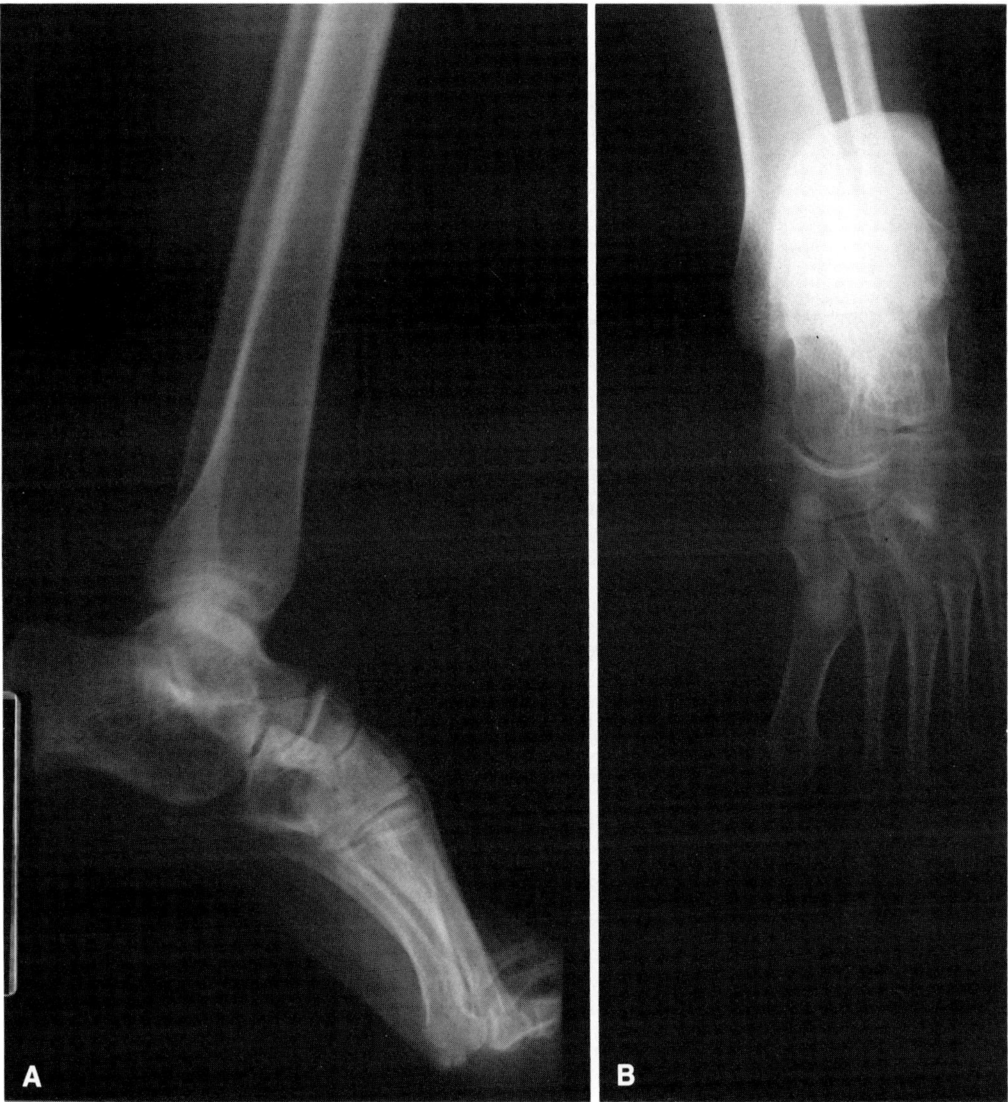

FIG. 21-12. Postoperative two-stage correction. *(A)* Note the normal talocalcaneal angle and proper relationship between the talus and the calcaneus. *(B)* The talus now presents a normal relationship to the long axis of the tibia.

were not treated. Thirty-eight cases were treated by open reduction. Naviculectomy was done in 11 cases, soft-tissue release in 3 cases, and serial corrective casts in 6 instances. The children treated by serial casts and open reduction obtained the best results.

The authors prefer the operative correction of congenital vertical talus as described by Coleman, Stelling, and Jarrett.[129] We would differ, in that it is thought that a subtalar bone block is an essential part of the operative correction in all children. It has been our experience that the talus is not likely to retain its upright position unless the bone block is done (Fig. 21-12).

Triple arthrodesis is necessary in a child of 12 years or more, and it may require possible excision of a portion of the head of the talus combined with lengthening of the Achilles tendon and the anterior structures. An axial pin traversing the talocalcaneal and ankle joint as well as a pin transfixing the talonavicular joint are usually necessary until the fusion is solid.

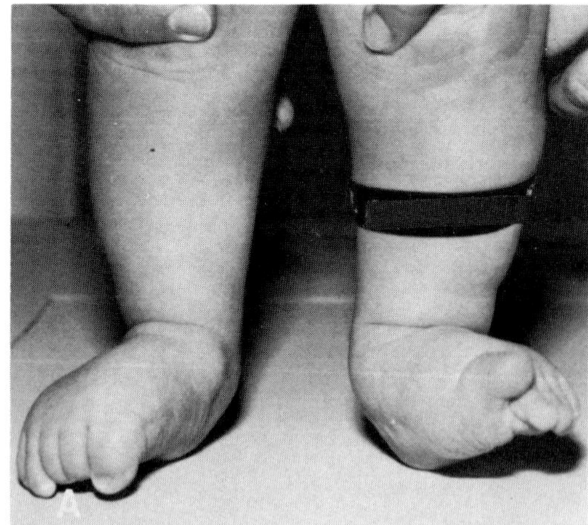

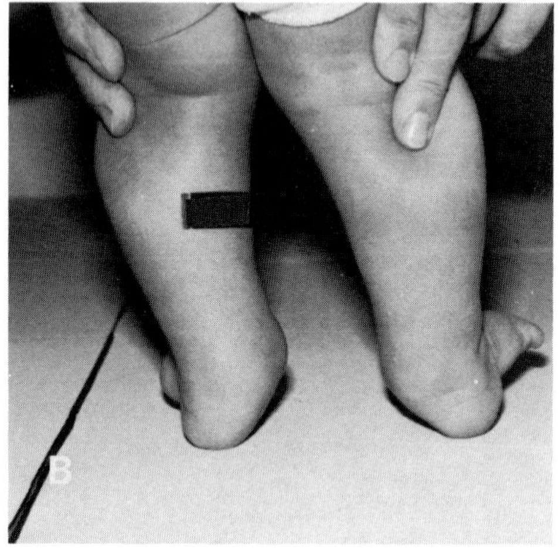

FIG. 21-13. *(A and B)* A 3-month-old child with flexible calcaneovalgus deformities of the feet.

CALCANEOVALGUS FOOT

CLINICAL FEATURES

The calcaneovalgus foot is a relatively common finding in the newborn in its mild form (Fig. 21-13). The deformity is a flexible one, consisting of dorsiflexion of the forefoot and hindfoot. In more severe deformities, the foot may be found lying against the anterior aspect of the tibia. Even in the milder form, the foot can be further dorsiflexed without great resistance until it impinges upon the lower leg. In so doing, no luxation occurs at the talonavicular joint and the calcaneus accompanies the extension of the forefoot. This is in contradistinction to the rare congenital vertical talus deformity, which shows severe abduction and extension of the forefoot in association with dislocation of the talonavicular joint and an equinus contracture of the calcaneus. In severe calcaneovalgus deformities, one finds an increased valgus position of the heel. In other cases, the valgus is first demonstrable with maximum dorsiflexion of the foot. Abduction of the forefoot is usually of a mild degree. The foot can be returned to a more normal position without great difficulty. An important distinction between this foot and a congenital vertical talus foot is flexibility. The former is flexible and the latter is rigid.

Kite[155] has pointed out the association of this deformity and an external rotation contracture of the hips. He also emphasized the role that various sleeping patterns play in the persistence of these problems.[154] Children who sleep in a prone position with their hips flexed, abducted, and externally rotated are those to whom he was referring. Wynne-Davies[157] noted that the incidence of a calcaneovalgus foot is one per thousand live births. The sex ratio was 0.6 male to 1 female. She has found that the problem predominates among the firstborn of young mothers. On the basis of her work, she concluded that the problem is partly genetic in origin. She was unable to delineate any clear pattern of inheritance. Wetzenstein[156] studied 2735 consecutive newborn infants and followed them for 2 years. He appraised clinically the degree of valgus of the hindfoot when the foot was maximally dorsiflexed. There were 147 patients with at least 20° of heel valgus, 333 with 10° to 15°, 759 with 0° to 5°, and 1496 with no heel valgus. When seen at 2 years, 43% of the 147 with at least 20° of heel valgus were considered to have flatfeet, whereas 23% of the group who were originally considered to have normal heel valgus were found to have flatfeet. He concluded that severe degrees of calcaneovalgus deformity have an increased likelihood of being associated with flatfootedness in later life.

TREATMENT

When examining a child with such a deformity, one must be certain that active plantar flexion is possible. Various neurogenic disorders such as myelomeningocele can result in posturing of the foot in a similar way. For a mild deformity that can be easily brought into plantar flexion, stretching exercises are recommended. Kite[155] has advised that proper stretching is done by placing the heel in slight varus with one hand and plantar flexing and adducting the forefoot with the other. This is most easily accomplished with the thumb and index finger placed on the dorsal and plantar surfaces of the foot, respectively. The external rotation contractures of the hips must also be stretched, if present. He further recommends that children be encouraged to sleep on their side in order to aid in the correction of the external rotation contracture of the hips.

For the more severe deformity, a series of short-leg casts applied by molding the foot into equinus at the ankle, varus at the hindfoot, and adduction at the midfoot are recommended. These are changed weekly in the young child and continued until the deformity is corrected and active plantar flexion is present. Post-cast splinting is generally unnecessary.

FLEXIBLE FLATFOOT

Introduction

Throughout the medical literature, there has been much written about this relatively common problem. There have been many theories as to the etiology and to the proper treatment. Strikingly absent from the literature are long-term studies on those who have had no treatment and on those who have had various forms of conservative treatment. There is general belief that exercises have limited value. Most of those who advocate surgery emphasize the importance of operating on symptomatic feet only. In order to properly assess the need for treatment, one must have a clear understanding of the natural history of the problem without treatment. Helfet,[174] for example, has stated that the institution of shoe modifications in children increases the likelihood of symptoms later in life if these modifications are discontinued. However, there is no general agreement on this point.

Clinical Features

The flexible flatfoot may be defined as a foot that assumes a pronated posture when weight is borne on the extremity. Abduction of the forefoot and valgus of the heel result in loss of the longitudinal arch (Fig. 21-14). When weight is relieved, it assumes a normal contour. Subtalar motion is normal to increased. Often such patients have associated generalized ligamentous laxity. As Inman[178] has emphasized, the everted foot is mechanically

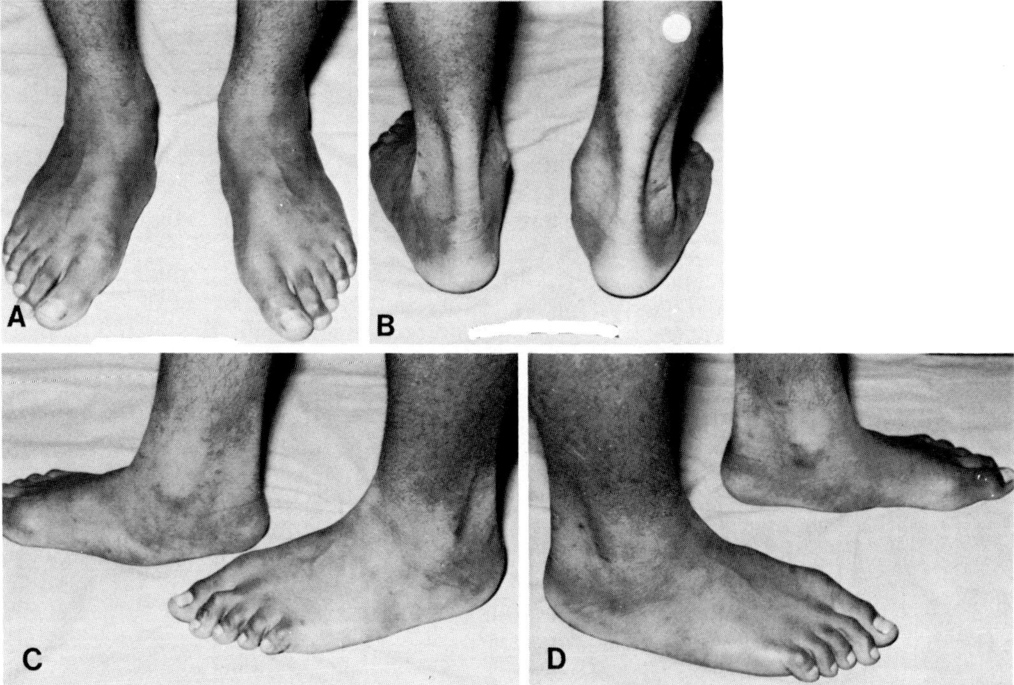

Fig. 21-14. *(A to D)* Clinical photographs of a 15-year-old male with severe flexible flatfeet.

weak. Much stress is put on the ligamentous support due to this posturing and the resultant medial shifting of the body weight. Normally, weight is borne over the lateral border of the foot and on the first and fifth metatarsal heads. Prolonged posturing of the foot in the everted position may result in a heelcord contracture. The vast majority of patients with a flexible flatfoot deformity are asymptomatic with regard to their feet.

Roentgenographic Features

Roentgenograms may be made in the standing position in the anteroposterior as well as the lateral projections. The degree of heel valgus may be assessed on the anteroposterior film by measuring the Kite talocalcaneal angle. Divergence of the talus and calcaneus of more than 35° should be considered roentgenographic evidence of heel valgus. A lateral projection will demonstrate the location of the loss of the longitudinal arch (Fig. 21-15).

Association With Congenital Pes Calcaneovalgus

The significance of congenital pes calcaneovalgus in the origin of flexible flatfoot was addressed by Wetzenstein.[212] He quotes Erlacher, Gocht, Mau, and Timmer as having indicated that it can give rise to flatfeet. He reports that the calcaneovalgus deformity is seen in up to 30% of live births and quotes reports citing incidences of up to 50%. In 2735 consecutive births, the degree of heel valgus was assessed. Those with heel valgus of greater than 20° were found in 147 cases. These children were followed for 2 years. At the end of that time, 43% of the original 147 and 23% of the previously normal group were judged to have a flexible flatfoot deformity. He concluded that those patients with severe valgus at birth have an increased risk of being flatfooted.

Etiology

Bone

There are several schools of thought as to the etiology of flatfeet. Harris and Beath[173] thought that the problem was related to weak support by the anterior portion of the calcaneus. They found it to be associated secondarily with a shortened Achilles tendon. With medial displacement of the head of the talus, or perhaps more accurately with lateral rotation of the calcaneus, the longitudinal arch can be maintained only by muscle and ligamentous support. Basmajian[159,160] noted that there is little or no muscular activity in the normal foot when standing at rest. Harris and Beath's[173] thesis is that the function of the foot and its shape under the stress of weightbearing depend chiefly on the design of the tarsal bones and their position in relation to each other. Support for the foot is provided both by passive factors (bone and ligament) and by active factors (muscle). These factors are reciprocal. In the strong foot, muscles are used to maintain balance, to adjust the foot to uneven ground, and to propel the body. In the weak foot, the muscles are called upon to maintain the normal shape of the foot at rest. Muscle cannot act unremittingly. The role of the os calcis in the production of the flatfoot was discussed by Percy Roberts in 1916 in an address to the American Orthopaedic Association.

Other early investigators who thought that the os calcis in its relation to the talus was important in the development of the flexible flatfoot were Gleich, Lord, and Chambers.[164] The rationale behind their operative procedures was that the weightbearing forces were directed medial to the foot. Surgery was designed to shift the center of weightbearing for the foot to a relatively more lateral position.

Chambers,[164] during his studies at the Daniel Baugh Institute of Anatomy, found that excessive heel valgus was associated with increased forefoot abduction. He found that the normal adolescent and adult foot had approximately 15° of what he termed *abduction*. Motion between the talus and calcaneus is what he was referring to. In the flexible flatfoot, this ranged to 35°. He thought that excessive abduction resulted in the characteristic flattening of the longitudinal arch and that stretching of the ligaments is a sequel and not the primary cause of the problem.

Milch[193] states that the term *balance* as applied to the foot structure does not refer to muscle activity but to the arrangement of the bones and ligaments that furnish a stable base upon which weight can be borne with the least demand for muscular exertion.

Muscle

Electromyographic studies of the foot have been used in recent years to elucidate the role of muscle in support of the longitudinal

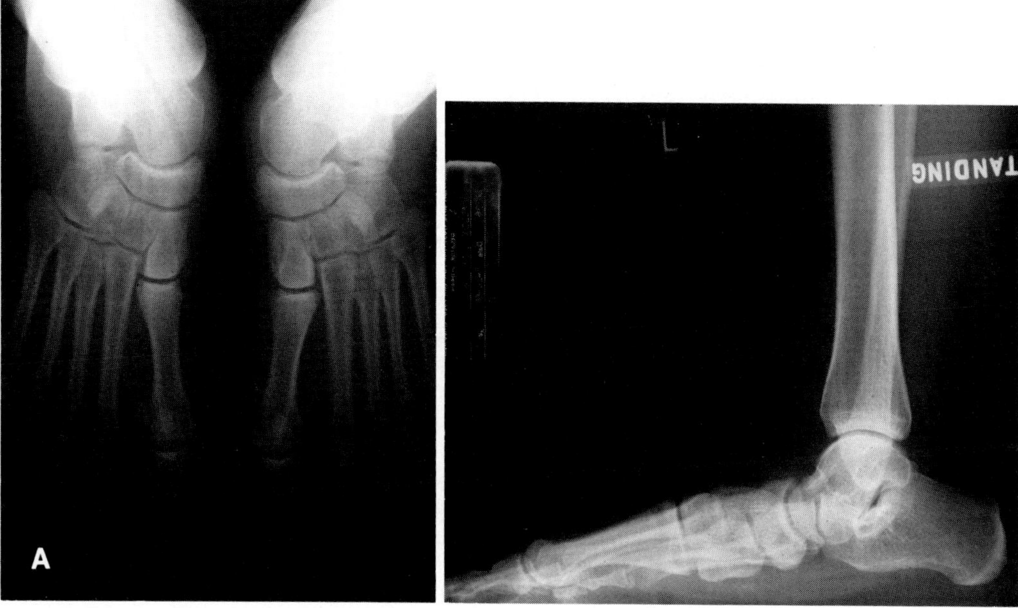

FIG. 21-15. A 13-year-old female with asymptomatic flexible flatfeet. *(A)* On this view can be seen a widened talocalcaneal angle. *(B)* Loss of the longitudinal arch is shown.

arch of the normal foot and flatfoot. Basmajian[159,160] quotes Duchenne, who 100 years ago stated that by faradization of the peroneus longus muscle in flatfooted children, he was able to produce the progressive formation of a normal plantar arch. Morton believed that the structural stability of the foot was not dependent upon muscles. He thought that appreciable muscle exertion was needed only when the center of gravity moved beyond the margins of structural stability. Only a slight controlling action by the muscles is required when the center of gravity remains between those margins. In 1952, he further showed that static foot strains are relatively low in intensity, following well within the capabilities of ligaments. His calculations showed that only acute, heavy, but transient forces, such as those in the take-off phase of walking, require the dynamic action of muscle.

In 1941, R. L. Jones, using the method of palpation in the living and direct observation in the cadaver, concluded that not more than 15% to 20% of the total tension stress on the foot is borne by the posterior tibial and peroneal muscles. A much greater part of this stress is borne by the plantar ligaments of the foot and to some extent by the short plantar muscles.

W. Jones, believed that maintenance of the normal arch of the foot resulted from the dual control exerted by passive elasticity of the ligaments and the active contractility of muscles. He concluded that the plantar aponeurosis and the plantar tarsal ligaments hold the anterior and posterior pillars of the arch together and that actively contracting intrinsic muscles between the aponeurosis and the tarsal ligaments also play an important role. In 1954, from electromyographic studies, Basmajian[159] concluded that the tibialis anterior, peroneus longus, and intrinsic muscles of the foot played no role in the normal static support of the longitudinal arch of the foot. Smith,[210] in 1954, using skin electrodes, confirmed this work.

In 1963, Basmajian[160] also concluded that after simultaneous study of the tibialis anterior, tibialis posterior, peroneus longus, flexor hallucis longus, abductor hallucis, and flexor digitorum brevis in 20 subjects, only heavy loading elicits muscle activity. In the relaxed standing position, the longitudinal arch is supported by bone and ligament. With loads of 400 pounds or more, the muscles do come into play, but, even then, muscles form a dynamic reserve.

Anatomic studies by J. H. Hicks[175,176] on the function of the plantar aponeurosis are interesting. He likens the human foot to a truss, which is a triangular structure composed of two rods and a tie. In the foot, the tie is the plantar aponeurosis, and there are five rods radiating from a common posterior rod. The plantar aponeurosis resists the deforming effect of body weight, and, in its absence, the foot loses it normal shape. The height of the triangle or truss increases when the base shortens. The shortening of the plantar aponeurosis is brought about by a windlass mechanism. The drum of the windlass is the metatarsal head; the cable that is wound around the drum is the plantar ligament of the metatarsophalangeal joint to which the plantar aponeurosis is firmly attached; and the handle, which winds the cable, is the proximal phalanx.

In 1954, Hicks[176] pointed out that when standing, passive extension of the great toe results in: (1) elevation of the longitudinal arch, (2) inversion of the hindfoot, (3) lateral rotation of the leg, and (4) tightening of the plantar aponeurosis. Elevation of the arch was accomplished without muscle forces.

It would be well to review the movements of the foot. Hicks,[175,176] Shephard,[207] Fick (1911), and Manter (1941) have demonstrated that the joint complex that makes up the hindfoot acts as a hinge. As in the cases of inversion and eversion, abduction and adduction are complex movements in the foot and involve motion in all the peritalar joints. Inversion and adduction are always combined in supination. Eversion and abduction are always combined in pronation. The peritalar and midtarsal joints are thus oblique hinge joints.

Inman[178] has shown that with eversion of the heel, as in pronation of the foot, all the articulations in the midfoot become unlocked and maximal motion in the talonavicular and calcaneocuboid joints occurs. If the heel is inverted and the forefoot is held firmly fixed, thus producing a twist in the foot, something happens to convert the entire foot into a rigid structure. Zadek[215] (1935) pointed out that loss of the longitudinal arch of the foot is secondary to abduction of the foot and heel valgus. A low longitudinal arch in a foot without abduction is often found in a strong stable foot that is symptom-free. Rose[200] believed that it was the limiting of extension at the midfoot of the joints of the metatarsals that was the main determinant of the posture that the foot assumed when standing, together with the relative lengths of the metatarsals. He stated that the posture of the foot is not dependent upon muscle.

Jack[179] based his work on two premises. First, he believed that severe degrees of flatfootedness were disabling. Second, he believed that the medial longitudinal arch of the foot and, therefore, the posture of the foot depended on the intrinsic structure of the bones and joints and the integrity of the plantar ligaments. Muscles are concerned solely with balance and protection of the ligaments from abnormal stress. They can lift the arch but cannot maintain it where there is a bony or ligamentous defect.

The strong arguments that have evolved against the longitudinal arch being supported by muscle have not always been accepted. While presenting the third H. O. Thomas Memorial Lecture in Liverpool, Sir Arthur Keith (1928)[182] said, "There is no need in Liverpool to insist that the longitudinal arch of the foot is dependent on properly and automatically balanced action of muscles in the leg and foot. Hugh Owen Thomas perceived this truth imperfectly but Sir Robert Jones has always taught it to his pupils with emphasis." Haraldsson[172] thought the etiology was an imbalance in the strength of muscles and ligaments of the foot and the weight to be carried. He quotes Niederecker (1950, 1959) as stressing the role of muscle anomalies in the causation of the condition and discussed a statically unfavorable insertion of the tibialis anterior and peroneus tertius as well as the occurrence of a peroneus quartus muscle. Hoke[177] (1931) based his procedure on a concept of muscle weakness as being the primary etiologic factor. Other thoughts on etiology have been voiced: Stracker (1953) believed that neurogenic factors are responsible. Priester (1958) postulated an endocrine disorder. Böhm (1930) was said to have been concerned with inhibition of the normal development of the ankle.

Treatment

Conservative Treatment

This is a difficult subject. Clearly, it can be assumed from the literature that conservative treatment is fundamental in the management of these patients. However, there is a great deal of controversy as to the definition of conservative management. Fremont Chandler[165] recommended exercises consisting of heelcord stretching and toe flexor strengthening. He thought that molded foot plates or prolonged use of plaster were rarely indicated. Yet, some would question this mode of treatment. Shaffer (1951) and Hackenbrock (1961) believed that some cases of flatfootedness in children spontaneously resolve without any form of treatment.

Various shoe modifications have been used in the management of this problem. Scaphoid pads, heel wedges, sole wedges, Thomas heels, extended medial counters, and others have been recommended and used by various authors in varying combinations.

Rose[199] believed that the scaphoid pad was unphysiologic. He considered that the heel valgus was the essential element to control and that the scaphoid pad was ineffectual in accomplishing this end. He recommended medial heel and sole wedges.

LeLièvre[189] agreed that arch supports were unsound. He said that with upward pressure on the plantar aspect of the tarsal navicular, the sole of the foot is then sheared between two antagonistic parallel forces. The infrascaphoid pressure is exerted upward from below, and, just posterior to it, the weight of the body is thrown on the medial border of the foot because of the valgus position of the os calcis. The result is stretching of the plantar musculature.

Lowman[192] and Milch[193] believed that exercises and shoe modifications were futile.

Helfet,[174] too, disagreed with the use of arch supports. He thought that once a child is accustomed to shoe modifications, it is difficult for him to give them up. Heel wedges, in his opinion, only lead to early wearing out of the shoes. He introduced heel seats and reported having used them in more than 500 children. After 2½ years of use, he found that an arch had formed. He did not report specific numbers but left the impression that success was rather uniform. Rose[200] reported on the meniscus that Schwartz designed to control heel valgus.

Penneau and associates[197] evaluated 10 children radiographically with flexible flatfeet. Films were taken barefoot, with a Thomas heel, with an over-the-counter scaphoid insert, and with specially molded plastic foot orthoses. The authors noted no significant change in the radiographic appearance of the feet with the shoe modifications.

The authors' treatment plan recognizes the difficulty in making the diagnosis of flatfootedness in a child younger than 18 to 24 months. The generalized ligamentous laxity of children must be kept in mind. One must be certain that the foot represents a flexible type of flatfoot and does not represent a prehallux syndrome.[184] Exercises are not thought to be useful. In the presence of heelcord contracture, stretching exercises are indicated. Avoidance of improper sitting when it results in external rotation of the foot and ankle is important. This position accentuates the forefoot abduction and heel valgus posture of the foot. Shoe modifications are instituted only in those patients with moderate to severe deformities. Parents should be counseled that the shoes being used are proper shoes but will not correct the deformity. The shoes should fit the heel well and provide adequate room for the forefoot. Various shoe modifications have been used. In the young child, a 3/16-inch scaphoid pad may be combined with a 1/8-inch medial heel wedge (Fig. 21-16). If shoe wear is excessive, an extended medial counter may be added. In the older child and in the younger child with more severe deformity, the Helfet heel seat, Schwartz meniscus, or the UCB heel cup may be used for better control of heel valgus. Modified shoes can prolong shoe life for the patient with severe deformity.

Surgical Treatment

When surgery is contemplated for this condition, there are several factors to observe. Jones[181] stated that pronated feet are a common occurrence in early childhood, at which time joint flexibility is greater than in later life. The feet may share in this laxity, and, to such structural immaturity, the pronated feet of this age group may reasonably be attributed. Rose[199,200] stated, "In most patients symptoms are absent, trivial or experienced only during times of exceptional stress and are then relieved by appropriate shoe modifications." Legg[187] advocated in 1907 that not all cases of flatfeet will become symptomatic. Crego and Ford[166] also caution that few patients with flexible flatfeet are symptomatic. Golding-Bird (1889),[170] when reporting his surgical procedure, advised his colleagues that surgery should be done only for the symptomatic foot. Leonard and colleagues[190] reported that of 1446 flatfeet seen over a 10-year period in his clinic,

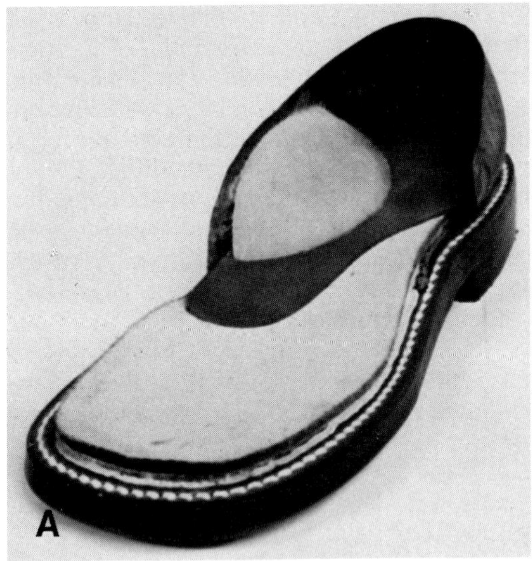

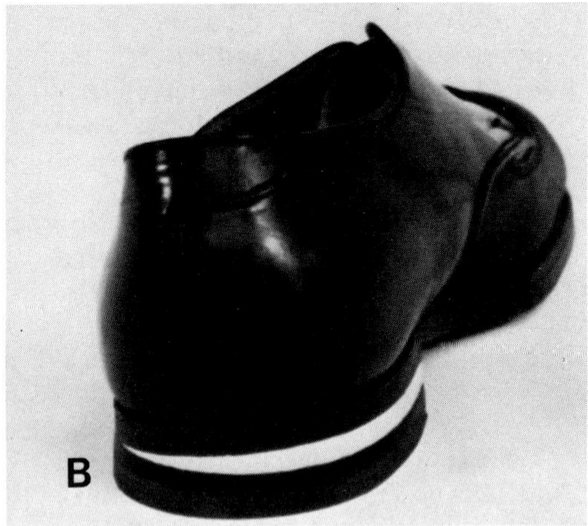

FIG. 21-16. *(A)* A 3⁄16-inch scaphoid pad with an extended medial counter. *(B)* Shoes with a 1⁄8-inch medial heel wedge.

25 were judged to be symptomatic enough to warrant surgical intervention.

The various types of surgical procedures advocated may be divided into three broad categories. Depending on the basic pathology perceived, procedures were designed to repair abnormal (1) ligaments, (2) tendons or (3) bone. Milch[193] and Schoolfield[203,204] reinforced or advanced the deltoid ligament. Jones[181] advocated reinforcement of incompetent plantar fascia by separating the inner half of the heelcord and attaching it to the neck of the first metatarsal. Phelps (1891) shortened all the structures on the medial aspect of the foot.

In 1905, Painter[196] reported resection of the peroneal tendons for severe rigid feet. Reyerson (1909)[202] transferred the peronei to the first cuneiform and reported that the results were similar to peroneal tendon section. Gocht (1905) advocated medialization of the Achilles tendon, and Hubscher (1910) shortened the flexor hallucis longus to which was sewn the posterior tibial tendon. Transfer of the anterior tibial tendon to the navicular was first done by Muller[214] in 1903. Lowman (1923)[192] and Young (1939)[214] incorporated this concept into their procedures. Zadek[215] stated that Achilles tendon lengthening alone was reported by Hoffer (1893), Kohler (1893), Hertle (1910), Els (1913), and Friebe (1920). He also reported that Wilson and Patterson in 1905 placed the extensor hallucis longus into a canal made in the navicular. Zadek also stated that Momberg (1912) used fascia lata, and, later, Fischer and Baron used peroneal tendon as a free graft and passed them from the navicular to the tibia. Thus, they acted as a passive force designed to elevate the arch.

There have been many bony procedures. Excision of the navicular was recommended by Golding-Bird (1878)[170] and later by Davy (1889).[167] Legg (1907)[187] reported 13 cases in which there had been 100% relief of pain 1 to 5 years postoperatively. Talectomy was also advocated by Weinhechner, Vogt, Morestin, and Eiselsberg.

Subtalar arthodesis has been done by several investigators on the premise that heel valgus was the primary problem. Soule (1921),[211] Leavitt (1943),[186] Rugtveit (1964),[201] and Haraldsson (1964)[172] have reported on the use of this procedure in the management of the flexible flatfoot. Some have used Grice's[171] original procedure and others have used variations of it. Variations of the Grice procedure have been reported by Dennyson and Fulford,[168] Seymour and Evans,[206] and Brown.[161]

Chambers[164] blocked the subtalar joint by raising a flap of bone in the sinus tarsi using a tibial bone graft–the basis of his operation being that the anterior lip of the body of the talus does not make contact with the floor of the sinus tarsi unless the posterior talocalcaneal facets fail to conform to what was called "the ideal pattern of normalcy." LeLièvre puts bone in the sinus tarsi. He does not necessarily attempt to obtain a fusion, but wants to prevent heel valgus. Zadek[215] does a transverse wedge resection based medially of the subtalar joint. Haraldsson[172] reported a series of 54 feet on whom surgery was done before age 12 years. Surgery was done between the ages of 4 and 11 years. Surgery was done on the younger children, because he thought that to be most effective, surgery must be done before the onset of symptoms—the premise being that pathologic displacement of the foot bones will, if untreated, result in structural changes in the skeleton and soft tissues with fixation of the distortion and increasing symptoms. A series by Brenning (1960) was quoted in which one half of 58 feet in 6- and 7-year-old patients had symptoms. Fifty of his patients had greater than 1 year follow-up; 34 had greater than 2 years follow-up. Twenty-one of 30 patients with preoperative symptoms were relieved of their symptoms by surgery. Overall, he reported 40 patients with good results, 10 who were considered improved, and 4 who had a poor result.

Supramalleolar tibial osteotomies have been done in the past for severe flatfeet. Trendelenberg (1889) used such a procedure for correction of deformity secondary to Pott's disease. Hahn (1889) and Meyer (1890) used it for the symptomatic rigid faltfoot.

Calcaneal osteotomy was first done by Gleich (1893). Whether he actually did the operation on living patients or just in the postmortem room is not clear. Zadek[215] credits Oblalinski (1895) for popularizing the operation. The procedure consisted of an oblique osteotomy of the calcaneus with the posterior fragment being displaced anteriorly. Lord[191] and Koutsogiannis[185] modified the original procedure by displacing the posterior fragment both anteriorly and medially.

Baker and Hill[158] and Silver and associates[208] have advocated calcaneal osteotomies for valgus deformities in the cerebral palsied patient. Evans[169] proposed a lateral opening wedge osteotomy to correct severe valgus deformity.

Phillips[198] reviewed 20 patients with 23 feet operated upon by Dillwyn Evans for symptomatic flexible flatfeet. The follow-up averaged 13 years. The procedure consisted of elongating the calcaneus by performing an osteotomy immediately posterior to the calcaneocuboid joint and inserting a tibial bone graft. At follow-up, 17 of 23 feet were considered to have either a good or very good result. It is interesting to speculate that the mechanism of pain in the flexible flatfoot is an abnormal weightbearing pattern. With either an osteotomy of the calcaneus or lengthening of the lateral column, the weightbearing forces are improved and symptoms are relieved.

Osteotomy of the neck of the talus of the closing wedge type was proposed by Sir William Stokes. Couchoix and Wachter also used this procedure. Perthes (1913) did a closing wedge osteotomy of the navicular and used the bone removed in doing an opening wedge osteotomy of the calcaneus. Wilms (1914) concurred with this approach.

Radical wedge resections have been done. Legg[187] stated that Larabrie removed the whole of the navicular, the head of the talus, a portion of the internal cuneiform, and a corner of the cuboid in very severe flatfeet.

Talonavicular fusions have been done in combination with other procedures for this problem. Soule (1921)[211] recognized that to correct forefoot abduction and heel valgus was to correct the depressed arch. Lowman (1923)[192] combined this with transfer of the anterior tibial tendon to the navicular. Ogston (1884)[195] was an early advocate of this procedure. Naviculocuneiform fusion has been used by many surgeons. Hoke (1931)[177] combined this with fusion of the navicular to the middle cuneiform. In 1953, Jack[179] reported the results in 46 feet in 25 patients aged 11 to 14 years with flatfeet 15 months to 5 years postoperatively. At the time, there were 54% excellent, 28% good, and 18% poor results. Seymour and Evans[206] reassessed 17 of 25 patients 16 to 19 years postoperatively and found 31% excellent, 19% good, and 50% unsatisfactory results. Tarsal degenerative changes developed in many. Butte[162] reviewed 72 patients who had had the Hoke procedure and found 50% satisfactory and 50% unsatisfactory results.

Surgeons frequently combined procedures, such as Haraldsson did in doing a Grice extra-articular arthrodesis together with a transfer of the anterior tibial tendon to the navicular. Caldwell[163] credits Durham in 1935 for devising a procedure that consists of: (1) division of the posterior tibial tendon at its insertion into the navicular; (2) elevation of a ligamentous capsular flap from the medial aspect of the foot; (3) naviculocuneiform fusion; and (4) insertion of a ligamentous flap into the susten-

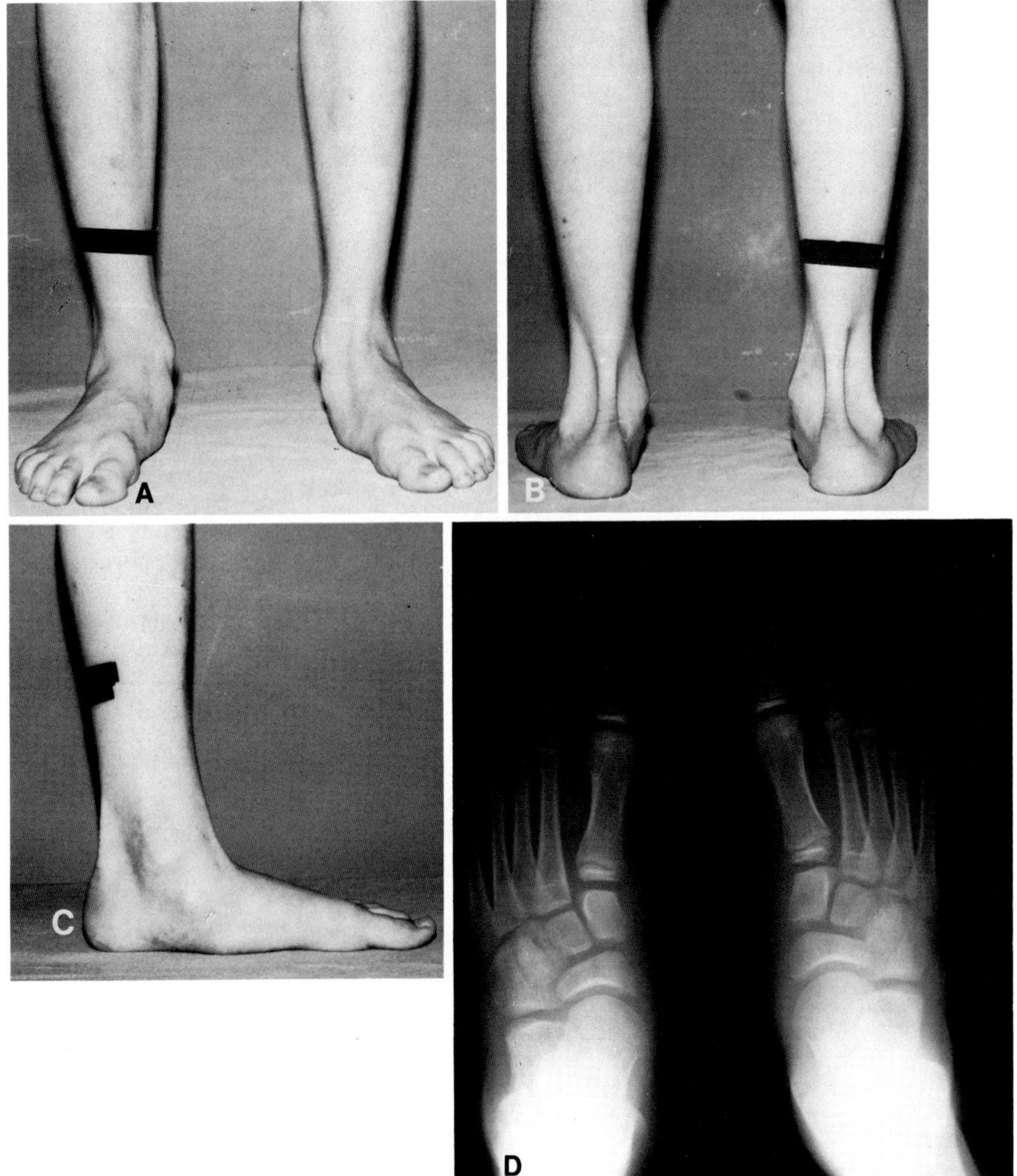

FIG. 21-17. A 12-year-old male with symptomatic flexible flatfeet not relieved by appropriate shoes and modifications. *(A, B, C)* Clinical photographs. *(D)* Roentgenogram showing the talocalcaneal angle.

taculum and reattachment of the posterior tibial tendon. Caldwell reported that this procedure had been done in 76 feet of 38 patients. He found 58 of 76% or 76% with excellent results, 14 of 76, or 18% with good, and 4 of 76, or 5% with poor results. Crego and Ford[166] reported the late results of various operative procedures in children. They estimated that surgery was done in one of 35 or 40 patients with flatfeet. All surgery had been done in patients younger than 15 years of age. They reiterated that this was a common problem and that most patients were asymptomatic with it. Indications for surgery were those feet that were flat and pronated with painful rocker-bottom deformities. They reviewed 102 feet (of 53 children) that had undergone 111 surgical procedures. Eighty-five feet were considered

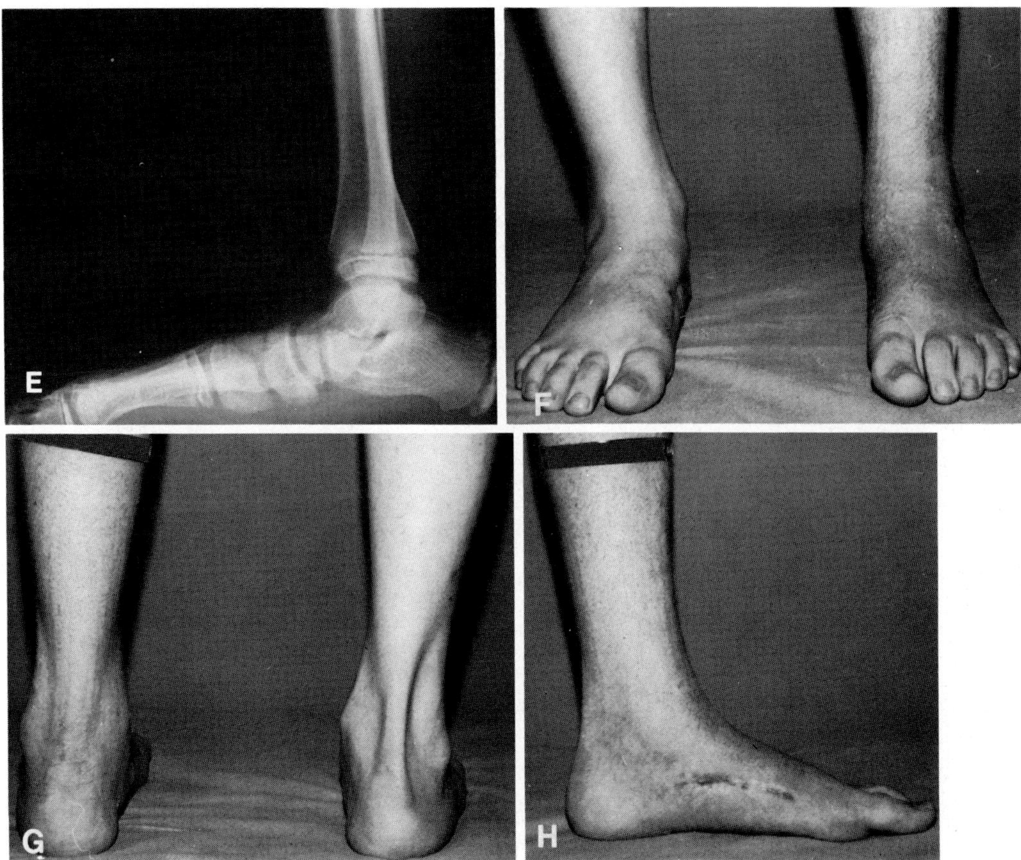

FIG. 21-17. *(Continued). (E)* Note the loss of the longitudinal arch. *(F* to *H)* Appearance of the feet following reconstructive surgery. *(Continued on overleaf)*

to have been flexible flatfeet. Accessory naviculars were found in 11.

Fusion between the talonavicular and naviculocuneiform joints was done 15 times between 1927 and 1935. Satisfactory results were obtained in 73%. The Hoke procedure was done in 9 with only two satisfactory results. Subtalar and talonavicular fusion was done in 24 feet between 1934 and 1944, with 78% satisfactory results. A modified Hoke procedure, consisting of talonavicular, naviculocuneiform, and sustentaculum tali and neck of talus fusion, was done 27 times, with 48% satisfactory results. The Hoke triple arthrodesis was done in 26 feet, with 77% acceptable results. They emphasized the need for subtalar fusion when symptoms were present. The authors favor a surgical procedure that is a modification of the Hoke and Miller procedures. It is indicated for the adolescent when there is pain in the foot not relieved by proper shoes, rapid abnormal shoe wear, and deformity. Surgery should be delayed until the skeletal age of 10 years.

In the adolescent who has a painful flexible flatfoot, there is loss of the longitudinal arch with a tight heelcord and a lax spring ligament. The posterior tibial tendon is also elongated and stretched. The surgical procedure preferred is as follows (Fig. 21-17):

1. An incision approximately 3 inches in length is made along the medial border of the foot, extending from the base of the first metatarsal to the navicular.
2. The anterior tibial tendon at its insertion into the base of the first metatarsal and first cuneiform is identified.
3. The posterior tibial tendon at its insertion into the navicular in the plantar aspect of the foot is identified.
4. An osteoperiosteal flap is then developed, with the flap beginning at the insertion of the anterior tibial tendon,

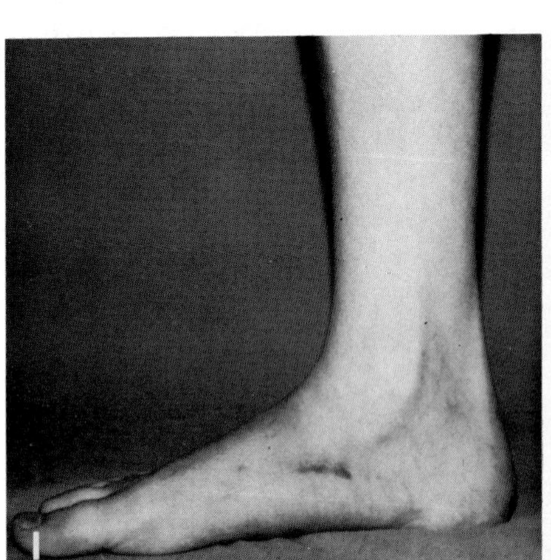

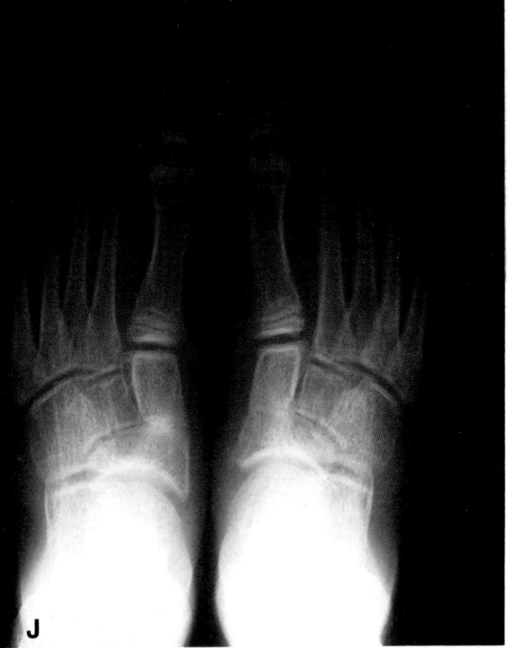

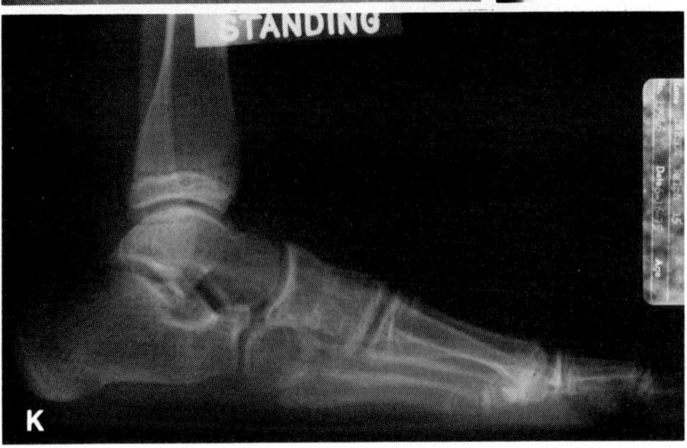

FIG. 21-17 *(Continued)*. *(I)* Appearance of the feet following reconstructive surgery. *(J)* Note the formal talocalcaneal angle and naviculocuneiform fusion. *(K)* Note the restoration of the longitudinal arch and the navicular cuneiform fusion.

and reflected posteriorly. The flap, which is ½ inch in width, extends from the posterior tibial insertion at the navicular to the anterior tibial tendon.

5. The capsule at the naviculocuneiform joint is incised, and the cartilage from the joint surface parallel to the bone is removed. Removal of a wedge with the base positioned medially should not be attempted.
6. The tubercle or prominence of the navicular should be excised and saved.
7. A dorsally based osteotomy is done, with an opening wedge dorsally at the first cuneiform. The inferior aspect of the cuneiform should be intact so that an opening wedge dorsally is formed.
8. The tubercle of the navicular is then wedged into the greenstick opening osteotomy of the first cuneiform. This, in effect, tends to elevate the arch.
9. The osteoperiosteal flap that has been created is passed under the anterior tibial tendon and sutured to itself with the sutures pulled toward the plantar aspect of the foot. This should be done with the foot in slight supination.
10. The spring ligament and the posterior tibial tendon plantar expansion are tightened with sutures into the osteoperiosteal flap.
11. A transfixation wire is used across the naviculocuneiform joint, with the foot in slight supination and slight varus with the ankle in slight equinus.

12. A cautious heelcord lengthening may in some instances be necessary.
13. The wound is closed, and the extremity is placed in a short-leg cast in the position described.
14. Total immobilization must continue for 3 months. A short-leg walking cast should be used for the final 6 weeks.

This procedure tends to do the following:

1. It elevates the depresssed equinus position of the talus.
2. It tightens the soft tissue on the plantar-medial aspect of the foot, creating dorsiflexion at the talonavicular joint, and elevates the arch.
3. It increases the supination of the first metatarsal-first cuneiform joint by tightening the anterior tibial tendon and placing the posterior tibial tendon insertion more distally.
4. It increases the lever arm (by fusion of the naviculocuneiform joint) on which the posterior tibial-anterior tibial tendons can work.
5. It shortens the medial column of the foot.
6. It corrects the abnormal talcalcaneal angle.
7. It corrects the talonavicular subluxation.

If there is excessive heel valgus, the authors recommend a Hoke triple arthrodesis. The skeletal age of 12 years must be attained before such a procedure may be performed. Subtalar fusion alone is of concern, because the peritalar joint complex acts as a unit. To restrict motion in one joint is likely to lead to premature degenerative changes in the others. The ability of a Grice extraarticular arthrodesis to withstand the stress placed upon it by an otherwise healthy individual is also a matter of concern.

TARSAL COALITION

Tarsal coalition was formerly known as peroneal spastic flatfoot, having first been described by Jones[238] in 1897. Blockley,[218] Cowell,[225] Harris,[233,234] Harris and Beath,[235] Lapidus,[242] and Webster and Roberts[259] have also used this term. Mitchell[245] prefers the term *spasmodic flatfoot*.

By definition, this condition represents a congenital synostosis or failure of segmentation between two or more tarsal bones. The resulting deformity almost always produces a rigid flatfoot. It has been known to exist for more than two centuries, having first been described in 1750.[219]

Slomann[251–253] made an important contribution to the recognition of calcaneonavicular coalition when he emphasized the need of oblique roentgenograms. In 1927, Badgley[216] discussed the treatment of this type of coalition and related it to the cause of peroneal spastic flatfoot. In 1948, Harris and Beath[235] identified the talocalcaneal coalition as another cause of peroneal spastic flatfoot.

Incidence

The incidence of this condition is unknown. Harris and Beath,[235] in their examination of 3,600 Canadian Army males, found that 2% had peroneal spastic flatfoot.

Cowell,[224] in studying more than 200 patients with tarsal coalition at the Alfred I. duPont Institute, stated that it is his impression that middle facet talocalcaneal coalition and calcaneonavicular coalition occur with the same incidence. However, he further states that if other abnormalities in the talocalcaneal area, including coalition in the area of the anterior facet and the posterior facet, are added, the incidence of talocalcaneal anomalies is higher than that of the calcaneonavicular bar alone.

Wynne-Davies[261] stated that the incidence of tarsal coalition is less than 1% in the general population.

According to Starmont and Peterson,[254] the overall incidence of tarsal coalition in the general population is unknown, but it is less than 1%. Most patients with tarsal coalition in their series did not have peroneal spastic flatfoot. In the 43 patients studied by Starmont and Peterson, 60 coalitions were found. Of the 60 tarsal coalitions, there were 32 calcaneonavicular coalitions, 22 talocalcaneal coalitions, 4 talonavicular coalitions, and 2 patients with multiple coalitions associated with multiple severe cogenital anomalies, including absent rays, deficient tibia, and pseudoarthrosis.

Classification

Tarsal coalition may exist in the following types: calcaneonavicular, talocalcaneal, talonavicular, naviculocuneiform, calcaneocuboid, cubonavicular, and block coalition.

In all the above types, the coalition may be fibrous, cartilaginous, or osseous.[232,235] The fibrous type may show only minimal restriction of inversion and eversion, whereas the cartilaginous and osseous types demonstrate no subtalar movement.

Mosier and Asher,[247] in an excellent review of this subject, emphasized that there are many conditions that may result in a peroneal spastic flatfoot. Calcaneonavicular coalitions and middle-facet talocalcaneal coalitions are commonly associated with the syndrome of peroneal spastic flatfoot.

The calcaneonavicular coalition is the most common type, with the talocalcaneal type being second in frequency of occurrence.[220,222,225,234,236,237]

Clark and Lovell[222] reviewed 94 tarsal coalitions representing 70 patients, with 24 patients having bilateral involvement. Sixty of the 94 tarsal coalitions were of the calcaneonavicular type, 31 were of the talocalcaneal type, two were of the talonavicular type, and one was of the naviculocuneiform type. The average age was 13.8 years, and there were 40 males and 30 females.

It is of interest that in the series described above, tarsal coalition was seen in Legg-Perthes disease, Blount's disease, cerebral palsy, dysplasia epiphysalis multiplex, idiopathic scoliosis, slipped capital femoral epiphysis, and Scheuermann's disease.

Tarsal coaltion associated with a ball and socket ankle joint was noted by Lamb.[240] The authors have seen one such case, which was symptomatic and necessitating treatment.

Naviculocuneiform coaltion has been reported in only two instances.[230,243] Figure 21-18

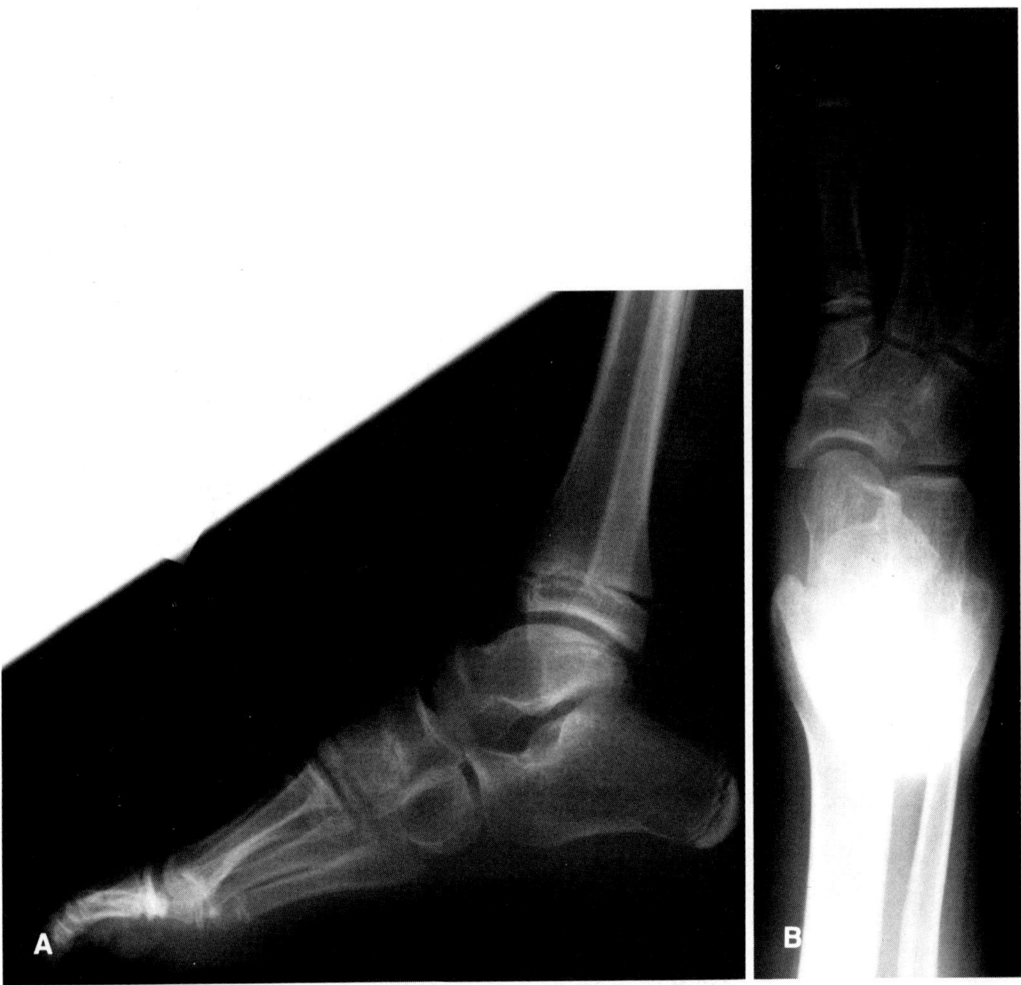

FIG. 21-18. *(A* and *B)* Roentgenogram showing navicular cuneiform coalition of the osseous type. This is a very rare coalition.

illustrates such a coalition recently seen because of a painful foot. Calcaneocuboid coalition, reported by Wagoner,[257] is rare and has not been seen by the authors. Mahaffey[244] has also described this condition. In the case reported by Veneruso,[256] there was complete absence of a metatarsal and toe. It apparently does not restrict subtalar motion, although it may be associated with pain. Cubonavicular coalition is also of infrequent occurrence.[226,227,258] Lapidus[242] described a case of bilateral congenital talonavicular fusion. The authors have seen one such case associated with a talocalcaneal coalition and a ball and socket ankle joint.

Etiology and Genetic Aspects

Etiology of tarsal coalition remains unknown. Harris and Beath[235] attributed this condition to the presence of an accessory bone that unites to adjacent tarsal bones. Badgley[216] stated that abnormal growth changes in the foot might possibly be a factor. Jack[237] suggested that coalition was due to an error in differentiation, which may result in a complete bony fusion at one extreme or to a small accessory bone at the other.

An autosomal dominant transmission is said to occur in this condition. Wray and Herndon[260] reported three cases of calcaneonavicular coalition in three successive generations of a family involving males. They concluded that some examples of calcaneonavicular coalition are caused by a specific gene mutation that behaves as an autosomal dominant trait with reduced penetrance. Webster and Roberts[259] reported talocalcaneal coalition occurring in two sisters. Massive familial tarsal synostosis has been noted by Bersante and Samilson.[217]

Clinical Features

The majority of patients with tarsal coalition at some time develop pain in the involved foot, and this usually follows injury or excessive activity.[218,220,223,231,249] The pain is described as being in the region of the sinus tarsi near the talonavicular joint or throughout the foot. The complaints are often aggravated by increased activity and may prevent further participation in athletics.

Symptoms are unlikely to appear until the second decade of life and are related to rapid ossification of the fibrous or cartilaginous coalition.[223] The increased activity associated with the early teens draws attention to the condition. Generally, the involved foot presents with pes planus and limited or absent subtalar motion. Very often, peroneal spasm may be noted, as well as spasm of the anterior tibial and common toe extensors. Simmons[250] has reported tarsal coalition accompanying pes cavus, and the authors have seen one such child.

The etiology of the pain in tarsal coalition has been debated. It has been suggested that the restriction of motion at the involved joints results in pain purely on a mechanical basis. Osteoarthritis may occur with narrowing of the talonavicular joint. The spasm of the peroneals and other tendons is probably secondary or possibly a reflex protective reaction to pain.

Outland and Murphy[248,249] called attention to the anatomic relationship between the calcaneus and navicular. These bones are held by the plantar calcaneonavicular ligament. The subtalar and the midtarsal joints, as a result, work synchronously. With forward movement of the calcaneus on the talus, the navicular glides over the head of the talus. If subtalar motion is eliminated as the result of a tarsal coalition, a reactive bone spur forms at the dorsal lateral aspect of the head of the talus.[223] Furthermore, if the restriction of motion is complete, alteration of the shape of the talar head may occur, and eventually there may be degenerative arthritis, with narrowing and irregularity of the talonavicular joint.

Roentgenographic Findings

A calcaneonavicular coalition is seldom demonstrated in routine anteroposterior and lateral views of the foot.[253] It is best seen in a 45° oblique projection as described by Slomann (Fig. 21-19).[252]

The width of the calcaneonavicular coalition extending from the anterior process of the calcaneus to the navicular may vary, with the average width being 1 cm. The osseous coalition is readily identified. The presence of a fissure associated with irregularity and sclerosis is indicative of a cartilaginous or fibrous coaliton. Another finding in the calcaneonavicular coalition is hypoplasia and smallness of the head of the talus.[223]

An axial view of the calcaneus, as described by Harris and Beath,[235] is essential to demonstrate talocalcaneal coalition (Fig. 21-20). These

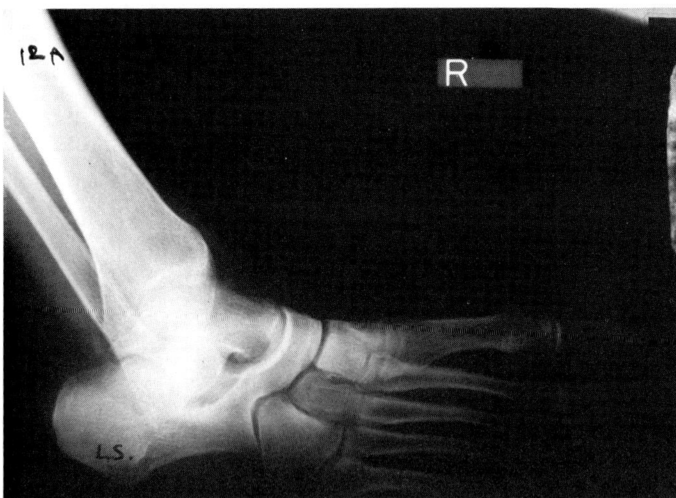

FIG. 21-19. An oblique film demonstrates a very large osseous calcaneonavicular coalition.

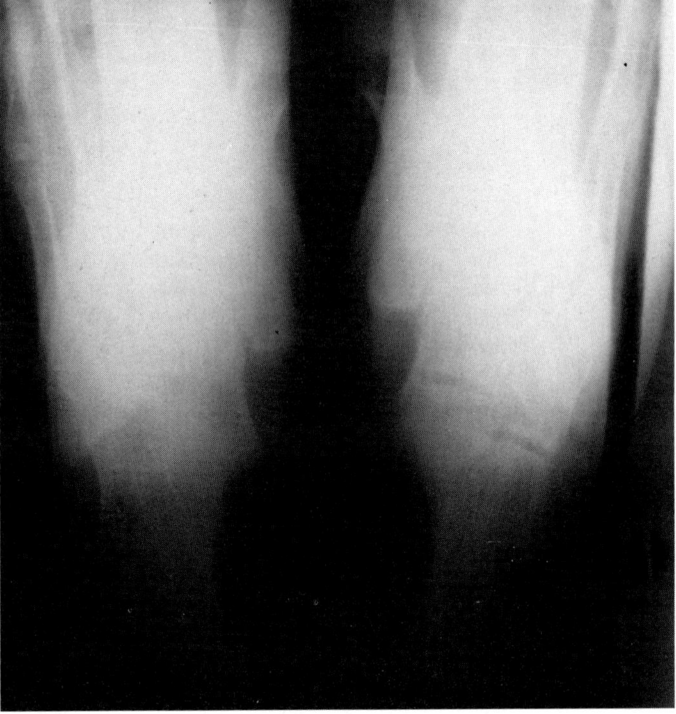

FIG. 21-20. Harris axial view demonstrating osseous coalition on the left and a normal medial facet on the right. This represents a left talocalcaneal coalition.

authors recommended a 45° angle axial view of the calcaneus. Conway and Cowell[223] have suggested that if there is difficulty in obtaining adequate visualization of the posterior and medial facets with this method, a lateral standing film of the foot should be made in order to determine the proper angle for the axial view. A line is drawn through the joint spaces of the posterior and middle facets, and the angle that this line forms with the horizontal is used as the x-ray beam angle for the axial view.

The middle facet talocalcaneal coalition occurs at the sustentaculum tali. If the coalition is osseous, the middle facet is completely obliterated. In the fibrous or cartilaginous coalition at this site, the joint is narrowed and irregular. The plane of the articulation between

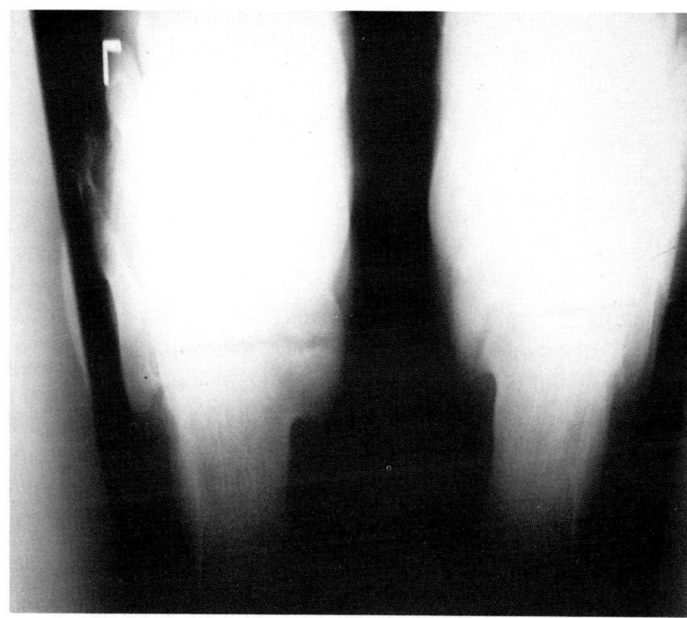

FIG. 21-21. Axial view showing obliquity of the medial facet, hypoplasia of the sustentaculum tali, and narrowing of the joint are pathognomonic of a cartilaginous talocalcaneal coalition. Contrast this to the transverse joint on the left with normally developed sustentaculum.

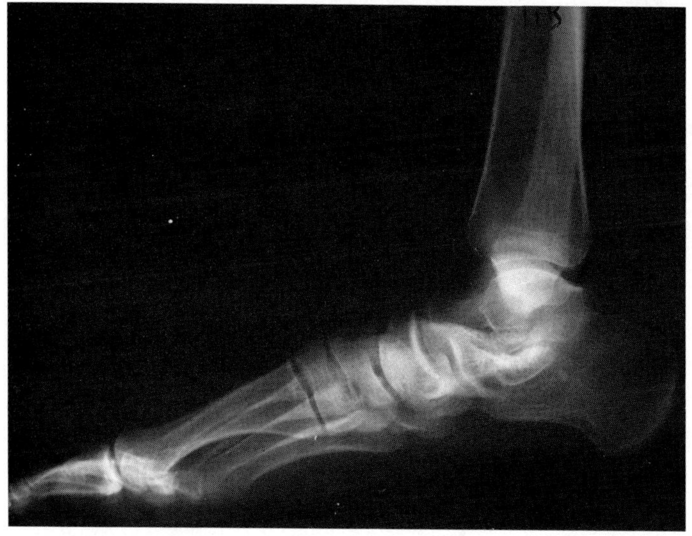

FIG. 21-22. Secondary signs of tarsal coalition are demonstrated in the lateral view of the foot and ankle. These include a broadened lateral process of the talus, narrowing of the posterior facet, and beaking of the head of the talus.

the talus and calcaneus is oblique rather than horizontal, and the sustentaculum tali is hypoplastic (Fig. 21-21). Secondary signs, as described by Cowell[225] include narrowing of the posterior subtalar joint, osteophyte formation of the talus, and broadening of the lateral process of the talus at the sulcus calcaneus (Fig. 21-22).

In 1969, Conway and Cowell[223] described anterior facet involvement resulting in a talocalcaneal coalition. They recommended that if the Harris view is negative for middle facet involvement, tomograms in the lateral projection should be secured to demonstrate the anterior facet. Anatomically, the anterior facet does not lie in the same plane as the middle and posterior facets; therefore, the routine axial view does not demonstrate this facet.

The authors have also noticed that peroneal spastic flatfoot may be associated with infections such as tuberculosis, rheumatoid arthritis, osteoid osteoma of the talus, and osteochondritis dissecans of the head of the talus. Cowell[225] has reported osteochondral fractures involving the under surface of the talar head as an additional cause of peroneal spastic flatfoot.

Goldman and colleagues[229] have developed a screening procedure for identifying symptomatic talocalcaneal coalition using bone-seeking nuclides.

Treatment

The treatment of a child with tarsal coalition must be individualized. If there is little discomfort, nothing other than restriction of excessive activities may be necessary. A pair of stout shoes with a long medial counter, Thomas heels, and ⅛-inch medial heel wedge may also be helpful in relieving symptoms.[222] A short-leg walking cast may be used for a period of 4 to 6 weeks in the more painful cases associated with peroneal muscle spasm. If pain is not relieved by the above measures, the authors have followed the recommendation of Cowell[223,225] in the cartilaginous calcaneonavicular coalition and have performed an arthroplasty using the extensor digitorum brevis muscle. Cowell emphasized that this procedure must be done before degenerative changes occur in a young patient. It is accompanied by resection of the coalition. A lateral Ollier incision is used and, after identifying the coalition, it is removed as a rectangular block of bone and the entire origin of the extensor digitorum brevis muscle is placed in the defect and tied over a button, medially. A cast is applied with the foot in a neutral position for 10 days. It is then removed, and range of motion exercises are instituted. Weightbearing should be delayed until motion in the subtalar joint is essentially normal. The purpose of the arthroplasty is to relieve pain and restore motion. Mitchell and Gibson[246] have also advised excision of the calcaneonavicular coalition.

Chambers and associates[221] evaluated the function of 19 patients 3 to 14 years after reconstructive surgery for calcaneonavicular coalition. It was found that better function correlated well with better postoperative subtalar motion.

A triple arthrodesis is indicated in all types of calcaneonavicular coalition if pain is not relieved by conservative measures or if degenerative changes are present.

Swiontkowski, Scranton, and Hansen[255] reviewed 40 patients with tarsal coalition who had 57 operations. Ten patients were treated for talocalcaneal coalition, with 4 having successful resections. Thirty patients had 39 calcaneonavicular resections. Only 2 patients in the entire series had a poor end result, which was due to either technically poor surgery or failed calcaneonavicular resection because of advanced degenerative changes. It was their belief that the talar beak when present did not in all instances preclude a resection arthroplasty. The presence of the talar beak may represent a traction process occurring secondary to increased motion and not necessarily a degenerative spur.

The statement was also made by these authors that tarsal coalition may involve any of the three talocalcaneal facets. Resection of such coalitions should be considered if there is absence of degenerative changes and if tomography shows the bar not to be markedly malaligned or excessively large.

ACCESSORY NAVICULAR

The accessory navicular is a supernumerary bone in the human foot. It may be found either attached to or fused with the medial border of the navicular. In relationship to the navicular, its usual position is posterior and inferior. The posterior tibial tendon attaches to the accessory navicular, the cuneiforms, and the metatarsal bases.

Kidner[262] credits Bauhin in 1605 for first describing the accessory navicular. In early writings, it was considered a sesamoid bone by some authors and a nonunion of a navicular fracture by others.

The accessory navicular appears in many lower mammals either as a part of a fully formed sixth ray or a remnant of such.

Zadek and Gold[265] stated that a separate cartilaginous center for the tuberosity of the navicular may be found in the fetus. He reports that the accessory navicular is present as a separate bone in approximately 10% of humans and that it persists as a separate bone in 2%.

Zadek[265] followed 14 patients into adult life who were seen as children with accessory naviculars. Fusion to the navicular occurred in five patients; partial fusion occurred in three patients; and failure to fuse in six patients.

Microscopic studies[265] carried out on removed surgical specimens demonstrated that the accessory navicular and navicular are joined by a layer of soft tissue. This soft-tissue plate consisted of hyaline cartilage, dense fibrocartilage, or a mixture of the two. The plate varied in thickness and frequently showed active ossification on each side. In no case studied was a well-developed freely movable joint found with smooth hyaline articular cartilage capping each bone and with the two articulating bones bound together by a synovial lined fibrous capsule, such as would be found in a true joint. Found in several specimens was evidence of trauma in the form of hemorrhages, organizing fibrous tissue containing giant cells, and callus-like reparative tissue. This would help to explain the acute symptoms and localized pain seen in some patients.

Clinical Signs and Symptoms

Patients present in late childhood and early adolescence with pain localized over the medial aspect of the foot and along the posterior tibial tendon. There will be a prominence over the medial aspect of the foot. Its size will vary. Frequently soft-tissue swelling and erythema are encountered over the prominence medially. On standing, there may be a loss of the longitudinal arch. The presence of an accessory navicular is not constantly related to loss of the longitudinal arch of the foot on weight-bearing.

Roentgenograms confirm the clinical impression of accessory navicular. The anteroposterior and lateral oblique views define the accessory navicular (Fig. 21-23).

Treatment

Nonoperative Treatment

Shoe modifications should be directed toward relieving pressure on the medial prominence. A doughnut pad placed over the prominence will allow more even pressure distribution and may relieve symptoms. Medial longitudinal arch supports and inserts are not likely to be helpful, because most patients do not have flatfeet. Inserts of plastozote/peolite can allow

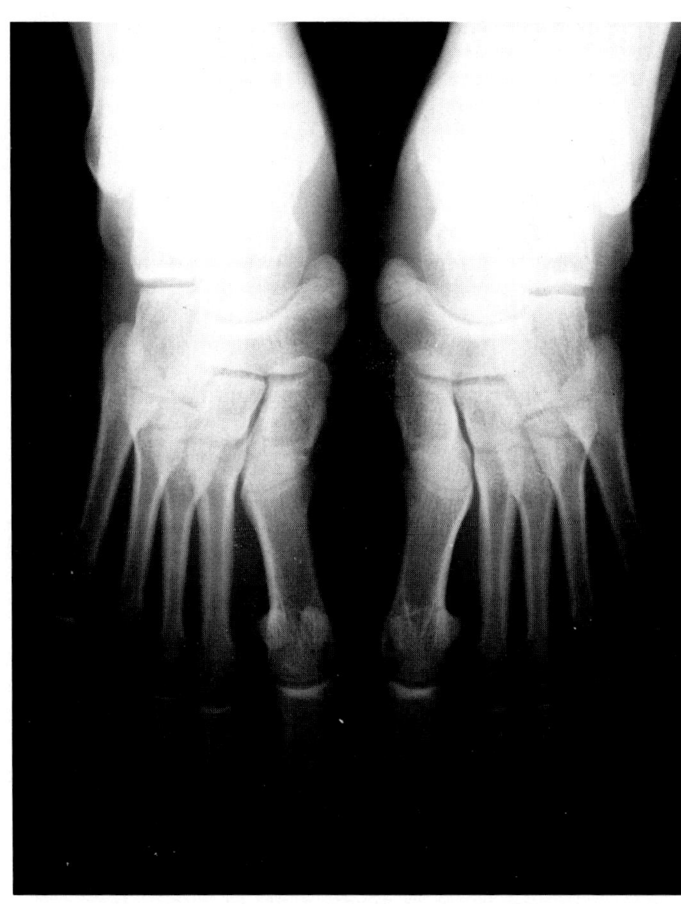

Fig. 21-23. A 15-year-old asymptomatic female with bilateral accessory naviculars.

relief of pressure symptoms and can be used in athletic footwear.

Surgical Treatment

Those patients not relieved by shoe modifications or those whose medial prominence is such that proper fitting is not possible are surgical candidates.

Veitch[264] reviewed 21 feet in 14 patients who had had a Kidner procedure. Follow-up was 5 years. The presenting complaint in all was pain over the medial prominence. Fifteen patients were described as having flatfeet preoperatively. Postoperatively, there was no objective evidence that the height of the longitudinal arch had been changed. The author felt that the success of the operation was related to removal of medial prominence.

Sullivan[263] reinforced these findings. He reviewed 18 patients who had simple excision of the medial prominence. All were considered to have had a satisfactory result at follow-up. All had their symptoms relieved.

Simple excision of the bony prominence is likely to relieve symptoms in most patients. Reattachment of the posterior tibial tendon to the navicular is probably not necessary for the majority of patients. If one does have a flatfoot deformity associated, reattachment of the tendon can be carried out, although one should not expect this to correct the flatfoot deformity.

PES CAVUS

Pes cavus means hollow-foot and commonly refers to pathologic elevation of the longitudinal arch. Identification of the apex of the deformity has therapeutic as well as etiologic implications.[309] To be as specific as possible, the term *pes cavus* should only refer to fixed equinus of the forefoot on the hindfoot. This may occur at the metatarsocuneiform joints or at the midtarsal joints. When the term *calcaneocavus* is used to describe the cavus foot, the calcaneus is fixed in a more vertical orientation. *Cavovarus* characterizes the cavus foot that assumes a varus position during weightbearing. Varus of the hindfoot may be fixed due to deformity of the calcaneus or may be flexible and secondary to excessive plantar flexion of the first ray.[272]

Table 21-2. Etiology of Pes Cavus

NEUROMUSCULAR
Charcot-Marie-Tooth disease
Spinal dysraphism
Roussy-Levy syndrome
Freidreich's ataxia
Cerebral palsy
Poliomyelitis
Spinal muscular atrophy
Syringomyelia
Diastematomyelia
Primary cerebellar disease
Guillain-Barré syndrome
Interstitial hypertrophic neuritis of childhood
Mollaret's spinocerebellar degeneration
Multiple sclerosis
Traumatic peroneal palsy
Spinal cord tumor
CONGENITAL
Residual clubfoot
Arthrogryposis
IDIOPATHIC
OTHER CAUSES
Traumatic
Infections
Ledeerhose disease (plantar fibromatosis)
Iatrogenic

ETIOLOGY

The etiology of pes cavus can be broken into four major categories: neuromuscular, congenital, idiopathic, and other causes (Table 21-2). Pes cavus is a frequent sign of underlying neurologic disease. The most common neuromuscular cause is Charcot-Marie-Tooth disease, followed in frequency by spinal dysrhaphism.[269,278,279,284,287,293] James and Lassman[293] emphasized that progressive cavovarus of the foot may be associated with spina bifida occulta. Abnormal gait and deformity of the foot may be the presenting complaint for extrinsic lesions of the cauda equina. External cutaneous manifestations such as excess hair, nevus, sacral dimples, or sacral lipoma may help establish the diagnosis. James and Lassman[293] further reported improvement in the foot abnormalities of 66% of the patients undergoing laminectomy and correction of the lesion. Brewerton, Sandifer, and Sweetnam[269] established a Pes Cavus Clinic at the Royal National

Table 21-3. Theories of Pathogenesis

INTRINSIC MUSCLE IMBALANCE	
Duchenne (1867)	Weakness of short muscles of hallux and interossei
Sherman (1905)	Paralysis of interossei and lumbricales
Mills (1924)	Paralysis of small muscles of foot supplied by lateral plantar nerve
Lambrinudi (1927)	Lumbrical and interosseous imbalance
Stamm (1948)	Lumbrical and interosseous imbalance
Garceau and Brahms (1956)	Overactivity of superficial plantar muscles
EXTRINSIC MUSCLE IMBALANCE	
Barwell (1865)	Weak gastroc with overactive posterior tibials
Fisher (1889)	Weak extensor digitorum longus with weakness of anterior tibials in severe cases
Golding-Bird (1883)	Weak peronei causing overactive anterior tibials and posterior tibials
Tubby (1896)	Overactive peroneus longus
Steindler (1917)	Weak gastroc and anterior tibial with overactive peroneus longus and toe flexors
Hibbs (1919)	Overactive long extensors acting against contracted calf and plantar fascia
Royle (1927)	Weakness of gastroc-soleus and overactive posterior tibial
Ollerenshaw (1927)	Overactive extensor digitorum longus
Altakoff (1931)	Overaction of calf muscles
Lowman	Strong extensor digitorum longus and peroneus longus with weak anterior tibial
Cole (1940)	Normal extensor digitorum longus with weak anterior tibial
Scheer and Crego (1946)	Weak gastrocnemius and soleus
Bentzon (1933)	Overactive peroneus longus
Karlholm and Nilsonne (1968)	Relatively strong posterior tibial
COMBINATION OF EXTRINSIC AND INTRINSIC MUSCLE IMBALANCE	
Ducroauet (1910)	Paresis of flexor hallucis brevis with overaction of extensor hallucis longus
Little (1938)	Insufficient interossei with weak extensor digitorum longus
Dickson and Diveley (1939)	Overaction of intrinsics caused by short tendo Achilles
Irwin (1958)	Several varieties of intrinsic-extrinsic imbalance lead to clawing
Chuinard (1973)	Imbalance of extensors, plantar flexors, or intrinsics cause deformity
Kirmisson (1906)	Primitive laxity of dorsal ligaments of foot
Tubby (1912)	Rheumatoid arthritis of tarsal joints
Rugh (1927	Primary contracture of plantar fascia
Gilroy (1929)	Congenital abnormality
Saunders (1935)	Loss of synergistic muscle control and ill-fitting shoes

Orthopaedic Hospital. In their initial group of 77 patients, 44% had roentgenographic evidence of a neural arch defect, and 75% were found to have underlying neurologic disease on the basis of the examination, electromyography, or nerve conduction studies.

Other than neuromuscular origin, cavus feet are also seen as a residual of clubfoot or arthrogryposis. Idiopathic pes cavus is probably an uncommon entity.

PATHOGENESIS

Numerous theories have been elaborated to explain the pathogenesis of pes cavus (Table 21-3). These causes may be subdivided into four categories: (1) intrinsic muscle imbalance, (2) extrinsic muscle imbalance, (3) combination of imbalance involving intrinsic and extrinsic muscles, and (4) nonmuscular causes.

Intrinsic muscle weakness as a cause of pes

cavus was first proposed by Duchenne (1867),[276] who thought that clawing of the foot was similar to clawhand. However, the intrinsic muscles of the foot are not anatomically the same as those in the hand.[274,295,301] The interossei of the foot insert mainly into the base of the proximal phalanx and do not send a slip to the extensor hood for interphalangeal joint extension as noted in the hand. Although electromyographic studies of the cavus foot have shown definite abnormalities in the intrinsic muscles and short toe flexors, interpretation of these findings has been difficult.[304] Coonrad and associates[273] postulated intrinsic overactivity rather than weakness as a cause of pes cavus. This was based on an observation of cavovarus in polio patients who had preservation of intrinsic and short toe flexors but an otherwise flail leg. Levik (1921)[298] had previously demonstrated the arch raising effect of the short toe flexors.

Extrinsic muscle imbalance has also been widely thought to be a cause of pes cavus. Golding-Bird (1883)[286] proposed that weakness of the peroneus longus was etiologic. Since then, Bentzon,[266] Steindler,[319] and others have believed that the condition was due to overactivity of the peroneus longus. Dwyer[278,279] pointed out that peroneal spasticity and overactivity produced flatfoot, not pes cavus. What is often regarded as overaction of the peroneus longus is actually secondary contracture after the metatarsals become flexed. Hibbs[289] attributed clawing and depression of the metatarsal head to overactive long extensors working against the contractured gastrocnemius and plantar fascia. Other theories of extrinsic imbalance have also been proposed.

The combination of intrinsic and extrinsic imbalance has been proposed by Irwin (1953),[291] who identified four possible pathogenetic mechanisms. Chuinard and Baskin[270] also favor a variety of possible mechanisms. They described the muscles of the ankle and foot as a right triangle (Fig. 21-24). The base consists of short flexors, abductors, and long toe flexors. The hypotenuse consists of extensor hallucis longus and anterior tibial muscles. The right angle is completed by the triceps surae. Imbalance in any portion of the triangle results in deformity.

Postulated nonmuscular causes of pes cavus include improper shoe wear, primary abnormality of bone, and weight of bed clothes during protracted illness.[285,300,306,307,312] Little and Rugh[300,306,307] postulated primary contracture of the plantar fascia. A tight plantar fascia is a uniquely consistent finding in the cavus foot. However, is contracture a primary or a secondary development? The primary contracture theory does not account for metatarsophalangeal joint dorsiflexion, because the plantar fascia inserts into the base of the proximal phalanges, and contracture should produce MP flexion.

The authors believe that the combination of intrinsic and extrinsic muscle imbalance is present in most cavus feet. No one pathomechanical process accounts for all varieties of pes cavus. Calcaneocavus primarily results from weakness of the triceps surae. Forefoot cavus may result from unopposed intrinsic muscle activity. Cavovarus is most frequently seen when there is relative weakness of the peroneal musculature as observed in Charcot-Marie-Tooth disease. Careful evaluation is necessary to determine appropriate treatment.

CLINICAL EVALUATION

Every evaluation should include a thorough search for the underlying etiology. A complete

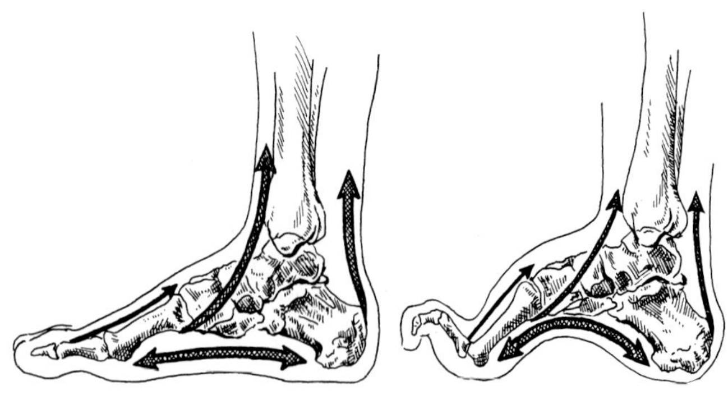

FIG. 21-24. The normal muscular balance of the foot is demonstrated on the left. A right triangle of muscle forces is generated by the gastrocnemius soleus group posteriorly, the plantar muscles distally, and the tibialis anticus anteriorly. Weakness, as demonstrated in the diagram on the right, causes imbalance in the foot with resultant pescavus. (Redrawn from Chuinard E, Baskin M: Clawfoot deformity. J Bone Joint Surg 55A:351–362, 1973)

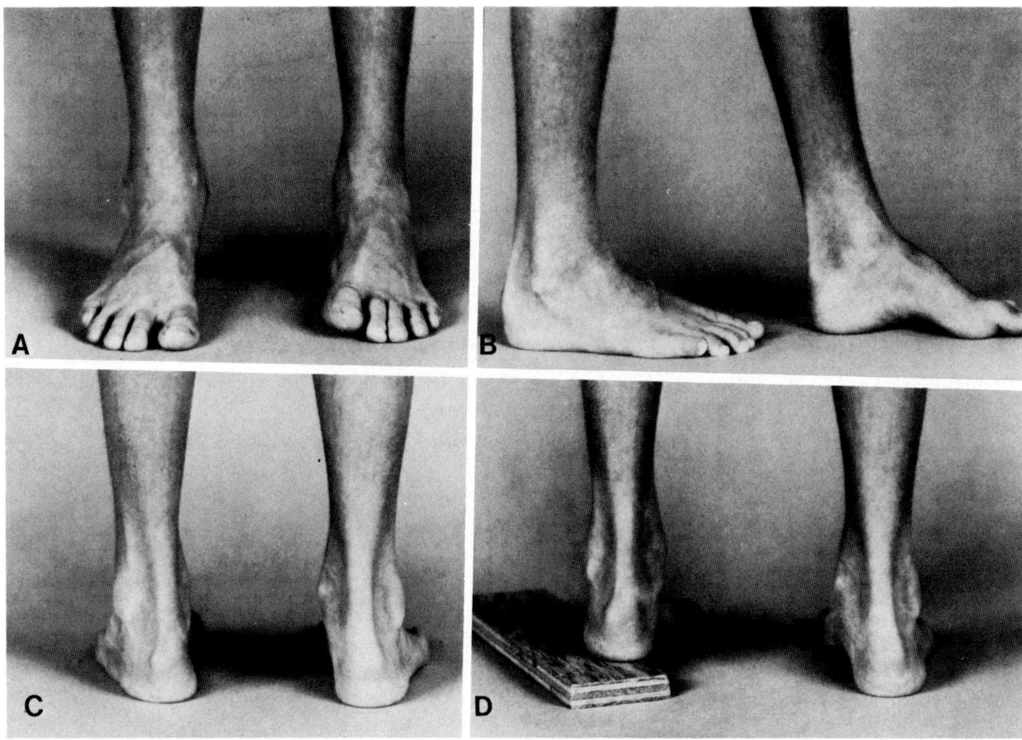

FIG. 21-25. *(A through D)* The typical appearance of a cavovarus foot is demonstrated in the standing position. The great toe is clawed, and the longitudinal arch is raised with apparent flexion and supination of the forefoot. The heel is in varus. In *(D)* is shown Coleman's block test. In this patient, the heel varus corrects when the hindfoot is elevated, evidence that the primary deformities are in the first and second metatarsals and can be corrected by a dorsal wedge osteotomy through the base of the metatarsals combined with a plantar release.

history and neurologic examination is essential. Roentgenograms of the entire spine, nerve conduction velocities, electromyographic studies, and appropriate blood chemistries are frequently helpful. Myelography and/or spinal computed tomographic (CT) scanning should be performed when indicated, particularly in the presence of spinal dysraphism. Muscle or nerve biopsy may also be required. Neurologic or neurosurgical consultation is frequently helpful.

Examination of the foot begins with observation of the apex of the deformity and assessment of the flexibility of the various components of the deformity. The plantar muscles and fascia are usually contracted. Coleman and Chestnut[272] have described a simple test for hindfoot flexibility in the cavovarus foot (Fig. 21-25). In this test, a 1-inch block is placed under the heel and lateral border of the weightbearing foot. This allows the first through third metatarsals to fall into pronation. If the heel varus corrects, it is flexible and will resolve with surgical correction of the forefoot pronation. If heel varus persists, hindfoot and forefoot procedures are necessary. Motor examination with detailed muscle grading is essential to assess possible tendon transfers and to prevent recurrence.

Roentgenograms of the feet should include a weightbearing lateral view to assess the apex of the deformity (Fig. 21-26). An assessment of the degree of calcaneus is provided by the posterior angle between the long axes of the tibia and the calcaneus. This is normally 120° or 130°. An angle greater than 130° demonstrates calcaneal deformity. Scheer and Crego[313] noted that the Tuber angle measures 50° to 70° in pes cavus and only 22° to 45° in the normal foot (Fig. 21-27). Hindfoot varus can be evaluated roentgenographically by a double exposure technique.[311] The first exposure is an anteroposterior view of the ankle mortise, and the second exposure is obtained with the beam

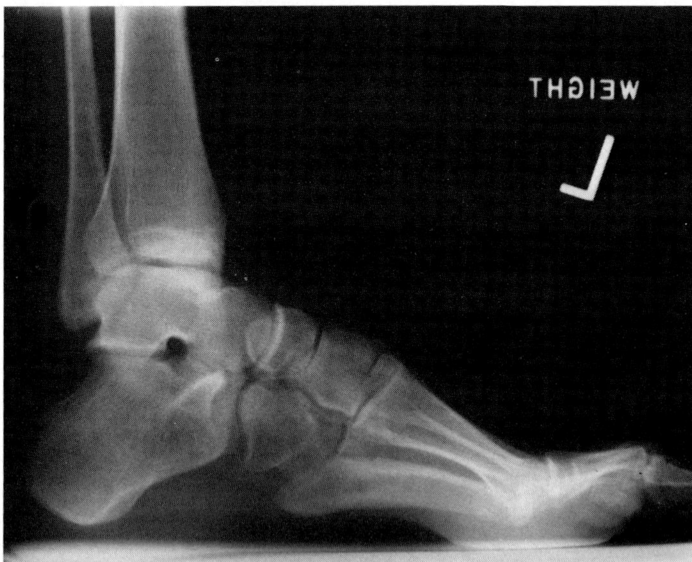

FIG. 21-26. Lateral weight bearing film showing cavus deformity with a higher arch, calcaneus position of the hindfoot, plantar flexion of the first metatarsal, and flexion deformity of the great toe. Note the open subtalar joint.

angled 20° cephalad and centered on the malleoli (Fig. 21-28). A perpendicular line is drawn, which intersects the superolateral talar dome. If the center of the os calcis is medial to this vertical line, heel varus is present.

TREATMENT

Nonsurgical management such as stretching exercises, orthotic devices, and shoe inserts will not correct the basic deformity but may provide symptomatic relief for patients with mild deformity. Soft-tissue procedures are usually performed in younger patients or in combination with bony operations. Procedures on bone are indicated in the adolescent and mature foot when deformity is fixed. Isolated deformities such as forefoot flexion (true pes cavus) or heel varus are best treated by specific procedures for each deformity. Triple arthrodesis is preferred when the deformity is severe, complex, or secondary to progressive neuromuscular disorder.

Two or more procedures are often combined to correct each component of the deformity. For example, the moderately severe cavovarus foot with fixed structural deformity of the forefoot and hindfoot may require plantar fasciotomy, closing lateral wedge osteotomy of the calcaneus, and osteotomy of the first and second metatarsals. Tendon transfers after correction of deformity may be indicated to correct claw toes and/or to prevent recurrence.

SOFT-TISSUE PROCEDURES

Tendo Achilles Lengthening

Tendo Achilles lengthening is rarely indicated for pes cavus except when equinus orientation of the calcaneus is present. This is most often seen with residual clubfoot deformity. Cavus with mild equinus angulation of the hindfoot from other causes may be treated by serial corrective casts following plantar release.[314]

The limited ankle dorsiflexion seen with calcaneocavus is caused by elongation of the os calcis secondary to triceps surae weakness. Therefore, tendo Achilles lengthening should not be performed in the calcaneocavus foot.

Plantar Release

Release of the plantar fascia, short flexor muscles, and abductors of the great and little toes from the os calcis was popularized by Steindler.[319] Steindler and others[289] warned against simultaneous plantar release and tendo Achilles lengthening, because tension against the os calcis is necessary to stretch the plantar contractures. Numerous variations of plantar fasciotomy have been described.[290,306,307,314,317]

Plantar release will correct hindfoot varus only if it is flexible and secondary to pronation of forefoot as demonstrated by Coleman's block test.[272] Sherman and Westin[314] reported an 83% success rate using plantar release alone to correct cavus deformity resulting from club-

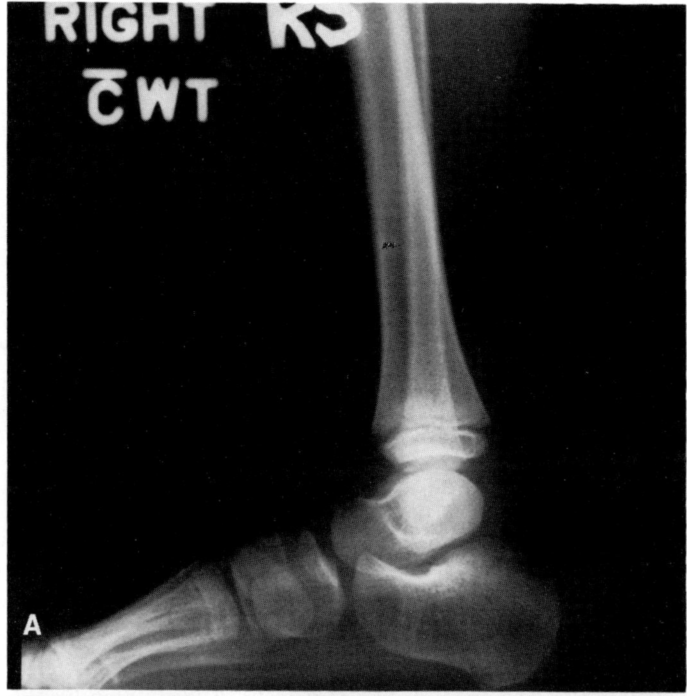

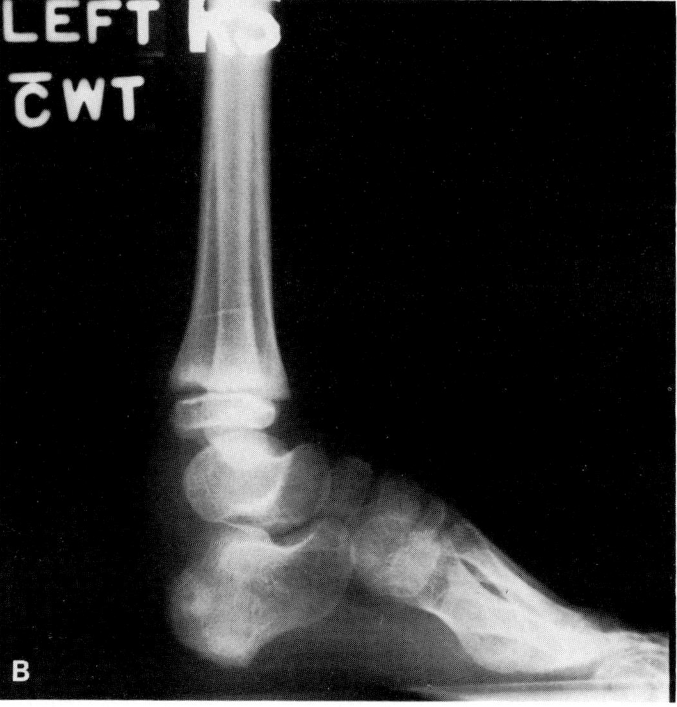

FIG. 21-27. *(A)* Lateral view of a normal foot showing a normal tuber angle. *(B)* Abnormal tuber angle in pes cavus. The tuber angle is formed by the intersection of a line along the subtalar articular surface of the calcaneus and a line from the posterior lip of the posterior articular facet of the calcaneal tuberosity.

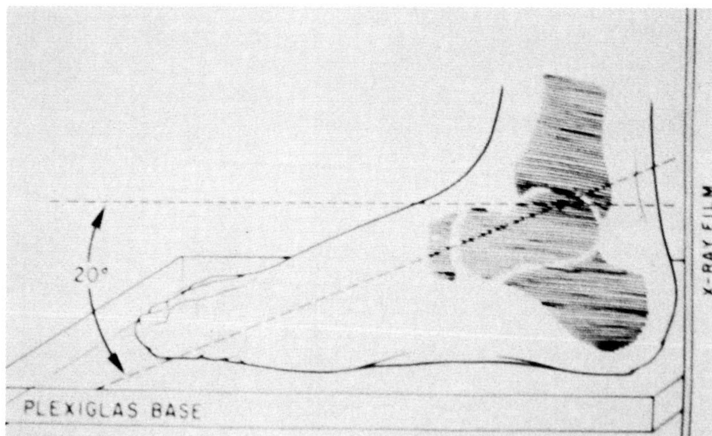

FIG. 21-28. Double exposure technique for determining hindfoot position. First exposure is made perpendicular to film plane. Second exposure is angled 20° cephalad. Both beams are centered on the malleoli. (Foot and Ankle I(5):286–288, 1981)

foot and poliomyelitis. The age of patients ranged from 1 to 16 years. The procedure was most successful for pure cavus deformity and equinocavus deformity from poliomyelitis. They concluded that the procedure is indicated in the clubfoot with residual cavovarus deformity only when there is no equinus angulation of the hindfoot. Plantar release was not effective for calcaneocavus deformity. However, others have successfully combined plantar fasciotomy with os calcis osteotomy to correct calcaneocavus.[268,278,305,308]

More extensive plantar releases have been described[277,303] and include sectioning of the posterior tibial tendon, the bifurcated Y-ligament (calcaneocuboid and calcaneonavicular ligaments), and the spring ligament. In general, these extensive releases have not been widely used.

The authors prefer the technique of Lucas as reported by Sherman and Westin.[314] A lateral incision is made opposite the tuberosity of the calcaneus just proximal to the plantar skin edge. The plantar fascia and complete expanse of the calcaneal origins of the abductor digiti quinti, flexor digitorum brevis, and abductor hallucis brevis muscles are exposed by blunt dissection. Complete release of the origins of the fascia and muscles is then accomplished. Serial casts are applied every 2 weeks, gradually stretching contracted soft tissues for 10 to 12 weeks after surgery. This is followed by night casts for 6 months.

Tendon Transfers

A tendon transfer should not be performed in the presence of fixed deformity. Appropriate transfers to balance the paralytic foot are discussed in the chapter on neuromuscular disorders.

Tendon transfers are recognized procedures for claw toes associated with pes cavus. Transplantation of the long extensor tendons to the metatarsal heads for claw toes and pes cavus was first described by Sherman[315] in 1905 and later by Forbes[280] in 1913. Ducroquet (1910) described transferring the extensor hallucis longus to the neck of the first metatarsal. In 1917, Robert Jones[294] described the same procedure, which today is known as the Jones procedure. In 1924, Stuart modified the procedure by adding fusion of the interphalangeal joint. Other modifications have since been described (Fig. 21-29).[271,281,288,289,298] The rationale for this type of transfer is that it removes the deforming force causing clawing and metatarsal head depression. The transferred tendon then can actively elevate the metatarsal head. Interphalangeal fusion gives the long flexor tendons a better lever arm to flex the metatarsophalangeal joint. Results with extensor tendon transfer to the metatarsal neck have generally been good when used in combination with other procedures.[270,281,302] However, Lambrinudi[297] believed that interphalangeal fusion alone was adequate. He stated that transferring the extensor tendons is not physiologic, because the muscles are not strong and the metatarsals are relatively fixed. The authors believe that interphalangeal fusion and extensor transfer is a satisfactory procedure for the relief of clawtoes. This procedure is usually combined with plantar release. Best results are obtained when the forefoot is supple and clawing corrects on passive elevations of the metatarsal heads.

Selective Neurectomy

Selective neurectomy of the motor branches of the medial and lateral plantar nerves has been advocated by Coonrad and co-workers[273] and by Garceau and Brahms.[283] This procedure may be indicated in the child with functioning intrinsics and an otherwise flail foot.

PROCEDURES IN BONE

Metatarsal Osteotomies

McElvenny and Caldwell[304] advocated correction of the cavus foot by elevating and supinating the first metatarsal. Fusion of the first metatarsocuneiform joint maintained the correction. If necessary, the naviculocuneiform joint was included also in the arthrodesis. They found the procedure to be excellent in the passively correctable pes cavus and a valuable adjunct to triple arthrodesis in rigid cavus.

The authors believe that first or first and second metatarsal osteotomy is successful as an isolated procedure when deformity is confined to pronation of the forefoot and hindfoot varus is supple as determined by Coleman's block test (see Fig. 21-25*D*). Osteotomy is accomplished by removing a dorsally based wedge from the proximal first and second metatarsals (Fig. 21-30). The osteotomy is closed and fixed with smooth Steinmann pins, and the leg is immobilized in a short-leg cast with the heel in valgus position.

In rigid pes cavus, proximal osteotomies through the base of all the metatarsals have been advocated.[282,283] Generally, this has not been an accepted procedure, because correction takes place distal to the deformity.

Tarsal Osteotomy

In 1921, Steindler[319] recommended a dorsally based tarsal wedge osteotomy through the cuboid and the neck of the talus. Saunders (1935)[312] proposed a more distal osteotomy at the level of the naviculocuneiform joint. This consists of excision of a dorsally based wedge of bone through the cuboid and naviculocuneiform joints. Other tarsal osteotomies have also been described.

Jahss[292] described a dorsally based truncated wedge arthrodesis of the tarsometatarsal joints to correct fixed cavus and cavovarus of the forefoot after skeletal maturity. Readers are referred to his article for specific indications and contraindications. Advantages of this procedure include preservation of subtalar motion and improved alignment of the forefoot by selective removal of bone from each tarsometatarsal joint. Disadvantages include possible undercorrection or overcorrection due to the exacting nature of the procedure.

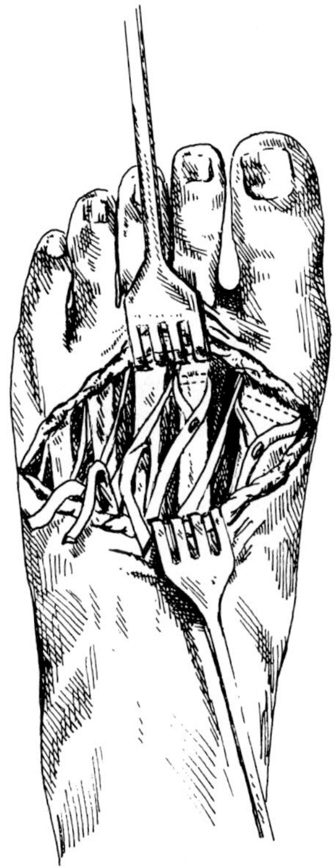

FIG. 21-29. A technique of transfer of the long extensors to the head of the metatarsals. (Redrawn from Chuinard E, Baskin M: Clawfoot deformity. J Bone Joint Surg 55A:360, 1973)

Osteotomy of the Calcaneus

Dwyer[278] described plantar fasciotomy and closing lateral wedge osteotomy of the calcaneus for cavovarus deformity. This is based on the theory that inversion of the heel causes the gastrocnemius-soleus muscle group to become active invertors. This force along with plantar fascia contracture leads to structural varus and cavus. Osteotomy to realign the hindfoot theoretically contributes to gradual stretching of the plantar structure. However, Dwyer himself reported good and excellent

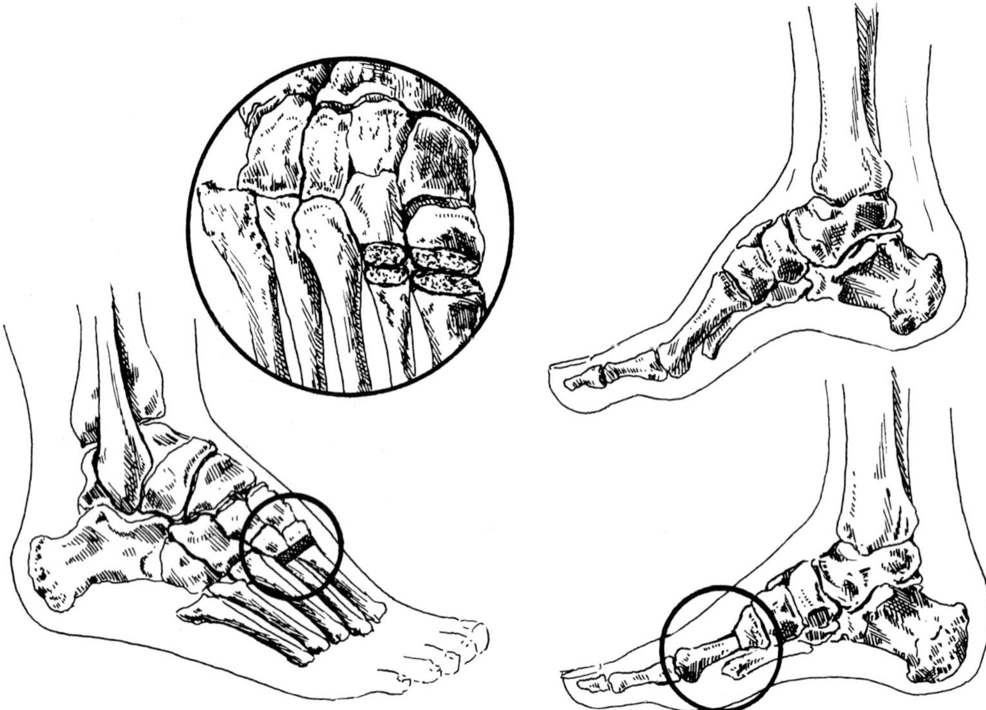

FIG. 21-30. Dorsal wedge osteotomy of the first and second metatarsals. This osteotomy may be performed through a single dorsal incision or through a medial and dorsal incision if plantar structures are released simultaneously. Care must be taken to avoid damage to the dorsalis pedis artery.

results in only 64% of 170 cases assessed after calcaneal osteotomy. Many of these feet had also required supplementary operations. The authors share the opinion of others[275,318] that the Dwyer osteotomy is useful for correcting fixed heel varus, but forefoot cavus must be corrected by other procedures.

Successful correction of calcaneocavus deformity has been accomplished by posterior displacement osteotomy of the calcaneus combined with plantar release (Fig. 21-31).[268,305,308,309] After correction, the osteotomy is fixed with a Steinmann pin, which is removed 3 to 4 weeks postoperatively. Immobilization is discontinued 8 to 10 weeks after surgery. Bradley and Coleman[268] recommended this procedure in children between the ages of 5 and 12 years as one stage of an operative program to correct deformity and prevent recurrence.

Triple Arthrodesis

Triple arthrodesis is a salvage procedure for correcting cavus feet and should be performed in the adolescent when deformity is severe or secondary to a progressive neuromuscular disorder. Triple arthrodesis is discussed in more depth in the chapter on neuromuscular disorders.

For severe calcaneocavus, Scheer and Crego[313] recommended a two-stage correction. At the first stage, the subtalar joint is approached posteriorly and a wedge of bone is removed. Four weeks later, through a sinus tarsi incision, a complete triple arthrodesis and plantar release is performed. At follow-up, an average of 2¾ years later, 24 of 27 patients had a satisfactory result. Siffert and associates[316] also described an arthrodesis for severe cavus in which the inferior half of the talar head and neck are resected, bringing the forefoot under the remaining talar "beak." Lambrinudi[296] arthrodesis is recommended for cavus deformity associated with equinus angulation of the hindfoot.

The most common cavus deformity requiring triple arthrodesis is cavovarus. For this,

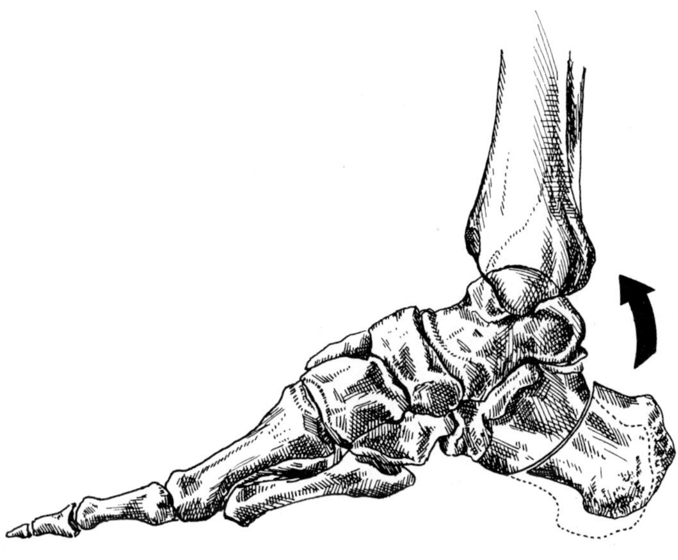

FIG. 21-31. Crescentic osteotomy of the calcaneus to correct calcaneocavus deformity. (Redrawn from Samilson RJ: Crescentic osteotomy of the calcaneus. In Bateman JE (ed): Foot Science, p. 20. Philadelphia, WB Saunders, 1976)

the authors prefer the method of Hoke as popularized by Kite. In a review of 104 triple arthrodesis procedures performed for a variety of conditions at the Scottish Rite Hospital between 1943 and 1975, Duncan and Lovell,[276a] 75% had satisfactory correction. The nonunion rate was 9%. Excision of wedges from the calcaneus rather than the talus has virtually eliminated avascular necrosis of the talus.

OSTEOCHONDROSES

The term *osteochondroses* refers to a group of conditions occurring in the juvenile age period. They are characterized by similar radiographic findings of increased density and fragmentation of the epiphyseal or apophyseal center. The lesions were all originally attributed to some form of avascular necrosis. Current evidence indicates that some are due to true osteonecrosis, whereas others are abnormalities of enchondral ossification. The causes of osteochondroses are unknown, but contributing factors probably include underlying constitutional predisposition and traumatic episodes.[321,322] Cases of familial and multiple joint involvement have been reported.[320,323,324,326] Each anatomic location is identified by its own eponym. Siffert[326] classified osteochondroses based on three anatomic sites of epiphyseal involvement: articular, nonarticular, and physeal.

FREIBERG'S INFARCTION (OSTEOCHONDRITIS OF THE METATARSAL HEAD)

Freiberg[330,331] presented a comprehensive description of this entity in 1913. He described an anterior form of metatarsalgia in which the pain was confined to the second metatarsal head and was associated with a "crushed in" roentgenographic appearance of the metatarsal head (Fig. 21-32).

The lesion is due to avascular necrosis of the metatarsal head. It generally involves the second metatarsal head but occasionally involves one of the lateral toes. Repetitive trauma from the stress of weightbearing may be etiologic.[329,335] Freiberg's infarction is more commonly seen in persons in whom the first metatarsal is shorter than the second. Maximum incidence is in the second decade of life, usually in adolescents.

The patient presents with pain localized under the second metatarsal head. There is usually local swelling and limitation of motion at the second metatarsophalangeal joint. Roentgenograms show the irregularity and flattening of the metatarsal head. Early in the disease, there is a sclerotic appearance. Later in the disease, the lesion is osteolytic, with hypertrophy of the metatarsal head.

Initial management consists of a low-heel shoe with a metatarsal bar or metatarsal pad. If pain is severe or persistent, the foot should

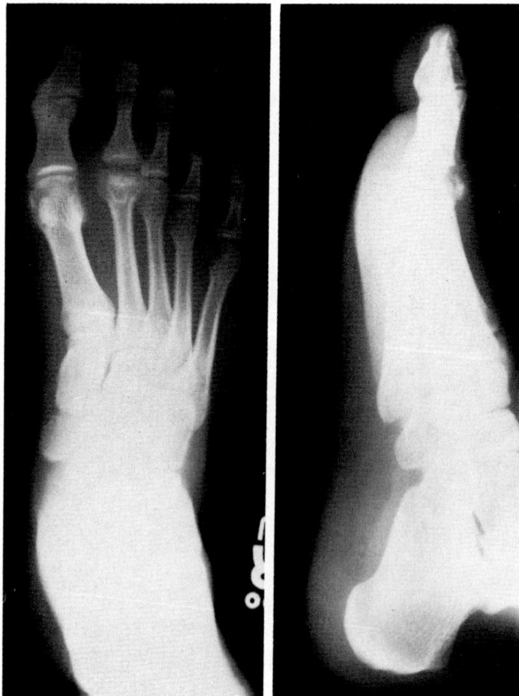

FIG. 21-32. Frieberg's infraction, right second metatarsal head.

be immobilized in a short-leg walking cast for 3 to 4 weeks. If conservative treatment fails, several surgical procedures have been advised, including resection of the metatarsal head, removal of loose bodies, and replacement with a silicone rubber prosthesis.[328,332–334]

KÖHLER'S DISEASE (OSTEOCHONDRITIS OF THE TARSAL NAVICULAR)

Köhler's disease is described as avascular necrosis of the tarsal navicular.[339,340] It is thought that repetitive compressive forces of the immature ossific nucleus leads to fragmentation and loss of blood supply. The navicular is the last tarsal bone to ossify, and it occupies a position at the apex of the longitudinal arch of the foot where it is at constant stress during weightbearing.[341] Some support for this theory is found in the fact that Köhler's disease is more common when navicular ossification is delayed beyond normal.[337] The process is also more common in boys, because the navicular ossifies later in boys than in girls. William and Cowell[343] suggest that the diagnosis of Köhler's disease be made only if the patient is symptomatic, because roentgenographic findings of increased density and fragmentation of the navicular in the asymptomatic foot represent a normal variant of ossification.[336,343] Bipartite tarsal scaphoid has also been described and should not be confused with Köhler's disease, because there is no increased density or collapse.[342]

Clinically, the child presents with pain and swelling in the region of the navicular. The average age of onset in females is 4 years, and, in males, it is 6 years. The onset may be precipitated by an incident of minor trauma following which the child is noted to limp and complain of pain. Two roentgenographic variations are seen (Fig. 21-33). A thin wafer of bone may be present with patchy increased density, giving the suggestion of collapse. In others, the navicular appears to have normal shape with minimal fragmentation and uniform increase in density.

The course is always benign and self-limited. Waugh[341] demonstrated that the navicular receives its blood supply peripherally from a circumferential leash of vessels. Revascularization is rapid, while surrounding reactive tissue and cartilage prevent deformity. Casting with a short-leg cast for a period of 8 weeks or more allows the patient to be pain free in the shortest possible time.[343]

SEVER'S DISEASE (CALCANEAL APOPHYSITIS)

Sever's syndrome is a self-limited apophysitis of the os calcis at the insertion of the Achilles tendon.[345–347] It is associated with pain and tenderness over the posterior aspect of the calcaneus. The condition is aggravated by activity. Increased density and partial fragmentation of the calcaneal apophysis may be noted roentgenographically, but this does not represent avascular necrosis. The heel of the opposite asymptomatic foot may have a similar roentgenographic appearance (Fig. 21-34).

The condition is most common in 6- to 10-year-old males, and treatment is symptomatic. Mild restriction of activities or elevation of the heel of the shoe or arch supports generally affords prompt relief.[344] Heelcord stretching exercises should be instituted to prevent recurrence. In severe cases, a short-leg walking cast may be indicated for 8 weeks duration.

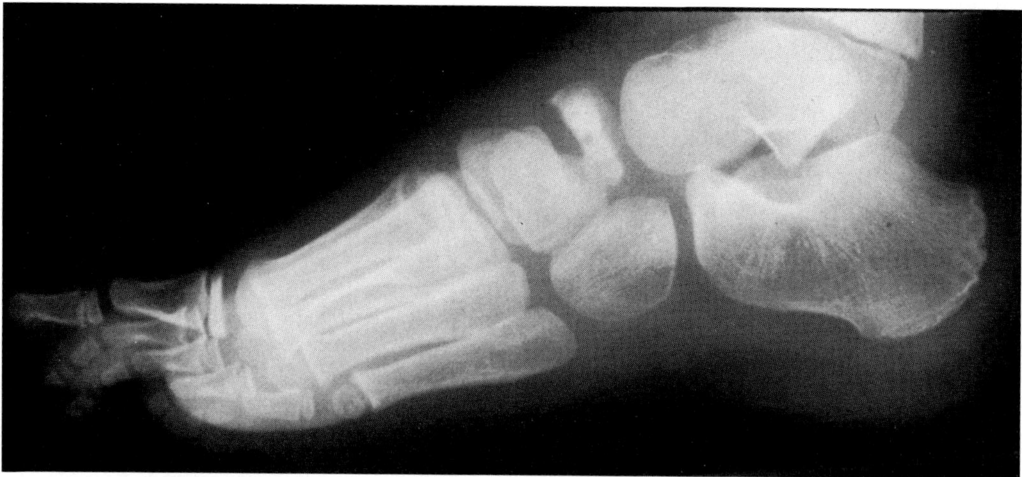

FIG. 21-33. Köhler's disease, showing increased density and collapse of the navicular.

OSTEOCHONDRITIS DISSECANS OF THE TALUS

This is an uncommon entity characterized by an avascular osteochondral fragment of the talus, which may separate from the underlying bone. Lesions of the superior medial aspect of the dome of the talus are most common and may be traumatic or atraumatic in origin. Lesions of the lateral portion of the talar dome are less common and are associated with inversion or inversion-dorsiflexion trauma.[349,351,353,355,356] Repetitive trauma with ischemic changes in the subchondral bone has been implicated in the etiology of osteochondritis dissecans of the talus, just as it has been implicated in osteochondritis affecting other joints.

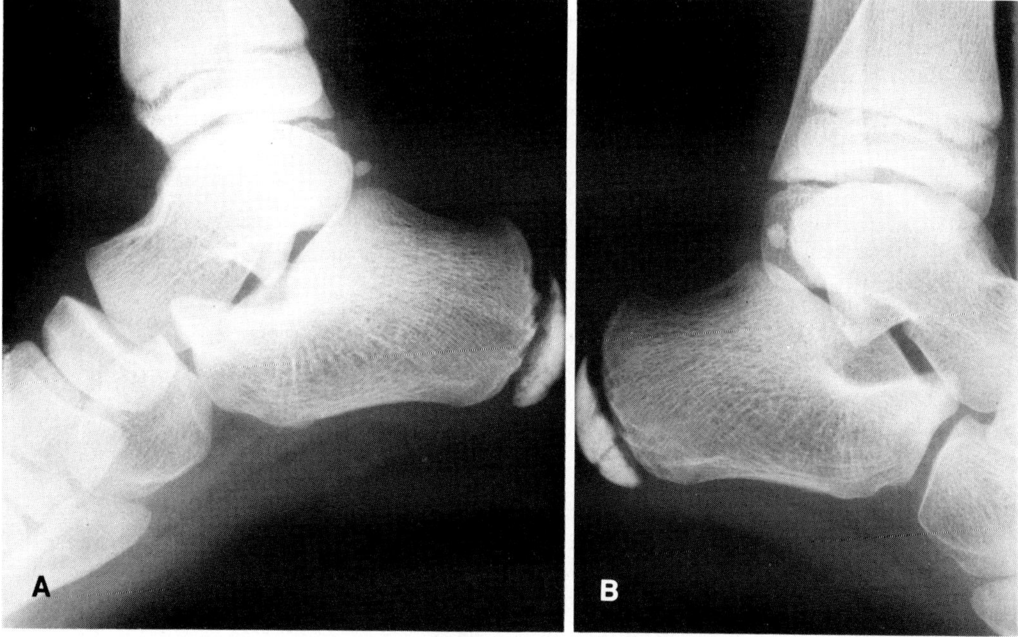

FIG. 21-34. *(A and B)* Apophysitis of the os calcis. There is increased density and partial fragmentation of the apophysis.

Clinically, the patient is usually an adolescent who complains of diffuse discomfort and swelling in the ankle joint.[352,357] The process is more common in males, and there is often a history of trauma. If conventional radiographs do not demonstrate a lesion, anteroposterior roentgenograms of the ankle mortise should be obtained in varying degrees of plantar flexion. CT or technetium scans may be necessary to identify a defect. Arthrography may be helpful in determining looseness of the fragment.[354] Arthroscopic evaluation has also been reported.[348]

If the fragment is not completely detached, treatment consists of immobilization and weight relief in a short-leg cast or patellar tendon weightbearing brace for 3 to 4 months.[350,351] Completely detached medial lesions that remain in the crater should be treated nonoperatively initially, but, if symptoms persist, surgical excision and curettage are indicated. Completely detached lateral lesions and all displaced fragments are best treated by early operation.[351]

At surgery for medial lesions, a transmalleolar approach provides optimal visualization. It is best to perform an oblique osteotomy of the medial malleolus after predrilling and partial insertion of the malleolar screw to facilitate later replacement of the malleolus. Lateral lesions can usually be visualized through an anterolateral approach without osteotomy of the fibula.[351] If the fragment is small or completely detached, it should be removed, and its bed should be curetted. If the articular cartilage is not severely damaged and the fragment is large enough, it should be preserved by pinning the fragment with smooth Kirschner wires. These wires should penetrate the opposite cortex of the talus so that they can be removed after the fragment has united with the underlying bone. Postoperatively, the leg should be immobilized in a short-leg cast until union is complete.

FOREFOOT DEFORMITIES

CONGENITAL DEFORMITIES

Congenital malformations of the forefoot and toes are not uncommon in childhood. Most of the deformities have a familial tendency. In general, toe deformities in children are unresponsive to nonoperative treatment. Some do not progress or cause symptoms in later life. With advancing age, however, the abnormality becomes more fixed while shoes become less accommodating. More severe deformity produces pressure symptoms in adulthood and should be surgically corrected. Examination during weightbearing is essential to help separate significant from insignificant deformity.

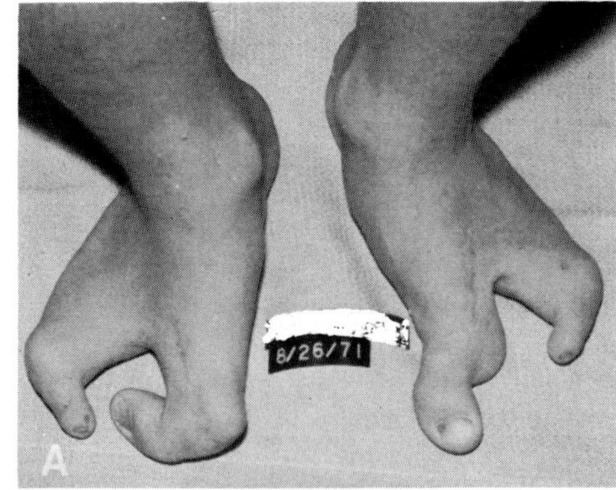

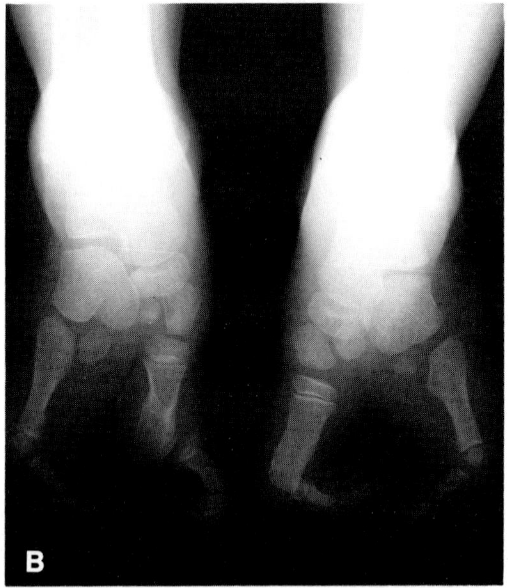

Fig. 21-35. A 9-year-old male with a cleft foot. *(A)* Clinical photograph. *(B)* Roentgenographic views.

Congenital Cleft Foot (Lobster Claw)

Congenital cleft foot is a rare deformity consisting of various combinations of deficiency of the central three rays. The first and fifth rays are often present, and the phalanges of these rays deviate toward the midline cleft (Fig. 21-35). The hindfoot is usually normal.

Cleft foot is generally accompanied by cleft hand or other digital anomalies. Typically, this deformity is bilateral and familial, being inherited as an autosomal dominant trait with incomplete penetrance.[358,362,363,365] Other associated abnormalities such as cleft lip and palate, deafness, and genitourinary tract anomalies have also been noted.[360,363] Because of the coincident development of genitourinary tract and limb buds during embryogenesis, an intravenous pyelogram is indicated in the evaluation of any child with congenital cleft foot.

Several types of correction have been described, depending on the extent of the deficit.[359,361,364,365,367] Onizuka[364,366] described a two-stage procedure that initially closes the defect with a local double-pedicled flap and approximation of the metatarsals with a fascia lata strip. After several weeks, five toes are created from the new central toe and the lateral toes. Cosmesis is improved, although flap lengthening may be required as the child grows. Function is satisfactory. Sumiya and Onizuka[366] recommend that surgery be performed before the child is 1 year of age, because weight-bearing on the uncorrected cleft foot may cause widening of the foot and more severe deformity.

Syndactyly

Syndactyly of the toes as an isolated deformity does not limit function and rarely becomes symptomatic.[369,375] Correction to improve cosmesis is inadvisable. Occasionally, surgery is indicated when multiple digits are webbed or if osseous structures are incompletely separated.

Surgical separation is accomplished by the same technique as that used for syndactyly of the fingers. Skin grafting is required.

Macrodactyly

Gigantism of one or more toes is a rare abnormality but creates a problem in shoe fitting and cosmesis (Fig. 21-36). Any child with localized gigantism should be evaluated to rule out the possibility of neurofibromatosis.[368,371]

Surgical correction is indicated when hypertrophy interferes with adequate shoe wear. To reduce the size of the forefoot or toes, total or partial osteoectomy with resection of an adequate amount of soft tissue should be performed.[370,372,374,376,378] Correction should be accomplished in two or three stages if necessary and should be carefully planned in advance. Epiphysiodesis is helpful in preventing longitudinal growth, but it does not limit circumferential growth.

Polydactyly

Polydactyly is a common malformation that varies widely in extent and is frequently associated with other anomalies. Duplication of the toes occurs more often in blacks than in Caucasians. The familial occurrence of polydactyly is not unusual. Venn-Watson (1976)[377] presented an excellent report on polydactyly of the foot based on a study of 72 patients.

The fibular side of the foot is involved most often.[373] The most common deformity is duplication of the fifth toe, with a Y-shaped metatarsal or a fifth metatarsal with a broad head (Fig. 21-37). Duplications of the hallux, which are less common, are often associated with a short-block first metatarsal.

Treatment consists of surgical excision of the most peripheral toe. If the accessory digit is entirely fleshy, a silk ligature about the base can be applied in the nursery and will accomplish the desired result.

When the duplication involves osseous structures, amputation of the accessory digits should be accomplished between the age of 10 and 15 months. Redundant skin and soft tissue should be excised to reduce the forefoot to normal dimensions. Duplicated metatarsals or bony protrusions of the common metatarsal should be removed. A wide metatarsal head should be narrowed surgically. Accessory tendons should be sutured to the adjacent tendon. The capsule and ligaments of the metatarsophalangeal joint must be carefully reconstructed to prevent varus or valgus deformity of the remaining toe. Polydactyly should be treated early to allow maximum time for remodeling of the foot. Excellent results can be anticipated except for a duplicated hallux with a short first metatarsal.

Congenital Hallux Varus

Congenital hallux varus consists of medial angulation of the great toe at the metatarsophalangeal joint.[386,387] This condition is due to an extra toe anlage in the medial part of the foot, which undergoes a developmental arrest and pulls the great toe into varus.[383] The anlage is frequently evident as a supranumerary bone

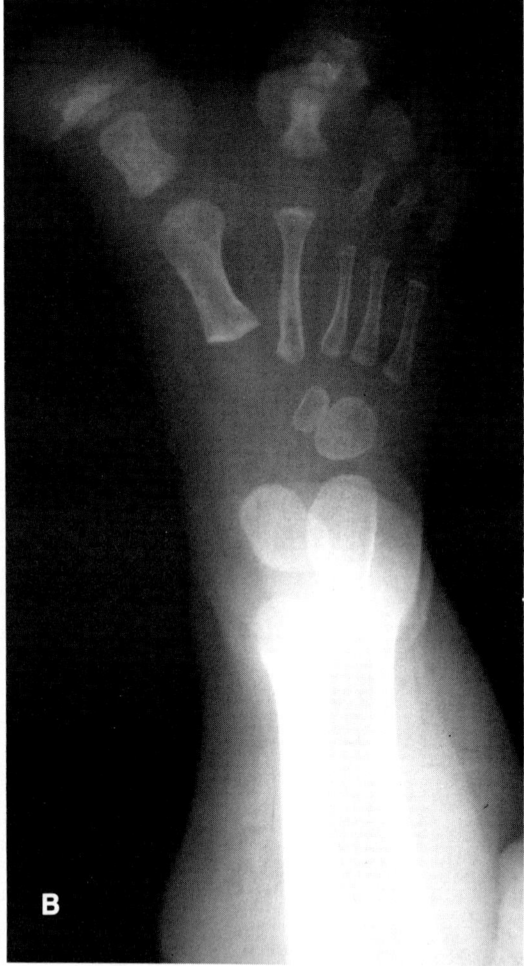

FIG. 21-36. *(A* and *B)* Macrodactyly.

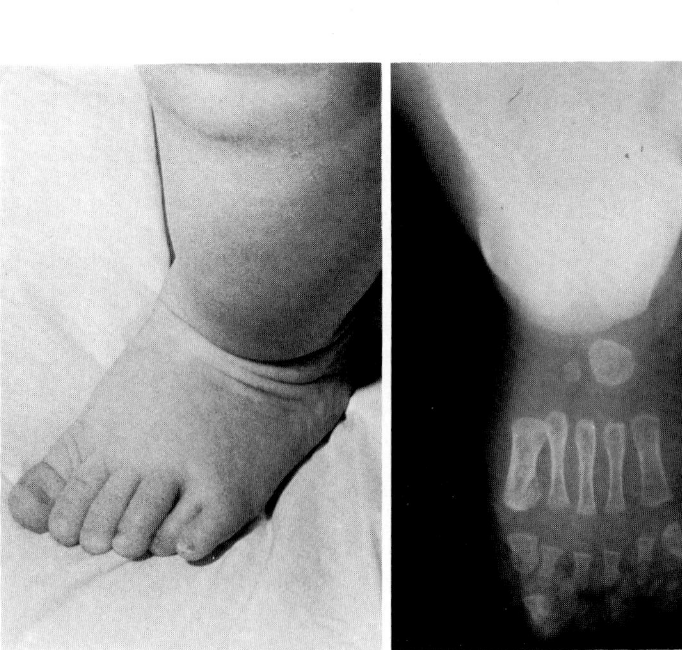

FIG. 21-37. Duplication of the fifth toe in which the proximal phalanx shares a broad fifth metatarsal head.

but may exist as a tight fibrous band. Frequently, the first metatarsal is broad and short. The lateral toes may also be pulled into varus. This congenital malformation, bilateral in 20% of patients, should be differentiated from medial deviation of the great toe associated with hallux varus or metatarsus primus varus.[381,384]

Nonoperative treatment is ineffective. Several authors have described operative procedures, which are best performed between 1 and 2 years of age.[379,380,382,383,385] Correction must include resection of the tethering band or bone, capsulotomy of the metatarsophalangeal joint, and syndactylization of the first to the second toe to prevent recurrence. McElvenny,[383] in addition, used the tendon of the extensor hallucis brevis to reinforce the lateral capsule. Framer[379] designed a rotational skin flap in order to lengthen the tight medial soft tissues. After any surgical correction, the joints should be held in the proper position with a Kirschner wire and cast for 3 weeks, and a cast alone for 3 more weeks.

Adolescent Bunion

Introduction

Although an uncommon problem for the surgeon dealing with children, this is a subject of some debate. There are several terms that are used to describe this problem, including *metatarsus primus varus, metatarsus primus adductus, hallux valgus,* and *adolescent bunion.* Its etiology and treatment remain a topic about which many disagree. Currently, the popularly held concept of metatarsus primus varus being the etiology is not accepted by all. In the early literature, it seems to have been assumed that bunion deformities resulted from improper footwear. It was reasoned that since the problem was seen primarily in the female and since the female often wore shoes that were more stylish than they were physiologic, the cause of the bunion deformity was improper footwear.[395] The concept of abnormal deviation of the first metatarsal has many proponents. Reidle was credited by Kleinberg[405] as being the first to suggest this as the primary problem. One of the earliest references in the English literature to metatarsus primus varus is by Truslow.[417] There have been many authors since who believe that it is etiologically related to adolescent bunion. Lapidus,[407] Kleinberg,[405] Mitchell,[398,410] Durman,[391] Hardy and Clapham,[397] Carr and Boyd,[390] and Bonney and McNab[389] are among those who share this view. Obliquity of the first cuneiform-metatarsal joint was observed by Truslow,[417] Lapidus,[407] Kleinberg,[405] Durman,[391] and Berntsen.[388] Hallux valgus was thought to be primary by Ewald[394] and Piggott.[412] Hiss[400] thought that muscle imbalance was primary.

Phylogenetically, the increased intermetatarsal angle is similar to that of other primates who use their feet for climbing. Hiss,[400] Lapidus,[407] and Truslow[417] have referred to this in their writings. During evolution, the foot had adapted itself from a grasping device to a supporting structure. In so doing, the human foot had to lose some of its mobility. The hallux straightened, and the lesser toes diminished. The hallux of primates resembles the human thumb in its greater range of motion and the larger angle formed by the first and second metatarsals.

Etiology

In an excellent article, Inman[401] made several interesting observations. He makes reference to the work of Wells,[418] who studied the feet of South African natives. He found abduction of the first metatarsal in association with hallux valgus. Engle and Morton[393] found hallux valgus in the West African population. These groups did not wear shoes. Lam Sim-Fook and Hodgson[406] found that 2% of non–shoe-wearing Chinese displayed definite hallux valgus. Inman[401] also describes mechanically the reasons why a pronated foot may develop a hallux valgus deformity. Hiss[400] reviewed 1812 cases involving 3092 bunions. He noted that 60% of his patients had what he termed *everted feet,* 32% had a loss of what was called the *spring arch,* and 82% had what was described as malposition of the arch bones.

Metatarsus Primus Varus. Support for the theory that metatarsus primus varus is the etiology of adolescent bunion deformity has come from several sources. Durman[391] studied 374 feet of 178 adult patients who stated that they had no foot problems. Nine of these patients were found to have significant bunion deformities. In 356 normal feet, the first intermetatarsal angle varied from 0° to 16°, and the metatarsophalangeal joint angle varied from 0° to 20°. He concluded that the ideal normal foot is one in which the first and second metatarsals are parallel and the great toe extends directly forward in the long axis of the first metatarsal. The average normal foot had a metatarsophalangeal angle of 20° and an intermetatarsal angle of 10°.

He then measured 18 feet with hallux valgus. The intermetatarsal angle ranged from 10° to 18° and the metatarsophalangeal angle ranged from 22° to 56°. Another group, consisting of 886 patients, was evaluated. In this group, there were 80 females and 102 males younger than 19 years of age. Twenty females and three males were found to have hallux valgus. Among the four hallux valgus feet in males, two had intermetatarsal angles of 10° or more. In the female group, of the 27 feet, 18, or 66%, had intermetatarsal angles of 10° or more.

There have been other detailed studies of feet with hallux valgus. Hardy and Clapham[397] studied several variables in the foot with hallux valgus. The intermetatarsal angle of 252 controlled feet was noted to range from 0° to 17°, with a mean of 8.5°. In 177 feet examined due to complaints referable to them, the angle ranged from 4° to 27°, with a mean of 13°. This widening of the intermetatarsal angle between these two groups was said to have been statistically significant. Also of interest was that 46% of the 177 had the onset of their symptoms before age 20 years. Thirty percent of these were symptomatic before age 15 years.

Another group, consisting of 125 controls, was examined. There were 73 males and 52 females. The first intermetatarsal angle was 1.3° greater in the females than in the males. This was a statistically significant difference.

Long First Metatarsal. An interesting facet to the work of Hardy and Clapham[397] was the finding that those patients with a high degree of hallux valgus and a low intermetatarsal angle had first metatarsals longer than the second. This difference was significant when compared with those who had a high degree of hallux valgus associated with a widened first intermetatarsal angle.

Cuneiform Variation. Abnormality of the first cuneiform has been discussed by many authors. In a group of Durham's,[391] 28 of 31 hallux valgus feet in adolescents were thought to have cuneiform abnormality. Of his original group of 886 patients, he found that 11% of normals had cuneiform variation and that 47% of those with hallux valgus had cuneiform variation. Ewald[394] in 1912 noted obliquity of the distal articulation of the first cuneiform in hallux valgus. In 1930, Berntsen[388] supported this observation when he reported cuneiform deformity in 67% of hallux valgus feet while noting this in only 6% of normal feet. Others have reported similar findings.[394]

In light of Inman's[401] observations, one wonders whether these variations are on the basis of rotation of the medial cunieform with pronation of the foot.

Os Intermetatarseum. The presence of the rare os intermetatarseum[406] has been described as a possible cause of metatarsus primus varus in some patients.

Associated Disease. Certain generalized diseases have been associated with hallux valgus. Neuromuscular disease, including cerebral palsy, poliomyelitis, and myelodysplasia may have concomitant bunion deformity. Adolescent bunion is also seen with such diverse and unrelated conditions as Sprengel's deformity, multiple osteochondromatosis, hemihypertrophy, juvenile rheumatoid arthritis, and otopalatal-digital syndrome.[416]

Family History

A familial incidence has been found. Johnston[402] studied one family through seven generations and concluded that hallux valgus was an autosomal dominant trait with incomplete penetrance. A family history was found in 63% by Hardy and Clapham[397] and in 58% by Mitchell.[398,410] Bonney and McNab[389] noted an increased incidence of an early onset of symptoms in those with a positive family history.

Anatomy

Haines and McDougall[396] give an excellent description of the anatomy of hallux valgus. Of particular interest was the discussion of the nature of the medial prominence. They credit Lane in 1887 for considering the medial prominence a part of the metatarsal that had originally articulated with a proximal phalanx of the great toe, and not a new growth. This area had lost contact with the articular cartilage of the proximal phalanx as it deviated laterally. The cartilage became soft and inelastic, losing its white color. In 1881, Anderson presented a cadaver preparation in which the great toe formed a right angle with the long axis of the first metatarsal. He found tissue destruction rather than new formation in the region of the medial prominence. Work by Payr in 1894 and Hewbach in 1897 supported Lane's theory. Stein in 1938 stated that the medial prominence was not an exostosis.

In mild cases, the cartilage over the eminence is well preserved but late; the eminence may even lose its cortical layer, exposing an uneven surface of spongy bone.

The sagittal groove was ascribed to pressure of the margin of the phalanx by Clarke in 1900 and Jordan and Brodsky in 1951. Hanes and McDougall[396] believe that it is more likely that it is formed by degeneration of the cartilage where cartilage-to-cartilage contact has been lost. The weakness of the bony trabeculae deep to the groove and their arrangement parallel to the surface suggest that the groove is a region of minimal pressure and that it is a fossa nudata due to lack of adequate stimulation rather than an erosion due to access.

Clinical Features

A patient may present in adolescence with painful feet. On examination, a prominent first metatarsal head with lateral deviation of the great toe is observed. When standing, these deformities are increased, and there is a widening of the forefoot. Secondary problems are related to hammertoe deformities and painful PIP joints, inflammation of the bursa overlying the first metatarsal head, and metatarsalgia involving the lesser metatarsals.

Symptomatic adolescent hallux valgus is different from that seen in the adult in several ways: (1) The degree of valgus of the great toe is usually less; (2) there are no arthritic changes in the metatarsophalangel joint; (3) the bursa overlying the medial prominence is not chronically thickened; and (4) frequently, epiphyseal plates are still viable, and further longitudinal growth is possible.[416]

Roentgenographic Features

Films are made with the patient standing in order to allow standard measurement of the first intermetatarsal angle. Intermetatarsal angles in excess of 10° are considered to be increased and to represent metatarsus primus varus (Fig. 21-38). The sesamoid bones are observed on standing anteroposterior roentgenogram to be laterally displaced, although, as Inman[401] has pointed out, this may only represent rotation of the first metatarsal. In advanced problems, the congruity of the metatarsophalangeal joint may become interrupted.

Treatment

Conservative management. Such treatment of the symptomatic foot includes footwear that properly fits the width of the forefoot. This may necessitate the purchasing of a shoe with a wider forefoot than hindfoot sections. One might also consider the use of a scaphoid pad if there is a loss of the longitudinal arch and heel wedges if there is excessive heel valgus.

Surgical Treatment. Indications for surgery include pain, failure to respond to proper shoes, difficulty obtaining proper shoes, and cosmesis.

Surgical procedures should be individualized. Those patients with metatarsus primus varus should have this corrected by metatarsal osteotomy. This can be done at the base,[405,407,414,417] midshaft[419] or distally.[388,398,410,411] Those who do not have metatarsus primus varus may need less extensive procedures.[395,408,413,445] Resection[404] or interposition[409] arthroplasty would not often be indicated in the adolescent, because degenerative changes are unlikely to be severe enough to warrant these procedures. Arthrodesis of the metatarsophalangeal is rarely to be considered in the adolescent. Ellis[392] has recommended stapling of the lateral portion of the first metatarsal growth plate. This would not seem to be a good choice in view of the difficulty with epiphyseal stapling done in more accessible areas. The Joplin[403] procedure is complicated but has given its proponents satisfactory results.

The authors favor either the Mitchell[389,398,410] or Wilson[419] procedures. The reader is referred to the original descriptions of the operative technique for details. These procedures have proved reliable (Figs. 21-39, 21-40). Postoperative care can be facilitated by the use of a toe spica cast. This is applied over the forefoot to include the great toe, using one roll of 2-inch plaster.

Operative correction should be delayed until skeletal maturity because there is the possibility of recurrence of the deformity if the procedure is performed before closure of the growth plates.

Complications. One must not underestimate these procedures. Bonney and McNab[389] reviewed the operative results in 54 adolescents. Twelve were in need of further surgery. In 34 of 54 feet operated upon, the metatarsus primus varus returned to its original state or to a larger intermetatarsal angle than before surgery. When permanent correction was obtained, the results were better. They concluded that primary failure may result from: (1) simple

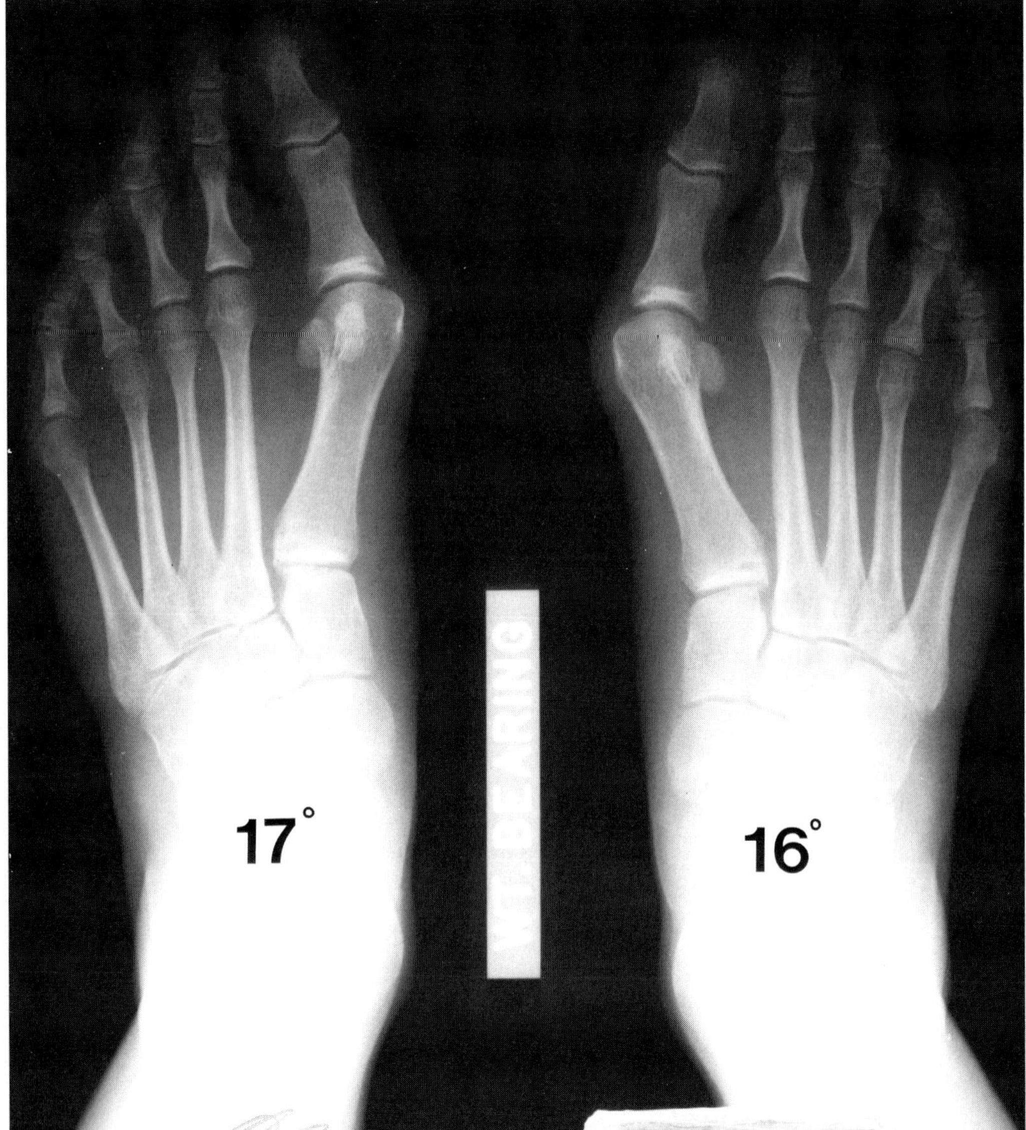

FIG. 21-38. Roentgenograms of the feet of a symptomatic 14-year-old female. Note the widened first intermetatarsal angle.

failure to swing the first metatarsal toward the second; (2) obtaining a "false" correction by soft-tissue compensation, with subsequent swinging out of the first metatarsal or removal of plaster; and (3) producing correction by swinging the proximal end of the first metatarsal medialward instead of having the distal end lateralward. Failure of maintenance of the initial correction was thought to be related to: (1) too early weightbearing, (2) inadequate immobilization during the critical period, and (3) osteotomy of the first metatarsal distal to a growing epiphysis with further bone growth occuring in a varus direction with consequent early recurrence of the deformity. In 14 feet that had good primary correction by osteotomy distal to the first metatarsal growth plate, 10 had recurrence. In 20 feet operated upon after the growth plate had closed that showed good results, 9 recurred. Other causes of failure, as cited by Bonney and McNab,[389] include: (1) operative production of an elevated or a de-

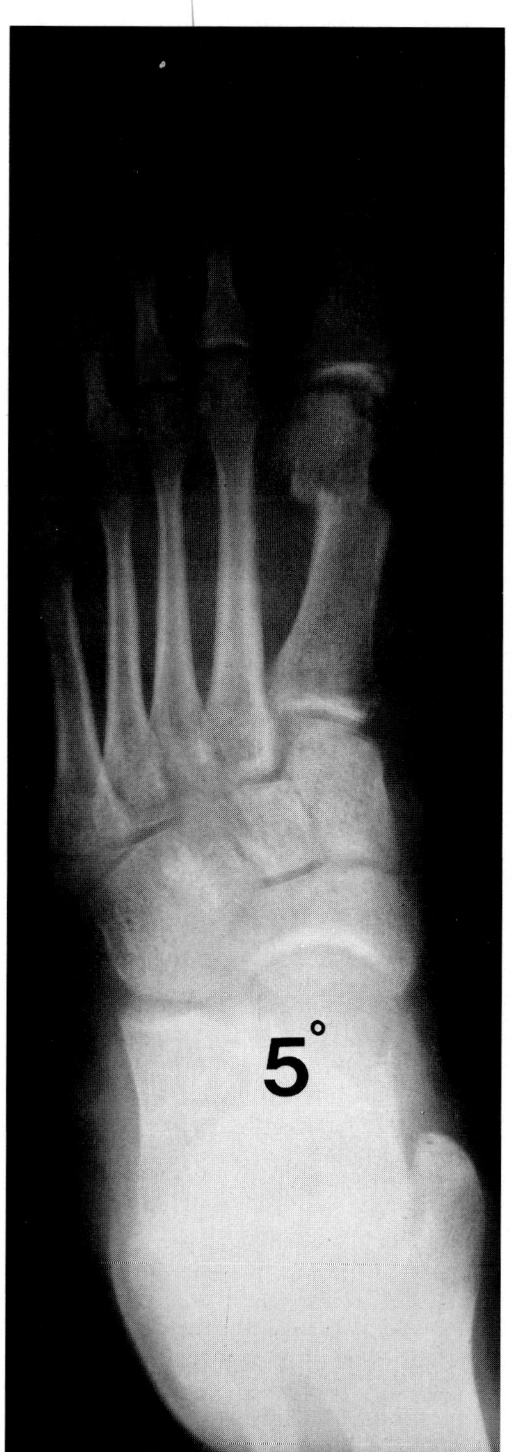

FIG. 21-39. Postoperative Mitchell bunionectomy showing a reduced intermetatarsal angle.

pressed first metatarsal; (2) long continued postoperative stiffness of the first metatarsophalangeal joint; (3) careless trimming of the medial prominence with a consequent increase of the hallux valgus; (4) failure to obtain correction of the hallux valgus due to unrelieved soft-tissue contracture; and (5) overcorrection of the metatarsus primus varus combined with trimming of the medial prominence, leading to medial subluxation of the first metatarsophalangeal joint.

Congenital Short First Metatarsal (Metatarsus Atavicus)

Congenital short first metatarsal is presented here only to point out that the condition is a variation of normal.[420] In 1927, Morton[422] described metatarsus atavicus (congenital short first metatarsal) as a specific cause of metatarsalgia. More recently, Viladot[423] revived the concept of first ray insufficiency due to short first metatarsal. Theoretically, metatarsalgia is due to increased weightbearing by the second metatarsal. The forefoot pronates so that more weight is borne on the first metatarsal. This pronation lowers the longitudinal arch and contributes to the metatarsalgia.

However, Harris and Beath[421] questioned this hypothesis and stated that the short first metatarsal can bear its share of weight simply by increased flexion at the metatarsotarsal joint. In a foot survey of the Canadian Army, Harris and Beath roentgenographically examined more than 7000 individual feet. They found that approximately 40% of these individuals had a short first metatarsal. In this group, there was no increased incidence of pes planus, callus formation, thickening of the second metatarsal, or foot symptoms due to strenuous activity.

Congenital Overriding of the Fifth Toe

This is a familial problem in which the fifth toe is in varus and overlaps the fourth toe. The capsule of the metatarsophalangeal joint is contracted, the extensor tendon is shortened, and there is a contracted band of skin between the fourth and fifth toes. The condition causes symptoms in approximately half of the feet involved.

Nonoperative treatment consisting of passive stretching of the little toe into plantar flexion and abduction is generally unsuccessful

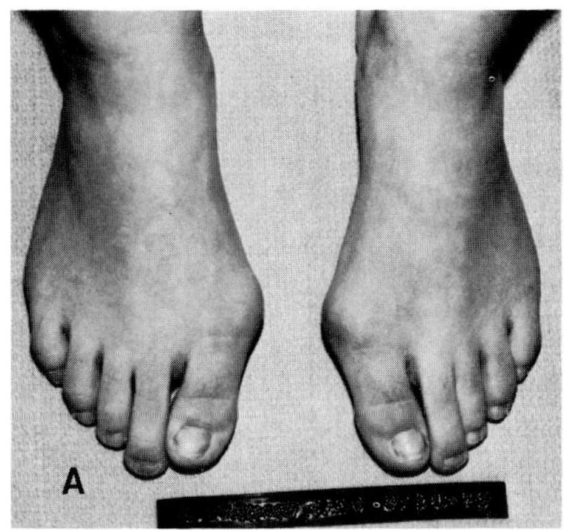

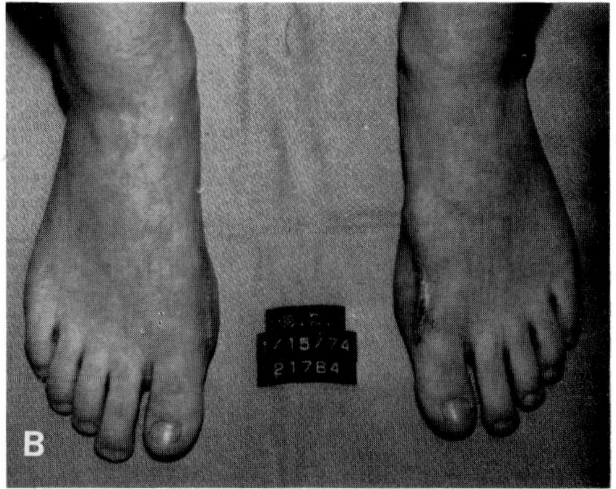

FIG. 21-40. Adolescent bunion, pre- and postoperatively. *(A)* Preoperative; *(B)* postoperative.

but may be used preoperatively or in infancy to decrease contracture. Splinting and taping have likewise been unsuccessful.[431] If symptoms warrant, operative correction is indicated. Several procedures have been described for the correction of the overriding fifth toe.

Lantzounis (1940)[429] recommended severing the extensor digitorum longus of the fifth toe and suturing it to the head of the fifth metatarsal. Lapidus (1942)[430] described a procedure in which the long extensor tendon of the fifth toe is severed proximally at the middle of the fifth metatarsal. The distal end of the tendon is drawn down to a second incision on the dorsal medial aspect of the fifth toe. Capsulotomy of the metatarsophalangeal joint is performed. Then the stump of the tendon is rerouted under the plantar aspect of the proximal phalanx and sutured to the abductor digiti quinti tendon under enough tension to correct the deformity.

Several procedures have been suggested for release of the extensor tendon and tight dorsal structures with plastic elongation of the skin fold that is created when the deformity is corrected. Goodwin and Swisher[426] recommended Y-advancement with capsulotomy and Z-lengthening of the long extensor tendon. Stamm[438] described a similar procedure but used V-Y advancement for the skin. Wilson[441] and Sharrard[437] also advocate the V-Y advancement in children. DuVries[425] described a similar procedure to Stamm's except "dog-ears" are excised after correction of the deformity. Scrase,[436] however, was dissatisfied with plastic elongation of the skin contracture and noted recurrence in a few cases.

Cockin[424] described an operation devised by R. W. Butler. This consists of a radical release of the metatarsophalangeal joint through a racket-shaped incision around the base of the fifth toe. There are both dorsal and plantar handles to the racket. Dorsal and plantar capsulotomies are performed with release of the extensor tendon. Lasting full correction of the deformity was obtained in 91% of 70 procedures. Tachdjian[439] has also found this procedure to be satisfactory.

McFarland (1950)[433] resected the base of the proximal phalanx and produced a surgical syndactyly between the fourth and fifth toes. Scrase[436] used this procedure in 42 patients with 39 good results. Leonard and Rising,[431] Kelikian,[428] and Tachdjian[439] have also advocated McFarland's procedure.

Proximal phalangectomy has been proposed by Ruiz-Mora[435] and others (Fig. 21-41). Ruiz-Mora described a plantar approach with excision of an elliptical segment of skin. The flexor tendons are severed and allowed to retract. Janecki and Wilde[427] recently reported results of 31 Ruiz-Mora procedures in patients followed for an average of 3½ years. All patients had complete correction of the deformity and relief of symptoms. However, 23% developed a painful prominent fifth metatarsal head on a bunionette deformity, and, in 32% symptomatic hammertoe deformity of the fourth toe developed. Based on their observation, Janecki and Wilde recommended resection of only the head and neck of the proximal phalanx. Sharrard[437] advised against excision of the proximal phalanx in children because of its effect on the growth of the little toe.

The authors believe that congenital overriding of the fifth toe is often asymptomatic and requires no treatment. When symptoms occur, surgery is indicated. Surgical correction is generally successful, and the procedures most widely used are those described by Ruiz-Mora[435] and McFarland.[433]

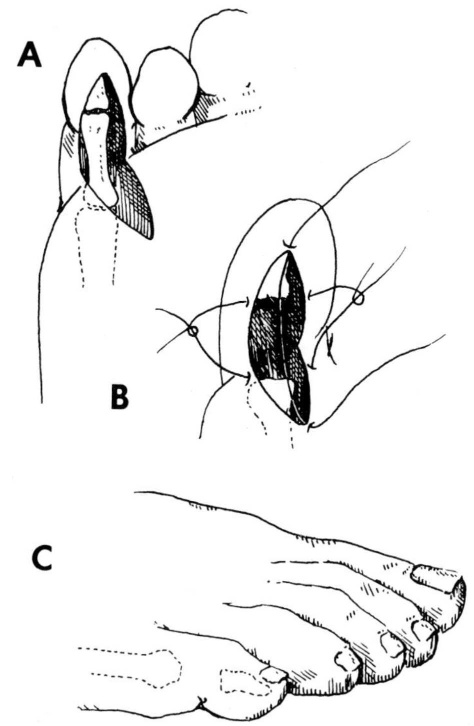

FIG. 21-41. Two methods of correcting congenital overriding of the fifth toe. *(A, B, and C)* the Ruiz-Mora procedure as described by Janecki and Wilde. (Redrawn from Janecki C, Wilde AH: Results of phlangectomy of the fifth toe. J Bone Joint Surg 58A:1005, 1976, and redrawn from Kelikian H: Hallux Valgus. Allied Deformities of the Forefoot and Metatarsalgia, p 328. Philadelphia, WB Saunders, 1965)

Congenital Curly Toes

This is the most common congenital deformity of the lesser toes. Usually mild, bilateral, and symmetrical, the abnormality consists of plantar flexion, varus deviation, and supination of the lateral two, three, or four toes. The terminal pulp may lie under the adjacent medial toe, resulting in abnormal pressure and callus formation under the adjacent medial metatarsal head.

The deformity, frequently familial, is present at birth and remains supple until adolescence. In infancy, Giannestras[442] recommends strapping the deformity between adjacent toes. Sweetnam[447] noted that 25% of 50 affected feet improved whether treated or untreated and the remainder did not respond to nonoperative methods. At an average age of 13 years, none of Sweetnam's patients were symptomatic. Therefore, most patients require no treatment. When the curly toe impinges on its adjacent toe, symptoms are likely to ensue after maturity, especially in women who wear tight shoes. For these unusually advanced deformities, surgical intervention is indicated.

Sharrard recommends transfer of the flexor digitorum longus to the lateral aspect of the extensor hood, as described by Girdlestone and Taylor.[448] This procedure can be performed at any age after 1 year. In older children, when the deformity is more rigid, Sharrard[445] recommends green-stick osteotomy of the middle phalanx of the toe as an adjunct to the tendon transfer.

Kelikian[443] recommended surgical syndactaly of the curly toe to a normal adjacent toe. In older adolescents and adults, he recommends partial proximal phalangectomy and syndactaly. Trethowan[449] advocated excision of the proximal interphalangeal joint with division of the extensor tendon. Specht[446] recommended wedge excision of the bone and joint at the apex of the curvature.

Giannestras[442] described a simpler procedure for children between the ages 2 and 12 years. He attributed this procedure to Eric Price of Melbourne, Australia. It consists of simple tenotomy of both flexor tendons through a longitudinal plantar incision. Pollard and Morrison[444] recently reported results of flexor tenotomy of 56 toes in 20 children. All maintained full passive range of motion and had cosmetic improvement with no disability at follow-up. They compared these results to 63 Girdlestone-Taylor procedures.[448] After the latter procedure, 58% had a stiff metatarsophalangeal joint and less than satisfactory cosmetic improvement.

In the authors' experience, surgical correction in childhood is only rarely indicated, but flexor tenotomy is preferred when the deformity is passively correctable. In adolescents with rigid deformity, resection arthrodesis of the PIP joint is performed.

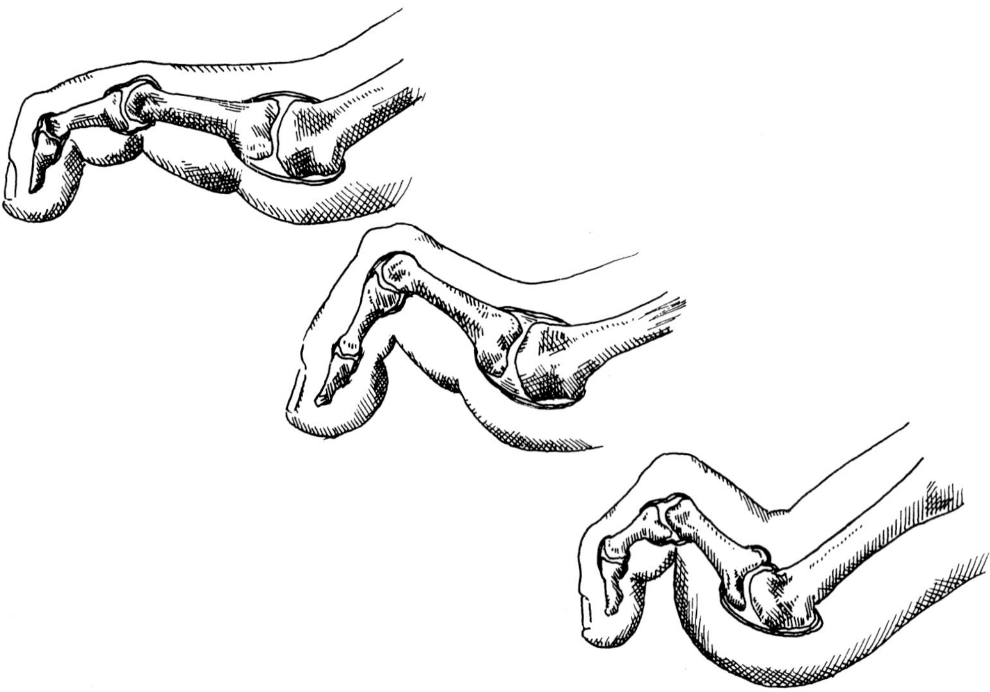

FIG. 21-42. *(Top left to bottom right)* A mallet toe with flexion deformity at the distal interphalangeal joint, a hammer toe with flexion contracture at the proximal interphalangeal joint, and a claw toe with flexion contractures of both interphalangeal joints and an extension contracture of the metatarsophalangeal joint. (Redrawn from Chuinard E, Baskin M: Clawfoot deformity. J Bone Joint Surg 55A:356, 1973)

CONGENITAL MALLET TOE

This congenital deformity consists of marked flexion at the distal interphalangeal joint, resulting from failure of development of the intrinsic extensor mechanism (Fig. 21-42). Only one or two toes are affected. The web space between the affected toes and normal adjacent toes is frequently shallow. Mallet toe is asymptomatic in childhood but develops a painful callus on the distal end of the toe in adolescence. An attempt should be made to differentiate this from the acquired mallet toe, which is rarely seen in childhood and results from ill-fitting shoes. Acquired deformity generally results in hammertoe rather than mallet-toe. Surgical correction, best performed after the age of 12 years, consists of resection arthrodesis of the distal interphalangeal joint.

ACQUIRED FOREFOOT DEFORMITIES

Acquired deformities of the forefoot are more common in adults than in children. The role of shoe wear in production or prevention of deformity is controversial. Only Sim-Fook and Hodgson have compared the feet of shod and unshod members of the same population. The relative incidence of various deformities reported by Sim-Fook and Hodgson are shown in Table 21-4. There is little doubt that restrictive, ill-fitting shoes can cause deformity and pain. However, many disorders have a familial tendency and suggest a genetic predisposition.

ADOLESCENT HALLUX RIGIDUS

Adolescent hallux rigidus is characterized by gradual onset of pain and limitation of dorsiflexion of the metatarsophalangeal joint of the great toe. Plantar flexion motion is often normal. Pain is present at toe-off and occurs with each step. Unilateral involvement is not uncommon.[468] Ages range from 12 to 20 years. Shoes with high heels are poorly tolerated, which may account for the female predominence.[451,468] Radiographs may reveal narrowing of the articular cartilage, osteophyte formation, and subchondral cyst formation. The most likely etiology is acute or repetitive

Table 21-4. Incidence of Foot Deformities in the Chinese Population

DEFORMITY	INCIDENCE IN SHOE-WEARING GROUP (%)	INCIDENCE IN UNSHOD GROUP (%)
Hallux valgux	33	1.9
Hallux rigidus	17	10.3
Overlapping fifth toe	14.4	3.7
Hammertoe	11	4.7
Flatfoot	10.1	7.5
Short first metatarsal	7.0	16.8
Metatarsus lactus	7.0	38
Metatarsus primus varus	6.0	24.3
Hypermobile metatarsus	0.9	13.1

trauma. However, foot shape may predispose certain patients to trauma. Patients with adolescent hallux rigidus usually have a long slender foot with an elongated first metatarsal.[468,469,471] Nilsonne[468] observed that the first metatarsal is longer than the second in 81.2% of the patients with adolescent hallux rigidus, but this variation was present in only 34.4% of 497 normal controls. Bonney and MacNab[451] noted that 50% of adolescent patients have a positive family history, whereas only 10% of adults with hallux rigidus have a positive family history. Other authors[450,464] believe that improper shoe wear exacerbates the condition. Pronation of the foot has been another frequent finding in patients with adolescent hallux rigidus, but the etiologic relationship is unclear.

Nonoperative treatment consists of properly fitted shoes of adequate length and breadth for the toes. A rigid sole or rocker-bottom sole may alleviate discomfort. Giannestras,[453] on the advice of F. R. Thompson, recommended intermittent home traction using a Chinese finger-trap for suspension. Despite conservative measures, surgical intervention is often necessary.

Cheilectomy has been advocated by several authors.[452,462,468] Mann, Coughlin and DuVries[462] recommended resection of proliferative bone at the metatarsophalangeal joint to allow for at least 45° of passive dorsiflexion. They reported satisfactory results in 20 patients with an average follow-up of 67.6 months.

Extension osteotomy at the base of the proximal phalanx[451,457,465] is often successful when dorsiflexion is limited but plantar flexion is normal. This converts the full range of plantar flexion to a functional range of dorsiflexion and plantar flexion. Prior to cessation of growth, the osteotomy should be performed through the neck of the first metatarsal[464,470] to avoid injury to the physis of the proximal phalanx.

Arthrodesis of the first metatarsophalangeal joint has been widely recommended.[451,454,455,459,462,467] This treatment, however, is unacceptable to most patients, particularly women who prefer variable heel heights. The authors agree with Mann and Oates[461] who recommend this procedure for patients with rheumatoid arthritis, muscle imbalance of the metatarsophalangeal joint, or as a salvage procedure when previous surgery has failed.

Resection arthroplasty,[451,456,460,466,469] silastic interposition arthroplasty,[472] and other procedures[452,469,471] have also been used, but they may not be successful in the adolescent age group.

HAMMERTOE

Hammertoe deformity was originally described by Blum (1883)[473] to include dorsiflexion of the metatarsophalangeal joint and plantar flexion of the proximal interphalangeal joint (Fig. 21-42). This deformity may be congenital or acquired. Growing children with hammertoe deformity can be managed by flexor-to-extensor tendon transfer.[481,483]

More often hammertoe deformity of the second toe is acquired and associated with hallux valgus.[482] Hallux valgus and overlapping second toe should be corrected at the same time. If the metatarsophalangeal joint of the second toe is not subluxed or dislocated, resection arthrodesis of the proximal interphalangeal joint as described by Jones[477] should be performed. When the metatarsophalangeal joint is subluxed or dislocated, Giannestras[476] recommends proximal interphalangeal arthrodesis combined with resection of the base of the proximal phalanx. These more severe deformities may also be treated by resection of the base of the proximal phalanx and surgical syndactylization, as described by Kelikian.[478]

Hammering of the third and fourth toes is less common but is treated in the same way as deformity of the second toe.[474,479,480,484]

Other procedures have been proposed for correction of hammertoe. Proximal phalangectomy has been advocated for severe deformity. This is, however, unnecessary and leaves a short useless toe. Cahill and Connor,[475] in a long-term follow-up of 74 patients with proximal phalangectomy, reported that 50% of the patients had objectively poor results and 25% were dissatisfied.

Clawtoes

In true clawing of the toes, the metatarsophalangeal joints are extended, and both interphalangeal joints are flexed. In contrast to hammertoe, which may involve only one or two toes, clawtoe deformity usually affects all the lesser toes and may involve the great toe. It is not seen before the age of 3 years and is unusual before the age of 7 years. Clawtoes are rarely symptomatic before the age of 10 years.

Clawing is usually associated with pes cavus and is frequently a manifestation of underlying neurologic disease. The theories regarding pathogenesis of clawing parallel those of pes cavus. DuVries[486] clearly demonstrated in cadavers that clawing results from simultaneous tension on long flexor *and* long extensor tendons.

In children, before the deformity becomes fixed, treatment should be directed toward the underlying disease. When varus or valgus are present, tendon transfer should be performed to restore balance to the foot. Other soft-tissue procedures may be indicated to retard the development of pes cavus (see pes cavus and Chapter 8).

Several soft-tissue procedures have been described for supple clawtoes. Forrester-Brown (1938)[487] described transfer of the flexor sublimus tendons into the extensor tendon for clawing of the great toe. Taylor[494] credited Girdlestone with the transfer of the flexor profundus tendon into the dorsal expansions of the extensor tendons. Taylor reported 50 good results in 68 patients. Pyper,[493] however, reported only 50% good results using the same procedure. Parrish[492] described a dynamic correction for clawtoes. The long flexor tendon is released distally and split longitudinally. The split tendon is then passed along each side of the midportion of the proximal phalanx. The halves are sutured together over the dorsum of the phalanx to create a sling, which flexes the metatarsophalangeal joint. Parrish[492] reported 40 good results in 46 procedures. The authors have not had experience with these procedures and prefer extensor tendon release or transfer to the metatarsal neck, combined with capsulotomy of deformed joints.

In general, soft-tissue procedures on the toes are not warranted in children who have supple deformity, and the procedures are ineffective in those with rigid deformity.

Rigid clawtoes are generally seen in older children. After allied deformities are corrected, clawing should be relieved by resection arthrodesis of the proximal interphalangeal joint and transfer of the long extensor tendon to the metatarsal neck. Other procedures have also been described for fixed clawing.[485,487–489,491] The authors have had no experience with these other procedures and have had satisfactory results after PIP joint arthrodesis and extensor tendon transfer.

ABNORMALITIES OF SKIN AND NAILS

VERRUCA PLANTARIS (PLANTAR WARTS)

Plantar warts are common lesions seen in children and adolescents. This condition should be distinguished from plantar keratosis. Generally, verrucae do not occur directly under the metatarsal heads and are painful to lateral pinch, whereas plantar keratosis is painful to direct pressure but not to pinch. A typical verruca is also circumscribed with either an oval or circular outline.

Plantar warts are histologically similar to warts found on other parts of the body except that the pressure of weightbearing causes them to become flattened. The etiology is viral.

Several modes of treatment have been advocated, including oral vitamin A, injection, irradiation therapy, psychotherapy, cautery, curettage, cryotherapy, and surgical excision. By whatever method, an attempt should be made to remove the lesion from the foot without scarring. Small lesions can be padded or ignored and occasionally resolve spontaneously. Larger, persistent, or painful lesions should be treated.

Caustic or keratolytic agents are poorly tolerated by children and should not be used. The simplest method of treatment involves the application of liquid nitrogen. When applying the liquid nitrogen, one must be certain to freeze the central core of the lesion.

If the lesion recurs, curettage should be performed. To do this, the foot is prepared and draped in a surgical field. Local Xylocaine is used as an anesthetic. The keratinized surface of the wart should be pared down with a #15 blade. The natural cleavage plane between the verruca and normal skin is then identified. A small, sharp curet is inserted into this plane, and the verruca may be enucleated with gentle pressure. After the lesion has been removed, the edges are trimmed slightly and a sterile dressing is applied. This gentle removal heals rapidly and seldom results in recurrence or scarring.

INGROWN TOENALIS

Ingrown toenails have been reported in infancy[496] but are much more common in the adolescent age group. The problem is usually initiated by trauma, improper shoe pressure, or improper nail cutting. Once penetration of an edge of the nail has begun, mechanical irritation causes hypertrophy of the nail fold with subsequent infection and formation of granulation tissue. The great toe becomes progressively swollen, tender, and reddened.

In the early stages of inflammation, treatment should be directed toward preserving the nail. This consists of elevation, soaks, and antibiotics. Gently inserting a few strands of cotton in the nail groove and underneath the tip of the nail may permit the nail to grow out

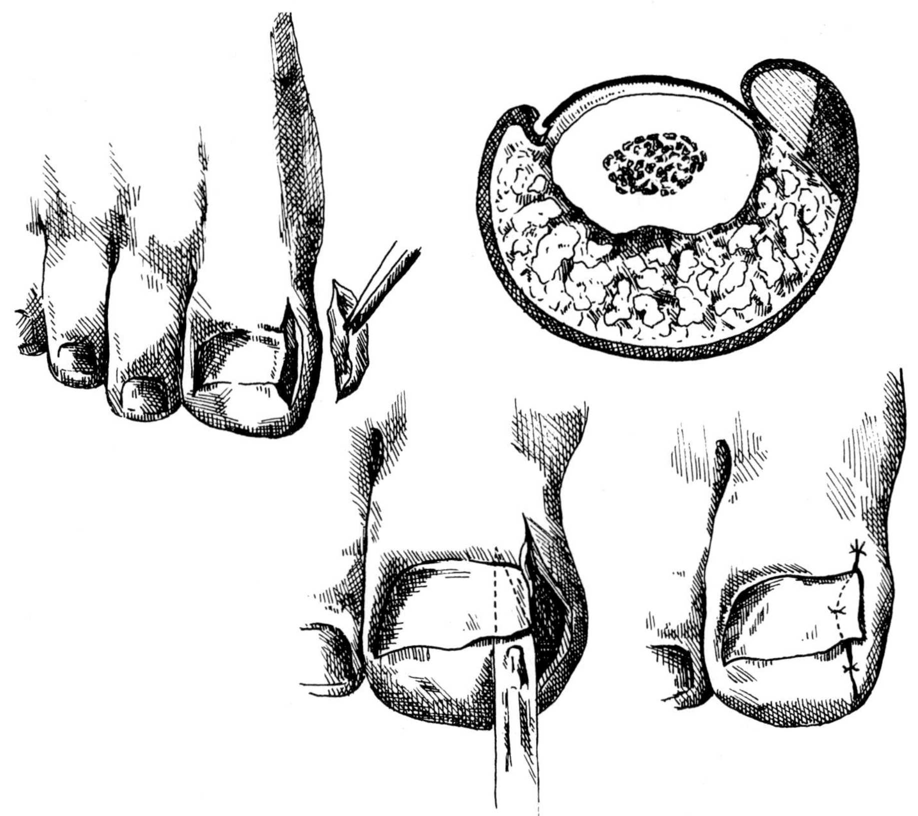

FIG. 21-43. Excision of hypertrophic nail lip and underlying fat, as described by DuVries. (Redrawn from DuVries HL: Disorder of the skin and toenails. In Inman VT (ed): DuVries' Surgery of the Foot, 3rd ed, pp 212, 213. St Louis, CV Mosby, 1973)

beyond the tip of the nail grove. Daily warm soaks are also recommended.

When infection is advanced, removal of the nail should be performed for control of the infection. No attempt should be made to perform definitive surgery on an infected toe. After the infection has subsided, the nail should be allowed to grow back.

If ingrowing recurs or if the nail is stunted and irregular, additional surgical procedures may be necessary. The simplest method of surgery involves elliptical excision of the hypertrophied nail lip and underlying fat, as described by DuVries[498] (Fig. 22-43). The lateral margin of the nail is then elevated, and the skin edge is sutured underneath the free nail margin (Fig. 21-43). Numerous other procedures have been described.[497]

REFERENCES

Structure and Function

1. Acton RK: Surgical anatomy of the foot. J Bone Joint Surg 49A:555, 1967
2. Basmajian JV, Stecko G: The role of muscles in arch support of the foot; an electromyographic study. J Bone Joint Surg 45A:1184, 1963
3. Ben-Menachem Y, Butler JE: Arteriography of the foot in congenital deformities. J Bone Joint Surg 56A:1625, 1974
4. Cunningham DJ: Text Book of Anatomy. London, Oxford University Press, 1953
5. Forster A: Considerations sur l'attitudes des orteils chez l'homme. Arch Anat Histol Embryol 7:247, 1927
6. Frazer JE: The Anatomy of the Human Skeleton. London, Churchill, 1920
7. Gardner E, Gray DL, O'Rahally R: The prenatal development of the skeleton and joints of the human foot. J Bone Joint Surg 41A:847, 1959
8. Gray H: Anatomy of the Human Body, 27th ed. Goss CM (ed).
9. Hicks JH: The mechanics of the foot. J Anat 87:345, 1953
10. Hollinshead WH: Anatomy for Surgeons, Vol 3. New York, Hoeber, 1958
11. Jones FW: Structure and Function as Seen in the Foot. London, Bailliere, Tindall and Cox, 1944
12. Kelekian H: Hallux Valgus, Allied Deformities of the Foot and Metatarsalgia. Philadelphia, WB Saunders, 1965
13. Kite JH: Flatfeet and lateral rotation of legs in young children. J Int Coll Surg 25:77, 1956
14. Kuhns JG: Changes in elastic adipose tissue. J Bone Joint Surg 31A:541, 1949
15. Lovett RW, Cotton FJ: Some practical points in the anatomy of the foot. Boston Med Surg J 139:101, 1898
16. Mann RA: Surgical implications of biomechanics of the foot and ankle. Clin Orthop 146:111, 1980
17. Mann R, Inman VT: Phasic activity of intrinsic muscles of the foot. J Bone Joint Surg 46A:469, 1964
18. Manter JT: Variations of the interosseous muscles of the human foot. Anat Rec 93:117, 1945
19. Smith JW: The ligamentous structures in the canalis and sinus tarsi. J Anat 92:616, 1958
20. Spalteholz W: Hand Atlas of Human Anatomy, 7th English ed. Borkev LF (trans). Philadelphia, JB Lippincott Company, 1957
21. White JW: Torsion of the achilles tendon, its surgical significance. Arch Surg 46:784, 1943
22. Willis TA: Orthopaedic anatomy of the foot and ankle. AAOS Instr Course Lect JW Edwards, 1947

Congenital Talipes Equinovarus

23. Abrams RC: Relapsed clubfoot. The early results of an evaluation of Dillwyn Evans operation. J Bone Joint Surg 51A:270, 1969
24. Adams W: Clubfoot, Its Causes, Pathology, and Treatment. London, Churchill, 1866
25. Addison A, Fixsen JA, Lloyd-Roberts GC: A review of the Dillwyn Evans–type collateral operation in severe clubfeet. J Bone Joint Surg 65–B:12, 1983
26. Attenborough CG: Severe congenital talipes equinovarus. J Bone Joint Surg 48B:31, 1966
27. Barrett JP, Lovell WW: Soft-tissue release for congenital talipes equinovarus. In preparation.
28. Beatson RR, Pearson JR: A method of assessing correction in clubfeet. J Bone Joint Surg 48B:40, 1966
29. Bechtol CO, Mossman HW: Clubfoot. Embryologic study and associated muscle abnormalities. J Bone Joint Surg 32A:827, 1950
30. Bell JF, Grice DS: Treatment of congenital talipes equinovarus with modified Denis Browne splint. J Bone Joint Surg 26:799, 1944
31. Bell PLA, Versfeld GA: Congenital clubfoot: An electromyographic study. J Pediatr Orthop II:139, 1982
32. Ben-Menachem Y, Butler JE: Arteriography of the foot in congenital deformities. J Bone Joint Surg 56A:1625, 1974
33. Berman A, Gartland JJ: Metatarsal osteotomy for the correction of adduction of the forepart of the foot in children. J Bone Joint Surg 53A:498, 1971
34. Böhm M: The embryologic origin of clubfoot. J Bone Joint Surg II:229, 1929
35. Böhm M: Das menschliche bein. Deutsch Orthop 9. Stuttgart, Enke, 1935
36. Bost FC, Schottstaedt ER, Larsen IJ: Plantar dissection. An operation to release the soft tissues in recurrent or recalcitrant talipes equinovarus. J Bone Joint Surg 42A:151, 1960
37. Brockman EP: Congenital Clubfoot (Talipes Equinovarus). Bristol, Wright and Sons, Ltd and New York, Wood and Co, 1930
38. Brockman EP: Modern methods of treatment of clubfoot. Br Med J 2:512, 1937
39. Cowell HR, Wein BK: Current concepts review genetics aspects of clubfoot. J Bone Joint Surg 62A:1381, 1980
40. Dunn N: Stabilizing operations in the treatment of paralytic deformities of the foot. Proc R Soc Med 15:15, 1922
41. Dwyer FC: Osteotomy of the calcaneus for pes cavus. J Bone Joint Surg 41B:80, 1959

42. Dwyer FC: The treatment of relapsed clubfoot by the insertion of a wedge into the calcaneus. J Bone Joint Surg 45B:67, 1963
43. Evans D: Relapsed clubfoot. J Bone Joint Surg 43B: 722, 1961
44. Flincheum D: Pathologic anatomy in talipes equinovarus. J Bone Joint Surg 35A:111, 1953
45. Fried A: Recurrent congenital club foot. The role of the M. tibialis posterior in etiology and treatment. J Bone Joint Surg 41A:243, 1959
46. Garceau GJ: Anterior tibial transposition in recurrent congenital clubfoot. J Bone Joint Surg 22:932, 1940
47. Garceau GJ, Manning KR: Transposition of the anterior tibial tendon in the treatment of recurrent congenital clubfoot. J Bone Joint Surg 29:1004, 1947
48. Garceau GJ, Palmer RM: Transfer of the anterior tibial tendon for recurrent clubfoot. A long-term follow-up. J Bone Joint Surg 49A:207, 1967
49. Garland JJ: Posterior tibial transplant in the surgical treatment of recurrent club foot. A preliminary report. J Bone Joint Surg 46A:1217, 1964
50. Ghali NN, Smith RB, Clayden AD, Silk FF: The result of plantar reduction in the management of congenital talipes equinovarus. J Bone Joint Surg 60–B:1, 1983
51. Gray DH, Katz JM: A histochemical study of muscle in clubfeet. J Bone Joint Surg 63B: 417, 1981
52. Handelsman JE, Badalamente MA: Neuromuscular studies in clubfoot. J Pediatr Orthop I(1):23, 1981
53. Harrold AJ, Walker CJ: Treatment and prognosis in congenital clubfeet. J Bone Joint Surg 65–B:8, 1983
54. Heyman CH, Herndon CH, Strong JM: Mobilization of the tarsometatarsal and intermetatarsal joints for the correction of resistant adduction of the forepart of the foot in congenital clubfoot or congenital metatarsus varus. J Bone Joint Surg 40A:299, 1958
55. Hirsch C: Observations on early operative treatment of congenital club foot. Bull Hosp Joint Dis 21:175, 1960
56. Hofmann AA, Constine RM, McBridge GG, Coleman SS: Osteotomy of the first cuneiform as treatment of residual adduction of the fore part of the foot in clubfoot. J Bone Joint Surg 66A:985, 1984
57. Hoke M: An operation for stabilizing paralytic feet. Am J Orthop Surg 3:494, 1921
58. Ippolito E, Ponseti IV: Congenital clubfoot in the human fetus. A histological study. J Bone Joint Surg 62A:8, 1980
59. Irani RN, Sherman MS: The pathological anatomy of club foot. J Bone Joint Surg 45A:45, 1963
60. Kendrick RE, Sharma NK, Hassler WL, Herndon CH: Tarsometatarsal mobilization for resistant adduction of the forepart of the foot. J Bone Joint Surg 52A:61, 1970
61. Kite JH: Nonoperative treatment of congenital club feet. South Med J 23:337, 1930
62. Kite JH: The surgical treatment of congenital clubfeet. Surg Gynecol Obstet 61:190, 1935
63. Kite JH: Principles involved in the treatment of clubfoot. J Bone Joint Surg 21:595, 1939
64. Kite JH: Congenital metatarsus varus. Report of 300 cases. J Bone Joint Surg 32A:500, 1950
65. Kite JH: Congenital metatarsus varus. AAOS, Instruc Course Lect Ann Arbor, JW Edwards, 1950
66. Kite JH: Some suggestions on the treatment of clubfoot by casts. J Bone Joint Surg 45A:406, 1963.
67. Kite JH: Conservative treatment of the resistant recurrent clubfoot. Clin Orthop 34:25, 1964
68. Kite JH: The Clubfoot. New York, Grune & Stratton, 1964
69. Kite JH: Congenital metatarsus varus. J Bone Joint Surg 49A:388, 1967
70. Kite JH: Errors and complications in treating foot conditions in children. Clin Orthop 53:31, 1967
71. Kite JH: Conservative treatment of the resistant recurrent clubfoot. Clin Orthop 70:93, 1970
72. Larsen EH: Congenital clubfoot. J Bone Joint Surg 45B:620, 1963
73. Lipmann KAW: The Kite method in the treatment of clubfoot. J Bone Joint Surg 33B:463, 1951
74. Lloyd-Roberts GC: Congenital clubfoot. J Bone Joint Surg 46B:369, 1964
75. Lovell WW, Hancock CI: Treament of congenital talipes equinovarus. Clin Orthop 70:79, 1970
76. Lucas LS: Surgical procedures in treatment of chronic clubfoot. West J Surg 56:542, 1948
77. McCauley JC Jr: Surgical treatment of clubfoot. Surg Clin North Am 31:561, 1951
78. McCauley JC Jr: Treatment of clubfoot. AAOS Instruc Course Lect 16:93, 1959
79. McCauley JC Jr: Triple arthrodesis for congenital talipes equinovarus deformities. Clin Orthop 34:25, 1964
80. McCauley JC Jr: Clubfoot. History of the development and the concepts of pathogenesis and treatment. Clin Orthop 44:51, 1966
81. McCauley JC Jr, Lusskin K, Bromley J: Recurrence in congenital metatarsus varus. J Bone Joint Surg 46A:525, 1964
82. McCormick DW, Blount WP: Metatarsus adductus. "Skewfoot." JAMA 141:449, 1949
83. McKay DW: New concept and approach to clubfoot treatment: Section I—Principles and morbid anatomy. J Pediatr Orthop 3:347, 1982
84. Orofino CF: The etiology of congenital clubfoot. Acta Orthop Scand 29:59, 1959
85. Peabody CW, Muro F: Congenital metatarsus varus. J Bone Joint Surg 15:171, 1933
86. Polo GV, Lechtman CP: Surgical treatment of congenital talipes equinovarus adductus. Clin Orthop 70:87, 1970
87. Ponseti IV, Becker JR: Congenital metatarsus adductus. The results of treatment. J Bone Joint Surg 48A:702, 1966
88. Ponseti IV, Smoley EM: Congenital clubfoot: The results of treatment. J Bone Joint Surg 45A:261, 1963
89. Preston ET, Fell TW Jr: Congenital idiopathic clubfeet. Clin Orthop 122:102, 1977
90. Price CT, Lovell WW: Nonoperative treatment of congenital clubfoot. In preparation.
91. Ryöppy S, Sairanen H: Neonatal operative treatment of clubfoot. J Bone Joint Surg 65–B:320, 1983
92. Scott WA, Hosking SW, Catterall A: Clubfoot observations on the surgical anatomy of dorsiflexion. J Bone Joint Surg 66–B:71, 1984
93. Settle FW: The anatomy of congenital talipes equinovarus. Sixteen dissected specimens. J Bone Joint Surg 45A:1341, 1963
94. Simon GW: Analytical radiography of club feet. J Bone Joint Surg 59B:485, 1977
95. Simon GW, Sarrafian S: The microsurgical dissection of a stillborn fetal clubfoot. Clin Orthop 173:275, 1983

96. Smith WA Jr, Campbell PD, Bonnett C: Early posterior ankle release in the treatment of congenital clubfoot. Orthop Clin North Am 7(4):889, 1976
97. Stewart SF: Club foot: Its incidence, cause and treatment. An anatomic-physiologic study. J Bone Joint Surg 33A:577, 1951
98. Turco VJ: Surgical correction of the resistant clubfoot. One-stage posteromedial release with internal fixation. A preliminary report. J Bone Joint Surg 53A:477, 1971
99. Turco VJ: Surgical correction of the resistant congenital clubfoot. One-stage release with internal fixation. The American Academy of Orthopaedic Surgeons Film Library, 1970.
100. Weinstein SL, Ponseti IV, Khoury GY, Ippolito E: A radiographic study of skeletal deformities in treated clubfeet. Orthop Trans 67(3):445, 1983
101. Westin GW: Personal communication, 1970
102. Wiley AM: Clubfoot. An anatomic and experimental study of muscle growth. J Bone Joint Surg 46B:464, 1964
103. Wynne-Davies R: Family studies and the course of congenital club foot. J Bone Joint Surg 46B:445, 1964
104. Wynne-Davies R: Talipes equinovarus. J Bone Joint Surg 46B:464, 1964
105. Wynne-Davies R: Heritable Disorders in Orthopaedic Practice. London, Blackwell, 1973
106. Yip A, Chu YC, Young LY, Ho KC: Congenital foot deformities: A review of 338 patients. J West Pacific Orthop Assoc 20(2):23, 1983

Congenital Metatarsus Varus

107. Berman A, Gartland JJ: Metatarsal osteotomy for the correction of adduction of the forepart of the foot in children. J Bone Joint Surg 53A:498, 1971
108. Bleck EE: Metatarsus adductus: Classification and relationship to outcomes of treatment. J Pediatr Orthop 3:2, 1983
109. Colonna PC: Care of the infant with congenital subluxation of the hip. JAMA 166:715, 1958
110. Ghali NN, Abberton MJ, Silk FF: The management of metatarsus adductus ET supinator. J Bone Joint Surg 66–B:376, 1984
111. Heyman CH, Herndon CH, Strong JM: Mobilization of the tarsometatarsal and intermetatarsal joints for the correction of resistant adduction of the forepart of the foot in congenital clubfoot or congenital metatarsus varus. J Bone Joint Surg 40A:299, 1958
112. Jacobs JE: Metatarsus varus and hip dysplasia. Clin Orthop 16:19, 203, 1960
113. Kendrick RE, Shorman NK, Hassler WL, Herndon CH: Tarsometatarsal mobilization for resistant adduction of the forepart of the foot. J Bone Joint Surg 52A:61, 1970
114. Kite JH: Congenital metatarsus varus. AAOS Instruc Course Lect Ann Arbor. JW Edwards, 1950
115. Kite JH: Congenital metatarsus varus: Report of 300 cases. J Bone Joint Surg 32A:500, 1950
116. Kite JH: Congenital metatarsus varus. J Bone Joint Surg 49A:388, 1967
117. McCauley JC Jr, Lusskin R, Bromley J: Recurrence in congenital metatarsus varus. J Bone Joint Surg 46A:525, 1964
118. McCormick DW, Blount WP: Metatarsus adductovarus, "Skewfoot." JAMA, 141:449, 1949
119. Mitchell G: Personal communication, 1973
120. Mitchell GP: Abductor hallucis release in congenital metatarsus varus. Internat Orthop 3:299, 1980
121. Peabody CW, Muro F: Congenital metatarsus varus. J Bone Joint Surg, 15:171, 1933
122. Ponseti IV, Becker JR: Congenital metatarsus adductus: The results of treatment. J Bone Joint Surg, 48A:702, 1966
123. Thompson SA: Hallux varus and metatarsus varus–a 5-year study. Clin Orthop 16:109, 1960
124. Wynne-Davies R: Family studies and the cause of congenital clubfoot–talipes equinovarus, talipes calcaneovalgus, and metatarsus varus. J Bone Joint Surg 46B:445, 1954

Habitual Toe Walkers (Congenital Short Tendo Calcaneus)

125. Griffin PP, Wheelhouse WW, Shiavi R, Bass W: Habitual toe walkers: A clinical and electromyographic gait analysis. J Bone Joint Surg 59A: 97, 1977
126. Hall JE, Salter RB, Bhalla SK: Congenital Short Tendo Calcaneus. J Bone Joint Surg 49B:695, 1967
127. Sutherland DH, Olshen R, Cooper L, Savio LYW: The development of mature gait. J Bone Joint Surg 62A: 336, 1980

Congenital Vertical Talus

128. Coleman SS, Martin AF, Jarrett J: Congenital vertical talus: Pathogenesis and treatment. J Bone Joint Surg, 48A: 1442, 1966
129. Coleman SS, Stelling FH III, Jarrett J: Congenital vertical talus: Pathomechanics and treatment. Clin Orthop 70:62, 1970
130. Drennan JC, Sharrard WJW: The pathologic anatomy of convex pes valgus. J Bone Joint Surg 53B:455, 1971
131. Eyre-Brook A: Congenital vertical talus. J Bone Joint Surg 49B:618, 1967
132. Grice DS: The role of subtalar fusion in the treatment of valgus deformities of the feet. Ann Arbor, JW Edwards, 16:127, 1950
133. Grice DS: Extra-articular arthrodesis of the subastragalar joints for correction of paralytic flatfeet in children. J Bone Joint Surg 34A:927, 1952
134. Hamanishi C: Congenital vertical talus: Classification with 69 cases and new measurement system. J Pediatr Orthop 4:318, 1984
135. Hark FW: Rocker-foot due to congenital subluxation of the talus. J Bone Joint Surg 34A:344, 1950
136. Harrold AJ: Congenital vertical talus in infancy. J Bone Joint Surg 49B:634, 1967
137. Henken R: Contribution a l'étude des formes osseuses du pied plat valgus congénital. Paris, Thèse de Lyon, 1914
138. Herndon CH, Heyman CH: Problems in the recognition and treatment of congenital convex pes planus. J Bone Joint Surg 45A:413, 1963
139. Heyman CH: The diagnosis and treatment of congenital convex pes valgus or vertical talus. St Louis, CV Mosby, AAOS Instructional Course Lectures 16:117, 1959
140. Hughes JR: Symposium on congenital vertical talus. J Bone Joint Surg 39B:580, 1957
141. Hughes JR: Pathologic anatomy and pathogenesis of

congenital vertical talus and its practical significance. J Bone Joint Surg 52B:777, 1970

142. Jacobsen ST, Crawford AH: Congenital vertical talus. J Pediatr Orthop 3:287, 1983
143. Lamy L, Weismann L: Congenital convex pes valgus. J Bone Joint Surg 21:79, 1939
144. Lloyd-Roberts GC, Spence AJ: Congenital vertical talus. J Bone Joint Surg 40B:33, 1958
145. Mead NC, Anast G: Vertical talus, congenital talonavicular dislocation. Clin Orthop 21:198, 1961
146. Osmond-Clark H: Congenital vertical talus. J Bone Joint Surg 38B:334, 1956
147. Outland T, Sherk HH: Congenital vertical talus. Clin Orthop 16:214, 1960
148. Parrish TF: Congenital convex pes valgus accompanied by previously undescribed anatomic derangements. South Med J 60:983, 1967
149. Patterson WR, Fitz DA, Smith WS: The pathologic anatomy of congenital convex pes valgus. J Bone Joint Surg 50B:456, 1968
150. Silk FF, Wainwright D: The recognition and treatment of congenital flat foot in infancy. J Bone Joint Surg 49B:628, 1967
151. Storen H: On the closed and open correction of congenital convex pes valgus with a vertical astragalus. Acta Orthop Scand 36:352, 1965
152. Storen H: Congenital convex pes valgus with vertical talus. Acta Orthop Scand (Suppl) 94, 1967
153. Tachdjian MO: Congenital convex pes valgus. Orthop Clin North Am 3:131, 1972

Calcaneovalgus Foot

154. Kite JH: The treatment of flatfeet in small children. Postgrad Med 15:75, 1954
155. Kite JH: Flatfeet and lateral rotation of legs in young children. J Int Coll Surg 25:77, 1956
156. Wetzenstein H: The significance of congenital pes calcaneovalgus in the origin of pes planovalgus in childhood. Acta Orthop Scand 30:64, 1960
157. Wynne-Davies R: Family studies and the cause of congenital clubfoot, talipes equinovarus, talipes calcaneovalgus, and metatarsus adductus. J Bone Joint Surg 46B:445, 1964

Flexible Flatfoot

158. Baker LD, Hill LM: Foot alignment in the cerebral palsy patient. J Bone Joint Surg 46A:1, 1964
159. Basmajian JV, Bentzon JW: An electromyographic study of certain muscles of the leg and foot in the standing position. Surg Gynecol Obstet 98:662, 1954
160. Basmajian JV, Stecko G: The role of muscles in arch support of the foot. J Bone Joint Surg 45A:1184, 1963
161. Brown A: A simple method of fusion of the subtalar joint in children. J Bone Joint Surg 50B:369, 1968
162. Butte FL: Naviculo-cuneiform arthrodesis for flatfoot. J Bone Joint Surg 19:496, 1937
163. Caldwell GD: Surgical correction of relaxed flatfoot by the Durham flatfoot plasty. Clin Orthop 2:221, 1953
164. Chambers EFS: An operation for the correction of flexible flatfeet of adolescents. West J Surg 54:77, 1946
165. Chandler FA: Children's feet; normal and presenting common abnormalities. Am J Dis Child 63:1136, 1942
166. Crego CH, Ford LT: An end-result study of various operative procedures for corrective flatfeet in children. J Bone Joint Surg 34A:183, 1952
167. Davy R: On excision of the scaphoid bone for the relief of confirmed flatfoot. Lancet 1:675, 1889
168. Dennyson WG, Fulford GE: Subtalar arthrodesis by cancellous grafts and metallic internal fixation. J Bone Joint Surg 58B:507, 1976
169. Evans D: Calcaneo-valgus deformity. J Bone Joint Surg 57B:270, 1975
170. Golding-Bird CH: Operations on the tarsus in confirmed flatfoot. Lancet 1:677, 1889
171. Grice DS: An extra-articular arthrodesis of the subastragalar joint for correction of paralytic flatfeet in children. J Bone Joint Surg 34A:927, 1952
172. Haraldsson S: Pes plano-valgus staticus juvenilis and its operative treatment. Acta Orthop Scand 35:234, 1964–1965
173. Harris RI, Beath T: Hypermobile flatfoot with short tendo Achilles. J Bone Joint Surg 30A:116, 1948
174. Helfet A: A new way of treating flatfeet in children. Lancet 1:262, 1956
175. Hicks JH: The function of the plantar aponeurosis. J Anat 85:414, 1951
176. Hicks JH: The mechanics of the foot. II. The plantar aponeurosis and the arch. J Anat 88:25, 1954
177. Hoke M: An operation for the correction of extremely relaxed flatfeet. J Bone Joint Surg 13:773, 1931
178. Inman VT: The human foot. Manitoba Med Rev 46:513, 1966
179. Jack EA: Naviculo-cuneiform fusion in the treatment of flatfoot. J Bone Joint Surg 35B:75, 1953
180. Johnston TB, Davies DV, Davies F: Gray's Anatomy, 32nd ed, pp 544–545 and 672–688. Toronto, Longmans Green, 1958
181. Jones BS: Flatfoot. J Bone Joint Surg 57B:279, 1975
182. Keith A: The history of the human foot and its bearing on orthopaedic practice. J Bone Joint Surg 11:10, 1929
183. Kidner FC: The prehallux (accessory scaphoid) and its relation to flatfoot. J Bone Joint Surg 11:831, 1929
184. Kidner FC: The prehallux in relation to flatfoot. JAMA 101:1539, 1933
185. Koutsogiannis E: Treatment of mobile flatfoot by displacement osteotomy of the calcaneous. J Bone Joint Surg 53B:96, 1971
186. Leavitt DG: Subastragaloid arthrodesis for the os calcis type of flatfoot. Am J Surg 59:501, 1943
187. Legg AT: Treatment of rigid flatfoot. Excision of scaphoid. Boston Med Surg J 156:(23):741,743, 1907
188. Legg AT: The treatment of congenital flatfoot by tendon transplantation. Am J Orthop Surg 10:584, 1912–1913
189. LeLièvre J: Current concepts and correction in the valgus foot. Clin Orthop 70:43, 1970
190. Leonard MH, et al.: Lateral transfer of the posterior tibial tendon in certain selected cases of pes planus (Kidner operation). Clin Orthop 40:139, 1965
191. Lord JP: Correction of extreme flatfoot. JAMA 81:1502, 1923
192. Lowman CL: An operative method for correction of certain forms of flatfoot. JAMA 81:1500, 1923
193. Milch H: Reinforcement of the deltoid ligament for pronated flatfoot. Surg Gynecol Obstet 74:876, 1942
194. Miller OL: A plastic flatfoot operation. J Bone Joint Surg 9:84, 1927
195. Ogston A: On flatfoot and its cure by operation. Br Med J 9:110, 1884

196. Painter CF: Peroneal resection as a means of correction in rigid valgus. Boston Med Surg J 153:164, 1905
197. Penneau K, Lutter, L, Winter R: Pes planus: Radiographic changes with foot orthoses and shoes. Foot Ankle 2:299, 1982
198. Phillips GE: A review of elongation of os calcis for flatfeet. J Bone Joint Surg 65B:15, 1983
199. Rose GK: Correction of the pronated foot. J Bone Joint Surg 40B:674, 1958
200. Rose GK: Correction of the pronated foot. J Bone Joint Surg 44B:642, 1962
201. Rugtveit A: Extra-articular subtalar arthrodesis, according to Green-Grice in flatfeet. Acta Orthop Scand 34:367, 1964
202. Reyerson Ed W: Tendon transplantation in flatfoot. Am J Orthop Surg 7:505, 1909
203. Schoolfield BI: An operation for the cure of flatfoot. Ann Surg 110:437, 1936
204. Schoolfield BI: Operative treatment of flatfoot. Surg Gynecol Obstet 94:136, 1952
205. Seymour N: The late results of naviculocuneiform fusion. 49B:558, 1967
206. Seymour N, Evans DK: A modification of the Grice subtalar arthrodesis. J Bone Joint Surg 50B:372, 1968
207. Shephard E: Tarsal movements. J Bone Joint Surg 33B:258, 1951
208. Silver CM, Simon SD, Spindell E, Litchman HM, Scala M: Calcaneal osteotomy for valgus and varus deformities of the foot in cerebral palsy. J Bone Joint Surg 49A:232, 1967
209. Smith JB, Westin GW: Follow-up notes on articles previously published, subtalar extra-articular arthrodesis. J Bone Joint Surg 50A:1027, 1968
210. Smith JW: Muscular control of the arches of the foot in standing, an electromyographic assessment. J Anat 88:152, 1954
211. Soule RI: Value of bone pin arthrodesis in the treatment of flatfoot. JAMA 77:1871, 1921
212. Wetzenstein H: The significance of congenital pes calcaneo-valgus in the origin of pes plano-valgus in childhood. Acta Orthop Scand 30:64, 1960
213. Wynne-Davies R: Family studies and the cause of congenital clubfoot, talipes equinovarus, talipes calcaneo-valgus, and metatarsus adductus. J Bone Joint Surg 46B:445, 1964
214. Young CS: Operative treatment of pes planus. Surg Gynecol Obstet 68:1099, 1939
215. Zadek I: Transverse-wedge arthrodesis for the relief of pain in rigid flatfoot. J Bone Joint Surg 17:453, 1935

Tarsal Coalition

216. Badgley CE: Coalition of the calcaneus and the navicular. Arch Surg 15:75, 1927
217. Bersante FA, Samilson RL: Massive familial tarsae synostosis. J Bone Joint Surg 39A:1187, 1957
218. Blockley NJ: Peroneal spastic flatfoot. J Bone Joint Surg 37B:191, 1955
219. Buffon GL: Histore naturelle avec la description du cabinet du roy. Tome 3:47, 1750
220. Chambers CH: Congenital anomalies of the tarsae navicular with particular reference to calcaneo-navicular coalition. Br J Radiol 23:580, 1950
221. Chambers RB, Cook TM, Cowell HR: Surgical reconstructive for calcaneonavicular coalition. Evaluation of function and gait. J Bone Joint Surg 64A:829, 1982
222. Clark NT, Lovell WW: Tarsal coalition. In preparation
223. Conway HR, Cowell HR: Tarsal coalition: Clinical significance and roentgenographic demonstration. Radiology 92:799, 1969
224. Cowell HR: Personal communication, 1984
225. Cowell HR: Talocalcaneal coalition and new causes of peroneal spastic flatfoot. Clin Orthop 85:16, 1972
226. Del Sel JM, Grand NE: Cubonavicular synostosis. A rare tarsal anomaly. J Bone Joint Surg 18:479, 1936
227. Del Sel JM, Grand NE: Cubonavicular synostosis. A rare tarsal anomaly. J Bone Joint Surg 41B:149, 1959
228. Glessner JR Jr, Davis GL: Bilateral calcaneonavicular coalition occurring in twin boys. A case report. Clin Orthop 47:173, 1966
229. Goldman AB, Pavlou H, Schneider R: Radionuclide bone screening in subtalar coalitions: Differential considerations. Am J Radiol 183:427, 1982
230. Gregersen HN: Naviculocuneiform coalition. J Bone Joint Surg 59A:128, 1977
231. Hark FW: Congenital anomalies of the tarsal bones. Clin Orthop 16:425, 1960
232. Harris RI: Rigid valgus due to talocalcaneal bridge. J Bone Joint Surg 37A:169, 1955
233. Harris RI: Peroneal spastic flatfoot. AAOS Instruc Course Lect 15:116, 1958
234. Harris RI: Retrospect: Peroneal spastic flatfoot (rigid valgus foot). J Bone Joint Surg 47A:1657, 1965
235. Harris RI, Beath T: Etiology of peroneal spastic flatfoot. J Bone Joint Surg 30B:624, 1948
236. Heikel HVA: Coalito calcaneo-navicularis and calcaneus secondarius. A clinical and radiographic study of 23 patients. Acta Orthop Scand 32:72, 1962
237. Jack EA: Bone abnormalities of the tarsus in relation to peroneal spastic flat foot. J Bone Joint Surg 36B:530, 1954
238. Jones, R: Peroneal spasm and its treatment. Report of meeting of Liverpool Medical Institution held 22nd April, 1897. Liverpool Med Chir J 17:442, 1897
239. Jones R: The soldier's foot and the treatment of common deformities of the foot. Br Med J 1:709, 1916
240. Lamb D: The ball and socket ankle joint—a congenital abnormality. J Bone Joint Surg 40B:240, 1958
241. Lapidus PW: Bilateral congenital talonavicular fusion. Report of a case. J Bone Joint Surg 20:775, 1938
242. Lapidus PW: Spastic flat foot. J Bone Joint Surg 28:126, 1946
243. Lusby HLJ: Navicular-cuneiform synostosis. J Bone Joint Surg 41B:150, 1959
244. Mahaffey HW: Bilateral congenital calcaneocuboid synostosis. J Bone Joint Surg 27:164, 1945
245. Mitchell G: Spasmodic flatfoot. Clin Orthop 70:73, 1970
246. Mitchell GP, Gibson JMC: Excision of calcaneonavicular bar for painful spasmodic flat foot. J Bone Joint Surg 49B:281, 1967
247. Mosier KM, Asher A: Tarsal coalition and peroneal spastic flatfoot. A review. J Bone Joint Surg 66A:976, 1984
248. Outland T, Murphy ID: Rotation of tarsal anomalies to spastic and rigid flat feet. Clin Orthop 1:217, 1953

249. Outland T, Murphy ID: The pathomechanics of peroneal spastic flat foot. Clin Orthop 16:64, 1960
250. Simmons EH: Tibialis spastic varus foot with tarsal coalition. J Bone Joint Surg 47B:53B, 1965
251. Slomann HC: On coalition calcaneonavicularis. J Orthop Surg 3:586, 1921
252. Slomann HC: On coalition calcaneonavicular coalition by roentgen examination. Acta Radiol 5:304, 1926
253. Slomann HC: On the demonstration and analysis of calcaneonavicular coalition by roentgen examination. Acta Radiol 5:304, 1926
254. Starmont DM, Peterson HA: The relative incidence of tarsal coalition. Clin Orthop RR 181:28, 1984
255. Swiontkowski MF, Scranton PE, Hansen S: Tarsal coalitions: Long-term results of surgical treatment. J Pediatr Orthop 1983:287, 1983
256. Veneruso LC: Unilateral congenital calcaneocuboid synostosis with complete absence of a metatarsal and toe. A case report. J Bone Joint Surg 27:718, 1945
257. Wagoner GW: A case of bilateral congenital fusion of the calcanei and cuboids. J Bone Joint Surg 10:220, 1928
258. Waugh W: Partial cubonavicular coalition as a cause of peroneal spastic flatfoot. J Bone Joint Surg 39B:520, 1957
259. Webster FS, Roberts WM: Tarsal anomalies and peroneal spastic flatfoot. JAMA 146:1099, 1951
260. Wray JB, Herndon CN: Hereditary transmission of congenital coalition of the calcaneus to the navicular. J Bone Joint Surg 45A:365, 1963
261. Wynne-Davies R: Heritable disorders in orthopedics. Orthop Clin North Am 9:3, 1978

Accessory Navicular

262. Kidner F: The prehallux (accessory scaphoid) in its relation to flatfoot. J Bone Joint Surg 11:831, 1929
263. Sullivan JA, Miller WA: The relationship of the accessory navicular to the development of the flatfoot. Clin Orthop 144:233, 1979
264. Veitch JM: Evaluation of the Kidner procedure in the treatment of symptomatic accessory tarsal scaphoid. Clin Orthop 131:210, 1978
265. Zadek I, Gold A: The accessory tarsal scaphoid. J Bone Joint Surg 30A:957, 1948

Pes Cavus

266. Bentzon PGK: Pes cavus and the M. peroneus longus. Acta Orthop Scand 4:50, 1933
267. Bernau A: Long-term results following Lambrinudi arthrodesis. J Bone Joint Surg 59A:473, 1977
268. Bradley GW, Coleman SS: Treatment of the calcaneocavus foot deformity. J Bone Joint Surg 63A:1159, 1981
269. Brewerton DA, Sandifer PH, Sweetnam DR: "Idiopathic" pes cavus. Br Med J 62:659, 1963
270. Chuinard EG, Baskin M: Clawfoot deformity. J Bone Joint Surg 55A:351, 1973
271. Cole WH: The treatment of clawfoot. J Bone Joint Surg 22:895, 1940
272. Coleman SS, Chestnut WJ: A simple test for hindfoot flexibility in the cavovarus foot. CORR 123:60, 1977
273. Coonrad RW, Irwin CE, Gucker T, Wray JB: The importance of plantar muscles in paralytic varus feet. J Bone Joint Surg 38A:563, 1956
274. Cralley J, Fitch K, McGonagle W: Lumbrical muscles and contracted toes. Anat Ang 138:348, 1975
275. Kekel S, Weissman SL (Tel-Aviv): Osteotomy of the calcaneus and concomitant plantar stripping with talipes cavovarus. J Bone Joint Surg 55B:802, 1973
276. Duchenne GB: Physiologie des Mouvements. Paris, Baillaire, 1867
276a. Duncan J, Lovell WW: Hoke triple arthrodesis. J Bone Joint Surg 60A:795, 1978
277. Dunn N: Stabilizing operations in the treatment of paralytic deformities of the foot. Proc R Soc Med 15:15, 1922
278. Dwyer FC: Osteotomy of the calcaneum for pes cavus. J Bone Joint Surg 41B:80, 1959
279. Dwyer FC: The present status of the problem of pes cavus. CORR 106:254, 1975
280. Forbes AM: Clawfoot and how to relieve it. Surg Gynecol Obstet 26:81, 1913
281. Frank GR, Johnson WM: The extensor shift procedure in the correction of clawtoe deformities in children. South Med J 59:889, 1966
282. Garceau GJ: Pes cavus. AAOS Instruc Course Lect 18:184, 1961
283. Garceau GJ, Brahms MA: A preliminary study of selective plantar muscle deviation for pes cavus. J Bone Joint Surg 38A:553, 1956
284. Giannestras NJ: Foot Disorders: Medical and Surgical Management, 2nd ed, pp 278–181, 506–514. Philadelphia, Lea & Febiger, 1976
285. Gilroy E: Pes cavus, clinical study with special reference to its etiology. Edinb Med J 36:749, 1929
286. Golding-Bird CH: Pes valgus, acquisitius, pes pronatus acquisitius, pes cavus. Guy's Hosp Rep 41:439, 1883
287. Heron JR: Neurologic syndromes associated with pes cavus. Proc R Soc Med 62:270, 1969
288. Heyman CH: Operative treatment of clawfoot. J Bone Joint Surg 14:335, 1932
289. Hibbs RA: An operation for "claw foot." JAMA 73:1583, 1919
290. Howard RJ: Operative treatment of early cavus feet. South Med J 64:558, 1971
291. Irwin CE: The calcaneus foot. Ann Arbor, JW Edwards Publishers, Inc, 15:135, 1958
292. Jahss MH: Tarsometatarsal truncated wedge arthrodesis for pes cavus and equinovarus deformity of the fore part of the foot. J Bone Joint Surg 62A:713, 1980
293. James CC, Lassman LP: The diagnosis and treatment of progressive lesions in spina bifida occulta. J Bone Joint Surg 44B:828, 1962
294. Jones R: Notes on Military Orthopaedics. New York, Hoeber, 1917
295. Kelikian H: Hallus Valgus, Allied Deformities of the Forefoot and Metatarsalgia, pp 305–326. Philadelphia, WB Saunders, 1965
296. Lambrinudi C: A new operation for drop-foot. Br J Bone Joint Surg 15:193, 1927
297. Lambrinudi C: An operation for clawtoes. Proc R Soc Med 21:239, 1927
298. Levick GM: The action of the intrinsic muscles of the foot and their treatment by electricity. Br Med J 1:381, 1921
299. Levitt RL, Canale ST, Cook AJ, Gartland JJ: The role of foot surgery in progressive neuromuscular disorders in children. J Bone Joint Surg 55A:1396, 1973

300. Little NJ: Clawfoot. Med J Aust 2:495, 1938
301. Mann R, Inman VT: Phasic activity of intrinsic muscles of the foot. J Bone Joint Surg 46A:469, 1964
302. M'Banali EI: Results of modified Robert Jones operation for clawed hallux. Br J Surg 62:647, 1975
303. McCauley JC Jr: Triple arthrodesis for congenital talipes equinovarus deformities. Clin Orthop 34:25, 1964
304. McElvenny RT, Caldwell GD: A new operation for correction of cavus foot. Clin Orthop 11:85, 1958
304a. Meary R: "Le Pied Creux Essential" Symposium. Rev Chir Orthop 53:389, 1967
305. Mitchell GP: Posterior displacement osteotomy of the calcaneus. J Bone Joint Surg 59B:233, 1977
306. Rugh JT: An operation for the correction of plantar and adduction contracture of the foot arch. J Bone Joint Surg 6:664, 1924
307. Rugh JT: The etiology of cavus and a new operation for its correction. Bull NY Acad Med 3:423, 1927
308. Samilson RL: Crescentic osteotomy of the calcaneus for calcaneocavus feet. In Bateman JE (ed): Foot Science. Philadelphia, WB Saunders, 1976
309. Samilson RL, Specht EE, DuVries HL: In Mann RA (ed): Surgery of the Foot, 4th ed, p 309. St Louis, CV Mosby, 1978
310. Samilson RL, Dillin W: Cavus, cavovarus, and calcaneocavus. CORR 177:125, 1983
311. Samuelson KM, Harrison R, Freeman MAR: A roentgenographic technique to evaluate and document hindfoot position. Foot Ankle 1:286, 1981
312. Saunders JT: Etiology and treatment of clawfoot. Arch Surg 30:179, 1935
313. Scheer GE, Crego CH: A two-state stabilization procedure for correction of calcaneocavus. J Bone Joint Surg 38A:1247, 1956
314. Sherman FC, Westin GW: Plantar release in the correction of deformities of the foot in childhood. J Bone Joint Surg 63A:1382, 1981
315. Sherman HM: The operative treatment of pes cavus. Am J Orthop Surg 2:374, 1905
316. Siffert RS, Forster RI, Nachamie B: Beak triple arthrodesis for correction of severe cavus deformity. CORR 45:101, 1966
317. Spitzy H: Operative correction of clawfoot. Surg Gynecol Obstet 45:813, 1927
318. Stauffer RN, Nelson GE, Gianco AJ: Calcaneal osteotomy in treatment of cavovarus foot. Mayo Clin Proc 45:624, 1970
319. Steindler A: Operative treatment of pes cavus. Surg Gynecol Obstet 24:612, 1917

Osteochondroses

320. Andren L, Carstam N, Linden B: Osteochondroses dissecans and brachymesophalangia: A hereditary syndrome. J Hand Surg 3(2):117, 1978
321. Douglas G, Rang M: The role of trauma in the pathogenesis of osteochondrosis. CORR 158:28, 1981
322. Duthie RB, Houghton GR: Constitutional apsects of osteochondrosis. CORR 158:19, 1981
323. Gardiner TB: Osteochondritis dissecans in three members of one family. J Bone Joint Surg 37B:139, 1955
324. Green WT, Banks HH: Osteochondritis dissecans in children. J Bone Joint Surg 35A:26, 1953
325. Siffert RS: Classification of the osteochondroses. CORR 158:10, 1981
326. Smith RB, Nevelos AM: Osteochondroses occurring at multiple sites. Acta Orthop Scand 51:445, 1980
327. Wagoner G, Cohn BNE: Osteochondritis dissecans. Arch Surg 23:1, 1931

Freiberg's Infraction

328. Bordelon RL: Silicone implant for Freiberg's disease. South Med J 70:1002, 1977
329. Braddock GTF: Experimental epiphyseal injury and Freiberg's disease. J Bone Joint Surg 41:154, 1959
330. Freiberg AH: Infraction of the second metatarsal bone: A typical injury. Surg Gynecol Obstet 19:191, 1914
331. Freiberg AH: The so-called infraction of the second metatarsal bone. J Bone Joint Surg 8:257, 1926
332. Gannestras NJ: Foot Disorders. Medical and Surgical Management, 2nd ed, pp 421–424. Philadelphia, Lea & Feibiger, 1973
333. Kelikian H: Hallux Valgus Allied Deformities of the Forefoot and Metatarsalgia, pp 372–379. Philadelphia and London, WB Saunders, 1965
334. Margo MK: Surgical treatment of conditions of the foot. J Bone Joint Surg 49A:1665, 1967
335. Smillie IS: Freiberg's infraction (Köhler's second disease). J Bone Joint Surg 37:580, 1955

Köhler's Disease

336. Brailsford JF: Osteochondritis of the adult trasal navicular. J Bone Joint Surg 21:111, 1939
337. Karp MG: Köhler's disease of the tarsal scaphoid. J Bone Joint Surg 19:84, 1937
338. Kidner FC, Muro F: Köhler's disease of the tarsal scaphoid or os naviculare pedis retardation. JAMA 83:1650, 1924
339. Köhler A: Uber enine haufige bisher anscheinend unbekannte Erkrankung einzelner kindlicher Knochen. Munch Med Wochen 55:1, 923, 1908
340. McCauley GK, Kahn PC: Osteochondritis of the tarsal navicular. Nuclear Medicine pp 705–706, 1977
341. Waugh W: The ossification and vascularization of the tarsal navicular and their relation to Köhler's disease. J Bone Joint Surg 40B:765, 1958
342. Wiley JJ, Brown DE: The bipartite tarsal scaphoid. J Bone Joint Surg 63B:583, 1981
343. William GA, Cowell HR: Köhler's disease of the tarsal navicular. Clin Orthop 158:53, 1981

Sever's Disease

344. Katz JF: Nonarticular osteochondroses. CORR 158:70, 1981
345. Pappas AM: The osteochondroses. Pediatr Clin North Am 14:549, 1967
346. Sever JW: Apophysities of the os calcis. NY Med J 95:1025, 1912
347. Sever JW: Apophysitis of the os calcis. Am J Orthop 15:659, 1917

Osteochondritis Dissecans of the Talus

348. Axe MJ, Casscells SW: Arthroscopic assistance in osteochondritis dissecans of the talus. Orthop Cons 4(2):1, 1983
349. Berndt AL, Harty M: Transchondral fractures (osteochondritis dissecans) of the talus. J Bone Joint Surg 41A:988, 1959

350. Cameron BM: Osteochondritis dissecans of the ankle joint. J Bone Joint Surg 38A:857, 1956
351. Canale ST, Belding RH: Osteochondral lesions of the talus. J Bone Joint Surg 62A:97, 1980
352. Fairbank HAT: Osteochondritis dissecans. Br J Surg 21:67, 1933
353. Mukherjee SK, Young AB: Dome fracture of the talus. J Bone Joint Surg 55B:319, 1973
354. Pappas AM: Osteochondritis dissecans. CORR 158:59, 1981
355. Ray RB, Coughlin EJ Jr: Osteochondritis of the talus. J Bone Joint Surg 55B:319, 1973
356. Scharling M: Osteochondritis dissecans of the talus. Acta Orthop Scand 49:89, 1978
357. Smyth FS: Local affections of the bones and soft tissues of the foot. In Surgery of the Foot. St Louis, CV Mosby, 1973

Congenital Cleft Foot

358. Barsky J: Cleft hand: Classification, incidence, and treatment. J Bone Joint Surg 46A:1707, 1964
359. Cowan R: Surgical problems associated with congenital malformations of the forefoot. Can J Surg 8:29, 1965
360. Leiter E, Lipson J: Genitourinary tract anomalies in lobster claw syndrome. J Urol 115:339, 1976
361. Maisels DO: Lobster claw deformities of the hands and feet. Br J Plast Surg 23:269, 1970
362. Myerding HW, Upshaw JE: Heredofamilial cleft foot deformity. Am J Surg 74:889, 1947
363. Mosavy SH, Vakhshuri P: Split hands and feet. South Afr Med J 49:1842, 1975
364. Onizuka T: Surgical correction of lobster claw feet. Plastic Reconstr Surg 57:98, 1976
365. Phillips RS: Congenital split foot (lobster claw) and triphalangeal thumb. J Bone Joint Surg 53B:247, 1971
366. Sumiya N, Onizuka T: Seven years' survey of our new cleft foot. Plastic Reconstr Surg 65:447, 1980
367. Weissman SL, Plaschkes Y: Surgical correction of lobster claw feet. Plast Reconstruct Surg 49:89, 1972

Syndactyly, Macrodactyly, Polydactyly

368. Charters AD: Local gigantism. J Bone Joint Surg 39B:542, 1957
369. Cowan RJ: Surgical problems associated with congenital malformations of the forefoot. Can J Surg 8:29, 1965
370. Dennyson WG, Bear JN, Bhoola KD: Macrodactyly in the foot. J Bone Joint Surg 59B: 355, 1977
371. Diammond LS, Gould VE: Marcodactyly of the foot. South Med J 67:645, 1974
372. Figura MA: Practical approach to a rare deformity: Macrodactyly. J Foot Surg 19(2):52, 1980
373. Kelikian H: Deformities of the Lesser Toes in Hallux Valgus: Allied Deformities of the Forefoot and Metatarsalgia. Philadelphia, WB Saunders, 1965
374. Sanchez AJ, Kamal B: Macrodactyly in the foot. Ann Acad Med 10(1):442, 1981
375. Specht EE: Minor congenital deformities and anomalies of the toes. In Inman V (ed): Surgery of the Foot. St Louis, CV Mosby, 1973
376. Tsuge K: Treatment of macrodactyly. Plast Reconstruct J 39:590, 1967
377. Venn-Watson EA: Problems in polydactyly of the foot. Orthop Clin North Am 7:909, 1976
378. Yaghma I, McKowne F, Alizadeh A: Macrodactylia fibrolipomatosis. South Med J 69:1565, 1976

Congenital Hallux Varus

379. Framer AW: Congenital hallux varus. Am J Surg 95:274, 1958
380. Haas SL: An operation for the correction of hallux varus. J Bone Joint Surg 20:705, 1938
381. Hawkins FB: Acquired hallux varus: Cause, prevention, and correction. CORR 76:169, 1971
382. Horwitz MT: Unusual hallux varus deformity and its surgical correction. J Bone Joint Surg 19:828, 1937
383. McElvenny RT: Hallux varus. Q Bull Northwest Med School 15:277, 1941
384. Miller JW: Acquired hallux varus: A preventable and correctable disorder. J Bone Joint Surg 57A:183, 1975
385. Myginal HB: Surgical treatment of congenital hallux varus. Nord Med 49:914, 1953
386. Sloane D: Congenital hallux varus. J Bone Joint Surg 17:209, 1935
387. Thomson SA: Hallux varus and metatarsus varus. CORR 16:109, 1960

Adolescent Bunion

388. Bernsten A: De l'hallux valgus, contribution à son etiologie et à son traitement. Rev Orthop 17:101, 1930
389. Bonney G, McNab I: Hallux valgus and hallux rigidus. J Bone Joint Surg 34B:366, 1952
390. Carr CR Boyd B: Correctional osteotomy for metatarsus primus varus and hallux valgus. J Bone Joint Surg 50A:1353, 1968
391. Durman DC: Metatarsus primus varus and hallux valgus. Arch Surg 74:128, 1957
392. Ellis VH: A method of correcting metatarsus primus varus. J Bone Joint Surg 33B:415, 1951
393. Engle ET, Morton DS: Notes on foot disorders among natives of the Belgian Congo. J Bone Joint Surg 13:311, 1931
394. Ewald P: Die atiologie des hallux valgus. Deutsch Z Chir 114:90, 1912
395. Fuld JE: Surgical treatment of hallux valgus and its complications. Am Med 25:536, 1919
396. Haines RW, McDougall A: The anatomy of hallux valgus. J Bone Joint Surg 36B:272, 1954
397. Hardy RH, Clapham JCR: Observations on hallux valgus. J Bone Joint Surg 33B:376, 1951
398. Hawkins FB, Mitchell L, Hedrick DW: Correction of hallux valgus by metatarsal osteotomy. J Bone Joint Surg 27:387, 1945
399. Henderson RS: Os intermetatarsium and a possible relationship to hallux valgus. J Bone Joint Surg 45B:117, 1963
400. Hiss JM: Hallux valgus: Its course and simplified treatment. Am J Surg 11:51, 1931
401. Inman VT: Hallux valgus: A review of etiologic factors Orthop Clin North Am 5(1):59, 1974
402. Johnston O: Further studies of the inheritance of hand and foot anomalies. Clin Orthop 8:146, 1956.
403. Joplin RJ: Sling procedure for correction of splayfoot, metatarsus primus varus, and hallux valgus. J Bone Joint Surg 32A:779, 1950
404. Keller WL: The surgical treatment of hallux valgus and bunion. NY Med J 80:741, 1904

405. Kleinberg S: The operative care of hallux valgus and bunions. Am J Surg 15:75, 1932
406. Lam S, Hodgson AR: A comparison of foot forms among the non-shoe and shoe-wearing Chinese population. J Bone Joint Surg 40A:1058, 1958
407. Lapidus PW: Operative correction of metatarsus varus primus in hallux valgus. Surg Obstet Gynecol 58:183, 1934
408. McBride ED: A conservative operation for bunions. J Bone Joint Surg 10:735, 1928
409. Mayo C: The surgical treatment of bunions. Ann Surg 48:300, 1908
410. Mitchell L, et al: Osteotomy-bunionectomy for hallux valgus. J Bone Joint Surg 40A:41, 1958
411. Peabody CW: The surgical cure of hallux valgus. J Bone Joint Surg 13:273, 1931
412. Piggott HH: The natural history of hallux valgus in adolescence and early adult life. J Bone Joint Surg 42B:749, 1960
413. Silver D: Hallux valgus, J Bone Joint Surg 5:225, 1923
414. Simmonds FA, Menelaus MD: Hallux valgus in adolescents. J Bone Joint Surg 42B:761, 1960
415. Stanley LL: Bunions. J Bone Joint Surg 17:961, 1935
416. Trott A: Hallux valgus in the adolescent. AAOS Instruc Course Lect 21:262, 1972
417. Truslow W: Metatarsus primus varus or hallux valgus? J Bone Joint Surg 7:98, 1925
418. Wells LH: The foot of the South African native. Am J Phys Anthropol 15:185, 1931
419. Wilson JN: Oblique displacement osteotomy for hallux valgus. J. Bone Joint Surg 45B:552, 1963.

Congenital Short First Metatarsal

420. Giannestras NJ: Foot Disorders. Philadelphia, Lea & Febiger, 1973
421. Harris RI, Beath T: The short first metatarsal. J Bone Joint Surg 31A: 553, 1949
422. Morton DJ: Metatarsus atavicus. J Bone Joint Surg 9:531, 1927
423. Viladot A: Metatarsalgia due to biomechanical alterations of the forefoot. Orthop Clin North Am 4:165, 1973

Congenital Overriding of the Fifth Toe

424. Cockin J: Butler's operations for an overriding fifth toe. J Bone Joint Surg 50B:78, 1960
425. DuVries HL: DuVries' Surgery of the Foot, 4th ed, pp 596–599. St Louis, CV Mosby, 1978
426. Goodwin FC, Swisher FM: The treatment of congenital hyperextension of the fifth toe. J Bone Joint Surg 25:193, 1943
427. Janecki CJ, Wilde AH: Results of phalangectomy of the fifth toe for hammertoe, the Ruiz-Mora procedure. J Bone Joint Surg 58A:1005, 1976
428. Kelikian H: Hallux Valgus, Allied Deformities of the Forefoot and Metatarsalgia. Philadelphia, WB Saunders, 1965
429. Lantzounis LA: Congenital subluxation of the fifth toe and its correction by a periosteocapsulotomy and tendon transplantation. J Bone Joint Surg 22:147, 1940
430. Lapidus PC: Transplantation of the extensor tendon for correction of the overlapping fifth toe. J Bone Joint Surg 24:555, 1942
431. Leonard MH, Rising EE: Syndactylization to maintain correction of overlapping fifth toe. Clin Orthop 43:241, 1965
432. Manter JT: Variations of the interosseous muscles of the human foot. Anat Rec 93:117, 1945
433. McFarland B: Congenital deformities of the spine and limbs. In Platt H (ed): Modern Trends in Orthopaedics, p 107. London, Butterworth, 1950
434. Michele AA, Krueger FJ: Operative correction for hammertoe. Milit Surg 103:52, 1948
435. Ruiz-Mora J: Plastic correction of overriding fifth toe. Orthopaedic Letters Club 6, 1954
436. Scrase WH: The treatment of dorsal adduction deformity of the fifth toe. J Bone Joint Surg 36B:146, 1954
437. Sharrard WJW: The surgery of deformed toes in children. Br J Clin Pract 17:263, 1963
438. Stamm TT: Surgery of the foot. In British Surgical Practice, Vol IV. London, Butterworth, 1918; St Louis, CV Mosby, 1948, p 160
439. Tachdjian MO: Pediatric Orthopaedics, pp 1416–1422. Philadelphia, WB Saunders, 1972
440. Thompson, CT: Surgical treatment of disorders of the fore part of the foot. J Bone Joint Surg 46A:1117, 1964
441. Wilson JN: V-Y correction for varus deformity of the fifth toe. Br J Surg 41:133, 1953

Congenital Curly Toes

442. Giannestras NJ: Foot Disorders, pp 102–107. Philadelphia, Lea & Febiger, 1973
443. Kelikian H: Hallux Valgus, Allied Deformities of the Forefoot and Metatarsalgia, p 330. Philadelphia, WB Saunders, 1965
444. Pollard JP, Morrison PJM: Flexor tenotomy in the treatment of curly toes. Proc R Soc Med 68:480, 1975
445. Sharrard WJW: The surgery of deformed toes in children. Br J Clin Pract 17:263, 1963
446. Specht EE: In Inman VT (ed): DuVries' Surgery of the Foot. St Louis, CV Mosby, 1973
447. Sweetnam R: Congenital curly toes, an investigation into the value of treatment. Lancet 2:398, 1958
448. Taylor RG: The treatment of clawtoes by multiple transfers of the flexor with extensor tendons. J Bone Joint Surg 33B:539, 1951
449. Trethowan WH: The treatment of hammertoe. Lancet I:1257, 1312, 1925

Adolescent Hallux Rigidus

450. Bingold AC, Collins DH: Hallux rigidus. J Bone Joint Surg 32B:214, 1950.
451. Bonney G, MacNab I: Hallux valgus and hallux rigidus. J Bone Joint Surg 34B:366, 1952
452. Cochrane WA: An operation for hallux rigidus. Br Med J 1:1095, 1927
453. Giannestras NJ: Foot Disorders, pp 400–402. Philadelphia, Lea & Febiger, 1973
454. Glissan DJ: Hallux valgus and hallux rigidus. Med J Aust 2:585, 1946
455. Harrison MHM, Harvey FL: Arthrodesis of the first metatarsophalangeal joint for hallux valgus and rigidus. J Bone Joint Surg 45A:471, 1963
456. Jansen M: Hallux valgus rigidus and mallens. J Orthop Surg 3:90, 1921

457. Kessel L, Bonney G: Hallux rigidus in the adolescent. J Bone Joint Surg 40B:668, 1958
458. Lambrinudi C: Metatarsus primus elevatus. Proc R Soc Med 31:1273, 1938
459. Lipscomb PR: Arthrodesis of the first metatarsophalangeal joint for severe bunions and hallux rigidus. CORR 142:48, 1979
460. Lloyd EL: The prognosis of hallux valgus and hallux rigidus. Lancet 2:263, 1935
461. Mann RA, Oates JC: Arthrodesis of the first metatarsophalangeal joint. Foot Ankle 1(3):159, 1980
462. Mann RA, Coughlin JJ, DuVries HL: Hallux rigidus: A review of the literature and a method of treatment. CORR 142:57, 1979
463. McMaster MJ: The pathogenesis of hallux rigidus. J Bone Joint Surg 60B:82, 1978
464. McMurray TP: Treatment of hallux valgus and rigidus. Br Med J 2:218, 1936
465. Moberg E: A simple operation for hallux rigidus. CORR 142:55, 1979
466. Monberg A: On the treatment of hallux rigidus. Acta Orthop Scand 6:239, 1935
467. Moynihan FJ: Arthrodesis of the metatarsophalangeal joint of the great toe. J Bone Joint Surg 49B:554, 1967
468. Nilsonne H: Hallux rigidus and its treatment. Acta Orthop Scand 1:295, 1930
469. Strombeck JP: Hallux rigidus und seine behandlung. Acta Chir Scand 73:53, 1934
470. Watermann H: Die Arthritis Deformans des Grosszehengrundgelenkes als selbstandiges Krankheitsbild. Z Orthop Chir 48:346, 1927
471. Watson-Jones R: Treatment of hallux rigidus (Reply letter to Mr. Cochrane). Br Med J 1:1165, 1927
472. Wenger RJJ, Whalley RC: Total replacement of the first metatarsophalangeal joint. J Bone Joint Surg 60B:88, 1978

Hammertoe

473. Blum A: De l'orteil en marteau. Bull Mem Soc Chir Paris 9:738, 1982
474. Brahams MA: Common foot problems. J Bone Joint Surg 49A:1653, 1967
475. Cahill BR, Connor DE: A long-term follow-up on proximal phalangectomy for hammertoes. Clin Orthop 86:191, 1972
476. Giannestras NJ: Foot Disorders: Medical and Surgical Management, pp 410–415. Philadelphia, Lea & Febiger, 1973
477. Jones R: Notes on Military Orthopaedics, pp 38–57. New York, Hoeber, 1917
478. Kelikian H: Hallux Valgus, Allied Deformities of the Forefoot and Metatarsalgia. Philadelphia, WB Saunders, 1965
479. McConnell BE: Hammertoe surgery. South Med J 68:595, 1975
480. Margo MK: Surgical treatment of conditions of the fore part of the foot. J Bone Joint Surg 49A:1665, 1976
481. Newman RJ Futton JM: An evaluation of operative procedures in the treatment of hammertoe. Acta Orthop Scand 50:709, 1979
482. Scheck M: Etiology of acquired hammertoe deformity. CORR 123:63, 1977
483. Taylor RG: The treatment of clawtoes by multiple transfers of the flexor into extensor tendons. J Bone Joint Surg 33B:539, 1951
484. Trethowan WH: The treatment of hammertoe. Lancet 1:1257, 1312, 1925

Claw Toes

485. Dickson FD, Dively RS: Functional Disorders of the Foot, pp 244–249. Philadelphia, JB Lippincott, 1944
486. DuVries HL: DuVries' Surgery of the Foot, 4th ed, pp 279–285. St Louis, CV Mosby, 1978
487. Forrester-Brown MF: Tendon transplantation for clawing of the great toe. J Bone Joint Surg 20:57, 1938
488. Frank GR, Johnson WM: The extensor shift procedure in the correction of clawtoe deformities in children. South Med J 59:889, 1966
489. Heyman CH: Operative treatment of clawfoot. J Bone Joint Surg 14:335, 1932
490. Hibbs RA: An operation for "claw foot." JAMA 73:1583, 1919
491. Lambrinudi C: An operation for clawtoes. Proc R Soc Med 21:239, 1927
492. Parrish TF: Dynamic correction of clawtoes. Orthop Clin North Am 4:97, 1973
493. Pyper JB: The flexor-extensor transplant operation for clawtoes. J Bone Joint Surg 40B:528, 1958
494. Taylor RG: The treatment of clawtoes by multiple transfers of the flexor into extensor tendons. J Bone Joint Surg 33B:539, 1951

Plantar Warts

495. Cracchiolo A: Toe disorders and plantar warts. Orthop Clin North Am 7(4):779, 1976

Ingrown Toenails

496. Bailie FB Evans DM: Ingrowing toenails in infancy. Br Med J 2:737, 1978
497. Dixon GL: Treatment of ingrown toenail. Foot Ankle 3:254, 1983
498. DuVries HL: Disorders of skin and toenails. In Surgery of the Foot, 4th ed. St Louis, CV Mosby, 1978

22

The Amputee

Robert E. Tooms

Although the number of juvenile amputees is relatively small, this group constitutes a significant segment of the pediatric population with major orthopaedic problems. The prosthetic and surgical management of these children, although similar in many respects to that of the adult amputee, may be extremely complex. Experience has proved that the child amputee is best managed in a specialized setting, separate and apart from the standard adult amputee clinic or the usual crippled children's clinic dealing with a variety of orthopaedic disabilities.[11,23,124]

By definition, the child amputee is skeletally immature and the epiphyses of his long bones are still open.[53] Not only are the limbs of a growing child increasing in length and in circumference, but the metabolism of all his tissues is progressing at a remarkably high rate, and he is rapidly maturing from a neuromuscular developmental standpoint.[3] This growth factor, or biologic dynamism, possessed by the child is the cardinal difference between child and adult amputees. Apart from these physiologic differences, it is further apparent that, in contrast to the adult, the child is emotionally immature, variably dependent upon others for his basic needs, and subject to the wishes of his parents and others in decision making.[10] All these factors may at times enhance the effectiveness of prosthetic and surgical care of the child amputee, or they may be detrimental to the ultimate success of the treatment program if not recognized and properly managed.

The rapidly growing child requires frequent adjustments of his prosthesis. Because he grows taller, length adjustment of the prosthesis is necessary at frequent intervals. Because his stump enlarges and changes in configuration, socket modification or replacement is also needed quite often. To maintain good cosmesis and ensure proper fit of clothing and footwear, prosthetic feet and other components must be frequently altered or replaced. Children engage in extremely vigorous play activities, often in environments hostile to the plastic, metal, and leather used in prosthetic fabrication. The child amputee is no different from his normal peers in this respect, and desirably so. In brief, rapid growth plus hard usage require that there are almost constant maintenance and frequent replacement of prosthetic devices used by children. Lambert has reported that children followed at the University of Illinois required a new lower limb prosthesis annually up to the age of 5 years, biennially from 5 to 12 years, and then one every 3 to 4 years until age 21 years.[100] The above facts are perhaps obvious but are cited to point out the need for the child amputee to be re-evaluated by all members of the clinic team on a regular and frequent basis. Experience has shown that such clinic visits should be made once every 3 to 4 months for optimal care.

Limb deficiencies in children have been divided into two broad catagories based on etiology: congenital and acquired. Since 1968, annual surveys of specialized child amputee clinics in the United States have consistently shown that approximately 60% of childhood amputations are congenital in origin and 40% are acquired.[81] A survey of prosthetic facilities across the country revealed significantly higher numbers of acquired limb deficiencies.[39] This discrepancy presumably indicates that the more complex congenital limb deficiencies are referred to specialized child amputee clinics for care, whereas the more conventional acquired amputation problems can be satisfactorily treated by clinicians in less specialized settings.

ACQUIRED AMPUTATIONS

ETIOLOGY

Acquired limb deficiencies in children are secondary to trauma or disease, with trauma being responsible for limb loss approximately twice as often as disease.[6,101] In the many traumatic incidents resulting in amputation, power tools and machinery are the worst offenders, followed closely by vehicular accidents, gunshot wounds and explosions, and railroad accidents, in that order. Smaller but significant numbers are the result of household accidents, thermal injuries, and injuries sustained in connection with childhood recreational activities (Fig. 22-1). As might be expected, vehicular accidents, gunshot wounds, and power tool injuries are the most common causes of limb loss in the older child (those of 12 to 21 years). In the toddler (ages 1 to 4 years), accidents with power tools such as lawn mowers and other household accidents are the most frequent causes of amputation.

Malignant tumors account for more than half the amputations performed for disease processes, with the largest number of cases occurring in the 12 to 21 year age group. Vascular malformations, neurogenic disor-

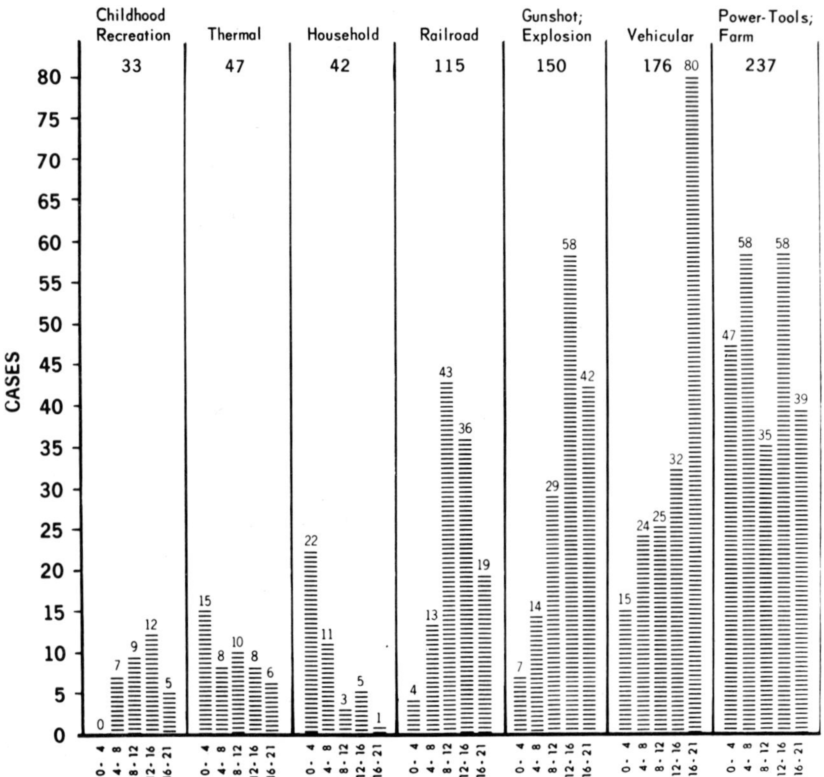

FIG. 22-1. Etiology of acquired amputations due to trauma. (From Northwestern University Medical School Prosthetic-Orthotic Program, Juvenile Amputee Course Manual.)

ders, and a large variety of miscellaneous disorders are responsible for the remainder of amputations in this category (Fig. 22-2).

In more than 90% of acquired amputations, only one limb is involved, and it is the lower limb that is involved in 60% of the cases. Males outnumber females in incidence of acquired limb loss by 3:2, a statistic probably attesting to the more hazardous work and recreational activities in which males engage.

SURGICAL PRINCIPLES

The well-established surgical principles for amputation surgery in the adult are just as applicable to amputations performed in children.[3,12,53,100] The cardinal dictum is to conserve all limb length possible, consistent with appropriate treatment for the condition necessitating the amputation. The biologic dynamism, or growth factor, present in the child may permit surgical techniques not successful in the adult. Skin grafts, firm traction, and wound closure under tension may be *judiciously* used in the child to conserve limb length without compromising wound healing or subsequent prosthetic use.[3,31,64,75]

In other ways, however, the growth factor may prove disadvantageous following amputations in children. One such disadvantage is relative loss of stump length due to epiphyseal loss.[3,31A,100] Loss of stump length is most marked in above-knee amputations in which the distal femoral epiphysis, accounting for approximately 70% of the length growth of the femur, is sacrificed. When a standard mid-thigh amputation is performed in a 5-year-old child, the above-knee stump present at age 16 years will be quite short and a considerably less than optimal lever for prosthetic use (Fig. 22-3). This complication points up the second major surgical dictum in amputation surgery in the child: Wherever possible, always perform a disarticulation rather than a supraepiphyseal or transdiaphyseal amputation in a growing child. Aside from the highly desirable preservation of epiphyseal growth, disarticulation provides a sturdy end-bearing stump and a long lever arm to enhance prosthetic use. In the growing child, prominent condyles or malleoli resulting from disarticulation undergo atrophy with the passage of time, eliminating the cosmetic objection to this type of surgery.[3,12,53,100] Furthermore, disarticulation precludes subsequent development of terminal

DISEASE – 423 PATIENTS

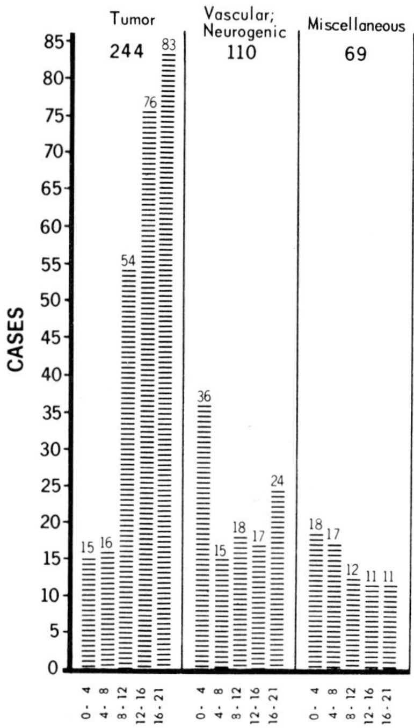

FIG. 22-2. Etiology of acquired amputations due to disease. (From Northwestern University Medical School Prosthetic-Orthotic Program, Juvenile Amputee Course Manual.)

overgrowth of bone, a complication discussed below.

COMPLICATIONS

Terminal Overgrowth

The most frequent complication of amputation surgery in children is terminal overgrowth. This is an appositional growth of bone at the transected end of a long bone in the skeletally immature individual,[152B] being seen most commonly in the humerus, fibula, tibia, and femur, in that order.[3] Although terminal overgrowth does not occur following disarticulation, it is in no way related to epiphyseal bone growth,[8A] and previous attempts to prevent this problem by epiphysiodesis have not been successful.[168] In this condition, the appositional growth of new bone exceeds the growth of the overlying soft tissues, and, if untreated, the bone end may actually penetrate

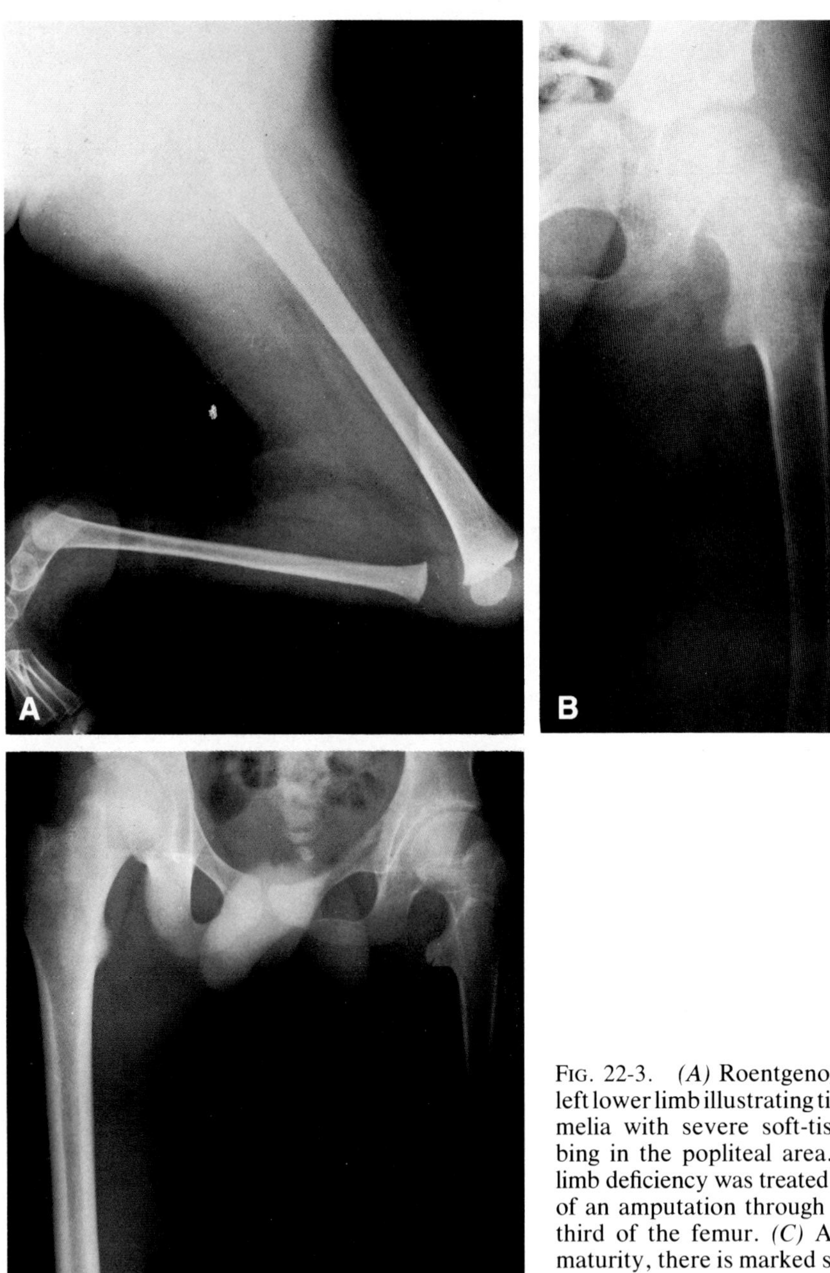

FIG. 22-3. *(A)* Roentgenogram of a left lower limb illustrating tibial hemimelia with severe soft-tissue webbing in the popliteal area. *(B)* This limb deficiency was treated by means of an amputation through the distal third of the femur. *(C)* At skeletal maturity, there is marked shortening of the femur on the amputated side due to loss of the distal femoral epiphysis, with a resultant very short amputation stump.

the skin (Fig. 22-4). Many surgical techniques have been devised in an attempt to prevent terminal overgrowth, but the best method at present is stump revision with appropriate resection of the bony overgrowth.[2,140] This has been necessary in 8% to 12% of most large reported series of acquired amputations in children.[2,3,6,11,12,53,133A] Once this condition occurs, recurrences are common and may necessitate repeated stump revisions at 2- to 3-year intervals until skeletal maturity. Techniques using intramedullary implants of silicone rubber[156,157] or porous polyethylene[122] to prevent terminal overgrowth initially appeared promising but have not proved sufficiently effective and trouble-free to gain wide-spread acceptance. Marquardt,[119A] has more recently described a technique for capping with autogenous cartilage–bone transplants those transected bone ends that have developed osseous overgrowth. Limited experience with this procedure has been encouraging. It was formerly believed that terminal overgrowth did not occur in congenital limb deficiencies, but it is now known that the condition does occur in a small percentage of this category of amputations. Aitken[2] has postulated that such cases may represent true instances of intrauterine amputation.[58,71,99] However, the rarity of true intrauterine amputation compared with the incidence of terminal overgrowth in congenital limb deficiencies, although low, would indicate some other etiology for this condition.

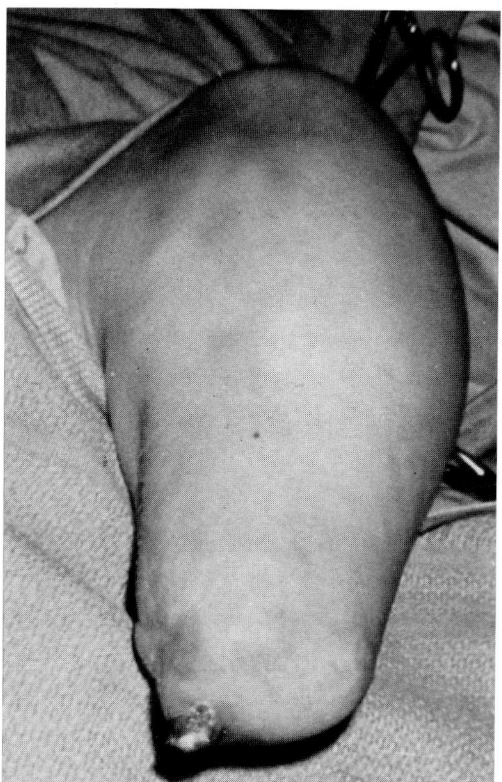

FIG. 22-4. Terminal overgrowth of the humerus in a post-traumatic above-elbow amputation. The bony overgrowth has actually penetrated the soft tissues at the end of the amputation stump.

Bursa Formation

Bursa formation may occur over any bony prominence subjected to recurrent pressure from a prosthetic socket, but it is most commonly seen overlying an area of terminal overgrowth (Fig. 22-5). Conservative treatment of these lesions by aspiration, corticosteroid injection, or stump wrapping has not been more than temporarily effective. Bursae are best managed by surgical excision of the bursal tissue, combined with appropriate resection of the underlying bone.[3,6,12] Surgery must be followed by socket adjustment or fitting with a new socket, as indicated.

Bony Spurs

These frequently form at the margin of transected bone in amputation stumps and are due to periosteal stimulation at the time of surgery. These spurs should be clearly distinguished from terminal overgrowth, because they are rarely an indication for stump revision.[3]

Stump Scarring

Extensive stump scarring from trauma or skin grafts is amazingly well tolerated by the child (Fig. 22-6). High tissue metabolism, exuberant vascularity, and tissue plasticity present in children permit prosthetic use in stumps that would quickly break down in the adult. Stump revision to higher levels is seldom indicated because of stump scarring or skin grafts unless other significant problems such as terminal overgrowth are coexistent.[3] However, prosthetic modification is often required to disperse weightbearing forces and to diminish shear at the stump-socket interface.[64]

Neuromas

These form in amputation stumps, as elsewhere, wherever a peripheral nerve is transected. A variety of surgical techniques have been used to prevent neuroma formation, without significant success. High, sharp transection of nerves at the time of amputation so the cut ends lie in normal tissue well away from the amputation site remains the most effective way to prevent painful neuroma formation. In a large series of acquired childhood amputations, Aitken found that slightly less than 4% required surgical treatment for neuromas, most being satisfactorily managed by socket adjust-

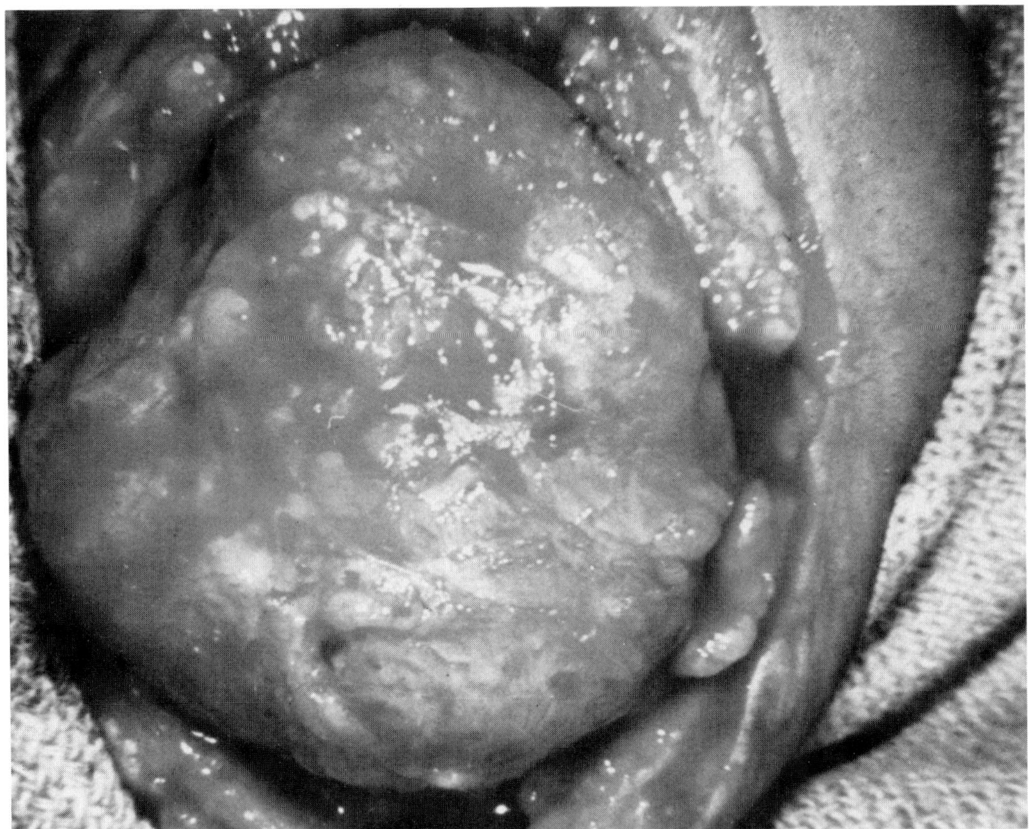

FIG. 22-5. This large bursa developed over the end of the humerus in an acquired above-elbow amputation. Surgical excision of the bursa as well as the underlying bony overgrowth is necessary to eradicate the problem.

ments.[3] Neuromas are not present in congenital limb deficiencies.

Phantom Limb

Phantom limb sensation always occurs following acquired amputations in children, as it does in adults. However, if the amputation is performed on a child younger than 10 years of age, the phantom sensation is rapidly lost.[100] This is in contrast to teenagers and adults whose phantom limb may persist indefinitely. *Painful phantom limb* does not occur in growing children but has been reported in teenagers. Neither phantom limb sensation nor painful phantom limbs occur in children with congenital limb deficiencies.[100]

PROSTHETIC MANAGEMENT

Although prosthetic devices used for the child amputee are remarkably similar to those used for adults, they are also strikingly different in many respects. Although it is quite obvious that the components used in fabricating a prosthesis for a child must be varied according to the age and size of the child, it is sometimes not so obvious that the length of the lever arms and, therefore, the resultant forces generated are radically different in a small child compared with an adult. It is, therefore, extremely important that established prosthetic principles be closely observed in fabricating a prosthesis for a child. Light-weight materials should be used in small amounts in prostheses for infants, and both the strength and weight should be increased as the child grows older and subjects his prosthesis to harder use.[163]

Upper Limb Prosthetic Fitting

Prosthetic fitting and training should be coordinated with the normal development of

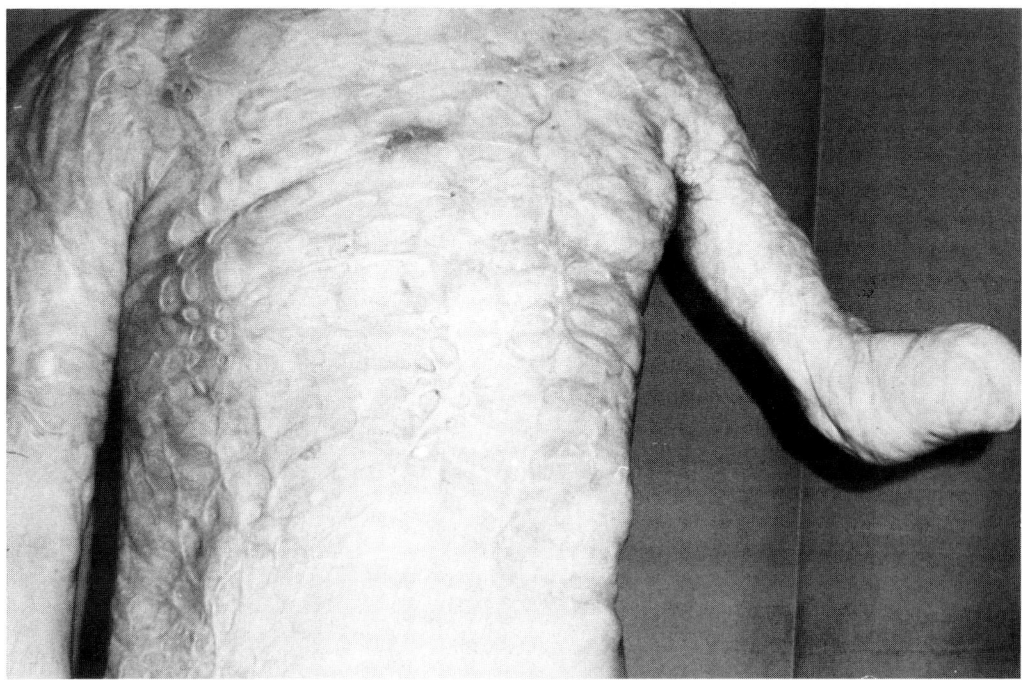

FIG. 22-6. Massive scarring and extensive skin grafting secondary to thermal burns present a very difficult prosthetic fitting problem in this child with a below-elbow amputation.

motor skills in the growing child.[31B] It is unreasonable to expect a 1-year-old infant to effectively use the complex harnessing and cable systems used in an adult above-elbow prosthesis. At this age, a child possesses neither the kinesthetic motor skills necessary to use the prosthesis actively nor a sufficiently long attention span to permit productive training sessions. Selection of prosthetic components compatible with the child's motor development and short frequent training sessions of sufficient simplicity are mandatory if child, parents, physician, and therapist are all to avoid frustration and achieve successful prosthetic use.

As a general rule, prosthetic fitting of the upper limb can be successfully initiated when the child has achieved adequate sitting balance. This will usually be at approximately 6 months of age. The terminal device is passive in this initial prosthesis and is not activated by cable control until the child exhibits interest in attempting to insert objects into the passive terminal device. This will occur in most children at some time during the second year of life but may be later in those children with higher levels of amputation. In an above-elbow or higher level prosthesis, the elbow lock may be activated by means of a pull-tab (used by the mouth or the sound opposite hand) incorporated into the prosthesis at the time of terminal device activation. However, a remotely controlled elbow lock should not be used until the child develops sufficient coordination to use this device successfully. This will usually be in the third year of life.

The primary purpose of the normal human upper limb is the appropriate placement of the hand in space. Likewise, the primary purpose of an upper limb prosthesis is to enable the wearer to position his terminal device in an appropriate position to achieve useful prehension. Prehensile activities in the infant are of the two-handed clasping variety, with subsequent progression to the more functional one-handed grasp, and then to finger-tip prehension as motor skills develop.[10] For this reason, many centers prefer to use a plastic mitten or plastisol-covered wafer as the initial terminal device for infants, thinking that this allows the child to use two-handed clasping activities more advantageously. Others believe the small plastisol-covered hook (No. 12-P) is equally effective in affording two-handed grasp and,

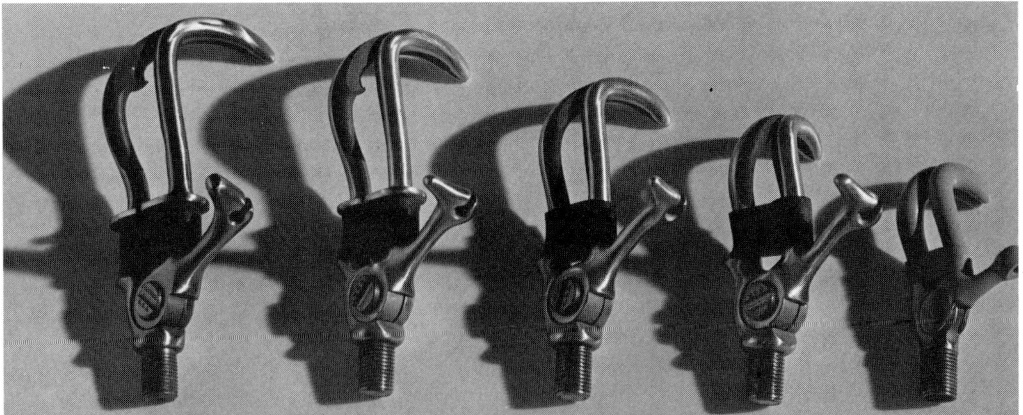

FIG. 22-7. Dorrance prosthetic hook terminal devices. From left to right are numbers 5-XA, 88, 99, 10, and 12-P.

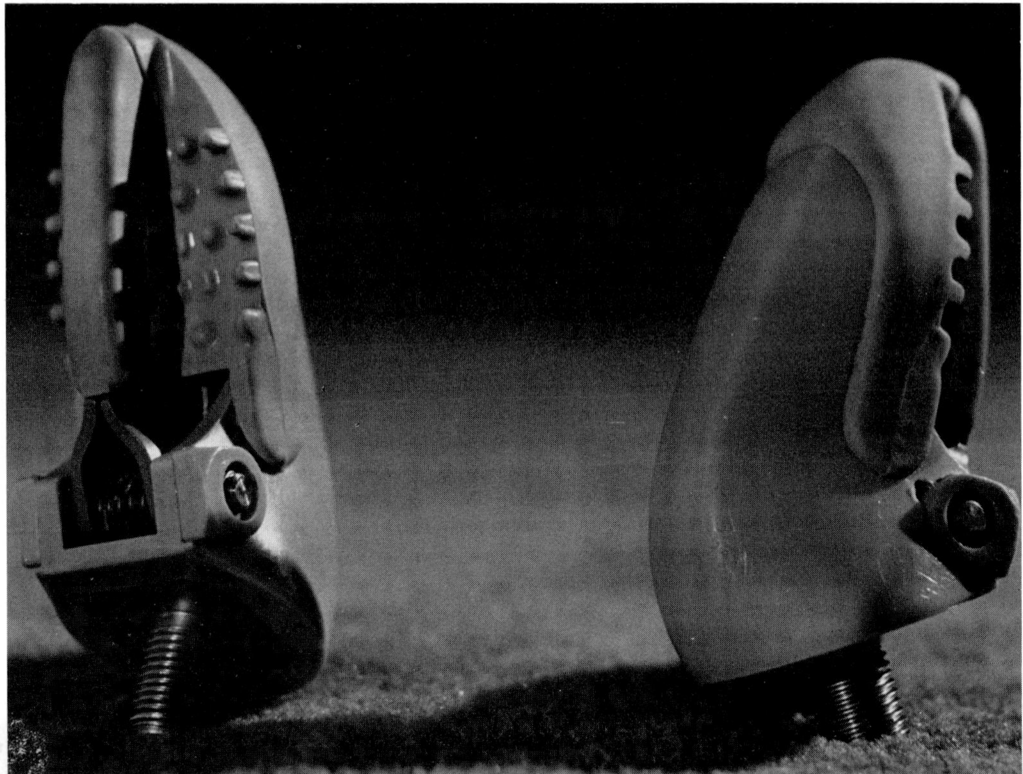

FIG. 22-8. The CAPP prosthetic terminal device is an innovative design originated at the Child Amputee Prosthetic Project at the University of California at Los Angeles. The large gripping surfaces provide the infant or small child with excellent friction for holding objects and are easily replaced as they become worn. A larger size is now available for the older child.

in addition, assists the child to pull up to the standing position (Fig. 22-7). Also, the hook can be cable activated at the appropriate time without the expense of purchasing a new terminal device. Another terminal device suitable for the initial fitting of infants and subsequent fitting of small children is the innovative Child Amputee Prosthetic Project (CAPP) terminal device[149A,149B] (Fig. 22-8), currently available in two sizes. Personal experience with this unique design indicates a significant improvement in both cosmesis and function over hook devices of similar sizes.

As the child grows older and larger, the original terminal device is progressively replaced with larger terminal devices (10-P, 99, and 88) and finally with the adult-sized 5X hook (see Fig. 22-7). As adolescence is approached, consideration is given to the use of a prosthetic hand. Presently available body-powered prosthetic hands come in a variety of sizes (Dorrance No. 2, No. 3, and No. 4) and are extremely functional (Fig. 22-9). Hands are considerably heavier than hooks, and their weight is disadvantageously positioned at the end of the prosthetic lever arm. This may prevent use of a hand in short below-elbow amputations and in higher level amputations where available forces for elbow flexion are minimal. Furthermore, the high initial cost of the hand, the most costly maintenance, and the necessity for frequent replacement of the cosmetic glove are economic deterrents to use of the hand in cases in which funds are limited. Quite often, however, the psychological benefits of wearing a prosthetic hand outweigh the economic considerations and some of the minor functional deficiencies of the devices. In Sweden, Sorbye[152A] demonstrated that children as young as 2 years of age can successfully use an EMG-controlled electrically powered prosthetic hand as the terminal device of a unilateral below-elbow prosthesis. His experience has been corroborated by clinicians in this country, as well as in other European centers.[39A,166A]

Prosthetic wrist units are usually of the manually controlled friction variety and provide passive substitution for pronation and supination in the prosthesis. Oval wrist units are cosmetically more pleasing than the standard round units. In the infant, the CAPP wrist

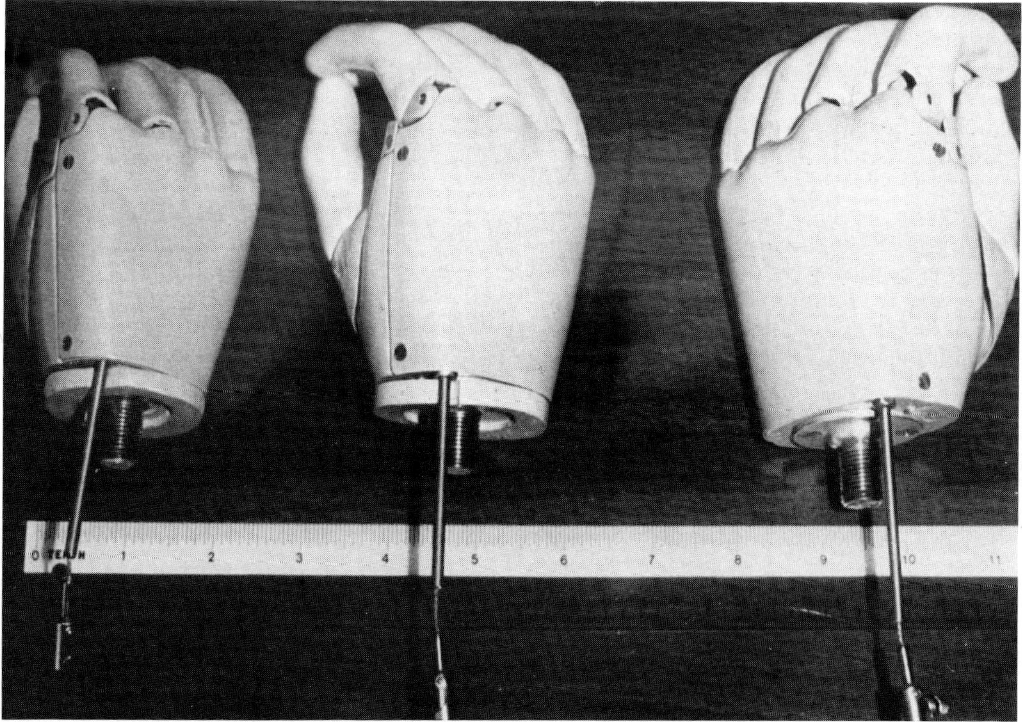

FIG. 22-9. Dorrance prosthetic hand terminal devices. From left to right are sizes No. 2, No. 3, and No. 4. (Photo courtesy of Hosmer-Dorrance Company.)

unit constructed of Delrin plastic has the advantage of lightness. Wrist flexion units should be considered in bilateral upper limb amputees to provide better prosthetic function for activities close to the face. Younger amputees will rarely use the flexion feature, however.

Elbow hinges are used with most types of prostheses for amputations distal to the elbow. The hinges are part of the suspension system, attaching to a triceps pad or half cuff. Flexible hinges are used in almost all cases to take advantage of any residual pronation and supination in the stump. Wrist disarticulation amputees retain 100% of pronation and supination unless the distal radioulnar joint has been damaged. Patients with shorter amputation levels retain progressively less pronation and supination. Whatever the level, only 50% or less of the available stump pronation and supination is actually transmitted through the prosthesis. In some infants, in very short stumps, and in certain older children using their prostheses for heavy lifting, rigid elbow hinges may be more effective for prosthetic suspension.

Outside elbow–locking mechanisms are used for the elbow disarticulation amputee where humeral rotation is readily transmitted through the socket and where length is a significant consideration. In the above-elbow and shoulder disarticulation amputee, a more sturdy inside elbow–locking mechanism is used with a manually controlled turntable, which provides passive substitution for humeral rotation. Electrically powered elbows are often beneficial for the shoulder disarticulation and forequarter level amputee.

A variety of passive prosthetic shoulder joints are available for the shoulder-disarticulation–type amputation and the forequarter amputation, each with its advantages and disadvantages. Newer research models have been introduced that incorporate universal or flexion-abduction joints.

Harnessing provides suspension of the prosthesis and, combined with the Bowden cable system, uses body motion for terminal device and elbow operation and for control of the elbow-lock mechanism. A figure-of-eight harness is most often used with both above- and below-elbow prostheses, but a shoulder saddle and chest strap may be required in patients who have skin problems or who for other reasons cannot comfortably wear a figure-of-eight harness. Harnessing for shoulder disarticulation and forequarter prostheses is highly individualized. Body-powered prostheses for these higher amputation levels are inefficient, and externally powered prostheses are highly desirable for such patients. (Externally powered prostheses are discussed in detail in the section on congenital limb deficiencies.) Teflon lining is frequently used in the cable housing to diminish friction and to increase the longevity of the cable. This is especially beneficial to small children and high level amputees.

The following are brief descriptions of the various prostheses used for the major levels of upper limb amputations in children.

Wrist Disarticulation. The double wall socket of this prosthesis is fabricated with a channel for the distal ulna in order to allow the bulbous end of the stump to enter the socket more readily (Fig. 22-10). Flexible elbow hinges are necessary to take advantage of the full pronation and supination normally present in these stumps. Harnessing is by means of a standard below-elbow figure-of-eight harness with a single-control Bowden cable.

Below-Elbow Amputations. Long and medium length stumps are fitted with a socket of standard double-wall construction with slight

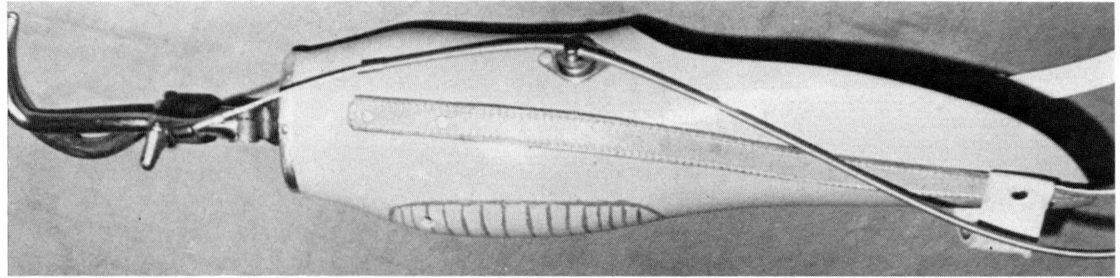

FIG. 22-10. The lined area on this wrist-disarticulation prosthesis indicates the channel fabricated for the distal ulna. This allows the bulbus end of the amputation stump to enter this socket more easily.

preflexion of the socket. Short stumps and especially very short below-elbow stumps present problems of socket suspension and retention of the stump in the socket when the elbow is flexed above 90°. These stumps are fitted in one of three ways, the most standard of which is with a markedly preflexed socket, the so-called banana arm. This allows positioning of the terminal device near the face with only limited elbow flexion, but it is cosmetically objectionable to some. A second choice is to use a split socket with step-up hinges (Fig. 22-11). These hinges provide approximately 10° of forearm flexion for each 5° of stump flexion. Durability of these joints is poor, and live lift is markedly decreased. This type of fitting is used primarily in bilateral cases. Standard below-elbow figure-of-eight harnessing is used with both of the above fittings. The third choice is the highly successful modified Muenster prosthesis.[51,61] This design originated with Drs. Hepp and Kuhn in Muenster, Germany and consists of a self-suspending socket fitted with the elbow in 35° of flexion (Fig. 22-12). Further flexion is possible to only 90° or 100°. The excellent cosmesis plus the outstanding live lift and axial loading capabilities provided by this prosthesis have made it quite successful in many clinics.[47,57] A further advantage is harnessing with a solitary axillary loop, the so-called figure-of-nine harness. The primary disadvantage of the Muenster prosthesis is limited elbow flexion, which precludes its use in bilateral cases. Neither the snug fit of this socket in the growing child nor excessive clothing wear because of the low take-off of the terminal device control cable has been a significant problem in our personal series of Muenster fittings, but these have been reported as troublesome problems in some clinics.[56,133]

Elbow Disarticulation. The socket is constructed with a large anterior biceps window to allow easier insertion of the bulbous stump end, and the entire trim line of the socket brim is level with the axilla (Fig. 22-13). These modifications from the standard fitting allow for growth accommodation, provide better ventilation, and make the prosthesis more easily donned and doffed.[165A] An outside elbow lock must be used at this level. Harnessing is with a standard *below-elbow* figure-of-eight harness to which is attached an elbow-lock control strap. A standard *above-elbow* dual control Bowden cable provides elbow flexion and terminal device operation.

Above-Elbow Amputations. The socket is of standard double-wall construction with a standard trimline. An inside elbow joint is used. A standard above-elbow figure-of-eight

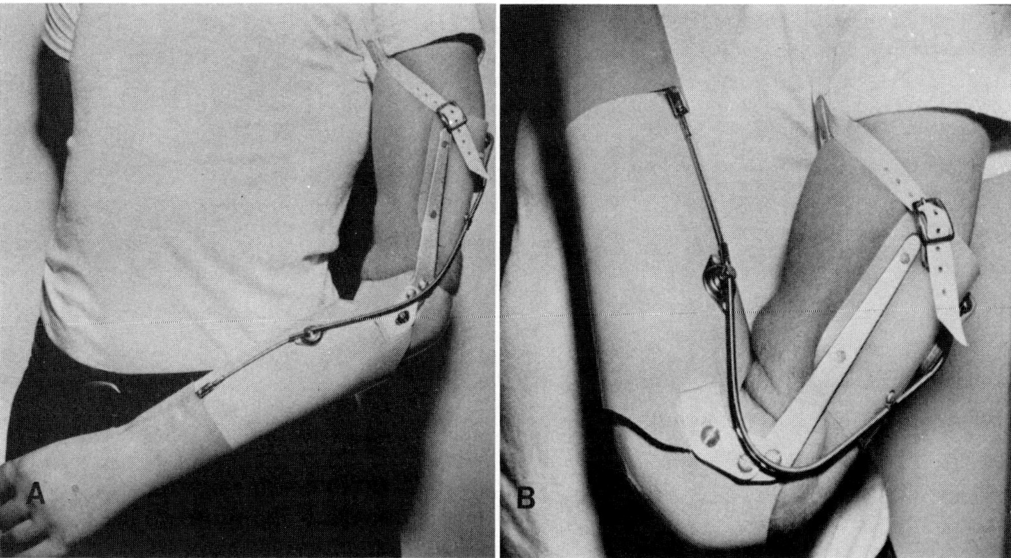

FIG. 22-11. *(A)* The split-socket prosthesis is designed for the very short below-elbow amputation. *(B)* Step-up elbow hinges provide 10° of forearm flexion for each 5° of stump flexion. (From The child with an acquired amputation. With the permission of the National Academy of Sciences, Washington, DC)

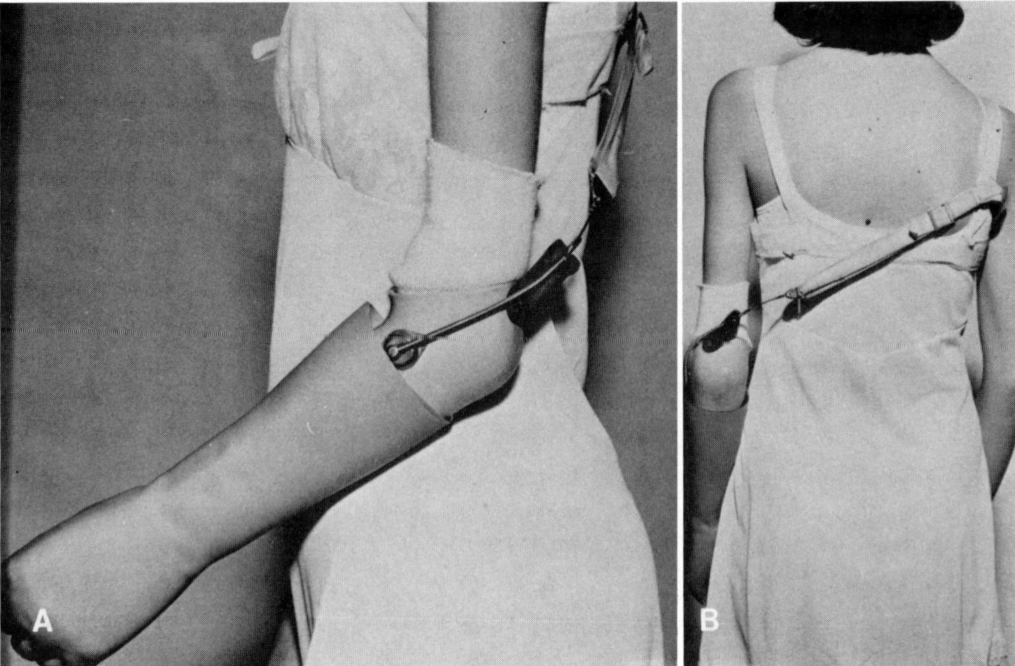

FIG. 22-12. *(A)* The modified Muenster prosthesis incorporates a self-suspending socket for the very short below-elbow amputation stump. *(B)* Harnessing for the Muenster prosthesis is of the simplified "figure-of-nine" variety. (From The child with an acquired amputation. With the permission of the National Academy of Sciences, Washington, DC)

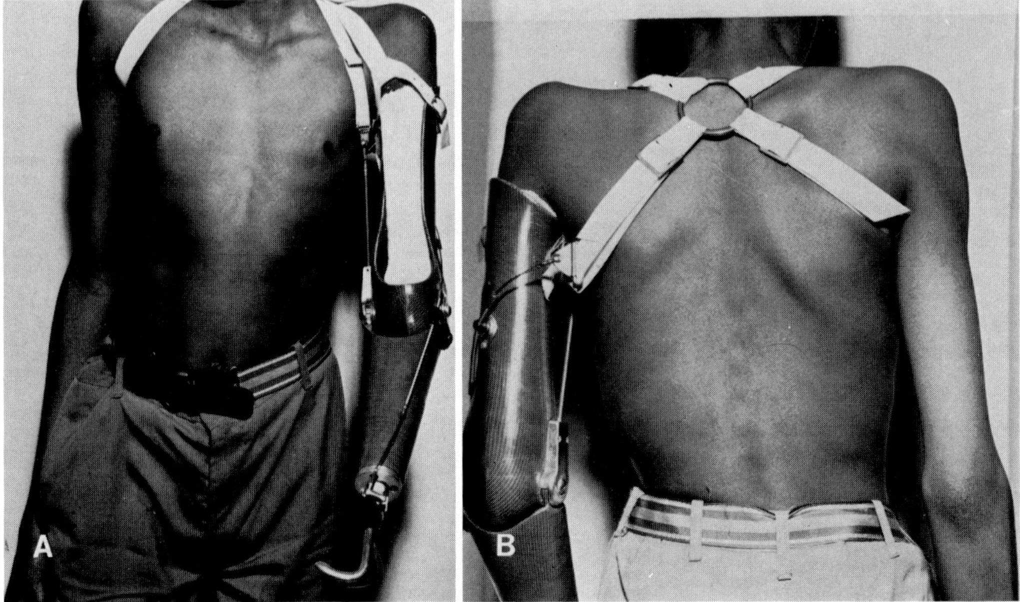

FIG. 22-13. *(A)* The elbow disarticulation prosthesis incorporates a large anterior biceps window to allow easy insertion of the bulbus stump. *(B)* An outside elbow lock is placed on the medial side of the socket at the elbow joint level and harnessing is of the "figure-of-eight" variety. (From The child with an acquired amputation. With the permission of the National Academy of Sciences, Washington, DC)

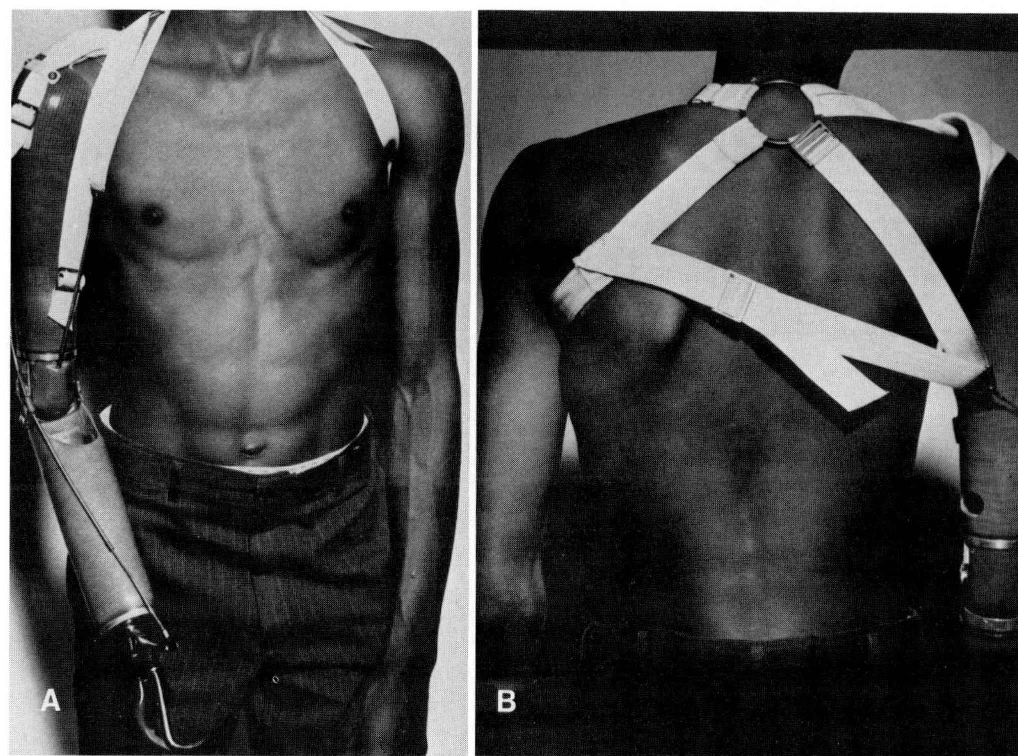

FIG. 22-14. *(A)* The above-elbow prosthesis incorporates an inside elbow joint mounted on the end of the socket by means of a turntable, which provides substitution for humeral rotation. *(B)* harnessing is of the above-elbow, "figure-of-eight" type with an across-the-back strap to take advantage of biscapular motion as well as humeral flexion in the control system. (From The child with an acquired amputation. With the permission of the National Academy of Sciences, Washington, DC)

harness with a dual-control Bowden cable is the harness of choice (Fig. 22-14). An across-the-back strap is used almost routinely to take advantage of biscapular motion as well as humeral flexion in the control system and to prevent upward sliding of the control attachment straps. In attaching the cable, the location and length of the forearm lift loop must be varied to coincide with the size of the child for maximum efficiency. For short stumps, the use of anterior and posterior wings on the socket enhances rotational stability, and a spring-lift assist for the forearm is advantageous.

Shoulder Disarticulation. The distal portions of this prosthesis are the same as those used for the above-elbow amputee. The humeral section is flattened on the medial side to allow room for bulky clothing in cold weather. Selection of the shoulder joint is variable, but we have used the passive abduction joint most often (Fig. 22-15). Harnessing for body-powered prostheses is the greatest problem at this level, and, where available, external power is preferable. When body power is used, harnessing must be individualized and must take into account both the excursion and force that can be generated by a specific control motion. In larger children, the control motion for elbow flexion and terminal device operation is scapular abduction with chest strap suspension. Elbow-lock control is usually achieved by means of shoulder elevation, with the anchor point for the control strap being a waist belt. In younger children, because of limited excursion in scapular abduction, shoulder elevation is normally used as the control motion for elbow flexion and terminal device operation, the anchor point being provided by a perineal strap. With this system, trunk rotation is usually used for elbow-lock control motion. As one may imagine, body gyration is often

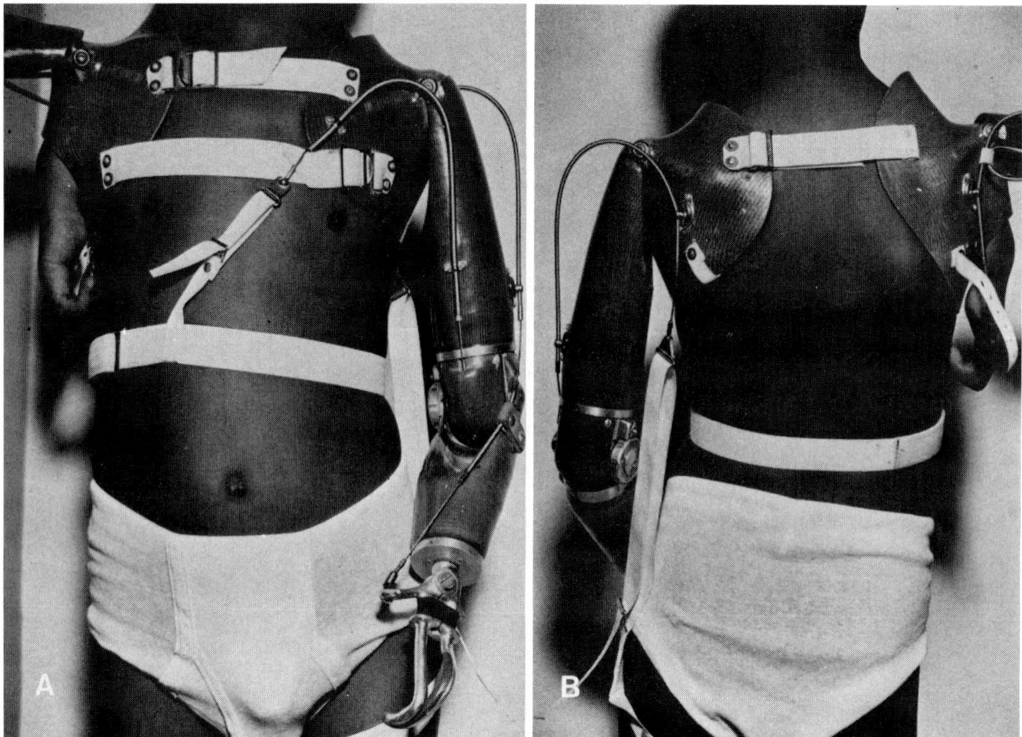

FIG. 22-15. *(A)* This young boy is fitted with a fairly typical shoulder disarticulation prosthesis on the left side. The inside elbow lock is controlled by means of a waist band. *(B)* Elbow flexion and terminal device operation are provided by shoulder elevation with the central strap being anchored to a perineal loop. Body-powered prostheses for this level of amputation necessitate a great deal of body gyration in order to achieve the desired prosthetic function. (From The child with an acquired amputation. With the permission of the National Academy of Sciences, Washington, DC)

quite marked in using a body-powered prosthesis at this amputation level, and prosthetic rejection and non-use is frequent. Externally powered prostheses, as will be discussed in the section on congenital limb deficiencies, have done much to improve prosthetic function and acceptance at this level of limb loss.

Forequarter Amputations. All components in the prosthesis for this level of amputation are the same as those used in the shoulder disarticulation prosthesis up to the socket. Socket suspension may be difficult and often requires an extension of the socket behind the neck and over the opposite shoulder (Fig. 22-16). Effective control motions of sufficient force and excursion are extremely difficult to find in children, and truly functional operation requires the use of external power. Terminal device operation and elbow flexion of a limited degree can be obtained by harnessing the opposite shoulder for control motion. Elbow-lock control is achieved by using chin nudges or mouth straps.

Lower Limb Prosthetic Fitting

In the lower limb, as in the upper limb, prosthetic fitting and training should be coordinated with the normal development of motor skills in the growing child.[10–12,32,48,141A] The average infant develops sitting balance at approximately 6 months of age and begins crawling on all fours at about the same time. Between 8 and 12 months of age, he learns to pull himself up and stand with support. Independent ambulation is usually achieved at approximately 12 months of age. Initial ambulation is carried out with the feet widely spread to achieve a more stable base of support, the lower limbs are usually externally rotated at the hip to enhance knee stability (by rotating the knee axis of motion away from the line of progression), and the arms are

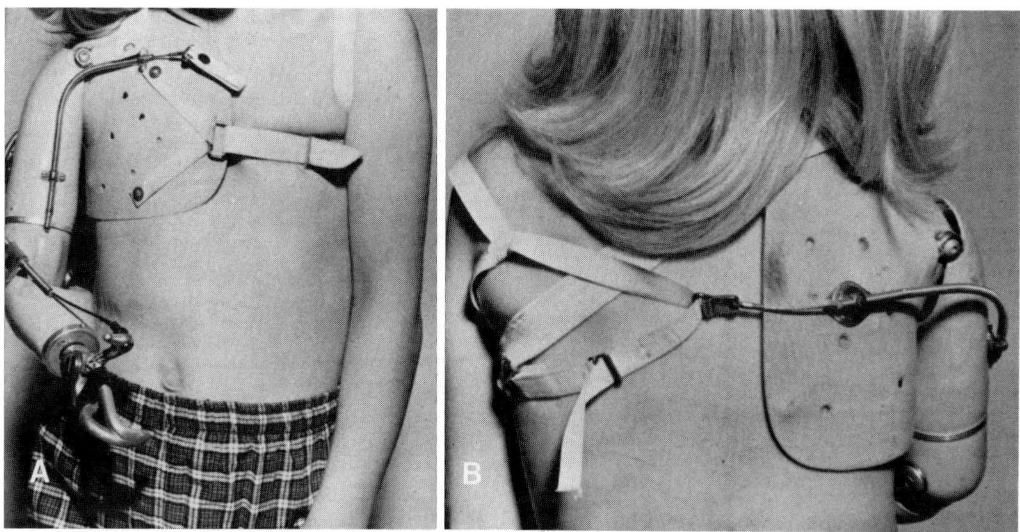

FIG. 22-16. *(A)* Elbow-lock control in this forequarter prosthesis is by means of a pull strap activated by the opposite hand or the mouth. *(B)* Elbow flexion and terminal device operation are achieved by harnessing the opposite shoulder for control motion. (From The child with an acquired amputation. With the permission of the National Academy of Sciences, Washington, DC)

typically held away from the trunk to enhance balance. With continuing neuromuscular maturation, the child's gait progressively improves, but it is not until approximately 5 years of age that his gait really reaches the heel-strike, mid-stance, and toe-off gait typical of the adult.

From the foregoing synopsis of lower limb functional development, it is evident that lower limb prosthetic fitting need not be attempted until the child amputee begins pulling himself up to the erect position between 8 and 12 months of age. It is only at this point that having two lower limbs of equal length becomes necessary. In bilateral lower limb deficiencies, the age of fitting will be a more arbitrary decision based on the time when a normal child would be expected to stand. In the above-knee amputee, stabilizing the prosthetic knee by means of locking mechanisms will be necessary until the child demonstrates adequate control of the prosthetic knee joint. Knee stability is conveniently obtained by attaching an adjustable strap-and-buckle device across the anterior aspect of the knee joint. Finally, it should be obvious that very young lower limb amputees cannot be expected to walk with the normal heel-strike, mid-stance, toe-off gait seen in older amputees, and training efforts expended to achieve this type of prosthetic gait prior to age 5 or 6 years will be fruitless.

The normal human lower limb is designed to provide weightbearing stability and locomotion. In the prosthetic lower limb, stance phase stability is achieved by proper prosthetic alignment, and locomotion is attained by proper sequential body and stump motion acting on prosthetic levers and joints.[10] The young child is not concerned with the appearance of his gait, only with progression from one point to another with the greatest expediency. Children will walk in some manner with the most maligned and malfunctioning prostheses imaginable, provided that there is minimal stability and adequate suspension. Judicious selection of prosthetic components, skillful prosthetic fabrication, and intelligent training combined with frequent follow-up by all members of the clinic team are necessary to achieve excellent prosthetic gait in the child.

The following are brief descriptions of the various prostheses used for the major levels of lower limb amputations in children.

Syme's-Type Ankle Disarticulation. This level of amputation is a true ankle disarticulation combined with a Syme's-type soft-tissue closure.[38,70,120] This provides an end-bearing stump and yet preserves epiphyses and avoids bone transection. In young children, the stump

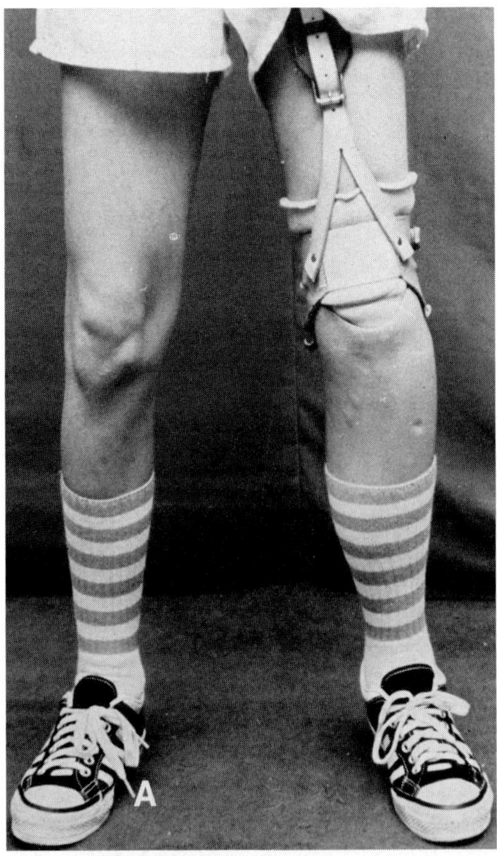

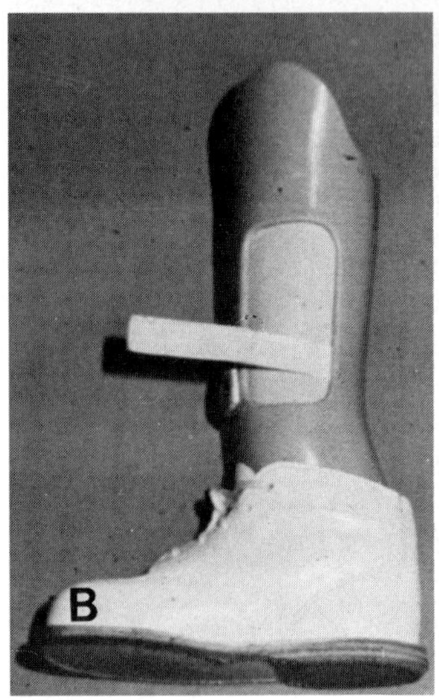

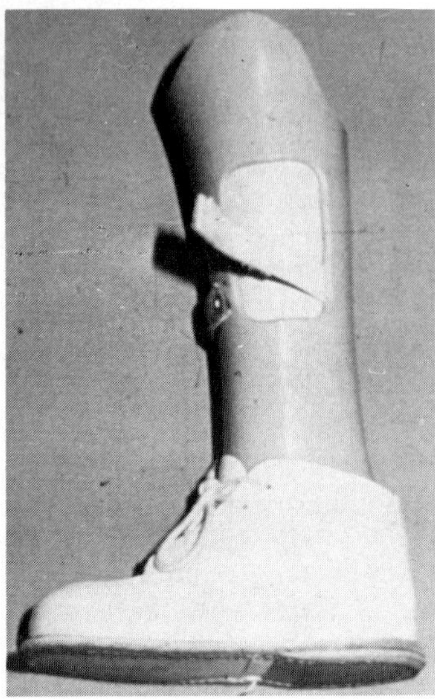

FIG. 22-17. *(A)* A cosmetically acceptable Syme prosthesis can be fabricated after the bulbus stump end has atrophied with growth of the child. *(B)* In most instances, the Syme prosthesis will have a medial opening window to allow entrance of the bulbus distal end of the stump into the prosthetic socket.

is not often bulbous, and, with growth of the child, the malleoli atrophy and an excellent cosmetic prosthesis can be fabricated.[3,53,100] In such instances, a hard (unlined) plastic laminate socket comparable to a long below-knee socket is used, incorporating end-bearing features and using supracondylar strap suspension (Fig. 22-17*A*). A solid ankle-cushion heel (SACH) prosthetic foot is used at this level, as it is for almost all lower limb amputation levels in the child. In older children, fitting with either an expandable socket or a socket with a removable medial window may be necessary to accomodate bulbous distal ends (Fig. 22-17*B*). These sockets are usually self-suspending.

Below-Knee Amputations. The patellar tendon–bearing (PTB) prosthesis is the standard prosthesis for this amputation level (Fig. 22-18*A*). The hard socket is generally preferred, but soft inserts may be used if desired. A SACH foot is standard and suspension is achieved by a supracondylar strap. Side joints and leather thigh lacers may occasionally be indicated for infants, for very short or extremely tapered stumps, for patients with ligamentous laxity of the knee, or for markedly scarred stumps (Fig. 22-18*B*). The so-called PTB variants are often helpful in the prosthetic management of certain stump problems or may

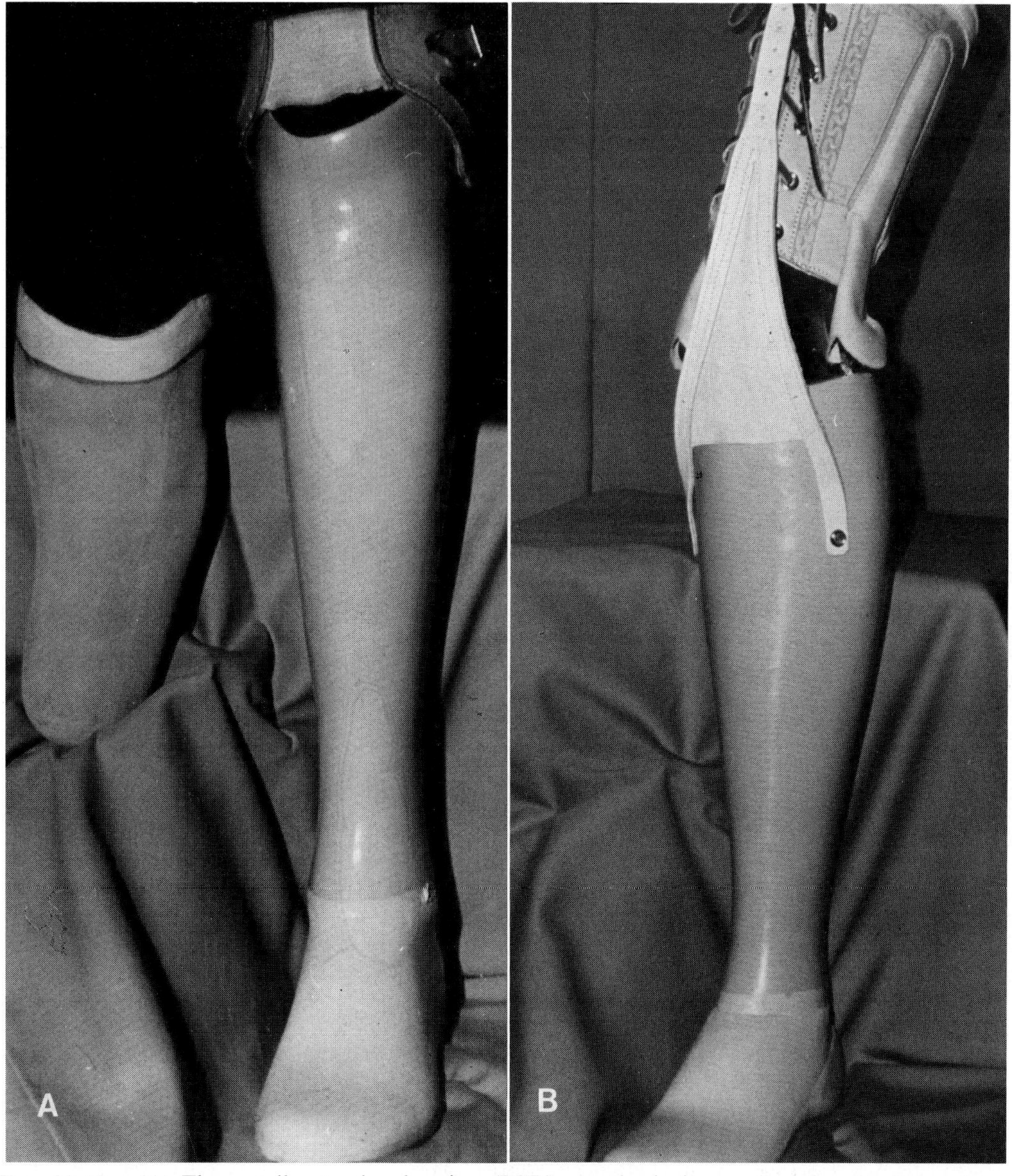

FIG. 22-18. *(A)* The patellar tendon–bearing (PTB) prosthesis is standard for the below-knee amputation and may be unlined or may incorporate a soft insert. *(B)* Side joints and a thigh corset added to the PTB prosthesis provide additional stability for very short or extremely tapered stumps or for patients with ligamentous laxity of the knee.

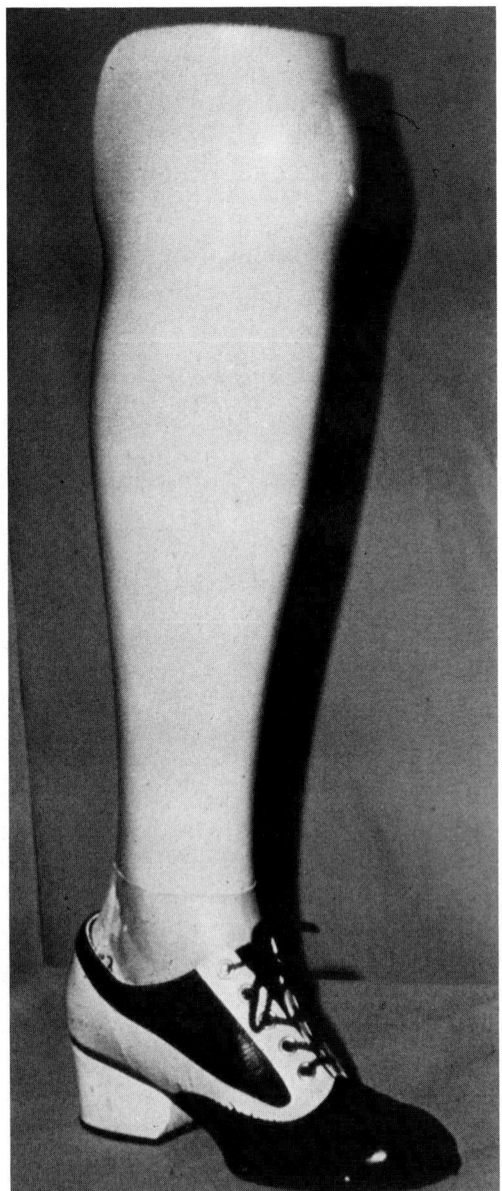

FIG. 22-19. The patellar tendon–supracondylar (PTS) prosthesis is self-suspending and provides excellent cosmesis when the child is standing. This type of fitting also provides good mediolateral socket stability and is helpful in fitting patients with significant genu recurvatum.

be preferred by the older child for cosmetic reasons or by virtue of their self-suspending characteristics. Where mediolateral socket instability from a variety of causes is a problem or where there is genu recurvatum, the patellar tendon–supracondylar (PTS) prosthesis is valuable (Fig. 22-19). The cosmesis of this prosthesis is excellent when the amputee is standing, but there is often an objectionable anterior gap between socket and stump when the amputee is seated. This has been a cause for rejection of this type of fitting in a number of patients. The supracondylar wedge (of several varieties) method of suspension provides good cosmesis and suspension plus mediolateral socket stability for the older amputee with minimal stump changes due to growth (Fig. 22-20).

Knee Disarticulation. The bulbous stump produced by amputation at this level in the older child and adult is not so pronounced in the very young child, and the condyles tend to atrophy with age, as mentioned with the Syme's-type ankle disarticulation. Younger children can usually be fitted with a solid plastic socket of either quadrilateral contour or "plug-fit," incorporating end-bearing (Fig. 22-21). Supplementary suspension with a Silesian belt may be necessary where the femoral condyles are quite atrophic. In the older child with prominent condyles, the socket may incorporate a removable panel or leather lacer opening to permit donning and doffing, or an expandable socket may be used in some cases. Outside knee joints must be used at this level, precluding the advantage of swing phase frictional knee control. The four-bar linkage knee (Fig. 22-22) may be used in larger children, and it does allow swing phase frictional or hydraulic knee control while properly positioning the knee axis of rotation in relation to the sound limb. A SACH foot is used with all knee disarticulation prostheses.

Above-Knee Amputations. The prosthetic socket used for the above-knee amputation is of total contact plastic laminate and is quadrilateral in contour. An inside-knee mechanism of the single axis, constant friction variety is standard in younger children (Fig. 22–23). In the infant, knee stability should be provided by a locking mechanism until the child demonstrates adequate control of the prosthetic knee. This is best accomplished by means of a strap-and-buckle device attached across the anterior aspect of the prosthetic knee joint. Gradual loosening of this device allows progressive knee flexion at the discretion of the therapist as the child develops knee control. The very active teenager may use a hydraulic or pneumatic swing phase knee control sufficiently well to justify the cost of this compo-

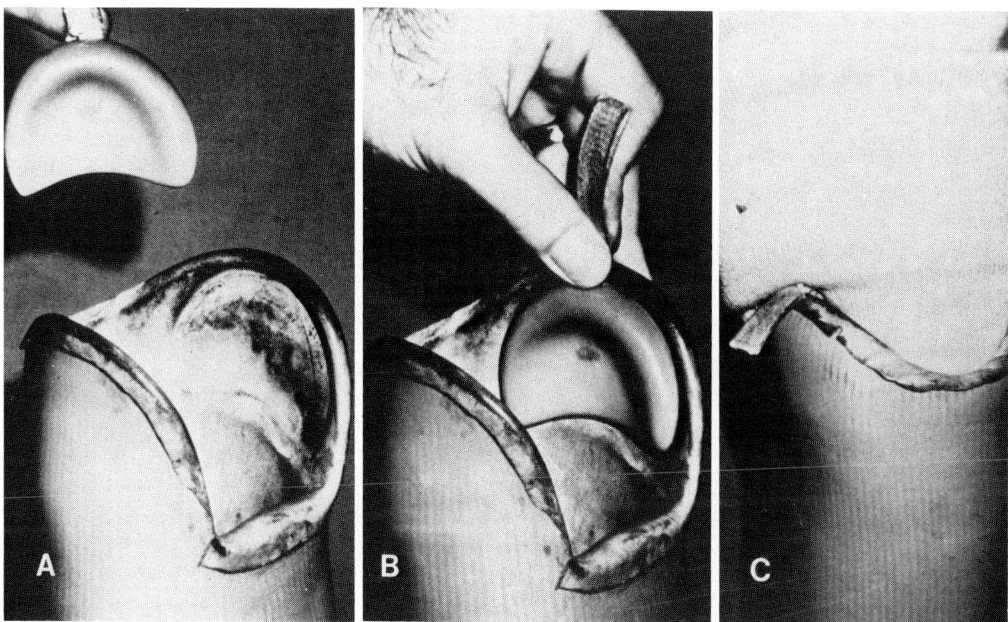

FIG. 22-20. *(A)* Suspension of the below-knee prosthesis may be accomplished by means of a removable wedge. *(B)* This wedge fits into a recess fabricated in the medial brim of the socket. *(C)* When in place, the wedge fits snugly over the medial epicondyle of the femur and provides stable suspension and excellent cosmesis.

nent. Prosthetic suspension is most often achieved by a Silesian bandage or by a hip joint with pelvic belt in the younger child. Suction suspension can be successfully incorporated into the prosthesis when the child is old enough to independently don and doff the prosthesis, and it affords benefits of secure suspension and increased cosmesis. A SACH foot is prescribed for above-knee amputees unless the additional knee stability afforded by an articulated wooden foot is needed with extremely short stumps. Endoskeletal construction incorporating a cosmetic cover of soft plastic foam should be considered in teenage girls, in whom cosmesis is quite important and hard usage is not anticipated (Fig. 22–24).

Hip Disarticulation. Prosthetic components at this level are the same as those used in the above-knee prosthesis except, of course, for a thigh section used in lieu of the above-knee socket. The socket is a plastic laminate pelvic "bucket" encasing the amputated side and extending around the pelvis on the sound side. Front opening with Velcro closures is provided for easy donning and doffing (Fig. 22–25). The hip joint is placed inferior and anterior to the axis of rotation of the anatomic hip joint to provide excellent prosthetic stability in midstance. SACH feet are usually used in children, but an articulated wooden foot may be selected to enhance knee stability. As with the above-knee amputation level, endoskeletal prostheses should be considered in teenage girls because of the marked improvement in cosmesis provided (Fig. 22–26).

Hemipelvectomy. The prosthesis used at this level is identical to the hip disarticulation prosthesis, with appropriate modifications made in the socket to accomodate the anatomic loss.

Immediate Postsurgical Prosthetic Fitting

The technique of immediate postsurgical prosthetic fitting is as applicable for the juvenile amputee as it is for the adult.[28,32,139,141]

Rapid stump maturation, early ambulation and resumption of normal activities, and a diminution of the psychological impact of limb loss are highly desirable benefits accrued by children from this technique. The only significant problem that has been observed in our experience is the tendency for the young child to attempt unprotected weightbearing too early. Appropriate supervision of ambulation and proper gait training will minimize this problem.

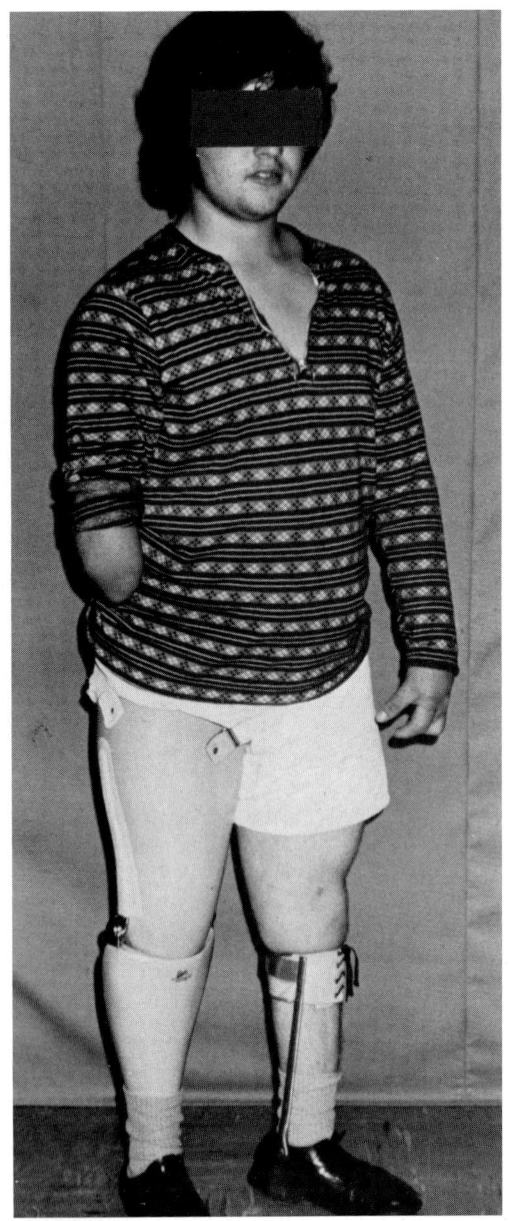

FIG. 22-21. The older child with a knee disarticulation can often be fitted with a solid plastic laminate socket, because the femoral condyles tend to atrophy with age. This end-bearing prosthesis is suspended by means of a Silesian belt.

It has frequently been reported that the very young child will often not fully appreciate the loss of a limb until the time of first cast change.

LIMB LOSS FROM MALIGNANCY

A separate section on prosthetic fitting following limb loss from malignancy seems appropriate in order to strongly emphasize the need to proceed promptly with prosthetic care in these children. In the past, the prevalent attitude of both physicians and lay administrators of state-sponsored crippled children's services was to delay prosthetic fitting of such children for 12 to 18 months in order to minimize the cost of fitting prostheses on children who would die from early metastases and not use them. Because most amputations for malignancy are in the lower limb, failure to provide prompt prosthetic substitution condemns the unfortunate victim to a level of limited ambulation and prevents resumption of normal school, social, and recreational activities at a time when the psychological benefit of these normal activities is so badly needed.

A number of reports in the literature has shown conclusively that at least two thirds of patients with limb loss from malignancy will use their prostheses for a year or longer if there is prompt early fitting.[5,102,161] Early results of new chemotherapeutic programs for malignant bone tumors indicate a marked improvement in survival rates for these lesions.[116,135,166] The widespread use of immediate postsurgical prosthetic fitting, coupled with the use of adjustable socket intermediate prostheses[168A] and/or early definitive prosthetic fitting in children, is of proven psychological and functional benefit. Most physicians and lay administrators have heeded these findings and have responded appropriately by authorizing early prosthetic fitting for children with limb loss due to malignancy, and the benefits have been apparent.

CONGENITAL LIMB DEFICIENCIES

Numerous surveys of the child amputee population have indicated that congenital limb deficiencies account for a larger percentage of children with limb loss than do acquired amputations. As mentioned earlier, for a number of years the relative frequency in new patients seen in a nationwide network of cooperative child amputee clinics has been reported as approximately 60% congenital and 40% acquired.

In contrast to acquired childhood amputations, congenital limb deficiencies occur with almost equal frequency in males and females, and the upper limb is involved twice as often as the lower limb.[1A,79] Multiple limb involvement occurs in approximately 30% of children with congenital limb deficiency compared with

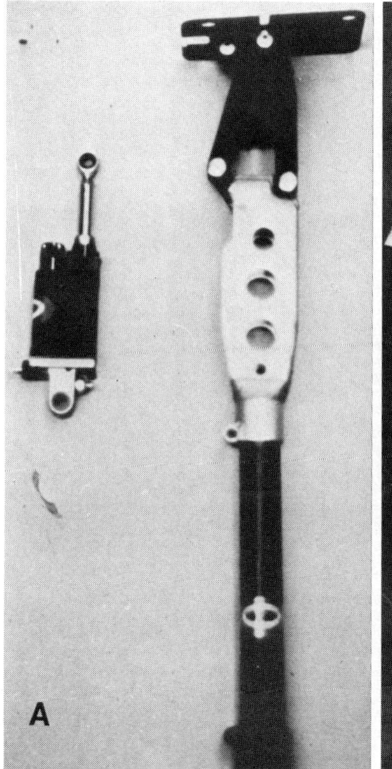

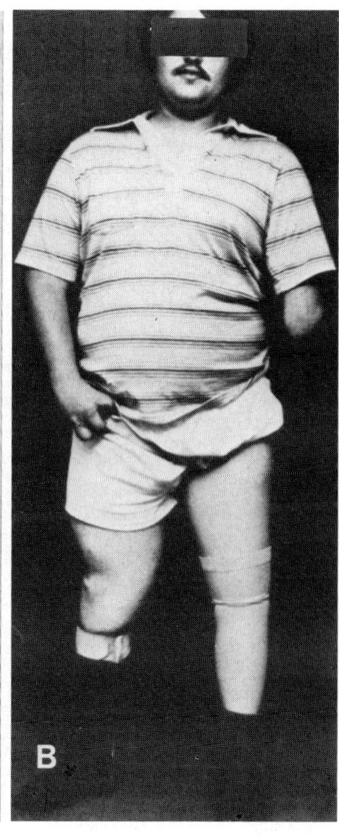

FIG. 22-22. *(A)* The four-bar linkage prosthetic knee allows incorporation of swing phase control of the knee while properly positioning the knee axis of rotation in relation to the sound limb. *(B)* Cosmesis is achieved by placing a foam rubber covering over the endoskeletal knee mechanism and shank.

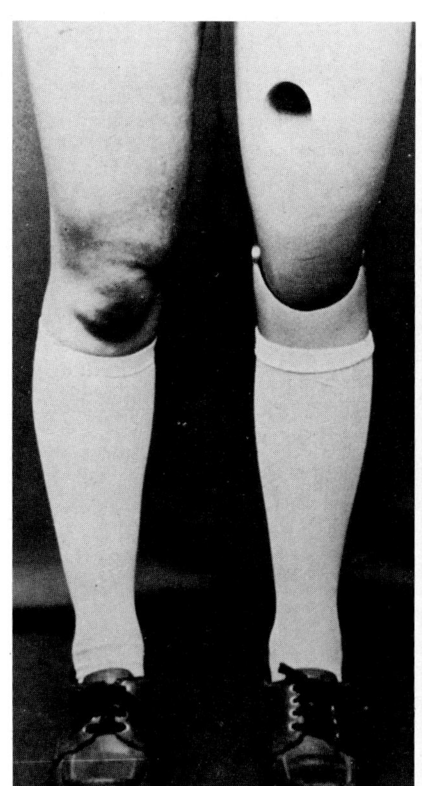

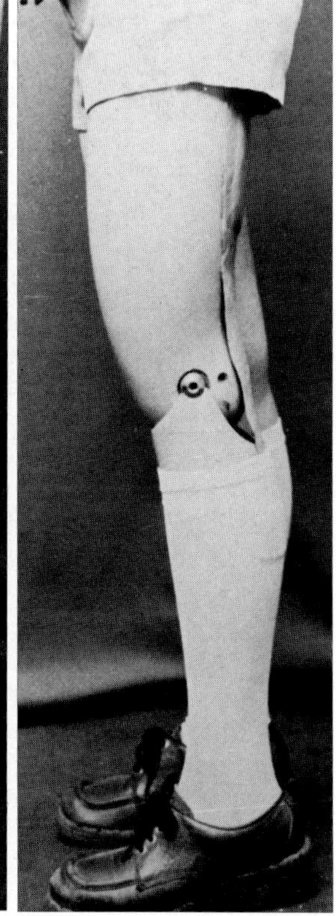

FIG. 22-23. The above-knee prosthesis has a quadrilateral socket and an inside knee joint, which provides constant or variable swing phase control. In this prosthesis, suspension is provided by means of suction.

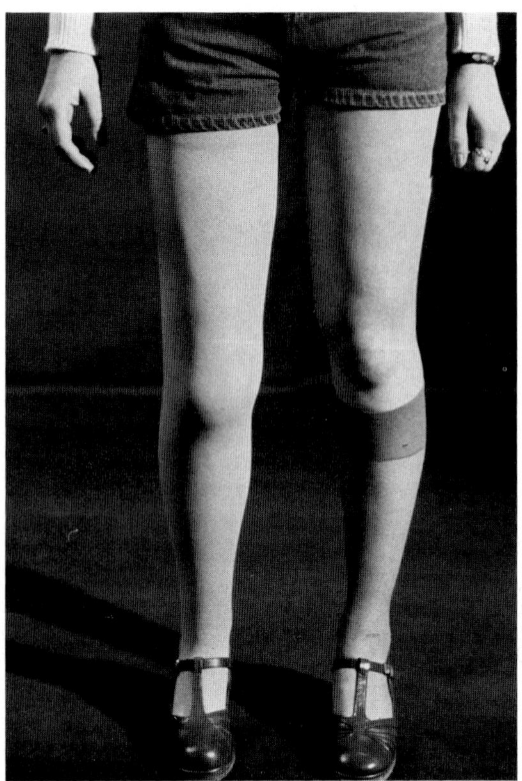

FIG. 22-24. The endoskeletal construction of this above-knee prosthesis provides outstanding cosmesis and may be the prosthesis of choice in the teenage female.

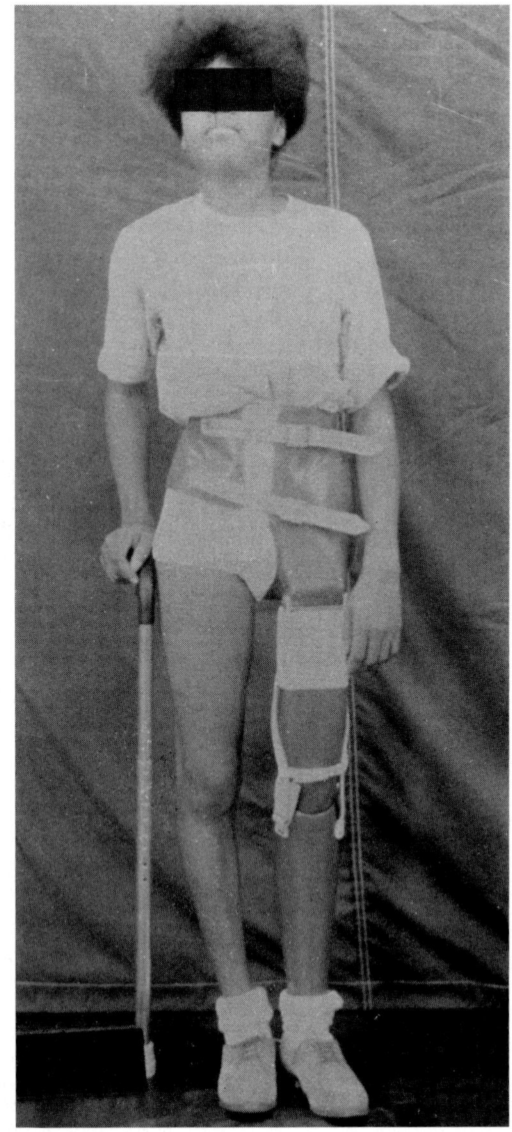

FIG. 22-25. The socket of the hip disarticulation prosthesis encases the amputated side and extends around the pelvis on the sound side. The hip joint is located inferior and anterior to the axis of rotation of the anatomic hip joint in order to provide stance phase stability.

10% of children with acquired amputations; bimembral involvement in 15%, trimembral in 5%, and quadrimembral in 10%.

ETIOLOGY

In order to comprehend the various theories concerning the production of skeletal limb deficiencies, it is necessary to have an understanding of the normal embryologic development of the human limb.[16,62,123,131,143] At 4 postovulatory weeks, the origins of the upper and lower limbs can be detected on the lateral body wall of the growing embryo as small buds of mesenchymal tissue. During the next 3 weeks, these limb buds grow larger and differentiate into the distinctly identifiable limb segments of arm, forearm, and hand in the upper limb buds, and thigh, leg, and foot in the lower limb buds. The development of the various limb segments is in a proximodistal sequence, so that the arm and thigh appear before the forearm and leg, which in turn appear before the hand and foot. The mesenchymal tissue within the limb buds condenses into detectable skeletal elements, which then chondrify and become cartilaginous models of individual bones. Ossification of these cartilaginous models rapidly follows in a regular sequence. Clefts occur in the cartilaginous

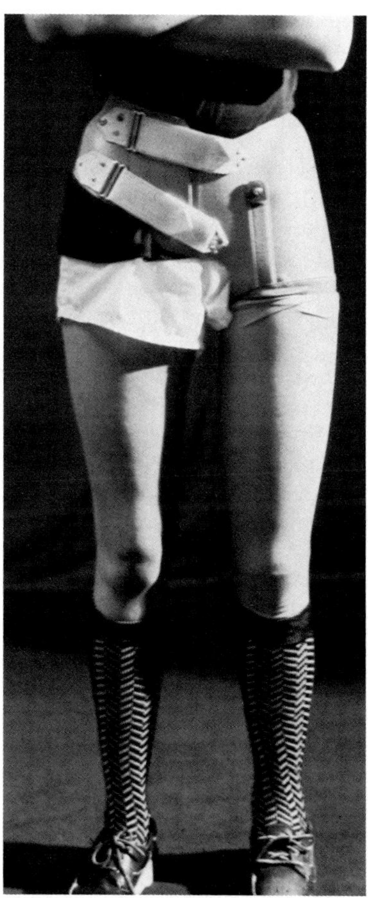

FIG. 22-26. This endoskeletal hip disarticulation prosthesis is markedly superior in appearance to the standard exoskeletal prosthesis illustrated in Figure 22-25.

skeleton and, with further cavitation, differentiate into articulations or joints. By 7 postovulatory weeks, the embryonic skeleton is well formed and is a readily recognizable replica of the postnatal skeleton. From the foregoing, it is apparent that, regardless of the nature of the factors responsible for congenital limb deficiencies, they must act upon the differentiating embryo some time between the third and the seventh postovulatory week.

Numerous theories concerning the mechanism of production of congenital defects have been proposed, and a veritable host of environmental factors capable of producing such defects has been identified, both experimentally and clinically.[33,43,44] To review such material is beyond the scope of this discussion. Suffice it to say that most theories indicate either a mechanism responsible for an arrest in the development of the embryonic limb or some form of destructive process of structures already formed. Such mechanisms or processes must act upon the embryo during narrowly defined time limits, as noted above.

CLASSIFICATION

Beginning as early as 1837, Saint-Hilaire devised a classification of skeletal limb deficiencies, and, in the subsequent literature on embryology, many others have been recorded. The terms used in these classifications were cumbersome and unwieldly and lent themselves very poorly to clinical application in orthopaedic surgery. It was not until 1951 when O'Rahilly[129] identified a consistent morphologic pattern in skeletal limb deficiencies that a clinically functional classification of these defects was devised. This classification was further expanded in the classic publication by Frantz and O'Rahilly in 1961[54] and has remained the most widely used classification for skeletal limb deficiencies in the United States. The Frantz and O'Rahilly classification will be used in this chapter. In this classification, only *absent* skeletal parts are described. Deficiencies are divided into two major types: (1) *terminal*, where there are no unaffected parts distal to and in line with the deficient portion, and (2) *intercalary*, where the middle part of a limb component is deficient but those portions proximal and distal to it are present. Each of these main groups is in turn divided into two groups: (1) *transverse*, where the defect extends transversely across the entire width of the limb, and (2) *longitudinal* (paraxial), where only the preaxial or postaxial portion of the limb component is absent.

There are seven terms of Greek derivation used to describe the various anomalies; three are based on the word *melos* (limb) combined with familiar medical prefixes: *amelia* refers to complete absence of a limb, *hemimelia* (literally ''half a limb') refers to absence of the major portion of a limb, and *phocomelia* (seal-limb) is when the terminal portion of a limb (hand or foot) is attached more or less directly to the trunk in a foreshortened manner. The remaining four terms are *acheiria* (absent hand), *apodia* (absent foot), *adactylia* (absent digit), and *aphalangia* (absent phalanx).

Hemimelia is further subdivided into *complete hemimelia*, where the entire distal half of a limb is absent; *incomplete hemimelia*, where the greater portion of the distal half of a limb is absent; and *paraxial hemimelia*, where the preaxial or postaxial portion of the distal half of a limb is absent. Paraxial hemimelia may be either terminal or intercalary. (Fig. 22–27 illustrates the Frantz-O'Rahilly classification of congenital limb deficiencies.)

Approximately 85% of congenital limb deficiencies can be easily and accurately classified by the Frantz and O'Rahilly method.[130] However, the European orthopaedic community has evolved yet another classification,[74] and there have been several modifications of the Frantz and O'Rahilly classification in the United States.[21,29,63] Most recently, the International Society of Prosthetics and Orthotics sponsored a new classification based on the Frantz and O'Rahilly system, which will hopefully be acceptable to both United States and European clinicians.[79,80]

MEDICAL MANAGEMENT

In addition to the high incidence of multimembral involvement, children with congenital limb deficiencies also have a high incidence of associated congenital defects of other organ systems, such as genitourinary anomalies, cardiac defects, and cleft palate. All these children should have a complete medical evaluation to detect and treat such lesions. Musculoskeletal problems other than skeletal limb deficiencies may occur, which can alter medical and prosthetic management. One such problem is radial head dislocation, which is seen in a high percentage of children with transverse partial hemimelia of the upper limb.[94,160] Another is idiopathic scoliosis, which has been reported in as many as 48% of children with upper limb deficiencies and which is apparently unrelated to either prosthetic use or nonuse.[45,68,104,115] The presence or potential development of such associated medical problems mandate that clinicians possess the knowledge that such associated conditions may occur and that they maintain a continuing high index of suspicion to detect them.

Because terminal transverse deficiencies are really homologues of acquired amputations[2] and are generally treated as such,[92,159] the medical and prosthetic management of these

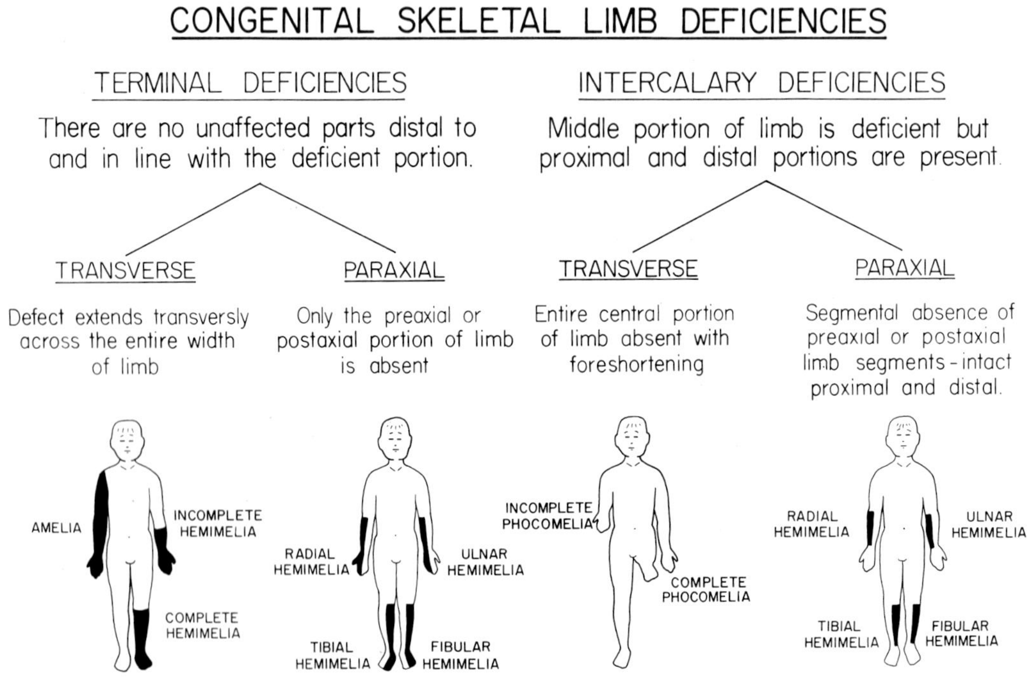

CONGENITAL SKELETAL LIMB DEFICIENCIES

TERMINAL DEFICIENCIES
There are no unaffected parts distal to and in line with the deficient portion.

INTERCALARY DEFICIENCIES
Middle portion of limb is deficient but proximal and distal portions are present.

TRANSVERSE
Defect extends transversly across the entire width of limb

PARAXIAL
Only the preaxial or postaxial portion of limb is absent

TRANSVERSE
Entire central portion of limb absent with foreshortening

PARAXIAL
Segmental absence of preaxial or postaxial limb segments - intact proximal and distal.

AMELIA
INCOMPLETE HEMIMELIA
COMPLETE HEMIMELIA
RADIAL HEMIMELIA
ULNAR HEMIMELIA
TIBIAL HEMIMELIA
FIBULAR HEMIMELIA
INCOMPLETE PHOCOMELIA
COMPLETE PHOCOMELIA
RADIAL HEMIMELIA
ULNAR HEMIMELIA
TIBIAL HEMIMELIA
FIBULAR HEMIMELIA

FIG. 22-27. The Frantz-O'Rahilly classification of congenital limb deficiencies. (Redrawn from Hall CB, Brooks MB, Dennis JF: Congenital skeletal deficiencies of the extremities. Classification and fundamentals of treatment. JAMA 181:590, 1962)

deficiencies will not be discussed except for bilateral amelia. This section will deal primarily with terminal paraxial hemimelia, intercalary paraxial hemimelia, and phocomelia.

Aitken[10] has enumerated the biomechanical losses occurring in intercalary and terminal paraxial lower limb deficiencies as: (1) limb length inequality, (2) malrotation, (3) inadequate proximal musculature, and (4) unstable proximal joints. In upper limb deficiencies, the same biomechanical losses are present, plus varying degrees of loss of prehension. An analysis of such deformities reveals that each deformity can be envisioned as a homologue of an acquired amputation. By determining the most distal stable joint beyond which there is adequate tissue to function as an amputation stump, one may then determine the proper prosthetic fitting level (*i.e.*, below-knee, above-knee, below-elbow, *etc*). At this point, a decision must be made to either proceed with prosthetic fitting, as determined above, or to perform a surgical conversion to provide a better stump and enhance prosthetic fitting. Prostheses used for anomalous limbs must often be quite atypical, and they frequently present problems in fabrication and in function.

SURGICAL MANAGEMENT

Surgical conversions of anomalous limbs are performed as either primary or secondary procedures.[10] Primary conversions are done in limb deficiencies whose life history is so well known that one can predict that a conversion will eventually become necessary. Secondary conversions are those performed after a period of prosthetic fitting around the deformity has proved that a conversion will undoubtedly provide better prosthetic use and overall function. Aitken believes that there are no indications for primary conversion in upper limb deficiencies and has found that only 8% to 10% of these cases need secondary conversion. However, in lower limb deficiencies, there are definite indications for primary conversion, and slightly more than half of these cases require either primary or secondary conversion. A clear understanding of this treatment philosophy will eliminate many frustrating uncertainties when the clinician is confronted with formulating a treatment program for the unusual and oftentimes bizarre congenital skeletal limb deficiencies.

UPPER LIMB DEFICIENCIES

Paraxial Radial Hemimelia

Radial hemimelia is second only to fibular hemimelia in frequency of occurrence among congenital deficiencies of the long bones.[129] However, the condition is not often seen as a primary or solitary presenting problem in child amputee clinics, because this skeletal limb deficiency is basically treated as a surgical problem rather than as a condition requiring prosthetic restoration. Furthermore, even untreated cases can develop a high degree of independent function. Nonetheless, the nature of the problem and its relative frequency appear to justify its inclusion in this section.

Radial hemimelia (often referred to as radial club hand) is characterized by radial deviation of the hand, marked shortening of the forearm, and a generalized underdevelopment of the limb.[136] The ulna is usually bowed with the concave side toward the radial side of the forearm (Fig. 22-28). Absence or abnormality of muscles, tendons, nerves, and blood vessels of the forearm are common.[152] There is often atrophy or absence of shoulder girdle muscles, and the scapula and clavicle may be hypoplastic. The humerus is often short, and either end may be deformed. The hand almost always exhibits absence of the thumb and first metacarpal, and the radial portion of the carpus is usually absent. The radius is completely absent in more than 50% of cases, but the proximal portion (and occasionally the distal portion) may be present. More than half the cases are bilateral.

Suggested treatment has varied from no treatment at all or simple casting to correct the hand deformity, to very aggressive surgical programs.[40,52,59,78,132,136,137] The most widely accepted treatment program at present consists of casting very early in infancy to stretch the soft tissues on the radial side of the wrist, followed by soft-tissue surgical releases on both the radial and ulnar sides of the wrist. A second surgical procedure is then done to centralize the carpus over the distal end of the radius, using temporary internal fixation with Kirschner wires, followed by casting or bracing until skeletal growth is complete. Most authors also advocate tendon transfers at the wrist to provide dynamic stabilization of the hand and osteotomy of the ulna, if indicated.[19,22,154] All authors emphasize that good elbow motion and satisfactory hand function

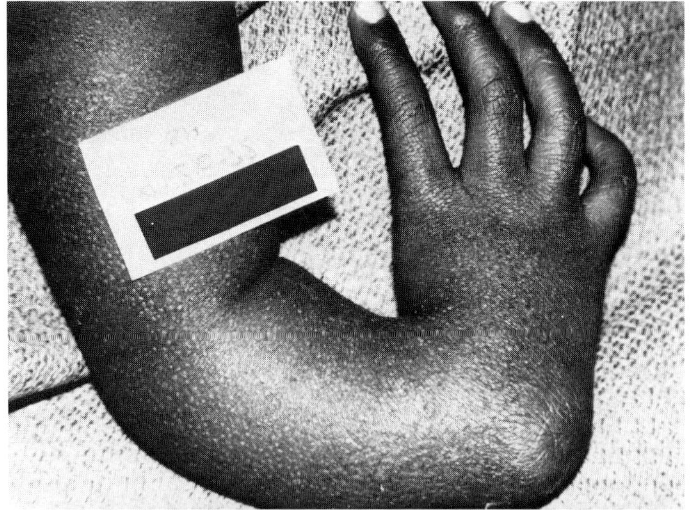

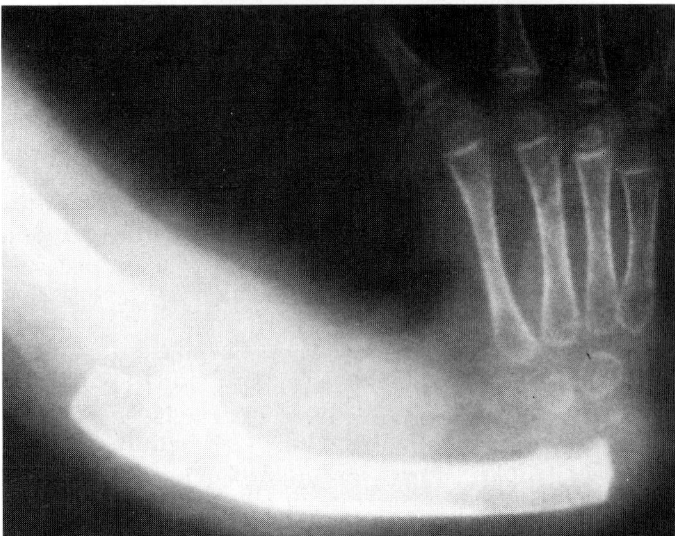

FIG. 22-28. Radial hemimelia is characterized by radial deviation of the hand together with a marked shortening of the forearm. The ulna is usually bowed, with the concave side toward the radial side of the forearm. The hand almost always exhibits absence of the thumb and first metacarpal as well as the radial portion of the carpus.

are prerequisites for surgery. In bilateral cases, the ability of the child to get his hand to his mouth following surgery is of prime importance. If this cannot be accomplished, surgery should not be done.

Paraxial Ulnar Hemimelia

Ulnar hemimelia is the second rarest type of congenital deficiency of a long bone, the rarest type being an isolated complete deficiency of the humerus (proximal phocomelia).[105,129] Most cases are unilateral, and males are involved twice as often as females. Because this deficiency presents as either a terminal or an intercalary deficiency and may be partial or complete, the clinical appearance of the limb is markedly variable.[55] The hand may have five digits, but, most commonly, the two ulnar rays are absent. A monodigital hand is the second most common hand deformity (Fig. 22-29). Partial deficiency of the ulna is more common than complete absence, and, when incomplete, the proximal remnant is usually late in ossifying. In such cases, early roentgenograms may give rise to a false diagnosis of a complete deficiency.[105,128A] At the elbow, the proximal radius may articulate with the capitellum in a normal manner, the radiohumeral joint may be fused, or the radial head may be completely dislocated. The position of the elbow varies from fusion in full extension to a severe flexion contracture, accompanied

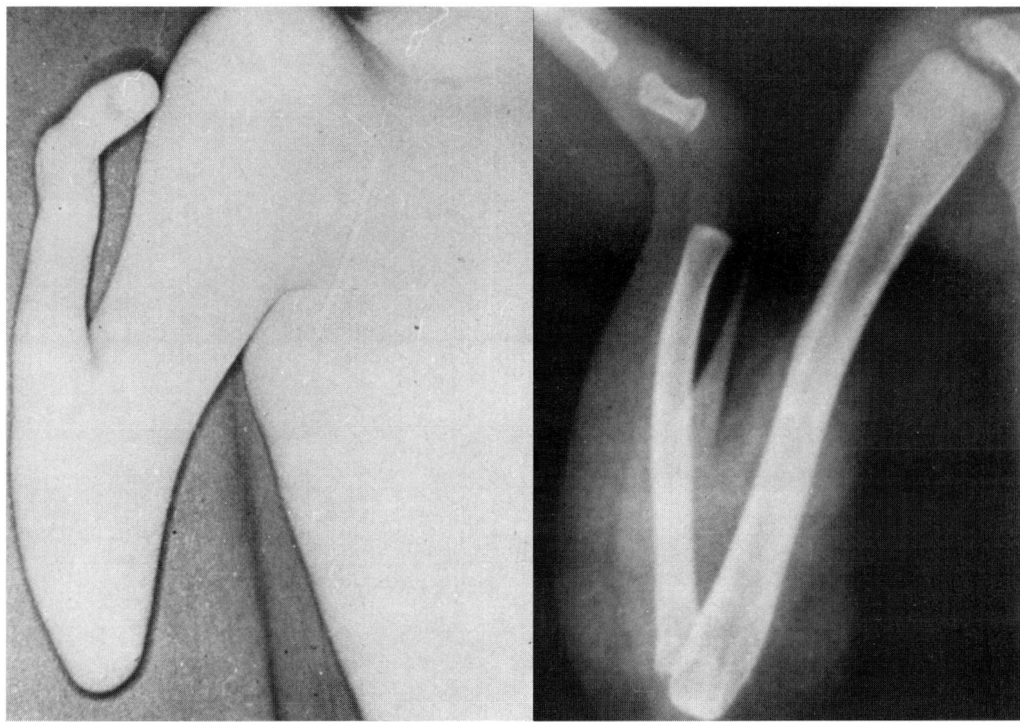

FIG. 22-29. In ulnar hemimelia, the hand is frequently monodigital, and in this instance, there is a severe flexion contracture of the elbow with marked soft-tissue webbing in the antecubital area.

by marked soft-tissue webbing in the antecubital area. Weakness and atrophy of the proximal arm and shoulder girdle musculature is common.

Treatment for ulnar hemimelia will obviously vary with the clinical picture presented.[55,154] Most patients can be managed without surgery and some without any form of prosthetic fitting. Prime considerations in designing a treatment program for children with this condition are the presence of bilateral involvement, the range of elbow motion, the number of digits present, and their prehensile capacity. If elbow motion of at least 90° of extension is present, fitting with a standard below-elbow prosthesis will provide prehension and equalize limb lengths. In the presence of severe antecubital soft-tissue webbing, experience has shown that surgical release of the soft tissues is ineffective in achieving functional elbow extension.[10] In such cases, where the elbow is severly flexed, the limb may be fitted prosthetically as an elbow disarticulation with the flexed forearm segment and the humerus encased within the socket and the digit or digits present used to control the elbow lock. If there is insufficient force or excursion in the digit to control the elbow lock, surgical conversion to an elbow disarticulation followed by appropriate prosphetic fitting may provide better function and cosmesis than any atypical prosthetic fitting (Fig. 22-30). In cases in which the elbow is fused in extension, there are reports of performing either a resection arthroplasty of the elbow or an angulation osteotomy of the humerus to improve elbow position.[129,154] There is no good follow-up data on the few such cases reported in the literature.

Phocomelia

Prior to the thalidomide tragedy that occurred in Europe in the latter part of the 1950s, phocomelia was an uncommon congenital limb deficiency. In Schleswig-Holstein, only three phocomelias occurred in 266,599 live births between 1949 and 1956. In September, 1961, at the height of occurrence of thalidomide-induced limb deformities, the rate had risen to five phocomelias per 1000 births. Upper limb phocomelia is bilateral in more than 50% of cases, and, in cases due to thalidomide, it is almost always bilateral.[125] Complete pho-

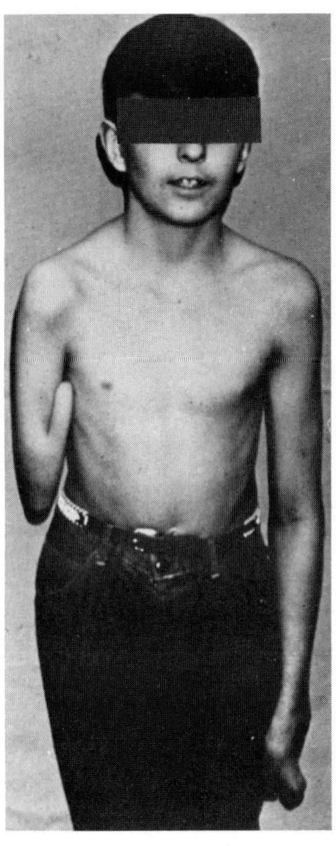
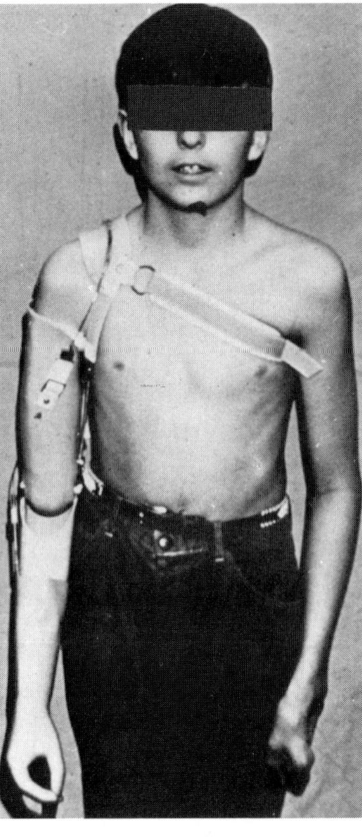

FIG. 22-30. In those instances of ulnar hemimelia with a nonfunctional monodigital hand and severe flexion contracture at the elbow, surgical conversion to an elbow disarticulation followed by appropriate fitting may be appropriate.

comelia occurs more commonly than either the proximal or distal forms.

The typical clinical picture of complete upper limb phocomelia is the child with a hand attached directly to the trunk at the level of the shoulder, more often bilaterally.[10,54,63,98] The hand may consist of five digits, but it more frequently has less, with the thumb being the digit most often absent (Fig. 22-31). Strength and function in these hands are rarely normal, but they tend to improve with growth of the child. However, prehension is usually possible to a greater or lesser degree except, of course, in monodigital hands. The chief biomechanical deficiency in such cases is loss of limb length. In bilateral cases, the affected children commonly develop independence in feeding and in writing but are unable to perform activities such as dressing and toileting because of the severe limb shortening. Children with proximal or distal forms of the defect obviously have less limb shortening and correspondingly less difficulty with dressing and toileting. Other skeletal limb deficiencies are frequently seen in association with phocomelia, especially amelia involving the contralateral limb.

Children with unilateral phocomelia of the proximal or distal variety and a sound opposite upper limb rarely use prostheses.[10] Their sound upper limb is used for most functional activities. The comparatively long phocomelic limb is more assistive than a prosthesis and, in addition, possesses normal sensation. Unilateral prosthetic fitting of the least functional limb in bilateral cases enhances dressing and toileting and may be desirable, although most such children prefer to use assistive devices rather than a prosthesis for these activities.

Children with unilateral complete upper limb phocomelia and a sound opposite upper limb may likewise reject conventional prosthetic fitting, but they often find an externally powered prosthesis beneficial. Bilateral cases require prostheses in order to achieve maximal function, although some older children prefer assistive devices rather than their prostheses. Prostheses should be fenestrated to allow maximal unrestricted use of the phocomelic hand. If conventional body-powered prostheses are used, fitting should be unilateral and the phocomelic hand should be used for elbow-lock operation, if possible.[10,111] A few highly skillful

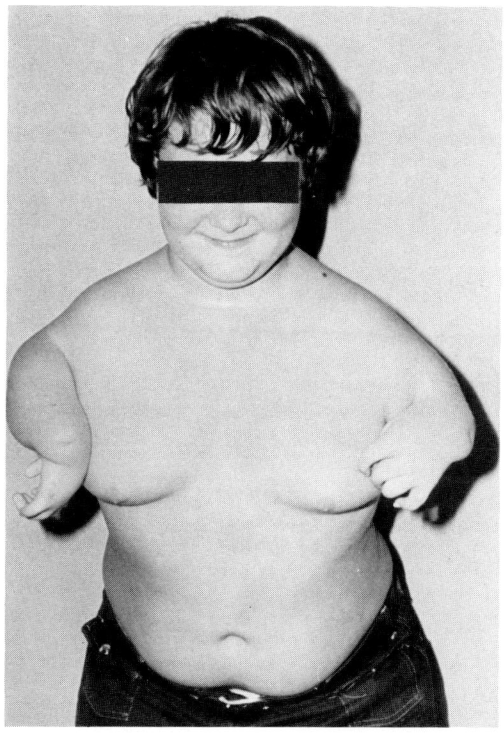

FIG. 22-31. In bilateral complete upper limb phocomelia, the hands are attached directly to the trunk at the level of the shoulder. Although prehension is possible, hand strength and function are rarely normal. Severe foreshortening of the limbs prevents independence in dressing and toileting.

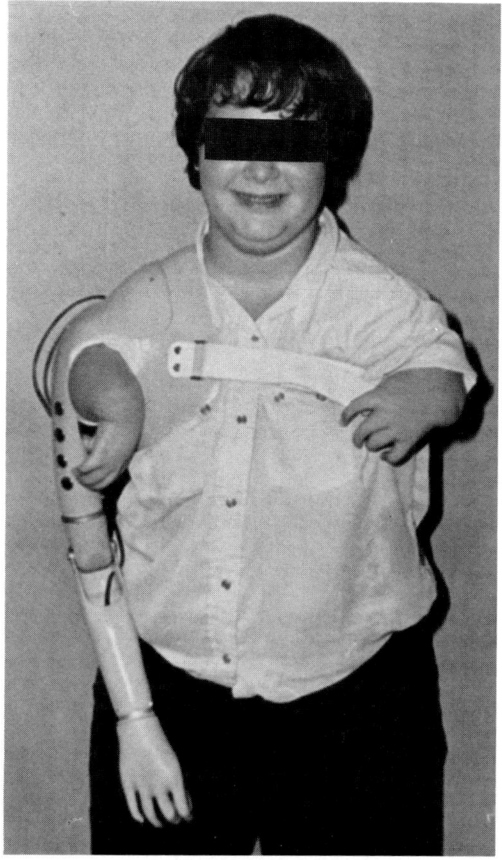

FIG. 22-32. This child with bilateral complete upper limb phocomelia has been fitted with an electrically powered prosthesis. The phocomelic hand is used to manipulate a series of switches in the arm segment to control various prosthetic functions.

children may successfully use bilateral prostheses of this type. Externally powered prostheses are highly desirable for these children. With such devices, the phocomelic hand can usually manipulate several switches and thereby can control a variety of prosthetic functions (Fig. 22-32).

Amelia

Amelia is the absence of all skeletal elements of the entire limb. The shoulder girdle (both scapula and clavicle) is present and is usually normal, although often hypermobile. Excessive fat is sometimes present about the shoulder, either in the form of fat pads or as a diffuse subcutaneous collection. In other instances, there is a paucity of subcutaneous fat and the acromioclavicular joint is quite prominent. Amelia occurs somewhat more often in males, and the condition is bilateral in approximately half the cases. A phocomelia, often of the monodigital type, may involve the opposite upper limb in unilateral amelia[54] (Fig. 22-33).

Being a terminal transverse deficiency, upper limb amelia is the congenital homologue of an acquired shoulder disarticulation. Unilateral cases may be fit prosthetically as described in the section dealing with acquired amputations, bearing in mind that conventional body-powered prostheses are less efficient in the high level upper limb amputee and that externally powered prostheses are preferable, if available.

Bilateral amelia presents the most severe functional loss of all upper limb skeletal deficiences.[10,98] The intelligent, highly motivated, and well-trained child with this defect can achieve near-normal levels of independence with a combination of good prosthetic man-

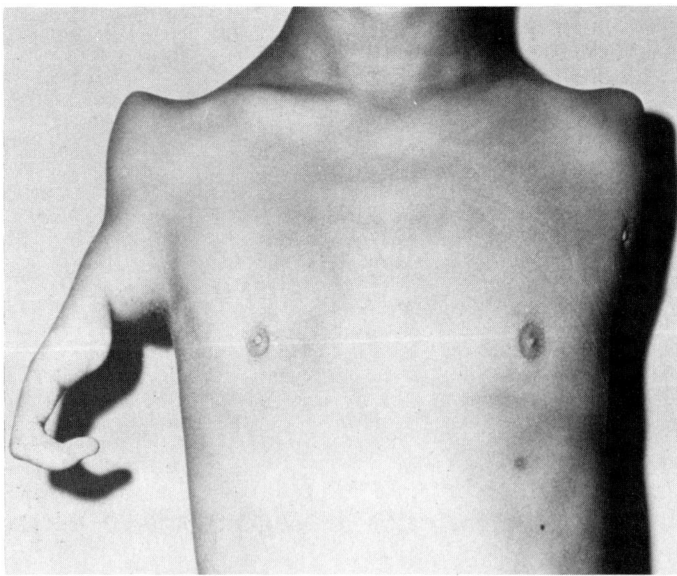

FIG. 22-33. In instances of unilateral upper limb amelia, the opposite upper limb often presents a monodigital type of phocomelia.

agement, excellent prehensile use of the feet, and certain adaptive devices such as modified clothing and dressing hooks.[4] The degree of prehensile foot capability that these children can attain is remarkable, and early and continuous use of the feet for assistance in self-care activities in the home should be encouraged.

Prosthetic fitting of the bilateral upper limb amelic is initiated by applying bilateral shoulder caps at approximately 6 months of age or whenever sitting balance is attained.[4,10] A passive articulated prosthesis can be applied on one side after the child becomes accustomed to the shoulder caps, and activation of the terminal device can be accomplished when the child evinces interest in attempting to insert objects into the hook—usually at 1 year of age or slightly older (Fig. 22-34). Voluntary control of the prosthetic elbow can rarely be accomplished before the age of 2 years. Unilateral prosthetic fitting of these children should be continued until their intellectual capacity and coordination matures enough for them to comprehend the complexity of bilateral control systems. This rarely occurs before age 6 years and may never be practical with body-powered prostheses.

When external power is used, bilateral fitting of extremely simple devices designed to provide two-handed clasping activity by means of powered humeral rotation has been successfully accomplished by children of 2 years of age and some even younger.[117] More sophisticated powered prostheses providing elbow motion, forearm rotation, and prehension should be fitted unilaterally when the child is sufficiently mature to operate them effectively.[112,118,144,151] In the past, powered prostheses designed to provide coordinated "feeding motions" of the shoulder, elbow, forearm, and terminal device[114] were used for feeding activities in the young child. These prosthetic devices are no longer available, and it is currently believed that feeding, dressing, and toileting activities are better performed by using powered components that allow selective, rather than synchronized, motions and by encouraging use of the feet and assistive devices.

Externally Powered Upper Limb Prostheses

During the late 1950s, the extensive use of thalidomide, a tranquilizing agent, by women in the early weeks of their pregnancy resulted in the birth of large numbers of infants with severe skeletal limb deficiences, especially bilateral phocomelia. This tragic event was directly responsible for the rapid development of externally powered upper limb prostheses for children. Body-powered prostheses for high level upper limb loss are functionally ineffective, especially in bilateral limb involvement. This functional ineffectiveness is most apparent in children, where both amplitude of power and cable excursion are limited.

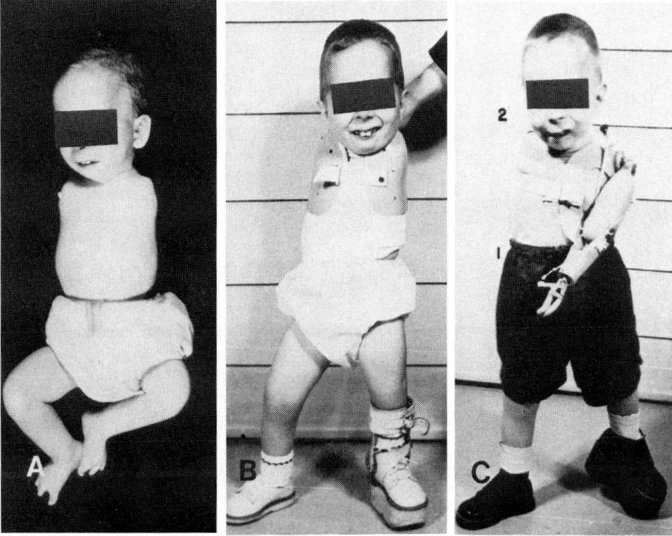

FIG. 22-34. *(A)* Bilateral upper limb amelia presents the most severe functional loss of all upper limb skeletal deficiencies. *(B)* Early prosthetic fitting is by means of shoulder caps. *(C)* Subsequent unilateral fitting with an articulated prosthesis. (Photographs courtesy of Dr. G. T. Aitken, Area Child Amputee Center, Grand Rapids, Michigan)

Thalidomide was not marketed in the United States but was widely prescribed in Europe. During the height of the thalidomide tragedy, European prosthetic centers were literally inundated with children with severe upper limb skeletal deficiences. Recognizing the limitation of body-powered prostheses in providing function for the high level, bilateral upper limb amputee, many of these centers began to experiment with pneumatic prostheses. Pressurized carbon dioxide was selected as the power source, being nonflammable, inexpensive, easily stored under pressure, and reasonably available. Prosthetic systems and components were developed, control techniques were designed, and training programs were devised to incorporate pneumatic-powered prostheses into the management program of these children. By 1962, Marquardt reported fitting children in the second year of life with a Co_2-powered prosthetic system that provided basic two-handed clasping function—the now famous "patty-cake" prosthesis.[118] More sophisticated systems providing elbow motion, wrist rotation, and terminal device operation were developed for older children.[118] Other centers in continental Europe, in Great Britain, and in Canada rapidly adopted the Heidleberg system, developed modifications, or designed entirely new systems for their own patients.[34,60,73,96,109,125,150,151] Electricity was selected as a power source by some centers, and prostheses were designed that used electronic components powered by nickel-cadmium batteries (Fig. 22-35).[50,56A,164] Control of these sophisticated and sometimes complex externally powered prostheses proved to be a major problem for some of the severely limb-deficient children, and a number of investigators began using amplified electrical signals generated by muscle contraction to activate powered components—a technique termed *myoelectric control.*[30,41A,80,145A,146]

As electronic components became more sophisticated and dependable during the ensuing years, pneumatic control systems gradually fell from favor and are rarely used at the present time. Electrically powered components and control systems, in spite of continuing refinements, still exhibit certain shortcomings. The high cost of these devices and the relatively small market for them has hampered their widespread availability. Furthermore, these sophisticated systems are less durable than conventional prostheses and when electronic or mechanical failure occurs, very few prosthetic facilities are able to repair them. This leads to a prolonged "downtime" when the child is unable to use the prosthesis, which, in turn, produces discouragement in the child, parent, and clinic staff. These difficulties clearly illustrate the need for a network of specialized fitting centers in this country and for governmental fiscal support for treating the severely involved limb-deficient child.

A detailed discussion of externally powered prostheses is obviously beyond the scope of this chapter, but it is appropriate to briefly

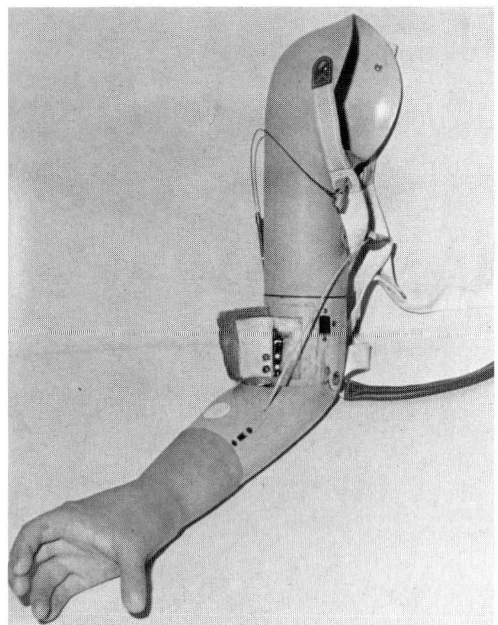

FIG. 22-35. Rechargeable nickel-cadmium batteries are the power source for both the elbow and the terminal device in this above-elbow prosthesis.

review the more commonly used electric power systems.[35,106,112,113,126,127]

Almost all electrically powered prosthetic systems use highly efficient rechargeable nickel-cadmium batteries as an energy source. These small batteries can be connected in series to provide a large amount of electrical energy in a small-sized, light-weight pack that can be suspended from the prosthesis or incorporated into the prosthesis in a variety of ways. Such battery packs are generally capable of providing sufficient energy for a full day of prosthetic operation. They are easily recharged overnight by a simple recharger, which is plugged into an ordinary 110-volt household electric outlet. Either switches controlled by body motion or myoelectric control systems may be used to release energy from the battery to the prosthetic components. Any of a variety of body motions of small amplitude and excursion can be used to operate biomechanically controlled switches such as pull switches or pushbutton switches. Appropriate pressure on the switch allows electrical energy to flow from the battery through wires to the actuator, which is most commonly a small 12-volt electric motor of the permanent magnet, direct current type. These motors produce the desired motion of prosthetic components through a variety of gear or screw mechanisms. When pressure is released from the switch, prosthetic motion ceases. Pressure on other switches (or variations in pressure on the initial switch) produces reverse motion of the prosthetic component. Various braking and cutoff mechanisms are incorporated into the design of these electrical components to prevent motors from burning out when switches are held down after the prosthetic component has achieved maximum excursion.

Control of electrically powered prostheses by means of myoelectric signals is a highly attractive option, and, in certain centers in North America, Great Britain, and continental Europe it has proved to be quite effective. Most commonly, myoelectric control systems use surface electrodes located over muscle remnants in the amputation stumps to pick up electric signals generated when these muscle fibers are contracted at the patient's volition (Fig. 22-36). These minute electrical signals are then amplified electronically to a level that is sufficiently high to control a switch that releases a flow of current from a battery pack to an electric motor, thereby activating a prosthetic component. Usually, two separate muscles are used to produce the signals that control opposing functions of a prosthetic component (*e.g.*, opening and closing of a prosthetic hand). However, it is possible to use multiple signals from the same muscle for this purpose, or even to use weak and strong signals from one muscle to control opposing functions. Furthermore, proportional control of a prosthetic component has been accomplished by using progressively more intense signals to produce more rapid motion or more powerful function. Unfortunately, the most successful applications of myoelectric control have been in that group of patients who need it least—the below-elbow amputees.[108,110,134] However, high-level upper limb amputees are successfully using such systems in a number of child amputee centers in the United States and abroad.[37,41,144,145,153]

When external power is used in prosthetics, the need for sensory feedback becomes even more apparent than when conventional body-powered systems are used. Biomechanical control of externally powered prostheses results in at least some pressure on sensitive body areas, and this produces a certain amount of feedback. Visual and even auditory feed-

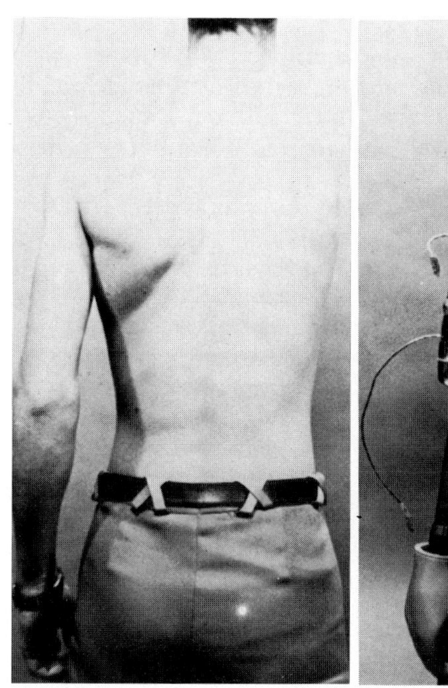
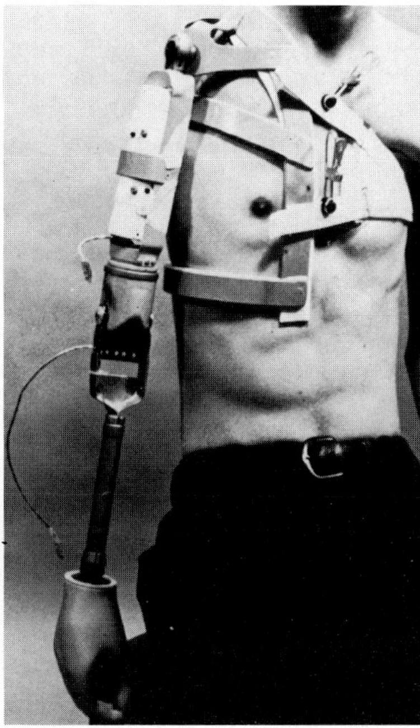
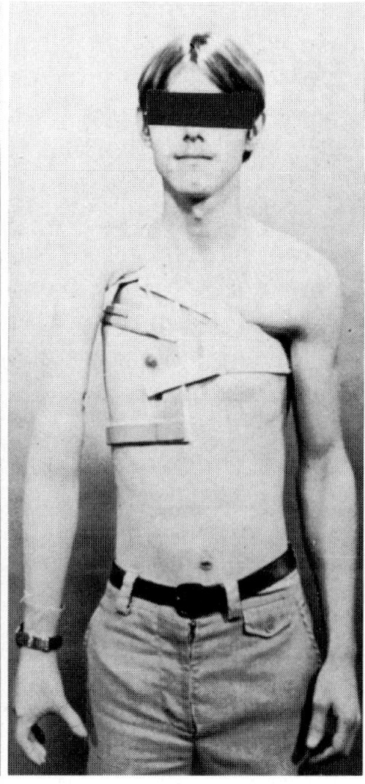

FIG. 22-36. Electromyelographic signals generated from muscle remnants are used to control the motions of the electrically powered forequarter prosthesis in this young man with an acquired forequarter amputation. The soft polyurethane foam covering of the endoskeletal system provides excellent cosmesis for the finished prosthesis.

back from the noise of prosthetic operation are important cues, especially in myoelectrically controlled systems. Sophisticated research to enhance sensory feedback in prosthetic use is in progress in several centers on this continent, among them the University of New Brunswick, Duke University,[31C] and the Massachusetts Institute of Technology.[138]

The need for and potential use of external power in children's prostheses is obviously great. In response to this demonstrated need, there are a number of electrically powered components of proven efficacy and durability currently available in sizes appropriate for the child amputee. Powered prosthetic hands are available in the United States from Swedish, Canadian, German, and English manufacturers in a variety of sizes to fit children from age 2 years to the young adult. Child-sized–powered elbows are available from Canadian and United States manufacturers, and, for larger children and young adults, two electric elbows with proportional control are available from United States manufacturers. A variety of dependable pull switches and pushbutton switches are on the market for biomechanical control of powered systems, and a number of two-state and three-state electrodes are available for EMG-controlled systems. This variety of dependable electric components is a marked improvement compared with the paucity of commercially available powered components available just a few years ago, and it is most gratifying to those providing care to the child amputee.

LOWER LIMB DEFICIENCIES

Paraxial Fibular Hemimelia

Fibular hemimelia is the most frequently occurring congenital deficiency of the long bones.[129,171] The deficiency may be of either the terminal or the intercalary type and may be either partial or complete. It is most commonly seen as a complete terminal deficiency and is more often unilateral, although a significant percentage of cases is bilateral. Males are affected almost twice as often as females in most reported series.

Although fibular hemimelia is often referred to as a congenital absence of the fibula, the condition is actually a total limb involvement rather than a simple absence of one bone.[1,49] Although the foot may be normal in the intercalary type, the typical patient exhibits a foot in which one or more of the lateral rays are absent and the lateral tarsal bones are absent or fused. The distal tibial epiphysis is abnormal, the tibia is markedly shortened, and there is a characteristic anteromedial tibial bowing. In more than half the cases, there is some degree of femoral shortening, varying from minor shortening to severe proximal femoral focal deficiency (Fig. 22-37). This combination of skeletal defects results in a limb with a very characteristic clinical appearance—the leg segment is short and bowed, there is a skin dimple overlying the apex of the bow, the foot is fixed in a pronounced equinovalgus position, and one or two lateral rays are commonly absent in the foot (Fig. 22-38).

The major clinical problems in unilateral fibular hemimelia are: (1) the severe leg length discrepancy, and (2) the foot deformity.[49,170A] Analyses of several large series have shown that leg length discrepancy is present in all cases and that it is progressive, the average discrepancy at skeletal maturity being approximately 5 inches.[14,49,93,171] Unfortunately, those children with intercalary deficiencies who present a normal foot tend to have greater leg length inequality than children with terminal deficiencies, who, of course, have more severe foot deformities.[95] Bilateral cases present the problem of foot deformities plus disproportionate dwarfism. Most authors now agree that the tibial bowing rarely requires active treatment by osteotomy, and they find that the bowing decreases with age and is not a significant clinical problem.[14,49] Where fibular hemimelia is associated with proximal femoral focal deficiency, the treatment should focus on the femoral deficiency rather than on the fibular hemimelia.[95]

In the past, the foot deformities seen in fibular hemimelia have been treated with various soft-tissue releases designed to place the foot beneath the tibia in a normal weightbearing position, sometimes followed by tarsal arthrodesis. The leg length inequality has been treated by leg lengthening procedures, epiphysiodesis of the sound limb, or a combination of such procedures.[17,36,147,162] The end result of these multiple operations has been unsatisfactory in essentially all large review series. The leg length inequality was not adequately corrected, and the foot was not often satisfactory for weightbearing. High shoe lifts, with or without braces, have been used to correct the leg length inequality. These devices are not only ungainly but are unsightly. In view of the current knowledge of the life history of this deficiency, at present, the preferred method of treatment is early ablation of the foot by an ankle disarticulation with a Syme's-type closure.[1A,14,49,93,93A,94,171] This produces a sturdy end-bearing stump at the below-knee level that can be nicely fit with an end-bearing below-knee prosthesis, which increases function and is cosmetically pleasing (Fig. 22-39). These children can ambulate without their prostheses when necessary in the home or in an emer-

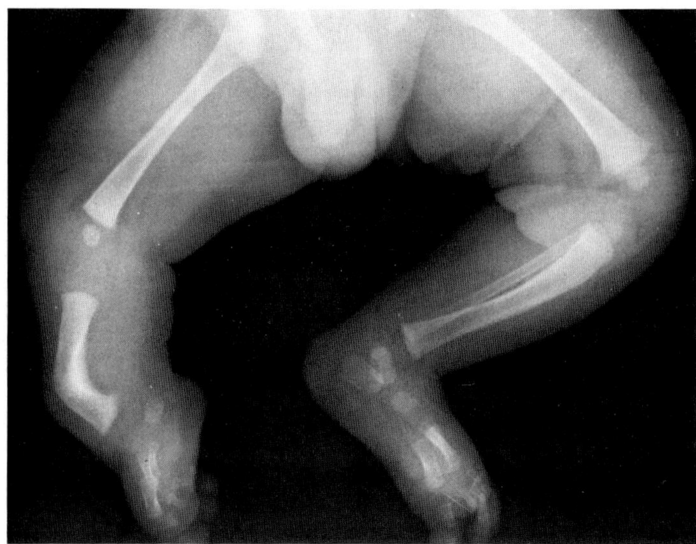

Fig. 22-37. In this roentgenogram of an infant with fibular hemimelia, not only is there an obvious complete absence of the fibula, but also the marked shortening of the tibia and the characteristic anteromedial tibial bowing are clearly seen.

gency situation, and their function remains excellent in adulthood. Even in the bilateral case, foot ablation and prosthetic fitting is preferable to the rather severe disproportionate dwarfism that such children exhibit at skeletal maturity.

Paraxial Tibial Hemimelia

Tibial hemimelia is unique among the congenital limb deficiencies in that it is the only such skeletal deficiency with a documented familial occurrence.[142] Furthermore, approximately three-fourths of all cases have accompanying skeletal anomalies, especially central aphalangia (lobster-claw hand) and reduplication of toes.[9] As many as 20% of these children have congenital hip dislocations.[10]

Exclusive of the terminal transverse deficiencies, tibial hemimelia is one of the more frequently occurring skeletal deficiencies in the lower limb. Its incidence has been estimated at one case per one million persons in the United States.[25]

Tibial hemimelia may occur as either a terminal or an intercalary deficiency and may be either complete or incomplete. Approximately 30% of cases have bilateral involvement.[25] The clinical picture varies with the exact type of deficiency. In all cases, however, the leg segment is markedly shortened and the foot is fixed in a severe varus position, with the sole of the foot facing the perineum (Fig. 22-40). The knee joint is unstable, with the degree of instability related to the presence or absence of a proximal tibial remnant (incomplete or complete deficiency). In some instances, there is a severe flexion contracture of the knee associated with a popliteal web. In terminal deficiencies, there is absence of one or more of the medial rays of the foot. In intercalary deficiencies, the foot may be nor-

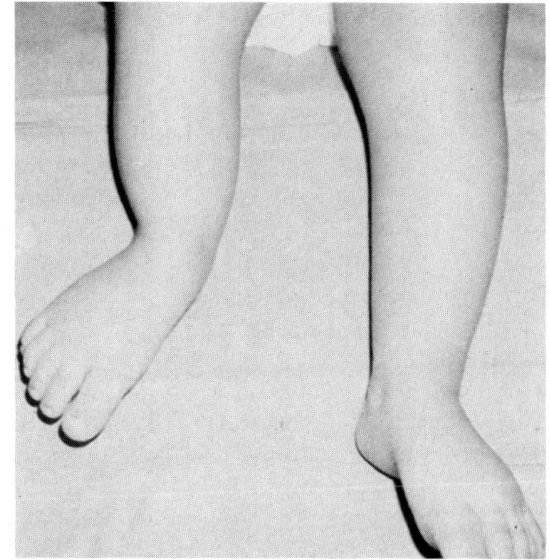

FIG. 22-38. The typical clinical appearance of fibular hemimelia is a limb in which the leg segment is quite short and bowed anteriorly and the foot is held in an equinovalgus position. The skin dimple overlying the apex of the tibial bow can be discerned in this photograph. In this instance of intercalary deficiency, all the rays of the foot are present.

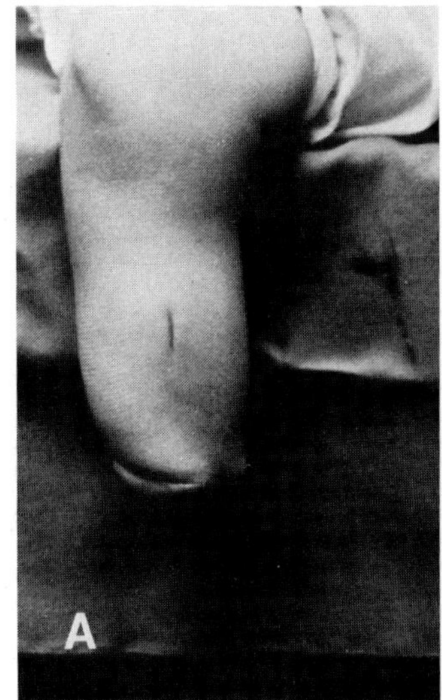

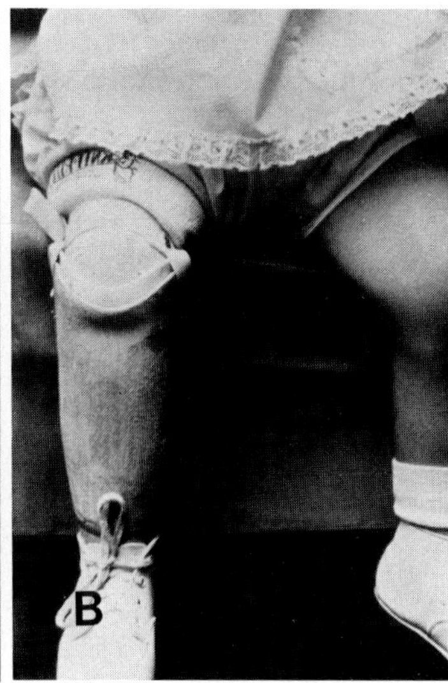

FIG. 22-39. *(A)* This child with fibular hemimelia has been treated by ankle disarticulation with Syme's-type closure. *(B)* Subsequent prosthetic fitting is with a patellar tendon–bearing prosthesis.

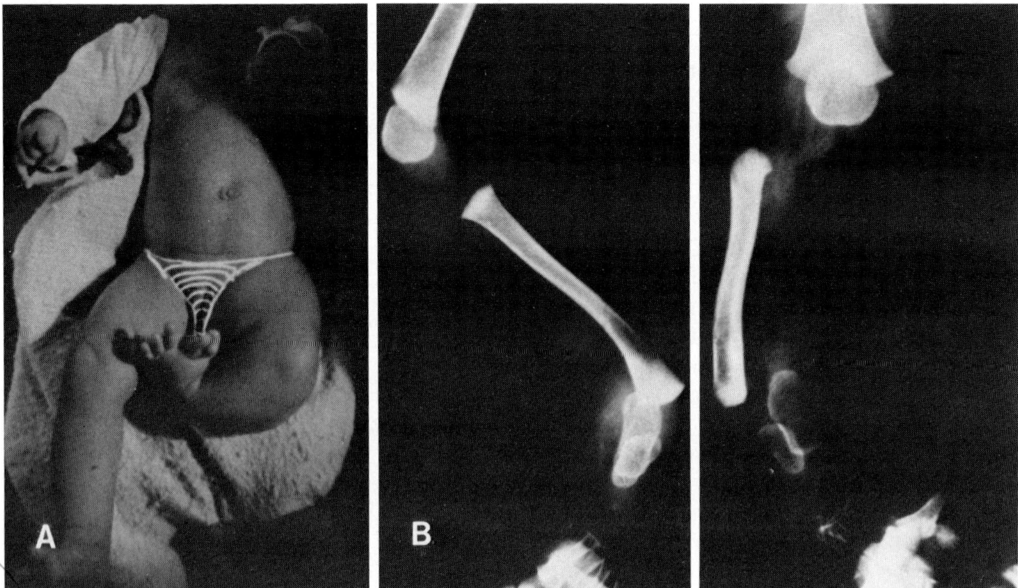

FIG. 22-40. *(A)* In tibial hemimelia, there is not only marked shortening of the leg segment, but also the foot is fixed in such a severe varus position that the sole of the foot is actually facing the perineum. Reduplication of toes is present in this particular infant. *(B)* Roentgenographically, the tibia is entirely absent, with lateral displacement of the fibula and marked varus positioning of the foot.

mal or there may be reduplication with more than five rays present.

The major clinical problems in tibial hemimelia are the severe shortening of the leg segment, the malrotation of the foot, and the instability and contracture of the knee. Traditional reconstructive surgical procedures are inadequate to satisfactorily correct these problems, and there is general agreement that this condition is best managed by primary surgical conversion of the defects into an acceptable amputation stump, followed by appropriate prosthetic fitting. The type of surgical conversion performed is determined by the exact nature of the deformity. If there is a severe flexion contracture of the knee with popliteal webbing, knee disarticulation is the procedure of choice.[9] This is followed by prosthetic fitting with a knee-disarticulation prosthesis (Fig. 22-41).

In complete deficiencies of either the terminal or intercalary type where the knee is not severely contracted, the upper end of the fibula may be centralized beneath the femur and the foot ablated—the Fredrick Brown procedure (Fig. 22-42).[24] This is followed by fitting with a below-knee prosthesis with side joints and a thigh corset to help stabilize the knee. There is remarkable hypertrophy of the fibula following transposition into a weight-bearing position, and excellent results have been achieved with this operation in properly selected cases.[9,158] Brown has emphasized that this surgery should be done during the first year of life and has pointed out the residual mediolateral knee instability and the tendency for recurrent knee flexion contracture that occurs following surgery.[25,26]

In incomplete deficiencies where the proximal tibial remnant articulates with the femur, a synostosis may be performed between the distal end of the tibial remnant and the fibula, followed by ablation of the foot and fitting with a below-knee prosthesis (Fig. 22-43).[9,69,77A] Side joints and a thigh corset are also needed in these cases because of mediolateral knee instability.

Proximal Femoral Focal Deficiency

If terminal transverse skeletal limb deficiencies are ruled out, the three most commonly encountered lower limb deficiencies are fibular hemimelia, tibial hemimelia, and that group of deficiencies wherein there is a sharply localized absence of the proximal end of the femur involving the iliofemoral joint.[10] This latter group has been extensively analyzed by Aitken[7,8] and others,[15,18,46,86,128,131A] and is known as

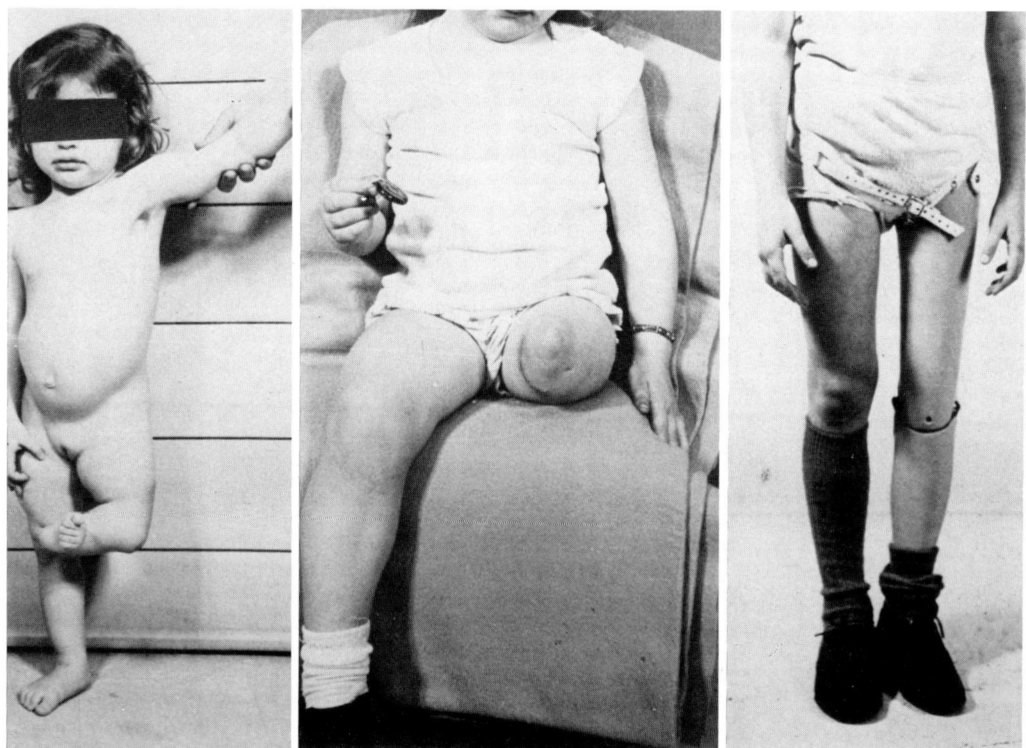

FIG. 22-41. In instances of tibial hemimelia with severe flexion contracture and webbing at the knee, knee disarticulation and fitting with a knee disarticulation prosthesis is the procedure of choice. (Photographs courtesy of Dr. G. T. Aitken, Area Child Amputee Center, Grand Rapids, Michigan)

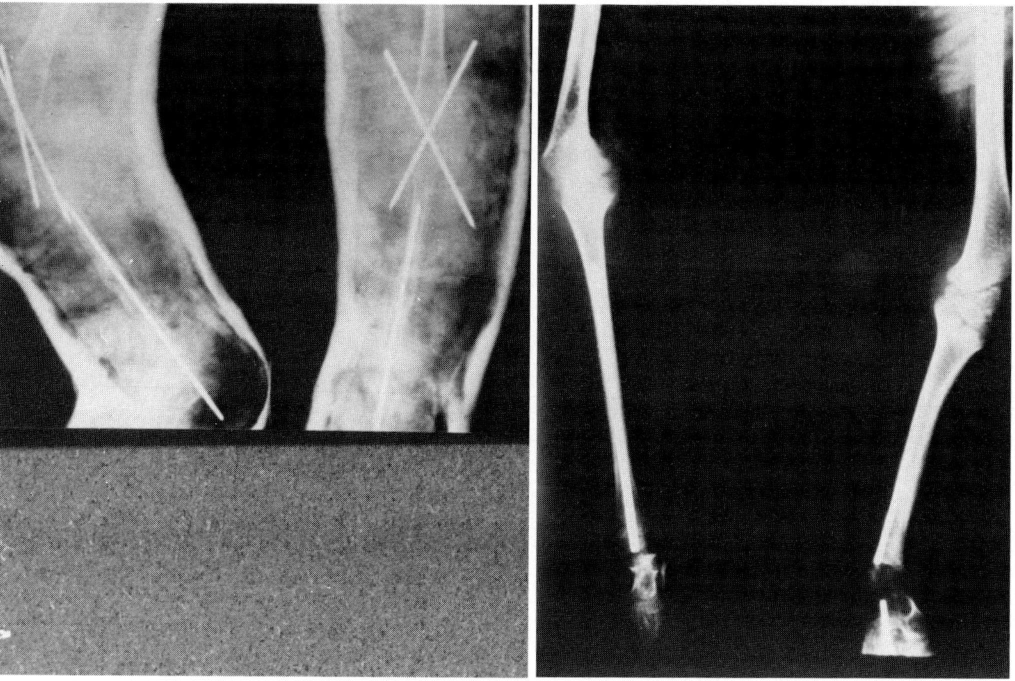

FIG. 22-42. In those instances of tibial hemimelia in which the knee is not severely contracted, the upper end of the fibula may be centralized beneath the femur—the Fredrick Brown procedure. In this instance, the foot was centralized beneath the fibula, but, in most instances, ablation of the foot is preferable because of the severe limb shortening present in this skeletal limb deficiency.

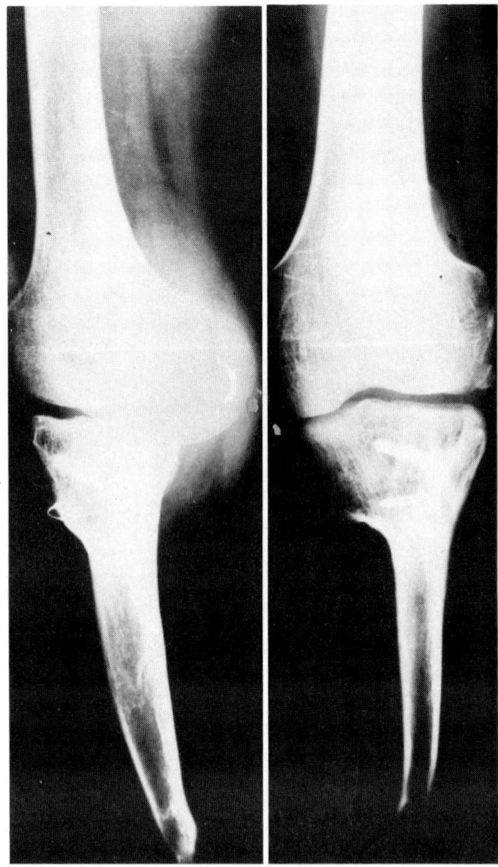

FIG. 22-43. The father of the patient illustrated in Figure 22-42 exhibited an incomplete tibial hemimelia with preservation of the proximal end of the tibia. His limb deficiency had been treated years earlier by a synostosing operation between the fibula and the upper end of the tibia with subsequent ablation of the foot and an excellent long-term surgical result.

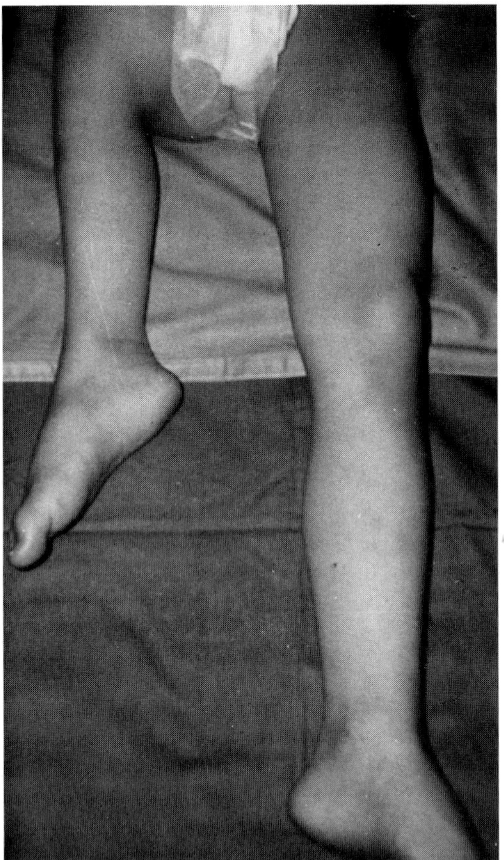

FIG. 22-44. The characteristic clinical picture of a child with proximal femoral focal deficiency. The thigh segment of the involved limb is quite short and is held in a flexed, abducted, and externally rotated position at the hip. The bulky soft tissues of the upper thigh taper sharply toward the knee, giving rise to the so-called ship's funnel appearance. The ankle joint of the involved limb often lies at approximately the level of the knee joint of the sound side.

proximal femoral focal deficiency (PFFD). In the past, this form of skeletal deficiency was frequently confused with other types of femoral dysgenesis, such as congenital coxa vara, congenital bowing of the femur, congenital shortening of the femur, and even phocomelia. However, PFFD is now recognized as a uniquely separate and distinct type of skeletal limb deficiency.

Children with this entity present a rather chararcteristic clinical picture (Fig. 22-44)[7,10] The thigh segment of the involved limb is quite short and is held in a flexed, abducted, and externally rotated position at the hip. The bulky soft tissues of the upper thigh taper sharply toward the knee, giving the thigh segment a "ship's funnel" appearance. The knee is carried in flexion but can usually be extended. Almost two thirds of these cases have an ipsilateral fibular hemimelia with the accompanying shortening of the leg segment and foot deformity anticipated in this condition. The foot on the affected limb usually lies at or near the level of the knee of the sound limb. Roughly 15% of cases have bilateral involvement and present as instances of profound asymmetrical dwarfism, with each lower limb exhibiting the above-described appearance.

Aitken[7] has classified proximal femoral focal

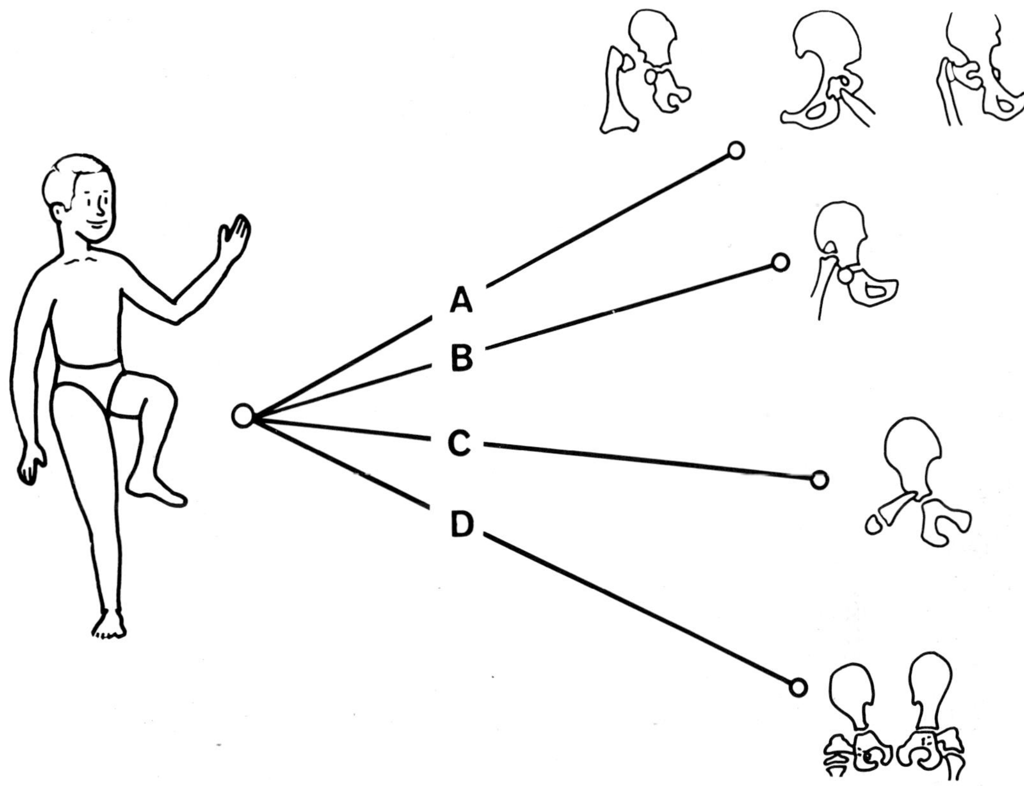

FIG. 22-45. Aitken classification of proximal femoral focal deficiency. (From Aitken GT: Proximal femoral focal deficiency. Definition, classification, and management. In A Symposium on Proximal Femoral Focal Deficiency—A Congenital Anomaly. National Academy of Sciences, Washington, DC, 1969)

deficiency into four subclasses, based on the roentgenographic appearance of the lesion (Fig. 22-45). In Class A, a head of the femur is present, together with an adequate acetabulum and a very short femoral segment. Initially, there is no bony connection between the shaft segment and the head of the femur. At skeletal maturity, a bony connection is present between the shaft of the femur and the head, neck, and trochanteric component. In most instances, a pseudarthrosis is evident at their point of connection, and this defect does not usually heal (Fig. 22-46*A*). In Class B, a head of the femur is present, and there is an adequate acetabulum. There is a short femur, usually with a small bony tuft on its proximal end. At skeletal maturity, there is no osseous connection between the femoral head and shaft (Fig. 22-46*B*). In Class C, there is no femoral head, and the acetabulum is severely dysplastic. The shaft of the femur is short with an ossified tuft at its proximal end (Fig. 22-46*C*). In Class D, the femoral head and the acetabulum are completely absent. The femoral shaft is deformed and very short, and there is no tuft of bone at its proximal end (Fig. 22-46*D*).

As with most skeletal limb deficiencies, treatment of proximal femoral focal deficiency is determined by the specific problems presented by each individual case. However, some general rules can be given for treating each specific subtype of the deficiency. All cases of unilateral PFFD exhibit the biomechanical losses of limb length inequality, malrotation, instability of proximal joints, and inadequacy of proximal musculature.[7] Bilateral cases do not present significant limb length inequality but manifest the other biomechanical deficiencies plus disproportionate dwarfism. It is of interest that almost all reported bilateral cases of PFFD are of the Class D subtype.[7]

Unilateral PFFD may be treated nonsurgi-

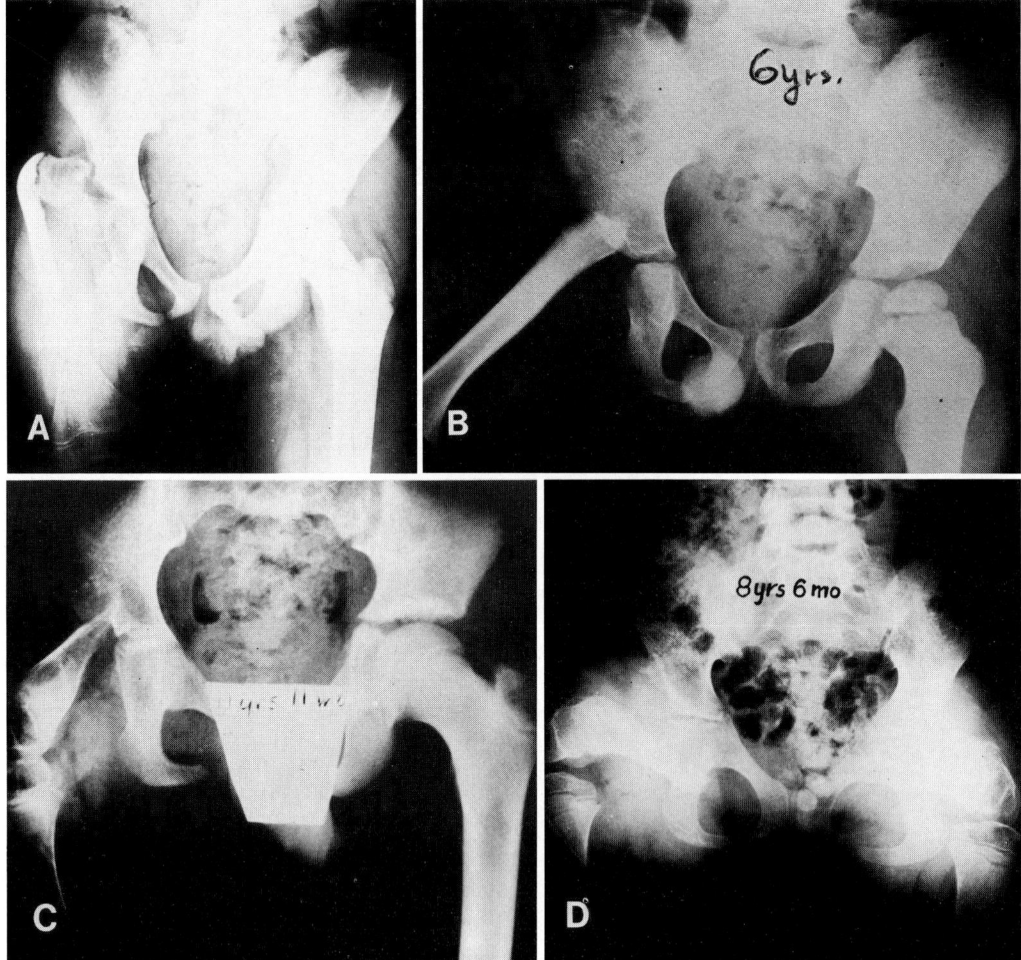

FIG. 22-46. *(A)* Type A proximal femoral focal deficiency. The femoral head is present within an adequate acetabulum, and, although the femur is quite short, there is an obvious connection between the shaft segment and the head and neck of the femur. A pseudarthrosis is evident at the point of connection. *(B)* Type B proximal femoral focal deficiency. A femoral head is present as well as an adequate acetabulum. The femur is quite short, and there is a small bony tuft at the proximal end. *(C)* Type C proximal femoral focal deficiency. The femoral head is absent, and the acetabulum is severely dysplastic. The shaft of the femur is quite short, and there is an ossified tuft at its proximal end. *(D)* Type D proximal femoral focal deficiency. The femoral head and the acetabulum are completely absent, the femoral shaft is markedly shortened, and no tuft of bone is noted at the proximal end. The majority of cases falling in the Type D category are bilateral. (Roentgenograms courtesy of Dr G. T. Aitken, Area Child Amputee Center, Grand Rapids, Michigan)

cally by a nonstandard prosthesis, which is fitted around the child's plantarflexed foot and incorporates a prosthetic knee joint just beneath the anatomic foot (Fig. 22-47). Such prosthetic fitting will immediately equalize leg lengths, and, by appropriate fabrication and alignment, it can minimize limb malrotation and instability of the hip and knee. A prosthesis will obviously have no effect on the inadequate proximal musculature. Ambulation in such prostheses is reasonably good, but the cosmetic effect leaves much to be desired.

Children with bilateral PFFD generally walk quite well without any form of prosthetic restoration, and surgical procedures almost always detract from their ambulatory inde-

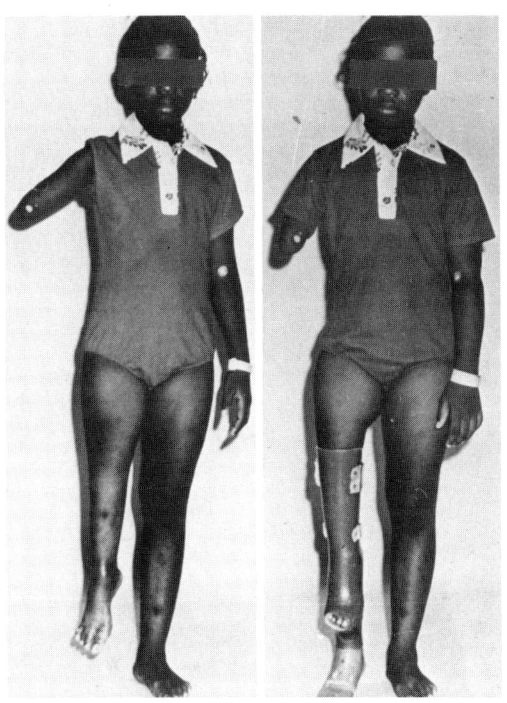

FIG. 22-47. This child with a unilateral proximal femoral focal deficiency also has a transverse terminal hemimelia of the ipsilateral upper limb. She has been fitted with a nonstandard prosthesis in order to equalize her limb lengths.

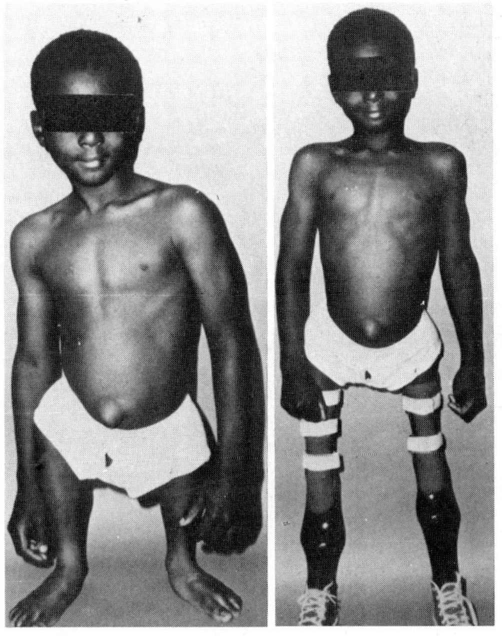

FIG. 22-48. Children with bilateral proximal femoral focal deficiency should not be treated surgically unless they have such severe foot deformities that they cannot ambulate without prostheses. Nonstandard prostheses are used outside of the home to correct the disproportionate dwarfism of these children and to raise them to peer height.

pendence rather than benefit them.[76] It is widely accepted that chlildren with bilateral PFFD should not be treated surgically unless they have such severe foot deformities that they cannot ambulate without prostheses.[7,66,91] Nonstandard prostheses, as described above, are used outside the home to correct the disproportionate dwarfism of these chldren and to raise them to peer height (Fig. 22-48).

When properly selected surgical procedures are carried out in the child with unilateral PFFD, subsequent prosthetic fit and function can be significantly improved. Standard orthopaedic reconstructive procedures have proved totally ineffective in correcting the leg length inequality seen in unilateral PFFD, especially where there is an accompanying ipsilateral fibular hemimelia.[7,88A,121,170] The preferred treatment is surgical conversion to the homologue of either an acquired below-knee or an above-knee amputation with appropriate prosthetic fitting. Whether to attempt conversion and prosthetic fitting as a below-knee amputee or to convert and fit as an above-knee amputee is a decision that is best made on the basis of the anticipated leg length discrepancy at skeletal maturity. Amstutz[13] has demonstrated that there is a constant percentage of growth retardation of the involved limb. By obtaining serial leg length roentgenograms and performing the appropriate calculations, a reasonably accurate prediction of limb length discrepancy at skeletal maturity can be made in a young child. If it is anticipated that the foot of the affected limb will lie proximal to or at the level of the knee of the sound limb, ablation of the foot by ankle disarticulation with Syme's closure and prosthetic fitting as an above-knee amputee is indicated (Fig. 22-49).[7,121,170] If calculations indicate that the foot of the affected limb will be significantly distal to the level of the knee of the sound limb, consideration should be given to performing a Van Nes rotational osteotomy[167] through the leg, removing enough bone to allow a full 180° rotation of the foot without creating tension on the neurovascular structures of the leg. The ankle joint of the rotated limb should then

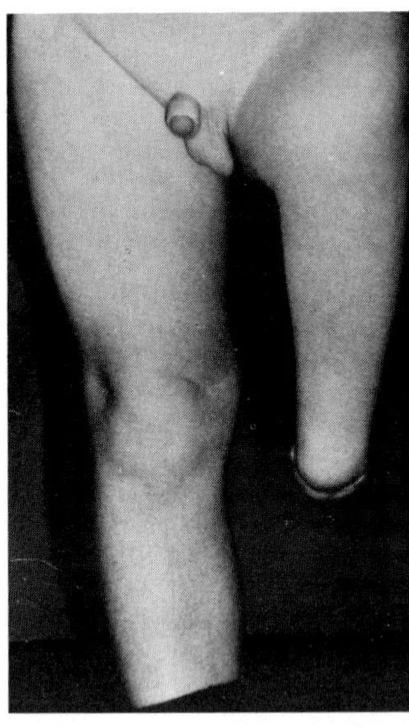
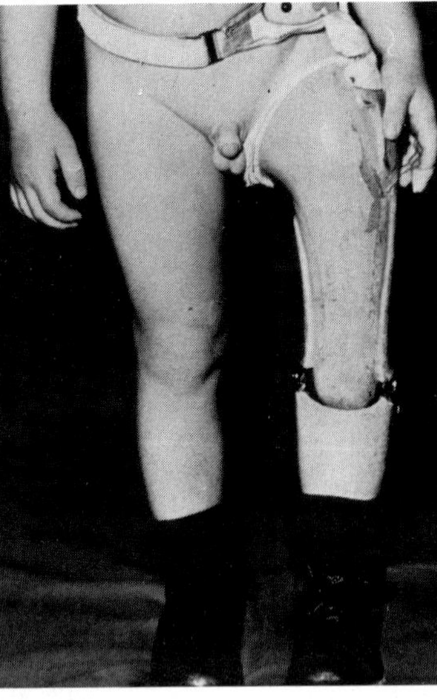

FIG. 22-49. In those children with unilateral proximal femoral focal deficiency in which the ankle joint of the involved limb lies approximately at the level of the knee joint of the sound limb, surgical conversion by means of an ankle disarticulation and Syme's-type closure with subsequent prosthetic fitting with a nonstandard above-knee prosthesis is appropriate.

lie at the level of the knee on the sound limb and will function as a knee joint, and the foot will function as a below-knee amputation stump[7,65,66,89,89A,90] Following surgery, these children are prosthetically fit as below-knee amputees, with the prosthesis having side joints and a thigh shell to encase and stabilize the true anatomic knee (Fig. 22-50). When the Van Nes procedure is performed in very young children, the twisted leg muscles tend to derotate the limb, and additional surgery is often necessary to restore proper rotation. For this reason, Hall[89] has suggested that the Van Nes procedure not be done on children younger than 12 years of age.

Following either ankle disarticulation and above-knee prosthetic fitting or rotation-plasty and below-knee prosthetic fitting, considera-

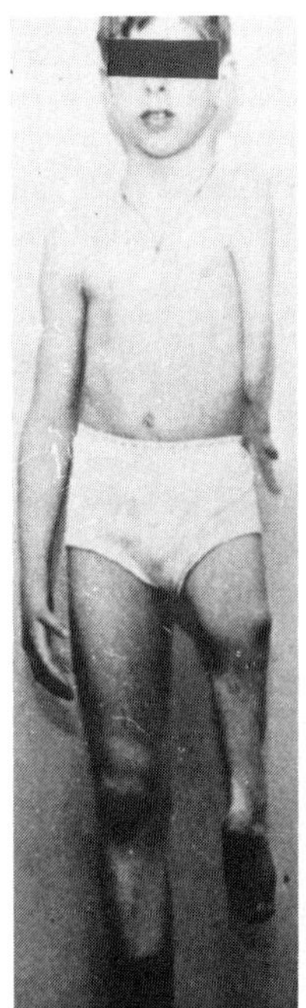
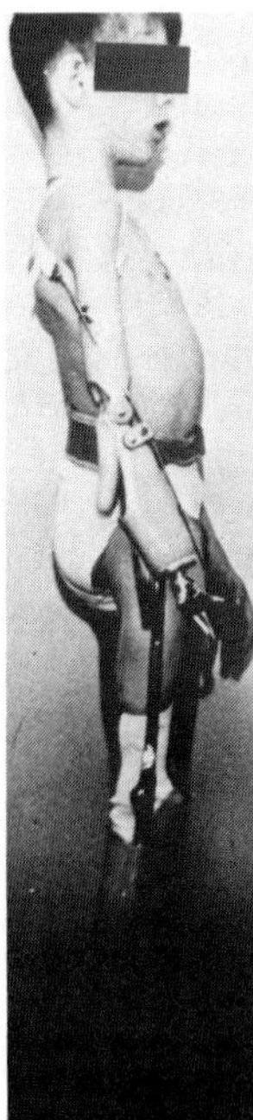
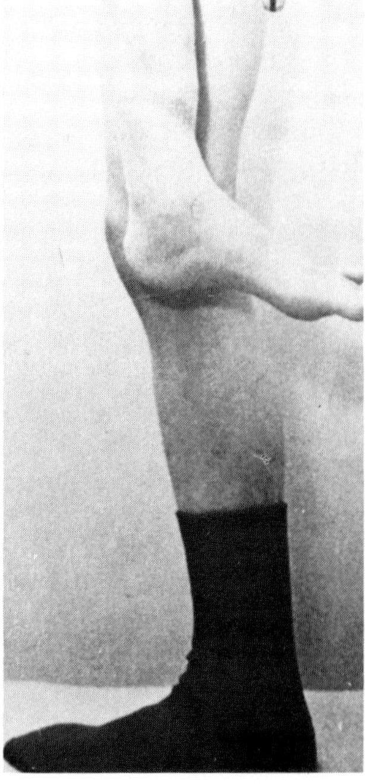

FIG. 22-50. In unilateral instances of proximal femoral focal deficiency in which the foot of the affected limb lies significantly distal to the level of the knee of the sound limb, a Van Nes rotational osteotomy through the leg may be performed. The foot is rotated 180°, and the leg segment is shortened so that the ankle joint of the involved limb lies at approximately the level of the knee joint of the sound limb. Prosthetic fitting as a below-knee amputation can then be satisfactorily accomplished. (Photographs courtesy of Dr. Al Kritter, Waukesha, Wisconsin)

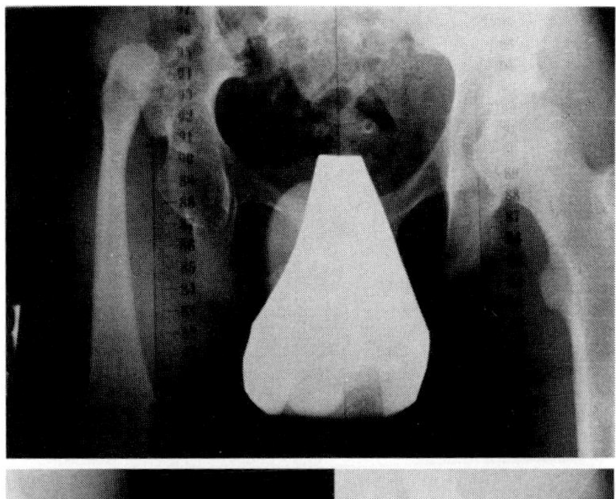

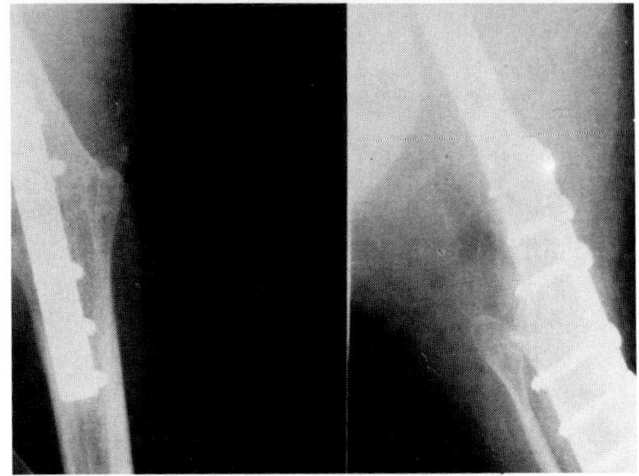

FIG. 22-51. This child with unilateral proximal femoral focal deficiency was treated by ankle disarticulation with Syme's closure and subsequent prosthetic fitting as an above-knee amputee. Subsequent arthrodesis of the knee joint of the involved limb with appropriate bone resection allowed equalization of knee centers and enhanced prosthetic fitting.

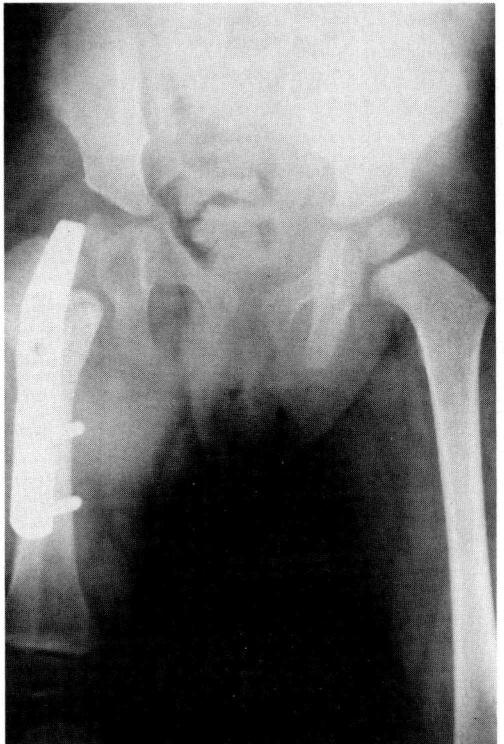

FIG. 22-52. In Type A or B proximal femoral focal deficiency, subtrochanteric osteotomy to achieve continuity between the femoral head-neck segment and the shaft segment may be beneficial.

tion should be given to arthrodesis of the knee in order to provide a more stable stump and to enhance prosthetic fitting.[7,13,20,121,170] Proper timing and technique of knee arthrodesis is essential to ensure that the growth potential of the distal femoral and proximal tibial epiphyses is not prematurely destroyed and desirable stump length is not lost. Knee arthrodesis can help to overcome the flexion-abduction-external rotation deformity at the hip and, when necessary, can affect rotational loss following a Van Nes procedure in the younger child (Fig. 22-51).

Reconstructive surgery about the hip can improve hip stability and can enhance the function of the hip musculature. However, hip surgery should only be undertaken in those subtypes in which a femoral head is present and the acetabulum is adequate—Classes A and B.[7,13,27,107] Reconstructive procedures of various types in Classes C and D have rarely been successful and have usually resulted in functional loss.[20,121,169,170] Subtrochanteric osteotomy of Class A and B hips has been beneficial when bony continuity between the femoral head–neck segment and the shaft segments can be obtained. (Fig. 22-52).

King[82–85,87] has achieved a significant degree of success in attaining hip stability and a single skeletal lever for prosthetic use by performing a two-stage surgical procedure in selected cases of unilateral PFFD. In Class B cases, he advises performing a concomitant knee arthrodesis and subtrochanteric osteotomy by using a single intramedullary nail for internal fixation at both the knee and the hip. At a second stage, the nail is removed, and the foot ablated by ankle disarticulation. These children are then prosthetically fit as above-knee amputees. Surgery can be done at an early age, because the knee epiphyses are not disturbed by the intramedullary nail.

Phocomelia

In complete lower limb phocomelia, all proximal portions of the limb are absent and the foot attaches directly to the trunk (Fig. 22-53). Tarsal elements may be absent or present in varying degrees in the foot, and the toes are variable in number. There is usually some degree of toe flexion. The condition is seen more often in males than in females and is bilateral in 20% to 30% of cases.[54]

Functionally, complete lower limb phocomelia may be considered the homologue of an acquired hip disarticulation and prosthetically treated with a hip disarticulation prosthesis, as discussed in the section on acquired lower limb amputation. The socket portion of the prosthesis must be appropriately modified to accommodate the phocomelic foot (Fig. 22-54). In spite of the bizarre appearance of a foot attached directly to the trunk, surgical removal of the foot is contraindicated, because it affords an excellent weightbearing surface, enhances socket suspension, and provides sensory feedback concerning the position of the prosthesis.[2]

In bilateral cases, treatment measures are initiated during infancy to develop head and trunk control. At approximately age 6 months, the child is placed in the upright position in a plastic laminate bucket mounted on a stable base to facilitate sitting balance. After 3 or 4 months, the child has usually achieved sufficient balance to graduate to an OCCC swivel walker.[10,67,97,119,144] This device was designed at the Ontario Crippled Children's Center to provide a limited degree of ambulation by converting lateral sway motion of the child's trunk to forward progression of the swivel walker (Fig. 22-55). Initially, the pylons of the swivel walker are quite short in order to maintain the child's center of gravity close to the floor and to enhance standing stability. As the child's balance and agility increase, the pylons may be progressively lengthened to bring the child up to peer height. The child with normal upper limbs who can use crutches may be fit with standard bilateral hip disarticulation prostheses at approximately 2 years of age and may be trained to walk with a swing-to or swing-through crutch gait. The child whose upper limbs will not accomodate crutches can be fit with more cosmetic articulated prostheses, incorporating swivel-walker ankle joints for short distance ambulation over level surfaces (Fig. 22-56). Such children will require some form of electrically powered cart or wheelchair for independent mobility over longer distances or over uneven surfaces.

Amelia

Lower limb amelia is the complete absence of all bony elements of the lower limb. There

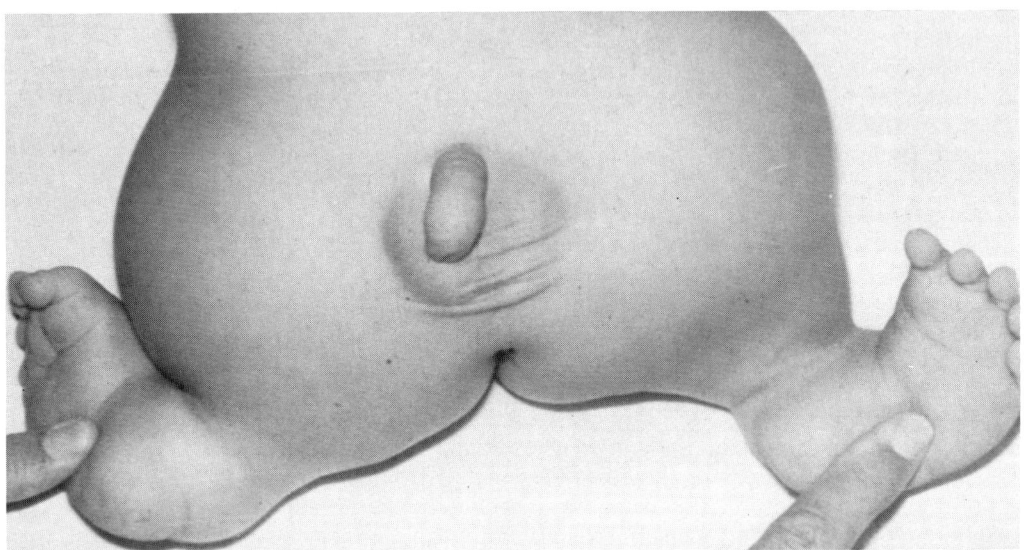

FIG. 22-53. Complete bilateral lower limb phocomelia. The foot attaches directly to the trunk, is usually deformed, and has very limited muscle function.

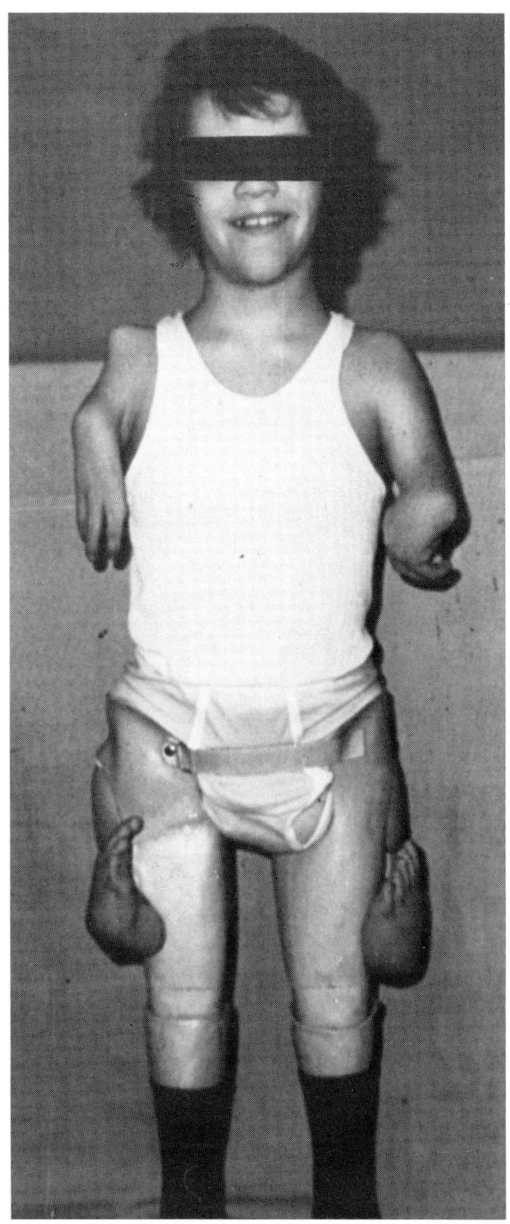

FIG. 22-54. In complete lower limb phocomelia, surgical removal of the foot is contraindicated, because the foot enhances socket suspension and provides sensory feedback concerning the position of the prosthesis. The socket portion of the prosthesis must be modified to accommodate for these phocomelic feet.

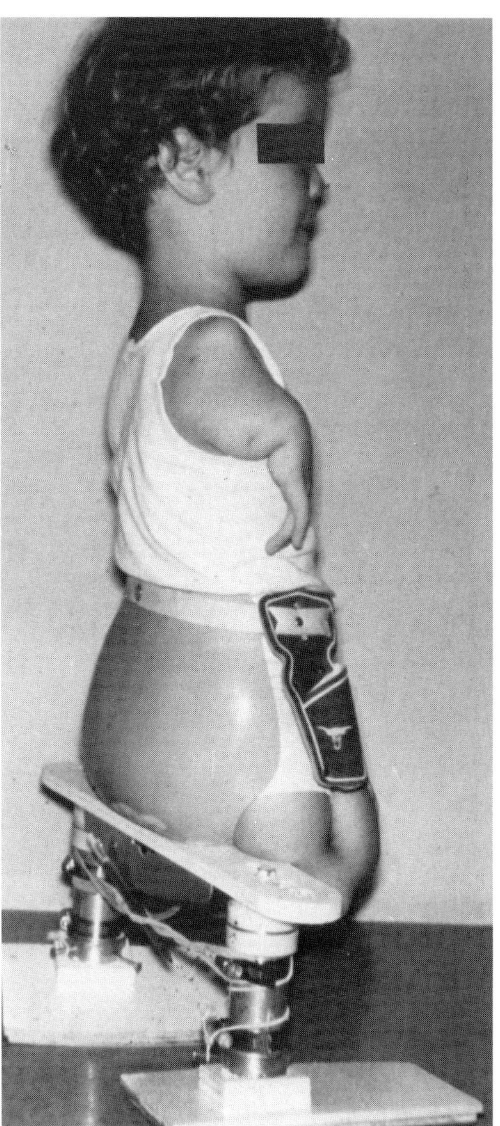

FIG. 22-55. The Ontario Crippled Children's Center swivel walker provides the bilateral lower limb phocomelic child with a limited degree of ambulation by converting lateral sway motion of the trunk to forward progression of the swivel walker.

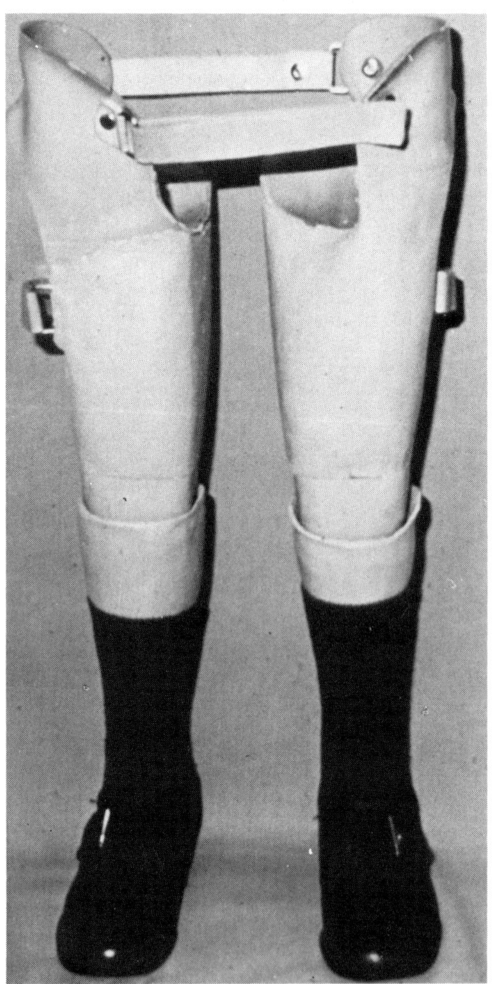

FIG. 22-56. Cosmetic articulated prostheses that incorporate swivel walker ankle joints can be fabricated for the older child with bilateral lower limb phocomelia to allow short-distance ambulation over level surfaces.

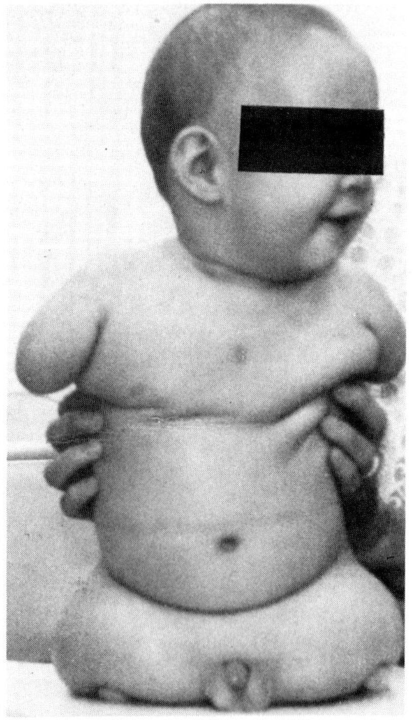

FIG. 22-57. In lower limb amelia, there is complete absence of all bony elements of the lower limb. A lobule of fat is present at the normal site of lower limb attachment, and the pelvis is characteristically widened due to a local accumulation of subcutaneous fat. This child has not only bilateral lower limb amelia but also bilateral transverse terminal hemimelia of his upper limbs.

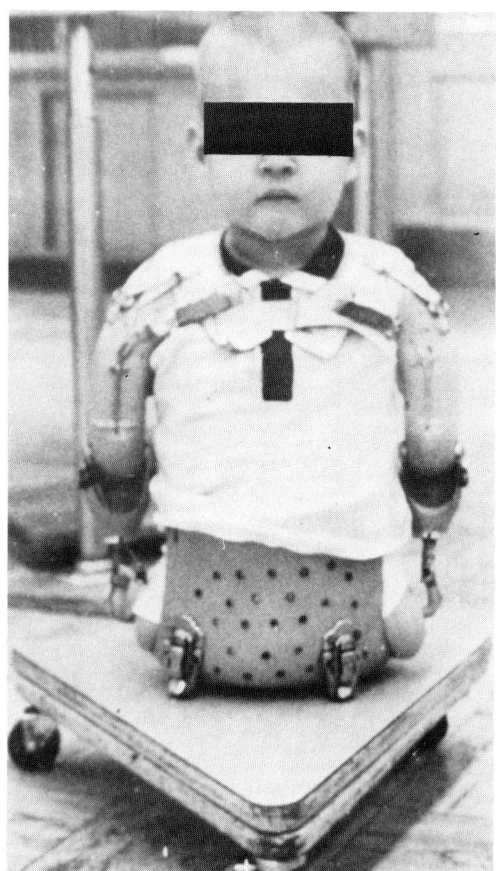

FIG. 22-58. Children with bilateral lower limb amelia are fitted with a plastic laminate "bucket" in infancy to allow them to achieve good sitting balance.

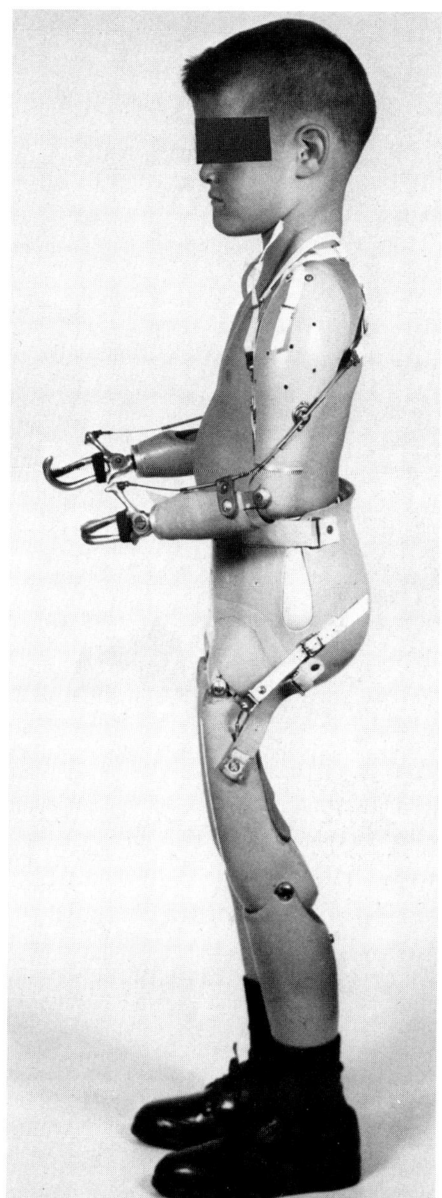

FIG. 22-59. Final prosthetic fitting of the bilateral lower limb amelic child is by means of articulated hip disarticulation prostheses.

may be a lobule of fat or a deep dimple present on the pelvis at the normal site of lower limb attachment. The pelvis is characteristically widened due to a local accumulation of subcutaneous fat (Fig. 22-57). The condition occurs more often in males than in females and is bilateral in 50% of cases.[54]

Amelia is a terminal transverse deficiency, and, in the lower limb, it is the congenital homologue of an acquired hip disarticulation. Unilateral cases are fit with a standard hip disarticulation prosthesis. As with the bilateral phocomelic, bilateral cases require the use of a stable plastic laminate bucket to achieve good sitting balance in infancy (Fig. 22-58). These children are then graduated to a swivel walker and subsequently to articulated hip disarticulation prostheses (Fig. 22-59). Those with good upper limb function will achieve a satisfactory swing-to or swing-through crutch gait, but those with upper limb deficiencies of such severity to preclude the use of crutches will require swivel walker ankle joints in their prostheses for limited walking on level surfaces and a powered cart (Fig. 22-60) or wheelchair for independent mobility over longer distances or over uneven surfaces.[10,42,72,165]

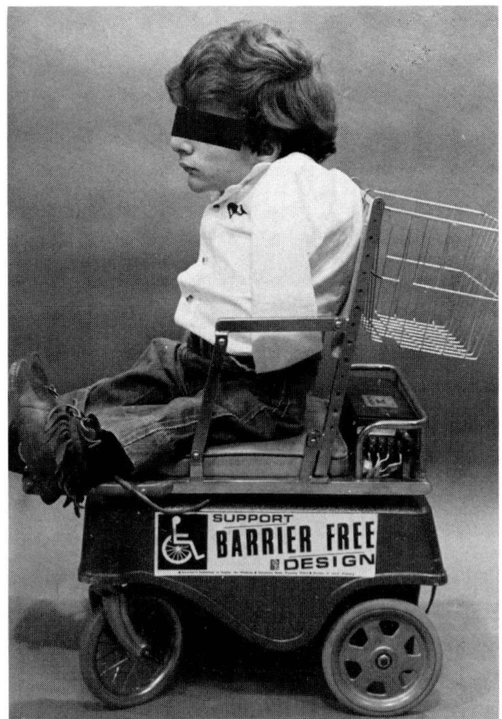

FIG. 22-60. The child Amputee Prosthetic Project electrically powered cart provides the severely involved lower limb or multimembral amputee with independent mobility over long distances.

REFERENCES

1. Achterman C, Kalamchi A: Congenital deficiency of the fibula. J Bone Joint Surg 61B:133, 1979
1A. Aitken GT: Amputation as a treatment for certain lower-extremity congenital abnormalities. J Bone Joint Surg 41A:1267, 1959
2. Aitken GT: Overgrowth of the amputation stump. ICIB 1(11):1, 1962
3. Aitken GT: Surgical amputation in children. J Bone Joint Surg 45A:1735, 1963
4. Aitken GT: Management of severe bilateral upper limb deficiencies. Clin Orthop 37:53, 1964
5. Aitken GT: Prosthetic fitting following amputation for bone tumors. ICIB 3(5):1, 1964
6. Aitken GT: The child with an acquired amputation. ICIB 7(8):1, 1968
7. Aitken GT: Proximal femoral focal deficiency—Definition, classification, and management. In A Symposium on Proximal Femoral Focal Deficiency—A Congenital Anomaly. Washington, DC, National Academy of Sciences, 1969
8. Aitken GT: Proximal femoral focal deficiency. In Limb Development and Deformity; Problems of Evaluation and Rehabilitation. Springfield, IL, Charles C Thomas, 1969
8A. Aitken GT: Osseous overgrowth in amputations in children. In Swinyard CA (Ed): Limb Development and Deformity, pp 448–456, Springfield, IL, Charles C Thomas, 1969
9. Aitken GT: Tibial hemimelia. In A Symposium on Selected Lower Limb Anomalies, Surgical and Prosthetic Management. Washington, DC, National Academy of Sciences, 1971
10. Aitken GT: The child amputee—An overview. Orthop Clin North Am 3(2):447, 1972
11. Aitken GT, Frantz CH: The juvenile amputee. J Bone Joint Surg 35A:659, 1953
12. Aitken GT, Frantz CH: Management of the child amputee. AAOS Instruc Course Lect 17:246, 1960
13. Amstutz HC: The morphology, natural history, and treatment of proximal femoral focal deficiency. In A Symposium on Proximal Femoral Focal Deficiency—A Congenital Anomaly. Washington, DC, National Academy of Sciences, 1969
14. Amstutz HC: Natural history and treatment of congenital absence of the fibula. J Bone Joint Surg 54A:1349, 1972
15. Amstutz HC, Wilson PD Jr: Dysgenesis of the proximal femur (coxa vara) and its surgical management. J Bone Joint Surg 44A:1, 1962
16. Arey LB: Developmental Anatomy. Philadelphia, WB Saunders, 1965
17. Arnold WD: Congenital absence of the fibula. Clin Orthop 17:20, 1959
18. Badger VM, Lambert CN: Differential diagnosis of an apparent proximal femoral focal deficiency. ICIB 5(1):3, 1965
19. Bayne LG, Lovell WW, Marks TW: The radial clubhand. J Bone Joint Surg 52A:1065, 1970
20. Bevan-Thomas WH, Millar EA: A review of proximal focal femoral deficiencies. J Bone Joint Surg 49A:1378, 1967
21. Blakeslee B: The limb-deficient child. Berkeley, Univ. of Calif. Press, 1963
22. Bora FW, Nicholson JT, Cheema HM: Radial meromelia: The deformity and its treatment. J Bone Joint Surg 52A:966, 1970
23. Brooks MB, Mazet R: Prosthetics in child amputees. Clin Orthop 9:190, 1957
24. Brown FW: Construction of a knee joint in congenital total absence of the tibia (paraxial hemimelia tibia). A preliminary report. J Bone Joint Surg 47A:695, 1965
25. Brown FW: The Brown operation for total hemimelia tibia. In A Symposium on Selected Lower Limb Anomalies, Surgical and Prosthetics Management. Washington, DC, National Academy of Sciences, 1971
26. Brown FW, Pohnert WH: Construction of a knee joint in meromelia tibia (congenital absence of the tibia). A 15-year follow-up study. J Bone Joint Surg 54A:1333, 1972
27. Burgess E: The surgical means of obtaining hip stability with motion in congenital proximal femoral focal deficiency. ICIB 1(3):1, 1961
28. Burgess EM, Romano RJ: Immediate postsurgical prosthetic fitting of children and adolescents following lower-extremity amputations. ICIB 7(3):1, 1967
29. Burtch RL, Fishman S, Kay HW: Nomenclature for congenital skeletal limb deficiencies, a revision of the Frantz and O'Rahilly classification. Artif Limbs 10:24, 1966
30. Buttomley AH: Myoelectric control of powered prostheses. J Bone Joint Surg 47B:411, 1965
31. Cary JM: Traumatic amputation in childhood—Primary management. ICIB 14(6):1, 1975

31A. Christie J, Lamb DW, McDonald JM, Britten S: A study of stump growth for children with below-knee amputations. J Bone Joint Surg 61B:464, 1979
31B. Clarke SD, Patton JC: Occupational therapy for the limb-deficient child. Clin Orthop 148:47, 1980
31C. Clippinger FW: A sensory feedback system for an upper limb prosthesis. Bull Prosthet Res 10:247, 1974
32. Clippinger FW Jr, Titus BR: Prosthetic principles—lower limb. In The Child With An Acquired Amputation. Washington, DC, National Academy of Sciences, 1972
33. Cohlan SO: Environmental factors in human teratology. In Normal and Abnormal Embryologic Development. Washington, DC, National Research Council, 1967
34. Corrivean C: Prostheses powered by carbon-dioxide. ICIB 7(5):13, 1968
35. Corrivean C: Prosthetic principles in upper-limb externally powered prostheses. In The Child With An Acquired Amputation. Washington, DC, National Academy of Sciences, 1972
36. Coventry MB, Johnson EW: Congenital absence of the fibula. J Bone Joint Surg 34A:941, 1952
37. Dankmeyer CH Sr, Dankmeyer CH Jr, Massey MD: An externally powered modular system for upper limb prostheses. Orthot Prosthet 26:36, 1972
38. Davidson WH, Bohne WHO: The Syme amputation in children. J Bone Joint Surg 57A:905, 1975
39. Davies EJ, Friz BR, Clippinger FW Jr: Children with amputations. ICIB 9(3):6, 1969
39A. Day HJB: The United Kingdom trial of the Swedish myoelectric hand for young children: An interim report. ICIB 17:5, 1980
40. Delorme TD: Treatment of congenital absence of the radius by transepiphyseal fixation. J Bone Joint Surg 51A:117, 1969
41. Dorcas DS, Dunfield VA, O'Shea BJ: A myoelectric prosthesis for a forequarter amputation. ICIB 7(11):15, 1968
41A. Dorcas DS, Scott RN: A three-state myoelectric control. Med Biol Engl 4:367, 1966
42. Dresher CS, Macdonell JA: Total amelia. J Bone Joint Surg 47A:511, 1965
43. Duraiswami PK: Experimental causation of congenital skeletal defects and its significance in orthopedic surgery. J Bone Joint Surg 34B:646, 1952
44. Duraiswami PK: Comparison of congenital defects induced in developing chickens by certain teratogenic agents with those caused by insulin. J Bone Joint Surg 27A:277, 1955
45. Epps CH: Upper-extremity limb deficiency with concomitant infantile structural scoliosis. ICIB 5(2):1, 1965
46. Epps CH: Proximal femoral focal deficiency: A case report of a necropsy. ICIB 6(5):1, 1967
47. Epps CH, Haile JH: Experience with the Muenster-type below-elbow prosthesis. ICIB 7(10):1, 1968
48. Epps CH, Vaughn HH: Training the child with a lower-limb amputation. In The Child With An Acquired Amputation. Washington, DC, National Academy of Sciences, 1972
49. Farmer AW, Laurin CA: Congenital absence of the fibula. J Bone Joint Surg 42A:1, 1960
50. Fisher AG, Childress DS: The Michigan electric hook: A preliminary report on a new electrically powered hook for children. ICIB 12(9):1, 1973
51. Fishman S, Kay HW: The Muenster-type below-elbow socket, an evaluation. Artif Limbs 8:4, 1964
52. Frankel ME, Goldner JL, Stelling FH: Radial club hand: Is centralization necessary: A rational surgical approach. J Bone Joint Surg 53A:1026, 1971
53. Frantz CH, Aitken GT: Management of the juvenile amputee. Clin Orthop 9:30, 1959
54. Frantz CH, O'Rahilly R: Congenital skeletal limb deficiencies. J Bone Joint Surg 43A:1202, 1961
55. Frantz CH, O'Rahilly R: Ulnar hemimelia. Artif Limbs 15:25, 1971
56. Friedman L: Should the Muenster below-elbow prosthesis be prescribed for children? ICIB 11(7):7, 1972
56A. Furgeson S: Electric power in upper limb prosthetics: The Michigan experience. ICIB 18:1, 1983
57. Gazeley WE, Ey MD, Sampson W: Follow-up experiences with Muenster prostheses. ICIB 7(10):7, 1968
58. Glassner JR: Spontaneous intrauterine amputation. J Bone Joint Surg 45A:351, 1963
59. Goldner JL: Congenital absence of the radius and digital deformities: "Club hand" (paraxial hemimelia radialis). ICIB 4(9):1, 1965
60. Goldner JL, Titus BR: An experience with externally powered prostheses for children. ICIB 7(2):1, 1967
61. Gorton A: Field study of the Muenster-type below-elbow prosthesis. ICIB 6(8):8, 1967
62. Hall CB: Recent concepts in the treatment of the limb-deficient child. Artif Limbs 10:36, 1966
63. Hall CB, Brooks MB, Dennis JF: Congenital skeletal deficiencies of the extremities. Classification and fundamentals of treatment. JAMA 181:590, 1962
64. Hall CB, Rosenfelder R, Tabloda C: The juvenile amputee with a scarred stump. In The Child With An Acquired Amputation. Washington, DC, National Academy of Sciences, 1972
65. Hall JE: Rotation of congenitally hypoplastic lower limbs to use the ankle joint as a knee. ICIB 6(2):3, 1966
66. Hall JE, Bochmann D: The surgical and prosthetic management of proximal femoral focal deficiency. In A Symposium: Proximal Femoral Focal Deficiency—A Congenital Anomaly. Washington, DC, National Academy of Sciences, 1969
67. Hall JE, Sauter WF: Surgical and prosthetic management of three congenital child amputees. ICIB 7(2):9, 1967
68. Hammond NL III, Levitt RL, Hunter JM: Scoliosis combined with congenital deficiencies of the upper limb: The effect of prosthesis wearing. ICIB 12(3):30, 1972
69. Hancock CI, King RE: The one-bone leg. ICIB 7(3):11, 1967
70. Harris RI: Syme's amputation. The technical details essential for success. J Bone Joint Surg 38B:614, 1956
71. Haslam ET: Intrauterine gangrene of the forefoot. ICIB 3(5):3, 1964
72. Haslam ET, Hayden J, Dutro J: The habilitation of a congenital quadruple amputee. ICIB 6(9):1, 1967
73. Hauberg G, John H: Treatment at Abteilung 10—Dysmelien. ICIB 5(6):4, 1966
74. Henkel L, Wilbert HG: Dysmelia. J Bone Joint Surg 51B:399, 1969
75. Herndon JH, LaNone AM: Salvage of a short below-elbow amputation with pedicle flap coverage. ICIB 12(7):5, 1973

76. Hussain T, Emmerson A: Conservative management of bilateral proximal femoral focal deficiency. ICIB 13(9):9, 1974
77. Hutchison J: The training of upper limb amputees with conventional and externally powered prostheses. In The child With An Acquired Amputation. Washington, DC, National Academy of Sciences, 1972
77A. Jones D, Barnes J, Lloyd-Roberts GC: Congenital aplasia and dysplasia of the tibia with intact fibula. J Bone Joint Surg 60B:31, 1978
78. Kato K: Congenital absence of the radius. J Bone Joint Surg 6:589, 1924
79. Kay HW: A proposed international terminology for the classification of congenital limb deficiencies. ICIB 13(7):1, 1974
80. Kay HW: Clinical applications of the new international terminology for the classification of congenital limb deficiencies. ICIB 14(3):1, 1975
81. Kay HW, Fishman S: 1018 Children With Skeletal Limb Deficiencies. New York Univ. Post-Graduate Medical School, Prosthetics and Orthotics, 1967
82. King RE: Concepts of proximal femoral focal deficiencies. ICIB 1(2):1, 1961
83. King RE: Surgical correction of proximal femoral focal deficiency. ICIB 4(11):1, 1965
84. King RE: Providing a single skeletal lever in proximal femoral focal deficiency. ICIB 6(2):23, 1966
85. King RE: Some concepts of proximal femoral focal deficiency. In A Symposium: Proximal Femoral Focal Deficiency—A Congenital Anomaly. Washington, DC, National Academy of Sciences, 1969
86. King RE, McCraney T: Proximal femoral focal deficiency—Quo vadis? ICIB 12(8):1, 1973
87. King RE, Marks TW: Follow-up findings on the skeletal lever in the surgical management of proximal femoral focal deficiency. ICIB 11(3):1, 1971
88. Knowles JB, Stevens BJ, Howe L: Myoelectric control of a hand prosthesis. J Bone Joint Surg 47B:416, 1965
88A. Korman LA, Meyer LC, Warren FH: Proximal femoral focal deficiency: A 50-year experience. Dev Med Child Neurol 24:344, 1982
89. Kostuik JP, Gillespie R, Hall JE, Hubbard S: Van Nes rotational osteotomy for treatment of proximal femoral focal deficiency and congenital short femur. J Bone Joint Surg 57A:1039, 1975
89A. Kritter AE: Tibial rotation–plasty for proximal femoral focal deficiency. J Bone Joint Surg 59A:927, 1977
90. Kritter A, Becker D: Proximal femoral focal deficiency and amelia: A case report. ICIB 14(4):1, 1975
91. Kritter AE, Gillespie T: Bilateral proximal femoral focal deficiency and bilateral paraxial fibular hemimelia. ICIB 11(12):1, 1972
92. Kruger LM: Classification and prosthetic management of limb-deficient children. ICIB 7(12):1, 1968
93. Kruger LM: Fibular hemimelia. In A Symposium on Lower Limb Anomalies, Surgical and Prosthetic Management. Washington, DC, National Academy of Sciences, 1971
93A. Kruger LM: Recent advances in surgery of lower limb deficiencies. Clin Orthop 148:97, 1980
94. Kruger LM, Bregan NR: A study of radial head dislocation in children with transverse partial hemimelia of the upper limb. ICIB 10(1):1, 1970
95. Kruger LM, Talbott RD: Amputation and prosthesis as definitive treatment in congenital absence of the fibula. J Bone Joint Surg 43A:625, 1961
96. Kuhn GC: Treatment of the child with severe limb deficiencies. ICIB 10(3):1, 1970
97. Lamb DW, Simpson DC, Pirie RB: The management of lower limb phocomelia. J Bone Joint Surg 52B:688, 1970
98. Lamb DW, Simpson DC, Schutt WH, Spiers NI, Baker G: The management of upper limb deficiencies in the thalidomide type syndrome. JR Coll Surg Edinb 10(2):102, 1965
99. Lambert CN: An unusual case. ICIB 6(7):20, 1967
100. Lambert CN: Amputation surgery in the child. Surg Clin North Am 3(2):473, 1972
101. Lambert CN: Etiology. In The Child With An Acquired Amputation. Washington, DC, National Academy of Sciences, 1972
102. Lambert CN: Limb loss through malignancy. In The Child With An Acquired Amputation. Washington, DC, National Academy of Sciences, 1972
103. Lambert CN, Hamilton RC, Pellicore RH: The juvenile amputee program: Its social and economic value. J Bone Joint Surg 51A:1135, 1969
104. Lambert CN, Sciora J: The incidence of scoliosis in the juvenile amputee population. ICIB 11(2):1, 1971
105. Laurin CA, Farmer AW: Congenital absence of ulna. Can J Surg 2:204, 1959
106. Lippay AL: External power and the amputee: An engineer's view. ICIB 7(5):7, 1968
107. Lloyd-Roberts GC, Stone KH: Congenital hypoplasia of the upper femur. J Bone Joint Surg 45B:557, 1963
108. Lozac'h Y: An improved and more versatile myoelectric control. ICIB 11(8):13, 1972
109. Lundberg C, Paul SW, Van Derwerker EE, Allen JC: Experience with carbon dioxide-power-assisted prostheses. ICIB 12(1):1, 1972
110. Lyttle D, Sweitzer R, Steinke T, Treffler E, Hobson D: Experiences with myoelectric below-elbow fittings in teenagers. ICIB 13(6):11, 1974
111. McKenzie DS: The prosthetic management of congenital deformities of the extremities. J Bone Joint Surg 39B:233, 1957
112. McKenzie DS: The clinical application of externally powered artificial arms. J Bone Joint Surg 47B:399, 1965
113. McLaurin CA: External power in upper extremity prosthetics and orthotics. ICIB 6(1):19, 1966
114. McLaurin CA: On the use of electricity in upper extremity prostheses. J Bone Joint Surg 47B:448, 1965
115. Makley JT, Heiple KG: Scoliosis associated with congenital deficiencies of the upper extremity. J Bone Joint Surg 52A:279, 1970
116. Malpas JS: Advancements in the treatment of osteogenic sarcoma. J Bone Joint Surg 57B:267, 1975
117. Marquardt E: Aktive Prosthesenversorgung eines Armlosen Kleinkindes im 2. Lebensjahr. Jahrbuch dur Fursorge fur Korperbehinderte, 1962 (Reprinted in ICIB 3(4):1964
118. Marquardt E: The Heidleberg pneumatic arm prosthesis. J Bone Joint Surg 47B:425, 1965
119. Matlock WM, Elliott J: Fitting and training children with swivel walker. Artif Limbs 10:27, 1966
119A. Marquardt E: The multiple limb-deficient child. In American Academy of Orthopaedic Surgeons: Atlas of Limb Prosthetics. St Louis, CV Mosby, 1981
120. Mazet R Jr: Syme's amputation. A follow-up study of 51 adults and 32 children. J Bone Joint Surg 50A:1549, 1968

121. Meyer LC, Friddle D, Pratt RW: Problems of treating and fitting the patient with proximal femoral focal deficiency. ICIB 10(12):1, 1971
122. Meyer LC, Sauer BW: The use of porous high-density polyethelene caps in the prevention of appositional bone growth in the juvenile amputee: A preliminary report. ICIB 14(9,10):1, 1975
123. Milaire J: The contribution of histochemistry to our understanding of limb morphogenesis and some of its congenital deviations. In Normal and Abnormal Embryologic Development. Washington, DC, National Research Council, 1967
124. Mongeau M: An approach to the rehabilitation of the child amputee. ICIB 6(4):1, 1967
125. Mongeau M: Our experience with the thalidomide children. An interim report. ICIB 6(4):3, 1967
126. Mongeau M: New hope for the patient with several upper extremity deficiencies: externally powered prostheses. ICIB 7(5):1, 1968
127. Mongeau M: General principles in the rehabilitation of upper limb amputees with conventional or externally powered prostheses. In The Child With an Acquired Amputation. Washington, DC, National Academy of Sciences, 1972
128. Morgan JD, Somerville EW: Normal and abnormal growth at the upper end of the femur. J Bone Joint Surg 42B:264, 1960
128A. Ogden JA, Watson HK, Bohne W: Ulnar dysmelia. J Bone Joint Surg 58A:467, 1976
129. O'Rahilly R: Morphologic patterns in limb deficiencies and duplications. Am J Anat 89:135, 1951
130. O'Rahilly R: The Nomenclature and Classification of Limb Anomalies. In Bergsma D (ed): Limb Malformations. New York, Birth Defects Original Article Series, The National Foundation, 1969
131. O'Rahilly R: Normal development of the human embryo. In Normal and Abnormal Embryologic Development. Washington, DC, National Research Council, 1967
131A. Panting AL, Williams PF: Proximal femoral focal deficiency. J Bone Joint Surg 60B:46, 1978
132. Pardini AG Jr: Radial dysplasia. Clin Orthop 57:152, 1968
133. Pellicore RJ, Mier S, Hamilton RC, Lambert CN: Experiences with the Hepp-Kuhn below-elbow prosthesis. ICIB 8(6):9, 1969
133A. Pellicore RJ, et al: Incidence of bone overgrowth in the juvenile amputee population. ICIB 13:1, 1974
134. Popov B: The bioelectrically controlled prosthesis. J Bone Joint Surg 47B:421, 1965
135. Price CHG et al: Osteosarcoma in children. J Bone Joint Surg 57B:341, 1975
136. Riordan DC: Congenital absence of the radius. J Bone Joint Surg 37A:1129, 1955
137. Riordan DC: Congenital absence of the radius: A 15-year follow-up. J Bone Joint Surg 45A: 1783, 1963
138. Rohland TA: Sensory feedback in upper limb prosthetic systems. ICIB 13(9):1, 1974
139. Romano RL: Immediate Postsurgical Prosthetic Fitting of the Child With an Acquired Amputation. Washington, DC, National Academy of Sciences, 1972
140. Romano RL, Burgess EM: Extremity growth and overgrowth following amputation in children. ICIB 5(4):11, 1966
141. Romano RL, Burgess EM: The immediate postsurgical prosthetic fitting technique applied to child amputees. ICIB 9(9):1, 1970
141A. Rosenfelder R: Infant amputees: Early growth and care. Clin Orthop 148:41, 1980
142. Russell JE: Tibial hemimelia: limb deficiency in siblings. ICIB 14(7,8):15, 1975
143. Saunders JW: Control of growth patterns in limb development. In Normal and Abnormal Embryologic Development. Washington, DC, National Research Council, 1967
144. Sauter WF: Prostheses for the child amputee. Surg Clin North Am 3(2):483, 1972
145. Schmeisser G, Seamone W, Hoshall CH: Early clinical experience with the Johns Hopkins externally powered modular system for upper limb prostheses. Orthot Prosthet 26:41, 1972
145A. Schmidl H: The INAIL experience fitting upper limb dysmelic patients with myoelectric control. Bull Prosthet Res 10:17, 1977
146. Scott RN: Surgical implications of myoelectric control. Clin Orthop 61:248, 1968
147. Serafin J: A new operation for congenital absence of the fibula. J Bone Joint Surg 49B:59, 1967
148. Setoguchi Y: School and the child amputee. In The Child With An Acquired Amputation. Washington, DC, National Academy of Sciences, 1972
149. Setoguchi Y, Shaperman J, Talbert D: Vocational considerations. In The Child With An Acquired Amputation. Washington, DC, National Academy of Sciences, 1972
149A. Shaperman J: The CAPP terminal device. ICIB 14:1, 1975
149B. Shaperman J, Sumida CT: Recent advances in research in prosthetics for children. Clin Orthop 148:26, 1980
150. Simpson DC: Gripping surfaces for artificial hands. ICIB 12(6):1, 1973
151. Simpson DC, Lamb DW: A system of powered prostheses for severe bilateral upper limb deficiency. J Bone Joint Surg 47B:442, 1965
152. Skerik SK, Flatt AE: The anatomy of congenital radial dysplasia. Clin Orthop 66:124, 143, 1969
152A. Sorbye R: Myoelectric prosthetic fitting in young children. Clin Orthop 148:34, 1980
152B. Speer DP: The pathogenesis of amputation stump overgrowth. Clin Orthop 159:294, 1981
153. Stern PH, Lanko T: A myoelectrically controlled prosthesis using remote muscle sites. ICIB 12(7):1, 1973
154. Straub LR: Congenital absence of the radius and of the ulna. J Bone Joint Surg 54A:907, 1972
155. Swanson AB: The Krukenberg procedure in the juvenile amputee. J Bone Joint Surg 46A:1540, 1964
156. Swanson AB: Bone overgrowth in the juvenile amputee and its control by the use of silicone rubber implants. ICIB 8(5):9, 1969
157. Swanson AB: Silicone-rubber implants to control the overgrowth phenomenon in the juvenile amputee. ICIB 11(9):5, 1972
158. Swanson AB, Polglase VN, Applegate W: The Brown procedure in congenital absence of the tibia: A report of two cases. ICIB 10(11):1, 1971
159. Sypniewski BL: The child with terminal transverse partial hemimelia: A review of the literature on prosthetic management. Artif Limbs 16:20, 1972
160. Tablada C, Clarke S: A fitting for the unilateral below-elbow amputee with a dislocated radial head. ICIB 13(8):1, 1974
161. Taft CB, Fishman S: Survival and prosthetic fitting

of children amputated for malignancy. ICIB 5(5):9, 1966
162. Thompson TC, Straub LR, Arnold WD: Congenital absence of the fibula. J Bone Joint Surg 39A:1229, 1957
163. Tooms RE, Snell RR: Prosthetic principles—Conventional upper limb prostheses. In The Child With An Acquired Amputation. Washington, DC, National Academy of Sciences, 1972
164. Tooms RE, Snell R, Speltz E: An electrically powered elbow unit. ICIB 6(10):1, 1967
165. Tooms RE, Snell R, Speltz E: Treating the quadrimembral amputee. ICIB 8(2):1, 1968
165A. Tooms RE, Speltz E, Snell R: A modified prosthesis for elbow disarticulation amputees. ICIB 5:1, 1966
166. Trifard A, Neary R: Prognostic et traitement des sarcomes osteogenigues. J Chir 104:185, 1972
166A. Trost FJ: A comparison of conventional and myoelectric below-elbow prosthetic use. ICIB 18:9, 1983
167. Van Nes CP: Rotation-plasty for congenital defects of the femur. Making use of the ankle of the shortened limb to control the knee joint of a prosthesis. J Bone Joint Surg 32B:12, 1950
168. Von Soal G: Epiphysiodesis combined with amputation. J Bone Joint Surg 21:442, 1939
168A. Watts HG, Carideo JF Jr, Marick MS: Variable volume sockets for above-knee amputees: Managing children following amputation for malignancy. ICIB 18:11, 1982
169. Wenzlaff EF: Surgical ablation of the remaining femoral segment in proximal femoral focal deficiency. ICIB 9(1):1, 1969
170. Westin GW, Gunderson GO: Proximal femoral focal deficiency—A review of treatment experiences. In A Symposium on Proximal Femoral Focal Deficiency—A Congenital Anomaly. Washington, DC, National Academy of Sciences, 1969
170A. Westin GW, Sakai DN, Wood WL: Congenital longitudinal deficiency of the fibula. J Bone Joint Surg 58A:492, 1976
171. Wood WL, Zlotsky N, Westin GW: Congenital absence of the fibula. Treatment by Syme amputation—indications and technique. J Bone Joint Surg 47A:1159, 1965

23

Orthotic Management

Newton C. McCollough III

The term *orthosis* refers to an external orthopaedic appliance used to control the motion of body segments. The motion controlled may be in the sagittal, coronal, or transverse planes. The types of motion controlled are rotary, as in most joint motion, or translatory, as in vertical displacement of a fractured long bone. Motion control may be of several different types. An orthosis may eliminate motion entirely in a joint by locking it in place, or it may impose varying degrees of assistance or resistance to joint motion. Another type of motion control is axial unloading, which is representative of translatory motion control, and it is frequently used in the lower limb.

Orthoses in children, as in adults, are prescribed to accomplish one or more specific functions. They may be used to prevent deformity, correct deformity, protect a joint or segment, or to improve function. It is important to identify the purpose or purposes of orthotic control at the time of prescription.

ORTHOTIC TERMINOLOGY

Until relatively recently, orthotic terminology has been in complete disarray. Harris has stated that it has in fact resembled "a mausoleum in which to record and honor the names of the departed."* A task force of the Committee on Prosthetic and Orthotic Education of the National Academy of Sciences has developed a simplified and internationally accepted terminology for describing classes of orthotic devices.[21] This terminology forms the basis for the Atlas of Orthotics recently published by the Committee on Prosthetics and Orthotics of the American Academy of Orthopaedic Surgeons.[1] The type or class of orthosis is now designated by the joints or segments of the body that it encompasses. Acronyms are used to abbreviate the designation for prescription writing. Thus, the device formerly known as a short-leg brace is now called an *ankle-foot orthosis* (AFO). A long-leg brace is described as a knee-ankle-foot orthosis (KAFO). A lumbosacral spine orthosis is designated as an LSO. The Milwaukee brace would be classified as a CTLSO. There are obviously many variations within each class or category of devices, and specific characteristics of each must be further described in the prescription. The new terminology, however, does introduce an orderly approach to identification of devices and to orthotic prescription.

RATIONALE FOR ORTHOTIC PRESCRIPTION

Much progress can be made in understanding the principles of orthotic prescription if it is possible to ignore many of our old concepts of "bracing." To "brace" confers the intention of shoring up or supporting by static means, whereas the term *orthotics* is used to include static as well as dynamic control of the limb. One of the erroneous concepts of "bracing" in the past has been the tendency to lock the extremity into a rigid static device

* Harris EE: Personal communication, 1973

for control of a particular undesirable motion, while at the same time inhibiting some of the remaining normal functions of the limb. For example, A KAFO to control genu valgum may also eliminate knee flexion and extension and limit eversion and inversion at the subtalar joint. The ideal orthosis would control *only* the genu valgum, while permitting normal biomechanical functions to continue unimpeded in the same limb.

One of the first major departures from conventional orthotic design was the functional long-leg brace developed at the University of California at Los Angeles.[4] This device with its quadrilateral socket, offset knee joints, and hydraulic resistance to plantar flexion provided knee stability during stance phase and free knee flexion during swing phase, thereby enabling the polio patient with a flail knee and ankle to walk with a more natural and less energy-consuming gait. This orthosis was designed on sound biomechanical principles to control a specific offending motion, that is, uncontrolled knee flexion during stance phase, but it permitted the normal and desirable function of knee motion during swing phase. Other investigational orthoses have been similarly designed to permit normal function, such as the dual axis ankle–foot orthosis developed at the University of California at Berkeley, which controls drop foot but permits subtalar motion.[24] A rational approach to orthotic prescription therefore involves approaching the problem on a biomechanical basis without preconceived ideas of conventional orthotic devices. This approach also tends to negate the concept of "disease bracing" or the automatic prescription of certain appliances identified with specific disease entities. Rather, one should approach each patient, regardless of the underlying disease, by analysis of the specific biomechanical deficits present, followed by translation of this information into the appropriate mechanical substitute.

Special forms have been developed and described elsewhere for diagrammatically illustrating the biomechanical deficits of the patient's limbs or spine.[1,37,49] Although these forms are helpful educational tools, they may be cumbersome to use for the average practitioner. However, the principle involved is an important one and serves as the basis for modern orthotic prescription. The approach to orthotic prescription should always follow a logical sequence: (1) a biomechanical analysis of the patient's deficits should be made; (2) the functional disability and the treatment objectives should be identified; (3) the desired orthotic control should be specified at each level; (4) the appropriate orthotic components should be selected to provide the desired control; and (5) the components should be combined in the prescription into an appropriate orthotic device.

ADVANCES IN ORTHOTICS

There have been many advances in orthotics during the past 15 years. Chief among them has been the increasing sophistication of the orthotic practitioner or certified orthotist, the advent of new materials for use in fabrication of orthotic devices, and the trend toward providing improved cosmesis and comfort in these devices.

New materials that have been introduced into the field of orthotics in the past 10 years are primarily plastics, including the thermosetting plastics and various thermoplastics. These plastic materials may be used alone or in combination with metal to produce lighter weight, more cosmetic, and, in many instances, more functional devices than were available in the past. Thermosetting plastics are those that require application of heat to cure or harden but that will not soften upon further heating. An example is the familiar plastic laminate used in prosthetic sockets. This type of material is useful in orthotics for quadrilateral brims of knee-ankle-foot orthoses, patellar tendon–bearing brims of ankle-foot orthoses, and for foot orthoses or shoe-insert designs. Thermoplastic materials are those that soften each time the temperature is raised to a critical level and harden upon lowering of the temperature. The most commonly used thermoplastics in orthotics are polypropylene, polyethylene, and polycarbonate. Of these, polypropylene has the widest application due to its unusual feature of extreme resistance to fatigue upon repeated bending. Recently, a copolymer of polyethylene and polypropylene has been widely used in situations that do not require the degree of rigidity offered by polypropylene alone. Although the fatigue resistance of the copolymer is not as great as polypropylene alone, it is sufficient for spinal orthoses as well as many lower limb orthoses. Thermoplastics are usually hand molded or vacuum molded over positive models of the limbs or trunk, giving a precise and intimate fit.

There has been an increasing trend toward providing better cosmesis and comfort in both limb and spinal orthotic devices. The more common use of plastics has had an enormous influence upon both of these factors. Although the objectives of cosmesis and comfort are probably secondary to providing adequate function or efficiency of the appliance, they are nevertheless important and are no less important in the child than in the adult. We have all known patients who will even sacrifice better function for comfort or cosmesis by refusing to wear a standard metal orthosis. The seemingly minor inconvenience of not being able to change shoes when an orthotic device is used is of major concern to many children. The advent of thermoplastic materials for use in orthoses to control inadequate dorsiflexion has obviated this problem by virtue of a shoe-insert design, while at the same time it has solved the problem of cosmesis. The physician should not neglect the importance of cosmesis and comfort when prescribing an orthosis for a child, because a much higher degree of acceptance may be obtained with less psychological trauma by appropriate utilization of newer materials in the design and fabrication of the device.

PHILOSOPHY OF ORTHOTIC PRESCRIPTION

Prescription of an orthosis for a child requires careful consideration of the purposes to be achieved, the biomechanical design, the length of time required for wear, the frequency of growth adjustments or frequency of replacement of the entire orthosis due to growth, and the impact of the device upon the child and his parents. The long-term effects of wearing an unsightly appliance may be much more devastating than the trauma of corrective or reconstructive surgery, if there is a choice between the two methods of treatment. The prescription of an appliance just to reassure the parents that something is being done for a mild or self-correcting deformity when the efficacy of the device is questionable is not fair to the child or to the parents.

The orthotic device prescribed should be the minimum amount of hardware required to accomplish the desired objective. Frequently, surgical correction of deformity may reduce or eliminate the need for orthotic prescription. A combination of surgical and orthotic management combined with a physical therapy program is frequently the best approach to a clinical problem, particularly in neuromuscular disorders.

In all cases, the feelings and emotional makeup of the child should be taken into consideration when prescribing a device. The physician should appreciate the impact on the child of having to wear an appliance for a long period of time during the formative years. Considerations as to alternative methods of treatment should be given, and, if orthotic management is the treatment of choice, the device prescribed should be as unencumbering as possible, controlling insofar as is possible only the particular problem in question. Consideration should also be given in the design of the device to provide optimum cosmesis and comfort insofar as is technically feasible.

LOWER LIMB ORTHOTICS

The most common site of application of orthotic devices in children is the lower limb. The purpose of orthotic management varies widely and includes prevention of deformity, correction of deformity, protection of a joint or limb segment, and improvement in function. Frequently, two or more of these purposes may be achieved by the same device, such as improvement in gait and prevention of ankle contracture by the use of an AFO, which positions the ankle at 90°.

The Foot and Ankle

Orthotic control of problems about the foot and ankle is accomplished by the use of proper shoes, foot orthoses (FO), or ankle-foot orthoses (AFO). Shoes are classified as orthotic devices when they are prescribed to perform specific orthotic functions. As the foundation for many lower limb orthoses, they also may be thought of as integral parts of the orthotic system.

Metatarus Adductus. The reverse-last or outflare shoe is indicated either as prewalker or closed-toe shoe. Shoes alone will not correct rigid deformities, but they are useful to maintain correction for a period of time following casting. Flexible deformities may be corrected over a period of several months with the use of this type of shoe worn 24 hours a day.

Pes Planovalgus. Mild degrees of flattening

of the longitudinal arch do not need treatment. Children usually do not develop a longitudinal arch until they are 5 to 6 years of age, so moderate flattening of the arch early in childhood is the rule rather than the exception. Children who have flattening of the arch associated with heel valgus may be treated with an inverted or supinated last shoe to adduct the forefoot, using Thomas heels with a ⅛- or 3⁄16-inch medial heel wedge and a medial arch support. Such children with hypermobile flat feet will always have the tendency to planovalgus deformity, regardless of how long the shoes are worn, but it may be possible to reduce the ultimate degree of deformity by prolonged corrective shoe wear.

Children who have more severe degrees of pes planovalgus and who are symptomatic may be treated with special foot orthoses. Today, the most commonly used devices are the molded leather shoe insert and the molded plastic shoe insert (UCB insert) developed at the University of California at Berkeley.[22] The molded leather insert is a custom-made, firm, longitudinal arch support fabricated from a cast of the foot. It provides good support for the longitudinal arch but does not control heel valgus. The molded plastic shoe insert not only provides an arch support but also grasps the heel of the foot to prevent heel valgus (Fig. 23-1). This device is fabricated over a positive plaster mold of the foot in the corrected position. Although the molded plastic insert foot orthosis is believed to be an effective positioning device for the foot, it is not known whether it will result in any permanent correction. The effectiveness of this device in repositioning the foot has recently been challenged, based on a radiographic evaluation in children.[43]

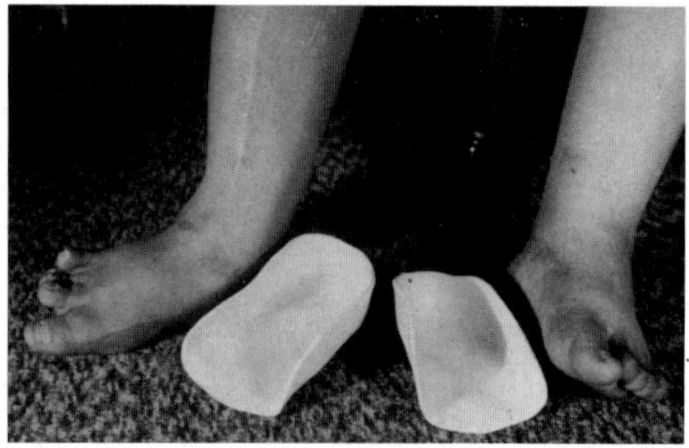

FIG. 23-1. The UCB (University of California at Berkeley) shoe insert for moderate to severe planovalgus. (Courtesy of Robert O. Nitschke, Rochester, New York)

Pes Calcaneovalgus. This common positional foot deformity in the newborn usually requires no specific treatment other than passive exercise by the mother. If severe, the Denis Browne bar foot orthosis may be used, angled with the apex cephalad and the feet in neutral rotation to accentuate inversion of the feet at the subtalar joint. The length of the bar in this instance should not exceed the width of the pelvis. Correction is usually observed within 2 months of night wear.

Talipes Equinovarus. Orthotic management of this condition is an adjunct to other nonsurgical and surgical methods of treatment and is used solely to maintain the correction achieved by these other methods. There is no corrective orthotic device for this deformity. Following correction in the infant, outflare or reverse-last prewalker shoes may be attached to a Denis Browne bar, which is angled with the apex caudad, the affected foot or feet being externally rotated on the bar to 70° to 80°. This arrangement produces a dorsiflexion-eversion force when the infant kicks and tends to prevent recurrent deformity. Another type of orthosis that may be used to maintain the foot in the corrected position is a single medial upright AFO with a 90° plantar flexion stop and a lateral T strap attached to a reverse-last prewalker shoe. For the ambulatory child, a reverse-last shoe with a ¼-inch lateral heel and sole wedge and a reverse Thomas heel should be used with or without the single-medial upright AFO, depending on the degree of concern regarding recurrence.

Dorsiflexion Insufficiency. Lack of adequate dorsiflexion of the foot results in a "drop foot," with inadequate clearance of the toes during the swing phase of gait. Secondary effects on gait occur from compensatory efforts to clear the foot, and include excessive hip and knee flexion (steppage gait), vaulting on the sound side, and circumduction of the affected limb. If inadequate dorsiflexion is combined with contracture of the heel-cord, a toe-heel gait during stance phase results, imparting an extension movement to the knee, resulting in genu recurvatum. If a varus component is present with inadequate dorsiflexion, foot contact occurs initially on the lateral border of the foot, perhaps producing initial stance phase instability. The orthotic approach to each of these three situations differs slightly.

Isolated Dorsiflexion Insufficiency. Pure loss of dorsiflexion power requires a dorsiflexion-assist AFO. The orthoses of choice are either the double-upright spring dorsiflexion-assist orthosis,[1] or the molded plastic-AFO-insert orthosis (Fig. 23-2).[49] Either of these devices will provide dorsiflexion assistance while permitting the normal function of plantar flexion at heel strike, thus providing the most optimal gait. If one were to use an AFO with a 90° plantar flexion stop, plantar flexion at heel strike would be restricted and an undesirable flexion movement would be imparted to the knee by the posterior calf band.

The molded plastic–insert AFO has the advantage of being lightweight and cosmetically appealing. However, there is no adjustability for growth; thus, the maximum period of use is about 2 years. If this device is selected, the trim lines at the ankle should be sufficiently posterior to allow flexible plantar flexion at heel strike.

Dorsiflexion Insufficiency With Dynamic Equinus. If inadequate dorsiflexion of the foot is associated with mild dynamic or spastic equinus, the orthoses described above may be used. If the spasticity is moderate to severe, the orthoses of choice are either the double-upright AFO with 90° plantar flexion stop, or the molded plastic–insert AFO fabricated with the ankle trim lines sufficiently anterior to provide stiff resistance to plantar flexion (Fig. 23-3). In cases that demonstrate significant hyperextension of the knee associated with the spastic equinus, modifying the plantar flexion stop to slightly above 90° or fabricating the plastic AFO in slight dorsiflexion is indicated. This modification will provide an increased flexion movement at the knee transmitted through the superior calf section.

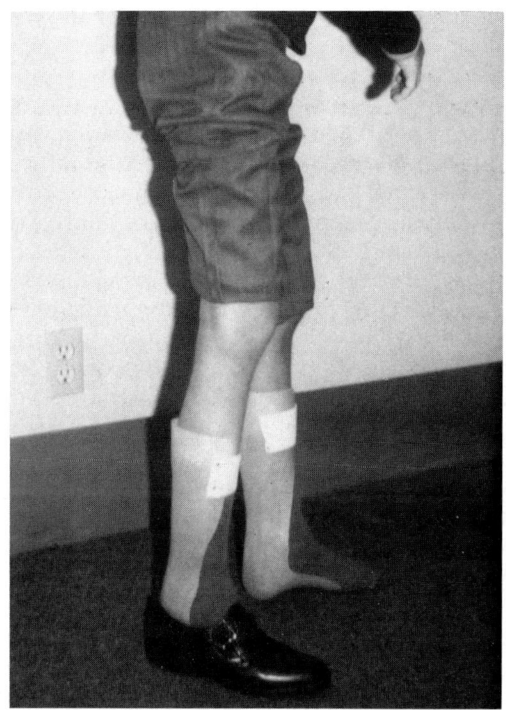

Fig. 23-3. Molded polypropylene AFO with ankle rigidity provided by extending the trim lines anterior to the malleoli.

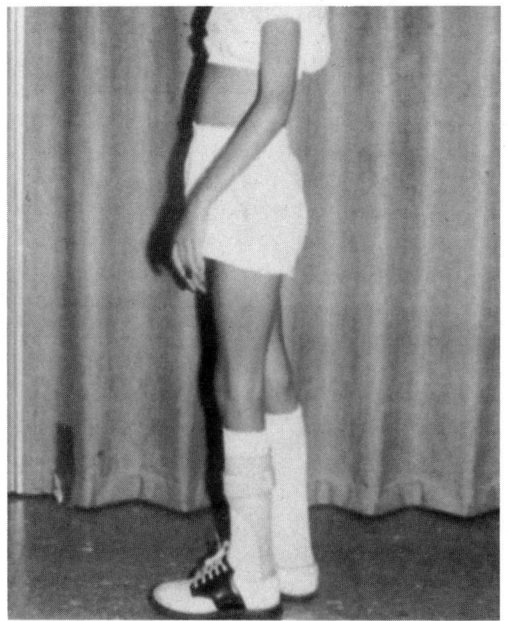

Fig. 23-2. Molded polypropylene AFO for foot and ankle control in a child with spastic left hemiparesis.

Dorsiflexion insufficiency combined with structural equinus requires surgical or serial-cast correction of the equinus deformity prior to bracing.

Dorsiflexion Insufficiency With Varus. Mild degrees of varus deformity during swing phase need no special consideration, and any orthoses used for isolated dorsiflexion insufficiency will be adequate. Moderate dynamic varus during swing phase may be controlled by the addition of a lateral T strap to the double-upright AFO or by extending the trim lines more anteriorly in the case of a polypropylene AFO. Severe varus deformity in swing phase cannot be controlled by orthotic means, and it requires surgical correction.

Dynamic Varus Deformity During Stance Phase. Orthotic management of dynamic varus deformity during stance phase of gait is difficult at best, and, frequently, it requires surgical correction as the preferred management. If the varus is mild during foot contact, a lateral T strap added to either a single-medial-upright or a double-upright AFO may be sufficient to provide stability in conjunction with a high-top shoe. Moderate degrees of dynamic varus deformity may be controlled by either the molded insert, double-upright AFO[9] (Fig. 23-4), or the molded plastic-insert AFO with the ankle trim lines anterior to the malleoli so as to provide mediolateral stability (see Fig. 23-3). Severe degrees of dynamic varus deformity or structural varus deformity are not amenable to orthotic control, and surgical correction is indicated.

Plantar Flexion Insufficiency. Inadequacy of ankle plantar flexion is usually caused by paralysis of the triceps surae. The effects on gait are excessive ankle dorsiflexion and knee flexion during stance phase, which may be exaggerated in the presence of a weak quadriceps and inadequate push-off. The former is subject to orthotic control, the latter is not. It is important to control excessive ankle dorsiflexion during stance phase in the growing child in order to minimize the development of the calcaneus deformity that invariably occurs.

The standard orthotic control for plantar flexion insufficiency is the double-upright AFO with 90° dorsiflexion (anterior) stops. There are two important considerations in the fabrication and application of this device. First, the calf band must be as high as possible to gain optimal mechanical advantage in preventing forward rotation of the tibia over the ankle. A more positive control may be gained by reversing the calf band to provide firm pressure over the proximal tibia. Second, in order to minimize motion between the orthosis and the shoe, an extended stirrup should be used, attached to a steel shank running the length of the shoe.

A molded plastic–insert AFO with a pretibial shell may also be used to provide control of excessive ankle dorsiflexion (Fig. 23-5).[19] It is essential that the ankle of this orthosis be made sufficiently rigid so that dorsiflexion is well controlled. This may be achieved either

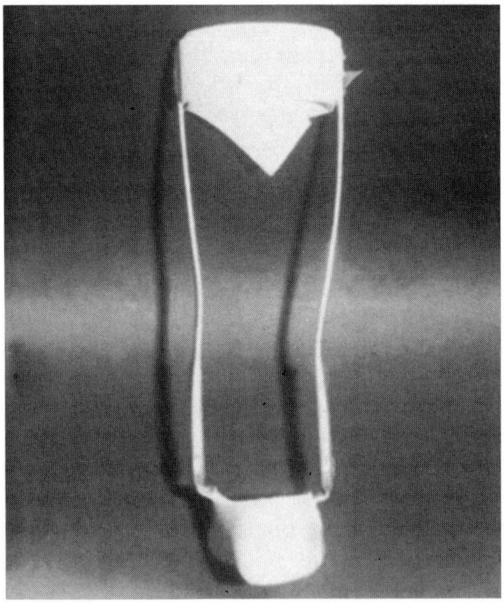

FIG. 23-4. NYU (New York University) AFO for foot and ankle control, viewed from the posterior.

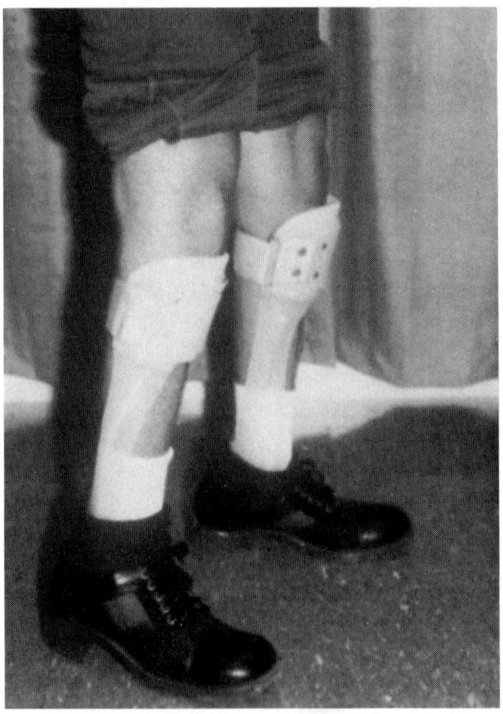

FIG. 23-5. Molded polypropylene AFO with a pretibial shell for control of excessive ankle dorsiflexion.

by corrugating the polypropylene at the ankle area or by the use of carbon inserts applied to the ankle area during fabrication.[19] This device, when properly constructed, gives excellent control of the foot and ankle and prevents excessive ankle dorsiflexion. The disadvantage of this orthosis in the growing child depends to a considerable degree on the height of the pretibial shell; a new orthosis may be required on a yearly basis.

The posterior-bar AFO is a relatively new device used to substitute for the plantar flexors of the ankle in preventing excessive ankle dorsiflexion (Fig. 23-6). The posterior bar may be made of spring steel or fiberglass material and must be attached securely to an extension or a steel shank in the sole of the shoe at the heel. The orthosis essentially provides a dynamic force to prevent forward rotation of the tibia over the ankle during stance phase of gait. A pretibial band with a lateral opening is preferred. This device is most effective in smaller children; the dynamic corrective force of the posterior bar may be insufficient for larger or older children.

The Flail Foot and Ankle. Total paralysis about the foot and ankle is best managed by an orthosis that provides some resistance to both plantar flexion and dorsiflexion, while providing adequate mediolateral stability for the subtalar joint. This may be accomplished by the use of a double-upright AFO with anterior and posterior spring-loaded resistance (Fig. 23-7) or by the molded plastic–insert AFO, using sufficiently thick material to provide the desired resistance.

The molded spiral AFO (Fig. 23-8)[31] also provides resistance to plantar flexion and dorsiflexion, but experience with this device in children has been limited.

The Painful Ankle. Hemophilia, rheumatoid arthritis, osteochondritis dissecans, and other abnormalities of the ankle joint may produce symptoms or potential conditions for which orthotic protection is indicated. In such situations, it may be desirable to eliminate all

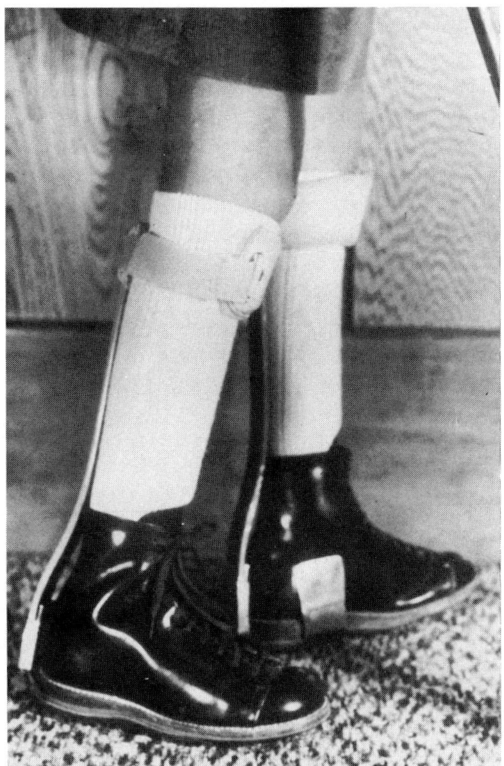

FIG. 23-6. Posterior-bar AFO for control of excessive ankle dorsiflexion. (Courtesy of Robert O. Nitschke, Rochester, New York)

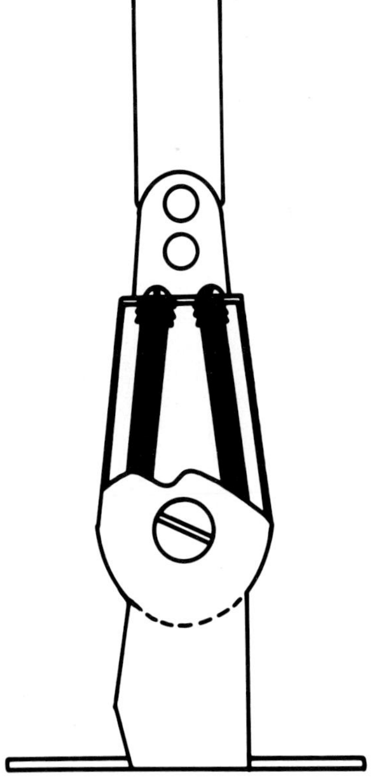

FIG. 23-7. Diagrammatic sketch of an ankle joint with anterior and posterior channels that may be used with stops or spring-loaded.

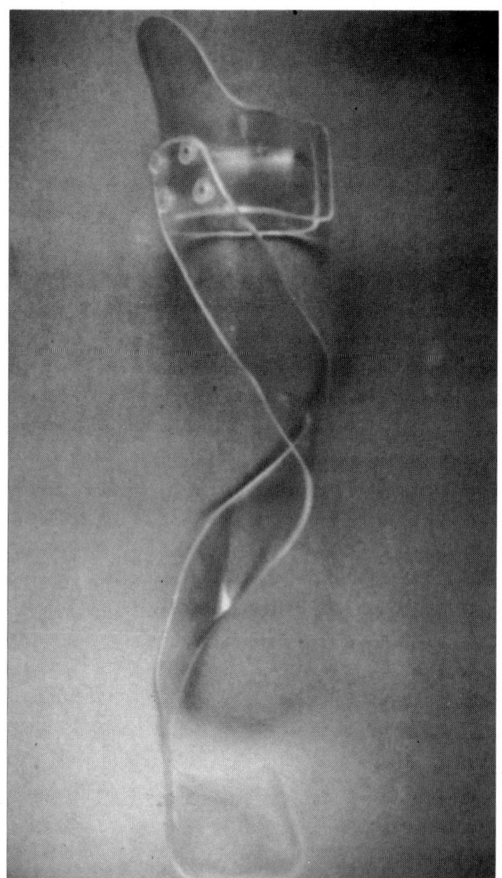

FIG. 23-8. Molded spiral AFO for resistance to both plantar flexion and dorsiflexion of the ankle.

motion in the ankle joint, or at least to reduce motion to a minimum. The molded plastic–insert AFO with trim lines that extend anterior to the malleoli (see Fig. 23-3) provides relatively rigid immobilization of the ankle joint. It should be used with special shoe modifications, consisting of a soft rubber heel (SACH heel) and a rocker bar on the sole. This permits simulated ankle motion by compression of the heel at heel strike followed by rolling over the rocker bar to achieve toe-off. As an alternative to the molded plastic–insert, AFO design, one may use a double-upright rigid-ankle AFO attached to a shoe with a steel shank and similar shoe modifications.

Axial unloading of the ankle joint, although highly desirable in many instances to relieve symptoms or to prevent joint compression, cannot be achieved effectively by orthotic means. The patellar tendon–bearing AFO[49] in theory reduces load-bearing forces on the ankle joint, but, in practice, it simply has not worked in the author's experience. Significant unloading of the ankle joint requires weight-bearing forces about the proximal tibia and patellar tendon that are more than the patient can tolerate.

The Leg

Tibial Torsion. Internal or external tibial torsion may occur as a developmental abnormality, but internal torsion of the tibia is by far the more common of the two. The decision to treat internal tibial torsion during infancy is highly individualized, and, among orthopaedic surgeons, a range of opinion can be found from "treat none" to "treat all." Clinical experience tells us that many, but not all, of these deformities spontaneously regress by the time the child begins to walk. If the deformity appears to be significant by the age of 4 to 6 months, treatment with the Denis Browne bar may be undertaken, and correction is usually apparent within 3 to 6 months. Prewalker shoes (reverse-last shoes if metatarsus adductus is also present) are attached to the bar and externally rotated from 45° to 60° or to the position at which slight resistance is felt to external rotation of the leg. The length of the bar should not exceed the width of the anterosuperior spines of the iluim by more than an inch or two; otherwise, the feet will be forced into pronation and a secondary deformity will be produced. This device may be used for treatment of internal tibial torsion during the first one and one half years of life as a night or sleeping brace. In the author's experience, it is poorly tolerated if instituted beyond that time, due to the fact that independent movement of the legs is prevented.

For the older child, a device has been developed that permits independent leg movement for the treatment of torsional deformities of the leg (Fig. 23-9). The design of this device was based on the experimental production of tibial torsion in the immature rabbit and the fact that torsion of the long bones may be influenced during growth by the application of external forces.[36] It consists of a posterior aluminum bar KAFO with a 90° bend at the knee and at the ankle. The shoe plate has a rotational adjustment permitting graduated external rotation. Placing the knee in flexion confines the rotational force to the leg segment, avoiding the dissipation of the force upward

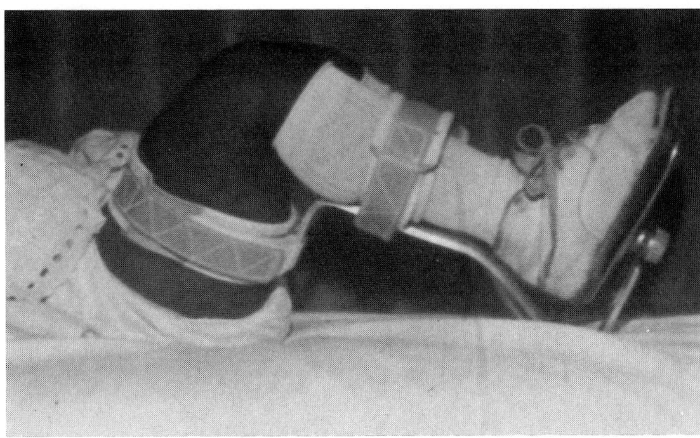

FIG. 23-9. This posterior-bar KAFO with a rotational adjustment at the foot is used as a night splint for internal tibial torsion.

to the hip, which occurs with the Denis Browne bar. The orthosis should be adjusted on the child, externally rotating the foot until resistance is encountered, then the foot plate should be locked in position. Further adjustments into external rotation are made monthly.

The HKAFO twister orthosis may also be used for the treatment of tibial torsion in the older child (Fig. 23-10). Because the torque force is not confined to the lower leg segment but is dissipated upward to the hip, it is not thought to be as effective as the orthosis just described. It consists of flexible hydraulic tubing or spring cables attached to a pelvic band and to the shoes with an adjustment to rotate the shoes outward or inward at the ankle. It produces essentially no restriction of motion of the limb other than the desired rotational control. It may be used as a nighttime device, or it may be worn during the waking hours as well. The device is well tolerated by children as a night splint, and successful results have been obtained up to 6 years of age with usage from 6 to 12 years.

Protection of the Leg. Protective orthoses for the leg segment may be indicated in the child with osteogenesis imperfecta, congenital pseudarthrosis of the tibia, or other pathologic states that compromise the integrity of bone structure. A lightweight protective device made of polypropylene or polyethylene and lined with polyethylene foam can be fabricated from a positive model of the leg (Fig. 23-11). It may be formed either as a leg cylinder or as an AFO, and it is of a "clamshell" design with anterior and posterior halves that are secured together with Velcro straps. Extension of the anterior, medial, and lateral portions to the supracondylar area of the femur will add rotational control and will still permit full flexion and extension of the knee.

Fractures of the Tibia and Fibula. Although the treatment of fractures is beyond the scope of this text, it should be pointed out that in the older child and adolescent, fractures of the tibia and fibula may be successfully managed by the use of fracture bracing (Fig. 23-12). The device may be fabricated from Orthoplast,* or commercially available prefabricated thermoplastic fracture braces may be used. The orthosis is applied after 2 weeks of immobilization in a long-leg cast, and full weight-bearing is permitted, as tolerated. Angular deformities must be corrected prior to application of the orthosis.

The Knee

Genu Varum. Bowing of the legs is a normal physiologic event in children up to 2 years of age and requires no treatment in children of this age group. Persistent genu varum that is not decreasing is pathologic in children older than 3 years of age, and it may be due to failure of spontaneous correction of developmental genu varum, tibia vara (Blount's disease), rickets, or other metabolic bone disease. Regardless of the cause, orthotic management is indicated in children older than 3 with varus deformities of the knee in excess of 10°, as measured by a standing roentgenogram. In the older child or adolescent, orthotic management is unlikely to be effective, and surgical correction is generally preferred.

---

* Johnson and Johnson, New Brunswick, New Jersey

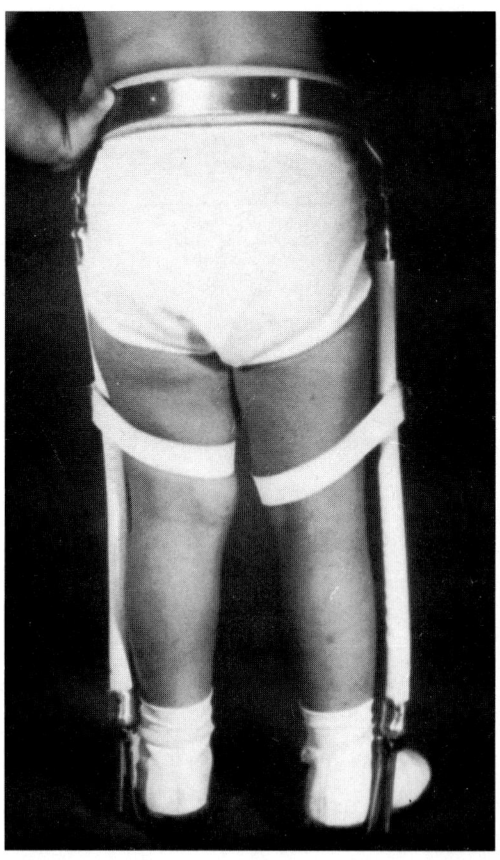

FIG. 23-10. HKAFO twister orthosis for dynamic control of limb rotation or tibial torsion. (From Staros A, LeBlanc M: Orthotic components and system. In American Academy of Orthopaedic Surgeons: Atlas of Orthotics. St Louis, CV Mosby, 1975

The degree to which orthotic management is effective in the management of pathologic genu varum is controversial. In principle, one hopes to influence epiphyseal growth at the distal femoral and proximal tibial growth plates by producing tension forces on the medial side of the knee joint and compressive forces on the lateral side. The extent to which this is possible is not known, nor is it known whether actual correction or simple arrest of progression of deformity can be achieved by orthotic means. In children who are braced for genu varum, it is important to obtain periodic standing roentgenograms out of the brace to measure the knee angle and assess the effect of orthosis wear. It has been the author's impression that gradual correction of genu varum deformity can occur with prolonged orthotic usage, although it is impossible to rule out spontaneous correction with growth or with vitamin D therapy in the case of rickets.

It is impossible to apply a corrective force at the knee and at the same time permit free knee motion. Therefore, orthoses used in the correction of genu varum must have locked knee joints or no knee joints at all. It is usually desirable to permit a few hours of freedom from the orthosis every day, using the device at night and about half of the waking hours.

Two orthotic designs for use in genu varum have been used. The more conventional system is an HKAFO with free ankle joints, a single-medial lower upright connected to a single-lateral upper upright by a posterior thigh band. The two lateral uprights are joined by a pelvic band with free hip joints (Fig. 23-13).

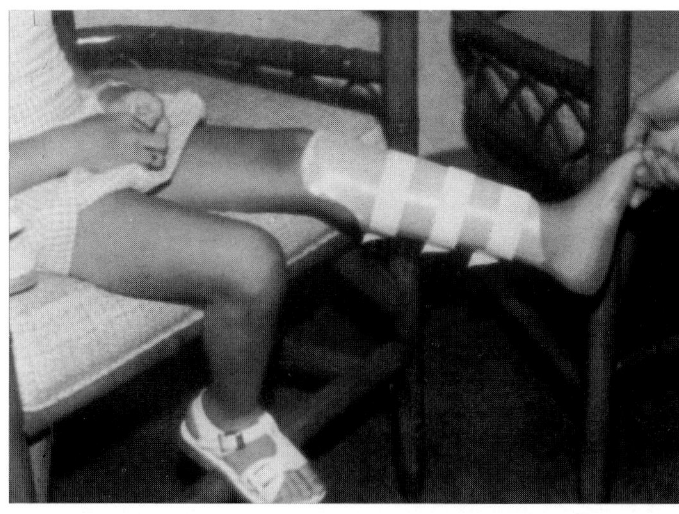

FIG. 23-11. Molded polypropylene AFO of a bivalve design with a shoe insert for protection of the tibia in a child with osteogenesis imperfecta.

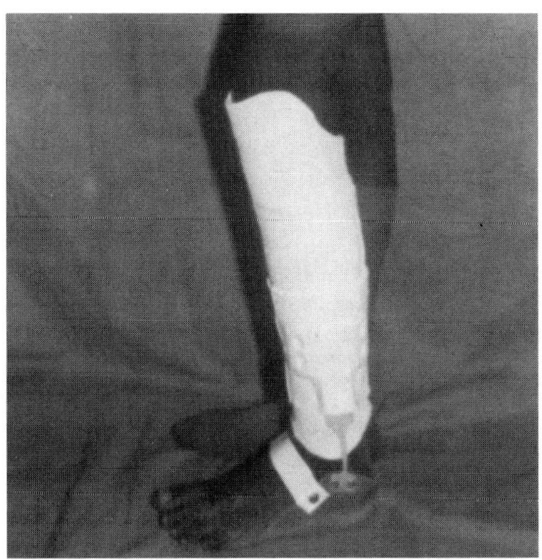

FIG. 23-12. Tibial fracture brace on a child 10 years of age.

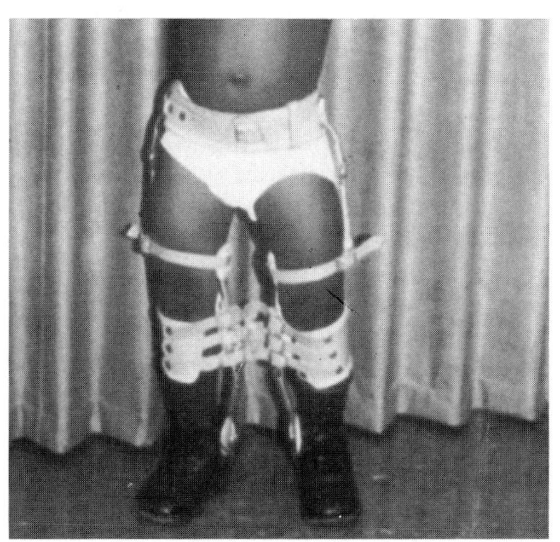

FIG. 23-13. A HKAFO for the correction of genu varum, with a pullover pad to a medial upright.

The corrective pullover pads are placed over the lateral aspect of the proximal tibiae and knee joints and are anchored to the medial uprights. The second design consists of a double-lateral-upright HKAFO with free ankle joints and hip joints and an adjustable pushover pad centered at the level of the knee joint (Fig. 23-14). Relief must be provided over the area of the peroneal nerve.

Salter has described a night splint for genu varum in children older than 2 years of age,

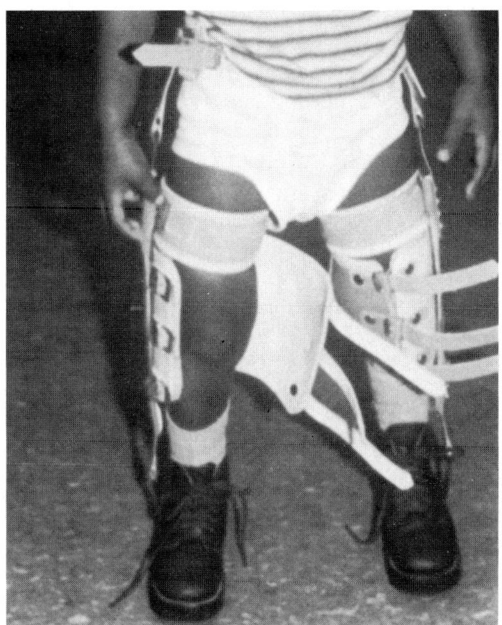

FIG. 23-14. A HKAFO for correction of genu varum, with lateral uprights and adjustable pads to provide a medially directed corrective force.

consisting of a Denis Browne bar to anchor the feet and an encircling leather or fabric gauntlet about the knees to produce the corrective force.[50] In the author's personal experience, this device is too confining to be tolerated well by the child.

Genu Valgum. Physiologic genu valgum occurs in many children between the ages of 2 and 8 years. Unfortunately, there is no available statistical information regarding the natural progression and resolution of this deformity. It has been the author's policy to consider genu valgum pathologic in this age group when it exceeds 15° as measured by a standing roentgenogram. In children older than the age of 8 years, genu valgum in excess of 10° is considered abnormal. Orthotic treatment is instituted in these two categories of patients and continued until correction is achieved or until the decision is made to treat surgically.

As in the case of genu varum, no available data exist as to the efficacy of orthotic treatment in this condition. The rationale for altering the deformity by orthotic means rests on the theory that it is possible to create tension forces on the lateral side of the knee joint and compressive forces on the medial side of the joint, thereby influencing epiphyseal growth.

It cannot be stated with certainty that the correction observed with the use of orthoses is due entirely to the effect of the appliance or whether some degree of natural correction with growth might be a factor. Significant correction of deformity by orthotic means in children over the age of 10 years is doubtful.

The recommended orthosis for genu valgum deformity is a single-lateral-upright KAFO with thigh and calf bands, a medial pullover pad anchored to the lateral upright, and a free ankle joint (Fig. 23-15). In order for the appliance to be effective, the knee must be maintained in full extension, so the device is fabricated either without a knee joint or with dropping knee locks. The orthoses should be worn as night splints and for one half of the waking hours, allowing some freedom of activity for the child during the day.

Genu valgum may also occur in conjunction with paralytic states in which muscles about the hip and knee are inadequate, and it is frequently seen in poliomyelitis. The management of this type of deformity will be discussed in the section entitled "Quadriceps Insufficiency," below.

Genu Recurvatum. In children, hyperextension of the knee during the stance phase of gait is most frequently observed in association with either spastic or flaccid paralysis. In the spastic state, the cause is usually related to overactivity of the triceps surae, producing a tethering effect upon normal forward rotation of the tibia over the ankle from foot flat to mid-stance. The use of either a rigid molded plastic–insert AFO fabricated in 10° of dorsiflexion or a double-upright AFO with the planter stop set at 10° above neutral frequently controls this gait defect, assuming that the quadriceps is of normal strength. If the deformity persists to a significant degree with the use of an AFO, a double-upright aluminum KAFO with free ankle and extension stops at the knees is indicated. If the quadriceps is also weak, drop-ring knee locks should be added to the orthosis to maintain knee stability.

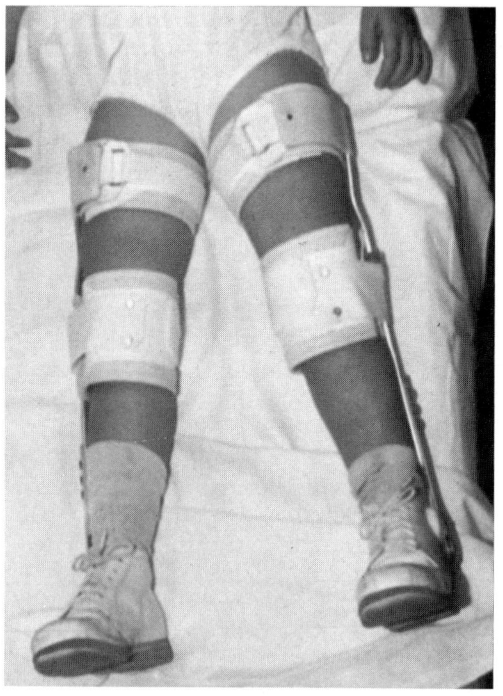

FIG. 23-15. Lateral-upright KAFO's with medial pullover pads for correction of genu valgum.

In the case of genu recurvatum due to flaccid paralysis, the cause is usually quadriceps insufficiency, and the knee is consciously placed in the hyperextended position to achieve knee stability. After a period of time, the recurvatum increases as a result of ligamentous stretching. The increasing pressures upon the anterior portions of the epiphyseal plates at the knee may cause accentuation of the deformity with growth. In this case, treatment with the appropriate KAFO for quadriceps insufficiency permits the knee to maintain a minimally extended or slightly flexed position during stance phase.

Quadriceps Insufficiency. Inadequacy of knee extension power as an isolated defect is rare, and paralysis of the quadriceps is usually associated with weakness in other portions of the limb. However, stabilization of the knee segment is the key to ambulation in extensive lower limb paralysis. Although it is possible for the child with a paralyzed quadriceps to walk without an orthosis if the hip extensors are adequate, he must maintain the knee in a hyperextended and locked position. Abnormal pressures are created on the epiphyseal plates at the knee, which can lead to progressive deformity. Therefore, it is important to provide knee stability in these children unless the natural course of their disease renders them nonambulatory in childhood.

The conventional orthosis used for quadriceps insufficiency is a double-upright aluminum KAFO with thigh and calf bands, drop-ring knee locks, an anterior knee pad, and an ankle joint that is appropriate to the biomechanical situation at the ankle. This device provides excellent knee stability and prevents hyperextension of the knee. In the case of bilateral involvement, the use of plunger knee locks may be preferred, so that manual operation of the knee locks can be performed at the hip level. If genu valgum is associated with quadriceps insufficiency, the anterior knee pad may be modified to pull the knee toward the lateral upright; or a pressure pad centered over the medial femoral condyle may be used.

Excellent knee stability may also be achieved in flaccid paralysis by the use of the single-lateral-upright KAFO with a pretibial shell and a posterior popliteal strap (Fig. 23-16).[42] This device is easier to don, lighter in weight, and more cosmetic than the double-upright KAFO. It incorporates a drop-ring knee lock and an ankle joint of choice, which may be attached to a shoe insert. The posterior cross strap effectively holds the knee forward into the pretibial shell, allowing the patient to kneel into the orthosis for stability. An accessory silesian belt can be added for rotational stability, if necessary. The device may be used in the case of bilateral quadriceps insufficiency in the younger or smaller child.

A third alternative for providing knee stability in the child is the molded plastic KAFO with drop-ring knee locks, which is fabricated from a positive model of the lower limb (Fig. 23-17). This device also provides excellent knee stability with the advantage of minimal weight, and it is particularly useful in situations of extreme general weakness where weight is an important consideration, such as in the patient with muscular dystrophy. The disadvantage of this orthosis is the relative lack of adjustability in the growing child. The maximum period of time before a completely new orthosis is needed is 2 years. The orthosis may be used without the drop-ring knee locks for control of genu recurvatum in the presence of an adequate quadriceps.

In spastic paralysis, weakness of knee extension is frequently associated with hamstring tightness or overactivity. The double-upright KAFO is usually indicated in this situation, because the single-lateral-upright and molded plastic designs do not provide sufficient control

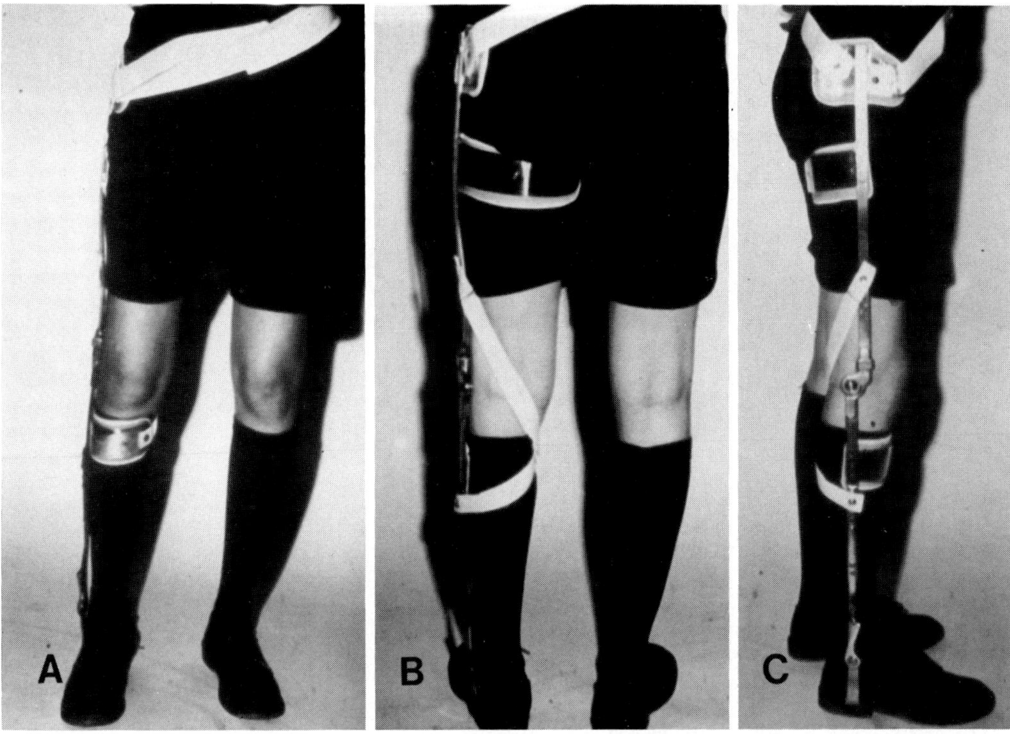

FIG. 23-16. *(A, B* and *C)* Single-lateral-upright KAFO with a pretibial shell and a silesian bandage for control of knee instability and flaccid paralysis.

of dynamic knee flexion. In many cases, it is preferable to improve quadricep function and knee extension by hamstring lengthening or transfer, thus reducing the orthotic requirements to that of an AFO.

Orthotic considerations with regard to hip control associated with quadricep insufficiency in cases with paralysis about the hip will be considered in the section entitled "The Hip."

Knee-flexion Contracture. The occurrence of knee-flexion contracture is common in flaccid paralysis, spastic paralysis, hemophiliac arthropathy, and rheumatoid arthritis. When a tendency to develop knee-flexion contracture is noted, the use of a night splint to control the deformity is indicated. The preferred splint is the three-point-extension knee orthosis (KO), which consists of double aluminum uprights attached to pivotal calf and thigh bands and an anterior knee pad. This device may also be used to correct mild knee-flexion deformities by gradually tightening the anterior knee pad as extension occurs.

In more severe knee-flexion deformities, attempting orthotic or plaster correction may result in posterior subluxation of the tibia on the femur. The dial-lock knee mechanism may be used on a double-upright KAFO, with shallow calf band placed under the proximal tibia to resist posterior displacement of the tibia. Graduated knee extension may then be achieved by progressive adjustment of the dial lock over a period of several weeks.

A more effective method of correcting knee-flexion contractures is the use of the extension-desubluxation hinge developed at Orthopaedic Hospital in Los Angeles for use in hemophiliac arthropathy.[34,54] This device is incorporated into a short-leg cast and a thigh cylinder, and it has adjustments to obtain knee extension as well as to obtain desubluxation of the tibia or to prevent subluxation of the tibia during correction of the flexion deformity (Fig. 23-18).

Protection of the Knee Joint. There are instances when one wishes to protect the knee joint from stress by the use of an orthotic device. Examples are hemophiliac arthropathy and post-traumatic situations.

The hinged knee cage may be used to provide minimal protection against flexion and extension as well as medial and lateral stresses. The most effective knee cage is custom-made from a positive model of the leg and is comprised of polypropylene thigh and calf cuffs connected by drop-ring knee locks.[12] Suspension may be achieved either by an elastic supercondylar strap or a soft medial wedge built into the orthosis over the medial femoral condyle.

The Lennox Hill knee orthosis is a special cage designed to prevent rotary stress as well as valgus stress following football injuries, and it may be useful in the older child and adolescent to prevent abduction, external rotation injuries of the knee joint.[1]

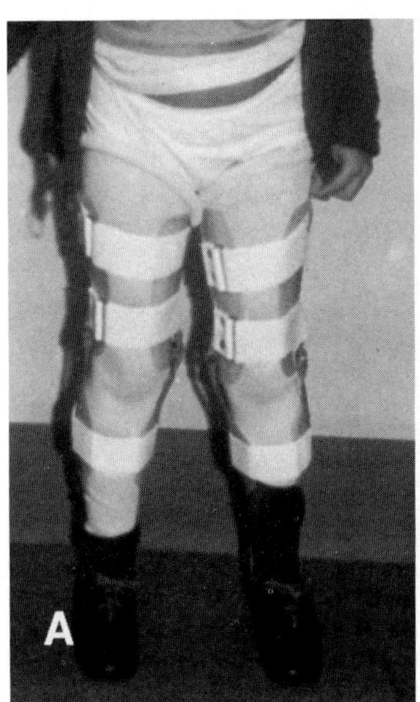

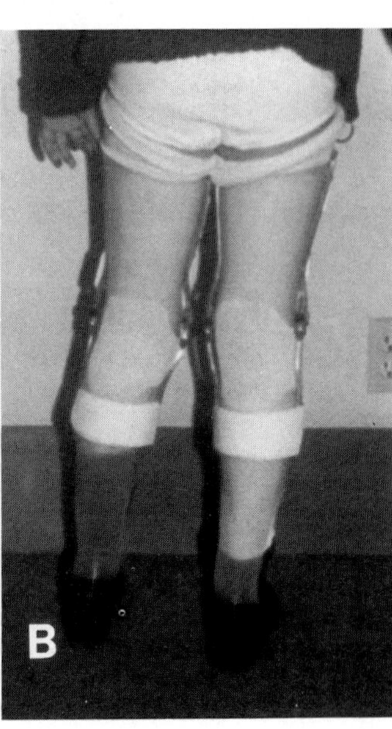

FIG. 23-17. *(A* and *B)* Molded polypropylene KAFO for control of knee instability used in a child with muscular dystrophy.

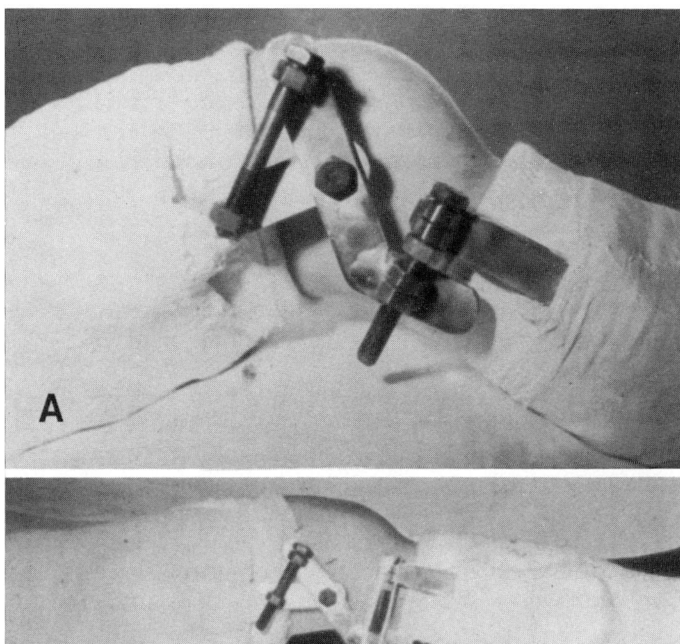

FIG. 23-18. *(A and B)* Extension-desubluxation hinge for correction of knee-flexion contracture associated with posterior subluxation of the tibia in hemophilia.

Maximal protection may be afforded the knee joint by the use of a full-length KAFO of either the single- or double-upright type with a drop-ring knee lock and a free ankle. As an alternative device for complete immobilization of the knee joint, a polypropylene knee cylinder may be used. Whenever the knee joint must be protected by an orthosis for a prolonged period of time, it is essential that the knee be mobilized at least a few hours each day and that a physical therapy program for quadriceps strengthening be instituted on a daily basis to prevent stiffness and atrophy.

The Hip

Orthotic control of hip motion in the swing phase of gait is reasonably effective, but the control of hip motion during stance phase to provide stability of the trunk on the femoral head is relatively ineffective. Stabilization of the trunk on the femur in both the anteroposterior and mediolateral directions can only be achieved by joining a lower limb orthosis to a spinal orthosis with an adequate hip lock. This situation renders the child so completely immobile as to defeat the purpose of orthotic use, which is to provide an ambulatory capacity. Children with extensive lower limb paralysis involving the hip who maintain a free range of hip motion can usually stabilize their hip joints by hyperextension, if knee stability is provided by the appropriate KAFO. Orthotic stabilization of the knees allows the child to shift his center of gravity posteriorly so that the floor reaction line is posterior to the hip joint, permitting stabilization of the hip by tension on the anterior capsule.

Adduction-Abduction Control. In flaccid paralytic states involving the musculature about the hip, a common gait defect is flailing of the lower limbs during swing phase due to inadequate control by the hip abductors and adductors to maintain the limb in the line of progression. An HKAFO consisting of a pelvic band with free hip joints in the sagittal plane attached to either a double- or single-upright KAFO controls unwanted adduction-abduction during the swing phase of gait. Hip rotation during swing phase is also prevented by this device. If some degree of flexion-extension control is also desirable, a hip lock may be used.

In the case of spastic paralysis, excessive adduction or "scissoring" is frequently present during swing phase, which may seriously interfere with the child's ability to walk. If knee instability is also present, the use of a similar HKAFO is indicated for control of excessive hip adduction. If knee stability is adequate, adduction control may be achieved by the use of the Rancho Los Amigos hip-control orthosis (Fig. 23-19).[1] This orthosis is designed to allow free hip flexion, extension and abduction, but it provides an adjustable stop against adduction. The advantage of using this device, even though AFOs are required, is that knee motion is preserved and a more natural gait can be achieved.

Stabilization of the pelvis on the femur during stance phase to prevent downward tilt of the pelvis is very difficult to achieve by orthotic means. Partial control may be obtained with a polypropylene girdle attached to a polypropylene thigh cylinder by a heavy-duty hip joint.

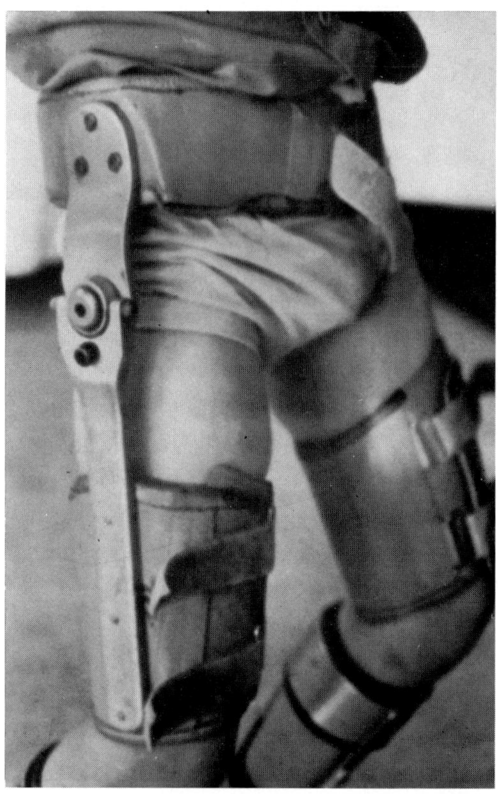

FIG. 23-19. HO for control of hip adduction in cerebral palsy. (From Staros A, LeBlanc M: Orthotic components and system. In American Academy of Orthopaedic Surgeons: Atlas of Orthotics. St Louis, CV Mosby, 1975)

Rotational Control. Control of unwanted rotation of the limbs during swing phase may be accomplished by use of the HKAFO with a pelvic band. If adequate knee stability is present and hip abduction–adduction control is adequate, a twister-cable orthosis from a pelvic band may be attached directly to the shoes or to the lateral uprights of the AFOs. This system selectively controls hip rotation while allowing all other hip motion and knee motion to remain free.

Flexion-Extension Control. Orthotic control of hip flexion and extension is frequently desirable in severe paralysis of the lower limbs, such as that which occurs in poliomyelitis and myelomeningocele, when the patient is unable to lock his hips by hyperextension. As has been noted previously, optimal control of undesired flexion of the hips due to extensor insufficiency during stance phase is difficult to achieve without rendering the patient completely immobile. Some degree of free hip flexion must be available to the child if he is to be able to advance the limbs in an alternating gait. This gait pattern can be achieved if the child has some strength in his hip flexors. Therefore, hip locks, when used to control flexion of the hips, should be modified to allow 10° to 15° of flexion-extension movement in children with available hip-flexion power to permit an alternating gait pattern.

In patients who exhibit excessive forward rotation of the pelvis and increased lumbar lordosis (commonly seen in myelomeningocele), the addition of a buttock sling to a modified pelvic band helps to reduce the tendency to hip flexion and improves the standing position (Fig. 23-20).

For children who have no motor power about the hips and who are unable to stabilize their hips by hyperextension to permit ambulation with KAFOs, complete immobilization of the hips for stability (may be) indicated. This also requires bracing of the trunk and limits ambulation to a swing-to type of gait. Children generally do not develop sufficient balance and coordination to perform this type of gait until they are 4 to 5 years of age. From the age of 1 to 5 years, an orthosis is used principally for standing rather than walking. The orthosis of choice is a standing frame of some type, which may be fitted between 1 and 2 years of age (Fig. 23-21). As the child approaches 3 to 4 years of age, the parapodium may be used for standing as well as for de-

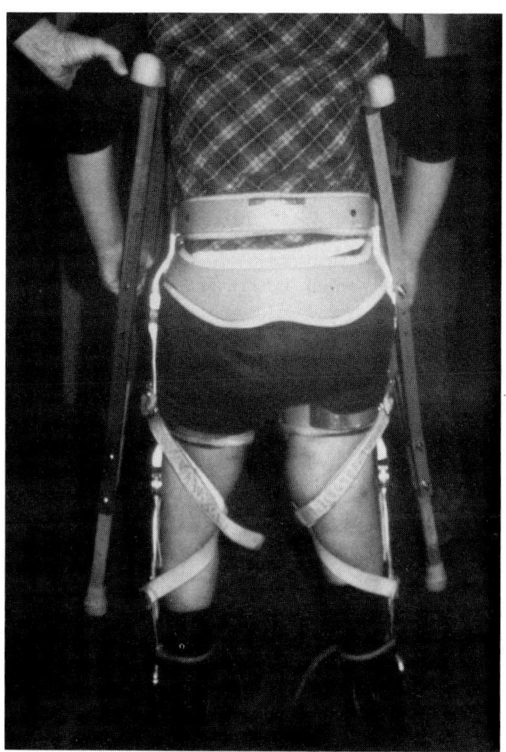

FIG. 23-20. HKAFO of single-lateral-upright design used in a child with myelomeningocele and absent hip extensors.

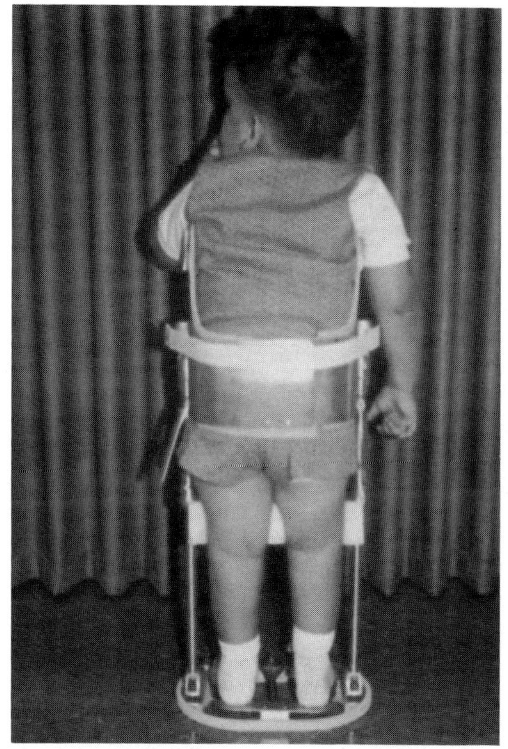

FIG. 23-22. Parapodium used for standing, as well as for a swing-to type of ambulation, in older children with extensive lower limb paralysis.

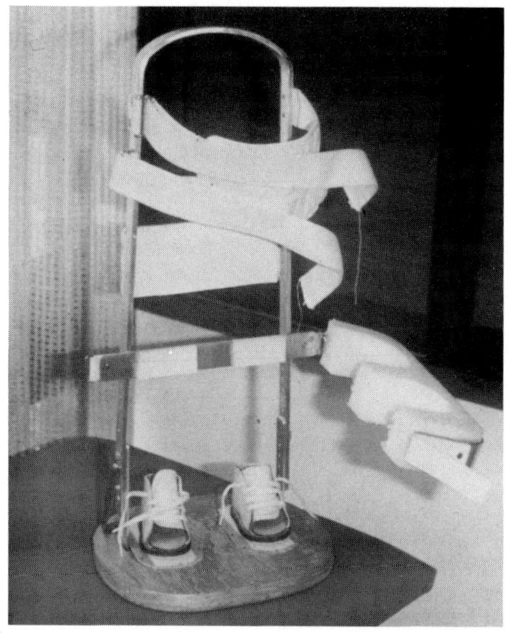

FIG. 23-21. Simple standing frame used for children ages 1 to 3 with extensive lower extremity paralysis.

veloping a swing-to gait (Fig. 23-22). The child learns this gait pattern on the parallel bars and then on crutches and must be taught how to fall and protect himself with his sound upper limbs so that he loses the fear of falling. When the swing-to gait has been mastered in the parapodium, an HKAFO can be prescribed with rigid hip locks and a spinal extension. Although the child may continue to ambulate with the parapodium, this device has the disadvantage of having to be worn over the clothing, which usually becomes objectionable by the age of 7 or 8 years. It should be emphasized that children who have such a severe level of paralysis are primarily wheelchair patients, and ambulation, such as it is, is purely for physiologic and psychologic reasons. Almost all children will discard their orthoses in favor of the wheelchair by the time of early adolescence.

Rose and associates[48] recently described their success with a swivel walker attached to a standing frame that enables children with thoracic level lesions to have limited mobility on smooth surfaces. For older children, they recommend a "hip guidance orthosis," which consists of a bilateral HKAFO with abducted hip joints that move freely in flexion and extension, enabling the child to walk with a four-point gait using crutches and body momentum.

Recent experience with a new version of the cable-driven reciprocating HKAFO has been rewarding in certain children with thoracic level paralysis (Fig. 23-23). Children fitted with this device are able to walk independently with a four-point gait using crutches or a walker but must have good intelligence, adequate motivation, and good coordination of the upper extremities and trunk.[13]

Femoral Anterversion. The entity of increased femoral anteversion, or excessive internal femoral torsion, is of clinical significance because it produces an intoeing gait. The long-term effects on the hip and knee joint are not known. Popular methods of treatment for this condition include various shoe modifications in an attempt to produce an out-toeing gait and orthotic devices for the purpose of producing external rotation of the limb such as the Denis Browne bar and the "twister" torsion orthosis. Although such devices may produce a change in the habit pattern of walking, there is no evidence that they have any effect upon the reduction of femoral torsion. Fabry and associates[15] have shown that little spontaneous reduction of increased femoral anteversion can be expected in children with a toeing-in gait, and, in fact, shoes, bars, and twisters have had no measurable effect upon femoral torsion after 5½ years.

In the case of the twister orthosis and the Denis Browne bar, the external rotation force applied to the foot is dissipated through the subtalar, ankle, and knee joints, and there is probably very little in the way of torque produced upon the femur. Therefore, until recently, it has been our policy either to not treat femoral anteversion by orthotic devices and allow compensatory mechanisms to de-

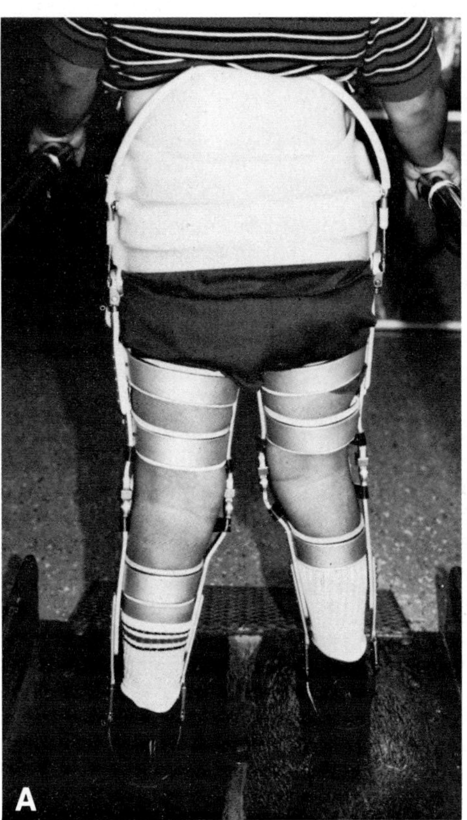

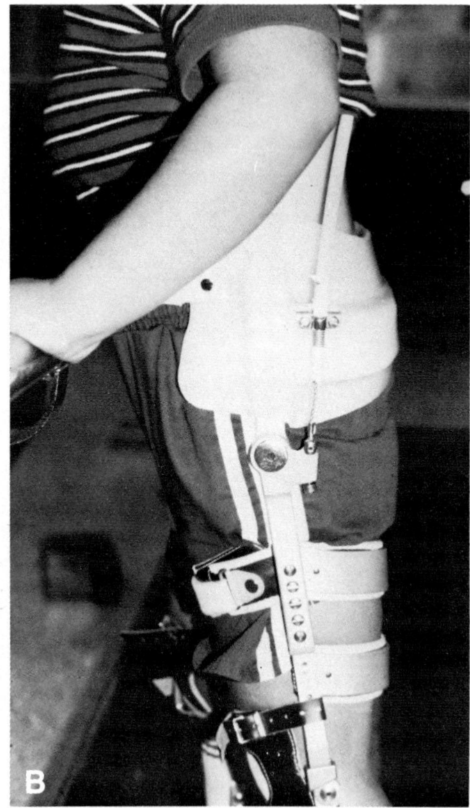

FIG. 23-23. *(A)* Cable-driven reciprocating HKAFO, posterior view. *(B)* Detail of hip joint and cable attachment.

velop, which eventually reduce intoeing, or, in the severe cases, to perform derotational femoral osteotomy.

A device developed at the University of Miami for use as a nighttime orthosis for femoral anteversion has been in use for the past 8 years. The "twister" principle is used, but the torsion force is confined to the femur by design of the orthosis. It consists of a pelvic band and twister cables attached to knee cages of thermoplastic design, which maintain the knees in the position of 20° to 30° of flexion (Fig. 23-24). In order to properly adjust this HKO on initial application, the femora are manually externally rotated until resistance is met, and the twister cables are locked in that position on the knee cages, thus preventing any further internal rotation. The orthosis is readjusted into further external rotation on a monthly basis, always locking the orthosis when resistance is met. Thus, a small amount of external torsional force is applied to the femur and across the femoral epiphyseal plates. After 6 to 12 months of night wear, a measurable increase in external rotation of the hips and a corresponding decrease in internal rotation will be noted, coinciding with reduction of the intoeing gait. This orthosis has been used in children up to 6 years of age with satisfactory results in about half the patients so treated.

Legg-Calvé-Perthes Disease. There is almost universal agreement that a basic principle in the orthotic management of Legg-Calvé-Perthes disease is concentric containment of the femoral head within the acetabulum.[7,11,22,27,44,51,56] There is less agreement about whether or not femoral head containment with weightbearing or without weightbearing is preferred.[29] In order to achieve equal distribution of pressures upon the head, the orthotic device used must position the hip in abduction and some degree of internal rotation. The old ischial weightbearing ring caliper with patten shoe has been condemned not only because it is ineffective but also because it is probably injurious to the femoral head due to its failure to position the hip in abduction and internal rotation.[10]

The earliest abduction ambulatory device used for treatment of Legg-Calvé-Perthes disease was the "broomstick plaster" described by Petrie.[44] Bilateral long-leg walking casts were connected by two broomsticks to fix the hips in 45° of abduction and 5° to 10° of internal rotation. The child ambulated with the use of crutches, and new plasters were applied every 3 to 4 months. The "Toronto orthosis" described by Bobechko and associates[7] obviates the need for casts and cast changes; it positions the hips in a similar degree of abduction and internal rotation (Fig. 23-25). Because the knees are permitted to flex in this device, the effects of prolonged joint immobility are eliminated, and it is possible to sit comfortably. A similar bilateral hip–abduction orthosis developed by Curtis and associates[11] at Newington Children's Hospital has been reported as giving 68% of patients with Perthes disease good results, with an average of 20 months' usage. It should be emphasized that all the devices mentioned above provide excellent positioning of the hips in abduction and internal rotation, with full weightbearing permitted. The disadvantages of this method of treatment are that both lower extremities must be braced and

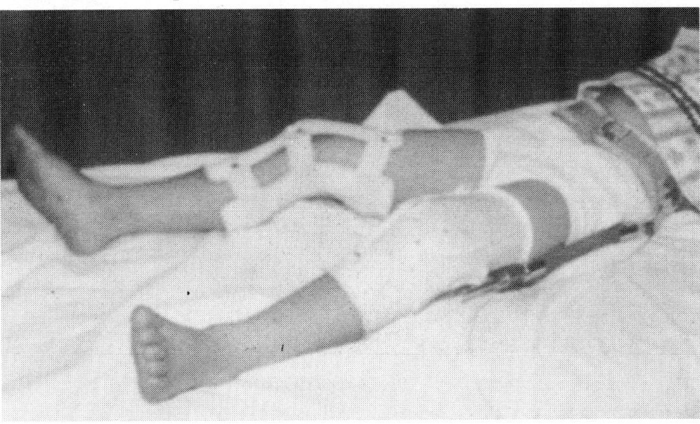

FIG. 23-24. HKO twister orthosis used as a night splint for control of internal femoral torsion.

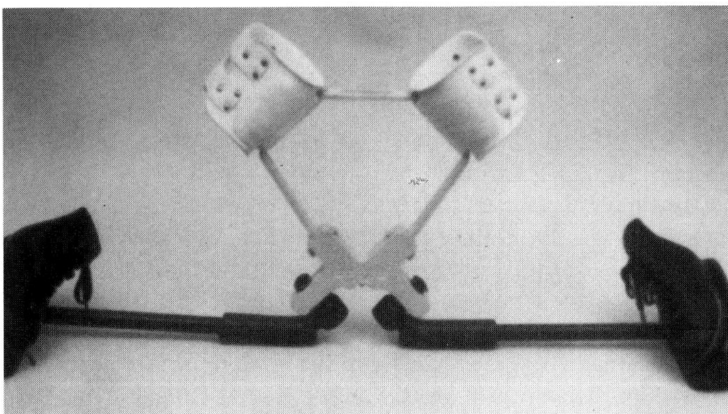

FIG. 23-25. Toronto-design KAFO for use in providing hip abduction and internal rotation in Legg-Calvé-Perthes disease. (From Staros A, LeBlanc M: Orthotic components and systems. In American Academy of Orthopaedic Surgeons: Atlas of Orthotics. St Louis, CV Mosby, 1975

crutches must be used to assist ambulation, which is awkward at best. In addition, unless adequate medial support is provided at the knees, genu valgum can be a complication due to forces upon the epiphyseal plates of the distal femur and proximal tibia.

Nonweightbearing hip-abduction internal rotation orthoses have been described by Harrison and associates.[22] Both of these devices position the femoral head within the acetabulum and maintain the knee on the affected side in about 90° of flexion. The opposite limb remains free, and a three-point gait is used with crutches. Due to the fact that the affected hip is positioned by fixing the relationship between the femur and the trunk, the hip is effectively immobilized. Although the forces of weightbearing on the hip are eliminated, the loss of hip motion is not conducive to the physiologic requirements of the joint, and this may be a theoretical disadvantage to this type of orthosis.

The trilateral-socket hip-abduction orthosis described by Tachdjian and Jouett[56] is an attempt to combine a reduction in weightbearing on the femoral head with adequate positioning of the head for acetabular containment. This is achieved in unilateral cases with a unilateral KAFO consisting of a trilateral socket of plastic laminate and a medial upright extending to a foot plate that suspends the limb from contact with the floor (Fig. 23-26). An elevated shoe is used on the sound side. Abduction is maintained by the shape of the socket and the ischial shelf, which is formed so as to be horizontal with the floor when the limb is in 30° of abduction. The advantages of this orthosis are that weightbearing on the femoral head is reduced while it is maintained in a position of containment,

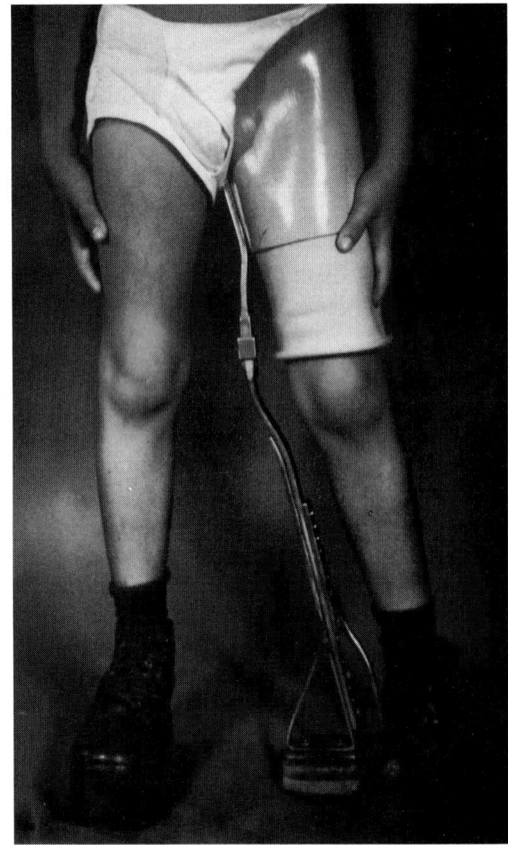

FIG. 23-26. Trilateral-socket hip-abduction orthosis for use in Legg-Calvé-Perthes disease. (From Staros A, LeBlanc M: Orthotic components and systems. In American Academy of Orthopaedic Surgeons: Atlas of Orthotics. St Louis, CV Mosby, 1975

the sound leg is not confined by the orthosis, and crutches are not required, allowing freedom of upper limb activity. The disadvantage of the device is that it does not provide as much abduction as the other devices mentioned, and, unless it is carefully constructed and maintained, it may not provide consistent femoral head containment.

The Scottish Rite Hospital orthosis for Legg-Calvé-Perthes disease has been described by Purvis, Dimon, Meehan, and Lovell.[46] This device, although maintaining sufficient abduction for femoral head containment, does not provide for internal rotation of the hip. However, the brace encourages a flexed posture at the hips during ambulation, which substitutes for internal rotation as a means of covering the anterior portion of the femoral head by the acetabulum (Fig. 23-27). Preliminary results with this device are encouraging.

In selecting the proper orthosis for the treatment of Legg-Calvé-Perthes disease, the physician must consider the relative importance of the amount of weightbearing on the femoral head, the degree of motion permitted at the hip, the degree of femoral head containment, the degree of freedom of activity permitted, and the psychologic impact of the device on the child. It is the orthopaedic surgeon's assessment of the relative importance of these parameters, combined with his assessment of the individual patient, that dictates the orthotic prescription. Whatever device is selected, adequate containment of the femoral head within the acetabulum is an essential prerequisite to optimal treatment. Periodic roentgenograms of the hip with the child standing in his orthosis should be obtained to assess the femoral head coverage.

The necessity for providing femoral head containment in younger patients and in patients with partial head involvement has been questioned in a long-term study by Kelly and colleagues.[28] At an average follow-up of 22.4 years in patients treated by use of a non-weightbearing sling that did not provide femoral head containment, they found that 91% of patients so treated had good or fair results.

Congenital Dislocation of the Hip. Orthotic devices have a prominent place in the early treatment of congenital dislocations of the hip. Many types of devices have been described, but all are designed to position the hip in flexion, abduction, and external rotation. Varying degrees of freedom of motion of the hip are permitted; even the static-type splints provide only relative immobilization of the hip joint.

There are two primary indications for the use of the hip orthosis in the management of congenital dislocation of the hip. The first and most common indication is for the treatment

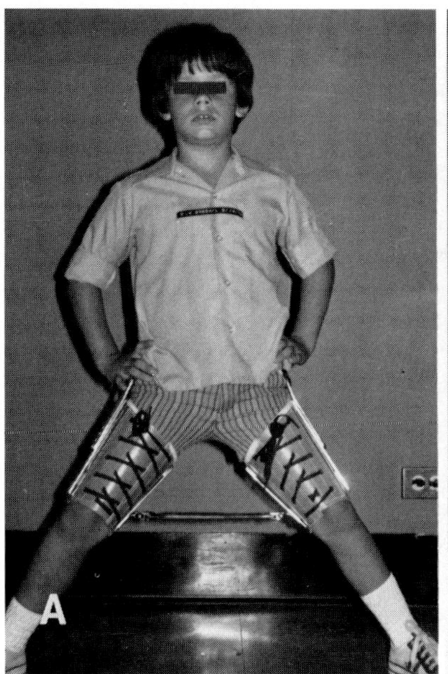

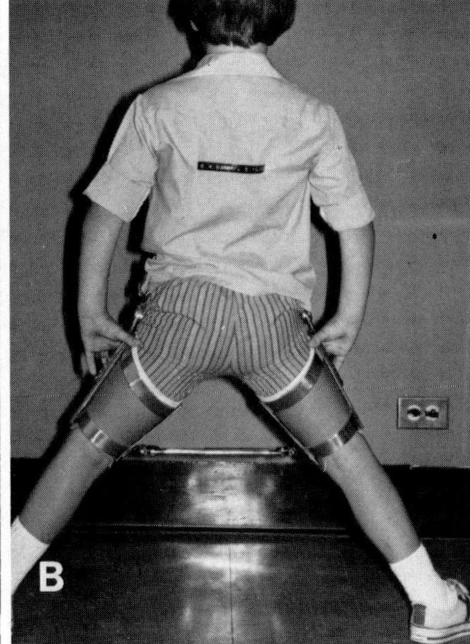

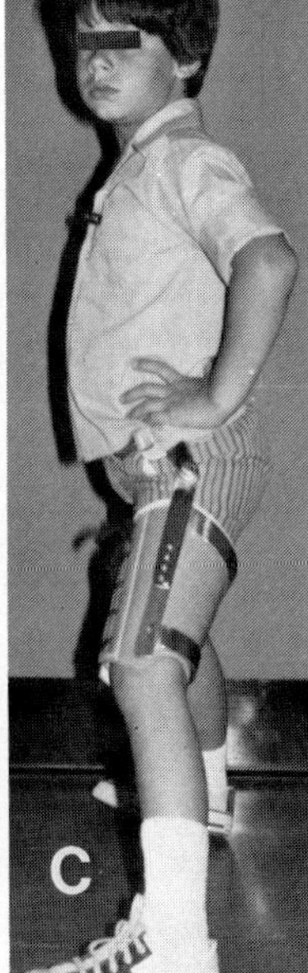

FIG. 23-27. The Scottish Rite Hospital orthosis for Legg-Calvé-Perthes disease.

of hip dysplasia in the newborn period. Prompt recognition of the disorder, followed by adequate positioning of the affected hip or hips by a splint of suitable design, usually results in a normal hip by 8 to 12 weeks of age.[6,57] The second indication is to reduce the period of cast immobilization following closed reduction of the dislocation in the older infant or child. Because the period of plaster immobilization may be 6 to 8 months in the child whose dislocation was recognized and treated at 6 months of age, the use of a suitable orthosis, in lieu of plaster, after the first 2 or 3 months of immobilization is thought to be highly desirable.[23]

The simplest splint for management of congenital dysplasia of the hip in the newborn is the pillow splint originally described by Frejka.[18] Commercially available, it is a waterproof pillow designed to be secured between the legs over the diapers so as to prevent adduction, extension, and internal rotation of the hips. Because it must be removed at each diaper change, it is recommended only for dysplastic and for subluxed hips, not for the treatment of truly dislocated hips in the newborn. A more modern version of the Frejka pillow is the Craig abduction splint, which is made of padded semirigid plastic, also worn over the diapers, necessitating removal with diaper change.[8]

A second class of orthotic devices developed for management of congenital dislocation of the hip in the infant is represented by the splints described by Von Rosen[57] and Barlow.[5] Both of these devices are made of thin, malleable aluminum strips that are covered by rubber or leather. They are designed so that the bulk of the splint cradles the child's back, and the terminal portions of the aluminum splints contour about the infant's thighs and shoulders, holding the hips in 90° of flexion, abduction, and external rotation. The degree of abduction as well as flexion can be adjusted by manual bending of the aluminum strips. Both of these splints, by their design, permit some motion of the hip joints but prevent an undesirable degree of extension, adduction, and internal rotation. Also, they have the advantage that the splint need not be removed when the diapers are changed; bathing the infant is even possible while the device is in place. Thus, they may be used effectively for dislocated hips, which when placed in the position of flexion, abduction, and external rotation are stable.

A third class of devices permits more active motion of the hips but confines the hip motion to a range that will not permit subluxation or dislocation of the hips. The device described by Ilfeld[23] consists of two metallic thigh cuffs with washable covers attached to an adjustable bar by universal joints. The design permits change of diapers without device removal, sitting, standing, and walking with adequate positional control of the hips. It has been used in children from 1½ to 30 months of age and for dislocation as well as for dysplasia. Ilfeld also reports good results with use after casting for 6 to 8 weeks following reduction of dislocations in the older infant, thus markedly reducing the time of plaster immobilization.

Currently, the most popular dynamic type of splint used for congenital hip dysplasia is the Pavlik harness.[25,26] This device restricts but does not severely inhibit motion of the hips while retaining adequate position. It may be used for the dislocated hip up to 6 months of age as well as for hip dysplasia. The incidence of complications using this device has been extremely low, but avascular necrosis of the femoral head has been reported as a complication of this treatment in a few instances.[16,40] Mubarak and associates[40] recently outlined the pitfalls in the use of this device, which include continued treatment of a dislocated hip with failure to obtain reduction, poor compliance of the patient, and poor quality and construction of the harness (Fig. 23-28).

The use of abduction bars between the feet is not recommended for treatment of congenital dislocation of the hip, because unless the degree of abduction is extremely wide, as described by Ponseti,[45] the child will be able to flex and adduct the hips to an undesirable degree. Such devices also tend to keep the hips in extension most of the time, which is not the optimal position for centralization of the femoral head within the acetabulum in infants.

With the exception of the Ilfeld splint, orthotic treatment of congenital dysplasia or dislocation of the hip may not be sufficiently effective beyond the age of 18 months to merit its use. Surgical approaches to centralization of the hip in patients older than 18 months are generally recommended.

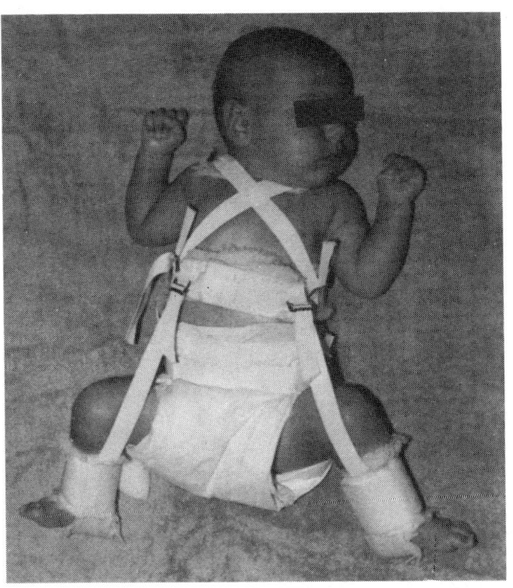

FIG. 23-28. Pavlik harness for control of hip extension and adduction in congenital dislocation of the hip.

UPPER LIMB ORTHOTICS

As in the lower limb, the application of orthotic devices in the upper limb may be used to prevent deformity, to correct deformity, or to improve function.

Prevention of deformity or protection of joint segments is usually accomplished by the use of static splinting devices designed of metal or thermoplastic material. Joint positioning prevents contracture, and, in some instances it may, in and of itself, improve function to a degree, such as positioning of the thumb in opposition. The greatest use of static splints is in the prevention of deformities following peripheral nerve injury and in temporary spastic states, as well as in the prevention of deformity due to juvenile rheumatoid arthritis.

Correction of deformity may be accomplished by adjustable static splints or by dynamic devices using elastic or spring force of mild but constant degree. Recent joint contractures associated with paralysis, arthritis, or hemarthrosis may be effectively corrected by such measures, but old or well-established contractures generally require surgical correction.

The task of restoring function by orthotic means to the defective upper limb has historically been fraught with difficulty. The problem of mechanically reduplicating the highly refined system of joints, levers, and motors present in the normal upper limb is enormous when compared with that of the lower limb. Added to this dilemma is the seemingly impossible task of providing an adequate sensory feedback system to allow coordination of motor skills to a degree necessary to restore upper limb function. Augmentation or restoration of motor power in the upper limb by orthotic means is gross at best, and when combined with a severe sensory deficit, it may be of little practical use to the patient. Substitution of motor activity may be accomplished by mechanical, electrical, or pneumatic devices subject to these limiting factors.

A major consideration in the use of upper limb orthoses in children is the degree of acceptance or tolerance of the device by the patient. If the orthosis is to be successful, it must be worn. Any orthosis that significantly impairs function rather than assisting it or any orthosis that gets in the way when performing certain activities will be doomed to failure. Children have very little "gadget tolerance" and reject a device if it is too encumbering or restrictive. Therefore, every effort should be made to keep the orthotic design simple, lightweight, and of a design that interferes as little as possible with remaining normal motor and sensory functions.

Upper limb orthoses are also designated by the joint levels that they encompass, that is, hand orthosis (HO), wrist-hand orthosis (WHO), and elbow orthosis (EO).

The Hand and Wrist

Prevention of Deformity. Orthoses designed to prevent deformity are most commonly used about the hand and wrist following musculoskeletal trauma, peripheral nerve injury, and burns and in rheumatoid arthritis. Usually they may be removed for several hours a day to permit therapy, bathing, and some freedom of activity. They are also considered relatively temporary devices, seldom having to be worn for more than a few months.

Basic positioning splints for the hand and wrist to maintain a functional position may be made of thermoplastic material, using either a dorsal or volar forearm section (Fig. 23-29). These splints are intended primarily for night use and limited daytime use, because they are

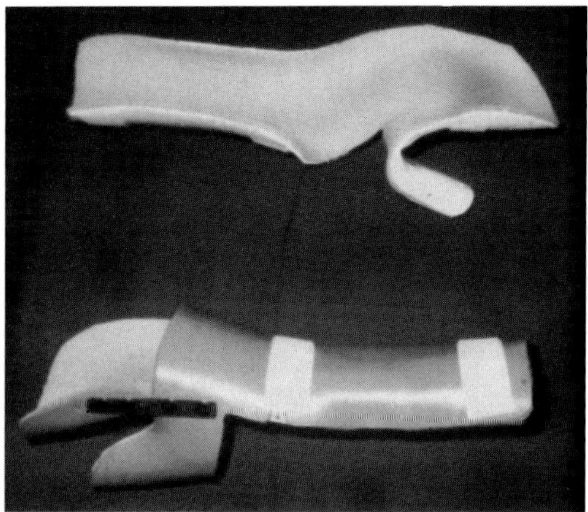

FIG. 23-29. Dorsal and volar WHO's for splinting of the wrist and hand.

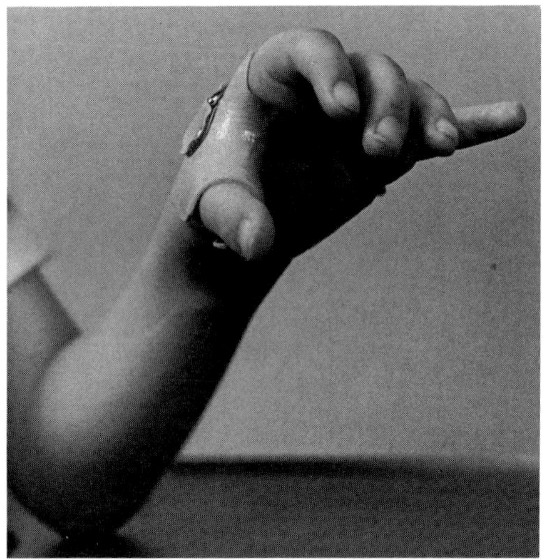

FIG. 23-30. Short opponens orthosis used for positioning the thumb in the functional position of opposition for grasp. (Courtesy of Thorkild Engen, C. O., Houston, Texas)

relatively encumbering. They are commonly indicated in juvenile rheumatoid arthritis.

Loss of thumb opposition and abduction requires the use of a short opponens splint, which maintains the thumb in a position of opposition and prevents contracture of the web space (Fig. 23-30). This splint also enhances function in cases of thenar paralysis, because it provides positioning for pinch activities. If wrist stabilization is also required, the long opponens splint, which also provides splinting and immobilization of the wrist, may be used (Fig. 23-31). In combined median and ulnar nerve loss with total loss of the intrinsic musculature, a dorsal bar over the proximal phalanges may be attached to maintain flexion of the metacarpophalangeal joints and to prevent an intrinsic minus contracture (extension contracture of the metacarpophalangeal joints). Associated flexion contractures of the interphalangeal joints may be prevented by the addition of an outrigger to this system to support rubberband slings for finger extension.

Loss of extensor power secondary to radial nerve palsy may be managed by use of the long opponens splint with a dorsal outrigger to provide rubberband sling extension assist to the metacarpophalangeal joints. The addition of a thumb-extension assist to the opposition post maintains the thumb in adequate position for a pinch type of grasp.

Detailed descriptions of these devices may be found in the recent Atlas of Orthotics published by the American Academy of Orthopaedic Surgeons.[1]

Correction of Deformity. Correction of mild deformities of the hand and wrist is possible by the use of orthotic devices, provided that the contractures are of relatively recent origin. A family of dynamic splints designed by the late Sterling Bunnel are available commercially as off- the-shelf items.* Included are extension and flexion assists for the interphalangeal joints and for the metacarpophalangeal joints. Dynamic extension assists for the metacarpophalangeal joints may also be provided by the use of rubberband slings for the fingers from an outrigger, which is based on a dorsal or long opponens wrist splint. Dynamic flexion assists for the metacarpophalangeal joints may be provided in a similar manner from an outrigger attachment based on a volar wrist splint. (Fig. 23-32). In the case of extension contractures of the metacarpophalangeal joints and flexion contractures of the interphalangeal joints associated with burns of the hand, this system may be modified by attaching the rubberbands to small metallic hooks that are glued to the fingernails. In this manner, direct contact of the slings with the burned fingers is avoided.

Flexion deformities of the wrist may best be corrected by serial casting into extension

*H. Weniger, Inc., 70 12th Street, San Francisco, California

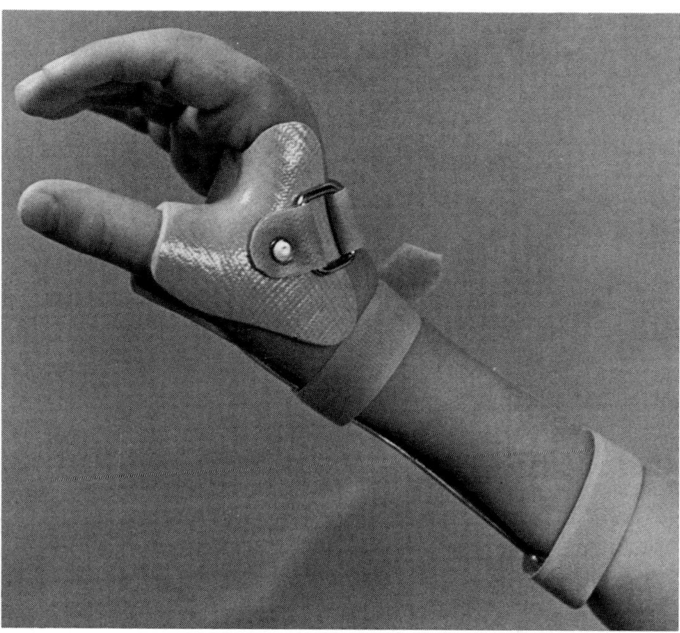

FIG. 23-31. Long opponens orthosis (WHO) for wrist stabilization as well as thumb opposition. (Courtesy of Thorkild Engen, C. O., Houston, Texas)

or by the use of a remoldable thermoplastic volar splint, which is periodically removed and heated, gradually bringing the wrist up into further extension.

Restoration of Function. Restoration of function about the hand and wrist may be accomplished by the use of simple positioning orthoses, by mechanical harnessing of wrist extensor power to provide two-digit flexion to a fixed thumb, or by the use of external power to drive a prehension-type orthosis. Regardless of the method used, the function provided by such devices is that of relatively gross prehension and release. There is at present no orthotic device that can provide the function of manipulation within the grasp.

Loss of wrist stability due to lack of extensor power or due to intrinsic joint disease will result in a weak and inefficient grasp. Wrist stabilization orthoses are indicated in this situation, and they considerably improve the strength of grip. The orthosis should be based dorsally on the wrist and forearm, and the palmar support section should be narrow so as to interfere minimally with the closing capacity of the hand and palmar sensation. The most effective wrist position for maximum strength of grasp is 35° of dorsiflexion. However, most day-to-day activities involving prehension are performed with the wrist in the neutral position.[30] Therefore, for optimal functional restoration, the wrist-hand orthosis should stabilize the wrist in the neutral or slightly dorsiflexed position.

Loss of thumb opposition, such as that seen in median nerve injuries and polio, is a severe functional handicap. Positioning of the thumb in opposition by means of an appropriate orthosis can restore fine prehension to a degree by allowing the mobile index and long fingers to approximate the fixed thumb. If wrist stability and extensor power are present, a short opponens splint in indicated (see Fig. 23-29).

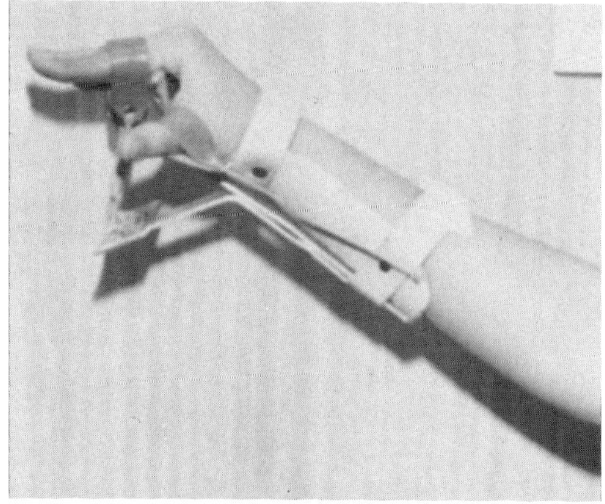

FIG. 23-32. Dynamic metacarpophalangeal joint flexion assist.

If the wrist is unstable or if wrist extensor power is inadequate, a long opponens splint should be used (see Fig. 23-30). Opponens splints may be made of aluminum,[3] plaster laminate,[14] or thermoplastic material. In the case of the younger child, custom-fabricated splints of thermoplastic material are generally required.

Loss of function of the thumb and the fingers, typified by the quadriplegia patient, is an even more severe disability, because grasp of any type is lacking. In those patients who retain wrist extension (for example, the C6 quadriplegic), gradual contracture of the finger flexors may provide return of gross grasp by a tenodesis effect. Finer prehension of a pinch type may be achieved by the use of the wrist-driven flexor-hinge orthosis or the "tenodesis splint."[3,14] This device uses a mechanical linkage to convert the excursion of wrist extension to flexion of the index and long fingers against the thumb, which is fixed in the position of opposition (Fig. 23-33). Thus, a "three-jawed chuck" type of prehension is produced by extension of the wrist, and release is accomplished by passive wrist flexion. It should be emphasized that although this type of prehension is useful for some activities, it is not useful for all, and the gross, natural tenodesis type of grasp is preferred much of the time. Wearing the orthosis also inhibits such activities as dressing and wheeling a wheelchair. Younger children tend to reject this orthosis due to these factors; older children use it for selected activities requiring a pinch type of prehension.

Combined loss of function of the thumb, fingers, and wrist, as exemplified by the C5 quadriplegic, requires the use of external power to restore the ability to grasp. In this situation, the basic wrist-driven flexor-hinge orthosis is used, but an external power source is used to activate the wrist extension mechanism of the orthosis (Fig. 23-34). The power source may be either electrical or pneumatic. In the case of electronically driven orthoses, a worm-gear mechanism is used, and, in the case of the pneumatically driven orthosis, the carbon dioxide artificial muscle is used.[3,14] Effective use of prehension-type orthoses requires sufficient proximal control of the limb segments to permit positioning of the hand in space, so that high-level quadriplegics who are devoid of shoulder and elbow movement are unable to benefit from this type of device. This device has application primarily in the older child who has sufficient coordination and skill developed in the proximal musculature and sufficient concentration and learning ability to be able to use the orthosis.

The Elbow and Shoulder

Prevention of Deformity. The majority of day-to-day activities are performed with the elbow flexed by 10° to 20° on either side of the 90° position. Therefore, splinting of the elbow is usually done with the elbow flexed

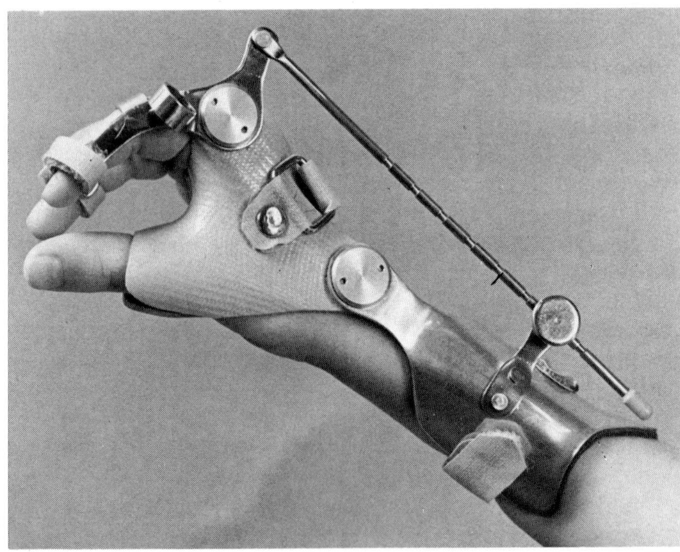

FIG. 23-33. The wrist-driven flexor-hinge orthosis converts the excursion of active wrist extension to finger flexion against the fixed thumb in opposition. The primary indication for this orthosis is in a child with a C6 quadriplegia. (Courtesy of Thorkild Engen, C. O., Houston, Texas)

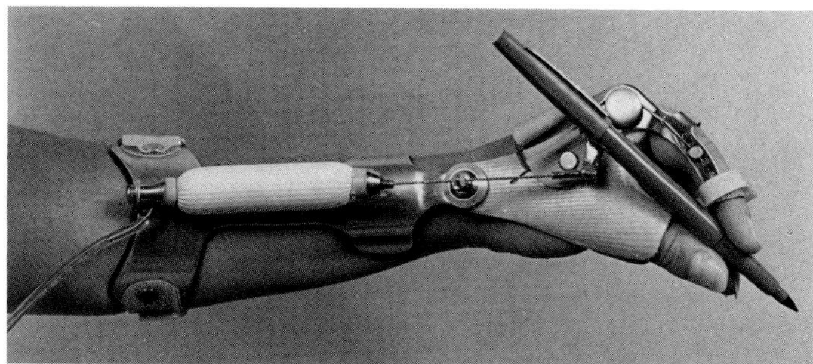

FIG. 23-34. Wrist-driven flexor-hinge orthosis using external power by means of a carbon dioxide artificial muscle. This device is indicated in quadriplegia when active wrist extension is absent but sufficient proximal arm control is present, as in the C5 quadriplegic. (Courtesy of Thorkild Engen, C. O., Houston, Texas)

at 90°. Various types of thermoplastic materials may be used to fabricate temporary elbow splints. A posterior splint is generally used, but anterior splints are useful in preventing flexion contracture in the burned child. Following injury of any type, the elbow joint tends to become stiff rapidly, so that whenever splinting of the elbow is used for immobilization alone, it is of the utmost importance that it be removed periodically for therapy and range-of-motion exercises.

Static splinting of the shoulder in abduction and external rotation may be accomplished by the "airplane splint." Such a position is commonly desirable in the management of children with burns involving the axilla to prevent the development of adduction and internal rotation contracture. The orthosis may be fabricated of aluminum covered by leather, or it may be made of thermoplastic material. In either case, the orthosis must derive its support from the iliac crest on the same side. Failure to base the device on the iliac crest results in instability and discomfort.

Correction of Deformity. Regaining lost elbow motion as a result of contracture is difficult and requires a combination of physical therapy and orthotic management. In contractures of long standing, surgical release of the contracture is usually indicated.

The simplest type of orthotic device used is the thermoplastic splint, which may be reheated and reformed to maintain the maximum correction obtained by physical therapy. The three-point extension orthosis may be used to gradually stretch the elbow into extension by progressive tightening of the elbow pad. The pivoted arm and forearm cuffs rotate to accommodate to the changing elbow position.

Hinged elbow orthoses may also be used in effecting reduction of either flexion or extension contractures. A turnbuckle may provide the corrective force, or dial-lock joints may be preferred. Dynamic hinged elbow orthoses have also been used to achieve elbow flexion, with rubber tubing or elastic straps providing the dynamic force.

Whenever an elbow orthosis is used for the purpose of correcting deformity, the correction should occur gradually over a long period of time, so that only minimal force is used and there is no discomfort produced by wearing the orthosis. A physical therapy program consisting of gentle passive and active assisted range of motion should be used concurrently.

Restoration of Function. Paralysis of elbow flexion may be substituted for by a dynamic elbow-flexion assist orthosis with arm and forearm cuffs connected by a single axis joint and elastic straps positioned anterior to the axis of the elbow joint.[32] The triceps is used to provide elbow extension against the dynamic flexion force.

When there is severe weakness of musculature about the shoulders and elbows but some residual strength remains in the poor-muscle-grade range, the mobile arm support is a most useful device.[2,32] This orthotic device is used primarily for wheelchair-confined patients with proximal upper limb weakness, as is seen frequently in polio, muscular dystrophy, and related disorders. It provides a support system for the upper limb, which counteracts and balances the forces of gravity, allowing the weakened muscles to function more efficiently by gravity assistance. The system is attached to the child's wheelchair, and it consists of a forearm trough that is balanced at an appropriate pivotal point on freely movable linkage rods. The pivotal point of attachment on the forearm trough is crucial to optimal function. With the system ideally balanced, weak external rotators and adductors of the shoulder produce elbow flexion and

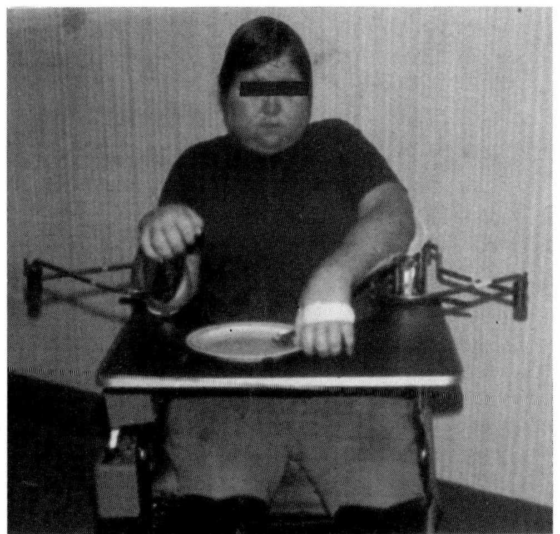

Fig. 23-35. Mobile arm supports as used in a child with severe Guillain-Barré syndrome.

some supination, and weak internal rotators of the shoulder are capable of providing elbow extension, pronation, and a downward type of reach (Fig. 23-35).

For the severely paralyzed shoulder and elbow, such as is seen in brachial plexus palsy or in poliomyelitis, restoration of function by orthotic means is essentially impossible. Elaborate orthotic devices such as the ratchet-type functional-arm orthosis[3] and the electric arm orthosis[41] have been described, but the amount of gadgetry required to accomplish relatively simple motion control is immense. Such orthoses are not well tolerated by children and are seldom tolerated even by adults, because the functional gains are minimal compared with the inconvenience of wearing the device.

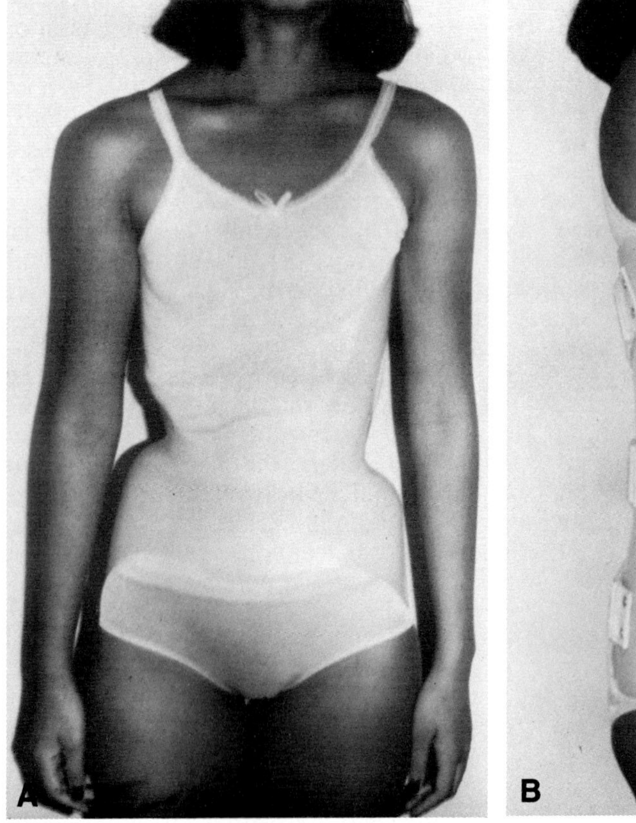

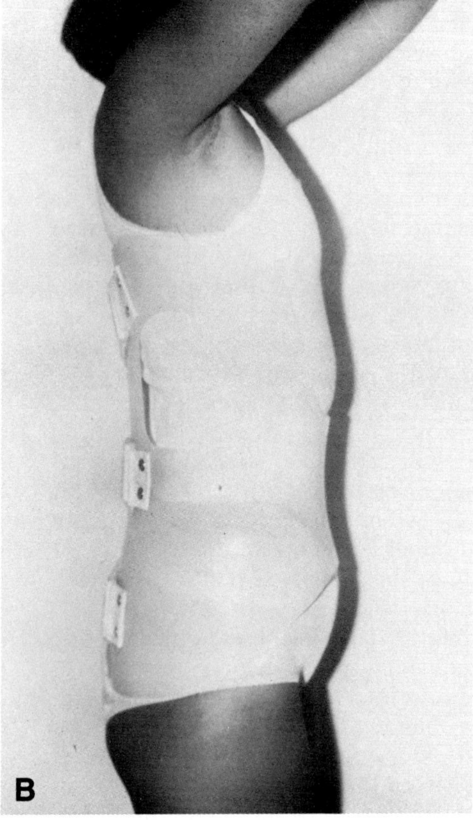

Fig. 23-36. *(A)* Anterior view of a molded polypropylene TLSO for control of idiopathic thoracolumbar scoliosis. *(B)* Side view of a polypropelene TLSO with a built-in corrective lumbar pad.

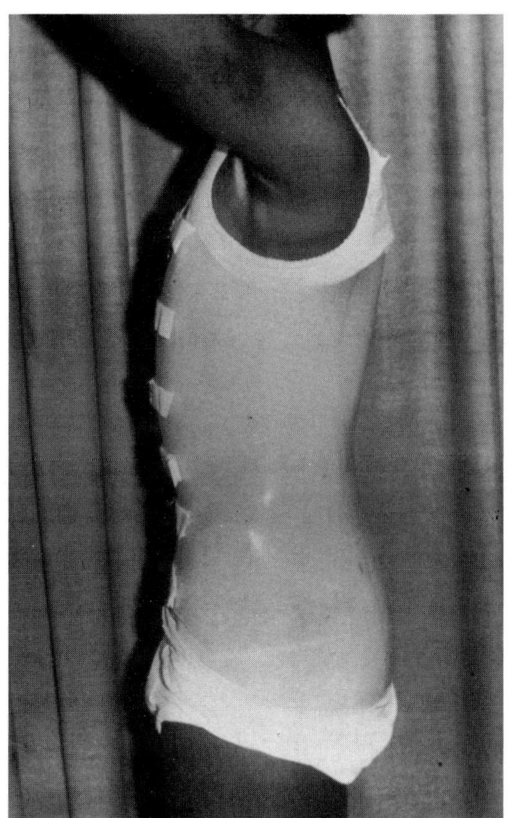

FIG. 23-37. Postoperative scoliosis jacket of polypropylene made from a positive plaster model.

THE SPINE

As in the extremities, orthoses for the spine are used to prevent and correct deformity. They may also be used to improve or restore function by stabilizing a collapsing paralytic spine, which, in turn, aids sitting balance and frees the arms from having to support the trunk.

Spinal orthoses in use for chldren today are vastly improved over those used years ago, due to the emergence of new materials and technology. Thermoplastics such as polypropylene, polyethylene, vitarathene, and Orthoplast are being used in the fabrication of the Milwaukee brace, LSO flexion jackets, and TLSO scoliosis jackets (Fig. 23-36). Postoperative scoliosis jackets made of thermoplastic material reduce the length of time in body casts, and, due to the intimate and total contact type of fit achieved, they provide excellent immobilization (Fig. 23-37).

In this text, the details of spinal orthotics in children can be found in Chapter 16.

REFERENCES

1. American Academy of Orthopaedic Surgeons. Atlas of Orthotics: Biomechanical principle and application, 2nd ed. St Louis, CV Mosby, 1985
2. Anderson MH: Functional Bracing of the Upper Extremities. Springfield, IL, Charles C Thomas, 1958
3. Anderson MH: Upper Extremity Orthotics. Springfield, IL, Charles C Thomas, 1965
4. Anderson MH, Bray JJ: Biomechanical considerations in the design of a functional long-leg brace. Biomed Sci Instrum 1:385, 1963 (Reprinted Orthot Prosthet Appl J 18:273, 1964)
5. Barlow TG: Early diagnosis and treatment of congenital dislocation of the hip. J Bone Surg 44B:292, 1962
6. Barlow TG: Congenital dislocation of the hip: Early diagnosis and treatment. Lond Clin Med J 5:47, 1964
7. Bobechko WP, McLaurin CA, Motlock WM: Toronto orthosis for Legg-Perthes disease. Artif Limbs 12:36, 1968
8. Coleman SS: Treatment of congenital dislocation of the hip in the infant. J Bone Joint Surg 47A:590, 1965
9. Committee on Prosthetics Research and Development: A Clinical Evaluation of Four Lower Limb Orthoses (Report E-5). Washington, DC, National Academy of Sciences, 1972
10. Committee on Prosthetics Research and Development: Report of a Workshop on the Child with an Orthopaedic Disability: His Orthotic Needs, and How to Meet Them. Washington, DC, National Academy of Sciences, 1973
11. Curtis BH, Gunther ST, Gossling HR, Paul SW: Treatment for Legg-Perthes disease with the Newington ambulation-abduction brace. J Bone Joint Surg 56A:1135, 1974
12. Dixon MA, Palumbo RL: Polypropylene knee orthosis with latex suprapatellar strap suspension. Orthot Prosthet 29:29, 1985
13. Douglas R, Larson PF, D'Ambrosia R, McCall RE: The LSU reciprocation-gait orthosis. Orthopaedics 6:834, 1983
14. Engen TJ: Development of upper extremity orthotics. I and II. Orthot Prosthet (March and June) 1970
15. Fabry G, MacEwen D, Shands AR Jr: Torsion of the femur. J Bone Joint Surg 55A:1726, 1973
16. Filipe G, Carlioz H: Use of the Pavlik harness in treating congenital dislocation of the hip. J Pediatr Orthop 2:357, 1982
17. Fillauer C: A new ankle-foot orthosis with a moldable carbon composite insert. Orthot Prosthet 35:13, 1981
18. Frejka MB: Treatment of congenital dislocation of the hip. Unpublished paper presented at the Annual Meeting of the American Academy of Orthopaedic Surgeons, Chicago, 1947
19. Glancy J, Lindseth RE: The polypropylene solid ankle orthosis. Orthot Prosthet 26:14, 1972
20. Hall JE, Miller WE, Schumann W, Stanish W: A refined concept in the orthotic management of scoliosis: A preliminary report. Orthot Prosthet 29(4):7, 1975
21. Harris EE: A new orthotic terminology. Orthot Prosthet 27:6, 1973

22. Harrison MHM, Turner MH, Nicholson TJ: Coxa plana—Results of a splinting. J Bone Joint Surg 51A:1057, 1969
23. Ilfeld FW: The management of congenital dislocation and dysplasia of the hip by means of the special splint. J Bone Joint Surg 39A:99, 1957
24. Inman VT: UC-BL dual axis control system and UC-BL shoe insert. Bull Prosthet Res 10:11, 1969
25. Johnson AH, Aadalen RJ, Eilers VE, Winter RB: Treatment of congenital hip dislocation and dysplasia with the Pavlik harness. Clin Orthop 155:25, 1981
26. Kalamachi A, MacFarlane R: The Pavlik harness: Results in patients over 3 months of age. J Pediatr Orthop 2:3, 1982
27. Karadinas JE: Conservaitve treatment of coxa plana: A comparison of the early results of different methods. J Bone Joint Surg 53A:315, 1971
28. Kelly FB Jr, Canale ST, Jones RR: Legg-Calvé-Perthes disease. Long-term evaluation of noncontainment treatment. J Bone Joint Surg 62:400, 1980
29. Kins EW, Fisher RL, Gage JR, Gossling HR: Ambulation-abduction treatment in Legg-Calvé-Perthes disease. Clin Orthop 150:43, 1980
30. Klopsteg PE, Wilson PD: Human limbs and their substitutes. New York, Hafner, 1968
31. Lehneis HR: New developments in lower limb orthotics through bioengineering. Arch Phys Med Rehab 53(7):303, 1972
32. Long C: Upper Limb Bracing in Orthotics Etc. Baltimore, Waverly Press, 1966
33. Lovell WW: Personal communication, 1978
34. McCollough NC III: Comprehensive management of musculoskeletal disorders in hemophilia. Committee on Prosthetics Research and Devlopment, Washington, DC, National Academy of Sciences, 1973
35. McCollough NC III: Current status of lower limb orthotics. Orthop Digest 3:17, 1975
36. McCollough NCIII: Experimental production of tibial torsion and its clinical relevance. Orthop Trans 4:60, 1980
37. McCollough NC III: Rationale for orthotic prescription in the lower extremity. Clin Orthop 102:32, 1974
38. McCollough NC III, Fryer CM, Glancy J: A new approach to patient analysis for orthotic prescription. Artif Limbs 14:68, 1970
39. McIlmurray WJ, Greenbaum W: A below-knee weightbearing brace. Orthop Prosthet Appl J 12(2):81, 1958
40. Mubarak S, Garfin S, Vance R, McKinnon B, Sutherland D: Pitfalls in the use of the Pavlik harness for treatment of congenital dysplasia, subluxation, and dislocation of the hip. J Bone Joint Surg 63A:1239, 1981
41. Nickel VL, Allen JR, Karshak A Jr: Control systems for externally powered orthotic devices, final project report. Rancho Los Amigos Hospital, Downey, California, May 1, 1960 to July 31, 1970, Professional Staff Association
42. Nitschke RO: A single-bar above-knee orthosis. Orthot Prosthet 25:4, 1971
43. Penneau K, Lutter LD, Winter RD: Pes planus: Radiographic changes with foot orthoses and shoes. Foot-Ankle 2:299, 1982
44. Petrie JG, Bitenc I: The abduction weightbearing treatment in Legg-Perthes disease. J Bone Joint Surg 53B:54, 1971
45. Ponseti I: Causes of failure in the treatment of congenital dislocation of the hip. J Bone Joint Surg 26:775, 1944
46. Purvis JM, Dimon JH III, Meehan PL, Lovell WW: Preliminary experience with the Scottish Rite Hospital abduction orthosis for Legg-Perthes disease. Clin Orthop 150:49, 1980
47. Rose GK, Sankarankutty M, Stallard J: A clinical review of the orthotic treatment of myelomeningocele patients. J Bone Joint Surg (Br) 65:242, 1983
48. Rose GK, Stallard J, Sankarankutty M: Clinical evaluation of spina bifida patients using hip guidance orthosis. Dev Med Child Neurol 23:30, 1981
49. Rubin G, Dixon M: The modern ankle foot orthoses (AFO's). Bull Prosthet Res 10 (19):20, 1973
50. Salter RB: Textbook of Disorders and Injuries of the Musculoskeletal System. Baltimore, Williams & Wilkins, 1970
51. Sanders JA: A long-term follow-up on coxa plana at the Alfred I. Dupont Institute. South Med J 62:1042, 1969
52. Sarmiento A: A functional below-the-knee brace for tibial fractures. J Bone Joint Surg 52A:295, 1970
53. Schultz M, McCollough NC III: Polypropylene in spinal orthotics. Orthot Prosthet 28(3):43, 1974
54. Smith CF: Long-term management and rehabilitation in hemophilia. Project Report. Los Angeles, Orthopaedic Hospital, 1969
55. Smith EM, Juvinall RC: Theory of feeder mechanics. Am J Phys Med 42:3, 1963
56. Tachdjian MO, Jouett LO: Trilateral socket hip abduction orthosis for the treatment of Legg-Perthes disease. Orthot Prosthet 22(2):49, 1968
57. Von Rosen S: Diagnosis and treatment of congenital dislocation of the hip joint in the new born. J Bone Joint Surg 44B:284, 1962

24

Assessment of Gait in Children and Adolescents

Chester M. Tylkowski

Most diseases affecting the neuromusculoskeletal system of children and adolescents will have an impact on walking ability. The orthopaedist must assess this ability, as well as joint mobility, muscle status, neurologic status, and roentgenographic information, during a clinical examination. The functional assessment, however, is often a simple walk across a room or a question directed to the patient or parent concerning walking performance. Classification of the observed walk into various limps may be the only attempt at gait classification. The ability to recognize the antalgic gait, gluteus medius limp, or spastic gait may be the extent of the functional assessment. Subjective assessment of walking ability by patient or parent is not easily translated into objective terms to allow the documentation of a gait pattern.

From observation with a stopwatch to the most sophisticated, computerized motion analysis laboratory, a range of technologies is available to describe and document an observed gait pattern. Whatever the method may be, a disciplined, structured approach with well-defined terminology is essential if a meaningful interpretation is to be achieved.

The study of gait may be divided into several discrete areas, including kinematics, kinetics, dynamic electromyography (EMG), and energy utilization. Each may be addressed independently, but, when integrated, they result in a comprehensive description and explanation of human motion. Each area will be defined and reviewed in the next few sections, with an attempt to enable a better understanding of human walking. This will be followed by a discussion of the maturation of gait, the interpretation of normal gait patterns, and a discussion of the methods of gait assessment. The information should offer a more critical method of describing and analyzing gait abnormalities.

KINEMATICS

Kinematics is the study of motion, which in gait analysis refers to body segment displacements and their relation to time. It is essential to first understand the kinematics of normal mature gait before discussing the maturation of gait or its pathologic deviations. Structuring the walk into definable terms facilitates the understanding of gait and the subsequent description and interpretation of complex patterns.

EVENTS IN THE GAIT CYCLE

The walking cycle is first described in terms of foot placement (Fig. 24-1). The cycle begins with right foot strike, followed by left toe-off, left foot strike, right toe-off, and ends with right foot strike. These five events in the gait cycle define stance and swing phase. Stance

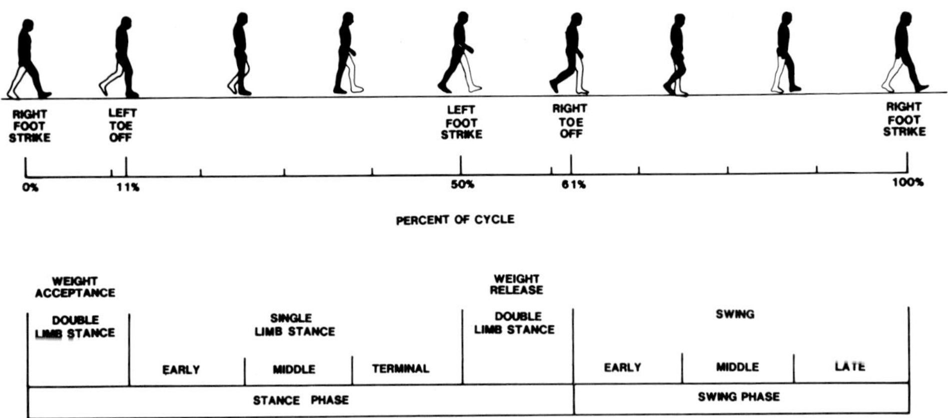

FIG. 24-1. Definition of phases and events of the gait cycle and their approximate percent time of occurrence.

phase is the period of time when one or two feet are on the ground. Swing phase is the portion of the gait cycle when a limb is being advanced forward without ground contact.

Stance phase may be divided into single limb stance and two periods of double limb stance. The first episode of double limb stance occurs when the swinging limb contacts the floor. Weight is transferred to this limb and defines the weight acceptance period of gait. As the opposite foot leaves the ground, the stance phase limb becomes the sole support of the body and is considered to be in single limb stance. With opposite foot strike, body weight is transferred from the first to the opposite limb, which defines the weight release period of gait.

Swing phase may be conveniently divided into early, middle, and late periods of swing. It is also useful to divide single limb stance into early, middle, and terminal single limb stance. It can be seen that by applying these definitions to the gait cycle, a framework is produced into which detailed descriptions of body segment motion, muscle activity, and other data may be inserted. Instead of describing an entire gait pattern in a phrase, a description of the events occurring in each portion of the gait cycle defines the particular pattern. Understanding of the pattern is facilitated by a segment-by-segment understanding of the action occurring. In the sections that follow, this concept will be developed and the convenience of dividing the gait cycle should become apparent.

Measuring the duration of a gait cycle allows the calculation of the time required for each phase of gait. Because a full cycle may not occupy exactly the same amount of time when repeated, when walking at different speeds or in pathologic situations, a special technique must be used to allow direct comparisons of gait cycles. The cycle is normalized by setting its total length of time to 100% and calculating each event and phase as a percentage of the total gait cycle (see Fig. 24-1). During normal relaxed walking, reasonable average values for each parameter are as follows: weight acceptance, 11%; single limb stance, 39%; weight release, 11%; and swing phase, 39% of the gait cycle.[10,31,32,34] These parameters have been shown to be remarkably constant when a natural pace (free speed) is assumed and correlates with the lowest energy consumption of any gait velocity. In terms of the events of the cycle, right foot strike begins at 0%, left toe-off occurs at 11%, left heel strike occurs at 50%, right toe-off occurs at 61%, with the cycle terminating at right foot strike, or 100% of the cycle. This framework serves as a convenient nomenclature for the graphic representation of joint or body segment motion during a gait cycle. Figure 24-2 is a motion graph in which the X-axis represents the percent normalized cycle time and the Y-axis represents motion of the hip joint.

Several meaningful parameters may be calculated from the timed and measured parameters of a gait cycle. These include velocity, cadence, step length, stride length, and step width. Single limb stance, double limb stance, and swing, previously described, are other

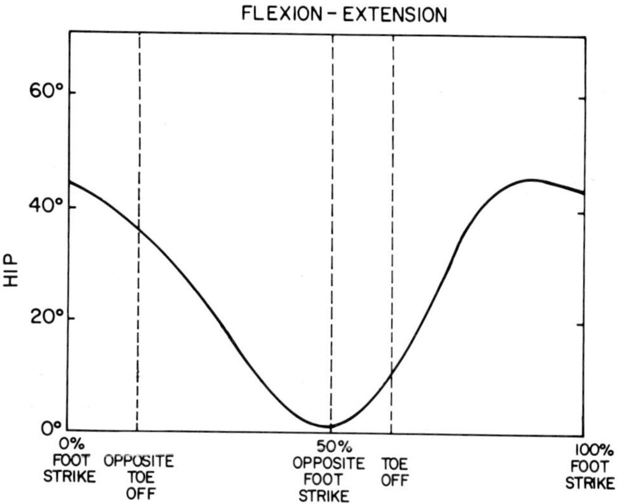

FIG. 24-2. Example of a motion graph of hip flexion-extension showing the change in degrees during each percent of the gait cycle.

parameters calculated from the time and distance parameters of the gait cycle. Velocity is the distance traversed by the person per unit of time. Step length is the distance between the feet in double limb stance. Stride length is the right plus the left step lengths within a single cycle. Cadence is the number of steps per unit of time. Step width is the distance between the feet in the frontal plane during a gait cycle. The normal values for these parameters are listed in Table 24-1. These values will change, however, with variations in velocity.[2,9,21,33]

BODY SEGMENT MOTION

Because body segment, or joint motion, is described within each of the three perpendicular planes dividing the body, a clear understanding of the coronal (frontal), sagittal, and transverse planes is essential (Fig. 24-3). Standard terms are applied to the joint range

Table 24-1. Average values for adult normal gait parameters*

Velocity	1.5 ± .2
Cadence	116 ± 10
Step length	0.78 ± 0.065
Stride length	1.56 ± 0.13
Step width	0.08 ± .01

*Velocities in meters per second, cadence in steps per minute, step lengths and stride lengths in meters.

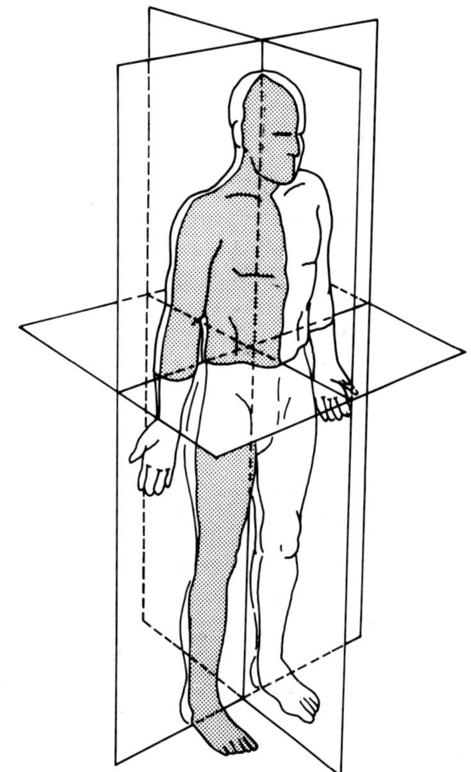

FIG. 24-3. Definition of the coronal, sagittal, and transverse planes of the body.

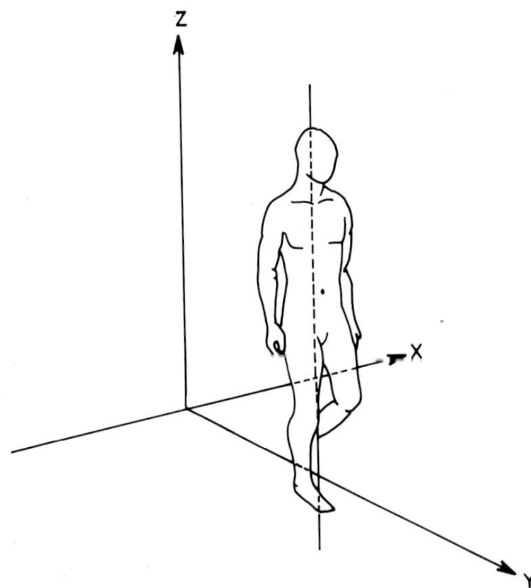

FIG. 24-4. X, Y, and Z axes of the laboratory, serving as a point of reference for body segment positions and motions.

of motion, that is flexion, extension, abduction, and so on.[17]

Depending on the methods used for data acquisition, various joint dynamic ranges of motion and/or body segment motions may be displayed. Gait laboratories using photographic or video techniques have the ability to display body segment as well as joint motions in all planes. Those relying on electrogoniometers may record only specific joint motions. The motions of the shoulder girdle, spine, pelvis, femur, tibia, and foot have been categorized and used to calculate joint motions.

The graphic display of segment motion uses certain conventions that define the positive or negative direction of segment motions. These are based on X, Y and Z axes embedded in the space in which the person walks (Fig. 24-4).[47,55,60] The positive Y-axis is in the direction of walking, the positive Z-axis is directed upward, and the positive X-axis is directed from right to left in the frontal plane. The direction assignments of these axes may vary among researchers and should be carefully noted to avoid confusion when interpreting the resultant data. Whether a positive direction on a motion graph denotes flexion or extension is dependent upon the axis direction assignment. The direction of the vector, the consequences of rotation about it as an axis, and the representation of that motion on a plot as positive or negative is related to the "right hand rule." If one visualized the thumb of the right hand pointing in the direction of the vector, the direction that the fingers point as they wrap around the line defines the positive direction of rotation. Pelvic obliquity is a motion defined as rotation of the pelvis in the coronal plane, about the forward directed Y-axis; with application of the "right hand rule," a positive plot on the graph is noted when the left side of the pelvis is elevated (Fig. 24-5). Most often, the plots will be labeled with the

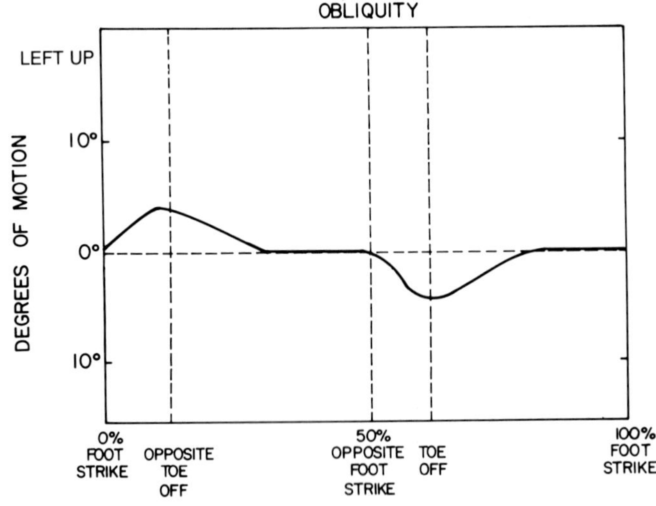

FIG. 24-5. Motion of the pelvis in the coronal plane defined as degrees of obliquity and plotted against the percent of the gait cycle.

particular joint motion simplifying interpretation.

SPECIFIC JOINT MOTIONS

Based on the above descriptions of the methods of data organization, kinematics will be explained by reference to standard motion graphs. Several investigators have contributed to the development of a normal motion database.[31,32,57] The following discussion will focus on data generated during normal, relaxed (free speed) walking. The velocity of relaxed walking has been determined to be remarkably consistent among individuals and reflects a person's attempt to use the least energy.[30,67,68] Variations in the motion patterns seen with changes in velocity will not be considered in this discussion but may be explored in the appropriate literature.[2,9,21,33]

Pelvic Motion. The motion of the pelvic segment of the body may be described in the three body planes as pelvic tilt, pelvic obliquity, and pelvic rotation. Pelvic tilt (Fig. 24-6) is recorded in the sagittal plane. The pelvis is tilted anteriorly during gait about 20° from the horizontal. During free speed-walking, the range of motion is about 3° to 4°. Minimal anterior tilt (maximal posterior tilt) occurs at about the time of toe-off, whereas maximal anterior tilt (minimal posterior tilt) occurs just prior to heel strike.

Pelvic obliquity (Fig. 24-5) is measured in the coronal plane. As right weight acceptance begins, the left side of the pelvis becomes higher than the right, reaching a maximum at left toe-off, then dropping to neutral by about 25% of the cycle. A neutral pelvic obliquity is maintained until left heel strike, at which time the right side of the pelvis begins to elevate (negative on the graph because of the Y-axis defined previously). Right pelvic elevation reaches a maximum at right toe-off and is once again level at neutral and remains so through left single limb stance. It is important to note that if our graph had started at left heel strike, the first deflection in the curve would have been down.

Pelvic rotation (Fig. 24-7) is measured in the transverse plane. The conventions of the adopted X, Y, and Z axes are once again important in the recognition of the side of the pelvis forward or behind while interpreting the motion graph. In this situation, a positive value on the graph indicates that the right side of the pelvis is forward. The motion graph indicates that the right side of the pelvis is maximally ahead just after left toe-off and the left is maximally ahead at right toe-off.

Hip Motion. Hip flexion and extension are defined by the vector sum of the pelvis and the femur positions in the sagittal plane (Fig. 24-8). The recognition that two segments contribute to joint motion is important, because more anterior tilt of the pelvis may increase flexion of the hip joint, as can greater upward rotation of the femur. A child with myelodysplasia with no hip extensor power may

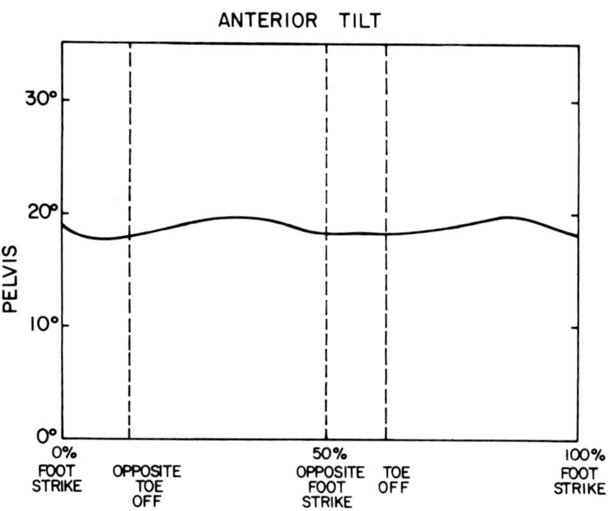

FIG. 24-6. Motion of the pelvis as viewed in the sagittal plane defined as degrees of anterior tilt.

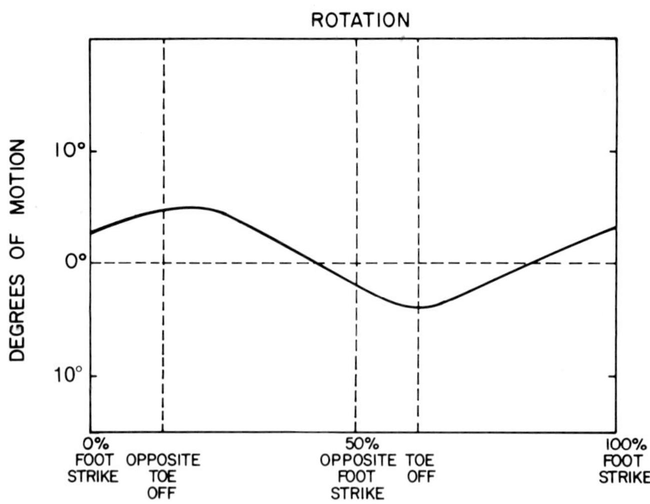

FIG. 24-7. Rotation of the pelvis in the transverse plane, plotted against percent of the gait cycle.

present with a marked lumbar lordosis compensatory to maximal anterior pelvic tilt. The anterior tilt of the pelvis on the femur increases hip flexion and contributes to the development of fixed hip contracture. In the normal cycle, hip flexion is about 40° at foot strike, diminishing to almost full extension at opposite heel strike (50% of the cycle), and reaching maximal flexion just prior to heel strike.

Abduction-adduction motion of the hip is determined by the vector sum of the pelvic and thigh motions in the coronal plane (Fig. 24-9). During right weight acceptance, adduction starts at about 7° and increases to approximately 12°. During right single limb stance, the adduction gradually decreases to about 5° at the initiation of right weight release. Neutral adduction-abduction of the right limb is attained at the beginning of right swing phase, and adduction once again increases during swing to about 5°.[58]

Rotation of the hip is defined by the vector sum of the rotation of the pelvis and the femur in the transverse plane (Fig. 24-10). The hip is in a slight amount of internal rotation during weight acceptance, exhibits about 5° of exter-

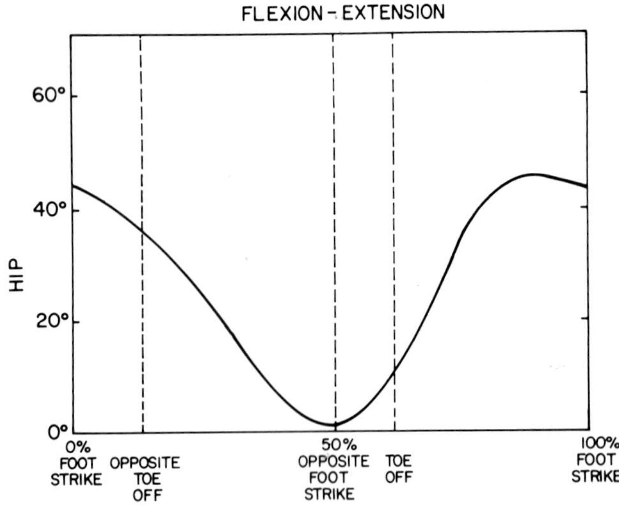

FIG. 24-8. The flexion-extension of the hip joint in the sagittal plane during one gait cycle.

FIG. 24-9. The abduction-adduction motion of the hip as defined by the vector sum of the pelvic and femur motions in the coronal plane during one gait cycle.

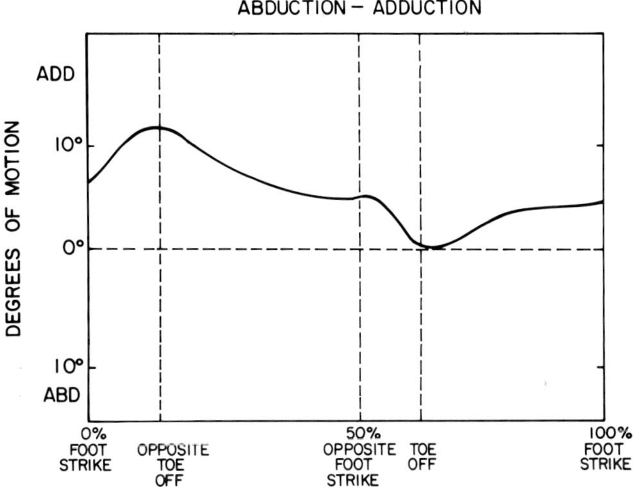

nal rotation during single limb stance, and attains neutral rotation during weight release. During the first half of swing, internal rotation is noted, followed by a slight amount of external rotation, and finally internal rotation at the completion of swing.

Femur and Tibia Motion. The motion of the femur in the sagittal plane describes hip flexion when discussed with the pelvic segment. When discussed with the tibia, it defines knee flexion and extension. In the coronal plane, motion of the pelvis and femur describe hip abduction-adduction. Comparison of femoral and tibial translation in the coronal plane can be used to define knee varus-valgus motion, not commonly reported. The above statements can be made more clear in relation to the motion plots by applying the "right hand rule." Hip flexion would be positive on the graph because the vector directed along the pelvis in the coronal plane from left to right, when grasped with the thumb in the direction of the vector, shows the fingers pointing in the direction of flexion, which is positive.

The motion of the femur and pelvis in the transverse plane is used to define hip rotation.

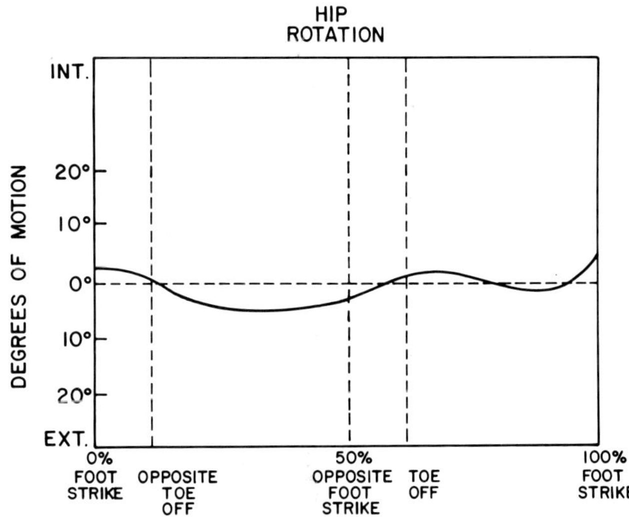

FIG. 24-10. Rotation of the hip as defined by the vector sum of the pelvis and femur in the transverse plane through one gait cycle.

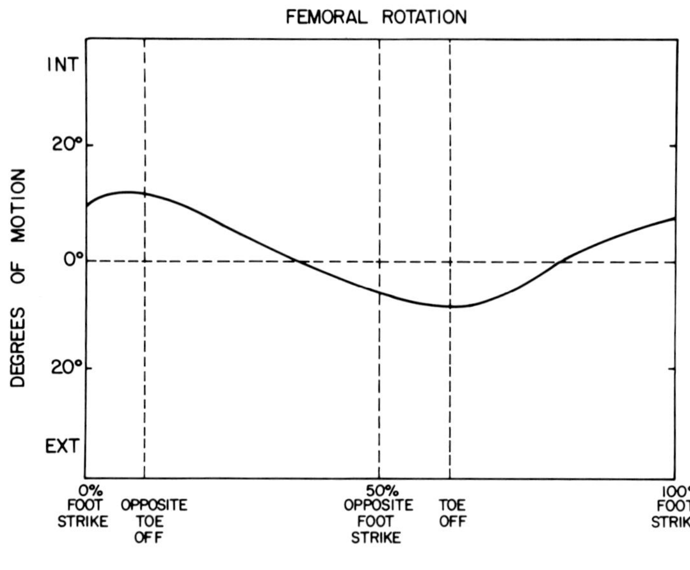

FIG. 24-11. Rotation of femur segment in the transverse plane through one gait cycle.

Knee rotation is the motion of the femoral and tibial segments in the transverse plane.[57] Rotation of the femur in the transverse plane (Fig. 24-11) reaches maximal internal rotation at the end of weight acceptance and maximal external rotation during early swing. The Z-axis of the femur directed from distal to proximal along the shaft, with application of the "right hand rule," explains the positive direction of the graph for internal femoral rotation. The motion graph of tibial rotation, less commonly reported, is shown in Figure 24-12.[57]

The pattern of knee flexion-extension in the sagittal plane is shown in Figure 24-13. At heel strike, the knee is at about 10° of flexion. This increases to about 15° during weight acceptance, extends toward zero during single limb stance, and begins to flex prior to and during weight release. Rapid and maximal knee flexion is noted in early swing, diminishing during the remainder of the swing phase. A knee flexion contracture of 40° would show maintenance of the value through all of weight acceptance, single limb stance, and weight

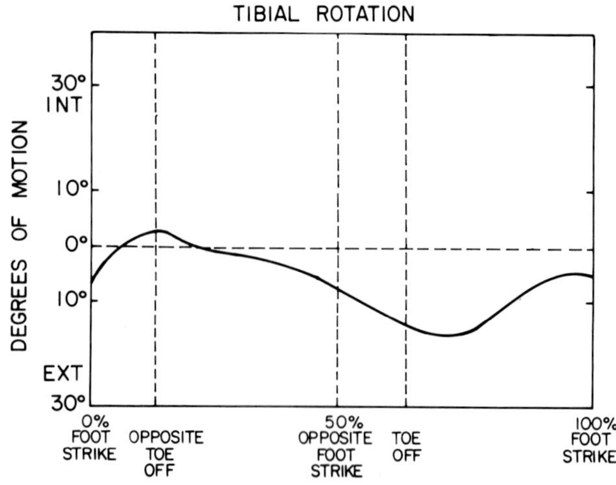

FIG. 24-12. Rotation of the tibia in the transverse plane through one gait cycle as reported by Sutherland.

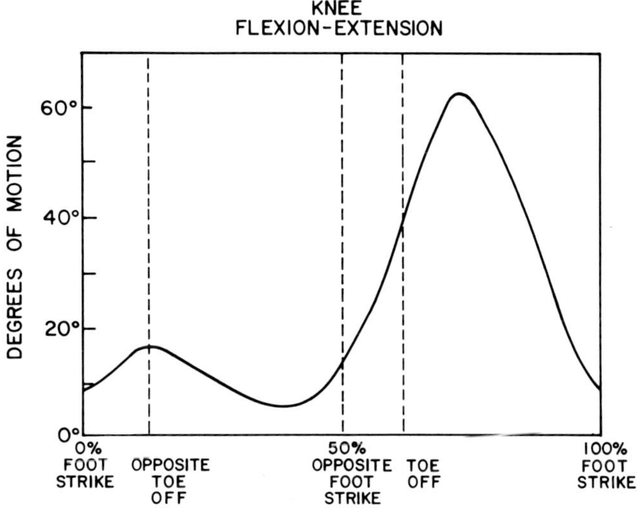

Fig. 24-13. The pattern of knee flexion-extension in the sagittal plane through one gait cycle.

release, with an increase in flexion occurring only during swing phase.

Ankle Motion. Ankle plantarflexion-dorsiflexion is measured in the sagittal plane (Fig. 24-14). The ankle is at about 5° of plantarflexion at heel strike, reaches a maximum of 10° during weight acceptance, and, at the beginning of single limb stance, is near neutral. Dorsiflexion is seen during single limb stance. The ankle returns to neutral at the beginning of weight release, showing maximal plantarflexion at the beginning of swing phase. There is rapid dorsiflexion to neutral during swing.

Shoulder And Trunk Motion. The shoulder girdle rotates in the transverse plane in a manner similar to the first thoracic vertebra.[15] This rotation, when compared with the pelvic motion (Fig. 24-15), is seen to be opposite in direction in each phase of the gait cycle.[21] This reciprocal transverse rotation is carried through the vertebrae such that maximal rotation occurs at the sixth or seventh thoracic verte-

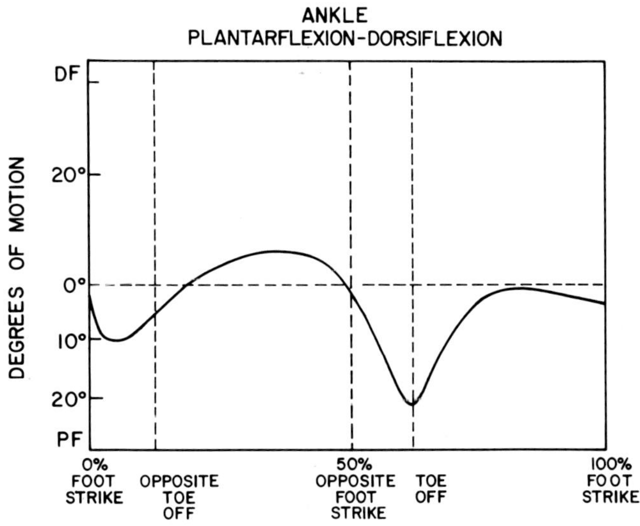

Fig. 24-14. Ankle plantarflexion-dorsiflexion measured in the sagittal plane during one gait cycle.

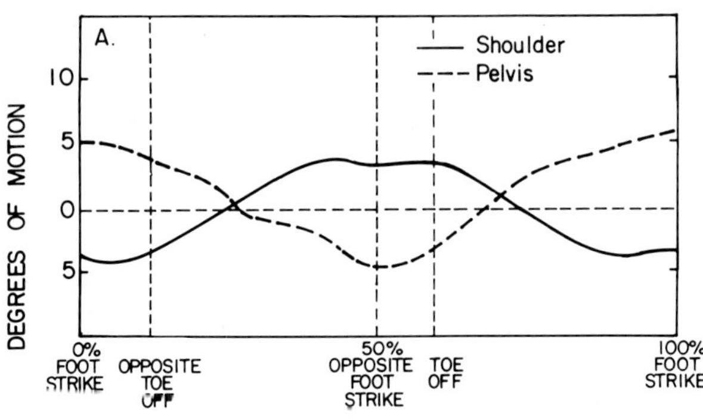

FIG. 24-15. The rotation of the shoulder contrasted to the rotation of the pelvis in the transverse plane, showing the reciprocal nature of the motions.

bra.[15] This correlates well with the observation of reciprocal upper and lower extremity swing. Thurston[59] has analyzed the motion of the lumbar spine in relation to the pelvis and has found it to be reciprocal in the coronal, transverse, and sagittal planes. He did not observe the sagittal and coronal plane motions. The trunk and the pelvis do undergo lateral and vertical displacements throughout the gait cycle. The description of these motions, although not referenced to motion differences between pelvis and spine, is important for an understanding of the mechanism of energy conservation in walking. The attempt by the body to minimize this motion and thus expend less energy in advancing the body has been described by Saunders and associates.[46]

MUSCLE ACTIVITY

During normal, relaxed walking, the major function of the skeletal muscles is to accelerate, decelerate, and stabilize the body segments in motion. This activity is accomplished not only by contraction with shortening of the muscle but also by elongation occurring during contraction. A muscle that is active while elongating is undergoing eccentric contraction and is exemplified by the action of the gastrocnemius-soleus musculature during single limb stance to control the forward progression of the tibia.[48,56] Concentric contraction of a muscle occurs with shortening and is exemplified by the action of the anterior tibial muscle to dorsiflex the foot during the swing phase of gait.

Muscles are mainly active to control the forward momentum of the body segments. In this sense, we do not use our muscles to initiate each segment movement, but rather to counteract the inertial loading on the segment or to resist the effects of gravity. The firing of the hamstring musculature at the termination of swing is used to control and decelerate the forward swinging limb in preparation for foot contact. The firing of the quadriceps musculature at heel strike and during weight acceptance is to resist the flexion moment present about the flexed knee and thereby to prevent further flexion and collapse.

EMG is the monitoring of the electrical activity of muscles. Fine wire electrodes may be inserted percutaneously to precisely monitor each muscle's activity. In some studies, it is crucial to monitor each muscle's contribution to the observed motion.[35,40,43] In studying the muscle activity during walking in children, however, it is often difficult to use needle electrodes and obtain meaningful results.[58] This is related to the discomfort of multiple electrode insertions required to effectively monitor a large group of muscles. The increased amount of time required to properly insert and position the electrodes may compromise the examiner's rapport with a young patient when it is time to examine the walking pattern. If the purpose of the study is to gather information on the overall effect of a muscle group, the monitoring by surface EMG is a reasonable method.[27,49,57,60]

Caution must be used in the collection and processing of EMG signals.[19,64] Knowledge as to the proper areas for needle insertion or electrode placement is crucial.[1,7] The use of "raw" EMG signals, which may contain artifacts, may not reveal meaningful information, whereas appropriate filtering may display a specific pattern of activity.[50] Muscle activity may be viewed as being on or off without an attempt to describe the changing intensity within a single EMG tracing. This is possible by setting a minimal signal intensity to indicate activity and by recording the muscle as active when that level is reached. It is also possible to integrate the area within an EMG signal, allowing a qualitative judgment of the intensity of muscle activity.[64] Unfortunately, it is not currently possible to quantify a signal and calculate the force of muscle contraction.[20,36,61]

Most investigators have contributed information pertaining to normal phasic activity of the musculature during free speed-walking.[4,10,25,42,52,57] Figure 24-16 depicts the surface electrode–monitored activity of muscle groups most useful in the overall assessment of gait.[1,21,37,38,57] If the muscle activity for specific muscles must be recorded by fine wire–inserted electrodes, appropriate references may be consulted. The intent of the diagram is not to show the variations in intensity that may be present during muscle activity, but to report the muscle as being active or not active. Waters and Morris[62] have reported on the electrical activity of the trunk musculature using needle electrodes during standing and walking.

KINETICS

Kinetics is the study of the forces that produce movement. The muscles may impart energy to a body segment; however, the subsequent movement of that segment will also depend on the effects of gravity and inertia. Inertia is that property of an object (mass) that makes it resist a change in its motion. The gastrocnemius-soleus muscle may contract during single limb stance, but it does not pull the tibia and the body backward; it counteracts the tendencies of gravity and forward inertia to dorsiflex the ankle.

The device commonly used to measure the forces on the body during gait is the force plate. It is mounted in the floor to record the forces generated during the stance phase of gait (Fig. 24-17). The force plate system can record the forces produced along the X, Y, and Z axes used previously to record motion in the three body planes. Force is described by magnitude and direction and is thus a vector. During stance phase, the force vector components generated by the body can be described in terms of the X, Y, and Z axes as the medial-lateral, fore-aft, and vertical forces, respectively (Fig. 24-18). These three components result in the ground reaction forces. For every force that the body applies against the floor, there is an equal and opposite reaction, an example of Newton's third law.

The manner in which the forces are distributed between the three axes is used as a method of documenting the gait pattern. Figure 24-19 represents the vertical ground reaction force

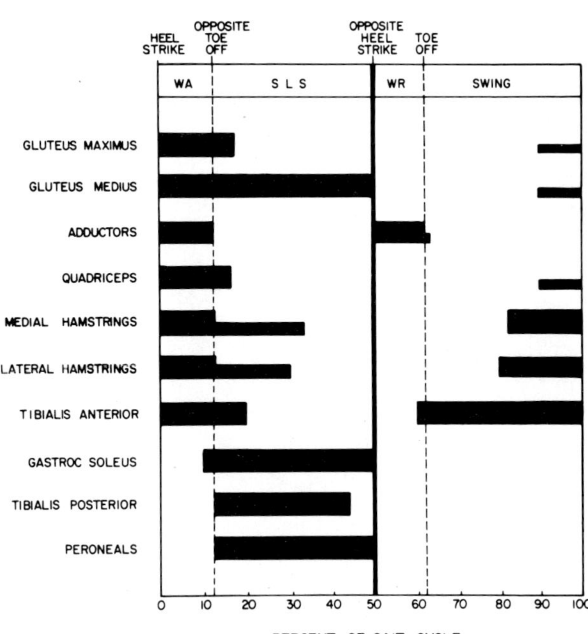

FIG. 24-16. The lines mark the time of the observed muscle electromyographic activity during one gait cycle of the most commonly analyzed muscles.

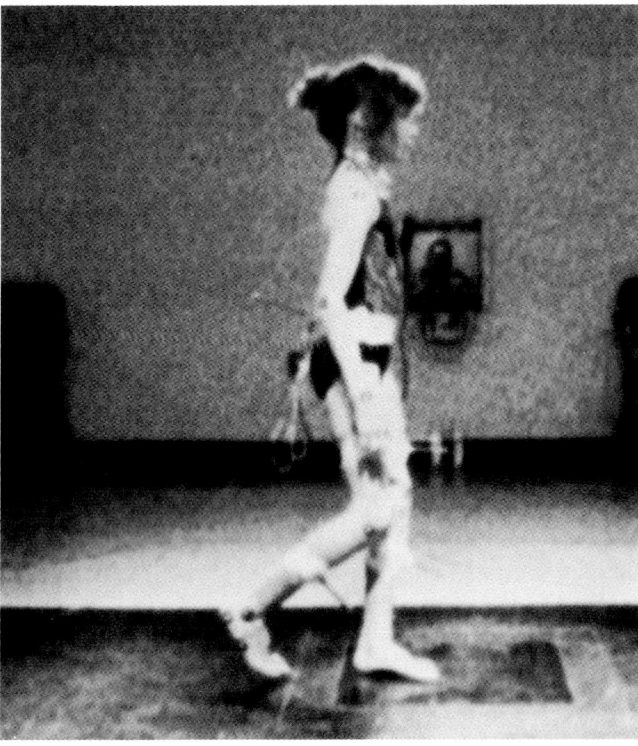

FIG. 24-17. A child at the University of Florida Gait Analysis Laboratory is seen stepping on a floor-mounted force plate as one of the three cameras record her body motions and surface electrodes monitor muscle activity.

plot during a gait cycle. Although the usual term for force is the Dyne, Newton, or Pound, the force is normalized to the percent of body weight to allow comparison among subjects. The force rises most rapidly after initial foot contact to about 60% of body weight in early weight acceptance. A less rapid rise is seen thereafter, reaching a maximal above body weight at the beginning of single limb stance. There is a decrease to below body weight seen at its minimum in mid-single limb stance, suggesting some "unloading" as a result of knee flexion.[64] As the knee extends prior to opposite foot strike, the force again rises to above body weight. As the limb goes into weight release, there is a rapid decline of the recorded force.

Figure 24-20 is a plot of the forward-aft force

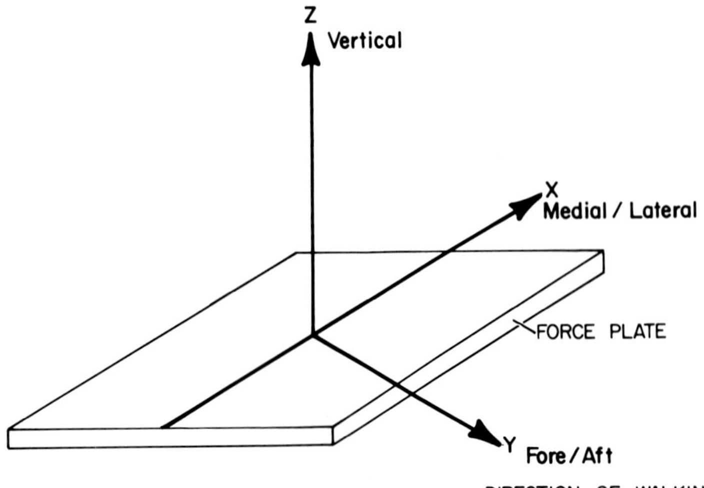

FIG. 24-18. Forces as they might be distributed on the X, Y, and Z axes of a floor-mounted force plate and their direction.

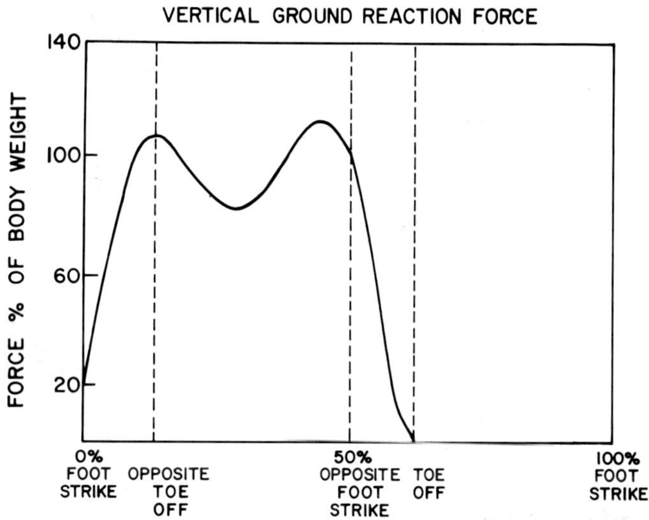

FIG. 24-19. A graphic display of the vertical ground reaction force as recorded in the Z axis of the force plate.

during one gait cycle. A forward peak is recorded during weight acceptance, representing the forward directed force imparted as a consequence of the arrest of forward body movement. After mid-stance, the direction reverses, showing the effect of the forward acceleration of the body's center of gravity.

The medial-lateral force plot is reproduced in Figure 24-21. At initial heel contact, there is a medially directed force representing the adduction and internal rotation of the limb as it enters weight acceptance. The rapid shift to the laterally directed force represents the lateral shift of the pelvis and trunk as well as the effects of hip extension and decreasing adduction.[4,38]

THE GROUND REACTION FORCE AND JOINT MOMENTS

The ground reaction force vector components may be added to produce a resultant vector in the sagittal or coronal plane. Summation of the vertical and forward-aft components will yield the sagittal plane vector reproduced in Figure 24-22. This vector is

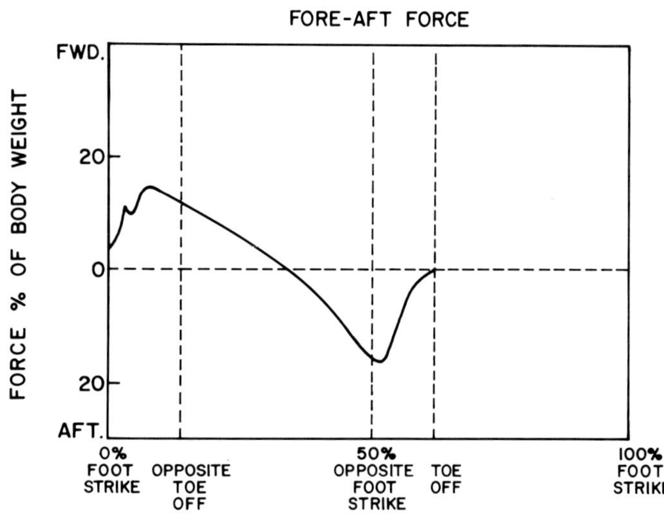

FIG. 24-20. A graphic display of the forward-aft force recorded during one gait cycle from a floor-mounted force plate.

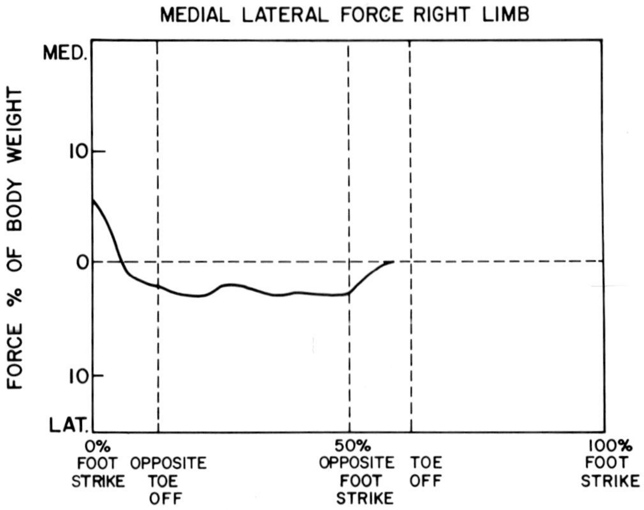

FIG. 24-21. Medial-lateral forces recorded from a floor-mounted force plate during one gait cycle.

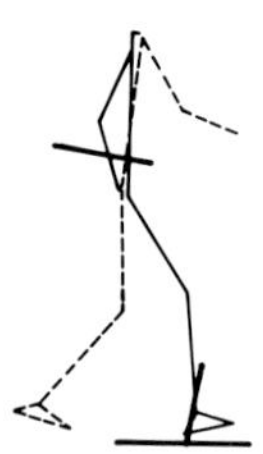
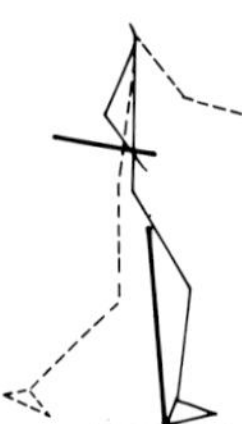
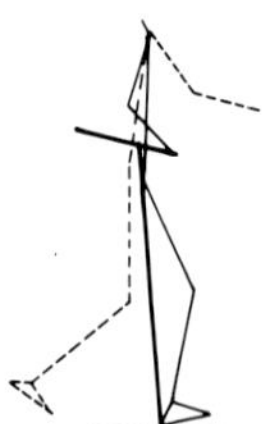
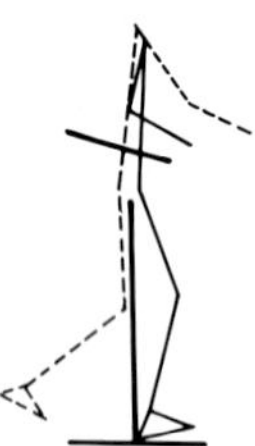

FIG. 24-22. A sagittal view of a person's walk in which selected segments of the gait cycle have been reproduced in stick figure form. The solid line indicates the right side of the body, stepping on the horizontal line indicating the force plate. The vertical and foreward-aft components of the ground reaction force vectors have been added to yield the sagittal plane vector superimposed over the stick figure.

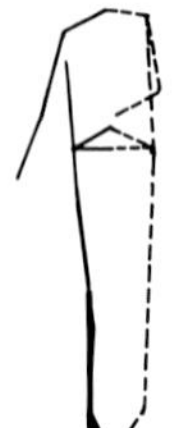
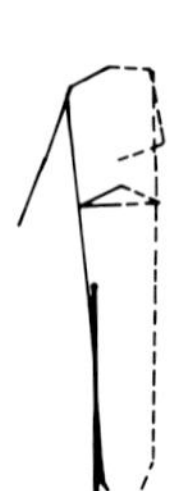
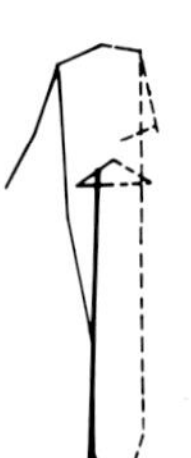
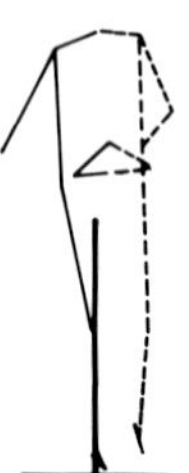

FIG. 24-23. The coronal view of segments of a person's walk in stick figure form. The solid line indicates the right side of the body, a vertical directed line indicates the sum of the vertical and medial-lateral force vectors superimposed on the stick figure.

superimposed over stick figure representations gathered from the kinematic data of a person's gait cycle. This technique serves as a useful method of displaying the ground reaction force across body segments. The changing length of the line represents the magnitude of the force, and its relation to the joint may be used to calculate the joint moment, which will be defined shortly. Summation of the vertical and medial-lateral force vectors produces the coronal plane resultant vector superimposed on the stick figure of Figure 24-23. These vector sums are a representation of the external forces acting across the mobile joints in the two body planes.[11]

The product of the ground reaction force magnitude and the perpendicular distance from the vector to the joint's center of rotation is the torque or moment of force (Fig. 24-24). The application of this torque, if unopposed, would create rotation about the joint; it is resisted by muscular activity, joint capsules, or ligaments. The study of the changing magnitude of the torque about each joint, correlated with EMG evidence of muscle activity, is a useful tool to define the mechanisms by which the body is dynamically stabilized during gait.[3] Figure 24-25 is an example of the torques generated about the ankle, knee, and hip during one gait cycle.

The visual examination of the relation of the ground reaction force to a joint is a useful method of assessment, without the need for analysis of joint moment plots. When the ground reaction force vector passes behind

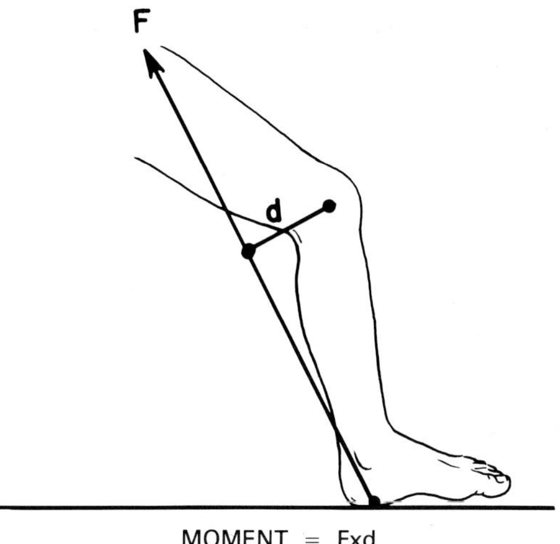

FIG. 24-24. The ground reaction force magnitude (F) multiplied by the perpendicular distance (d) from the vector to the joint's center of rotation equals torque or moment of force.

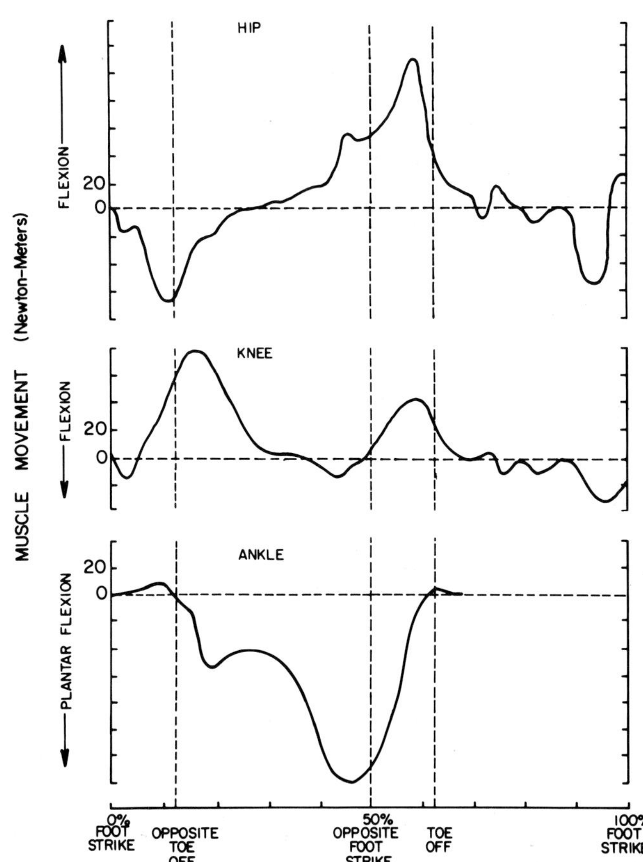

FIG. 24-25. Representative plot of the torques as generated across the hip, knee, and ankle over the entire gait cycle.

the knee joint (see Fig. 24-24), a flexion moment about the knee is produced. If this force was unopposed by quadriceps muscle activity, knee flexion would increase. When the vector passes in front of the knee, it creates an extension moment. The knee capsule and ligaments oppose further extension. The use of calculated moments allow a more precise and quantitative assessment of gait to be performed, but much useful information can also be gathered from a vector drawn over the stick figure and assessed in the above manner.[3,22]

DEVELOPMENT OF MATURE GAIT

The maturation of the central nervous system responsible for the recognized developmental milestones in infancy and childhood has been well documented in the literature.[14,24,28] The progressive control of reflex patterns leading to head and trunk control, the ability to sit, pull to stand, crawl, and cruise are known to occur at specific ages. A child's ability to attain the postural control necessary to stand unsupported and begin independent ambulation does not imply that a mature form of gait is immediately established. At each age, specific characteristics may be noted that differ from the mature gait pattern.[5,6,12,18,45,51] Many of these characteristics may be attributable to central nervous system maturation,[57] whereas others are more directly related to stature.[2,16]

Sutherland[57] has amplified the observations of Burnett and Johnson[5,6] by defining the kinematics of childhood gait in his study of 186 children, ages 1 through 7 years. The 1-year-old children (Fig. 24-26) were shown to walk at a slower velocity, with a shorter step length and increased cadence in comparison with adults. They spent less time in single limb stance, did not display reciprocal swing of the upper and lower limbs, and had a wider step width. The knee was maintained in flexion during stance phase, there was ankle plantarflexion at foot strike (flat foot gait), as well as less ankle dorsiflexion during swing. During the swing phase of gait, there was more hip flexion, abduction, and pelvic tilt. Throughout

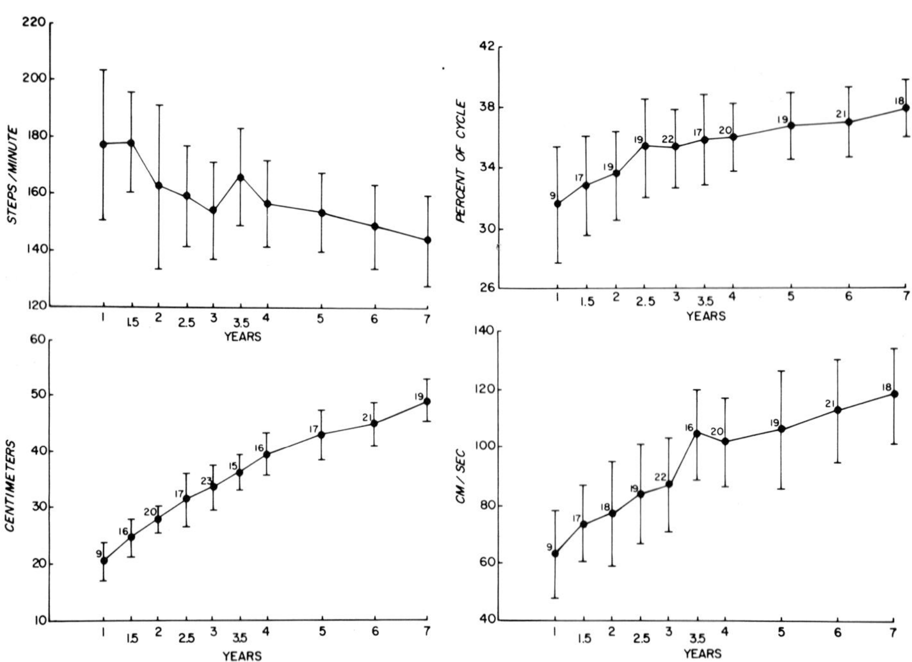

FIG. 24-26. The graphs as reproduced from Sutherland's article. In a clockwise direction: Cadence as steps per minute versus age, the duration of single limb stance versus age, the velocity versus age, and the step length in centimeters versus age. The vertical bars are plus and minus one standard deviation. (Reproduced from Sutherland DH et al: The development of the mature gait. Bone Joint Surg 62A:336–353, 1980.)

the cycle, pelvic rotation, hip rotation, and knee rotation were increased. The hip was maintained in greater external rotation.

Children in the 2-year-old group (see Fig. 24-26) showed increased velocity, step length, and diminished cadence when compared with 1-year-old children. They spent an increased percentage of time in single limb stance and showed a greater tendency to have a reciprocal swing of the upper and lower limbs. Heel strike was more common, and the ankle was dorsiflexed during swing phase. Increased knee flexion after foot strike followed by extension prior to toe-off demonstrated the adult pattern of motion. Pelvic tilt, hip abduction, and external rotation were diminished from that observed in the 1-year-old children. Most of the adult motion patterns were present by the age of 3 years, with changes in velocity, stride, and cadence continuing to 7 years of age (see Fig. 24-26). The gait characteristics of the 7-year-old children were similar to those of the adult population.

EMG by surface electrodes showed changes, when compared with adult normals, in the length of muscle activity through the gait cycle. The gluteus maximus showed less activity extending into single limb stance with advancing age. The gluteus medius maintained the adult pattern of activity. The quadriceps musculature showed decreased length of activity in stance and swing, whereas the anterior tibialis showed less activity into stance. The medial and lateral hamstring muscles were noted to lessen their time of stance phase activity, and the activity of the gastrocnemius-soleus group in swing and weight acceptance diminished with advancing age.[57]

Sutherland's analysis of the data generated from the gait of children aged 1 through 7 years led to the conclusion that there are five important determinants of mature gait. The five determinants are (1) duration of single limb stance, (2) walking velocity, (3) cadence, (4) step length, (5) and the relation of pelvic span to ankle spread. Appearance of adult values for these parameters is the best indicator of maturity, because joint motions show mature patterns at a much earlier age.

The relation of step length to limb length and its influence on velocity and cadence has been documented.[16] Beck and colleagues[2] have assessed the relationship of stride length, cadence, stance and swing times, and the ground reaction forces to changes in the velocity of gait in the growing child. Reference to their work allows one to calculate normal values for the above parameters based on the velocity of gait. Their analysis of the three ground reaction forces showed a pattern similar to the adult, but with an increased normalized amplitude persisting until about the age of 5 years.

In summary, the motion patterns of children after the age of 3 years are similar to an adult. The ground reaction forces seem to differ only in normalized amplitude until the age of 5 years. There is extension of the phasic activity of some muscles within the first 3 years of life. The velocity, stride length, cadence, and step width change until about the age of 7 years, at which time they achieve adult values. Normal values must be modified if the child does not walk at free speed. The interpretation of pathologic gait must be based on age-appropriate normal data before meaningful conclusions can be drawn from the data.

INTERPRETATION OF NORMAL GAIT

The accumulation of data on walking becomes useful when it is synthesized to explain the interrelationships among observations. Teleologically, each component contributes to an efficient form of ambulation. The rotation of the shoulders, trunk, pelvis, femur, and tibia in the transverse plane offer a good example of the interrelated motions of the body. During right weight acceptance, as the left shoulder is rotating forward, the right side of the pelvis is also advancing. The right femur and tibia are at the same time internally rotating, each at a slightly more rapid rate and over a smaller arc of motion. During single limb stance, the process reverses, as the right shoulder begins to come forward, the left pelvis comes forward, and the stance phase femur and tibia each begin to externally rotate. This process reaches its maximum at the end of weight release. Right swing phase shows the left shoulder behind, the right pelvis ahead, and the femur and tibia, having externally rotated in the first half of swing, begin to internally rotate in the last half of swing phase. The reciprocal motion of the shoulder girdle to the pelvis and the individual rotational patterns of the femur and tibia have been described in the section on specific joint motions. Perturbations of this rotational sequence are recognized as the internal rotation crouch gait pattern in cerebral palsy.[60] The importance of transverse rotations of body segments on the energy conservation in gait has been delineated.[26]

Saunders, Inman, and Eberhart were among the first investigators to attempt to correlate kinematic and kinetic data.[46] Their concentration on the influence of body segment motion on the location of the body's center of gravity led to the description of the six elements or determinants of gait. Pelvic rotation, pelvic obliquity, knee flexion, stance-phase knee flexion with ankle motion, and the anatomic configuration of the limbs and pelvis to limit lateral displacements of the body were shown to minimize the path that the body's center of gravity must move in the horizontal and vertical planes. The motion of the body segments therefore combined to limit the vertical and horizontal displacements and thereby diminish the energy used in walking.

More recent studies have concentrated on the energy used in gait to define normal and pathologic patterns. Perry has reported on oxygen consumption; Winter,[65,66] Mansour, and co-workers[26] and others[23,44] have analyzed the mechanical energy involved in the motion of each segment of the body in normal walking. From these studies, an explanation of the observed data has been developed at a more sophisticated level. These data also more directly address the functional significance of the movements during gait. A gait pattern that requires a marked amount of compensation may use a great deal of energy and diminish velocity and/or endurance. A very good example of this is the compensations necessary to walk after an upper motor neuron lesion as in cerebral palsy. The combined muscular efforts and altered joint ranges of motion may be so taxing as to preclude walking except in a physical therapy setting or, perhaps, not at all.

METHODS OF GAIT ASSESSMENT

When analyzing a patient's gait, two factors become critical: (1) the equipment available to gather the data, and (2) the method used to arrive at an interpretation of a gait pattern.

OBSERVATIONAL ANALYSIS

Visual observation of an individual's walk can be more critical if an attempt is made to divide the walk into the phases of gait. Dividing the cycle into weight acceptance, single limb stance, weight release, and swing, while observing, will assist in structuring the walk. Subsequent description of the motion of each body segment within such a framework allows a more precise recognition of the pathologic events. An example of its usefulness would be in the assessment of a child with spastic hemiparesis demonstrating foot inversion during gait. If the foot is inverted in swing as well as in stance phase, a posterior tibial tendon lengthening procedure would be appropriate, whereas inversion only in swing might best be treated with a posterior tibial tendon transfer.

In addition to the written description of the walking pattern, if the walk is recorded on film or video, a permanent record may be established of the person's pattern over a period of time. This method alone does not allow one to quantify joint or segment motions, but it does supplement the written record.[5,6] The velocity may be calculated by timing the walk over a known distance. This one parameter documents function and can be easily followed over the course of the disease process or its treatment.

INSTRUMENT–ASSISTED ANALYSIS

The addition of foot–floor contact switches to mark and time stance and swing phase is a significant move toward documenting the gait cycle objectively.[41] Use of this method over a measured walkway allows the calculation of many critical gait parameters. Cadence, velocity, step and stride lengths, intervals of single limb stance, double limb stance, and swing phase may be documented. These may be used to comment upon the stability, efficiency, symmetry, and effectiveness of the gait pattern. With severe disorders, it is possible to quantitatively document the consequences of the course of the disease or the effects of treatment. Such devices are relatively inexpensive and, within their limits, offer an objective way of recording gait.

The addition of dynamic EMG to the foot switch system allows one to record the phasing of muscle activity and may assist in the planning of muscle transfer procedures.[39,53,63] The combination of time–distance parameters, dynamic EMG, and the recording of motion to document the positions of the body segments is helpful in making the analysis more complete. For example, recorded activity of the quadriceps mechanism with the knee in excess flexion during stance would call for a different interpretation than if the knee were in full extension. With the knee flexed in stance, the quadriceps might act to stabilize the knee and thereby compensate for an abnormal knee position. Quadriceps activity with an extended knee in stance might indicate abnormal muscle phasing as a result of an upper motor neuron lesion, because the extended knee is stabilized by the capsule and ligaments in single limb stance phase.

Recording of the kinematic data on videotape with automatic digitization[2,13] or on high-speed motion picture film[47,57,60] digitized into a computer, opens up many more possibilities for more specific and detailed computerized data analysis and presentation. The stored data may be used to calculate joint and body segment motions, the phases of gait, velocity, segment acceleration, and so on, without the need for encumbering foot switches or electrogoniometers. The graphics capabilities of current software allow data to be displayed in many different formats. Computer software may also be used to synchronize the EMG data with the kinematic data. Utilization of a force plate allows acquisition of kinetic information, which may be synchronized with EMG and kinematic data to allow a full assessment of gait.

With computer-aided data acquisition, synchronization, processing, and display, the most sophisticated analysis of walking is possible. The acquired flexibility is expensive and requires a staff to maintain the equipment. The analysis of gait with complex systems is most appropriately suited to research or the particularly difficult patient management problems. The complicated gait patterns of cerebral palsy or other neuromuscular disorders should be studied prior to initiating treatment. The application of gait analysis techniques to other neuromuscular disorders should be studied prior to initiating treatment. The application of gait analysis techniques to other walking disorders may offer a more detailed appreciation of the compensatory mechanisms used by the body. The more sophisticated the system, the greater the different types of information that may be gathered to aid in the management of complex gait problems.[8,29,49,54,58,60]

CONCLUSION

The amount of effort needed to assess a particular walking abnormality depends on its severity. The more complex the compensatory pattern used to overcome the insult producing the gait abnormality, the more difficult the categorization of the pattern. A child presenting to the physician with an abnormal gait may not require the full efforts of a computerized motion analysis laboratory but does require a trained observer to dissect the pattern. Prerequisite is the ability to apply the appropriate level of technology to best document the problem and, subsequently, the clinical acumen to analyze the data. Only when as much objective information as is appropriate has been gathered, can recommendations be made regarding the treatment of the gait problems.

REFERENCES

1. Basmajian JV: Muscles Alive, Their Functions Revealed by Electromyography, 4th ed. Baltimore, Williams & Wilkens, 4th ed. 1979
2. Beck RJ, Andriacchi TP, Kuo KN, Fermier RW, Galante JO: Changes in the gait patterns of growing children. J Bone Joint Surg 63A(9): Dec. 1981
3. Boccardi S, Pedotti A, Rodano R, Santambrogio GC: Evaluation of muscular moments at the lower limb joint by an on-line processing of kinematic data and ground reaction. J Biomechanics 14:35, 1980
4. Bowker JH, Hall CB: Normal Human Gait in Atlas of Orthotics. Biomechanical Principles and Application. American Academy of Orthopaedic Surgeons. St. Louis, CV Mosby, 1975
5. Burnett CN, Johnson EW: Development of gait in childhood. Part I. Dev Med Child Neurol 13:196, 1971
6. Burnett CN, Johnson EW: Development of gait in childhood. Part II. Dev Med Child Neurol 13:207, 1971
7. Delagi EF, Iazzetti J, Perotto A, Morrison D: Anatomic Guide for the Electromyographer, 2nd ed. Springfield, IL, Charles C Thomas, 1980
8. Demottaz JD, Mazur JM, Thomas WH, Sledge CB, Simon SR: Clinical study of total ankle replacement with gait analysis. J Bone Joint Surg 61-A(7):976, 1979
9. Drillis R: Objective recording and biomechanics of pathologic gait. Ann NY Acad Sci 17:86, 1958
10. Eberhart HD: The Principle Elements in Human Locomotion. In Kapster PE and Wilson PD (eds): Human Limbs and Their Substitutes, pp. 463–470. New York, Hufner Press, 1968
11. Elftman M: Forces and energy changes in the leg during walking. Am J Physiol 125:339, 1939
12. Foley CD, Quanbury AO, Steinke T: Kinematics of normal child locomotion—A statistical study based on TV data. J Biomechanics 12:1, 1978
13. Gage JR, Fabian O, Hicks R, Tashman S.: Pre- and postoperative gait analysis in patients with spastic diplegia: A preliminary report. J Pediatr Orthop 4(b):715, 1984

14. Gesell A: The First Five Years of Life. New York, Harper, 1940
15. Gregersen GG, Lucas DB: An *in vivo* study of the axial rotation of the human thoracolumbar spine. J Bone Joint Surg 49A, March 1967
16. Grieve DW, Gear RJ: The relationship between length of stride, step frequency, time of swing, and speed of walking for children and adults. Ergonomics 9:379, 1966
17. Heck CV, Hendryson IE, Rowe CR: Joint Motion, Method of Measuring and Recording. American Academy of Orthopaedic Surgeons, 1965
18. Hennessy M, Simon SR, Reed R: Development of Bipedal Gait in the African Child. Read at the Annual Meeting of the American Academy for Cerebral Palsy and Developmental Medicine. Atlanta, Georgia, Oct 1977
19. Herschler C, Milner M: An optimality criterion for processing electromyographic (EMG) signals relating to human locomotion. The Transaction on Biomedical Engineering BME-25 (5):413, 1978
20. Hof AL: EMG and muscle force: An introduction. Whiting HTA (ed): Human Movement Science. 3(½): 1984
21. Inman VT, Ralston HJ, Todd FL: Human Walking. Baltimore, Williams & Wilkins, 1981
22. Jacobs NA, Skorecki J: Analysis of the vertical component of force in normal and pathologic gait. J Biomechanics 5:11, 1972
23. Lamoreaux LW: Kinematic Measurements in the Study of Human Walking. Bulletin of Prosthetics Research, Spring, 1971
24. Longwerthy OR: Development of Behavior Patterns and Myelinization of the Nervous System in the Human Fetus and Infant. In Contributions to Embryology, Vol XXIC, No 139. Publication No 443:1–57. Washington, Carnegie Institute, 1933
25. Mann RA: Biomechanics of Gait: A Critical Visual Analysis. Prepared by Gait Anal Lab Shriners Hosp for Crippled Children. San Francisco, 1975
26. Mansour JM, Lesh MD, Nowak NC, Simon SR: A three-dimensional multi-segmental analysis of the energetics of normal and pathologic human gait. J Biomechanics 15 (1):51, 1982
27. Mazuur JM, Schwartz E, Simon SR: Ankle arthrodesis. Long-term follow-up with gait analysis. J Bone Joint Surg 61A (7):964, 1979
28. McGraw MB: Neuromuscular development of the human infant as exemplified in the achievement of erect locomotion. J Pediat 17:747, 1940
29. Mena D, Mansour JM, Simon SR: Analysis and synthesis of human swing leg motion during gait and its clinical applications. J Biomechanics 22:823, 1980
30. Molen HN, Rozendahl RH, Boon W: Graphic representation of the relationship between oxygen consumption and characteristics of normal gait of the human male. Proc Kow Ned Akad Wet Ser C 75:305, 1972
31. Murray MP: Walking pattern of normal men. J Bone Joint Surg 46A:335, 1964
32. Murray MP: Walking patterns in healthy old men. J Geront 24:169, 1969
33. Murray MP: Comparison of free and fast speed-walking patterns of normal men. Am J Phys Med 45:8, 1969
34. Murray MP: Walking patterns of normal women. Arch Phys Med Rehab Nov 637, 1970
35. Pare EB, Stern JT, Schwartz JM: Functional differentiation within the tensor fasciae latae. J Bone Joint Surg 63-A (9): Dec 1981
36. Patriacot AG, Mann RW, Simons SR, Mansour JM: An evaluation of the approaches of optimization models in the prediction of muscle forces during human gait. J Biomechanics 14 (8):513, 1981
37. Perry J: Pathologic Gait in Atlas of Orthotics. Biomechanical Principles and Application. American Academy of Orthopaedic Surgeons, CV Mosby, 1975
38. Perry J: Kinesiology of lower extremity bracing. Clin Orthop Rel Res 102:18, 1974
39. Perry J, Hoffer MM, Antonelli D, Plut J, Lewis G, Greenberg R: Electromyography before and after surgery for hip deformity in children with cerebral palsy. J Bone Joint Surg 58-A (2):201, 1976
40. Perry J, Hoffer M: Preoperative and postoperative dynamic electromyography as an aid in planning tendon transfers in children with cerebral palsy. J Bone Joint Surg 59-A (4):531, 1977
41. Perry J, Bontrager E: Development of a gait analyzer for clinical use. Trans Orthop Res Soc 2:48, 1977
42. Perry J: Pre-op and post-op dynamic EMG as an aid in planning tendon transfers in children with CP. J Bone Joint Surg 59A:531, 1977
43. Perry J, Fox JM, Boitano MA, Skinner SR, Barnes LA, Cerny K: Functional evaluation of the pes anserinus transfer by electromyography and gait analysis. J Bone Joint Surg 52A (6):973, 1980
44. Robertson GD, Winter DA: Mechanical energy generation, absorption and transfer amongst segments during walking. J Biomechanics 13:845, 1980
45. Rose-Jacobs R: Development of gait at slow, free, and fast speeds in 3- and 5-year-old children. Research 63 (8):1251, 1983
46. Saunders JB, Inman VT, Eberhart HD: The major determinants in normal and pathologic gait. J Bone Joint Surg 35-A (3):543, 1953
47. Simon SR, Nuzzo RM, Koshinen MF: A Comprehensive Clinical System for Four-Dimensional Motion Analysis. Bulletin of the Hospital for Joint Diseases, Vol XXXVIII, No 1, April 1977
48. Simon SR, Mann RA, Hagy JL, Larsen LJ: Role of the posterior calf muscles in normal gait. J Bone Joint Surg 60-A (4):465, 1978
49. Simon SR, Deutsch SD, Nuzzo RM, Mansour MJ, Jackson JL, Koskinene M, Rosenthal RK: Genu recurvatum in spastic cerebral palsy. J Bone Joint Surg 60-A (7):882, 1978
50. Simon SR: Kinesiology—Its measurement and importance to rehabilitation. In Orthopaedic Rehabilitation. New York, Churchill Livingstone, 1982
51. Statham L, Murray MP: Early walking patterns of normal chldren. Clin Orthop 79:8, 1971
52. Sutherland DH: An electromyographic study of the plantar flexors of the ankle in normal walking on the level. J Bone Joint Surg 48A:66, 1966
53. Sutherland DH, Schottstaedt ER, Larsen LJ, Ashley RK, Callander JN, James PM: Clinical and electromyographic study of seven spastic children with internal rotation gait. J Bone Joint Surg 51-A (6):1070, 1969
54. Sutherland DH, Cooper L: The pathomechanics of progressive crouch gait in spastic diplegia. Orthop Clin North Am 9 (1):143, 1978
55. Sutherland DH, Olshen R, Cooper L, Woo SLY: The

development of mature gait. J Bone Joint Surg 62-A (3): April, 1980

56. Sutherland DH, Cooper L, Daniel D: The role of ankle plantar flexors in normal walking. J Bone Joint Surg 62-A (3): April, 1980
57. Sutherland DH: The development of natural gait. J Bone Joint Surg 62A:336, 1980
58. Sutherland DH: Gait Disorders in Childhood and Adolescence. Baltimore, Williams & Wilkins, 1984
59. Thurston AJ: Normal kinematics of the lumbar spine and pelvis. Spine 8:199, 1983
60. Tylkowski CM, Simon SR, Mansour JM: Internal Rotation Gait in Spastic Cerebral Palsy. In The Hip Society: The Hip: Proceedings of the Tenth Open Scientific Meeting of the Hip Society, 1982. CV Mosby, 1982
61. Van Leemputte MF, Spaepen AJ, Willems EJ: Quantification of EMG Using a Differentiation Technique. Biomaterials and Biomechanics, pp 103–107. 1983
62. Waters RL, Morris JM: Electrical activity of muscles of the trunk during walking. J Anatomy III (2):191, 1972
63. Waters RL, Perry J, Garland D: Surgical correction of gait abnormalities following stroke. Clin Orthop Rel Res 131:54, 1978
64. Winter DA: Biomechanics of Human Movement. New York, John Wiley & Sons, 1979
65. Winter DA: Overall principle of lower limb support during stance phase of gait. J Biomechanics 13:923, 1980
66. Winter DA: Kinematic and kinetic patterns in human gait: Variability and compensating effects. In Whiting HTA (ed): Human Movement Science. 3(½): 1984
67. Zarrugh MY, Todd FN, Ralston HJ: Optimization of energy expenditure during level walking. Eur J Appl Physiol 33:293, 1974
68. Zarrugh MY: Power requirements and mechanical efficiency of treadmill walking. J Biomechanics 14 (3):157, 1981

25

Partial Growth Plate Arrest and Its Treatment

Hamlet A. Peterson

Premature partial arrest of growth of an epiphyseal growth plate (physis) produces angular and length growth abnormalities of the involved bone. The arrest is produced when a bridge of bone forms from metaphysis to epiphysis, thereby crossing the physis. This continuity of bone has become known as a *bone bridge* or a *bone bar*. The bar tethers growth. As the remaining physis grows, angular deformity occurs (Fig. 25-1). The size and location of the bar determine the clinical deformity. If the bar is located laterally in a physis, for example, the distal femur, the normal physis medially continues to grow, producing genu valgus deformity.[8,9,12,19,26] If the bone bar is anterior, the normal physis posteriorly grows, producing genu recurvatum. If the bar is central, the periphery may grow causing "cupping," "tenting," or "dip deformity" of the metaphysis combined with relative shortening of the bone but little, if any, angular deformity.[1,6,7,27,41]

Bone bars may result after any injury to physeal cells. The most common cause is fracture, although bars may occur after other types of physeal damage such as infection, tumors (with or without surgery), irradiation, thermal burns, and the iatrogenic insertion of metal across the physis. Neural and vascular abnormalities have been shown to alter physeal growth in a manner simulating bar formation.[36] Theoretical possibilities include reduced vascular supply from any cause (*e.g.*, an adjacent metaphyseal osteotomy, localized vascular occlusion, arterial embolization, altered blood flow from a cast or immobilization), frost bite, electrical burns, and metabolic abnormality (vitamin A intoxication[27]).[6,41,] Some cases have been found in which no etiology was apparent, and these have been called *congenital* or *developmental* (Blount's disease would be an example). However, none has ever been found at birth.

Bone bars can occur after any type of fracture that involves the physis. Growth arrests have been reported after all five Salter-Harris[31] types of injuries. Because the type IV injury is the only one that crosses the metaphysis and epiphysis as well as the physis, it has the greatest potential to form a bone bar. A bone bar will usually develop after a displaced and unreduced type IV injury. Even with anatomic reduction, a bar may form. All compression type V injuries reported in the literature have resulted in complete rather than partial closure of the physis. Because there is no remaining open physis, none has been treated by bar excision. Although a compression injury of the physis theoretically could produce a partial closure, none has been reported in the literature, and there is some question that such a lesion exists.[30]

All bone bars are a result of damage of the physeal cells and, in this sense, cannot be prevented. An exception is the iatrogenic placement of metal pins and screws across the physis (Fig. 25-2). Many factors are involved (*e.g.*, pin size, location, obliquity to the physis

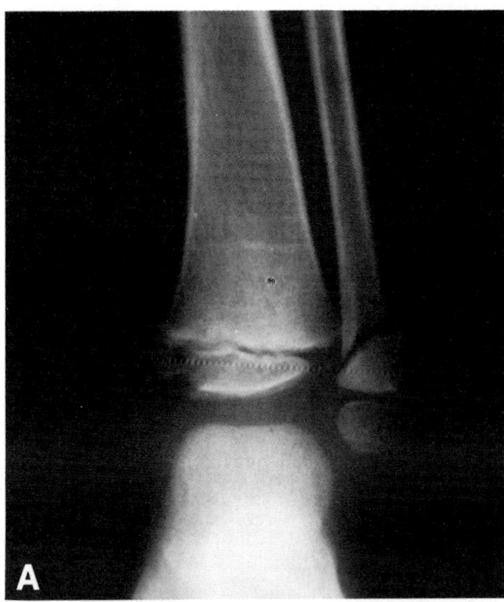

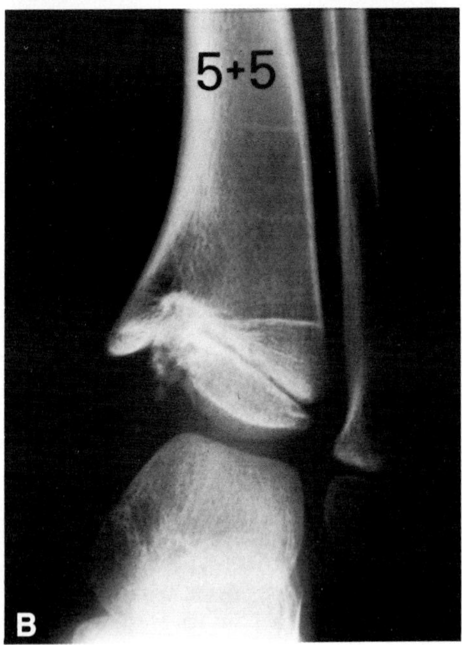

FIG. 25-1. Boy (3 years 7 months old) who fell from a tree. *(A)* Distal tibial physeal Salter-Harris-type IV injury with proximal displacement of medial malleolar fragment. This was treated by cast immobilization without reduction. *(B)* Same child 22 months later (age 5 years 5 months). Note physeal bar medially, growth arrest line perpendicular to longitudinal axis of the tibia, asymmetric growth of remaining normal physis producing 45° varus angulation of the physis, and adaptive contouring of the lateral edge of the tibial epiphysis, allowing the ankle varus to be less than the physeal varus. The medial malleolus is present but not yet ossified. Long-term follow-up of this case has been published.[29]

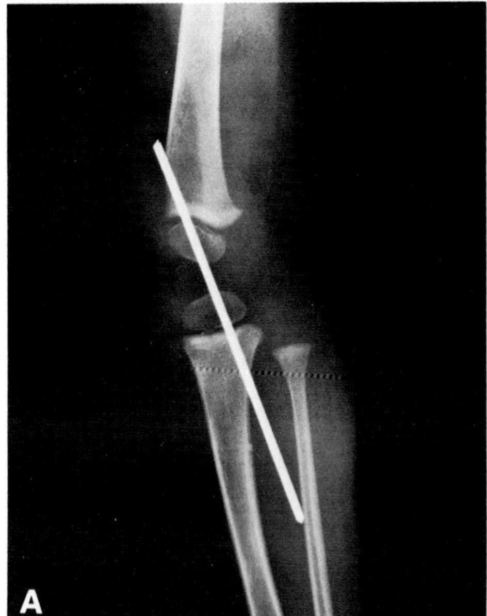

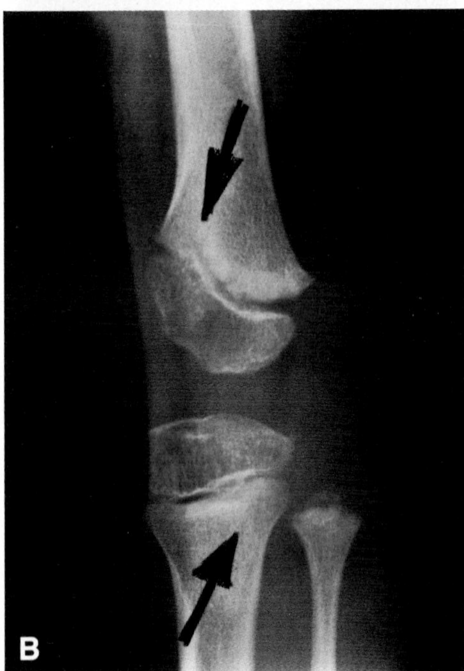

FIG. 25-2. Boy (age 2 years 3 months) whose left knee was severely lacerated by a lawn mower. There was complete disruption of the patellar tendon, joint capsule, and collateral and cruciate ligaments but no fracture. *(A)* Joint stability achieved by fixation with a single longitudinal threaded Steinmann pin. *(B)* Two years two months later (age 4 years 5 months). Note bar formation with angular growth of distal femur. The mild growth disturbance of the proximal tibia did not form a physeal bar and corrected spontaneously.

duration left in place, and whether the pin is smooth or threaded). A smooth pin of small diameter placed perpendicularly across the center of the physis for a short period of time (*e.g.*, 2 to 3 weeks) rarely causes a growth arrest.[12] On the other hand, a threaded wire of any diameter placed obliquely across a physis and left in place for a few weeks will usually result in a bone bar. Of all these factors, the presence or absence of threads on the pin appears to be the most important.

The development of bone bars can be anticipated after comminuted type IV injuries and, if followed closely, can be detected as early as a few weeks after the injury. Some bone bars do not become clinically evident until years after the injury and underscore the need to follow any significant physeal injury for years, if not until maturity. This is particularly true after metaphyseal osteomyelitis (Fig. 25-3A–G).

Anatomic differences between the various physes are also important in the production of bone bars. Factors include the size of the physis, the rate of growth, and the contour of the physis (*i.e.*, whether the physis lies on one plane or is irregular). Although the proximal radius is by far the most frequently injured physis,[28] it is an uncommon site of a bone bar.[4,13,18] The proximal tibia and distal femur account for only 3% of all physeal injuries,[28] but they are responsible for the majority of bone bars.[4,13,18] These physes are both large in area and irregular in contour, and they account for 60% to 70% of the growth of their respective bones.

The age of the patient at the time of physeal injury is perhaps the paramount factor. Injury of the physis of a 14- or 15-year-old girl or a 16- or 17-year-old boy is of little consequence, because these teenagers have so little growth remaining that deformity is not likely to become clinically manifest. Because most type III fractures occur near skeletal maturity, they infrequently produce bone bars with clinical deformity. Any bone bar in an infant or young child, however, is a significant problem with wide-ranging clinical effects. Clinical follow-up until maturity is mandatory in these children.

EVALUATION

Bone bars are usually first noted clinically because of angular deformity or relative shortening of the involved extremity. History, physical examination, and routine roentgenograms will localize the involved physis. Evaluate the relationship of the growth arrest line, physis, and joint surface carefully (see Fig. 25-1*B*).

Tomograms determine both the configuration and the area of bar involvement and, perhaps more important, determine the configuration and area of the remaining normal physis (see Fig. 25-3*F, G*). Tomograms may be either linear, circular, spiral, ellipsoidal, or hypocycloidal (sometimes incorrectly termed *trispiral*). For purposes of evaluating the physis, hypocycloidal tomograms are superior, because the cuts may be as small as 1 mm thick and give sharp focus. False-positive and false-negative findings have been reported with standard tomography.[37] Thin cuts (1 mm) taken every 3 mm in both the anteroposterior and lateral planes are used to construct both the area and configuration of the bar on a piece of paper. This may be referred to as a "map" of the bar. This aids in determining whether or not the bar is resectable and the surgical approach.

Lengths of both the involved and the uninvolved extremity should be documented radiographically. Three methods are in common use: teloroentgenography, orthoroentgenography, and scanography. Scanograms are superior because the distance may be measured directly on the film, the measurement is not affected by the thickness of the extremity, there is no magnification, there is no chance of technical error (if the child moves during the examination, the image on the film will be wavy and the examination should be repeated), and the true measurements can be compared with previous and future scanograms in longitudinal studies (see Fig. 25-3*B, C, E, J*). Scanograms become even more valuable when analyzing growth between two metal markers after treatment (see Fig. 25-3*I, K*).

Bone age must be determined to assess the potential for remaining growth. Of the methods available, comparison of a roentgenogram of the hand with an atlas is the most commonly used.[35] Because most bars occur in the knee, perhaps a method using the knee would have more direct applicability.

Computed tomographic (CT) scans are of little value in assessing the bar because of the irregularity of the physis. Even cuts as thin as 1 mm will not pass through only physeal tissue of most normal physes because of undulations

(*Text continues on page 1089*)

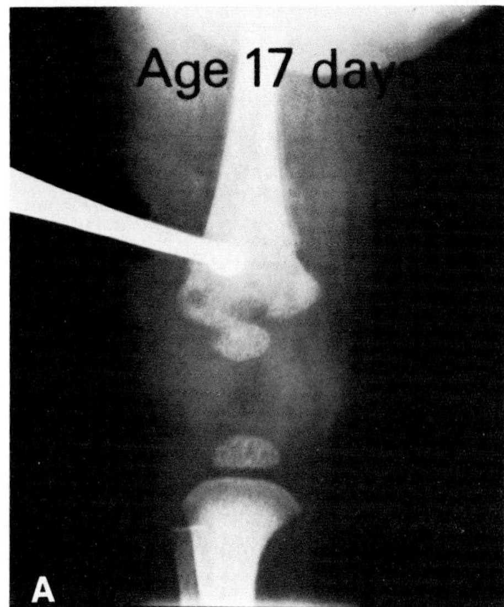

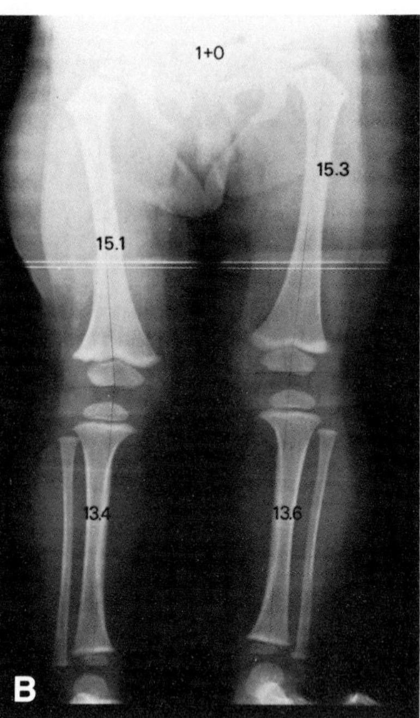

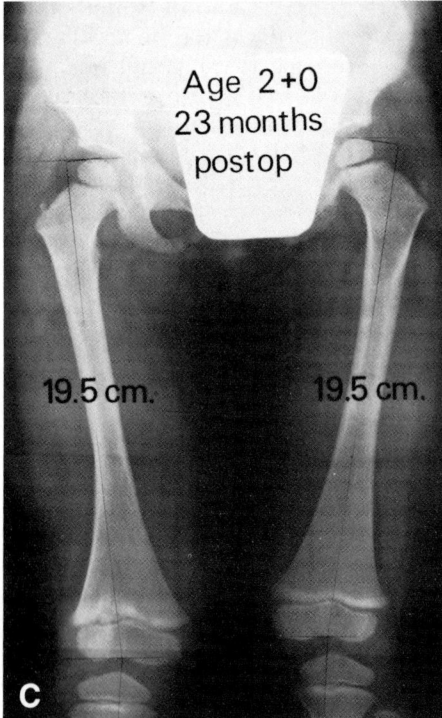

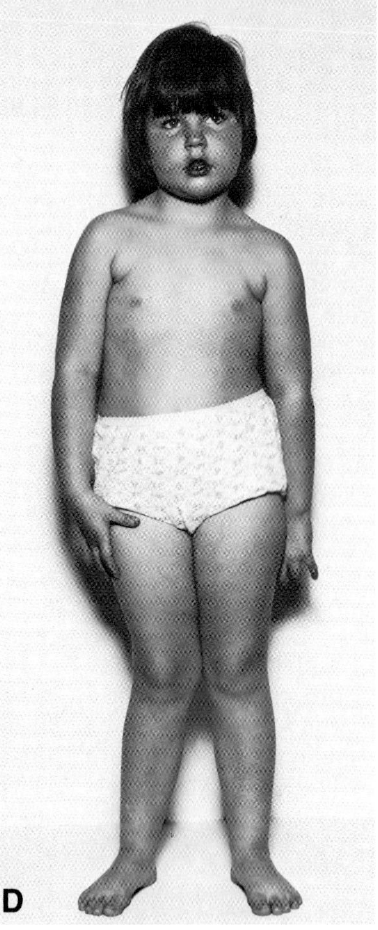

FIG. 25-3. Infant girl had a cutdown inserted into right ankle saphenous vein on second day of life. *(A)* Staphylococcus osteomyelitis distal right femur treated by incision and drainage on day 17 of life. Care was taken to avoid contact of curet with physis. *(B)* Scanogram 1 year later shows both femora and tibiae growing normally. Right metaphysis is only slightly more wide and irregular than left. *(C)* Scanogram 2 years later shows both femora growing normally, but metaphysis and physis are more irregular on right than left. *(D)* Photograph at age 4 years 11 months shows right leg genu valgum with relative shortening.

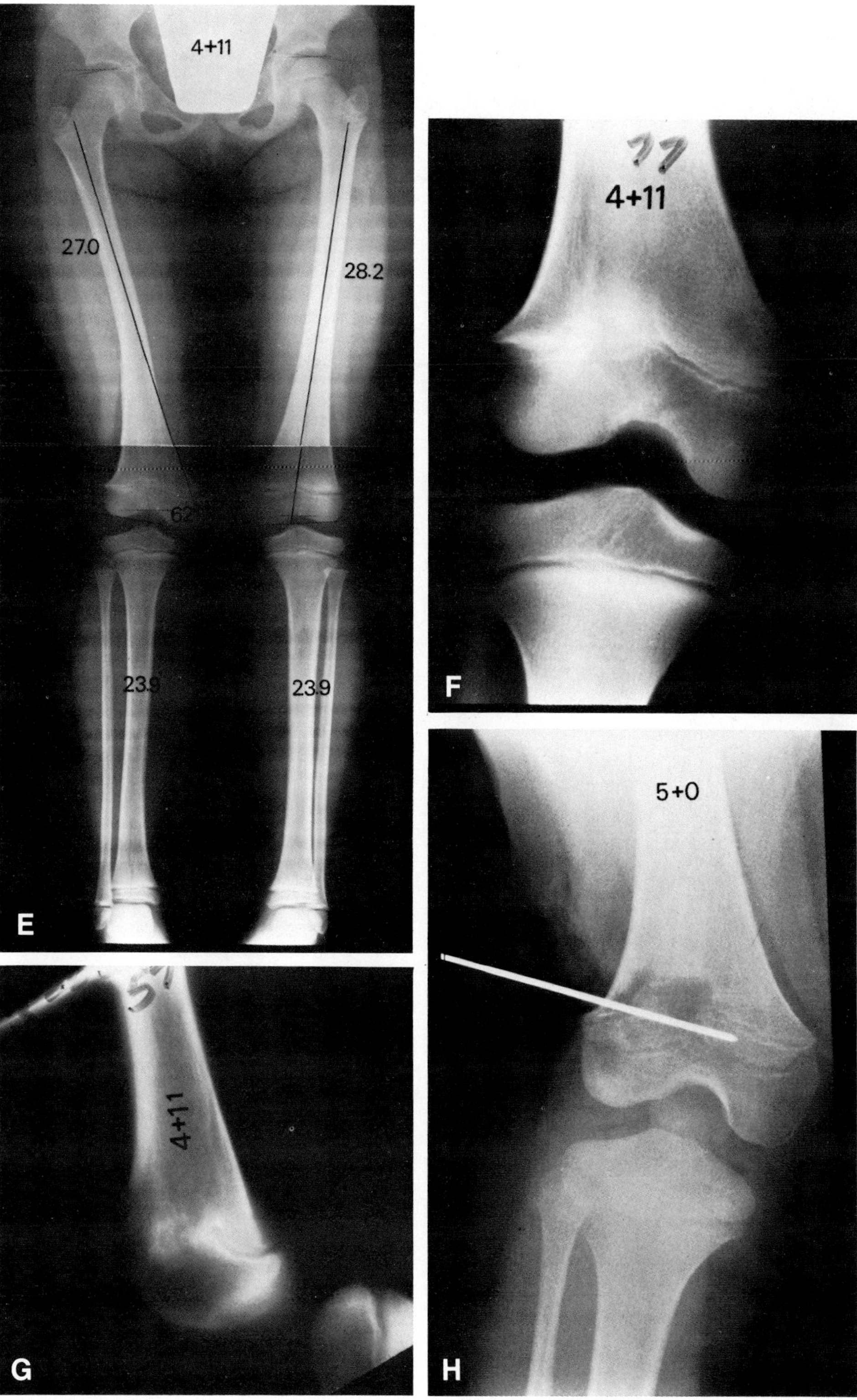

FIG. 25-3. *(Cont.)* *(E)* Scanogram 4 years 11 months postoperatively shows right distal femoral valgus angulation and relative shortening of femur (1.2 cm). Note femoral shaft–femoral condyle angle of 62°. *(F)* Anteroposterior tomogram of right knee shows central bar with "tenting" or "cupping" of remaining physis. *(G)* Lateral tomogram shows central bar. *(H)* Operative anteroposterior roentgenogram during removal of a window of cortex in the metaphysis to approach the central bar from above (age 5 years 0 months). This avoids damage of normal peripheral physis. The metal pin was used to determine medial extent of the bar excision and was removed after completion of the roentgenogram.

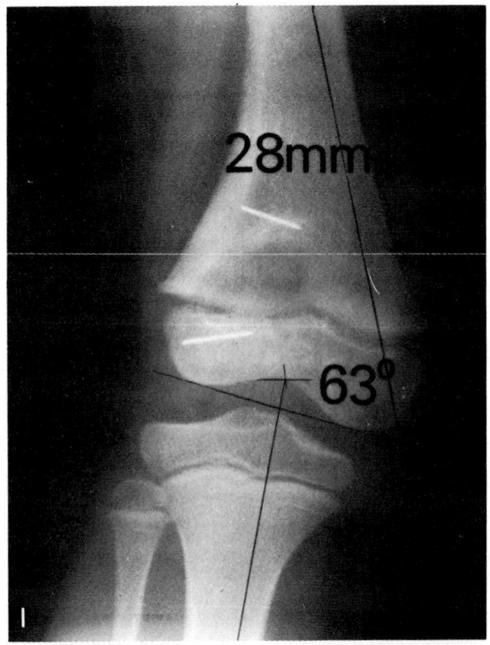

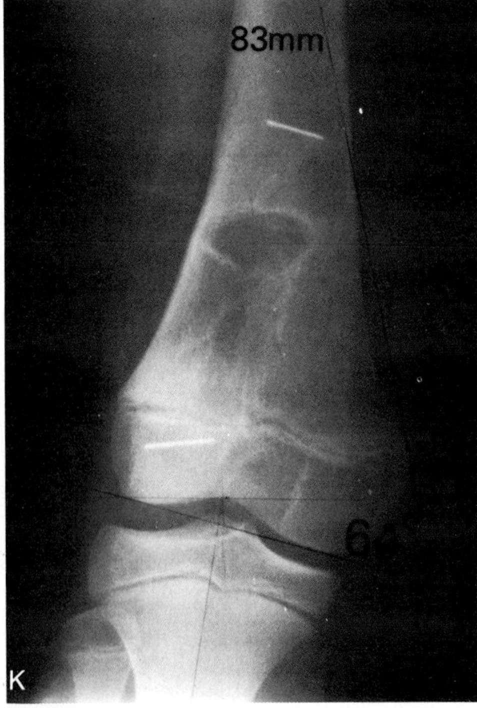

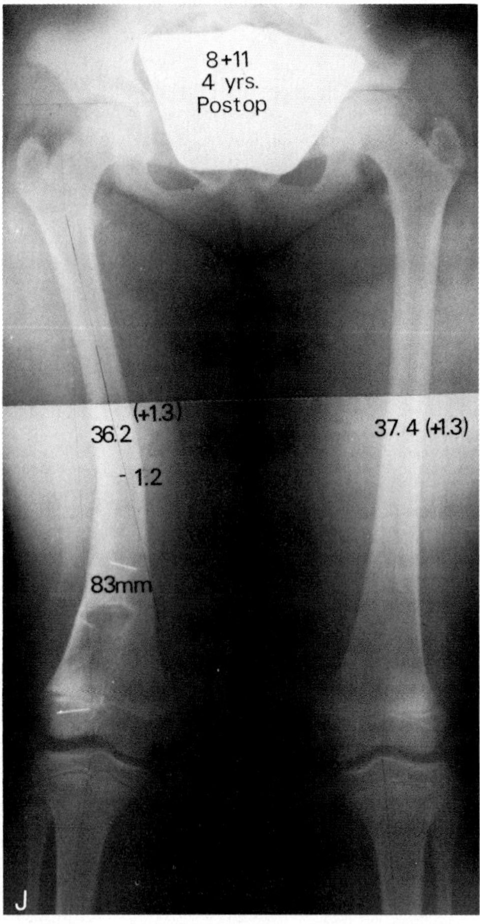

FIG. 25-3. *(Cont.)* *(I)* Close-up of scanogram 5 months postoperatively. The physis remained open. The two metal markers inserted at the time of the operation are 28 mm apart. Femoral shaft–femoral condyle angle has increased from 62° to 63°. Note that the cranioplast lucency is very close to the proximal marker. *(J)* Scanogram 4 years postoperatively shows metal markers 83 mm apart. Both femora have grown equally since operation (discrepancy remains 12 mm). The femoral shaft–femoral condyle has increased only 1° to 64°, and the orientation of the metal markers to each other remains unchanged. *(K)* Close-up of scanogram of right knee 4 years postoperatively. Because this is taken from a scanogram, there is no magnification of the distance between the two metal markers. Note that the cranioplast plug initially stayed with the epiphysis (as evidenced by the increased distance of the plug from the proximal metal marker; compare with Fig. 25-3*I*). Later, the epiphysis grew away from the plug (as evidenced by the increased distance of the plug from the distal metal marker).

of the physis. Any projection of bone from undulation could be interpreted as a bone bar. Multiple projections of bone could not be differentiated from multifocal or "satellite" bars.

Scintigraphy at the time of injury and shortly thereafter has recently been proposed as an investigative modality to aid in detecting compression injuries that might lead to bar formation.[40] For this concept to become useful clinically, further investigation is necessary.

TREATMENT

Premature partial closure of the physis may be treated in many ways. If the patient is a teenager approaching maturity and little growth remains in the involved physis, no treatment may be necessary. If the patient is young with significant growth remaining, a combination of many modalities may be used.

1. Shoe lift. This is applicable when a lower extremity bar is central and causes no angular deformity and the leg length discrepancy is anticipated to be minor at maturity (*e.g.*, 2 cm or less).
2. Arrest the remaining growth of the injured physis. This should be considered in an older child with a beginning angular deformity when limb length inequality will be minor (lower extremity) or of relatively little functional consequence (upper extremity).
3. Arrest the remaining growth of the injured physis and the physis of the adjacent bone (in the case of forearm and lower leg).[15]
4. Arrest the remaining growth of the injured physis, the physis of the adjacent bone if one is present, and the corresponding physis or physes of the contralateral bone or bones.[15]
5. Modality 2, 3, or 4 combined with open- or closed-wedge osteotomy to correct angular deformity.
6. Open- or closed-wedge osteotomy to correct angular deformity without operative arrest of the remaining normal physis. The untreated bone bar would reproduce angular deformity after osteotomy. Repeat osteotomy may be required several times prior to attainment of full growth if this method is used alone. Some final relative shortening of the involved bone should be expected.
7. Bone lengthening or bone shortening.
8. Transplantation of an epiphysis and physis from another part of the body to fill a defect in a physis. This has been attempted[33] but was unsuccessful. (This is different from transplantation of an entire epiphysis to take the place of nonexistent epiphysis, which has been performed many times.) With recent advances in microvascular techniques, this method might be reconsidered in isolated cases in the future.
9. Excision of the physeal bar (to be discussed below).
10. Combinations of the above. It is unusual for a patient to be treated optimally by only one of the above modalities. Even when bar excision allows several inches of longitudinal growth, some other modality, such as a shoe lift or closure of the contralateral physis near maturity, is often beneficial.

Leg length discrepancy of 2 cm or less usually causes little if any functional impairment or low back pain and can be left untreated, particularly in a tall person. A shoe lift may be applied on the short side. Leg length discrepancy anticipated to be 5 cm or less at maturity may be managed by arrest of growth of the contralateral bone if the child has sufficient growth remaining to correct the discrepancy. Bone shortening on the contralateral side may be considered if all physes are closed or the child is nearing maturity. Bone shortening should be considered only for the femur, because shortening of the tibia is usually accompanied by uncorrectable muscle weakness, especially of foot dorsiflection. Lengthening of the femur or tibia, or repeated lengthenings, may be considered for shortenings of 5 cm or greater. The anticipated height of the patient at maturity is a factor in making a decision in all these instances, because short people do not readily accept being made shorter.

Arm length discrepancy results in functional impairment only when the discrepancy is extreme. Discrepancies of 9 cm or less are best left untreated. Shortening of the contralateral upper extremity has never been reported and, to my knowledge, has no application. Lengthening of the humerus and forearm has been reported but carries significant potential morbidity and should be done only by surgeons with experience in the procedure.

All the above treatment options have been used in the management of physeal bars and should be considered in every case. When successful, excision of the bar, however, avoids the use of the other modalities and their potential morbidities. If it is used and is unsuccessful, the other options may still be used.

EXCISION OF PHYSEAL BARS

History. Many investigators have performed animal experiments attempting to prevent the formation of a physeal bar (Table 25-1). These experiments have included removal of a portion of the physis from the periphery or the creation of a type IV injury by osteotomy, the interposition of material to prevent physeal bar formation, and observation of subsequent growth.[7–9,12,21,32,39] Although the results have been varied, there has been enough success to suggest that bar formation can be prevented or inhibited. When no interposition material is inserted, bar formation occurs consistently.[21] Cartilage appears to be superior to fat as an interposition material.[21] There are no reports of this procedure being used for humans (*i.e.*, the operative insertion of an interposition material at the time of acute physeal injury in an attempt to prevent subsequent bar formation). Its first application might occur during open reduction of a comminuted type IV injury or when excision of a benign tumor includes loss of normal physis.

Treatment of physeal bars by excision of the bar has an experimental basis. The presence of injured or dead portions of cartilage in an epiphyseal plate has been shown to prevent the formation of a physeal bar following injury.[10,19] It is assumed that the injured portion of the cartilage regenerated from adjacent parts of the growth plate.

Animal experiments have also been performed to excise a bone bar after the creation of it (Table 25-2).[2,8,24,26,34] In all these experiments, a defect was created operatively across the physis to produce a bar at a primary operation, and the bar was resected at a secondary operation. Various interposition materials were used with variable success.

The first case in a human was reported in 1967 by Langenskiöld.[14] It involved a 15-year-old boy with genu recurvatum secondary to a bone bar in the anterior proximal tibia; the etiology was unknown. The bone bar was excised, and the space was filled with autogenous fat. During the 1.5 year follow-up, the angle of genu recurvatum improved 10°, but there was no documentation of longitudinal growth. The first case documenting longitudinal growth was presented more recently.[29] In this case, a tibia grew 16.7 cm after excision of a distal tibial bar in 1968 in a boy 5 years of age; follow-up was for 10 years. Sheet Silastic and Gelfoam were used as interposition materials.

Multiple series of cases have since been reported in which several different interposition materials were used. Fat,[14,16–18,20,38] bone wax and fat,[37] Silastic,[3,4] and methyl methacrylate[13,22,23,37] appear to be the most popular. There are not enough cases followed to maturity in these studies to permit assessment of superiority of one interposition material over the others.

Table 25-1. Experimental Insertion of an Interposition Material Across a Defect in the Physis to Prevent Bone Bar Formation

Year	Investigator	Interposition Material	Animal	Site
1878	Vogt[39]	Gold leaf	Goat	Proximal tibia
		Rubber film	Dog	Distal radius
1956	Ford and Key[7]	Gelfoam	Rabbit	Distal femur
1956	Friedenberg and Brashear[9]	Bone wax	Rabbit	Distal femur
1957	Friedenberg[8]	Bone wax	Rabbit	Distal femur
		Methyl methacrylate	Rabbit	Distal femur
1958	Key and Ford[12]	Bone wax	Rabbit	Distal femur
1970	Serafin[32]	Bone wax	Rabbit	Distal femur
		Muscle	Rabbit	Distal femur
1983	Lennox *et al*[21]	None	Rabbit	Distal femur
		Fat	Rabbit	Distal femur
		Cartilage	Rabbit	Distal femur

Table 25-2. Experimental Insertion of an Interposition Material After Excision of a Bone Bar to Prevent Bar Reformation

Year	Investigator	Interposition Material	Animal	Site
1957	Friedenberg[8]	Bone wax	Rabbit	Distal femur
1969	Nordentoft[24]	None	Rabbit	Proximal tibia
1972	Österman[26]	Fat	Rabbit	Distal femur
		Cartilage	Rabbit	Distal femur
		Bone wax	Rabbit	Distal femur
1974	Bright[2]	Silicone-rubber	Dog	Distal femur
		Silicone-adhesive	Dog	Distal femur
		Isobutyl cyanoacrylate	Dog	Distal femur
1982	Sudmann *et al*[34]	None	Rabbit	Distal femur

Interposition Materials. Fat has the distinct advantage of being autogenous. Usually, enough fat can be found in the same incision to fill the defect, although sometimes additional fat must be obtained from another site of the body, such as the buttocks. No foreign material is inserted. Fat has the disadvantage of lack of hemostasis in the resected cavity. When the tourniquet is released, fat tends to float out of the cavity. Closing periosteum over the cavity to contain the fat predisposes to new bone formation peripherally. This is undesirable because it tends to tether growth again. The operative defect weakens the structure of the bone, and it is best to protect a weightbearing bone from fracture.[37] The final fate of large cavities in the metaphysis filled with fat is not yet known. One, in a distal femur, resulted in pathologic fracture.[18] Gradual ossification seems to occur.

Silastic is inert, nonreactive, and virtually unaffected by long-term exposure within the body. When mixed with a catalyst, silicone-rubber monomer vulcanizes. While it is in the semipolymerized state, the silicone-rubber can be molded and pressed into the surgical defect so as to assume the exact form of the cavity. It must remain in direct contact with the exposed physis to prevent bar re-formation. Sterilization of both the monomer and the catalyst is done by recipe the night before. A culture is taken of the Silastic after mxing but before insertion during the operation. Postoperative infection has been reported.[4] The implant is free-floating and easily removed later. It is a Food and Drug Administration (FDA)–controlled substance, and its use requires authorization (Investigational New Drug Number must be obtained) and detailed postoperative follow-up records. The substance recommended by Bright[3,4] is Silastic elastomer No. 382 (Dow Corning).

Methyl methacrylate is light, thermally nonconductive, transparent, and easy to mold. Both the liquid (monomer) and the powder (polymer) are sterile as packaged and may be mixed in the operating room. It is unnecessary to take cultures. It has had wide clinical trial in both neurosurgery and orthopaedics since its first use in humans in 1940. When used as an isolated substance, it has caused no rejection, infection, or neoplastic change.[5] Because the solid substance fills the cavity, there is excellent hemostasis. There is no bone weakening, thus no postoperative protection of the extremity is necessary. It may be the material of choice to support the epiphysis after considerable excavation of a bone bar.[37] Barium has been added to the methyl methacrylate used by most orthopaedists for ease in identifying it radiographically. For bar resection, cranioplast* has the advantage of not containing barium, thus being radiolucent. Postoperative bar re-formation, therefore, can be more easily identified. It is easily obtainable and is not an FDA–controlled substance.

A recent study of rabbits suggests that reformation of a bar after excision can be inhibited by the use of indomethacin given orally without the use of an interposition material.[34] Indomethacin has been shown to result in a nonspecific inhibition of the osteoblastic activity that is triggered by fracture or postoperative inflammation. Whether indomethacin can be

*Cranioplastic, manufactured by L.D. Caulk Company (Milford, DE, 19963); distributed by Codman and Shurtleff, Inc. (Randolph, MA, 02368)

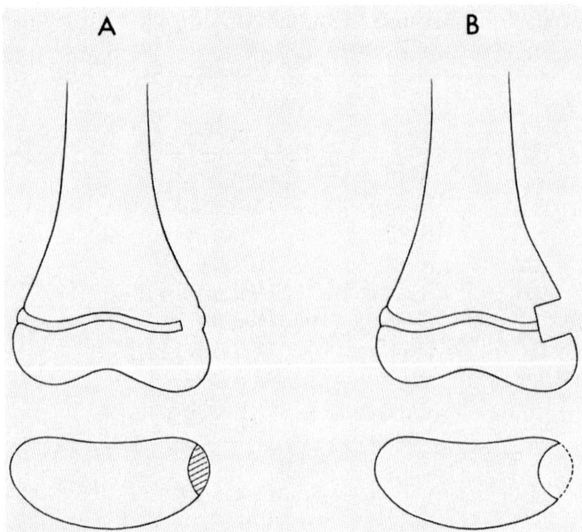

Fig. 25-4. Peripheral bar shown in anteroposterior view above transverse section through physis *(below)*. *(A)* With map of bar composed from tomograms. *(B)* Bar excised by direct approach.

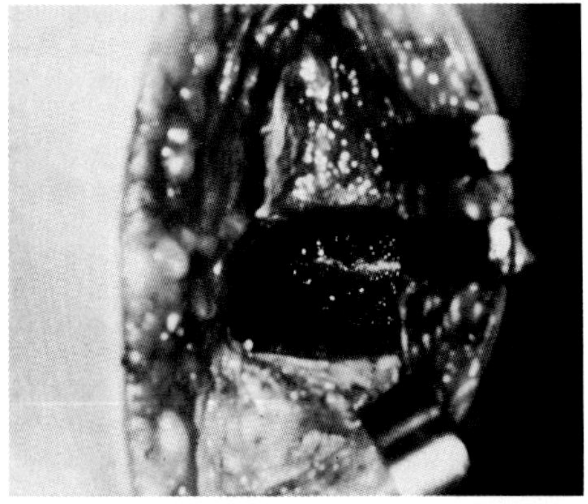

Fig. 25-5. Operative photograph. The thin transverse white line in the depth of the cavity is the physis, with adjacent metaphysis and epiphysis.

given in sufficient doses in humans to prevent bone bar re-formation without inhibiting normal bone growth remains to be seen.

Technique. The objectives of surgical excision of a bone bar are to remove the bar completely and to preserve as much of the normal remaining physis as possible. This requires careful preoperative evaluation and planning and may be difficult if the bar is irregular or if there are multiple or satellite bars.

Peripherally located bars should be approached directly from the periphery (Fig. 25-4). Any periosteum overlying the bar should be excised. Under direct vision, the bar can be removed from inside-out until normal physis can be visualized on all sides of the cavity (Fig. 25-5). Although an operating microscope has been used,[16,18,20,37] I have not found this to be helpful. Some surgeons may prefer optical loupes. The bone bar may be removed by using an osteotome, curet, and rongeur but is most precisely removed with a motorized burr. This allows excellent visualization of the physis, removal of as little normal physis as necessary, and removal of as little metaphyseal bone as necessary, and it facilitates contouring of the cavity in the epiphysis. The heat from the burr has no apparent deleterious effect on the viability of the remaining physis.

Bars that extend completely across the physis (common after type IV fractures) require careful evaluation of the tomographic maps to determine surgical approach and to ensure complete removal of the bar (Fig. 25-6).

Centrally located bars that have normal physis peripherally and an intact perichondrial ring of Ranvier should not be approached from the periphery so that an attempt is made to save these structures (Fig. 25-7*A*). These bars should be approached through the metaphysis or the epiphysis. Although theoretically desirable because it has the potential to leave little if any interposition material in the metaphysis, the transepiphyseal approach is seldom used, particulary if there is tenting or cupping, because the bar is not readily accessible and because this usually requires traversing the joint. The transmetaphyseal approach requires removing a window of cortical bone and a fair amount of cancellous metaphyseal bone before the physeal bar can be reached (Fig. 25-7*B*). After removal of the entire bar, the normal physis must be visualized circumferentially in the cavity. This may be accomplished by the use of a small (5 mm diameter) dental mirror (Fig. 25-8*A*). The use of an operating microscope would be technically difficult in these cases. An intracavity light is often helpful.*

Metal markers should be placed in the metaphysis and epiphysis (Fig. 25-9*A*). This is the only way to measure subsequent growth of the involved physis accurately. Without these markers, overgrowth of the physis at the other end of the bone may falsely enhance the result. These markers should be placed in

*Flexi-Lum, flexible surgical light from Concept, Inc. (12707 U.S. 19 South, Clearwater, FL 33519)

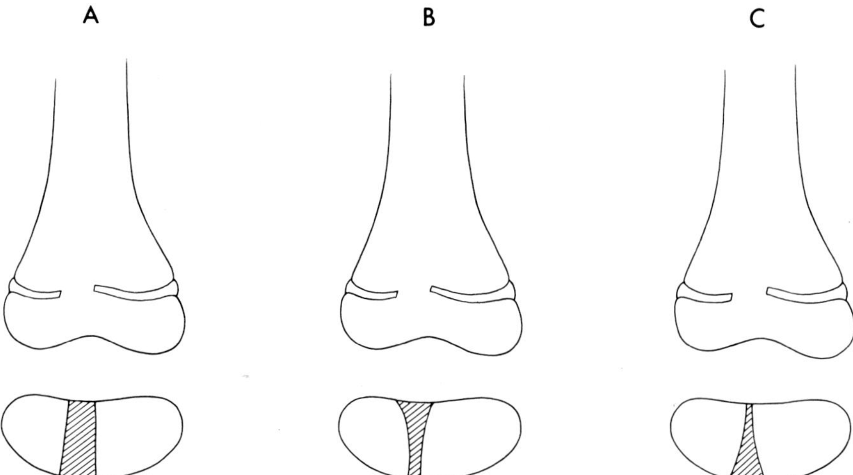

FIG. 25-6. Elongated bar extending from anterior to posterior surfaces. Although these three bars have the same appearance on the anteroposterior view *(above)*, they have different contours and areas on the transverse sections *(below)*. In order to achieve complete bar removal with retention of as much normal physis as possible, the bar in *C* would optimally be approached anteriorly, and that in *B*, posteriorly.

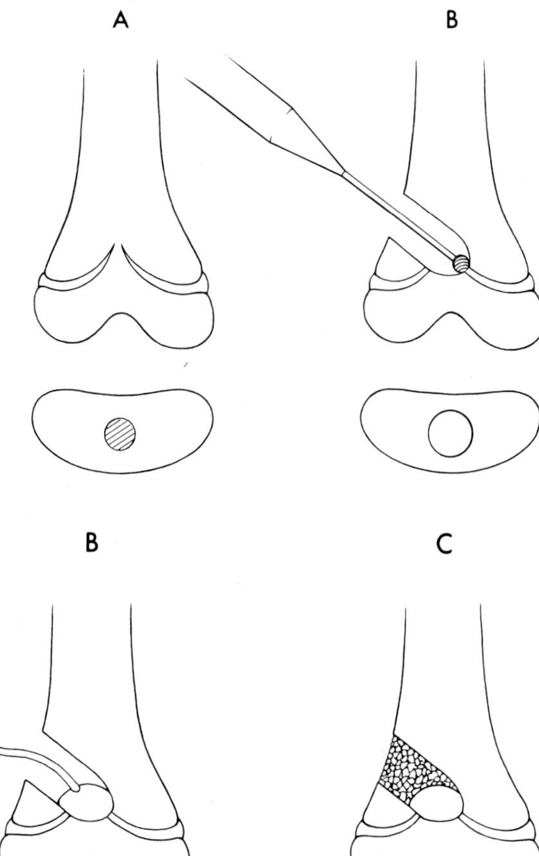

FIG. 25-7. Central bar. *(A)* Bar in center with growth peripherally results in "tenting" or "cupping" of the physis. *(B)* Excision of central bar through window in metaphysis.

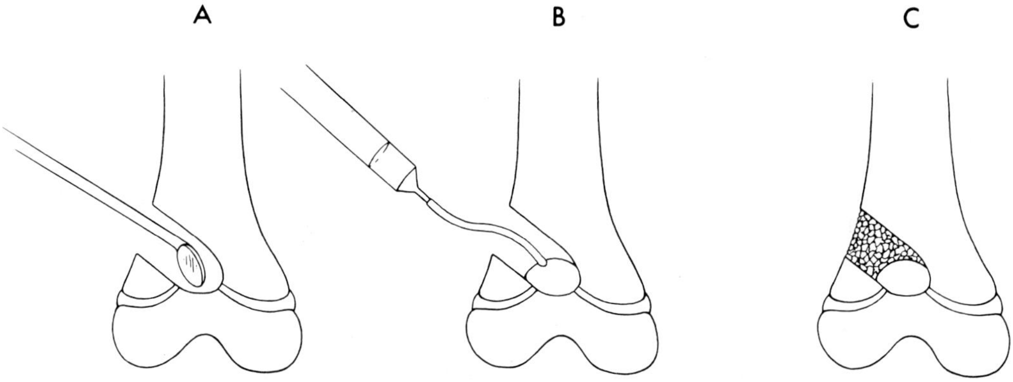

A B C

FIG. 25-8. Technique of excision of central bar. *(A)* Visualization of entire physis with dental mirror. *(B)* Insertion of only enough cranioplast, by use of syringe and catheter, to bridge all physeal surfaces. *(C)* Remainder of defect filled with bone grafts.

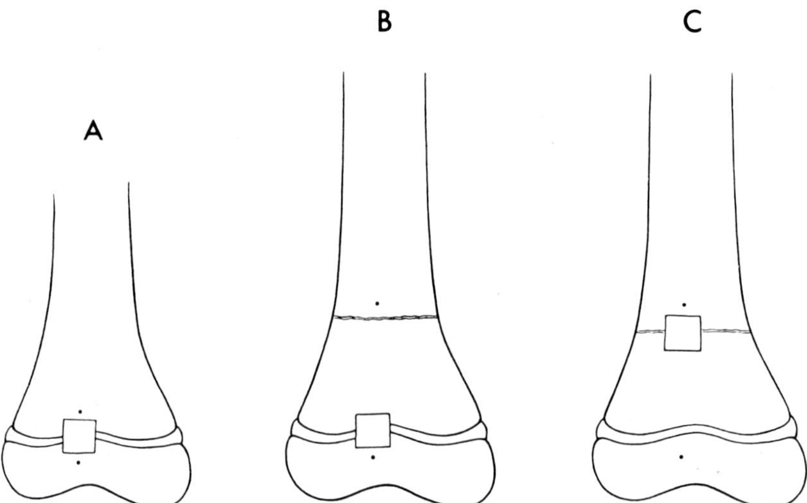

FIG. 25-9. Metal markers. *(A)* Placement of markers in cancellous bone of metaphysis and epiphysis away from the interposition plug and longitudinally oriented to each other. *(B)* The plug has stayed with the epiphysis, growing away from the proximal marker and growth arrest line. *(C)* The plug stayed with the metaphysis as the epiphysis grew.

cancellous bone, not in contact with the cavity, because they might become attached to the interposition material or, if fat is used, they might migrate into the cavity. The markers should be in the same longitudinal plane proximally and distally to the defect. Any metal marker will do; half of a silver clip works nicely. Transversely oriented Kirschner wires parallel with each other and with the physis, one in the metaphysis and one in the epiphysis, allow more accurate assessment of angular growth (see Fig. 3*I, J, K*).

For an interposition material, I prefer cranioplast because of its easy availability (no second incision is needed as for fat; no FDA control, as for Silastic), handling properties, hemostasis (by virtue of occupying the entire desired portion of the cavity), strength, and absence of side effects.

In a large cavity that is gravity-dependent, cranioplast can be poured in a liquid state. If the cavity is not in a dependent position, the cranioplast may be placed in a syringe and pushed into the defect through a short polyethylene tube (Fig. 25-8*B*). The cranioplast can also be allowed to set partially and then be pushed into the defect like putty. As little cranioplast as possible should be allowed to remain in the metaphysis. After the cranioplast has set, the remainder of the metaphyseal cavity should be filled with cancellous bone previously removed (Fig. 25-8*C*).

The sides of the cavity should be flat and smooth (Fig. 25-10*A*). Undermining the metaphyseal and epiphyseal bone away from the physis, as advocated by Odgen,[25] may be beneficial in reducing the likelihood of bar re-formation if fat is used as interposition material but would only act as a tether when a solid interposition is used (Fig. 25-10*C*). In addition, the protruding physis would be deprived of its blood supply, and more of the physis would have been removed than is necessary.

The contour of the cavity may be important. Bar re-formation is less likely when the interposition material (plug) remains in the epiphysis (Fig. 25-9*B* and 25-11) than when the epiphysis grows away from it; Figs. 25-9*C* and 25-12).* Therefore, various techniques have been used in attempts to keep the plug in the epiphysis. Drill holes in the cavity of the epiphysis allow "pods" of cranioplast to act as anchors (Fig. 25-10*B*). Perhaps the easiest technique is to enlarge the cavity in the epiphysis like half of a collar button, maintaining a rim of bone next to the physis for vascular nourishment (Fig. 25-13*A*). Placing Kirschner wires through methacrylate, as it is setting,

*Klassen RA, Peterson HA: Unpublished data

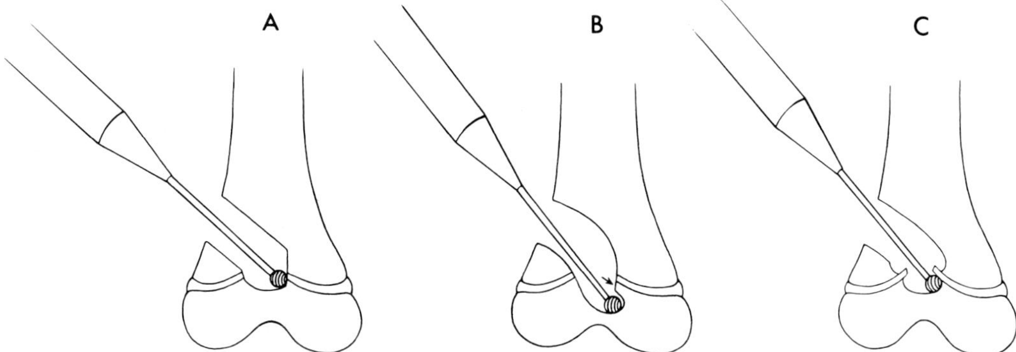

FIG. 25-10. Contour of cavity. *(A)* As normal physis is exposed, the adjacent metaphyseal bone surface should be smoothed to help prevent the plug from staying with the metaphysis. *(B)* Bone in the epiphysis is undermined in an attempt to allow the plug to stay with the epiphysis. If this is done, a small rim of epiphyseal bone should be preserved to maintain viability of the physis *(arrow)*. *(C)* Undermining bone away from the physis should be avoided, because the protruding physis would be deprived of its blood supply and prevented from growing inward over the plug as the epiphysis grows distally.

into the epiphysis is effective in keeping the plug with the epiphysis but makes removal of the plug at a later time very difficult, if this should become necessary. I therefore would not recommend it.

The most important feature of the technique involves the growth of the remaining physis. Presumably, as the epiphysis and its retained interposition material advance, the edges of the physis in contact with the plug grow inward over the top of the plug (Fig. 25-13*B*). This has never been proved because biopsy of this area would be contraindicated if it is growing. Thus, it becomes important to have the metaphyseal portion of the plug as small, smooth, and regular in outline as possible. A large metaphyseal portion of plug predisposes to the epiphysis growing away from the plug (Fig. 25-13*C*). Theoretically, an elongated, tapered plug would require less physeal cartilage ingrowth as the plug moves with the epiphysis (Fig. 25-13*D*). Because of the difficulty in creating such a defect in living bone, this has not yet been attempted.

Mild angular deformity secondary to peripheral bars often corrects spontaneously with growth after excision of the bar (Figs. 25-11*E*, 25-12*G*). Angular deformities greater than 20° will probably not correct spontaneously and usually require osteotomy.[13] This may be performed at the same time as bar excision or later.

Postoperatively, joint motion may be begun immediately if cranioplast is inserted. In the absence of concomitant osteotomy, no cast or other immobilization is necessary. Weight-bearing is encouraged on the day of operation or as soon as operative discomfort subsides.

Follow-up. Follow-up must be continued until maturity. Re-established physeal growth may cease at any time. Recurrent bar formation has been successfully treated by re-excision of the bar.* If a bar re-forms near maturity or if the entire physis ceases growing on the injured side earlier than its contralateral counterpart (a fairly frequent finding), physeal arrest on the contralateral side may be considered.

Scanograms are the most precise way to measure the increasing distance between the two metal markers. As the child grows, the circumference of the extremity enlarges, allowing magnification of the distance between the markers on regular roentgenograms, teloroentgenograms, and orthoroentgenograms. Scanograms have no magnification. In addition, as the markers grow further apart, regular roentgenograms, teloroentgenograms, and orthoroentgenograms magnify this distance, falsely enhancing the result.

It is suspected that the physis on the opposite end of an injured or operated bone will sometimes "overgrow" to compensate for any damage at the other end.[11] Although the amount of growth of bone attributable to each physis has been fairly well established (distal femur,

*Klassen RA, Peterson HA: Unpublished data

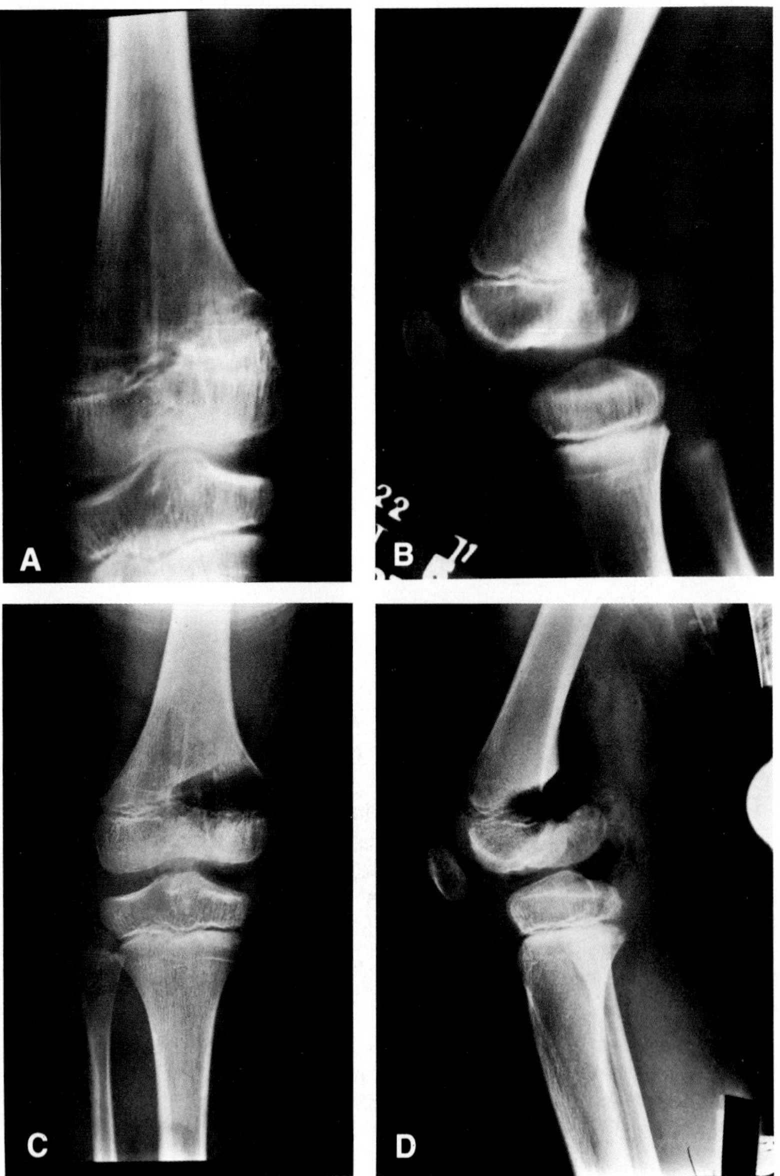

FIG. 25-11. Boy (age 8 years 8 months) sustained an undisplaced Salter-Harris-type III fracture of the right medial condyle. After subsequent bar formation and excision, the plug stayed with the epiphysis (see Fig. 25-9*B*). No metal markers were inserted in this early case. (*A* and *B*) Right knee 1 year 2 months after injury (age 9 years 10 months) shows physeal bar posteromedially with varus and posterior angulation of the physes. (*C* and *D*) Excision of peripheral bar (age 9 years 11 months) by direct approach (see Fig. 25-4). Drill holes into the epiphysis helped to anchor the plug in the epiphysis; the metaphyseal surface was made smooth. No cast was used postoperatively.

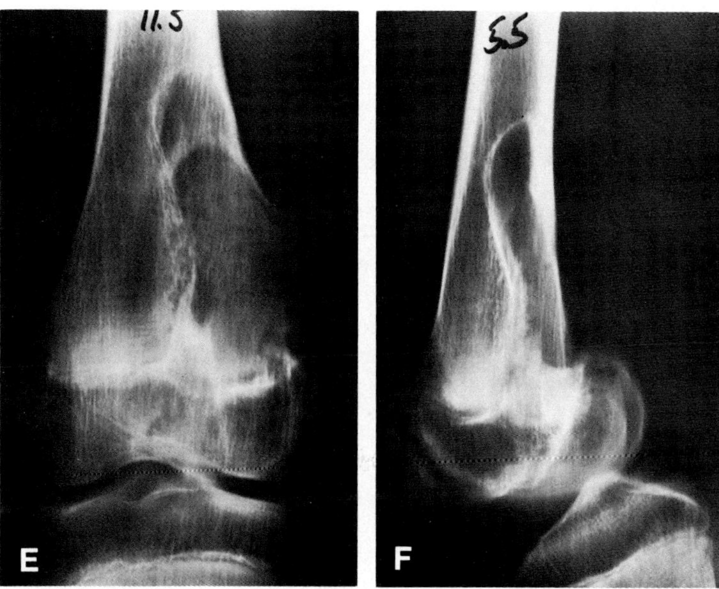

FIG. 25-11. *(Cont.) (E* and *F)* At 4 years 6 months after bar excision (age 14 years 5 months), the right femur has grown 10.9 cm and the normal left femur has grown 11.5 cm (the right has grown 94% as much as the left). Note that the plug has remained with the epiphysis, leaving a trail of lytic-appearing bone (presumably fibrous tissue) behind. No fracture has occurred in this or similar cases. The lytic-appearing bone gradually assumed a normal appearance. Note the spontaneous correction of the varus angulation without osteotomy (compare with Fig. 25-11*A*).

70%; proximal tibia, 60%; distal tibia, 40%; etc.), the only way to determine precisely the amount and percentage of growth contributed by each physis of a bone after bar excision, compared with its contralateral member, is to place a single metal marker in the diaphysis of the normal contralateral bone. This has been performed in two cases, but it will take years of follow-up to determine whether this will be useful clinical information.*

Results From 1968 through 1982, 71 cases have been treated by bar excision at the Mayo Clinic.* Cranioplast was used for the interposition material in 68 cases, bone wax and fat in 2 cases, and sheet Silastic and Gelfoam in 1 case (this case has been reported[29]). All operations were performed by three staff pediatric orthopaedists with little variation in technique.

In one case of both proximal and distal tibial bar formation following irradiation for sarcoma of the fibula, there was no growth after bar excision at each site. Although the remaining physis appeared normal radiographically, it may have had no potential for growth due to radiation damage. In all other cases, there was some growth after bar excision. This has also been found to be true by other investigators.[18,37] This renewed growth may diminish the angular deformity and the rate of progression of limb length inequality, and, occasionally, there may even be reduction of the length inequality (the treated limb growing faster than the normal limb).

Excision of bars constituting 50% or more of the entire physis does not give good results. It appears that the remaining physis cannot grow inward completely across the defect to allow predictably satisfactory longitudinal growth. It is now my preference to perform bar excision only if the area of the bar is 50% or less of the entire physis.

The growth of the bone operated on as a percentage of the growth of the normal bone has varied from 0 to 200%, with a mean average of 94%.[13] if only those cases that are followed to maturity are included, the mean value is 84%. It appeared that some physes, although

*Klassen RA, Peterson HA: Unpublished data

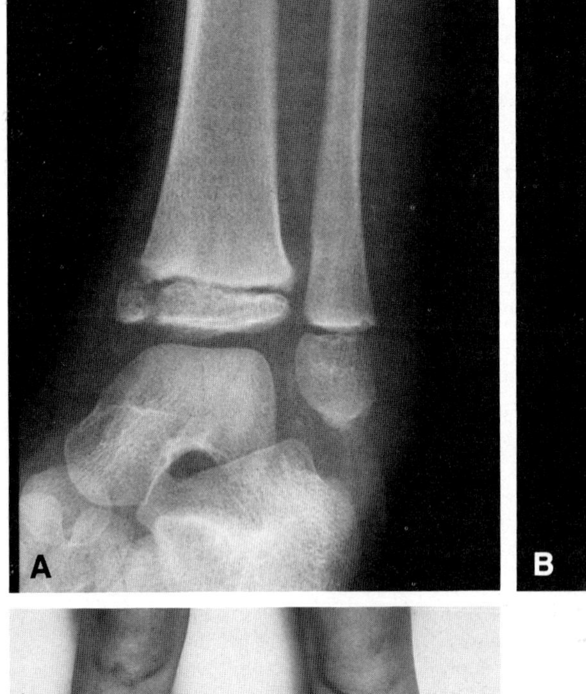

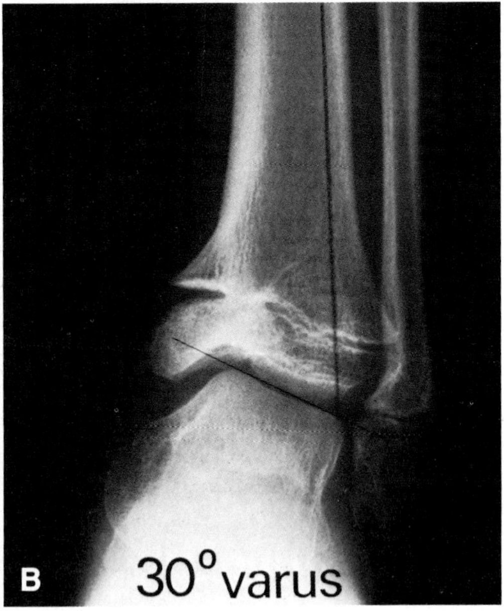

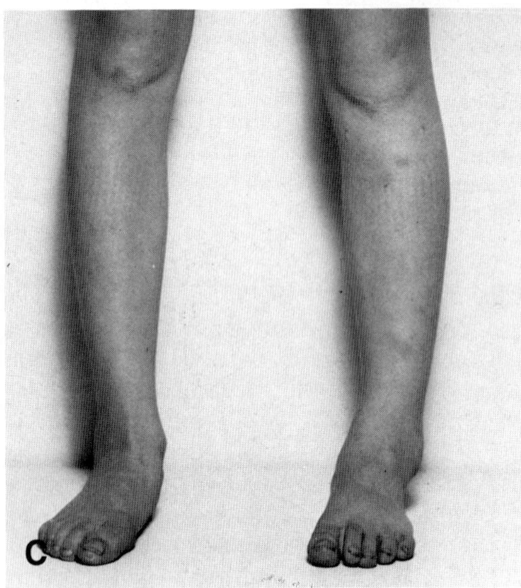

FIG. 25-12 Girl (age 7 years 5 months) sustained a mildly displaced Salter-Harris-type IV fracture of the distal left tibia. After subsequent bar formation and excision, the plug stayed with the metaphysis (see Fig. 25-9*C*). *(A)* Fracture of medial malleolus at age 7 years 5 months, treated by cast for 6 weeks. *(B)* Bar formation with 30° ankle valgus, 2 years 6 months later (age 10 years 1 month). *(C)* Clinical appearance at same time as *B*. Left tibia was 12 mm shorter than the right by scanogram.

growing well during active growth, closed earlier than their contralateral physes near the end of growth. In some of these cases, there was operative physeal arrest of the contralateral bone toward the end of growth to produce the final length equalization. This favorably influences the result expressed as a percentage. Cases in which metal markers were inserted (which gives the absolute growth following bar excision) are currently being analyzed.

A troublesome and undesirable occurrence is bar re-formation. This tends to occur more frequently in cases in which the physis grows away from the plug (see Fig. 25-9*C*) than when the plug stays with the physis (see Fig. 25-9*B*). Perhaps the use of oral indomethacin therapy in conjunction with an interposition material would decrease this occurrence.

Criteria for subsequent removal of interposition material have not been established. If the physis grows away from the interposition material, the material becomes embedded in the metaphysis. As the metaphysis remodels, the interposition material, although remaining the same size, occupies a greater proportion of the transverse plane of the shaft of the

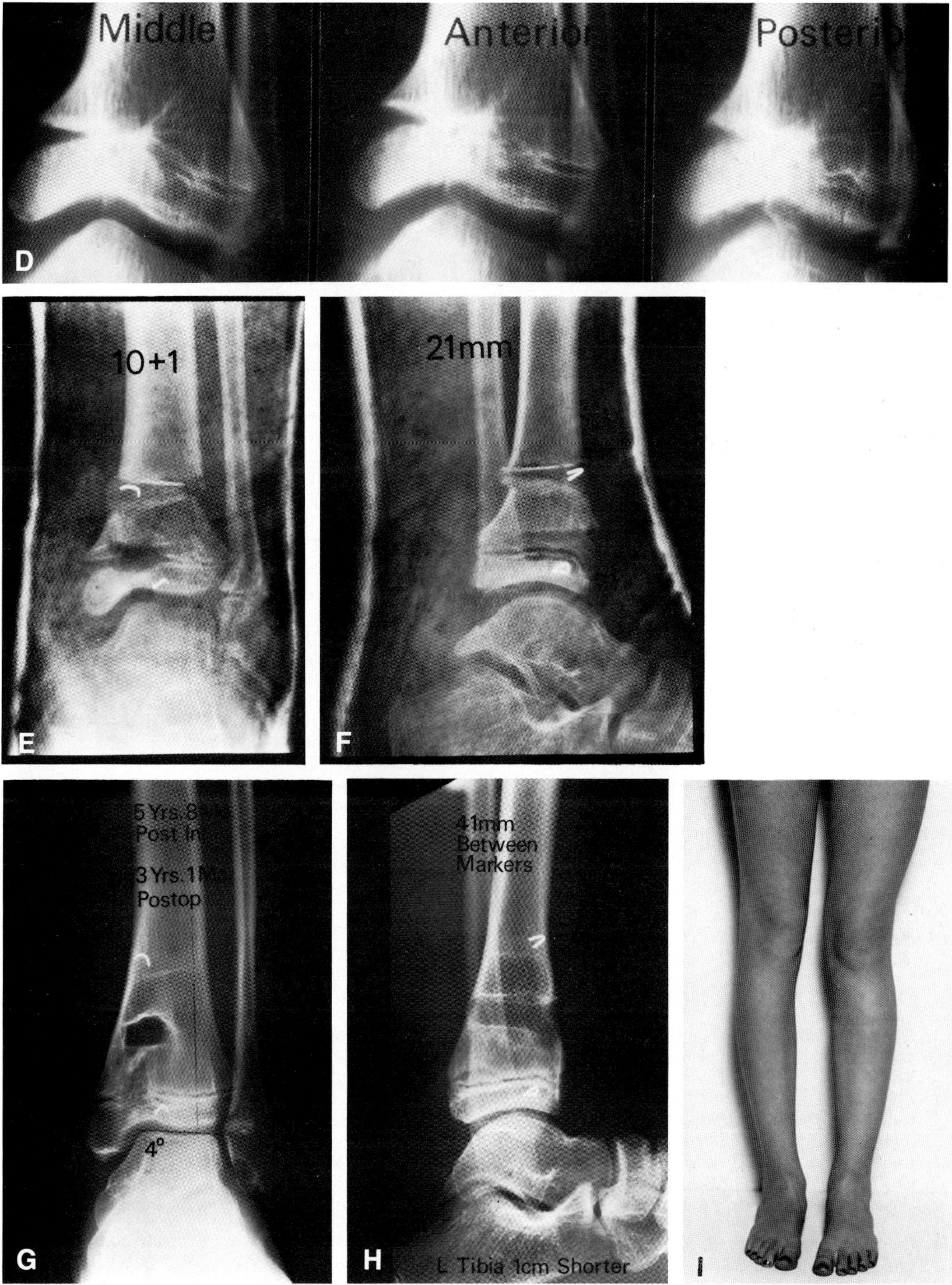

FIG. 25-12 (Cont.) *(D)* Tomograms show elongated bar from anterior to posterior (see Fig. 25-6*A*). *(E* and *F)* Bar excision by tunnel technique from periphery to periphery at age 10 years 1 month. Distal tibial open-wedge osteotomy, held open with autogenous iliac crest bone, corrected 20° of the 30° varus angulation. The metal markers are 21 mm apart. A cast was used because of the osteotomy. *(G* and *H)* At 3 years 1 month postoperatively (age 13 years 3 months), the plug remains in the metaphysis (see Fig. 25-9*C*), the metal markers are 41 mm apart, and the varus has diminished from 10° to 4° (the contralateral normal ankle also measured 4° varus). *(I)* Clinical appearance at age 13 years 4 months. Scanograms show the left tibia to be 10 mm shorter than the right.

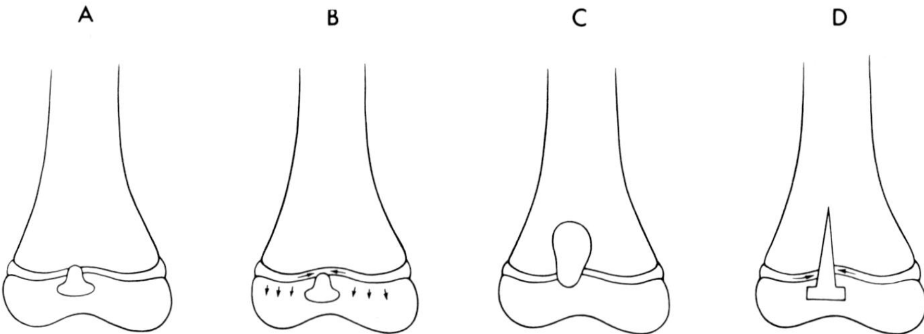

FIG. 25-13. Contour of plug *(A)* "Collar button" contour anchors bone in epiphysis and leaves as little plug as in metaphysis. *(B)* As the epiphysis grows distally, the physis grows inward over the metaphyseal portion of the plug. *(C)* The metaphyseal portion of the plug is larger than the epiphyseal portion; it will stay with the metaphysis. *(D)* Elongated contour (theoretical) would require slow physeal ingrowth as the plug, anchored in the epiphysis, moves with the epiphysis.

bone. Theoretically, this may predispose to pathologic fracture, but it has not yet been observed to do so. Patients should be advised that the interposition material may have to be removed in the future. All cranioplast plugs have been firmly embedded in the bone; there has been no loosening as is seen when used with a prosthesis. In the few that have been removed, histologic evaluation has revealed only a thin surrounding layer of fibrous tissue and no untoward reaction. The material is not easily removed, and usually a thin area of surrounding bone must be excised. The Midas Rex burr has been used to remove craniplast plugs from inside-out in a few recent cases.

REFERENCES

1. Barash ES, Siffert RS: The potential for growth of experimentally produced hemiepiphysis. J Bone Joint Surg [Am] 48:1548, 1966
2. Bright RW: Operative correction of partial epiphyseal plate closure by osseous-bridge resection and silicone-rubber implant: an experimental study in dogs. J Bone Joint Surg [Am] 56:655, 1974
3. Bright RW: Surgical correction of partial growth plate closure, laboratory and clinical experience. Orthop Rev 8:149, 1978
4. Bright RW: Partial growth arrest: identification, classification, and results of treatment (Abstr). Orthop Trans 6:65, 1982
5. Cabanela ME, Coventry MB, MacCarty CS, Miller WE: The fate of patients with methyl methacrylate cranioplasty. J Bone Joint Surg [Am] 54:278, 1972
6. Caffey J: Traumatic cupping of the metaphyses of growing bones. Am J Roentgenol 108:451, 1970
7. Ford LT, Key JA: A study of experimental trauma to the distal femoral epiphysis in rabbits. J Bone Joint Surg [Am] 38:84, 1956
8. Friedenberg ZB: Reaction of the epiphysis to partial surgical resection. J Bone Joint Surg [Am] 39:332, 1957
9. Friedenberg ZB, Brashear R: Bone growth following partial resection of the epiphyseal cartilage. Am J Surg 91:362, 1956
10. Heikel HVA: Experimental epiphyseal transplantation. Part II. Histological observations. Acta Orthop Scand 30:1, 1960–1961
11. Heikel HVA: Has epiphyseodesis in one end of a long bone a growth-stimulating effect on the other end? An experimental study. Acta Orthop Scand 31:18, 1961
12. Key JA, Ford LT: A study of experimental trauma to the distal femoral epiphysis in rabbits—II. J Bone Joint Surg [Am] 40:887, 1958
13. Klassen RA, Peterson HA: Excision of physeal bars: the Mayo Clinic experience 1968–1978 (Abstr). Orthop Trans 6:65, 1982
14. Langenskiöld A: The possibilities of eliminating premature partial closure of an epiphyseal plate caused by trauma or disease. Acta Orthop Scand 38:267, 1967
15. Langenskiöld A: Traumatic premature closure of the distal tibial epiphyseal plate. Acta Orthop Scand 38:520, 1967
16. Langenskiöld A: An operation for partial closure of an epiphyseal plate in children and its experimental basis. J Bone Joint Surg [Br] 57:325, 1975
17. Langenskiöld A: Partial closure of epiphyseal plate: principles of treatment. Int Orthop 2:95, 1978
18. Langenskiöld A: Surgical treatment of partial closure of the growth plate. J Pediatr Orthop 1:3, 1981
19. Langenskiöld A, Edgren W: Imitation of chondrodysplasia by localized roentgen ray injury—an experimental study of bone growth. Acta Chir Scand 99:353, 1949–1950
20. Langenskiöld A, Österman K: Surgical treatment of partial closure of the epiphyseal plate. Reconstr Surg Traumatol 17:48, 1979
21. Lennox DW, Goldner RD, Sussman MD: Cartilage as an interposition material to prevent transphyseal bone bridge formation: an experimental model. J Pediatr Orthop 3:207, 1983

22. Mallet J: Les épiphysiodèses partielles traumatiques de l'extrémetié inférieure du tibia chez l'enfant: leur traitement avec désépiphysiodèse. Rev Chir Orthop 61:5, 1975
23. Mallet J, Rey JC: Traitement des épiphysiodèses partielles traumatiques chez l'enfant par désépiphysiodèse. Int Orthop 1:309, 1978
24. Nordentoft EL: Experimental epiphyseal injuries: grading of traumas and attempts at treating traumatic epiphyseal arrest in animals. Acta Orthop Scand 40:176, 1969
25. Ogden JA: Skeletal Injury in the Child. Philadelphia, Lea & Febiger, 1982
26. Österman K: Operative elimination of partial premature epiphyseal closure: an experimental study. Acta Orthop Scand [Suppl] 147:1, 1972
27. Pease CN: Focal retardation and arrestment of growth of bones due to vitamin A intoxication. JAMA 182:980, 1962
28. Peterson CA, Peterson HA: Analysis of the incidence of injuries to the epiphyseal growth plate. J Trauma 12:275, 1972
29. Peterson HA: Operative correction of post-fracture arrest of the epiphyseal plate: case report with 10-year follow-up. J Bone Joint Surg [Am] 62:1018, 1980
30. Peterson HA, Burkhart SS: Compression injury of the epiphyseal growth plate: fact or fiction? J Pediatr Orthop 1:377, 1981
31. Salter RB, Harris WR: Injuries involving the epiphyseal plate. J Bone Joint Surg [Am] 45:587, 1963
32. Serafin J: Zaburzenia wzrostu po doświadczalnym podużnym przecieciu nasady i przynasady rosnacej kości dugiej. Chir Narsadow Ruchu Orthop Pol 35:325, 1970
33. Spira E, Farin I: Epiphyseal transplantation: a case report. J Bone Joint Surg [Am] 46:1278, 1964
34. Sudmann E, Husby OS, Bang G: Inhibition of partial closure of epiphyseal plate in rabbits by indomethacin. Acta Orthop Scand 53:507, 1982
35. Tanner JM, Whitehouse RH, Marshall WA, Heally MJR, Goldstein H: Assessment of Skeletal Maturity and Prediction of Adult Height (TW2 Method). London, Academic Press, 1975
36. Troupp H: Nervous and vascular influence on longitudinal growth of bone: an experimental study on rabbits. Acta Orthop Scand [Suppl] 51:1, 1961
37. Vickers DW: Premature incomplete fusion of the growth plate: causes and treatment by resection (physolysis) in 15 cases. Aust NZ J Surg 50:393, 1980
38. Visser JD, Nielsen HKL: Operative correction of abnormal central epiphyseal closure by transmetaphyseal bone-bridge resection and implantation of fat. Netherlands J Surg 33 (3):140, 1981
39. Vogt P: Die traumatische Epiphysentrennung und deren Einfluss auf das Längenwachsthum der Röhrenknochen. Arch Klin Chir 22:343, 1878
40. Walter E, Feine U, Anger K, Schweizer P, Neugebauer W: Szintigraphische Diagnostik und Verlaufskontrolle bei Epiphysenfugenverletzungen. Fortschr Geb Rontgenstr Nuklearmed Erganzungsband 132:309, 1980
41. Wiss DA: Metaphyseal cupping: a case report. Orthopedics 4:649, 1981

26

Overuse Injuries In Children

Lyle J. Micheli

Musculoskeletal injuries to children have traditionally been the result of single-impact macrotrauma, such as a fall or twist resulting in injuries to bones, joints, and soft tissues of the extremities or axial skeleton. The more traditional approach to trauma in children has invariably assumed this mechanism of injury. A text on pediatric trauma will review injuries resulting from motor vehicle accidents, falls, and biking accidents and equate these, in a reflex fashion, with pediatric injury.

More recently, however, there has been a growing incidence of a whole new genre of injuries occurring in children. These have as a common factor their mechanism of injury. These injuries are the result of repetitive microtrauma, such as repetitively swinging an arm back and forth over the head as in painting or throwing, and repetitive movements of the lower extremities, such as bending and rising in work activities or running along the ground in sports activities. As a group, these injuries have been labeled the "overuse" injuries.

There is no question that the increased involvement of people of all ages, sizes, and shapes in organized sports and fitness activities has dramatically increased the incidence of overuse injuries.[5] In the past, these overuse injuries were the bane of the recreational adult athlete but were rarely encountered in the child. The assumption was that these injuries reflected a breakdown of the "aged" tissues of the often inadequately trained or maintained adult, who often participated in athletics at infrequent intervals, without regular training—the "weekend warrior" syndrome.

In the pediatric age group, the growing involvement of children in organized sports and fitness activities has also been paralleled by an increased number and, in some cases, new types of these overuse injuries. Unfortunately, good epidemiologic data are not yet available to compare the rates of injuries in sports with the rates in free-play activities for children.[27,47] When impact or single macrotrauma injuries are compared, there is certainly no clear evidence that organized sports are more dangerous or safer than free play. Children can break their arms while playing football or by falling out of a tree, and the relative risk may be similar.[11]

When the overuse injuries are compared, however, there is no doubt whatsoever that the repetitive training activities of children engaged in organized sports or fitness have resulted in a whole new genre of injuries that have rarely occurred in the free-play situation. These overuse injuries—the tendonitis of the shoulder, elbow, ankles, or hips; the stress fractures; and, in particular, the patellofemoral stress syndromes about the knee—are invariably related to repetitive training activities that are usually encountered in the organized sports situation.

As with similar adult injuries, the role of maltraining, usually too much over too short a period of time, appears to be common to most of these pediatric overuse injuries. It now appears that this overuse phenomenon can even affect the very young child. Aging, although perhaps still a factor in susceptibility to overuse injury, is probably less important than it was once thought.

The physician dealing with young athletes

must become intimately aware of the stresses and special potential for injury inherent in each particular sport. The sport that can be used as an example of this process is gymnastics. High-impact traumatic injuries can certainly occur in gymnastics. Snook[55] found that approximately two thirds of gymnastics injuries in a collegiate level competition were traumatic in origin. However, repetitive microtrauma from gymnastics training also results in a significant number of overuse injuries to these young athletes. The physician dealing with these gymnastics-injured children must be particularly aware of the potential for this type of injury.

Goldberg,[16] in a recent review of gymnastics injuries, found a great variety of special overuse-induced injuries, including stress fractures of the carpal bone, dorsal capsulitis of the wrist, medial epicondylitis of the elbow, and a variety of lower extremity overuse injuries, including Osgood-Schlatter disease, stress fractures, and os calcis apophysitis. Kirby and colleagues[31] reviewed overuse injuries in female gymnasts and compared them with age- and height-matched groups of sedentary girls. He found that the gymnasts had a significantly higher incidence of wrist, low back, shin, and foot symptoms. In addition, several studies have suggested that female gymnasts have a much higher incidence of spondylolytic stress fractures of the lumbar spine.[26] The suggested mechanism in these children was a fracture of the pars intra-articularis caused by repetitive flexion or extension of the lumbar spine. Axial rotation of the lumbar spine may also play a role in the occurrence of lesions in these young gymnasts. It is evident that the physician dealing with young gymnasts must be aware of the particular potential for overuse injuries in this population if they are to be diagnosed and managed effectively.

ETIOLOGY: RISK FACTORS

In our own sports medicine clinic, we have found the use of the following checklist of risk factors helpful in determining the etiology of a given overuse injury and as a first step in determining ways of preventing the occurrence or recurrence of other overuse injuries in the young athlete.

1. Training errors, including abrupt changes in intensity, duration, and frequency of training.
2. Musculotendinous imbalance of strength, flexibility, or bulk.
3. Anatomic malalignment of the lower extremities, including differences in leg length, abnormalities or rotation of the hips, position of the kneecap, bowlegs, knock-knees, or flatfeet.
4. Footwear—improper fit, inadequate impact absorbing material, excessive stiffness of the sole, or insufficient support of hindfoot.
5. Playing surface—concrete pavement versus asphalt, running track, dirt, or grass.
6. Associated disease state of the lower extremity, including previous Perthes' disease, old fracture, or other injury.
7. Growth—in particular, the growth spurt.

It is noteworthy that risk factor growth and, in particular, the growth spurt, must be added when assessing the occurrence of overuse injury in the young athlete.

Training Errors

As with the adult athlete, training error is frequently encountered when the etiology of a child's overuse injury is assessed. This is often dramatic, as when a child playing backyard basketball or pickup hockey for an hour a day is sent off to basketball or hockey camp where he or she must train for 6 to 8 hours a day.

The evolution of the summer camp experience from a 2- to 4-week recreational activity involving camping, archery, canoeing, and art to a specialized, often intensive, experience in one sport such as basketball, hockey, football, wrestling, soccer, or dance appears to have dramatically increased the incidence of childhood overuse injuries.

Muscle-Tendon Imbalance

Muscle-tendon imbalance is the second risk factor. This can be an imbalance of strength, flexibility, or bulk and is certainly also a factor in many of these childhood injuries. In the past, little attention was paid to specific muscle conditioning exercises for children. Although this laissez-faire attitude may have been appropriate for children involved in free-play activities, children playing organized sports are often subject to predictable repetitive demands that may result in imbalances of strength or range of motion about certain joints.

As an example, children engaged in repetitive throwing or in the performance of certain swimming strokes, such as the breast stroke, may develop an external rotation contracture of the shoulder, most probably reflecting a tight posterior capsule and loose anterior capsule. Persistence of this imbalance may result in an impingement syndrome or even anterior subluxation of the shoulder. Early recognition and appropriate exercises may help to avoid these problems by restoring the muscle balance to the shoulder.

Repetitive training, including running training, can result in imbalance about the lower extremities. We know from studies of running that a characteristic pattern of tight, strong quadriceps; tight and strong gastro-soleus; and tight, weak hamstrings results from running training alone.[4] Now that young runners are training at distances and speeds unheard of even 5 to 10 years ago, similar imbalances are being noted in them, and a specific stretching program must be used to reverse this tendency.[57] In children, the factor of growth further contributes to this tendency for muscle imbalance, particularly about the joints of the lower extremity; this will be discussed later in the chapter.

Anatomic Malalignment

Anatomic malalignment can be a factor in the occurrence of an overuse injury in the child, as in the adult, and can often be difficult to compensate for. Excessive femoral anteversion in a young dancer can severely limit turn out, all important in ballet technique, and result in knee pain if excessive external tibial rotation and foot pronation are substituted for natural hip turn out. Although there is some evidence that ballet training that is started before the child is 10 years old may result in the development of increased external rotation of the hip, femoral anteversion may result in a child not being able to be a part of this activity.[46]

Other postural or anatomic alignment problems, such as excessive lumbar lordosis or hyperextension at the knees, can be corrected by careful, directed exercise programs.[62] However, some rather dramatic malalignments about the knee, lower leg, or foot may be completely compatible with injury-free participation. Some of the better runners we have seen have dramatic lower leg bowing and can run without problems. Similarly, flat or pronated feet are often indicted as a cause of overuse injury in the adult athlete and are treated with compensatory orthoses in the shoe.[60] In the young athlete, we sometimes prescribe orthotics for the child with symptomatic flatfeet but take care to rule out associated growth-related muscle-tendon imbalances, such as tight heelcords or peroneii muscles. Frequently, directed exercises can relieve symptoms completely. We will occasionally use prophylactic semirigid orthotics in an athletically active child with very flat feet but certainly do not believe that this should be a routine procedure.

Another anatomic malalignment that has received considerable attention in the management of adult athletes is that of leg length discrepancy. Although a leg length discrepancy of as little as 0.5 cm may affect an elite adult runner, discrepancies, unless quite severe, are rarely associated with symptoms in the young athlete. We will however, use a built-up shoe or inset type of orthosis for a discrepancy of 1.0 cm or greater.

Footwear and Playing Surface

Shoewear and playing surface can be important in the occurrence of overuse injuries in children's lower extremities. A child involved in regular running should wear well-fitted running shoes. Some of the major manufacturers are now making well-designed, but less expensive, shoes for children. Characteristics of an acceptable running shoe for children are a firm heel counter, an elevated heel, and both flexibility and impact-absorbing materials in the forefoot as well as the heel. The playing surface can sometimes have a rather dramatic role in overuse injury. Knee pain in the young tennis player who plays on an asphalt court may disappear when the athlete switches to a clay court.

Associated Disease State

The sixth risk factor, an associated or preexistent injury or disease state, can occasionally be a factor in the child, as in a child with previous Perthes' disease of the hip who has had loss of rotation about the hip and subsequently develops knee pain with running. Similarly, some children with tarsal coalition may develop foot pain with vigorous sports training.

Growth

The final risk factor, growth, appears to have a twofold role in the occurrence of children's overuse injuries. There is clinical and some biomechanical evidence that the growth cartilage, particularly the growing articular cartilage, is less resistant to repetitive microtrauma than is adult cartilage.[3]

Growth cartilage is located at three sites in the child: the epiphyseal plate, the joint surface, and the apophyseal insertions of major muscle-tendon units. Injuries to the growth plate from the repetitive trauma of athletic activities have been suggested as an etiologic factor in adult onset arthritis of the hip, presumably as a result of minimal capital femoral epiphyseal displacement from this repetitive microtrauma.[48] Retrospective studies by Stulberg and associates[59] support this view. Whether or not other growth plates of the lower extremity are subject to injury and subsequent deformation from repetitive microtrauma is still a matter of debate. Kato and Ishiko[30] suggested that early heavy work by children could result in bony deformation from growth plate injury. Recently, Chantraine[8] reported that a long-term follow-up of soccer players suggested that they had a increased incidence of bilateral genu varum and osteoarthritis at the knee when compared with the general population.

In the upper extremity, nondisplaced but symptomatic microfractures at the growth plate of the proximal humerus are seen after the repetitive trauma of throwing a ball and have been dubbed "Little League shoulder."[6]

The growing articular surface of the child is also susceptible to overuse injury. There is increased evidence that the child's articular surface is more susceptible to shearing than is adult cartilage, particularly at the elbow, knee, and ankle. Repetitive trauma appears to be responsible for many cases of osteochondritis dissecans, certainly at the elbow in the child pitcher, with an increased incidence of osteochondritis of the capitellum resulting.[1,35,37] Recurrent microtrauma has been implicated in the etiology of osteochondritis dissecans of the proximal and distal femur and the talus.[7] In the future, particular attention must be paid to children involved in distance running, particularly those engaged in marathon competitions, to ensure that subtle overuse injuries at the joint surfaces or even the growth plates are not resulting.[40]

The third site of growth cartilage, the traction apophyses, can also be the site of overuse injury. Osgood-Schlatter disease is the best known of these, but certainly os calcis apophysitis is frequently seen in the young athlete, particularly in those who play such sports as soccer or baseball.[49] Although in the past the etiology of these entities has been debated and they have been included in the general category of the osteochondroses, there is increasing evidence that they are the result of tiny avulsion fractures and the body's resultant healing processes. These conditions are usually associated with tight muscle-tendon units in the affected children.[49] Although rare, similar entities can be seen about the pelvis, at the site of rectus femoris or sartorius insertion, usually as a result of overtraining, as in the new young runner or gymnast.

The second aspect of growth as a risk factor in children's overuse injuries, and one that has received less emphasis in the past, is the growth process itself and its subsequent effect on the tissues at risk. Longitudinal growth, of course, occurs in the bones of the extremities and spine only with the soft tissue—muscle-tendon units, ligaments, and neurovascular elements—secondarily elongating in response to this growth. During periods of rapid growth, the growth spurts, there can be a real increase in muscle-tendon tightness about the joints, loss of flexibility, and an enhanced environment for overuse injury. This loss of flexibility during the adolescent growth spurt was well documented more than 30 years ago, and, certainly, the traditional assessment of "growing pains" has been known to us much longer than that.[18]

At the present time, we are seeing a coincidence of growth spurt, and perhaps even an enhanced growth spurt, in our current generations of larger and stronger children at exactly the time when many of these children are first being exposed to repetitive training and conditioning in sports and in an environment of susceptible growth tissue sites.[20]

TYPES OF INJURY

Overuse injuries can occur to any of the major structural components of the body, including the bones, ligaments, muscle-tendon units, and articular cartilage.

STRESS FRACTURES

Stress fractures or fatigue fractures of bone have a most interesting history. In adults, the first large reports of these overuse or fatigue fractures were noted in military recruits, who were frequently being maltrained, with too much training over too short a period of time and with inadequate time allowed for the musculoskeletal system to condition itself to the new patterns of stress applied, in particular, to the bones. These "march" fractures were rarely encountered in the civilian population until repetitive training activities of lower extremities, most notably with distance running, began to be practiced by the general population. Certainly, the only additional reports related to stress fractures were found in the sports medicine literature and, were, of course, occurring in fully maturc individuals.

The first published reports of stress fractures occurring in children were not seen until the advent of organized sports training for younger children—a post World War II phenomenon.[12,13] Stress fractures in children are now well known and, as noted above, invariably occur in the child participating in organized sports training. Although most often seen in the long bones of the lower leg, particularly the tibia and fibula, a stress fracture is the "great masquerader." With any persistent, activity-related pain of an extremity, whether of the foot, hip, knee, or ankle, stress fracture must be suspected, with the involved bones ranging from pubic ramus to the tarsal navicular. Again reflecting the sports training–specific nature of this overuse injury, stress fractures of the forearm bones are a frequent occurrence in gymnastics.

We have learned much more about the etiologic factors involved in all overuse injuries from studies of stress fractures. During a 7-month period in our own Sports Medicine clinic, a total of 53 stress fractures of the lower extremity were diagnosed, including five hip fractures.[44] When etiologic factors thought to be related to the occurrence of these stress fractures were determined for each fracture, the occurrence of stress fracture appeared to be most frequently associated with maltraining, particularly with inappropriate rate and intensity of training. In addition, imbalance of muscle tendon units, anatomic malalignment, shoewear, and surface were all assessed. Anatomic alignment appeared to be particularly important in stress fractures about the ankle and foot. Otherwise, maltraining remained the most frequently associated risk factor in the occurrence of these stress fractures.

With increased experience and a high index of suspicion, particularly when the all important history is obtained of repetitive sports training activities, the diagnosis of stress fracture can usually be made clinically. A technetium 99 bone scan is usually reserved for the situation in which absolute certainty of diagnosis is required prior to a high level or elite amateur competition, or when there is important clinical necessity for making the diagnosis, such as when the possibility of a stress fracture of the femoral neck exists, or in a situation where there is lower leg pain in which compartment syndrome is also part of the differential diagnosis (Fig. 26-1*A*,*B*).[53]

The management of stress fractures, once diagnosed, is relatively simple. Cast immobilization is rarely required except, perhaps, in certain stress fractures in the feet. The concept of "relative" rest is useful. The basic goal of treatment is to render the child asymptomatic and free of pain and have him remain so for at least 6 weeks. A young ballet dancer with a tibial stress fracture may be rendered pain-free simply by avoiding jumping for that period of time. A young basketball player with a distal femoral stress fracture may require 6 weeks of crutch gait ambulation and swimming.

The management of stress fractures of the hip is somewhat controversial. Much of the experience with this fracture has been gained in young adults, particularly military recruits, and recommendations have included open pin fixation and stabilization, even if the stress fracture has not displaced. In our own experience, this has not been necessary in the young athlete with a stress fracture. At the most, particularly in the unreliable adolescent, we have used spica cast immobilization. In other cases, simple crutch ambulation has been sufficient.

TENDONITIS

Tendonitis may also occur in the child who is doing repetitive activities, although the incidence is much lower than that in the adult. Usually the site of tendon insertion, the apophysis, becomes symptomatic before the tendon itself, although both may become painful and inflamed. Because frank tendonitis occurs infrequently in the child, this diagnosis should be made cautiously and only after other possible etiologies, including stress fracture, osteochondritis, or even neoplasm or infection, have been ruled out.

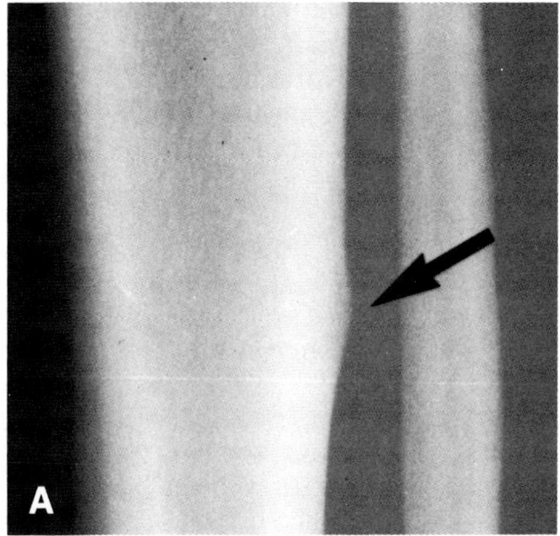

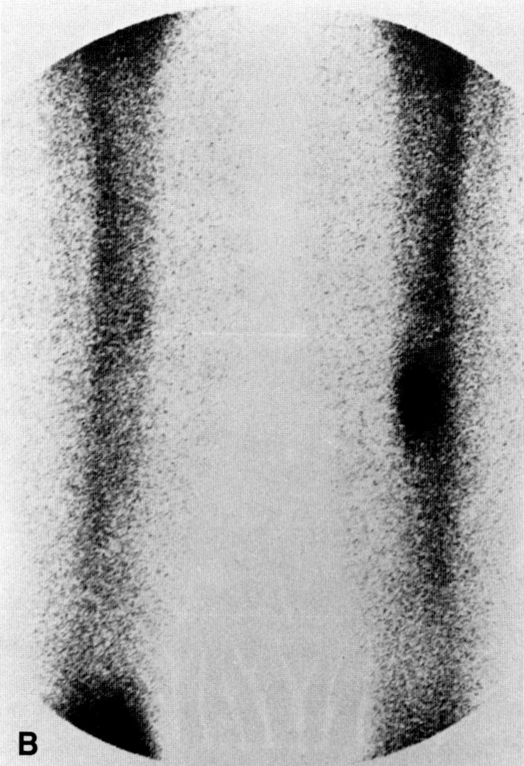

FIG. 26-1. *(A)* This stress fracture of the tibia is identifiable on plain radiographs only by this late appearance of periosteal callus formation. *(B)* Technetium bone scan with area of increased uptake in the tibia, confirming recent stress fracture.

It is important to remember that the inflammatory phase of a tendonitis is really the body's healing response to micro tears of the tendon fibers, and we must respect this response. Rest is an important part of the initial management, particularly in children. It is rarely necessary to completely rest or immobilize the injured extremity, however, and complete rest may actually delay healing. Recent work by Curwin and Stanish[10] has suggested that even during the period of acute inflammation, careful, directed eccentric exercise may be helpful in restoring the strength and function of the inflamed tendon unit.

A period of "relative" rest is useful, during which the extremity is used but with a very different stress pattern. A runner with an acute achilles tendonitis who is swimming for an hour a day may not be running, but he or she is certainly not resting. Similarly, a young ballet dancer who is doing carefully controlled barre work but avoiding jumping that will exacerbate her tibialis anterior tendonitis is again undergoing "relative" rest as part of the treatment program.

Ice and gentle compression are useful in the acute stages of a tendonitis. In particular, ice massage, in which water frozen in a styrofoam type of coffee cup with the rim removed is used to massage the area of inflammation, is a very useful technique, and can be easily taught to the child with tendonitis.

Nonsteroidal anti-inflammatories can also be useful in the management of acute tendonitis in the child. Because the safety of many of these more complex agents has not been demonstrated in children, we usually prescribe buffered aspirin and have found this agent to be satisfactory. We do not use corticosteroid injections in a young athlete, in particular, because we believe that they are generally not useful or needed and may have serious side effects.

In addition to the aforementioned basic conservative techniques for management in the early stages of a tendonitis, rehabilitation and restoration of the strength and flexibility of the muscle tendon unit are particularly important if the child expects to resume repetitive training techniques. Unfortunately, the importance of rehabilitation after injury has not been adequately appreciated in this age group. Just as a relatively tight or weak muscle tendon unit may be the pre-condition for the occurrence of injury and secondary inflammation of the tendon, it becomes additionally important to restore this strength and flexibility to normal or even increased normal ranges, depending on the demands that will be placed on it by the activity in question, in order to prevent re-injury.[41]

In addition to tendonitis, we have seen some cases of "tendonosis" in the young athlete, specifically in the achilles tendon and the patellar tendon. As Puddu and associates[51] noted, this appears to be an aseptic necrosis of the tendon, and even the young athlete may require surgery in order to promote revascularization.

BURSITIS

Overuse injury of joint capsule or ligament is frequently expressed or diagnosed as bursitis. A bursae is, of course, only a potential space and becomes swollen or inflamed when adjacent tissues, such as tendon or ligament, sustain injury or irritation. As with tendonitis, bursitis in young athletes usually responds quite rapidly to relative rest or conservative management. Both management and prevention include determination and correction of the factor responsible for its initial occurrence. These are most frequently training errors or muscle tendon imbalance.

JOINT DISORDERS

Disorders of the joints or articular cartilage can also result from overuse injury. Osteochondral injuries, in particular, appear to be a common result of overuse injury in a young athlete and will be discussed when disorders of the elbow joint or knee are reviewed. Patellofemoral pain may also be a reflection of an overuse injury, particularly in the athletically active child. In addition, frank subluxations about the shoulder joint appear to be occurring with increasing frequency in association with swimming and throwing training. We have seen a number of cases of recurrent subluxation of the shoulder in young swimmers, which appear to be a result of swimming training.

SITES OF OVERUSE INJURY

SPINE

The incidence of back injuries in association with children's sports is increasing dramatically, and many of these injuries are the result of recurrent microtrauma occurring at the time of the adolescent growth spurt, when there appears to be a particular risk of injury.

With growth, especially during the growth spurt, there appears to be a tendency to develop lordosis of the lumbar spine. This may be due to increased growth anteriorly and in the vertebral bodies and the secondary tethering of the spine posteriorly by the heavy lumbodorsal fascia. We have observed a growth-related pattern of posture developing at this time, with tight lumbar lordosis, a relative flexion contracture at the hips with associated tight hamstrings, and, because normal forward excursion of the lumbar spine is limited, a tendency to develop thoracic kyphosis, where forward bending must now occur.

If at the time that this malposturing is occurring, repetitive sports training is done that requires repetitive flexion, extension, or rotation of the spine, a characteristic pattern of injuries may develop.

Research on lumbar spine mechanics has suggested that increased lumbar lordosis increases the tendency toward both posterior element failure at the pars interarticularis and disc failure.[32]

This theoretical concern appears to be consistent with clinical observations. The overuse back problems seen in the young athlete generally fall into one of three categories: stress fracture of the pars interarticularis (spondylolysis), hyperlordotic mechanical low back pain, or disc herniation, all of which appear to be helped to a greater or lesser extent by an anti-lordotic program of exercises and, sometimes, bracing (Figs. 26-2 and 26-3).[42]

At the thoracolumbar junction, back pain can develop that is associated with radiographic deformation of one or more vertebral bodies anteriorly. Although the etiology of this "atypical" Scheuermann's disease is still being debated, the time of onset and the frequent association with repetitive microtrauma suggest that this may actually be a compression fracture of the vertebral bodies anteriorly, the result of excessive flexion at this site because of limited motion of the tight lordotic lumbar

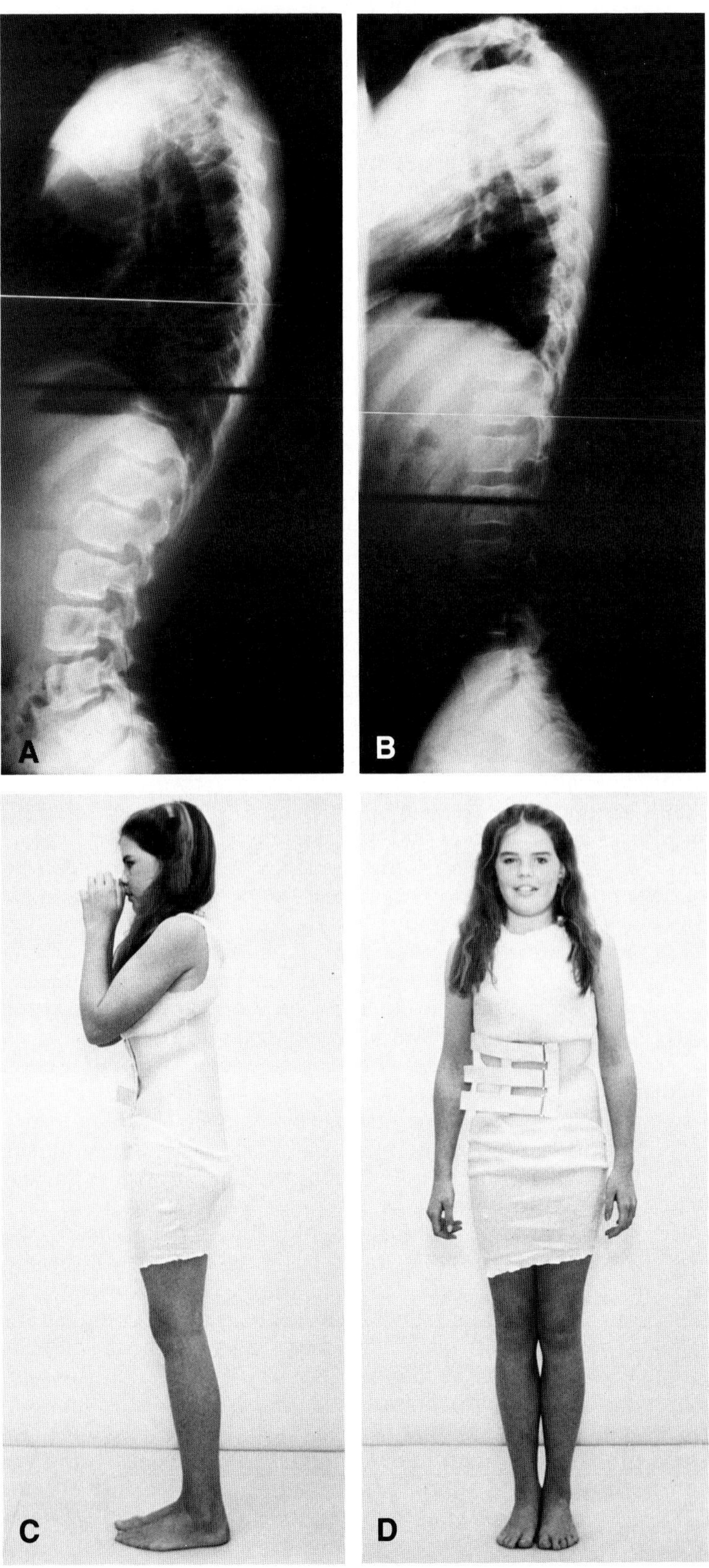

FIG. 26-2. *(A)* Lateral radiograph of the spine in an adolescent with hyperlordotic low back pain. *(B)* Lateral radiograph of the same child in an anti-lordotic thermoplastic brace. *(C* and *D)* Thermoplastic brace designed to decrease lumbar lordosis as an aid in the treatment of adolescent back pain.

In clinical practice, three different types of injury appear to be the result of repetitive overhand throwing activities at the elbow in the immature child: (1) osteochondral injuries of the capitellum, with or without associated loose bodies in the joint; (2) injury and premature closure of the proximal radial epiphysis, sometimes with associated overgrowth of the radial head; and (3) medially, irritation or even frank avulsion of the medial epicondyle. The mechanism of injury to these structures appears to be the result of a repetitive valgus strain applied to the elbow with throwing, with compression medially, and with traction laterally.[1,15]

The management of these overuse injuries of the elbow in the young active athlete depends to a large degree on the stage at which they are detected. If this problem is detected early, relative rest and exercise to improve the strength of the entire arm, as well as attention to throwing techniques that minimize the valgus strain at the elbow, can halt the process. It is our own belief that the very first stage in this entire process may include a relative flexion contracture at the elbow with tightening of the anterior capsular structures and a relative weakening of the triceps. In the child who is complaining of elbow pain from repetitive throwing, we believe that it is particularly important that a careful and directed program of rehabilitation be used in which the anterior structures of the elbow are stretched and the triceps is strengthened with progressive resistive exercises, in addition to rest. If osteochondral lesions have already developed, particularly with the formation of a loose body, and if there is an associated elbow contracture, surgical débridement followed by thorough rehabilitation seems to give the best result.[37]

HIP AND PELVIS

Interestingly, it has been hypothesized that childhood sports activity may predispose the individual to adult primary osteoarthritis of the hip because of small, undetected slipping of the capital femoral epiphysis in association particularly with running or jumping activities, resulting in deformation of the femoral head and progressive, slow deterioration of the hip joint itself. Certainly, more careful study and documentation are necessary.[48]

In an attempt to determine whether there appeared to be a greater incidence of osteoarthritis at the hip in patients who had partici-

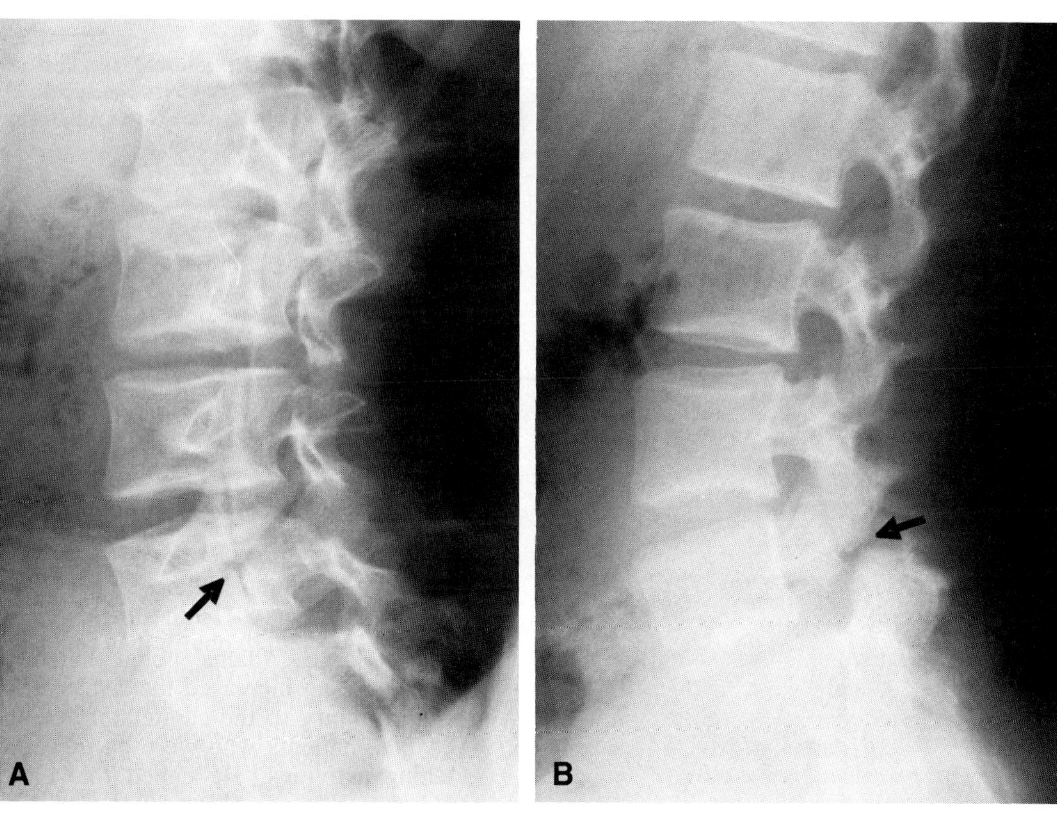

FIG. 26-3. *(A and B)* Spondylolysis in the adolescent athlete may be an overuse stress fracture, the result of repetitive hyperflexion or hyperextension of the lumbar spine.

spine below.[23] With early recognition and, usually, bracing, rapid healing and bony reconstitution can be seen.

Juvenile roundback, or even some cases of Scheuermann's kyphosis, may have a similar pathogenesis, particularly in boys. Again, the consistent finding of tight lumbodorsal fascia and rapid reversal, with bony reconstitution of the vertebral bodies if early bracing is instituted, supports this theory.[2] As with disorders of the lumbar spine noted earlier, a good low back and hamstring flexibility program is an essential part of the treatment program.

SHOULDER

Overuse injuries of the shoulder can be a reflection of injury to joint surface, muscle tendon units, or even a frank subluxation of the shoulder. The term *Little League* shoulder refers to a stress fracture of the proximal humeral physis from repetitive throwing.[6] Recently, an increased number of impingement syndromes have been noted in young athletes involved in throwing or swimming. It is hypothesized that impingement occurs between the rotator cuff muscle in the humeral head and the coracoacromial ligament or acromion itself above.[22,52] Satisfactory results have been reported from coracoacromial ligament resection.[25]

It is our own belief that this particular overuse injury is actually a result of the development of a muscle tendon and capsule imbalance about the shoulder. We have found that these children, usually as the result of repetitive swimming or throwing activities, develop a characteristic contracture above the shoulder, with loss of internal rotation at the 90° abduction position and an associated increase in external rotation (Fig. 26-4). We believe that this reflects a tightened posterior shoulder capsule and relatively loosened anterior capsule, with a secondary-associated repetitive partial anterior subluxation of the shoulder.

This repetitive tendency toward anterior

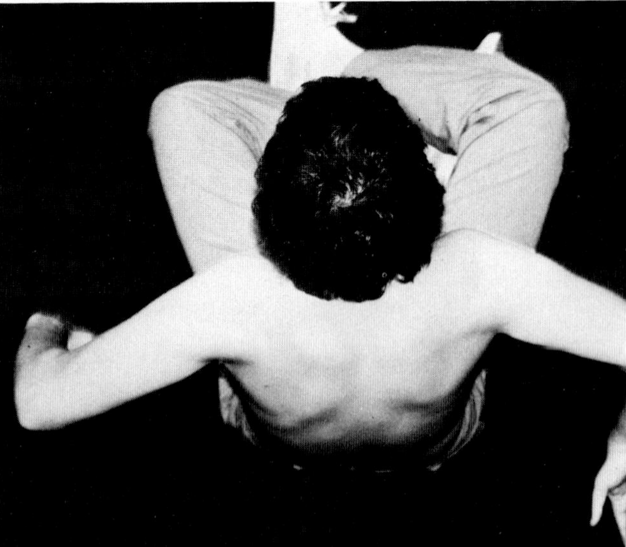

luxation at the shoulder with repeated throwing or swimming becomes a vicious cycle—the posterior capsule becomes tighter, and the anterior capsule becomes relatively more lax. In association with this, there may be a secondary impingement of the rotator cuff musculature or the biceps anteriorly at the coracoacromial ligament, but this is not really the primary problem. We have been very pleased with the response in these cases to a directed exercise program aimed at restoring a full range of motion with good strength to the involved shoulder. This exercise program includes, in particular, active-resisted internal rotation when the shoulder is held in the 90° abduction position. In addition, stretching of the posterior capsule by translation of the involved extremity across the torso is also important.

An interesting clinical observation has been made by Dr. Frank Jobe,[29] a well-known authority on shoulder problems in athletes. He has observed that there appears to be a much higher incidence of impingement syndrome of the shoulder in adult professional pitchers who have pitched as children, and he has suggested that this early repetitive stress in the child's immature articular cartilage at the proximal humerus may result in hypertrophy of the humeral head and secondary decreased capacity for excusion of the rotator cuff tendons.

ELBOW

Historically, the elbow was one of the first sites of overuse injury to be noted in children.

In 196
appea
teoch
of his
in pit
Little
a con
the te
incide
is uni
petiti
surve
Orego
dence
these
with

In
unde
chon
throv
signi
high
to re
but
year
sugg
entit
dary
the
quie
frag
with
bod
off,
mov

very tight in the musculature about the hip, particularly during the growth spurt. These injuries usually respond rapidly to appropriate training and rehabilitation techniques, as outlined in the section on tendonitis (Fig. 26-5).

KNEE

In addition to being the most common site of macrotrauma injury in the young North American athlete, the knee is often the most frequent site of overuse injury. The vast majority of these overuse injuries involve the extensor mechanism, however, whereas the macrotrauma injuries about the knee usually involve the ligaments or internal structures.

With growth, particularly with the growth spurt, the muscles spanning the knee joint must adjust to the most rapidly growing bones in the body. The presence of a strong fascia lata laterally and relatively weaker tissues medially results not only in longitudinal traction but also lateral deviation forces on the growth of the knee and, in particular, on the quadriceps mechanism and its sesamoid bone, the patella (Fig. 26-6).

If this tendency toward proximal and lateral deviation of the quadriceps mechanism is excessive, lateral luxation or even a dislocation of the patella may occur. Lesser degrees of this growth-related deviation of the extensor mechanism and patella may be expressed as low-grade kneeache, made worse by stair-climbing and prolonged sitting in one place (the "theatre sign").

This parapatellar pain may often begin after a particular episode of overuse, such as double basketball practices, dancing on an unsprung wooden floor, or suddenly beginning hill running. This entity has been labeled *patellofemoral stress syndrome*. We find this a useful classification and prefer it to the frequently used diagnosis of chondromalacia. Chondromalacia refers to a pathologic condition of articular cartilage, including the patella, in which there is softening, fibrillation, or frank erosion of the cartilage. Although parapatellar knee pain, or the patellofemoral stress syndrome, may result in chondromalacia of the patella or underlying femoral articular cartilage, particularly if it is allowed to persist for a prolonged period of time, there is by no means a direct or necessary relationship.

There is also more recent evidence that deformations of the shape of the patella itself, which are frequently seen with these lateral deformation conditions, may be secondary to the soft-tissue contractures that result from this growth process, and therefore, these bony deformations can actually be prevented if the soft-tissue imbalances about the knee and extensor mechanism are reversed at the time of the growth spurt.

Based on this hypothesized pathogenesis of the patellofemoral stress syndrome, a useful clinical approach has been to attempt to

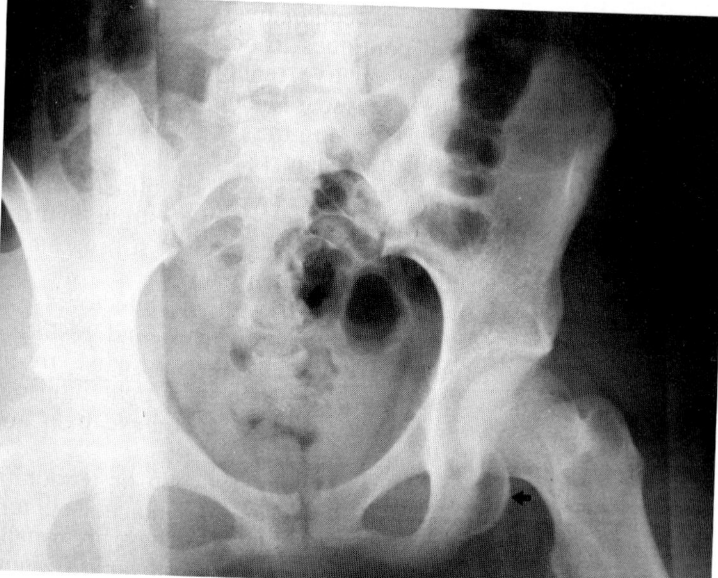

FIG. 26-5. Avulsion of the ischial tuberosity in a young figure skater. The child has had low-grade pain at the site for several months before one episode of acute pain and frank avulsion.

strengthen the medial structures of the quadriceps mechanism and upper leg and to stretch the lateral structures. We have found this to be a very successful approach, with progressive resistive adductor and quadriceps muscle strengthening, done with the knee extended, combined with stretching exercises of the fascia lata and hamstrings. In our opinion, it is essential that this exercise program be of the progressive resistive straight-leg raising type. Although initially a child may only be able to lift the weight of the leg itself, carefully directed exercises to slowly increase the resistance can result in dramatic increases in strength. We have found that the ability to lift 5.4 kg in a straight-leg raising manner, done in three sets of 10 repetitions, is usually associated with the disappearance of symptoms.[41] This level is approached in a slow and progressive manner, of course, and without pain, because, at times, the quadriceps, and particularly the vastus medialis, which is specific to determine extension, may be quite weak. Both legs are strengthened, and, although 5.4 kg seems to be the minimum level at which symptoms will usually disappear, the goal for a given child or adolescent may be as high as 9.9 kg or even 11.25 kg (Fig. 26-7).

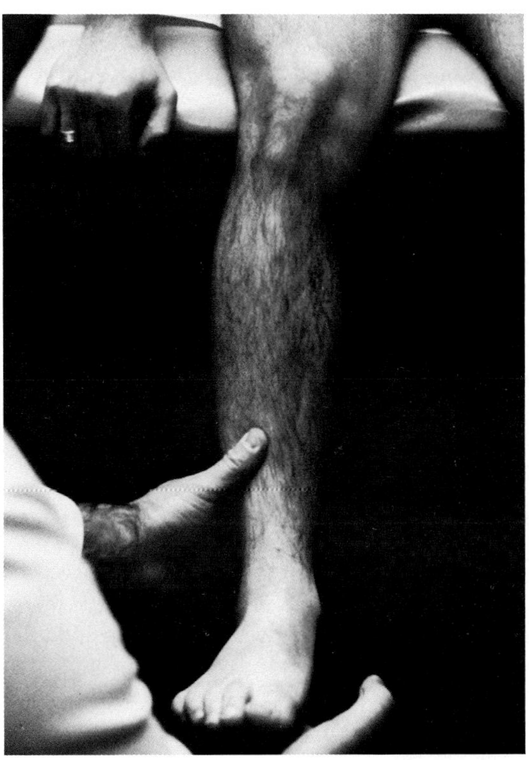

FIG. 26-6. Increased Q-angle, reflecting lateral deviation tendency of the patella, in a young athlete.

If, after 6 months of exercise, the knee remains painful and 5.4 kg is not reached, a lateral release of the retinaculum is performed and exercise is then resumed. With this ap-

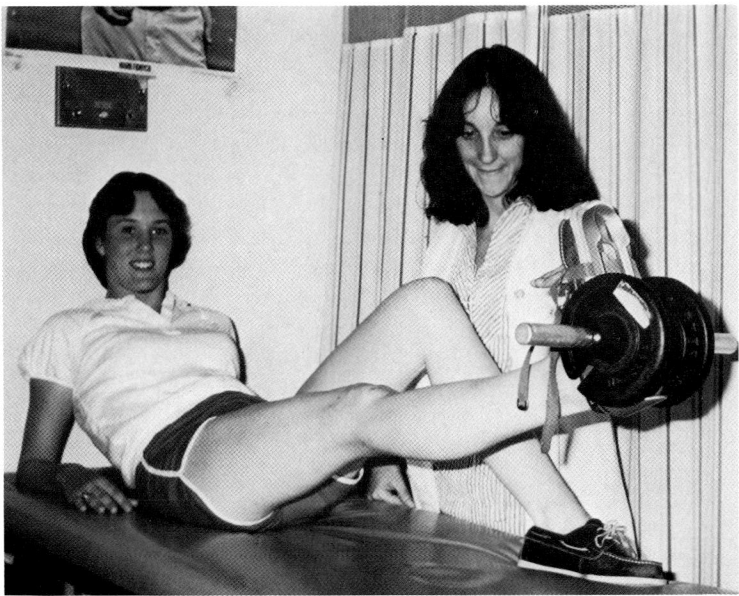

FIG. 26-7. Straight-leg raising with progressive resistance added to foot or ankle is effective in treating many overuse injuries of the knee.

proach, 92% of our children were satisfactorily treated with exercise alone, and, of the remaining 8% who were treated surgically with lateral release, 82% were able to restore strength and resume activities free of pain.[45]

Clinically, Osgood-Schlatter disease appears to follow a similar pattern. In the past, this was primarily a condition encountered in young boys and appeared to generally have its onset in conjunction with the adolescent growth spurt.[49] Recently, however, we have noted a new population presenting with Osgood-Schlatter symptoms—younger girls 10 to 12 years of age who are involved in vigorous jumping training as in figure skating or gymnastics (Fig. 26-8).[43] Interestingly, the onset of this condition is also occurring at the time of the adolescent growth spurt in these young girls and is really an equivalent stage of skeletal development when compared with the boys. Although the etiology of this condition requires further investigation, we have assumed that this entity is also a relative overgrowth syndrome, reflecting imbalance of tension and lateral deviation of quadriceps structure and have used a similar static straight-leg raising strengthening program for treatment and rehabilitation, as well as a stretching program for the tight and weak quadriceps. In addition, these children appear to invariably have tight hamstring and gastroc-soleus mechanisms. A good directed stretching program for these structures also appears to be essential.

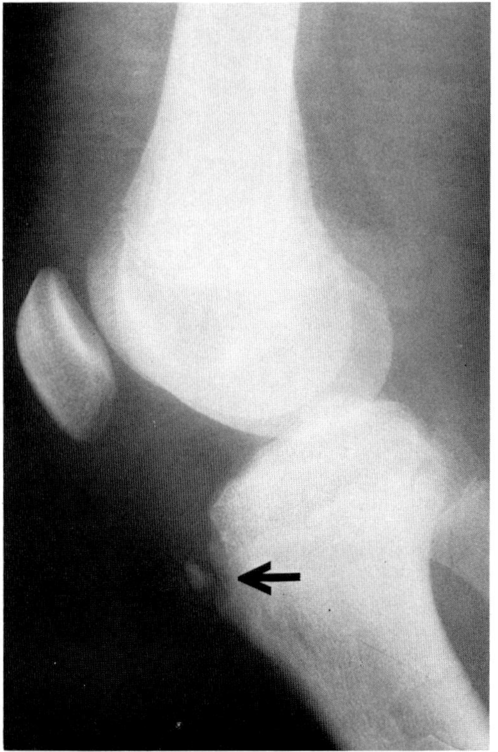

Fig. 26-8. A painful and tender tibial tubercle may reflect repetitive microavulsion of the quadriceps apoplysis.

One of the traditional approaches to Osgood Schlatter disease has been to use a preliminary stage of casting with the knee in full extension. We now think that this is rarely necessary and believe that it may actually be contraindicated, in so far as the muscle tendon units are still relatively tight and weak after cast removal, despite the fact that the avulsion injury at tibial tubercle may have had an opportunity to heal. If the child is acutely painful with Osgood Schlatter disease, we may indeed use a period of crutch support, but we usually attempt to continue the knee on a rehabilitation exercise program and try to maintain the child in such activities as swimming or bicycling, while avoiding impacting activities such as running.

A third, and less common expression of the overgrowth syndrome at the knee, may result in small bony avulsions in the upper or lower pole of the patella. Children with this problem often also present with histories suggesting a patellofemoral stress syndrome but are usually discretely tender at one site on the patella and often have a history of one particular episode of pain onset superimposed upon repetitive microtrauma activities.[13] In these injuries, we will generally use a period of cylinder cast immobilization. We have found that 4 weeks is usually a sufficient period of time for healing of these lesions to occur, although we will sometimes then begin using a knee immobilizer that allows the initiation of quadriceps strengthening and stretching while the child's knee still remains in extension for most of the day (Fig. 26-9).

In all three of these conditions, envelopment braces that leave the patella open, such as the Marshall or Palumbo brace, can have a very useful role in the early stages of management of these conditions. In addition, they can be used to allow relatively early return to painless activity (Fig. 26-10).

As noted earlier, osteochondritis dissecans may, in some instances, be the result of repetitive microtrauma at the knee. The characteristic location is at the inner aspect of the

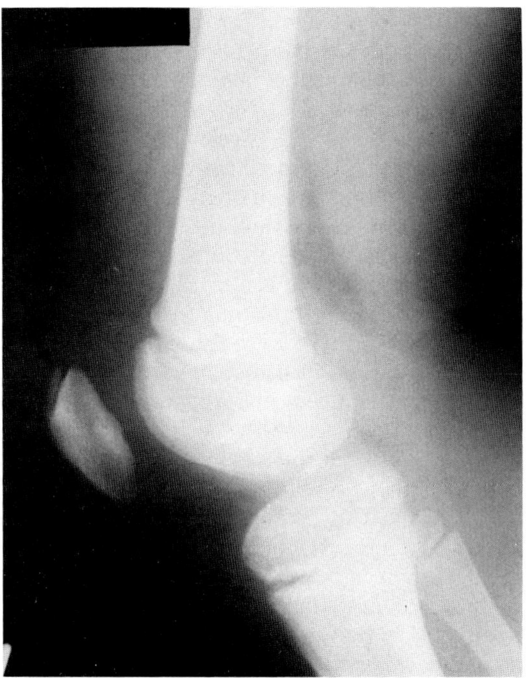

FIG. 26-9. Traumatic avulsion of the proximal margin of the patella resulting from repetitive microtrauma in a young male basketball player, initially misdiagnosed as an accessory ossification center.

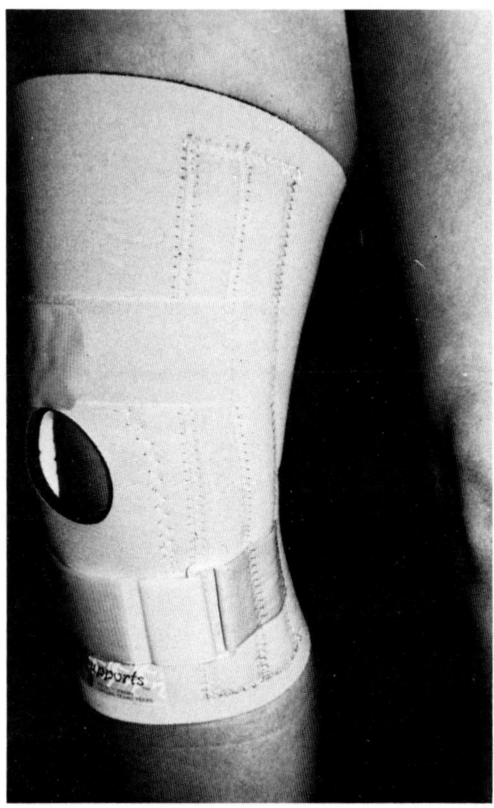

FIG. 26-10. The Marshall-type knee brace with open patella is useful in treating many extensor mechanism overuse injuries.

medial femoral condyle, suggesting that impingement of the tibial spine may be the causative factor in this lesion. This clinical presentation can be indistinguishable from patellofemoral stress syndrome, thus, radiographs, including the tunnel view, are necessary in a child who has these complaints. In addition, the child with osteochondritis dissecans may be tender along the inferior and medial poles of the patella. Care must be taken not to confuse this or misdiagnose it as "plica" syndrome (Fig. 26-11).[50]

Although the more traditional management of this lesion includes a period of immobilization if it is nondisplaced, more recent techniques, which have been facilitated by the development of arthroscopy, include resection under arthroscopic control if the lesion is loose or transarticular drilling or pinning again under arthroscopic control if the lesion is intact.[17] More experience with this approach is needed before it can be recommended as a program that increases the rate or incidence of union.

A relatively newer diagnosis being made with increasing frequency in children and adolescents is that of "plica" syndrome.[50] Plica are, of course, evaginations of the joint capsule and synovium in the knee, which may, at times, become impinged between articular surface and rendered symptomatic. Plica may normally be present in as many as 70% of human knees. The most common site of symptomatic plica is on the inferior and medial margin of the patella. In our experience, plica may become symptomatic during periods of rapid growth—perhaps another example of overgrowth syndrome at the knee. Additionally, symptomatic plica will almost invariably respond to a well-directed exercise program of quadriceps strengthening and stretching. We believe that at least 6 months of extensor mechanism rehabilitation and treatment should be attempted before operative intervention and resection of plica should be considered, particularly in the adolescent.

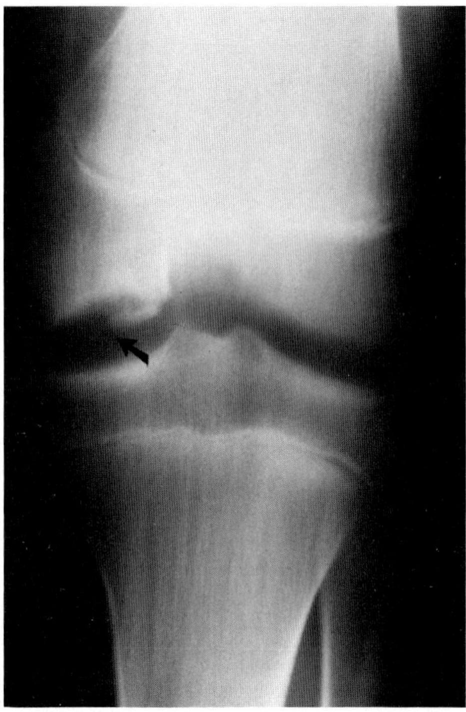

FIG. 26-11. The etiology of osteochondritis dissecans may be due to repetitive microtrauma to the joint surface.

ANKLE AND FOOT

Overuse injuries at the foot and ankle are not uncommon in children. The most common complaint is heel pain, often in a child involved in field sports such as soccer or lacrosse. Tenderness over the os calcis apophysis at the insertion of the achilles tendon, along with a tight gastroc-soleus mechanism are the characteristic findings in this condition. In the past, this condition has been labeled *Sever's disease* and has been classed as one of the osteochondroses. Radiographs have sometimes been used to confirm the diagnosis, with increased density in the os calcis apophysis noted. In our own experience, radiographs have generally not been helpful and the condition is most frequently diagnosed clinically.

Although the primary etiologic factor in os calcis apophysitis appears to be a tight achilles, usually associated with a growth spurt, maltraining is often also indicated. In addition, inspection of the playing shoe will often reveal a shoe with a "negative cant," with the heel actually lower than the toe, as a result of cleat wear or shoe design. Although the design of running shoes has included a raised heel of ¼ to ⅜ inch, many soccer, football, tennis, and basketball shoes have low heels, which increase the chance of achilles tendon strain, particularly in a rapidly growing adolescent.

This condition usually responds very rapidly to a program of directed heelcord stretching and dorsiflexion strengthening exercises, as well as a temporary heel lift. We have found a new synthetic impact absorbing material, sorbothane, used as a heel insert, to be particularly useful in this condition. A short program of intermittent icing and mild anti-inflammatories may also be indicated.

A stress fracture of the os calcis can present similarly but can usually be ruled out by the presence of tenderness on the sides of the os calcis, rather than directly over the site of tendo Achillis insertion. If there is any doubt as to the diagnosis, radiographs, including the axial Harris view of the os calcis should be obtained. Occasionally, a bone scan may be necessary to distinguish the cause of foot pain in a child. Rarities such as stress fractures of the navicular encountered in the sports active child may be diagnosed in this way.

Occasionally, the child athlete or dancer will develop tendonitis about the foot and ankle, most commonly of the tibialis posterior or peroneus muscles. These usually respond quite readily to conservative management, particularly if treatment is initiated early.

Pain on the sole of the foot in association with repetitive training activities is rare in the child. This is as opposed to the adult, in whom plantar fasciitis is one of the most common injuries of the adult runner in particular.[4] We have, however, observed stress fractures in young dancers and runners presenting as midfoot and plantar surface pain, and this must always be ruled out. Commonly, the shaft of the second metatarsal will be the site of the stress fracture. As noted earlier, although stress fractures were once rare in children, they are now being encountered with increasing frequency, and the diagnosis must always be considered.

In addition, we have seen a number of children involved in distance running who have presented with what appears to be an avulsion injury of the medial malleolus. This appears to be a relatively new condition in a child and one that may have an increased incidence with such activities as distance running.[58] This raises the spectrum of types of overuse injuries in the child engaged in heavy running and training and will deserve careful study in the future.

PREVENTION

It is evident from the previous discussion that overuse injuries in children are most frequently associated with repetitive training activities, particularly in training and preparation for sports or dance. The incidence of these types of injuries appears to be increasing rapidly and, in our own clinic, represent more than half of the sports injuries we now see in our child athletes. Because the etiology of these overuse injuries is often multifactorial, determination of which risk factors are specifically involved in a given overuse injury in a given child is important, not only as a help in instituting accurate and effective treatment but also as an aid in preventing the occurrence or recurrence of such injuries.

With prompt early recognition, techniques used to treat and manage these overuse injuries in children are actually quite simple. They may involve nothing more than very well-directed strengthening or stretching exercises. The importance of these well-directed exercises cannot be overemphasized. In the past, particularly in regard to stretching exercises, it was thought that the child needed little if any supplementary training exercises of this type. Such preventive exercises have rarely been incorporated in children's sports programs. The effectiveness of these techniques, however, in treating children's sports injuries has suggested their additional usefulness and advantage in the preparation of children for sports and training activities in order to prevent the occurrence of injury.

Additional steps that can be extremely helpful in preventing overuse injury may include changes in training intensity or duration, changes in sports or dance technique, and changes in, or additions to, protective or supplemental equipment. In each instance, the physician must be intimately aware of the demands and training techniques used in a given sport or fitness activity in order to suggest effective preventative measures to the parents and child.

Unfortunately, very little of this type of information has been incorporated into medical school or post graduate curricula. The physician dealing with such injuries must educate himself from the available sports medicine literature. The discipline of sports medicine is still emerging. In the past, it involved primarily the care of the elite or skilled adult athlete. Now it appears to have special application to the treatment and prevention of sports injuries in children.

As is evident from the examples that have been used throughout this text, there are usually a number of risk factors responsible for the occurrence of a given injury in a given child. One must be careful not to simply ascribe the occurrence of injury to the growth spurt or muscle tendon imbalance if it is possible that other etiologic factors such as anatomic malalignment or coexistent disease might be present. The child is at risk for an infectious process and neoplasms of the axial skeleton—in particular, osteogenic sarcoma. It would be a tragedy, indeed, if a child with a low-grade aching knee pain due to an osteogenic sarcoma of the proximal tibia were treated with straight-leg raising exercises and orthotics simply because this pain presented in the course of athletic activities.

Careful longitudinal studies are needed if we are to determine both the maximal and the minimal levels of athletic training and physical activity that should be done during childhood. In our opinion, this remains one of the most exciting and interesting areas of development in pediatric orthopaedics today.

REFERENCES

1. Adams JE: Injuries to the throwing arm: A study of traumatic changes in the elbow joints of boy baseball players. Cal Med 102:127, 1965
2. Bradford DS, Moe JH, Montalro FJ, *et al*: Scheurmann's kyphosis and roundback deformity: Results of Milwaukee brace treatment. J Bone Joint Surg 56A:740, 1974
3. Bright RW, Burstein AH, Elmore SM: Epiphyseal plate cartilage—a biomechanical and histologic analysis of failure modes. J Bone Joint Surg 56A:668, 1974
4. Brubaker GE, James SL: Injuries to runners. J Sports Med 2:189, 1974
5. Buxbaum R, Micheli LJ: Sports for Life. Boston, Beacon Press Publishers, 1979
6. Cahill BR, Tullos HS, Fain RH: Little league shoulder. J Sports Med 2:150, 1974
7. Canale ST, Belding RH: Osteochondral lesions of the talus. J Bone Joint Surg 62A:97, 1980
8. Chantraine A: Osteoarthritis and axis deviation of the knee joint in soccer players. Med Sci Sports Exerc 14:130, 1982
9. Conway FM: Osteochondritis dissecans: Description of the stages of the condition and its probable traumatic etiology. Am J Surg 38:691, 1937
10. Curwin S, Stanish WD: Tendonitis: It's Etiology and Treatment. Lexington, MA, Collamore Press, 1984
11. DeHaven KE: Athletic injuries in adolescents. Pediatr Ann 7:95, 1978
12. Devas MB: Stress fractures in children. J Bone Surg 45B:528, 1963
13. Dickason JM, Fox JM: Fracture of the patella [illegible] overuse injury in a child. Am J Sports Med [illegible] 1982

14. Ficat RP, Hungerford DS: Disorders of the patellofemoral joint. Baltimore, William & Wilkins, 1977
15. Gainor BJ, Piatrowski G, Puhl J, *et al*: The throw: Biomechanics and acute injury. Am J Sports Med 8:114, 1980
16. Goldberg MJ: Gymnastics Injuries. Orthop Clin North Am 11:717, 1980
17. Green WT, Bank HH: Osteochondritis dissecans in children. J Bone Joint Surg 35A:26, 1953
18. Guerewitsche AD, O'Neill M: Flexibility of healthy children. Arch Phys Ther 25:216, 1944
19. Gugenheim JJ Jr, Stanley RF, Woods GW, *et al*: Little league survey: The Houston study. Am J Sports Med 4:189, 1976
20. Hamill RVV, Johnson EE, Granes W: Height and weight of children. United States Vital Health Statistics, Series 11, No 104. Rockville, MD, US Dept of Health, Education, and Welfare, National Center for Health Statistics, 1970
21. Hamilton WH: Personal communication
22. Hawkins RJ, Kennedy JC: Impingement syndrome in athletes. Am J Sports Med 8:151, 1980
23. Hensinger RN: Back pain and vertebral changes simulating Scheuermann's disease. Orthop Trans 6:1, 1982
24. Herschman E, Micheli LJ: Chronic iliopsoas tendonitis in young athletes: Results of tenolysis in selected cases. Am J Sports Med (in press)
25. Jackson DB: Chronic rotator cuff impingement in the throwing athlete. Am J Sports Med 4:231, 1971
26. Jackson DW, Wiltse C, Cirincione RJ: Spondylolysis in the female gymnast. Clin Orthop 117:68, 1976
27. Jackson DW, Jarrett H, Bailey D, *et al*: Injury prediction in the young athlete: a preliminary report. Am J Sports Med 6:6, 1978
28. Jacobs M, Young R: Snapping hip phenomenon among dancers. Am Correct Ther J 32:92, 1973
29. Jobe F: Personal communication
30. Kato S, Ishiko T: Obstructed growth of children's bones due to excessive labor in remote corners. In Kato K (ed): Proceedings of International Congress of Sports Sciences. Tokyo, Japanese Union of Sports Sciences, 1976
31. Kirby RL, Simms FC, Symington BA, *et al*: Flexibility and musculoskeletal symptomatology in female gymnasts and age-matched controls. Am J Sports Med 9:160, 1981
32. Kraus H: Effect of lordosis on the stress in the lumbar spine. Clin Orthop 117:56, 1976
33. Larson RL: Epiphyseal injuries in the adolescent athlete. Orthop Clin North Am 4:839, 1973
34. Larsson L: Morphologic and functional characteristics of the aging skeletal muscle in man. Acta Physiol Scand (Suppl) Vol 457, 1978
35. Lipscomb AB: Baseball pitching in growing athletes. J Sports Med 3:25, 1975
36. Martens R: Joy and sadness in children's sports. Champaign, IL, Human Kinetics Publishing, 1978
37. McManama GB, Micheli LJ, Berry MV, Sohn RS: The surgical treatment of osteochondritis of the capitellum. Am J Sports Med 13, No. 1:11–20, 1985
38. Micheli LJ: Sports injuries in children and adolescents. In Strauss RH (ed): Sports Medicine and Physiology. Philadelphia, WB Saunders, 1979
39. Micheli LJ: Lower extremity injuries: Overuse injuries in the recreational adult athlete. In Cantu RC (ed): The Exercising Adult. Lexington, MA, Collamore Press, 1982
40. Micheli LJ: Young runners. Pediat Alert 6, 1981
41. Micheli LJ: Special considerations in children's rehabilitation programs. In Hunter L, Funk FJ (eds): Rehabilitation of the Injured Knee. St Louis, CV Mosby, (in press)
42. Micheli LJ, Hall JE, Miller ME: Use of modified Boston brace for back injuries in athletes. Am J Sports Med 8:351, 1980
43. Micheli LJ, Gerbino PG: The epidemiology of children's sports injuries. Orthop Trans 3:88, 1979
44. Micheli LJ, Santopietro FJ, Gerbino PG, *et al*: Etiologic assessment of overuse stress fracture in athletes. Nova Scotia Med Bull 59:43, 1980
45. Micheli LJ Stanitski CL: Lateral patellar retinacular release. Am J Sports Med 9:330, 1981
46. Miller EH, Schneider HJ, Bronson JL, *et al*: A new consideration in athletic injuries—the classical ballet dancer. Clin Orthop 11:181, 1975
47. Mueller F, Blyth C: Epidemiology of sports injuries in children. Clin Sports Med 1:343, 1982
48. Murray RO, Duncan C: Athletic activity in adolescence as an etiologic factor in degenerative hip disease. J Bone Joint Surg 53B:406, 1971
49. Ogden JA, Southwick WO: Osgood-Schlatter disease and tibial tubercle development. Clin Orthop 116:180, 1976
50. Patel D: Arthroscopy of the plicae-synovial folds and their significance. Am J Sports Med 6:217, 1978
51. Puddu G, Ippolito E, Pastacchini F: A classification of Achilles tendon disease. Am J Sports Med 4:145, 1976
52. Richardson AB, Jobe FW, Colins RH: The shoulder in competitive swimming. Am J Sports Med 8:159, 1980
53. Rosen PR, Micheli LJ, Treves S: Early scintigraphic diagnosis of bone stress and fractures in athletic adolescents. Pediatrics 70:11, 1982
54. Roser LA, Clawson DK: Football injuries in the very young athlete. Clin Orthop 69:212, 1970
55. Snook GA: Injuries in women's gymnastics. A 5-year study. Am J Sports Med 7(4):242, 1979
56. Sohn RS, Micheli LJ: The effect of running on the pathogenesis of osteoarthritis of the hips and knees. Clin Orthop 188:106–109, 1985
57. Squires W: Improving your running. Roxbury Crossing, MA, Running Systems, Inc, 1979
58. Stanitski CL, Micheli LJ: Medial malleolus avulsion injuries. Presented at Pediatric Orthopaedics Study Group Meeting, San Diego, CA, April 1982
59. Stulberg SD, Cordell LD, Harris WH, *et al*: Unrecognized childhood hip disease: A main course of idiopathic osteoarthritis of the hip. In The Hip: Proceedings of the Third Open Scientific Meeting of the Hip Society, Vol 3. St Louis, CV Mosby, 1975
60. Subotnick SL: Orthotic foot control and the overuse syndrome. Phys Sports Med 3:75, 1975
61. Teitz CC: Sports medicine concerns in dance and gymnastics. Pediatr Clin North Am 29:1399, 1982
62. Walaszek A: Physical therapy rehabilitation of dance injuries. In Gillespie WJ (ed): Sports Medicine, Sports Science, Bridging the Gap. Lexington, MA, Collamore Press, 1982
63. Walters NE, Wolf MD: Stress fractures in young athletes. Am J Sports Med 5:165, 1977

27

Neurofibromatosis

Alvin H. Crawford

HISTORICAL COMMENTS

Akenside, in 1768, first recorded a description of a patient with multiple neurofibromatoses.[98] However, credit is most frequently given to Wilhelm G. Telesius for contributing one of the earliest clinical descriptions of a patient with neurofibromatosis in 1793. Telesius was a good draftsman and was encouraged to make drawings of the patient by his teacher because of the peculiar soft, moist warts all over the patient's body. The well-executed drawings show a large number of skin tumors, some of them pedunculated, and the general appearance of the man ensures that the condition was neurofibromatosis. The patient was short in stature with a large head and a rather crooked back with one shoulder projecting (Fig. 27-1).

R.W. Smith, first professor of surgery at the Dublin Medical School and better known for his work on forearm fractures (reverse Colles), published a remarkable volume in 1849 in which he reported in great detail two cases of generalized neurofibromatosis with necropsy and completed the first review of the literature with 75 references. In 1863, Virchow described the pathology of peripheral nerve tumors, differentiated between nerve sheath tumors and nerve tumors. Genersich first reported a patient with kyphoscoliosis in 1870.

In 1882, Frederick Daniel von Recklinghausen published his book, *Uber die Multiplen Fibrome der haut und ihre Peziehung zur den Multiplen Neuromen*, dedicated to the pathologist Rudolf Virchow in honor of the 25th anniversary of the foundation of the Pathological Institute of Berlin. In this book, von Recklinghausen coined the term *neurofibroma*, and was able to demonstrate that a small cutaneous nerve was found to be connected to every one of the cutaneous and subcutaneous tumors. Prior to this, the term *dermal fibroma* or *false neuroma* had been applied to the nodules. Thus, von Recklinghausen was the first to demonstrate the origin of the tumors from nerve sheaths and his clinical and pathologic descriptions of the disease were epoch making.

Lisch, in 1937, substantiated the importance of Iris nodules first seen in patients with neurofibromatosis by Goldstein and Wexler to be associated with most patients with neurofibromatosis. Lisch nodules (melanocytic hamartomas of the iris) are thought by some investigators to be diagnostic of neurofibromatosis.

In 1956, Crowe, Schull, and Neil[33] described the diagnostic significance of multiple café-au-lait spots in reference to neurofibromatosis. The manifestations of neurofibromatosis in children have been reviewed by others.[23,28,30–32,42,43,105,125]

The original descriptions of the neurofibromatosis syndrome were by pathologists, and the neurofibroma occupied a central position in diagnosis. Through gradual increase in knowledge of other features of the disease such as pigmentary changes, dysplastic changes in bones, and inheritance, these manifestations of the disease have assumed an increasing role in diagnosis. As more and more cases of neurofibromatosis combined with other diseases have been recorded, so have more and

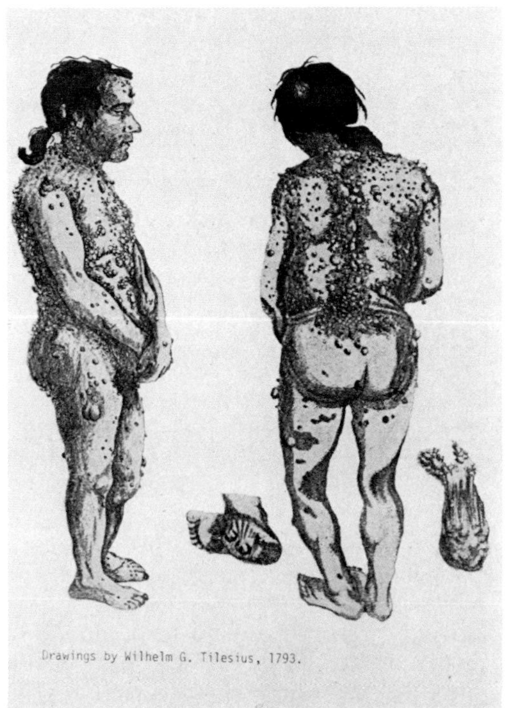

FIG. 27-1. Drawing of patient with neurofibromatosis. Note the elevation of the right shoulder and asymmetry of the trunk. (Reproduced from *Historia Pathologica Singularis Cutis Turpitudinus*. Leipzig, SL Crusis, 1793)

more diseases come to be recognized as being associated with neurofibromatosis, many of these showing strong evidence of the presence of neurofibromatosis.

Because of the multifarious facets of the disease, neurofibromatosis has stimulated many hypotheses as to its mechanism of origin. Neurofibromatosis was at one time defined as one of the neurocutaneous syndromes of unknown etiology, primarily of neuroectodermal origin. It, along with the hereditary syndromes of tuberous sclerosis, encephalotrigeminal angiomatosis, and cerebroretinal angiomatosis, is designated as a *phakomatosis* because of the hamartomatous lesions of the eye, skin, and brain. Other manifestations include café-au-lait spots and cutaneous and subcutaneous tumors, with secondary mesodermal defects responsible for various osseous abnormalities.

The condition is now considered to be a neurocristopathy or a hamartomatous disorder, probably of neural crest origin, not only involving the neuroectoderm and mesoderm but also involving the endoderm with the potential of appearing in almost all organ systems.[61] Four theories have been predominant. The oldest is the infection theory, later abandoned in favor of the endocrine, hormonal theory, which holds that neurofibromatosis may be due to widespread disturbance of the endocrine system, including, among other things, dysfunction of the hypothalamus.

More recently, the neurogenic theory and the dysontogenetic theory have gained increasing adherence. The neurogenic theory holds that the disease arises through a deviation in development of the primitive neuroblast, affecting its differentiation into other neurogenic cells, among them the Schwann cells. In the dysontogenic theory, which has gained most adherents, neurofibromatosis is seen as a congenital defect causing tendency to dysplasia of ectodermal and mesodermal tissue. More recently, Fisher and Vuzevski[44] provided electron-microscopic evidence of collagenous fibriles arising from interdigitating extension of the basement membrane of Schwann's cells in neurofibromatosis to connect mesenchymal and neuroectodermal elements of the disease. The true neurofibroma will show itself to be separated by a large extracellular compartment containing numerous bundles of collagen.[44] Cell bodies show slight variation in size and shape. In some cases, there has been noted to be a distribution of extracellular structures demonstrating a uniquely banded arrangement. Waggener[135] reported these structures as being comprised of thin, longitudinal filaments approximately 250 Å apart. The electron dense crossbands measured 400 to 500 Å in thickness and had a periodicity of 900 to 1500 Å. These cross-banded fibers frequently lay in close proximity to the mature collagen fibers or basement membrane. The practical significance for diagnostic value of these bands is limited, because they cannot be resolved with certainty by light microscope or routinely prepared sections.

DIAGNOSTIC PROBLEMS IN NEUROFIBROMATOSIS

In many cases, neurofibromatosis is typical in its development, with multiple café-au-lait spots and neurofibromata, leaving no doubt about the diagnosis. However, in certain cases, the manifestations of the disease are few and relatively uncommon, so that the diagnosis may be greatly in doubt. Difficulties may also arise through the nature of the disease which often shows slow clinical evolution over decades—the typical cutaneous neurofibromata developing at or after puberty or considerably later in life. Sharp and Young pointed out that it was difficult to classify the disease into different clinical forms because of its protean manifestation and also because of the occurrence of incomplete forms, for example, those patients with nothing more than café-au-lait spots on the skin or axillary freckling.

The fact that neurofibromatosis is probably of multiple cell origin has been substantiated by studies using the X-linked glucose 6-phosphate dehydrogenase mosaicism marker.[41] It may be influenced by increased nerve growth stimulating factor, although current conflicting evidence regarding this theory remains to be resolved.[115,116] The etiology is still unknown.

Having accepted the autosomal dominant theory of inheritance in neurofibromatosis, one has to be concerned about the high number of mutations (50%) occurring with the disorder. This spontaneous mutation rate has been challenged by Steg and co-workers,[123] with dermatoglyphic analysis using a computerized pattern analysis and classification system (PAC). Abnormal congenital dermatoglyphic patterns have been found in many parents of patients formerly classified as spontaneous mutations. When one considers the many different clinical presentations of the disease, one can more easily accept the autosomal dominant concept and appreciate the varying penetrance and expressivity. Such thinking also allows the possibility that rather than a skipped generation, there was a different mode of expression with the dominant gene present. Contrast those patients with multiple café-au-lait spots versus bilateral acoustic neuromata versus axillary freckling only.

Young and associates[145] classified neurofibromatosis into three hereditary forms: (1) the peripheral form, with café-au-lait spots and neurofibroma; (2) the central form, with multiple tumors in the central nervous system of a type consistent with neurofibromatosis; and (3) a mixed form, with both peripheral signs of neurofibromatosis and tumors in the central nervous system. These investigators further pointed out that the diseases often, although not always, are inherited in the same form in the next generation. Other investigators have considered the penetrance of the disease form to be related to maternal involvement and elderly paternity ages.

The study by Crowe and colleagues[33] included patients showing a typical clinical picture of neurofibromatosis in the form of peripheral neurofibromas, radiologic changes specific for neurofibromatosis, or a histologic diagnosis of neurofibroma. No particular change has yet been recognized that is pathognomic of Recklinghausen's neurofibromatosis. Crowe and co-workers included patients with two or more neurofibromata plus positive biopsy. However, several investigators have subsequently pointed out that solitary or very few neurofibromata alone do not justify diagnosis of neurofibromatosis. According to Clemis,[25] neurogenic tumors of exogenous causation can arise after injury or irradiation. For example, Knight and associates[70] reported 69 cases of solitary neurofibroma which exhibited no other signs of neurofibromatosis. Several authors have required one, two, and three neurofibromata as a minimum for diagnostic criteria for neurofibromatosis.[10,101,106,136]

During the past decade, several authors have constructed tables of the changes typical of neurofibromatosis and have required at least two of the criteria in the table to be met for establishment of the diagnosis. Riccardi and Kleiner[110] required the presence of neurofibromata plus at least one of the the three following criteria; multiple café-au-lait spots, more than one neurofibroma, or positive heredity. These authors would regard at least six café-au-lait spots measuring 1.5 cm or more in their greatest diameter as being adequate for the diagnosis of neurofibromatosis.

Crawford (1978)[30,31] presented 82 cases of neurofibromatosis with the diagnostic requirement that two of the following four criteria be present: café-au-lait spots (five in number with a diameter of at least 0.5 cm), positive family history, histologic diagnosis of neurofibroma, and a characteristic osseous lesion (hemihypertrophy, kyphoscoliosis, or congenital pseudoarthrosis tibia).

For the diagnosis of their 102 neurofibromatosis patients, Winter and colleagues[142] required the presence of two or more of the six classical criteria: six café-au-lait spots, multiple subcutaneous neurofibromata, elephantiasis neuromatosa, positive biopsies showing neurofibroma, positive heredity, and the osseous dystrophic changes specific for neurofibromatosis.

Most investigators now accept the two clinical forms of neurofibromatosis, that is, peripheral neurofibromatosis and central neurofibromatosis. The central form has been split into those with multiple central nervous system involvement such as neuraxial neoplasia, meningoneuroplasia, cranial schwannoma, optic glioma, and optic globe schwannoma. The exception to this concept is the patient with a special form of central neurofibromatosis, that is, bilateral acoustic neuroma occurring as the only sign of neurofibromatosis. Dermal lesions are uncommon in central neurofibromatosis. Young and associates,[145] in 1970, reported on 55 members of a single family studied over eight generations. Forty-two persons in this family were suspected of having bilateral acoustic neurinoma. Not more than two members of the family had café-au-lait spots, and only two members had more than one subcutaneous neurofibroma. This somewhat lengthy and extensive account illustrates the multiplicity of presentation of a multi-systemic disorder.

Recently, Rubenstein has contrasted hereditary patterns of families with dermal neurofibromas as opposed to plexiform neurofibromas and has found their hereditary pattern to be somewhat interchangeable. He also illustrated that in one generation, there might be as few as one café-au-lait spot and several dermal neurofibromas, whereas the next generation might have plexiform neurofibromas. In general, peripheral signs together with biopsies showing neurofibroma have been accorded great diagnostic significance, whereas central nervous system signs of neurofibromatosis have received considerably less emphasis.

GENETICS

Neurofibromatosis is the most common single gene disorder found in humans. It has been virtually unknown to the general public until the recent popularity of the Elephant Man, Joseph Carey MacDonald ("John") Merrick. It is much more common than other conditions that are well known to the general public such as muscular dystrophy, cystic fibrosis, and Down's syndrome. The occurrence of this disease in multiple family members was reported in Europe as early as 1847 by Virchow.[134] In 1901, Adrian[2] reported that 20% of 447 cases he reviewed exhibited direct transmission. Preiser and Davenport[105] first described the condition as an autosomal dominant trait in 1918. It is considered to be an autosomal dominant trait with variable penetrance and a very high rate of spontaneous mutation; however, the above discussion identifying the various forms that may propagate through several generations severely challenges the spontaneous mutation theory. Genetic heterogeneity is a key element in neurofibromatosis. There are likely to be multiple forms of the disorder, probably involving multiple alleles at a single locus and possibly several gene loci. The disorder has tremendous clinical variability, an aspect that must be taken into account in any discussion of pathogenesis.[109] It has been documented to have a frequency of 1 per 2500 to 3000 live births. Spontaneous abortion in patients with neurofibromatosis has not been studied to date.

CLINICAL FINDINGS

CAFÉ-AU-LAIT SPOTS

The café-au-lait type of pigmentation is a characteristic lesion of neurofibromatosis; however, von Recklinghausen did not consider it to be a part of the disorder. This pigmentation is tan, macular, and melanotic in origin and is located in and around the basal layer of the epidermis. The lesions may vary in shape, size, number, and location (Fig. 27-2*A*). In neurofibromatosis, they are frequently found in areas of the skin not exposed to the sun. The presence of a café-au-lait spot may be normal. McCarroll[86] examined normal nursing students and found that 20% had café-au-lait spots without associated anomalies. Crowe and associates[33] concluded that an adult who has more than six café-au-lait spots measuring 1.5 cm or more in diameter should be presumed to have neurofibromatosis. Whitehouse[141] evaluated 365 children younger than the age of 5 years and stated that two or less café-au-lait spots occur in only 0.75% of normal children and that five spots, with a diameter of at least 0.5 cm, should be diagnostic of neurofibromatosis until proved otherwise. Crawford[30,31] reported on patients younger than 12 years of age, conclusively diagnosed by his criteria as having neurofibromatosis, who occasionally did not have any café-au-lait spots on presentation but developed them at a later age. His young patients presenting with only a few café-au-lait spots showed an increase in number and size with increasing age. The lesions are usually present by 9 years of age. In men, the intensity of color of the spots increases up to puberty and then remains stable. In women, the areas become darker with pregnancy and remain dark throughout pregnancy. The geometric requirements for diagnosis, that is, smooth edges (coast of California) for neurofibromatosis in contrast with the jagged edges seen in fibrous dysplasia (coast of Maine) have been questioned. Undue emphasis on the number, size, and shape of café-au-lait spots can lead to underdiagnosis, overdiagnosis, or misdiagnosis.[109]

Recent investigators have attempted to make a qualitative distinction between the café-au-lait spots of neurofibromatosis and those of fibrous dysplasia as opposed to those occurring in normal subjects. Johnson and Charneco[65] described the presence of giant melanosomes in the melanocytes in café-au-lait spots in six of eight neurofibromatosis patients whom they examined. No similar changes were found in the so-called normally occurring café-au-lait spots. The café-au-lait spots in neurofibromatosis showed a higher number of melanocytes per square millimeter compared with the number of these cells in corresponding parts of the skin of healthy persons. Johnson and Charneco[65] and Takahashi[126] have noted an increased activity of melanocytes in neurofibromatosis; however, these findings have been of no pathognomonic value. The café-au-lait spots of children with neurofibromatosis rarely show giant melanosomes compared with those of adults with the disease that show large numbers of the pigment bodies.

Frenk[46] showed that in Albright's disease, café-au-lait spots did not contain giant melanosomes. Therefore, some differences that are quantitative and qualitative but not pathognomonic have thus been recognized, and these afford some possibility of distinguishing the café-au-lait spots of neurofibromatosis from those seen in other conditions.

NODULES

Cutaneous nodules (fibroma molluscum) are only found in post pubescent children. The lesions are now considered to be dermal neurofibromas. They are manifestations of long-standing or adult disease and do not occur with any frequency (12%) in childhood.[60] These soft tumors may grow under, be flush with, or be raised above the level of the skin (Fig. 27-2*B*). Although they are usually the color of normal skin, early lesions may be violaceous.[100] Ormsby and Montgomery[100] interpreted these tumors as true neurofibromas arising from peripheral nerves and their supporting structures, but this conclusion had not been proved. Rubenstein shares this theory. Stout[124] considered these tumors to be simple proliferation of fibrous tissue. Electron microscopy demonstrated the axons and the Schwann cells in these tumors; therefore, it is appropriate that they be included under the term *dermal neurofibroma*.[55] Dermal neurofibroma are rarely associated with central nervous system lesions, and only occasionally does one see skeletal involvement with this peripheral type of neurofibromatosis.

NEVUS

Nevi, or hyperpigmentation, may be present in up to 6% of children with neurofibromatosis. These lesions are dark brown–pigmented areas of the skin, which occasionally tend to isolate themselves to one side of the body (Fig. 27-2*C*). Patients may present with large nevi that cover broad areas of the skin, some of which are quite sensitive. The sensitivity is often related to an underlying subcutaneous plexiform neurofibroma. The plexiform neurofibromata have a "ropey," "bag of worms" feeling and are extremely sensitive. The areas of involvement may also have decreased sensation, thus allowing sores to develop under brace or cast without the patient's knowledge. When a plexiform neurofibroma is found underlying an area of cutaneous hyperpigmentation, especially when the tumor approaches or reaches the midline of the body, it appears to indicate that the tumor will be aggressive and/or involve the spinal cord. The plexiform neurofibroma is known for harboring the potential for malignant degeneration.

Surgical treatment during early childhood is recommended for pigmented nevi. The major reason for excising the lesions early is to eliminate the 10% chance of transformation of the underlying plexiform neuroma. Early excision may also decrease the secondary psychological effects of these cosmetically objectionable lesions and, at the same time, result in better healing.

ELEPHANTIASIS

Frequently, large soft-tissue masses are seen in neurofibromatosis. These masses have been termed *pachydermatocele* or *elephantiasis neuromatosa*. They are characterized by a

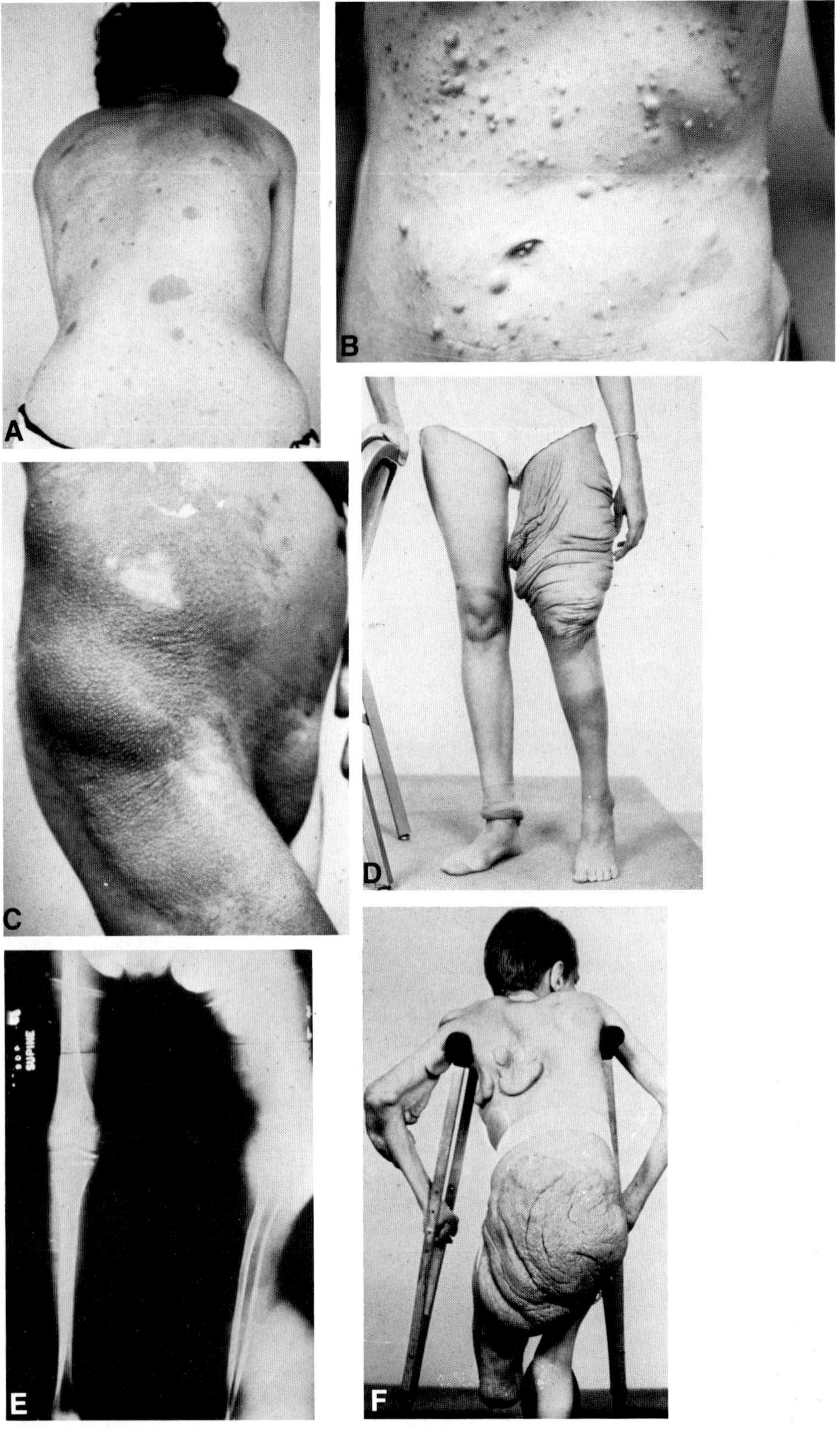
A
B
C
D
E
F

rough, raised villous type of skin hypertrophy presenting an unmistakable appearance. Although they occur more frequently in adults, approximately 10% occur in children, with varying degrees of involvement. Weiss[139] described this finding to be characteristic of neurofibromatosis. There may be dysplasia of the underlying bone (Fig. 27-2*D*).[63]

VERRUCOUS HYPERPLASIA

Verrucous hyperplasia is an infrequent but definite noncosmetic cutaneous lesion of neurofibromatosis. There is tremendous overgrowth of the skin, with thickening but a velvety soft papillary quality to it. Many crevices form in this disorder and tend to break down easily with some weeping occurring in the skin folds. The sites often become superficially infected and give rise to a foul odor. The lesion presents most often unilaterally and can be considered one of the most grotesque lesions of neurofibromatosis (Fig. 27-2*E*).

AXILLARY FRECKLING

Axillary freckles, which are diffuse small hyperpigmented spots up to 2 mm or 3 mm in diameter found in the armpits, are helpful diagnostic criteria for neurofibromatosis if present. Axillary freckling and an occasional dermal neurofibroma may be the only physical findings in the parent of a child who shows all the criteria required for the diagnosis of neurofibromatosis. Prior to our being aware of these presentations, the child would have been considered a spontaneous mutation.

SKELETAL MANIFESTATIONS

SCOLIOSIS

Scoliosis is the most common osseous defect associated with neurofibromatosis. Gould[49] and Weiss[139] were the first to point out the high incidence of spinal deformities in this disease. The spinal deformity may vary in severity from mild, nonprogressive forms to severe curvatures. Since Weiss', a dermatologist, first description in 1921, many authors have cited the association of the two conditions.[3,13,15,16,22,46,75,81,91,108,111,117,133,142]

The cause of spinal deformity is unknown, but it has been suggested to be secondary to osteomalacia, a localized neurofibromatous tumor eroding and infiltrating bone, endocrine disturbances, and mesodermal dysplasia.[20,49,50,56,115,118,139]

The relative incidence of spine deformities in neurofibromatosis is unknown. In a general orthopaedic clinic, 2% of the scoliosis population will have neurofibromatosis. In the scoliosis clinic population, approximately 3% will have neurofibromatosis, whereas in a neurofibromatosis population, 60% of patients will have some disorder of the spine.

Of approximately 10,000 patients with scoliosis seen by Winter *et al.*,[142] only 102 were found to fit the traditional criteria for diagnosis of neurofibromatosis. They thought it most

◀ Fig. 27-2. The cutaneous lesion of neurofibromatosis as seen in children. *(A)* Multiple café-au-lait spots in a young patient with a spinal deformity. Note the variation in size and shape of the lesions. These lesions tend to increase in size and number as the child matures. *(B)* Multiple dermal neurofibroma (fibroma molluscum). These pedunculated lesions occur in the post pubescent adolescent. They have no particular distribution and can be seen on the adjacent right forearm. Several subcutaneous neurofibroma and café-au-lait spots are also present on this photograph. *(C)* This large nevus overlies a plexiform neurofibroma. The plexiform neurofibroma was directly over the greater trochanter and iliac crest in this patient who had a spinal deformity but could not tolerate a Milwaukee brace over the area because of the extreme sensitivity. The lesion only occurred on one side of the body. The neurofibroma underneath these lesions will occasionally extend into the spinal canal. *(D* and *E)* Elephantiasis neuromatosis. This thickening of the skin with redundant folds gives a pachydermatocele appearance to this lesion. Several unsuccessful attempts have been made to perform epiphyseal arrests of the distal femur and proximal tibia. Anteroposterior roentgenogram of both lower extremities showing normal-appearing bone on the right and the dysplastic, narrow, elongated bone on the left; the soft-tissue shadows partially obliterate the femur on the left. The child subsequently succumbed to a retroperitoneal neurofibrosarcoma. *(F)* Verrucous hyperplasia of the skin over the left buttocks. This lesion was associated with elongation of the lower extremity. Note that the child has had a knee disarticulation but the femur extends far below its opposite knee joint. The pendulous skin lesions on the upper body are on one side only. Verrucous hyperplasia represents the most grotesque of all cutaneous lesions of neurofibromatosis. (*A, B,* and *C* reproduced with permission from Neurofibromatosis in the pediatric patient. Orthop Clin North Am 9, No. 1:11–23, 1978. *D* and *E* reproduced with permission from Neurofibromatosis in childhood. AAOS Instruc Course Lect 30:56–74, 1981) important to recognize the dysplastic or dystrophic curve and contrast it from the nondystrophic curve. They also believed that brace treatment was not effective in the management of the dystrophic curve and recommended an aggressive approach to management: "There is no justification for passively observing the progression of a spine deformity in neurofibromatosis". The truely good results in their series were in patients who had fusions promptly, before the curve became severe. Even in the young children, because the curves were usually short with very poor vertical growth potential in the involved vertebra, early fusion caused minimal stunting of trunk height. The stunting of trunk height was much less than would have occurred if the curve had been allowed to progress (Fig. 27-3*A* and *B*).

According to most investigators, the scoliosis is usually in the thoracic area and tends to produce a very short sharply angulated curvature, including 4 to 6 vertebrae, and is usually progressive. Miller[91] described the curvature of neurofibromatosis as a kyphoscoliosis with a site of predilection in the lower thoracic area, which may be noticed in early childhood. A characteristic feature is a sharp angulation at the apex of the gibbus. Scott[117] evaluated the spine deformities in 81 patients and found no evidence of any consistent pattern of scoliosis in neurofibromatosis. He noted that the severity of some of the curves resembled congenital scoliosis. Veliskakis and associates[133] noted in 43 of 55 patients a characteristic short curve composed of five or fewer segments with sharp apical wedging and rotation in the lower thoracic area. The wedging was occasionally so severe that it was mistaken for a hemivertebrae. They believed that the tendency of this curve to progress

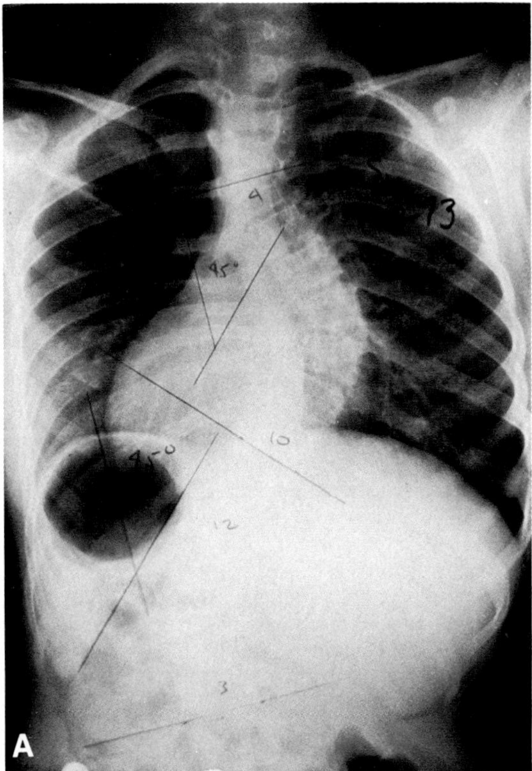

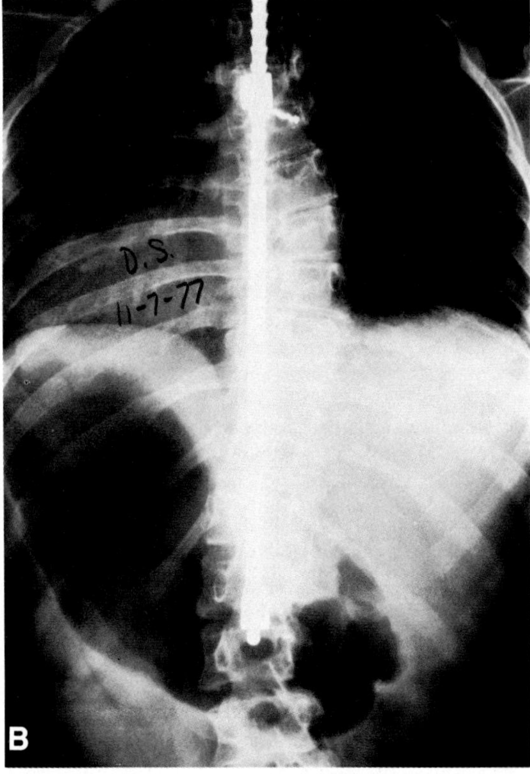

FIG. 27-3. Idiopathic lateral spinal deformity in a patient with neurofibromatosis. *(A)* Right dorsal T4–T10 scoliosis with compensatory lumbar curve in a 14-year-old female with neurofibromatosis. (Her 17-year-old brother had severe kyphosis requiring surgery.) There is no evidence of scalloping of vertebral margins or paraspinal masses. *(B)* Four years following spinal fusion and Harrington rod instrumentation showing maintenance of correction and solid fusion. (Reproduced with permission from Neurofibromatosis in childhood. AAOS Instruc Course Lect 30:56–74, 1981)

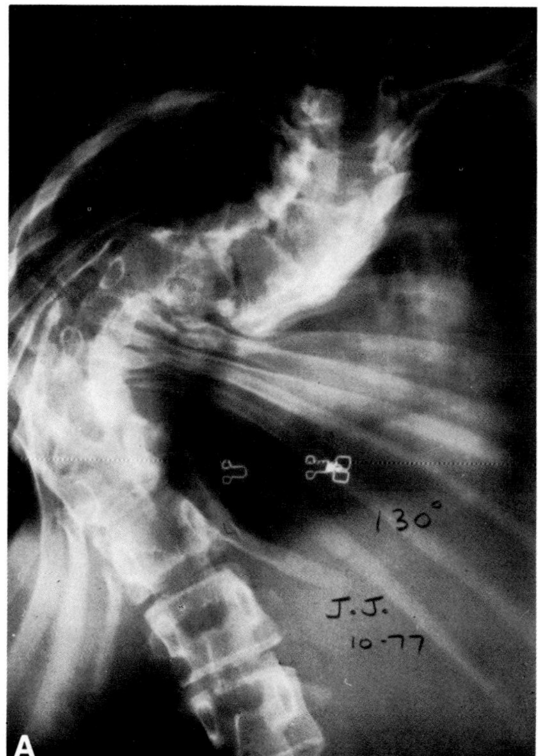

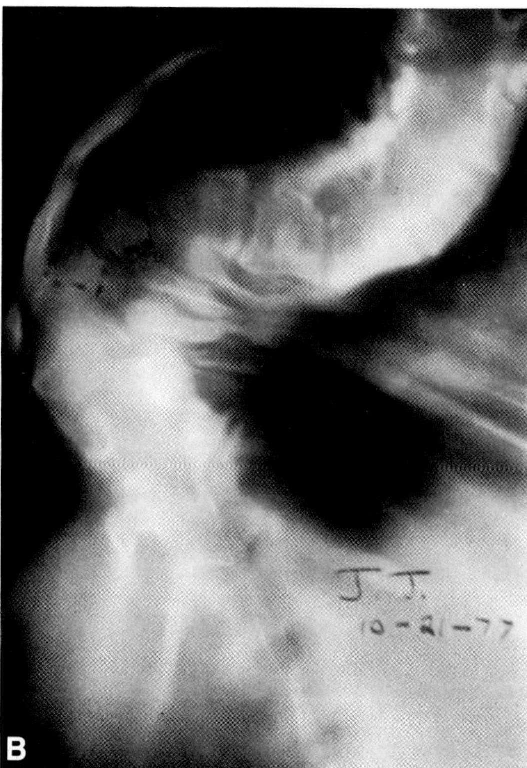

FIG. 27-4. Neurofibromatotic spinal deformity with short segmented, sharply angulated "kinky" spinal deformity: plain film and tomography. *(A)* Anteroposterior roentgenogram of spine associated with neurofibromatosis. There is scalloping of the vertebral margins, gross rotation of the apical vertebrae, relative appearance of a paraspinous mass, and penciling of the ribs in the concavity. *(B)* Plain polytomography reveals widening of the spinal canal in the upper thoracic region inferring dural ectasia. There appears to be a 180° vertebral body rotation between the upper thoracic vertebrae and the apical vertebrae. Note the proximity of the apical vertebrae to the ribs. (Courtesy of Dr. Michael Schafer, Chicago, Illinois. Reproduced with permission from Neurofibromatosis in childhood. AAOS Instruc Course Lect 30:56–74, 1981)

rapidly warranted early spine fusion of the involved segments to prevent progression. Other investigators have suggested that there is no standard pattern of spine deformity in neurofibromatosis and that the types of curvature found are quite variable.[22,52,117]

Cobb[26] was one of the first to recognize the serious nature of this spine deformity and especially the deleterious effect of laminectomy in the patient with neurofibromatosis and scoliosis. He also believed that a high proportion of scoliosis classified as idiopathic may be due to neurofibromatosis.

The consensus is that there are probably two patterns of scoliosis found in neurofibromatosis, that is, the characteristic short-segmented, dysplastic, sharply angulated curve and curves resembling idiopathic scoliosis. Right and left convex thoracic curves occur in about equal numbers. The dysplastic curvature is characterized by severe wedging of the apical vertebral bodies, strong rotation of apical vertebrae, scalloping of vertebral bodies, spindling of transverse processes, foraminal enlargement, and pencilling of the apical ribs (Fig. 27-4). Those curvatures resembling idiopathic scoliosis demonstrate the same tendency to progress as idiopathic curvatures and have no dysplastic changes of the vertebral bodies.

There have been relatively few clinical series pertaining to the treatment of spine deformities in patients with neurofibromatosis. Winter and associates[142] reviewed the natural history, associated anomalies, and response to operative and nonoperative treatment in 102 patients with neurofibromatosis and spine deformity. Eighty patients were found to have curvature associated with dystrophic changes in the vertebrae and ribs. The presence of dystrophic changes such as rib pencilling, spindling of the transverse processes, vertebral scalloping, severe apical vertebral rotation, foraminal enlargement, and adjacent soft-tissue neurofibroma, was found to be highly significant in the prognosis and management. Brace treatment of dystrophic curves was unsuccessful. Posterior fusion, with or without internal fixation, was the procedure of choice for problems due purely to scoliosis. Patients with dystrophic kyphoscoliosis required both anterior and posterior fusion to achieve stability. Sixteen patients had compression of the spinal cord or cauda equina.

Crawford reviewed 50 scoliotic patients who presented with scoliosis when they were younger than 12 years of age. Only 8 had the characteristic neurofibromatosis curve; the remainder had curves indistinguishable from the idiopathic type. The x-ray characteristics and response to treatment of curves in those young patients were similar to those of patients without neurofibromatosis. Forty-five of the 50 patients with spine deformities were female. Seven were detected because of an ongoing family study to determine the genetic aspect of scoliosis. The finding of neurofibromatosis in the family study of scoliosis reconfirms the genetic aspect. Thirty-six patients underwent posterior spinal fusion, and, of these, 9 required re-exploration for possible pseudarthrosis, of which 5 were found to have defects in the fusion mass (a 17% pseudarthrosis rate). One other patient was known to have a pseudarthrosis, but it had not been explored at the time of publication. The percentage of

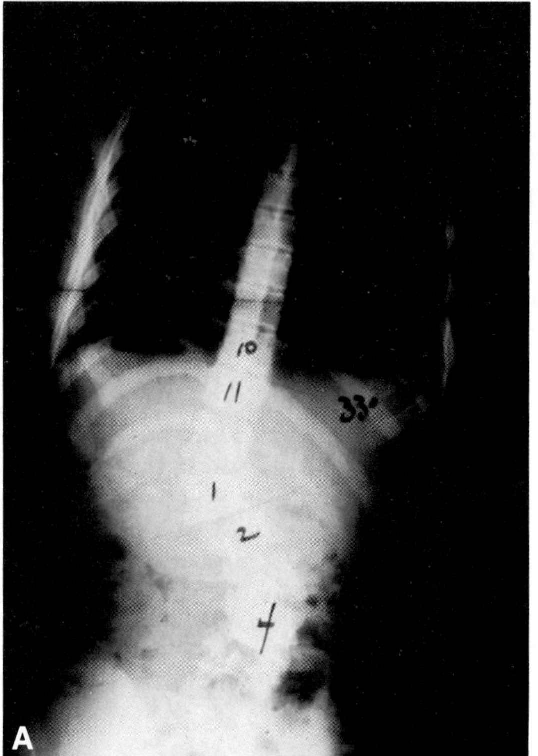

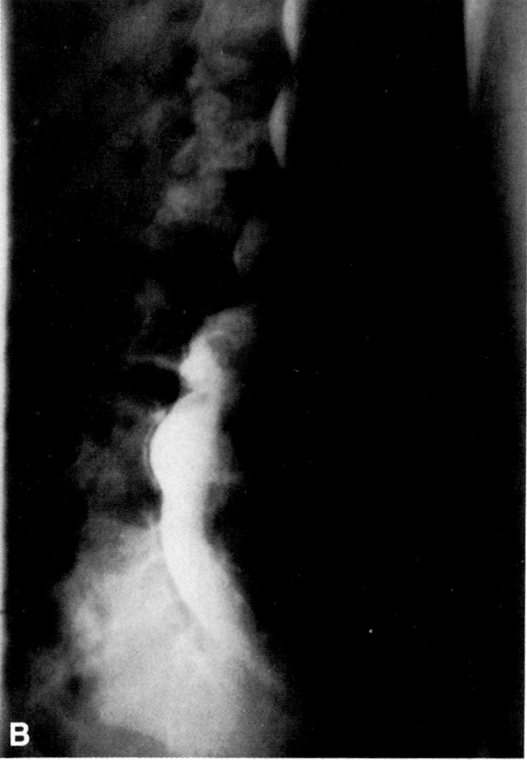

FIG. 27-5. A short segmented double primary scoliosis associated with neurofibromatosis. The lateral view showed significant scalloping of the posterior vertebral bodies and increase in the anteroposterior diameter of the neural formamina and spinal canal. *(A)* The double primary curvature extending from T11 to L4. Note the sharp wedge-shaped margins of the vertebral bodies suggesting extrinsic pressure. *(B)* An oblique view of the myelogram demonstrating the dural ectasia and pressure erosion of the vertebral bodies. (Referred from Dr. William Lonon, Oakland, CA)

pseudarthrosis in these patients was much higher than that for idiopathic curves treated during this same period of time.

Except for those patients with dystrophic spine deformity, a posterior spinal fusion with or without Harrington rod gave satisfactory results for patients with only scoliosis. Because of paraplegia encountered due to unsuspected posterior dural ectasia, it is strongly suggested that dystrophic patients have a complete high-volume myelography in the prone, lateral, and supine positions or comparable CT or MRI scan prior to surgical treatment (Fig. 27-5).[56]

KYPHOSCOLIOSIS

The severe kyphoscoliosis seen in neurofibromatosis is distinguished by the predominance of kyphosis over the scoliosis, with acute angulation being a typical sign. The vertebral bodies frequently are so deformed and attenuated at the apex that it may be impossible to identify them on routine roentgenograms. Curtis and associates[34] believe that the kyphosis contributed more to the production of paraplegia in their patients than did the scoliosis. This view is supported by the biomechanical studies of Breig,[17] which showed that flexion of the spine caused elongation of the spinal canal and deformation of the spinal cord. Pathologically increased spinal flexion, as by a kyphotic deformity, leads to excessive axial tension of the spinal cord parenchyma and may result in neurologic impairment. In 1936, Miller,[91] found that in 20 patients who had paraplegia associated with von Recklinghausen's disease, severe angulation of the spine was responsible for the paraplegia in more than half the patients. Lonstein and coworkers[80] reviewed 45 patients with cord compression due to spinal curvature and found neurofibromatosis to be secondary only to congenital kyphosis as a cause of the compression. Crawford presented four patients younger than 12 years of age with neurofibromatosis who had kyphoscoliosis. One patient, 6 years of age, underwent a posterior spinal fusion from T4 to T12 and an attempted anterior spinal fusion for progressive kyphosis. The anterior procedure was aborted because of pronounced local invasion of the soft tissue with neurofibromatous material. The soft tissue appeared to have directly invaded the spinal elements. Winter and colleagues[142] reported a 64% incidence of pseudarthrosis in patients with dystrophic scoliosis and kyphosis of more than 50°. It was their conclusion that dystrophic patients with angular kyphosis responded very poorly to posterior fusion alone, and posterior pseudarthrosis repair was not successful in achieving stabilization (Fig. 27-6*A* and *B*). Good results were consistently obtained only in those patients who had both anterior and posterior fusion. However, not every patient obtained solid fusion initially with both anterior and posterior procedures; several required repeat operative procedures. The investigators believed that technically inadequate anterior procedures were the usual reason for failure. Most important was the recommendation that the entire structural area of the deformity be fused anteriorly with complete disc excision and strong strut graft, preferably from the fibula as well as ribs and iliac crest graft. No soft tissue should be allowed to interpose between the grafts, and all grafts should have contact with each other and with the spine. Those grafts surrounded by soft tissue tended to resorb in the midportion.

Because of the association of paraplegia with kyphoscoliosis, there has been a tendency to perform laminectomy. Laminectomy for kyphoscoliotic cord compression is contraindicated. The inciting lesion is usually anterior, and the compression cannot be visualized from behind. Also, the removal of the posterior elements predisposes the patient to progressive postlaminectomy kyphosis and removes valuable bone stock that is required for posterior spinal fusion.[142]

CERVICAL SPINE DISORDERS

Klose[69] recorded the first case of cervical abnormality associated with neurofibromatosis. Until recently, only casual references to the cervical spine have been evident in studies of other manifestations of neurofibromatosis.

Yong-Hing and associates[144] reviewed 56 patients with neurofibromatosis from the Alfred I. Dupont Institute, specifically for abnormalities of the cervical spine, and found 17 to have lesions. Of 34 patients who had scoliosis or kyphoscoliosis, 15 (44%) had cervical spine lesions. Many of these patients were asymptomatic. Adkins and Ratvich[1] reviewed 85 patients with von Recklinghausen's neurofibromatosis at the Children's Hospital of Pittsburgh and found that head and neck masses

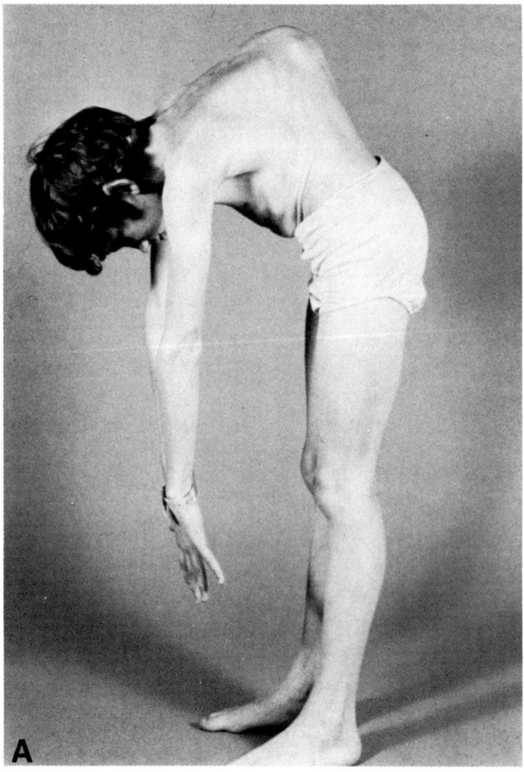

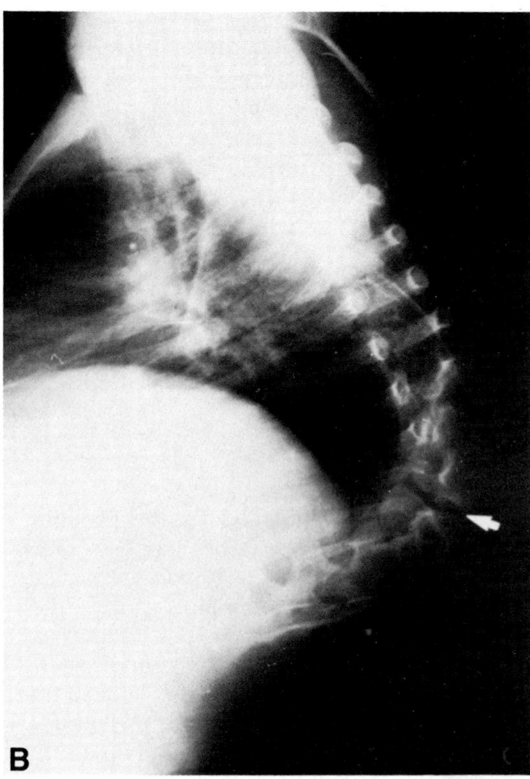

FIG. 27-6. A young boy with a kyphotic spinal deformity when seen following two attempts at posterior spinal fusion. *(A)* Clinical photograph of side view while bending shows severe gibbus or hump. The trunk is significantly foreshortened. *(B)* Lateral x-ray view of thoracic spine showing one of the areas of pseudarthrosis *(arrow)*. (Reproduced with permission from Neurofibromatosis in children. Am Fam Phys 17(3):163–170, 1978)

constituted 22% of the presenting problems (Fig. 27-7*A* and *B*).

Most patients presenting to the orthopaedist with cervical spine anomaly usually present secondarily after having undergone excision of a neck mass by the surgery service, the preceding work-up having included an x-ray of the cervical spine showing considerable bony anomaly. Other reasons for presentation include torticollis and dysphagia (Fig. 27-8).

Yong-Hing and associates[144] showed that the cervical spine in patients with neurofibromatosis was more likely to be abnormal if there was a thoracic spine curvature (44%) than if there was no thoracic spine curvature (9%). They believe that there is a frequent association of abnormalities of the cervical spine with scoliosis and kyphoscoliosis. Holt[61] found that cervical deformities were confined to young adults. Yong-Hing and co-workers[144] noted the occurrence of cervical spine deformities in nine of their patients who were younger than 15 years of age, including a 20-month-old girl with paraplegia. They believe that cervical spine deformities are not infrequent in childhood and that some may be evident during infancy. There was also a higher incidence of cervical spine abnormalities with the short, sharply angulated dysplastic thoracic spinal curve than with a long curve that resembled idiopathic scoliosis. Cervical spine x-ray examinations *are recommended* for all neurofibromatosis patients who are to have either general anesthesia or skull traction for the treatment of thoracic spine deformities.

SPONDYLOLISTHESIS

Only 11 cases of spondylolisthesis due to neurofibromatosis have been reported—2 by Hunt and Pugh,[63] 1 by Mandell,[82] and 1 by Winter and co-workers.[142] McCarroll[86] noted spondylolisthesis in four of his patients. Crawford noted only one of 82 patients with neurofibromatosis (50 of whom had spine deformity) to have spondylolisthesis, even though lateral x-ray films of the lumbar spine were taken on all patients. This represented a lower incidence of spondylolisthesis than that found either in the general population or a population of thoracic spine deformities.

Several patients have shown a tendency to marked increase in size of the lumbar spine neuroforamina with coexisting narrowing and elongation of the pedicle, which could predispose to "stress risers" or pathologic spondylolisthesis. Myelography may reveal dural ectasia and pseudomeningocele formation. Treatment of spondylolisthesic progression requires stabilization and massive bone grafting.

INTRATHORACIC MENINOGOCELE AND DUMBBELL LESIONS

An intrathoracic meningocele is relatively rare; fewer than 50 cases are reported in the English-speaking literature. Pohl[103] reported the first case of an intrathoracic meningocele associated with neurofibromatosis. Roentgenographically, with myelography, a soft-tissue mass is seen protruding from the spinal canal into the posterior mediastinum (Fig. 27-9). Structural defects in the pedicle, enlargements of the intervertebral foramina, and abnormalities of the vertebral bodies may accompany the masses. The occurrence of spinal meningoceles in patients with neurofibromatosis has been reported.[97,103,112] The association of meningoceles with enlarged intervertebral foramina and other vertebral deformities has seldom received comment. The scalloping of the vertebral body with deformity of the pedicles and widening of the intervertebral foramina could be caused either by the presence of dumbbell tumors (intraspinal neurofibromas) or saccular dilatations of the dura, *dural ectasia*. The dumbbell neurofibromata in the thoracic area may be associated with lateral

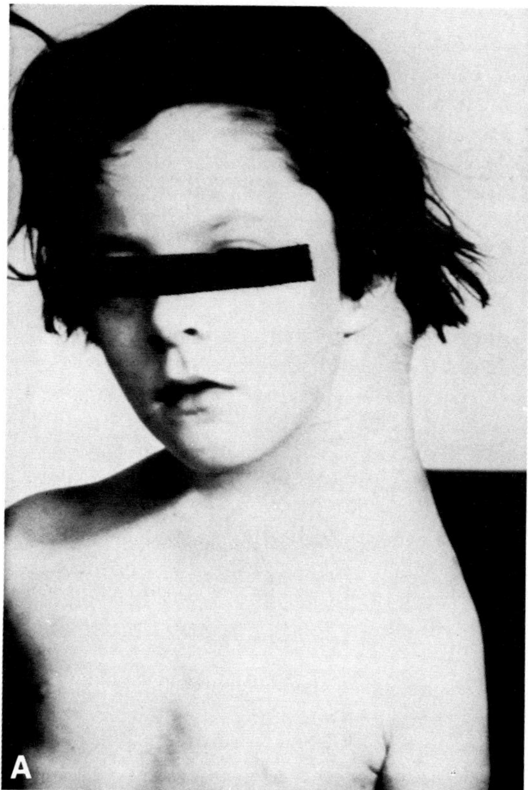

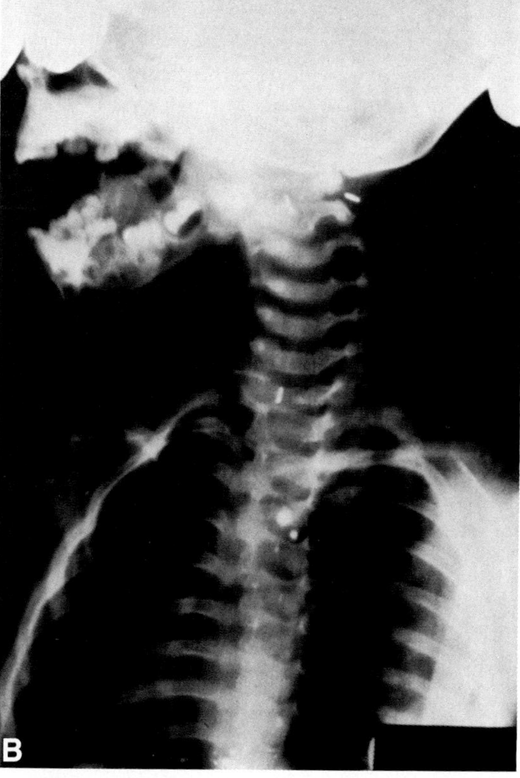

FIG. 27-7. This very young child presented with the chief complaint of a mass in her left cervical region and a torticollis. *(A)* Postexcision, the child continued to have moderate to severe torticollis. *(B)* Note the enlargement of the neural foramina and the vascular clips outlining the area of surgical excision of the mass. There is also retained contrast media in the spinal canal. The neural foraminal enlargement represents the exiting of intraspinal neurofibroma through this route, (*i.e.*, multiple dumbbell lesions).

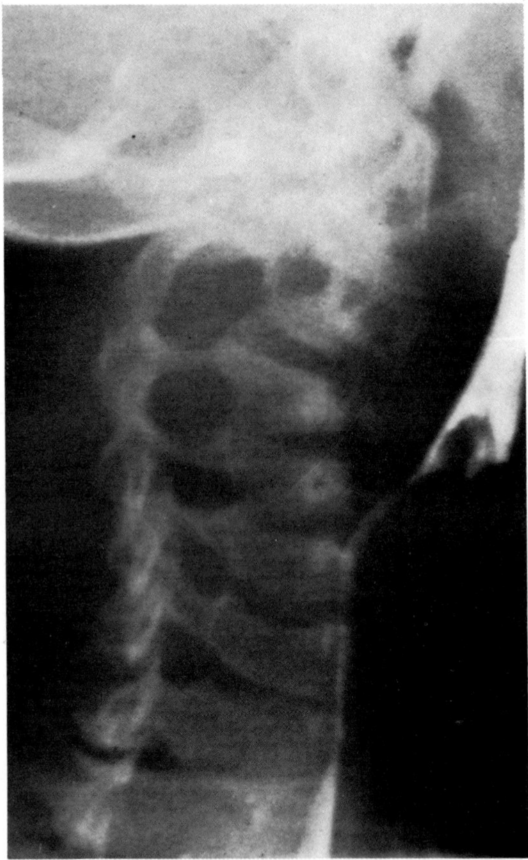

FIG. 27-8. This child presented 3 years following excision of a mass from the left side of her neck. The mass had recurred, and she had difficulty swallowing. An esophagram demonstrated the outline of a prevertebral retropharyngeal soft-tissue mass. The enlargement of the neural foraminae infers that the mass is exiting from the spinal canal at multiple locations and that it is presenting anterior. When the neurofibroma exits from the spinal canal through the neuroforamina, a constriction occurs giving it a bilobed or "dumbbell" appearance. The mass was surgically removed with a CO_2 laser. (Case referred from Dr. Dan Bethem, Akron, OH)

meningocele, possibly as a result of increased intraspinal tension associated with a scoliotic curve but not necessarily in the area of the tumor or the meningocele. Scalloping of the vertebral body has also been associated with intraspinal neurofibroma. This deformity may also occur with an expansion of the dural sac, suggesting erosion of the vertebral bodies. This particular bone defect has been carefully investigated, and it has been found that scalloping can exist without any of the aforementioned eroding factors. The implication is that the deformity was a primary vertebral or developmental defect associated with neurofibromatosis and was not dependent upon pressure erosion.[82] Because some intraspinal studies with myelography have shown the contrast material to not conform to the posterior scalloped surface of the vertebra, there is a suggestion of an intervening intradural mass. The vertebral scalloping and hyperplasia may be either signs of mesodermal dysplasia or indirect manifestations of a proximal tumor. Because of the two patients reported by Winter and associates[142] who developed paraplegia with dystrophic curve showing evidence of vertebral scalloping and possible dural ectasia, it is strongly recommended that high-volume myelography be performed on those patients with dystrophic curves requiring fusion.

DISORDERS OF BONE GROWTH

The "Elephant Man" was the most publicized patient with neurofibromatosis in medical history. Beginning in 1884, Sir Frederick Treves described this miserable, grotesque creature, repeatedly calling attention to his large misshapen head. Actually, Treves did not realize at the time that his patient had von Recklinghausen's disease.[128–131] It remained for Weber, the illustrious dermatologist, with remarks on the classification of incomplete and anomalous forms of Recklinghausen's disease to point this out in later writings.[136] Treves, the British surgeon, is renowned for his kind assistance to Joseph Carey MacDonald Merrick (called "John" Merrick in the movie). Merrick was afflicted by neurofibromatosis with a profound disorder of facial bone growth, and he traveled with freak shows as the Elephant Man. His deformity was touted to be the result of his mother being trampled by a carnival elephant when she was pregnant with him.

Disorders of bone growth are frequently associated with changes in the soft tissue overlying the bony deformity. Dermatologists, who often see these patients initially, should be encouraged to look for previously unrecognized bone manifestations of the disease.

The diffuse hypertrophy of an extremity may first demand the attention of the ortho-

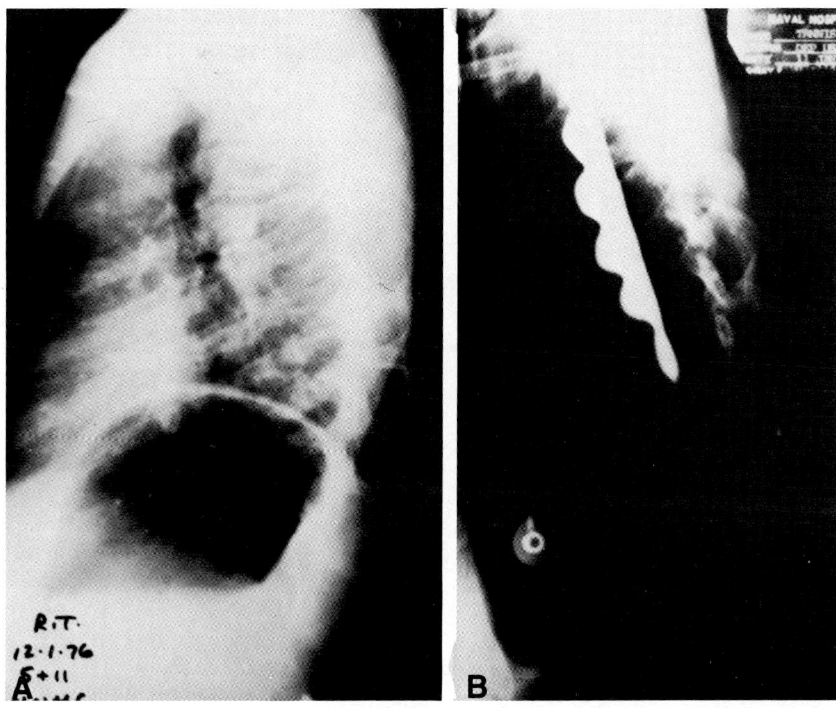

FIG. 27-9. Patient with erosive bone defects on the posterior aspect of the thoracic vertebrae. *(A)* Lateral view of the thoracic spine showing tremendous increase in the anteroposterior diameter of the spinal canal and scalloping of the posterior vertebral borders. *(B)* Myelogram showing the pseudomeningocoeles or "pouchings" of the contrast media as it lines the scalloped posterior margins of the vertebrae. (Patient referred by Dr. Peter Meehan, Atlanta, GA. Reproduced with permission from Neurofibromatosis in the pediatric patient. Orthop Clin North Am 9(1):11–23, 1978)

paedic surgeon (11 of Crawford's patients presented with limb length discrepancy, of which 4 had associated elphantoid changes) (Fig. 27-10).

The changes in the soft tissue are usually those of hemangiomatosis, lymphangiomatosis, elephantiasis, or occasionally beaded plexiform neuromas. The zones of overgrowth in bone and soft tissue are usually unilateral, involving the lower extremities or the head and neck. These osseous changes characteristically cause the bone to be elongated, with a wavy irregularity of the cortex, which may be thickened. Two of Crawford's patients subsequently developed retroperitoneal sarcoma.[32]

CONGENITAL BOWING AND PSEUDARTHROSIS

The relationship of pseudarthrosis of the tibia to neurofibromatosis was first described by Ducroquet.[36] Of his 11 patients with tibial pseudarthroses, 9 had manifestations of neurofibromatosis. The single bone most commonly affected by neurofibromatosis is the tibia.[5,6,9,30–32,37,54,85,87,88,93,94] The bowing of the tibia in neurofibromatosis is characteristically anterolateral and is usually evident within the first two years of life. The anterolateral bowing must be distinguished from posteromedial "kyphoscoliosis tibia" bowing, which is a relatively benign condition and not known to be associated with neurofibromatosis. Other affected bones have been reported such as the ulna,[27,83,93] femur[63,93] clavicle,[4,75,93] radius,[5,84,107] and humerus.[93] Pseudarthrosis may develop spontaneously after a fracture or after osteotomy.

Pseudarthrosis has also been reported as being familial.[140] Only one pseudarthrosis of the tibia has been reported in a patient presenting after 11 years of age.[12] This was a case of a fracture in a 41-year-old man. The cause

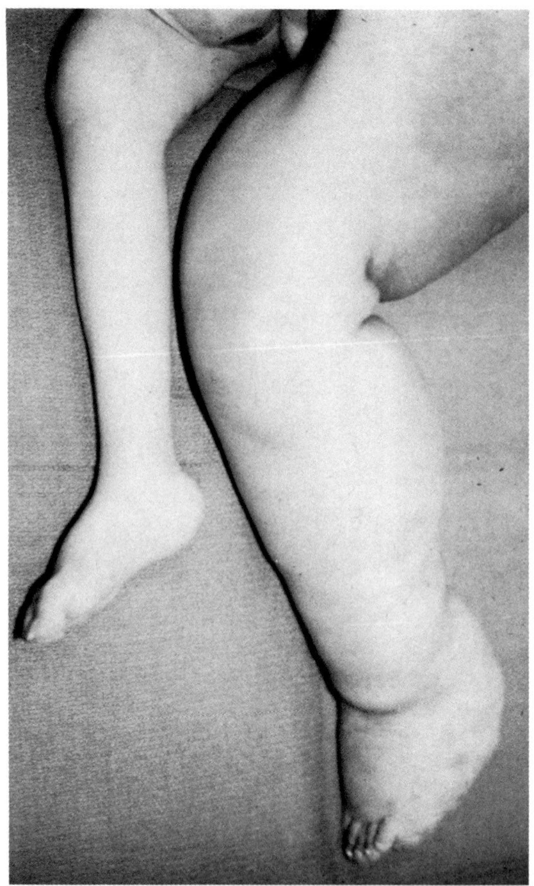

FIG. 27-10. This child presented to orthopaedics with hypertrophy of the left lower extremity after having undergone excision of a retroperitoneal neurofibroma and colostomy. The left lower extremity was approximately four times the size of its opposite side. The bulk and weight of the mass prevented the child from ambulating, and it was necessary to ablate the lower extremity. The fibrofatty changes under the sole of the foot are characteristic of neurofibromatosis. (Reproduced with permission from Neurofibromatosis in childhood. AAOS Instruc Course Lect 30:56–74, 1981)

of pseudarthrosis is questionable. At one time, it was thought that the mechanism that causes pseudarthrosis could be explained by the fact that neurofibroma growing within the bone cortex caused the fracture and interfered with union, eventually resulting in pseudarthrosis. Except for the case report of Green and Rudo,[50] in which the histologic studies showed neurofibromatotic tissue growing in the pseudarthrosis segment, surgical specimens have failed to show neurofibromatotic tissue at the pseudarthrosis site. Aegeter[3] believed that the basic lesion was in the surrounding soft tissue, with secondary bony involvement. He speculated that if all the tumor tissue were removed, normal callus tissue would still form. Briner and Yunis[19] examined the soft tissue removed from three patients with pseudarthrosis tibia by electron microscopy and found fibroblasts rather than Schwann cells or perineural cells. These findings differed from true neurofibromatosis and neurilemoma in which both Schwann cells and fibroblasts, as well as occasional unmyelinated axons, are found.

Congenital pseudarthrosis of the tibia poses a difficult problem in management for the orthopaedic surgeon. Those tibial pseudarthroses associated with skin dimples that are bilateral and have posteromedial bowing, skeletal deformity, and ring constrictions have no association with neurofibromatosis. Pseudarthrosis tibia in neurofibromatosis associated with other skeletal problems are rare, only 5% to 10% being found to have scoliosis. The diagnosis of congenital pseudarthrosis of the tibia is made quite early (when the child is younger than 2 years of age), with usually no other evidence of neurofibromatosis. Other manifestations may subsequently occur, such as café-au-lait spots and other bony or soft-tissue deformities. The sex distribution is equal in pseudarthrosis tibia with and without neurofibromatosis. The average age of tibial fracture is approximately 1.2 years. Fifty-five percent of patients with congenital pseudarthrosis can be diagnosed as having neurofibromatosis. Holt[61] found congenital pseudarthrosis of the tibia with anterolateral bowing to ultimately be associated with neurofibromatosis in 97% of his cases. Forty percent of patients with neurofibromatosis and pseudarthrosis tibia have relatives with neurofibromatosis.

The union rate for patients treated surgically for congenital pseudarthrosis tibia does not change with or without the diagnosis of neurofibromatosis. Many surgical procedures to improve alignment and to internally stabilize the bone fragments have been described. Few satisfy the basic requirements of stability of fixation and promotion of osteogenesis.[14,85,132] The widely used methods include massive onlay grafts,[58] dual autogenous only,[67] trough with chip graft,[53] delayed autogenous only,[67] bypass,[39] fragmentation, and turn-around plasty.[121]

Charnley[24] used an intramedullary nail for better fixation. Langenskiold[73] devised a procedure for stabilizing the ankle by fusion of the distal tibial and fibular metaphyses. Lloyd-Roberts and Shaw[78] suggested pre-fracture grafting of the kyphotic tibia as a means of preventing pseudarthrosis. Lavine and associates[74] reported on the application of pulsating electromagnetic fields to the pseudarthrosis defect. Both internal and external sources of current have been used. The success rates vary with the length of follow-up. The initial successes have not been substantiated.[11,18,71,74]

Recent advances in the field of microsurgery have permitted the transfer of massive segments of bone along with accompanying nutrient vessels to a distant recipient site, with preservation of the blood supply by microvascular anastomosis to recipient vessels. With the nutrient blood supply provided, osteocytes and osteoblasts in the graft can survive, and healing of the graft in the recipient site will be facilitated without the usual replacement of the graft by creeping substitution.[138] The contralateral fibula has been used in most cases, with early results being quite encouraging. Most recently, Leung[76] has used the vascularized iliac crest as a transplant for small defects of less than 7 cm, and the contralateral fibula for those defects greater than 7 cm. He believed that the technical ability to affect reimplantation and vascular anastomosis was easier with the pelvis bone because of the size of the vessels.

Most of the preliminary reports of microvascular bone transplants are encouraging; however, there has been a tendency for pseudarthrosis to recur above and/or below the united vascularized segment. Only time will tell whether or not the ultimate success of microvascular transplants will exceed conventional bone grafting.

Crawford reported on eight patients younger than 12 years of age with angular deformities of the tibia.[32] Seventeen surgical procedures were performed, including bone grafting, multiple osteotomies, plate fixations, below-knee amputations, and application of electrical current. He presented the following classification. [Fig. 27-11].

Type I. Anterolateral bowing with increased bone density and normal medullary canal. These patients have the best prognosis, can usually be followed without bracing, and may never have a fracture.

Type II. Anterolateral bowing with failure of retubulation and a sclerotic medullary canal. These patients inevitably have a fracture. They should be protected from the time the diagnosis is made and prepared for surgical intervention, possibly prophylactically.

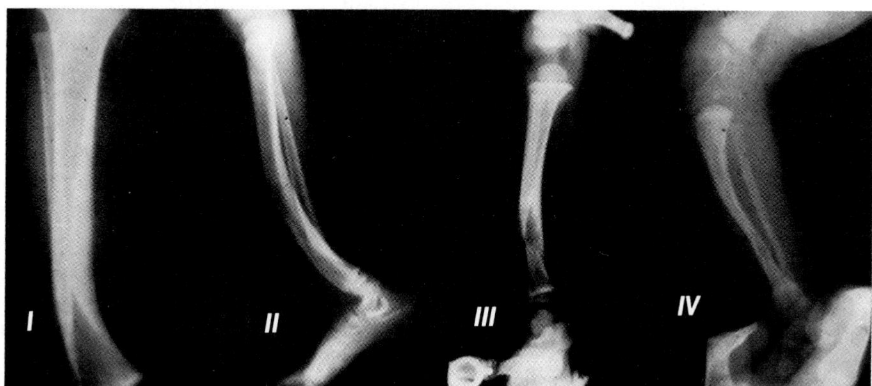

FIG. 27-11. Classification of congenital pseudarthrosis tibia: Type I—anterolateral bowing with increased bone density in the area of the medullary canal. These patients have the best prognosis, can usually be followed without bracing, and may never have a fracture. Type II—anterolateral bowing with failure of tubulation. These patients inevitably have a fracture. They should be protected from the time that the diagnosis is made. Type III—anterolateral bowing with cystic lesion. This is the cystic prefracture that may represent some early healing of a previous fracture. Type IV—anterolateral bowing with dysplastic constriction or frank pseudarthrosis of both the tibia and fibula. Types III and IV lesions characterize the dysplastic pseudarthrotic lesion and have been the most difficult lesions to obtain a lasting union by any means. (Reproduced with permission from Neurofibromatosis in children. Fam Phys 17(3):163–170, 1978)

Type III. Anterolateral bowing with cystic lesions. These patients should have a graft early in the course because of their tendency to early fracture, with the resulting dire consequences.

Type IV. Anterolateral bowing with fractures, cysts, or frank pseudarthrosis. These patients have the worst possible prognosis. All aspects of the patient must be considered in the eagerness to achieve union. The number of operations and length of hospitalization must be carefully considered in terms of whether the psychological costs are a fair price to pay for the anticipated results. Amputation should be considered early in the course of treatment. Some of the happiest patients had amputation early, particularly those who had experienced several operations requiring prolonged confinement. Observation of children with similar problems often helps the psychological effect on the patient and family.

Morrissey and associates[96] reviewed 40 patients who were treated over a period of 25 years by several different surgeons. One hundred sixty-two bone grafting operations were performed on the 40 patients; however, the investigators were not able to recommend one method as being superior to another. The chief difficulty they found was in achieving union between the graft and the short distal segment of tibia. They found it most difficult to decide when to abandon further attempts at achieving union and amputate the leg. Two factors emerged as statistically significant in separating acceptable from poor results: age and segment length.[95] The older the patient at the time of his last graft, the less likely he was to achieve union, and no patient who was still being grafted at age 13 years achieved an acceptable result. Other authors believe that the older the child at the time of bone grafting, the better the chance of success, and the later the fracture occurs, the better the result.[58,78] Significant shortening also represented an unacceptable result. The shortening is noted to be associated with abnormal growth of the distal tibial epiphysis. The fact that the graft usually failed distally and that there was decreased uptake by bone scan of the distal epiphysis suggested that there was a physiologic disturbance in the epiphyseal region of bone. The high incidence (25%) of subsequent development of central nervous system gliomas in Morrissey and associates[96] series caused them to reflect as to whether or not enthusiasm and continued attempts at bone grafting should be carried out as the patient grew older. Andersen[5] reported that for those patients with dysplastic anterolateral bowing and neurofibromatosis who achieved solid bony union, complaints centered around the leg length discrepancy, limitation of ankle motion, pain in the ankle joint, and atrophy of the leg and foot. If union was not achieved after three or four grafting procedures or before the age of 7 years, the benefit of further procedures should be questioned.[5]

Andersen[6] reviewed 21 cases of congenital pseudarthrosis of the tibia and found that all cases of the dysplastic type (Crawford Type III and IV) showed evidence of neurofibromatosis. His most significant observation concerned those patients without dysplastic changes (Crawford's Type I and II) who had positive diagnosis of neurofibromatosis and who underwent osteotomies. The x-ray films from before the osteotomy showed typical anterolateral bowing but no obvious dysplasia. In all three patients who underwent osteotomy, pseudarthrosis resulted. It should be emphasized that children with congenital anterolateral bowing of the lower leg *should not* have corrective osteotomy unless the indications are well substantiated and the extremely great risk of pseudarthrosis has been seriously considered. (Fig. 27-12).

It has often been stated that osteosynthesis could be achieved in those patients with a pseudarthrotic tibia lesion by ankle amputation and bone grafting.[38] It was thought that the ability to directly compress the pseudarthrotic site with direct weightbearing would lead to early union. Jacobsen and associates[64] recently reported on eight patients treated by through-the-ankle amputation, bone grafting, and direct weightbearing. None of the patients achieved a union by this method (Fig. 27-13). When amputation was inevitable, they did recommend ankle amputation rather than through-the-bone amputation because of the increased length having a greater biomechanical advantage for prosthetic wear and the avoidance of stump overgrowth found so commonly in skeletally immature amputees.

EROSIVE DEFECTS OF BONE FROM CONTIGUOUS NEUROGENIC TUMORS

Erosive defects are considered by some investigators as the most characteristic bone

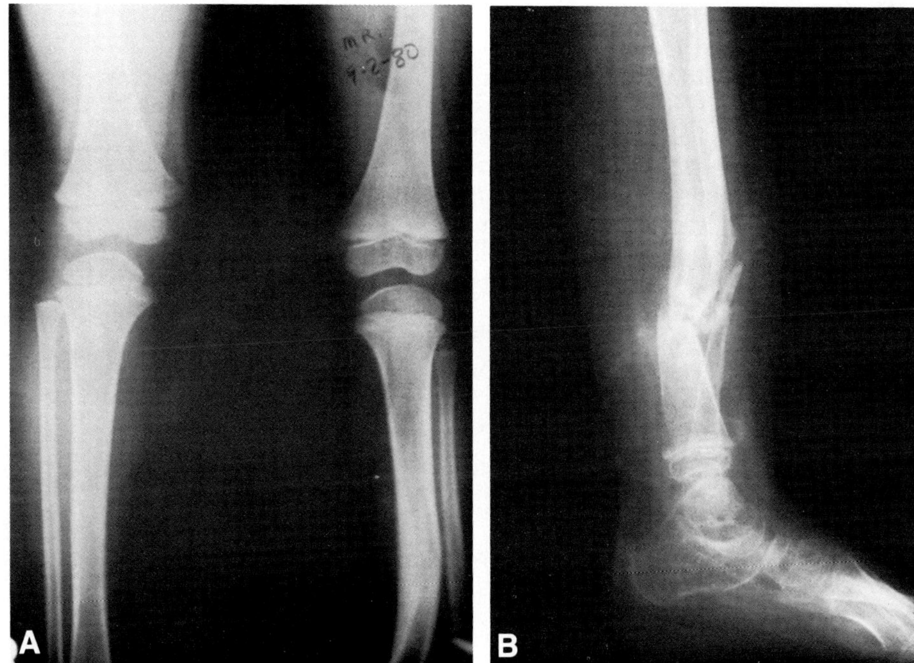

Fig. 27-12. This child was noted to have an anterior lateral bow of the left tibia and neurofibromatosis. Because of some concern for the bowing deformity, an osteotomy was performed. A pseudarthrosis developed following the osteotomy and has failed to unite, despite prolonged application of external pulsating electromagnetic fields. *(A)* Anterolateral bowing with increased bone density (Crawford I). *(B)* Following corrective osteotomy and bone graft, both the tibia and fibula went on to develop a frank pseudarthrosis. Note the development of sclerosis of the proximal and distal ends of both the tibia and fibula with osteopenia of the inferior tibial–fibular fragments and foot. Osteotomy for the correction of anterior lateral bowing of the tibia when associated with neurofibromatosis is to be *strongly condemned.*

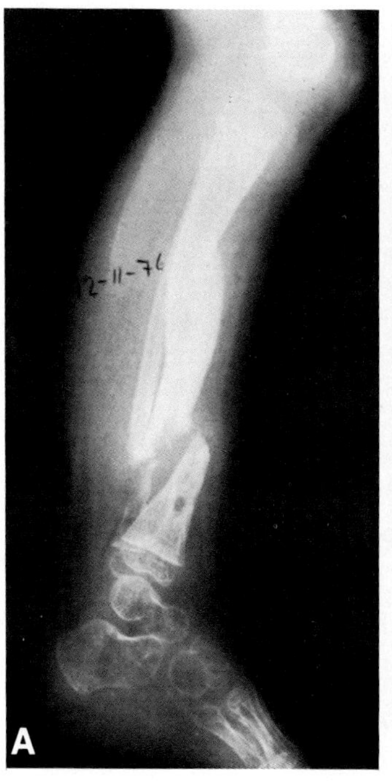

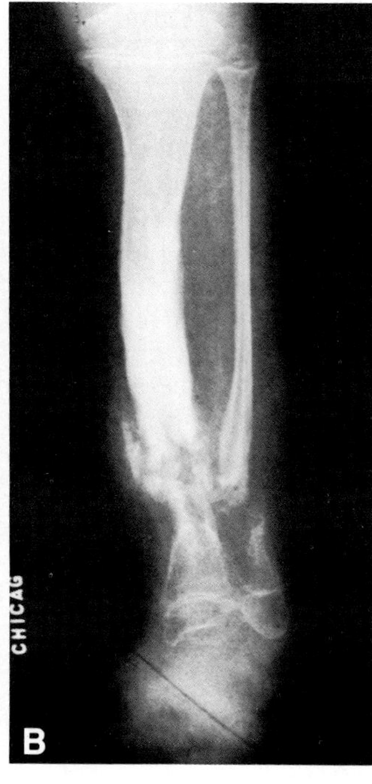

Fig. 27-13. This child presented with a dysplastic anterolateral bowing of the tibia associated with neurofibromatosis and underwent eight attempts at synostosis. It was thought that if the foot were amputated and bone grafting were carried out with immediate weightbearing, the lesion would finally heal. Three and one half years following foot amputation, bone grafting, and prosthetic fitting, the pseudarthrosis has shown no evidence of uniting. *(A)* A lateral x-ray showing the fixed pseudarthrosis after multiple attempts at bone grafting. *(B)* Three and one half years after final bone grafting and Boyd-Symes amputation had been performed. There has been no healing of the bone following the procedures.

change in neurofibromatosis.[20,47,48] Nogaard[99] described these erosions as a pit or caẃe in the bone. Crawford reported seven such cases of erosive defects in 82 patients younger than 12 years of age, with the defects ranging from gross enlargement of the vertebral neuroforamina to extrinsic cystic lesion of the tibia and femur.[32] Various radiolucent lesions occurring in conjunction with true neurofibromatosis (*e.g.*, the fibroxanthomas) are presently thought to be coincidental.[68] Lesions once thought to be cystic are now thought to be mechanical erosions of directly contiguous tumors.

SUBPERIOSTEAL BONE PROLIFERATION (SUBPERIOSTEAL CALCIFYING HEMATOMA)

Among the protean manifestations of multiple neurofibromatosis is the occurrence of the subperiosteal bone proliferation as described by Brooks and Lehman.[20] Two cases were described in their original report; other investigators reported similar lesions.[49,59,60,72,79,86,101,114] Most cases are thought to be initiated by minor fractures with subperiosteal bleeding followed by osseous dysplasia of the subperiosteal hematoma (Fig. 27-14 *A* and *B*). The lesion is quite rare, and its etiology is unknown. Yaghmai and Tafazoli[143] demonstrated angiograms that show only stretching and displacement of blood vessels. This tends to support Pitt's contention that the hemorrhage is due to a mesodermal dysplasia involving the periosteum rather than an intrinsic vascular abnormality. There is no evidence to prove that there is infiltration of the periosteum by plexiform neurofibroma as previously suspected. Crawford noted five such lesions in 82 patients,[32] three of which had been previously reported. All five patients had elephantoid overgrowth of soft tissue with pachydermatocele formation. All have overgrowth of the bone that initially started with cystic subperiosteal involvement.

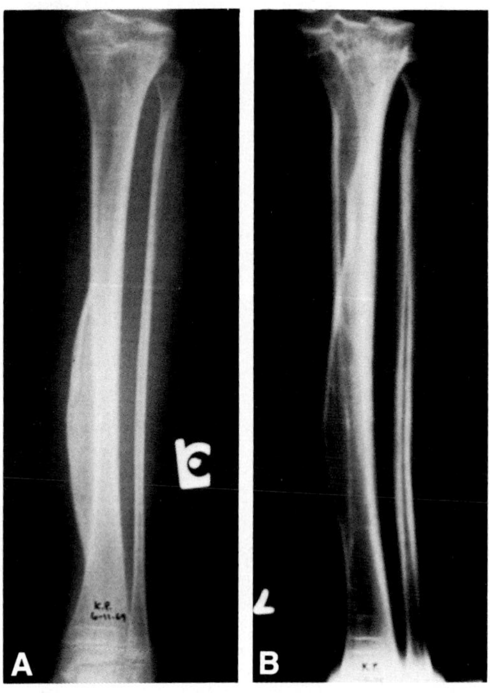

FIG. 27-14. Left tibia of child showing subperiosteal calcifying hematoma. *(A)* Initial presentation of lesion as a mass and a radiopaque density on the tibia. *(B)* Six years later, there is involvement of the entire tibia with what appears to be a double density from the proximal lateral aspect to mid-one third. There are also similar changes noted in the proximal fibula. (Referred from Dr. Robert Winter, Minneapolis, MN)

NEOPLASIA

Any study of a large series of patients diagnosed as having neurofibromatosis will reveal soft-tissue neoplasms. Despite the frequency of café-au-lait spots, the single most common criterion leading to a diagnosis of neurofibromatosis has been parental recognition of a growing mass that resulted in a surgical examination.[1,62,90,119] Most of the neoplasms are of neurogenic origin and are either central or peripheral in location. The tendency for these lesions to undergo malignant change has been cited by other investigators.[90,124]

The list of malignant tumors associated with neurofibromatosis is growing. Added to the list of non-neural crest malignancies known to be associated with neurofibromatosis are nonlymphocytic leukemia, Wilms' tumor, and urogenital rhabdomyosarcoma.[7,88,122] It has been suggested that the association of Wilms' tumor and neurofibromatosis reflects the geographic proximity of the metanephrogenic tubules and primitive neural elements and that chordoma in neurofibromatosis may reflect the embryonic proximity of the notochord and neural crest.[122] Hecht and McCaw[57] raised several questions concerning the relationship of malignancies and neurofibromatosis.

Is neurofibromatosis simply a neurocristopathy?[57] Is the malignant potential in neurofibromatosis restricted to tissues derived from the neural crest and to tissues that are near it? Or, as suggested by the Association of Leukemia, does the gene for neurofibromatosis simply increase the risk for a multiplicity of malignancies? Bader and Miller[7] suggested that the overall risk of cancer in patients with neurofibromatosis is unknown. The risk of cancer in the normal population is 25%, whereas the range of those patients being reported with neurofibromatosis who subsequently contract cancer is too wide of a range to be meaningful (3% to 48%). Furthermore, the data reported to date is biased, and the tumors that will cause problems cannot be readily identified. The data thus far reported were not obtained under appropriate controls for age, sex, race, and location. The current 14% incidence of malignancies in neurofibromatosis possibly represents a stop-frame in the life sequence and does not represent a true incidence. The most common cancers associated with neurofibromatosis in children are optic glioma, brain tumor, urogenital rhabdomyosarcoma, and nonlymphocytic leukemia.

The Mayo Clinic has reported a higher risk of cancer in those patients with neurofibromatosis who have undergone irradiation. It is probably important to conclude that no system in the entire body is exempt from neurofibromatosis.

Malignancy is a significant risk, and it increases with age from about 7% in the preadolescent to more than 20% in those older than 21 years of age.[110] A central lesion such as benign astrocytoma may be malignant purely because of its unresectible location in the substance of the brain. Crawford reported 13 of 82 patients to have neoplastic lesions.[32] Although all the benign tumors represented neural elements, they could not be considered functionally benign because of the impairment of the central nervous system at the target organs. Not only was the target organ intrinsically impaired, but attempts at resection of the lesion usually resulted in further neurologic loss.

What product of a single mutant gene could account for the diverse manifestations, from subtle scoliosis or a few café-au-lait spots to grotesque dysplasia or malignancy? Of the 3,000,000 annual births in the United States, 1 in 1000 to 1200 would be expected to have neurofibromatosis. Of these 250 to 300, 1 in 4 will develop cancer by chance in a lifetime. About 1% of cancer in the total population occurs in persons younger than 20 years of age. An overall frequency of 19% of hospitalized children with neurofibromatosis had malignancy, of which optic nerve glioma accounted for 11%, other brain tumors 3%. Of 4900 consecutive children younger than 15 years of age reported with cancer at 12 centers in the United States and Europe, neurofibromatosis, the most frequently mentioned single gene trait, was recorded in the charts of 38 patients (0.8%) who had 42 malignancies—25 central nervous system tumors, 10 other neural malignancies, and 7 non-neural malignancies. Astrocytoma is the most common intracranial tumor in children, and the most specific type is optic glioma. The acoustic neuroma associated with neurofibromatosis is much more common in adults. Optic gliomas associated with neurofibromatosis seem to have a distinct pattern of aggressive proliferation and infiltration in the perineural and subarachnoid spaces. Tumors arising from within nerve trunks presented an average of 13 years earlier than those arising outside neural sheaths, supporting the idea that a different process leads to the two tumor types.

In spite of the tendency toward bony involvement in association with neurogenic tumors, the occurrence of primary bone sarcomas in patients with neurofibromatosis seems to be a sporadic event. In a recent study from the Mayo Clinic, 65 cases of von Recklinghausen's disease in which malignant tumors of the peripheral nerve sheaths developed, no primary non-neurogenic tumor of bone was found. Of a total of 4774 malignant bone tumors, only 3 were in patients with known well-substantiated von Recklinghausen's disease.[35] Fawcett and Dahlin reviewed 3987 primary bone tumors; only 7 were neurilemomas, and only 1 patient had neurofibromatosis. No reliable statistics are available documenting the association of primary bone sarcomas and neurofibromatosis.

MISCELLANEOUS

Organic manifestations of neurofibromatosis previously reported in children, such as sexual precocity and retarded sexual development, malignant hypertension secondary to renal artery stenosis and a few small vessel changes, and mental retardation are beyond the scope of this chapter. Most series show patients with neurofibromatosis to have a definite trend toward learning disability, with about 50% of patients having a combination of being slow in comprehension with delayed speech and motor development when compared with their peers. Samuelsson[113] recently concluded a genetic and clinical study of 96 cases of neurofibromatosis in Goteborg, Sweden. These patients were all comprehensively reviewed by the Health, Education, and National Registration records. She noted significant reduction in the number of older patients in the age distribution, which she believed indicated an excess mortality in connection with neurofibromatosis. Mild mental retardation was detected in 45% of the patients, and mental illness was detected in 33%, of whom 67% had severe forms. No significant correlation was found between physical activity or neurofibromatosis and either mental illness or mental retardation.[113]

Malignant hypertension, noted in most series on neurofibromatosis in childhood, is thought to be related to renal artery stenosis and hyperplasia and is quite rare. When severe hypertension is seen in adults with neurofibromatosis, one has to rule out pheochromocytoma.[124]

The clinical diagnosis of neurofibromatosis in childhood will usually be based on the presence of numerous café-au-lait spots. However, short stature, macrocrania, seizures, endocrine disorders, neoplastic lesions of the central nervous system, Wilms' tumor, urogenital rhabdomyosarcoma, and nonlymphocytic leukemia may also occur. Early diagnosis allows for continuing follow-up and appropriate counseling. Symptomatic therapy can be provided when necessitated by the disease process. The disorder has a tendency via its mesodermal route to affect almost every system in the body; however, few laymen have even heard of the disorder and except for the Elephant Man's notoriety are totally unaware of it, whereas muscular dystrophy, cystic fibrosis, and mongoloidism, although occurring less frequently, are well known to the general public.[60] The management of neurofibromatosis in children covers an extremely broad spectrum—at times, the management appears to be simple, involving little more than clinical evaluation and simple investigations. However, in view of the protean manifestations of the condition, a complete history, including family history, is obligatory, and investigation must include radiologic studies of the abdomen, chest, spine, and skull, the latter to include special views of the orbits and optic foramina.[28] An aggressive surgical approach to the myriad of lesions associated with this disease is not always the answer; however, *early stabilization of spinal deformity* has proved to be more than moderately successful. The management of tumors of the brain and spinal cord, as well as limb hypertrophy and congenital pseudarthrosis tibia, is undergoing innovations at this time that may result in a better cure rate. The National Neurofibromatosis Foundation appears well on its way to obtaining the recognition for this disorder via the establishment of local as well as national chapters dedicated to the education of the medical practitioner and the public at large. Genetic counseling is a part of this educational process. The hereditary nature of the disease offers the prospect for prevention through family counseling, a prospect that can only be realized by recognition of its manifold expression in childhood.[60] In advising parents, the epidemiologic data provided by Crowe and colleagues[33] are preferable to the data presented in this chapter, which is biased toward the more serious manifestations, as was the study of Cole and Meyers.[28] It is most important to remember that at least 25% of affected patients have *café-au-lait spots as the only manifestation of the disease* throughout their lifetime.[33]

REFERENCES

1. Adkins JC, Ratvich MD: Children's Hospital of Pittsburgh, The operative management of von Recklinghausen's neurofibromatosis in children, with special reference to lesions of the head and neck. Surgery 82(3):343, 1977
2. Adrian C: Ueber neurofibromatose und ihre komplikationen. Beitr Klin Chir 31:1, 1901
3. Aegeter E: The possible relationship of neurofibromatosis, congenital pseudarthrosis, and fibrous dysplasia. J Bone Joint Surg 32A:618, 1950
4. Alldred AJ: Congenital pseudarthrosis of the clavicle. J Bone Joint Surg 45B:312, 1963
5. Andersen KS: Congenital pseudarthrosis of the leg. J Bone Joint Surg 58A:567, 1976
6. Andersen KS: Congenital pseudarthrosis of the tibia and neurofibromatosis. Acta Orthop Scand 47:108, 1976
7. Bader JL, Miller RW: Neurofibromatosis and childhood leukemia. J Pediatr 92:925, 1978
8. Baldwin DM, Weiner DS: Congenital bowing and intraosseous neurofibroma of the ulna. J Bone Joint Surg 56A:803, 1974

9. Barber CG: Congenital bowing and pseudoarthrosis of the lower leg. Manifestations of von Recklinghausen's neurofibromatosis. Surg Gynecol Obstet 69:618, 1939
10. Barone DA: Neurofibromatoses: A clinical overview. Postgrad Med 66(2):73–76, 79–81, 1979
11. Basset CAL, Caulo NP, Dort JS: Congenital pseudarthrosis of the tibia: Treatment with pulsating electromagnetic field. Presented at the American Academy of Orthopaedic Surgeons, Las Vegas, Nevada, 1981
12. Berk L, Mankin HJ: Spontaneous pseudoarthrosis of the tibia occurring in a patient with neurofibromatosis. Report of a case in a man 41 years old. J Bone Joint Surg 46A:619, 1964
13. Biot B, *et al.*: Les lesions vertebrales de la neurofibromatose. Rev Chir Orthop 60:607, 1974
14. Boyd HB, Sage FP: Congenital pseudarthrosis of the tibia. J Bone Joint Surg 40A:1245, 1958
15. Bradford DS: Neurofibromatosis in children. American Academy of Orthopaedic Surgeons, Instructional Course Lectures, Las Vegas, Nevada, 1976
16. Brasfield RD, Das Gupta TK: von Recklinghausen's disease: A clinicopathologic study. Ann Surg 175(1):86, 1972
17. Breig A: Biomechanics of the Central Nervous System: Some Basic and Normal Pathologic Phenomena Concerning Spine, Disk, and Cord. Stockholm, Almquist & Wiskel Printers and Publishers, 1960
18. Brighton CT, Friedenberg ZB, Zemski LM, Pollis BR: Direct current stimulation of non-union and congenital pseudoarthrosis. Exploration of its clinical application. J Bone Joint Surg 57A:368, 1975
19. Briner J, Yunis E: Ultrastructure of congenital pseudarthrosis of the tibia. Arch Pathol 95:97, 1973
20. Brooks B, Lehman EP: The bone changes in Recklinghausen's neurofibromatosis. Surg Gynecol Obstet 38:587–595, 1924
21. Casselman ES, Mandell GA: Vertebral scalloping in neurofibromatosis. Pediatr Radiol 131:89, 1979
22. Chaglassian JH, Riseborough EJ, Hall JL: Neurofibromatosis scoliosis: Natural history and results of treatment in 37 cases. J Bone Joint Surg 58A:695, 1976
23. Chao DH: Congenital neurocutaneous syndromes in childhood. Chapter I, Neurofibromatosis. J Pediatr 55:189, 1959
24. Charnley J: Congenital pseudarthrosis of the tibia treated by intramedullary nail. J Bone Joint Surg 38A:238, 1956
25. Clemis JD: The coexistence of acoustic neuroma and otosclerosis. Laryngoscope 83:1959, 1973
26. Cobb JN: Outline for the study of scoliosis. American Academy of Orthopedic Surgeons, Instructional Course Lectures, Ann Arbor, MI, JW Edwards Publishers, 5:261, 1948
27. Cobb N: Neurofibromatosis and pseudarthrosis of the ulna: A case report. J Bone Joint Surg 50B:146, 1968
28. Cole WG, Meyers NA: Neurofibromatosis in childhood. Aust NZ J Surg 48(4):360, 1978
29. Cowell HR, Hall JN, MacEwen GD: Genetic aspects of idiopathic scoliosis: A Nicholas Andry Award Essay, 1970. Clin Orthop 86:121, 1972.
30. Crawford AH: Neurofibromatosis in children. Am Fam Phys 17:163, 1978
31. Crawford AH: Neurofibromatosis in the pediatric patient. Orthop Clin North Am 9(1):11, 1978
32. Crawford AH: Neurofibromatosis in childhood. American Academy of Orthopedic Surgeons, Instructional Course Lectures. Chapter 3, pp 56–74, 1981
33. Crowe FW, Schull WJ, Neil JW: A Clinical, Pathologic, and Genetic Study of Multiple Neurofibromatosis. Springfield, IL, Charles C Thomas, 1956
34. Curtis BH, *et al:* Neurofibromatosis with paraplegia: Report of eight cases. J Bone Joint Surg 51A:843, 1969
35. Ducatman BS, Scheithaur BW, Dahlin DC: Malignant bone tumors associated with neurofibromatosis. Mayo Clin Proc 58:578, 1983
36. Ducroquet RL: A propos des pseudoarthroses et in flexions congenitales du tibia. Mem Acad Surg 63:863, 1937
37. Dunn AW: Case of overgrowth of leg and anterolateral bowing of tibia in neurofibromatosis. Am J Orthop 7:120, 1965
38. Edvardsen P: Resection osteosynthesis and Boyd amputation of congenital pseudarthrosis of the tibia. J Bone Joint Surg 55B:179, 1973
39. Eyre-Brook AL, Baily RAJ, Price CHG: Infantile pseudarthrosis of the tibia. J Bone Joint Surg 51B:604, 1969
40. Fairbank HAT: Neurofibromatosis: Atlas of general infections of the skeleton. J Bone Joint Surg 32B:266, 1950
41. Fiaklow PJ, Sagebeil RW, Gartler SM, Rimoin DL: Multiple cell origin or hereditary neurofibromatosis. N Engl J Med 284:298, 1971
42. Fienman NL Yakovac WC: Neurofibromatosis in childhood. J Pediatr 76(3):339, 1970
43. Fienman NL: Comprehensive Therapy. Pediatric neurofibromatosis: Review. Frontiers in Medicine 7(11):66, 1981
44. Fisher ER, Vuzevski VD: Cytogenesis of schwannoma (neurilemmoma), neurofibroma, dermatofibrosarcoma as revealed by electron microscopy. Am J Clin Pathol 49:141, 1968
45. Fleming MP, Miller WE: Renovascular hypertension due to neurofibromatosis. AJR Radium Ther Nucl Med 113:452, 1971
46. Frenk N: Ultrastructure of the pigment with Albright's syndrome. Dermatologica 143:12, 1971
47. Friedman M: Neurofibromatosis of bone. AJR 51:623, 1944
48. Goel MK: Osseous lesions in neurofibromatosis. Unpublished data
49. Gould EP: The bone changes occurring in von Recklinghausen's disease. Q J Med XI:221, 1918.
50. Green WT, Rudo N: Pseudarthrosis and neurofibromatosis. Arch Surg 46:639, 1943
51. Gregg PJ, Price BA, Ellis HA, Stevens J: Pseudarthrosis of the radius associated with neurofibromatosis. CORR 171:175, 1982
52. Hagelstrom L: Deformities of the spine and multiple neurofibromatoses (von Recklinghausen). Acta Chir Scand 93:169, 1946
53. Hallock H: The use of multiple small bone transplants in the treatment of pseudarthrosis of the tibia of congenital origin or following osteotomy for the correction of congenital deformity. J Bone Joint Surg 20A:646, 1938
54. Harding EK: Congenital anterior bowing of the tibia.

The significance of the different types in relation to pseudarthrosis. Ann R Coll Surg (English translation) 51:817, 1972
55. Harkin JC, Reed RJ: Tumors of the Peripheral Nervous System, Second Series, Fascicle 3. Washington, DC, Armed Forces Institute of Pathology, 1969
56. Heard GE, Ho JE, Naylor B: Cervical vertebral deformity in von Recklinghausen's disease of the nervous system. Review with necropsy finding. J Bone Joint Surg 10:483, 1978
57. Hecht F, McCaw BK: Neurofibromatosis and malignancy (letter to the editor). J Pediatr 94(6):1010, 1979
58. Henderson MS: Congenital pseudarthrosis of the tibia. J Bone Joint Surg 10:483, 1978
59. Hensley CD: The rapid development of a "subperiosteal bone cyst" in multiple neurofibromatosis. J Bone Joint Surg 35A:197, 1953
60. Holt JF, Wright EM: The radiologic features of neurofibromatosis. Radiology 51:647, 1948
61. Holt, JF: Neurofibromatosis in children. AJR 130:615, 1978
62. Hosoi K: Multiple neurofibromatosis (von Recklinghausen's disease) with special reference to malignant transformation. Arch Surg 22:258, 1931
63. Hunt JC, Pugh DC: Skeletal lesions in neurofibromatosis. Radiology 76(1):1, 1961
64. Jacobsen ST, Crawford AH, Millar EA, Steel HH: The Syme amputation in patients with congenital pseudarthrosis of the tibia. J Bone Joint Surg 65A:533, 1983
65. Johnson BL, Charneco DR: Café-au-lait spots in neurofibromatosis and in normal individuals. Arch Dermatol 102:442, 1970
66. Kessel AWL: Intrathoracic meningocele, spinal deformity, and multiple neurofibromatosis. J Bone Joint Surg 33B:87, 1951
67. Kite JH: Congenital pseudarthrosis of the tibia, fibula. Report of 15 cases. South Med J 34:1021, 1941
68. Klatte EC, Franken EA, Smith JA: The radiographic spectrum in neurofibromatosis. Semin Roentgenol 11:17, 1976
69. Klose J: Recklinghausen, neurofibromatosis. Clin Wochenschr 5:817, 1926
70. Knight WA, Murphy WK, Gottlieb JA: Neurofibromatosis associated with malignant neurofibromas. Arch Dermatol 107:747, 1973
71. Kort JS: Congenital pseudarthrosis of the tibia: Treatment with pulsating electromagnetic field. American Academy of Orthopaedic Surgeons, Instructional Course Lectures, Las Vegas, Nevada, 1981
72. Kullmann L, Wouters HW: Neurofibromatosis, gigantism, and subperiosteal hematoma: Report of two children with extensive subperiosteal bone formation. J Bone Joint Surg 54B:130, 1977
73. Langenskiold A: Pseudarthrosis of the fibula and progressive valgus deformity of the ankle in children: Treatment by fusion of the distal tibial and fibular metaphyses: Review of three cases. J Bone Joint Surg 49A:436, 1967
74. Lavine LS, Lustrin I, Shamos MH, Rinald RA, Liboff AR: Electric enhancement of bone healing. Science 175:118, 1972
75. Laws JW, Pallis C: Spinal deformities in neurofibromatosis. J Bone Joint Surg 45B:674, 1963
76. Leung PC: Congenital pseudarthrosis of the tibia. Three cases treated by free vascularized iliac crest graft. CORR 175:4550, 1983
77. Levine DB: Spondylolithesis, neurofibromatosis, and thoracic meningocele: A case report. J Bone Joint Surg 52A:403, 1970
78. Lloyd-Roberts GC, Shaw NE: The prevention of pseudarthrosis in congenital kyphosis of the tibia. J Bone Joint Surg 51B:100, 1969
79. Locht RC, Huebert HT, McFarland DF: Subperiosteal hemorrhage in cyst formation in neurofibromatosis. CORR 155:141, 1981
80. Lonstein JE, *et al:* Neurologic deficits secondary to spinal deformity. Spine 5(4):331, 1980.
81. Loop JW, Akeson WH, Clawson DK: Acquired thoracic abnormalities in neurofibromatosis. AJR 93:416, 1965
82. Mandell, GA: The pedicle in neurofibromatosis. AJR 130:675, 1978
83. Manske PR: Forearm pseudarthrosis and neurofibromatosis. CORR 139:125, 1979
84. Masihuz-Zaman: Pseudarthrosis of the radius associated with neurofibromatosis. J Bone Joint Surg 59A:977, 1977
85. Masserman RL, Peterson HA, Bianco A: Congenital pseudarthrosis of the tibia: A review of the literature and 52 cases from the Mayo Clinic. CORR 99:140, 1974
86. McCarroll HR: Clinical manifestations of congenital neurofibromatosis. J Bone Joint Surg 32A:601, 1950
87. McFarland B: Pseudarthrosis of the tibia in childhood. J Bone Joint Surg 33B:36, 1951
88. McKeen EA, Bodurtha J, Meadows AT, Douglass EC, Mulvihill JJ: Rhabdomyosarcoma complicating multiple neurofibromatosis. J Pediatr 93:992, 1978
89. McKellar CC: Congenital pseudarthrosis of the tibia: Treatment by tibial lengthening and corrective osteotomy seven years after successful bone graft: A case report. J Bone Joint Surg 55A:195, 1973
90. Merten DF, Gooding CA, Newton TH, Malamud N: Meningiomas of childhood and adolescence. J Pediatr 84(5):696, 1974
91. Miller A: Neurofibromatosis with reference to skeletal changes, compression myelitis, and malignant degeneration. Arch Surg 32:109, 1936
92. Moe JH: Scoliosis and other spinal deformities. Philadelphia, WB Saunders, 1978
93. Moore JR: Delayed autogenous bone graft in the treatment of congenital pseudarthrosis. J Bone Joint Surg 31:23, 1949
94. Moore JR: Congenital pseudarthrosis of the tibia. American Academy of Orthopaedic Surgeons, Instructional Course Lectures, pp 222–237. Ann Arbor, MI, JW Edwards Publishers, 1957
95. Morrissey RT: Congenital pseudarthrosis of the tibia. A long-term follow-up study. Clin Orthop 166:14, 1982
96. Morrissey RT, Riseborough EJ, Hall JE: Congenital pseudarthrosis of the tibia. J Bone Joint Surg 63B:367, 1981
97. Nanson EM: Thoracic meningocele associated with neurofibromatosis. J Thorac Surg 33:650, 1957
98. National Neurofibromatosis Foundation, Inc: Newsletter: Neurofibromatosis: An historical perspective. 6(1):8, 1983
99. Nogaard F: Osseous changes in Recklinghausen's neurofibromatosis. Acta Radiol 18:460, 1937.

100. Ormsby OS, Montgomery H: Diseases of the Skin, 8th ed. Philadelphia, Lea & Febiger, 1954
101. Pitt M, Mosher JF, Ediken J: Abnormal periosteum in bone in neurofibromatosis. Radiology 103:143, 1972
102. Pless J, Roed-Peterson K, Nielsen K: Microglossia neurofibromatosis. Ugeskr Laeger 139(11):655, 1977
103. Pohl R: Meningocele im brustraum unter dem bilde cine intrathorakalen rundschattens. Rontgen-praxis 5:747, 1933
104. Pollnitz R: Neurofibromatosis in childhood: A review of 25 cases. Med J Aust 2:49, 1976
105. Preiser SA, Davenport CB: Multiple neurofibromatosis (von Recklinghausen's disease and its inheritance). Am J Med Sci 156:507, 1918
106. Radhakrishnar S, Varadarajan V, Narenden S: Neurofibromatosis of the transverse colon and omentum. J Indian Med Assoc 71(11):287, 1978
107. Rankin E: Neurofibromatosis in the radius of a 9-year-old. Personal communication, 1975
108. Rezian SM: The incidence of scoliosis due to neurofibromatosis. Acta Orthop Scand 47:534, 1976
109. Riccardi VM: Neurofibromatosis. In Riccardi VM, Mulvihill JJ (eds): Advances in Neurology, Vol 29, New York, Raven Press, 1981
110. Riccardi VM, Kleiner B: Neurofibromatosis: A neoplastic birth defect with two age peaks of severe problems. Birth Defects 13:131, 1977
111. Robin GC: Scoliosis and neurologic disease. Isr J Med Sci 9:578, 1973
112. Sammons BP, Thomas DF: Extensive lumbar meningocele associated with neurofibromatosis. AJR 81:1021, 1959
113. Samuelsson B: Neurofibromatosis (von Recklinghausen's disease). A clinical, psychiatric, and genetic study. Goteborg, Sweden, University Press, 1981
114. Sane S, Yunis E, Greer R: Subperiosteal or cortical cyst and intramedullary neurofibromatosis: Uncommon manifestations of neurofibromatosis. A case report. J Bone Joint Surg 53A:1194, 1971.
115. Saville *et al:* In von Recklinghausen. Hirschwald, Heard & Holt Publishers, 1882
116. Schenkein I, Buerker ED, Helson L, Axelrod F, Dancer J: Increased nerve growth stimulating activity in disseminated neurofibromatosis. N Engl J Med 290:613, 1974
117. Scott JC: Scoliosis and neurofibromatosis. J Bone Joint Surg 47B:240, 1965
118. Seville PD, Nassim JR, Stevenson RH, Mulligan L, Carey M: Osteomalacia in von Recklinghausen's neurofibromatosis. Metabolic study of a case. Br Med J 1:1311, 1955
119. Sheklakov ND: A case of neurofibromatosis with 9242 tumors. Vstn Venerol Dermatol 3:51, 1950
120. Siggers DC: Nerve growth factor in some inherited neurologic conditions. Proc R Soc Med 69:183, 1976
121. Sofield HA, Millar EA: Fragmentation, realignment, and intramedullary rod fixation of deformities of the long bones in children: A 10-year appraisal. J Bone Joint Surg 41A:1371, 1959.
122. Stay EJ, Vawter G: The relationship between nephroblastoma and neurofibromatosis (von Recklinghausen's). Cancer 39:2550, 1977
123. Steg NL, Wong AKC, Bogel MS, Wang CC, Casey PA: The potential of computerized dermatoglyphia analysis as demonstrated through studies of patients with myelomeningoceles and neurofibromatosis. In Bergsma D, Lawry RB (eds): Numerical Taxonomy of Birth Defects and Polygenic Disorders. New York, Allan R. Liss Series, March of Dimes 13, No. 3A:158–159, 1977
124. Stout AP: Tumors of the peripheral nervous system. In Atlas of Tumor Pathology, Section Z, Fascicle 6. Washington, DC, Armed Forces Institute of Pathology, 1949
125. Suziki M, Tamura E, Kamoshita S, Saito M: Clinical observations of phacomatosis in infancy and childhood. Chapter I. von Recklinghausen's disease. Paediatr Univ Tokyo 9:23, 1963
126. Takahashi M: Studies in neurofibromatosis and pigmented macules of nevus spilus. Tohoku J Exp Med 118:255, 1976
127. Tilesius von Tilenau WG: Historia Pathologica Singularis Cutis Turpitudinus. Leipzig, SL Crusius, 1793
128. Treves F: Congenital deformity. Br Med J 2:1140, 1884
129. Treves F: Congenital deformity. Br Med J 1:595, 1885
130. Treves F: A case of congenital deformity. Trans Pathol Sec London 36:494, 1895
131. Treves F: The Elephant Man and Other Reminiscences. New York, Henry Holt, 1924
132. Vannes CP: Congenital pseudarthrosis of the leg. J Bone Joint Surg 48A:1467, 1966
133. Veliskakis KP, *et al:* Neurofibromatosis and scoliosis: Significance of the short angular spine curvature. J Bone Joint Surg 52A:883, 1970
134. Virchow R: Ueber de reform der pathologischen und therapeutischen anschauugen durch die midroskopischen untersuchungen. Arch Pathol Anata Phys Klin Med 1:207, 1847
135. Waggener JD: Ultrastructure of benign peripheral nerve sheath tumors. Cancer pp 699–709, May 1966
136. Weber FPl: Cutaneous pigmentation as an incomplete form of Recklinghausen's disease, with remarks on the classification of incomplete and anomalous forms of Recklinghausen's disease. Br J Dermatol 21:49, 1909
137. Weichert KA, Ding MS, Benton C, Silverman FN: Macrocranium and neurofibromatosis. Radiology 107:163, 1973
138. Weiland AJ, Daniel RK: Congenital pseudarthrosis tibia: Treatment with vascularized otogenous fibular grafts. A preliminary report. Johns Hopkins Med J 147:89, 1980
139. Weiss RS: (A) von Recklinghausen's disease in the Negro; (B) Curvature of the tibia in siblings with neurofibromatosis. J Bone Joint Surg 53B:314, 1971
140. Well JM, Bulmer JA, Graff DJC: Congenital defects of the tibia in siblings with neurofibromatosis. J Bone Joint Surg 53B:314, 1971.
141. Whitehouse D: Diagnostic value of the café-au-lait spot in children. Arch Dis Child 41:316, 1966
142. Winter RB, Moe JH, Bradford DS, *et al:* Spine deformity in neurofibromatosis. J Bone Joint Surg 61A:677, 1979.
143. Yaghmai I, Tafazoli M: Massive subperiosteal hemorrhage in neurofibromatosis. Radiology 122:439, 1977
144. Yong-Hing K, Kalamchi A, MacEwen GD: Cervical spine abnormalities in neurofibromatosis. J Bone Joint Surg 61A:695, 1979.
145. Young DF, Eldridge R, Gardner WJ: Bilateral acoustic neuroma in a large kindred. JAMA 214:347, 1970

28

The Role of the Orthopaedic Surgeon in Child Abuse

Behrooz A. Akbarnia

"The man does not remember the hand that struck him, the darkness that frightened him, as a child; nevertheless, the hand and the darkness remain with him, invisible from him forever, part of the passion that drives him wherever he thinks to take flight."

James Baldwin

There are few of us who can tolerate with equanimity the concept of a small and defenseless child, the weakest member of our species, deliberately and cruelly being harmed by those who care for him. Inflicted trauma is not a new occurrence. Over the centuries, parents have reacted to stress and frustration of everyday life by striking out at their children, causing soft-tissue and bone injuries. As for children, there has never been a golden age. Throughout the history of various societies, children have been killed, abandoned, beaten, and sexually abused. However, it has been only over the past two decades that the attention of the medical community has been focused on child abuse, one of the most dramatic manifestations of family violence.

HISTORY

Dr. John Caffey,[7] who was a pediatrician and pediatric radiologist in New York City, first reported, in 1946, the association of multiple fractures in long bones in six infants with chronic subdural hematoma, none of whom had a history of significant trauma or roentgenographic or clinical evidence of generalized or localized skeletal disease to explain the fractures. He recommended investigation for subdural hematoma in infants with long bone fractures as well as investigation for long bone fractures in patients with subdural hematoma. In 1953, Silverman[23] clearly implicated the parent or guardian as the cause of traumatic lesions and described as part of the syndrome, irregular fragmentation of one or more metaphyses in the tubular bones associated with new bone formation external to the shaft. In 1960, Altman and Smith[3] were the first to report cases of unrecognized trauma in infants and children in the orthopaedic literature.

Although many physicians have contributed to the understanding and recognition of child abuse, medicine as a profession did not officially recognize child abuse until the paper entitled "The Battered-Child Syndrome" was published in the Journal of the American Medical Association by C. Henry Kempe and associates in 1962.[17] The introduction of the term *battered-child syndrome* was helpful in attracting attention to this still neglected medical and social problem. Within a few years of the publication of this article, reporting laws were passed in all states mandating health professionals to report suspected cases of abuse. Increased public awareness finally resulted in the passage of the Child Abuse Prevention Act of 1974. Unfortunately, the syndrome still remains a major cause of death and physical and mental disability among children.

DEFINITION

In 1968, Helfer and Kempe[14] described child abuse as being physical injury inflicted upon children by persons caring for them. Since then, the concept of child abuse has been broadened to include physical and emotional neglect, physical abuse, as well as psychological and sexual abuse. Additionally, the list of professionals mandated to report has been increased to include virtually all who are responsible for the care of children.

PREVALENCE

The prevalence of child abuse has been difficult to determine. It has been estimated that 1% to 1.5% of all children are being abused each year. The number ranges from 70,000 to 2,000,000.[27] There were 750,000 reported cases in 1979. It has been estimated that 3000 children are killed each year by those who take care of them.[24] For every child who is reported, many cases remain unreported. The case reports and statistics are heavily biased toward poor and minority children. Children of the affluent may receive different diagnostic labels for their problems ("accidents" rather than "abuse"), and practitioners may feel an obligation to protect more affluent families from the stigma of reporting to public agencies.

DIAGNOSIS

In the spectrum of child abuse and maltreatment, orthopaedic surgeons are often involved in the cases of physical injury rather than the physical and emotional neglect. Approximately 30% of fractures in children younger than the age of 3 years are nonaccidental.[16] In a study of children younger than 1 year of age, it was found that 56% of their fractures were nonaccidental.[20] If child abuse is missed in the emergency room, there is a 35% chance of reabuse and a 5% to 10% chance of death.[1] Because the physical abuse as well as chronic neglect of young children tends to recur and often results in permanent sequelae, the orthopaedic surgeon must be satisfied that each injury seen in a child is adequately explained.

To differentiate those lesions resulting from inflicted trauma from those due to accidents, the physician, in addition to diagnostic skills, should have a high index of suspicion. Furthermore, he should be knowledgeable in the patterns of child growth and development as well as common injuries in children. The diagnosis of child abuse is seldom made without difficulty. Attention to the history, child and maternal behavior, and certain clinical manifestations serves as a practical guideline to differentiate the nonaccidental injury from that associated with pathologic conditions.

The history in a child abuse case is usually vague and does not correlate with the physical findings. Observation of the behavior of the parents and the child, as well as the history itself, are often more helpful in the diagnosis than the physical examination. The physician should be able to control his attitudes and feelings when faced with a suspected case of child abuse. Parents who are abusive may not readily volunteer information. They might be self-contradictory and display irritation at inquiries regarding the symptoms. They might show over-reaction with hostility or under-reaction with casualness or little evident concern. They might be unavailable or refuse to give information or consent to different tests. Many times, there might be inappropriate delays in seeking health care. When they interact with their child, they might seldom touch or look at the child or they may be critical and angry with the child and might never mention a positive or good quality of the child.

It is important to realize that, of course, no single behavior or combination of behaviors make a parent an abusive parent by definition. Ninety-five percent of the cases of child abuse involve the parents, and they are not often psychotic. Because a parent may have psychological difficulties does not automatically translate into the confirmation of child abuse, and, equally important, cases should not be dismissed because the parent does not seem sick.

As for the behavior of the abused child, he might be overly compliant and passive or extremely aggressive. There might be a delay in the development, and, finally, he might show a role reversal behavior as a response to the unspoken parental need for nurturing.

Some abusive parents were abused as children and never had their own nurturing needs met as a child. The history of stress, drug abuse, or family disruption is usually a hint.

CLINICAL MANIFESTATIONS

There is no great difference in the sex ratio, but premature babies and stepchildren are at greater risk. Boyfriends and stepparents are high-risk abusers. Most abused children are younger than the age of 3 years. Younger children are at greater risk because they are demanding, defenseless, and nonverbal. In a study of 231 abused children, it was found that 50% were younger than 1 year of age, and 78% were less than 3 years of age.[2]

When confronted with a traumatic lesion, one must examine the whole child and look for other possible clues. If there is any question regarding the general examination, help should be sought from medical colleagues, because frequently, the non-orthopaedic manifestations of child abuse lead the physician to the diagnosis.

Failure to thrive or growth retardation secondary to physical and emotional deprivation frequently occurs in the child who has been subjected to repeated abuse. This should be differentiated from usual causes of growth retardation.

SKIN LESIONS

A variety of skin lesions, including bruises, burns, welts, lacerations, and scars, are seen and are by far the most common finding in the cases of child abuse.[21] The typical toddler has bruises over the shins, knees, elbows, and brow. There may be a few old cuts or scars around the eye or a cheekbone resulting from the usual collisions. However, bruising of the buttocks, perineum, trunk, and the back of the legs or the back of the head or neck suggests inflicted trauma. They might be morphologically similar to the implement used to inflict the trauma (Fig. 28-1). Loop marks or scars on the skin are secondary to a doubled over cord or rope. Human bite marks are distinctive, paired, crescent-shaped bruises facing each other. The skin lesions might be in various stages of healing (Fig. 28-2). Wilson[28] suggests some guidelines to estimate the age of bruises from their colors. Between 0 to 3 days after injury, the color is usually red, blue, or purple. From 3 to 7 days, it is green or green yellow, and between 8 and 28 days, the color turns yellow or yellow brown. This guideline is often helpful in making a reasonable guess as to whether bruises are the result of one or more traumatic episodes. When bruises are present, other possibilities such as leukemia, idiopathic thrombocytopenic purpura, and hemophilia should be ruled out. Other cutaneous manifestations that have been identified include bruises in the shape of a hand print, alopecia or subgaleal hematoma from pulling of the hair, and areas of abrated skin that may be caused by being bound or restrained. Impetigo in its various forms may be confused with burns or inflicted injuries.

It may be helpful to have photographs of these lesions for the purpose of documentation. The significance of obtaining informed

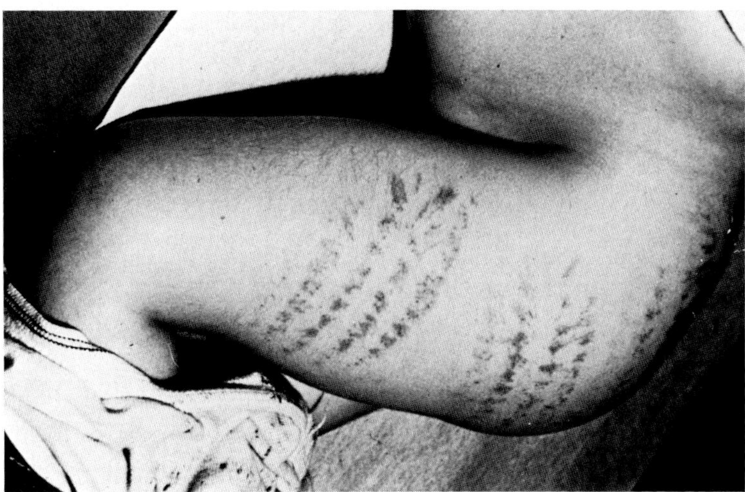

FIG. 28-1 Rope marks on an infant who was a victim of repeated physical abuse.

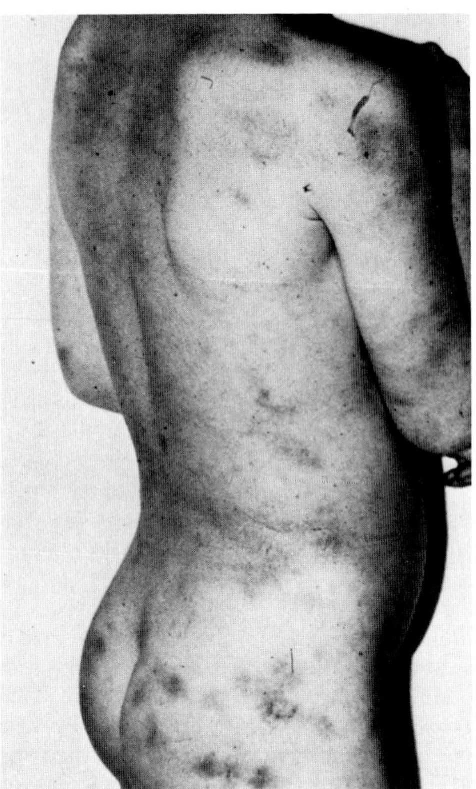

FIG. 28-2. Bruising of back and buttocks, typical of physical abuse. Bruises may be found in different stages of healing.

consent for such procedure cannot be over emphasized, and, if this interferes with having a good relationship with the parents, it might be advantageous to omit the pictures in the interest of building and sustaining a helpful relationship.

Cao-gio, "scratch the wind," is a Vietnamese folklore medical practice. It consists of using a boiled egg covered with hair, a coin, or a similar object, to scratch the skin previously massaged with hot oil. This leaves broad bruises or ecchymosis. It is believed that these scratching maneuvers help rid the body of "bad wind." These lesions should not be mistaken with nonaccidental lesions.[4]

Burn injuries are common and are seen in 10% of abused children.[1] These lesions may be scalding injuries, cigarette burns, or burns caused by flames. The most common age group for burns is from birth to 5 years of age. The pattern of deliberate immersion burns is often symmetrical with sharp lines between the burned and unburned skin. Accidental scald burns are usually asymmetrically distributed.[21]

HEAD INJURIES

The head is a convenient and vulnerable target. Because "the face represents the person", it is logical to strike the face in order to assail the person. The most convenient weapon for striking a child is the human hand. An open palm, knuckles, or a closed fist is sufficient to produce severe damage to the brain, skull, or scalp when used forcefully. Of 110 cases of physically abused children seen by O'Neill and associates,[22] 32 had evidence of cerebral trauma; of these, 6 died of brain injury and 6 suffered permanent neurologic damage. More than 60% of all abused fatalities and more than 50% of all cases of permanent disability occur among children younger than 2 years of age and result, in large part, from inflicted head injuries. The scalp might show swelling. Extension of the swelling and ecchymosis to the eyelids and face is a telltale sign of cranial trauma. The head injury might be so severe as to result in immediate death or less severe and result in various subtle neurologic impairments. Subdural hematoma can occur with or without skull fractures. Many children with brain injuries have no external evidence of trauma. Caffey[6] suggested that violent shaking may cause stretching and tearing to the veins, creating subdural hematoma. If the insult is repeated, each time causing minor brain injury, it may result in additional brain damage manifested by mental retardation, seizure disorders, and other motor and learning disabilities, some not apparent for months or years after the abusive behavior has ended. Careful neurologic assessment of all suspected cases of abuse or neglect is essential. Conversely, unexplained appearance of central nervous system symptoms in an infant should trigger suspicion of abuse. Fractures of the skull are not easy to produce in infants due to yielding elasticity of the thin cranial bones not yet fixed at the sutures. When present, they may be indicative of a forceful nonaccidental impact to the skull. There are a number of children with an inappropriate widening of the cranial sutures, which is believed to be due to increased intracranial pressure secondary to cerebral edema or subdural hematoma.[2]

INTERNAL INJURIES

Injuries to the internal organs can be produced and include rupture of the pancreas and pseudocyst formation, laceration of the liver and spleen, intramural hematoma of the bowel, retroperitoneal hemorrhage, renal laceration or contusion, intestinal perforation, and rupture of the ureter or bladder.[22] Of those fatalities resulting from child abuse, many are due to internal hemorrhage from rupture of abdominal organs caused by punches or kicks. Almost all these fatalities occur in children 3 years old or younger. The high death rate of these injuries is due not only to severity but also delay in seeking medical attention on the part of the abuser. Unfortunately, the lack of history of the trauma and failure of the physician to notice other signs of abuse often result in a delay of diagnosis.

ORTHOPAEDIC MANIFESTATIONS

Approximately one third of all physically abused children require orthopaedic management.[2] The consultation by orthopaedic surgeons is often critical from the legal standpoint and should be handled with utmost care. All the findings should be documented as clearly as possible in the medical record. Fractures can occur in almost any bone of the body. However, long bones, ribs, and the skull are common locations. Fractures may be classified as epiphyseal, metaphyseal, diaphyseal, and a group of miscellaneous fractures.[2]

The epiphyseal fractures, although rare, are most often seen in the femur, tibia, and humerus and are being recognized more often in recent years in cases of child abuse.[10,11] A fracture through a growth plate, especially when the epiphysis is not visible, may cause difficulty in diagnosis. Soft-tissue swelling might be the only finding in the radiologic examination. Arthrographic examination of the joint may be helpful in certain cases (Fig. 28-3).

The metaphyseal fractures are classified into impaction, buckle fractures, periosteal avulsion or corner fractures, and irregular metaphyseal deformity. The corner fractures are

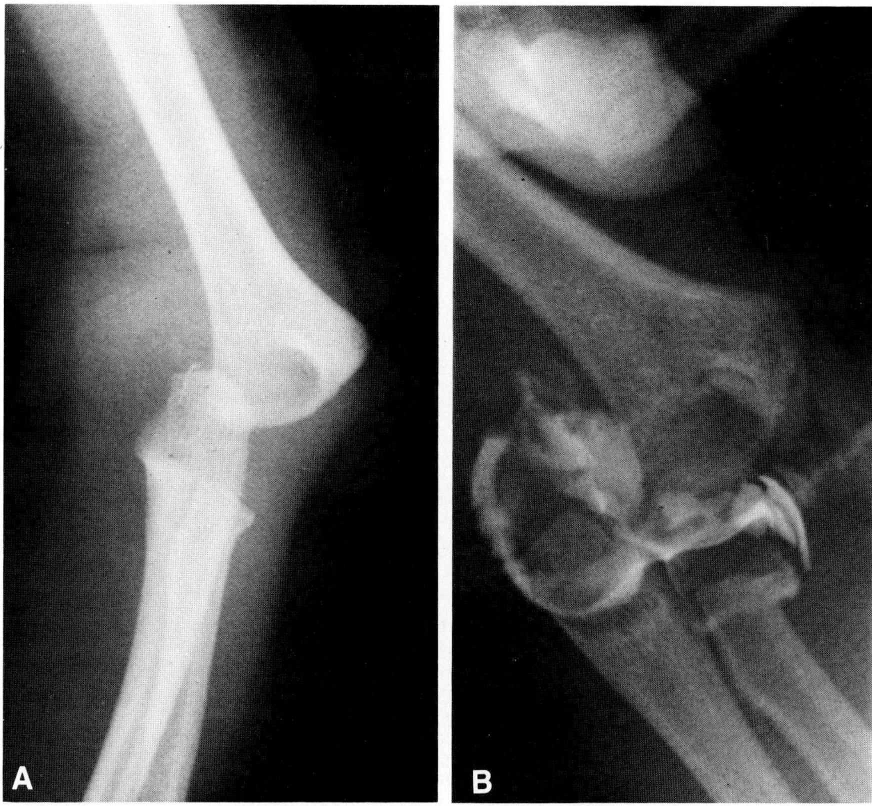

FIG. 28-3. A 15-month-old infant was seen in the emergency room because she was not able to move the right elbow. *(A)* The exact location and severity of the fracture of the distal humerus cannot be identified. *(B)* An arthrogram of the elbow showing the outline of the distal humeral epiphysis, which is separated.

caused by forceful downward pull of the extremity and are often bilateral. They may not be large enough to be visible in the first roentgenogram, but they result in periosteal separation and subperiosteal hemorrhage, with subsequent new bone formation external to the shaft. The periosteal new bone formation will be visible in about 7 to 10 days (Fig. 28-4). These patients often have swollen and painful extremities that refuse to move. If the lesion is already 7 to 10 days old, the picture of the swollen and warm extremity with periosteal new bone formation often associated with fever may be confused with osteomyelitis. In an impaction injury that is rather severe, the epiphysis is impacted into an expanded metaphysis and subsequently exuberant periosteal new bone formation occurs (Fig. 28-5). Buckle fractures are common in the metaphysis and are often multiple. Unlike other metaphyseal lesions, they do not produce a significant amount of callus (Fig. 28-6). Gross irregularity of the metaphysis is seen after repeated injuries and is often associated with deformity of the joint with limitation of motion.

The diaphyseal lesions are grouped into three categories: (1) spiral or oblique fractures of the shaft, sometimes associated with exuberant callus due to the delay in seeking medical help and lack of proper immobilization, (2) multiple lesions in various stages of healing, and, (3) gross bony deformity.

Spiral or oblique fractures, especially in the lower limbs and in nonambulatory children, are suggestive of abuse (Fig. 28-7). If fractures are repeated, the child may sustain fractures involving many bones, and these fractures may be in different stages of healing (Fig. 28-8). They may refracture through a previously fractured diaphysis. Many of these fractures leave permanent sequelae of gross deformities, which, in some patients, require reconstructive surgery during adult life.

Fractures involving the ribs are usually posterior or posterolateral, and they may be in various stages of healing (Fig. 28-9). Involvement of the spine consists of fractures, fracture-dislocations, paraplegia, extradural hemorrhage, and spine deformity.[8,26] The absence of neurologic signs or of obvious deformity

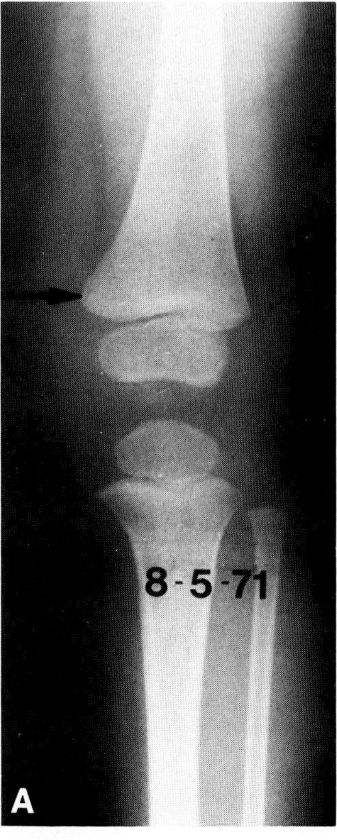

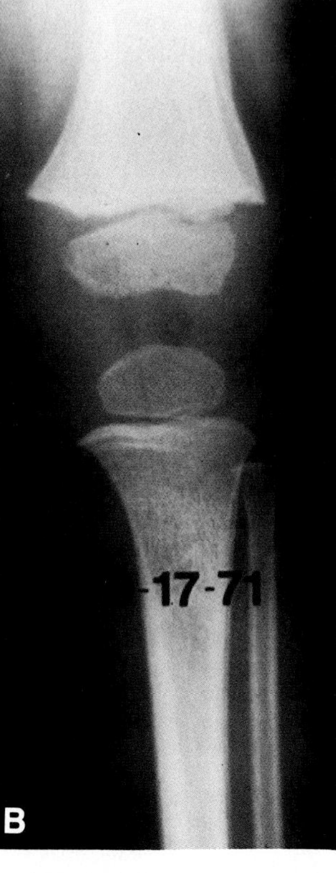

Fig. 28-4. A 15-month-old child was admitted with a painful and swollen left thigh. Infection was suspected. One week later, she was improved clinically. *(A)* An anteroposterior roentgenogram of the knee was interpreted as normal. *(B)* Subsequently, periosteal new bone secondary to periosteal avulsion and hemorrhage were observed. This sequence is a pathognomonic finding in physical abuse. (From Akbarnia BA *et al.* J Bone Joint Surg 56:1159, 1974)

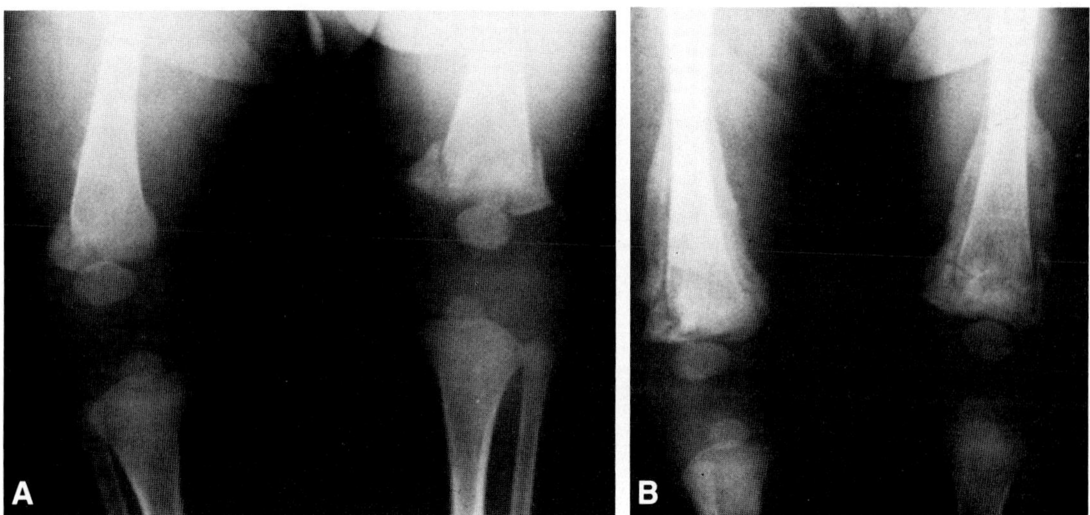

FIG. 28-5. *(A* and *B)* Bilateral impaction fracture of the distal end of the femur, with subsequent exuberant periosteal new-bone formation. (From Akbarnia BA *et al.* J Bone Joint Surg 56:1159, 1974)

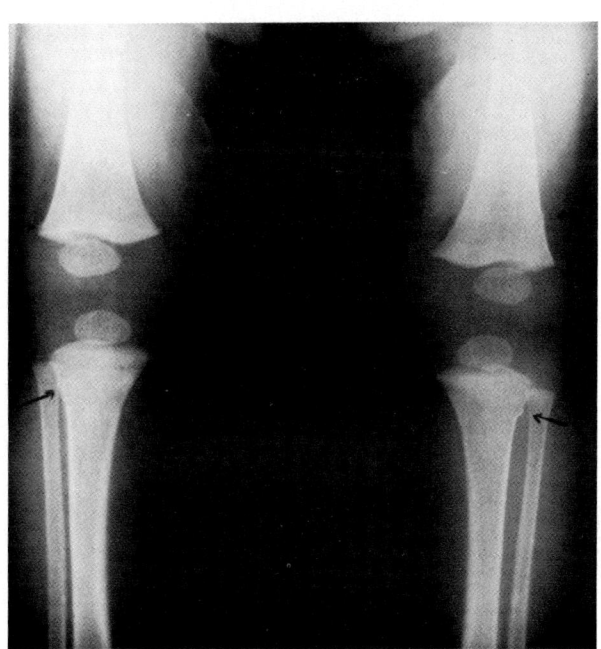

FIG. 28-6. Metaphyseal buckle fractures involving distal end of the femur and proximal part of the tibia. These fractures are often bilateral. (From Akbarnia BA *et al.* J Bone Joint Surg 56:1159, 1974)

may allow the spinal lesion to pass unrecognized. There may be narrowing of intervertebral disc space, anterior vertebral notching, and irregularities of the end-plate, which might be confused with developmental changes or disc space infection (Fig. 28-10). Fractures and fracture-dislocations may cause late spinal deformity in adult life, with subsequent severe disability (Fig. 28-11).

In a recent study of 89 fractures in 36 children,[11] it was suggested that the patterns of fractures are often more helpful in making the diagnosis of child abuse than is the finding of multiple fractures in various stages of healing. These patterns include metaphyseal corner fractures, lower extremity fractures in nonweightbearing children, bilaterality of acute fractures, fractures in special locations, and,

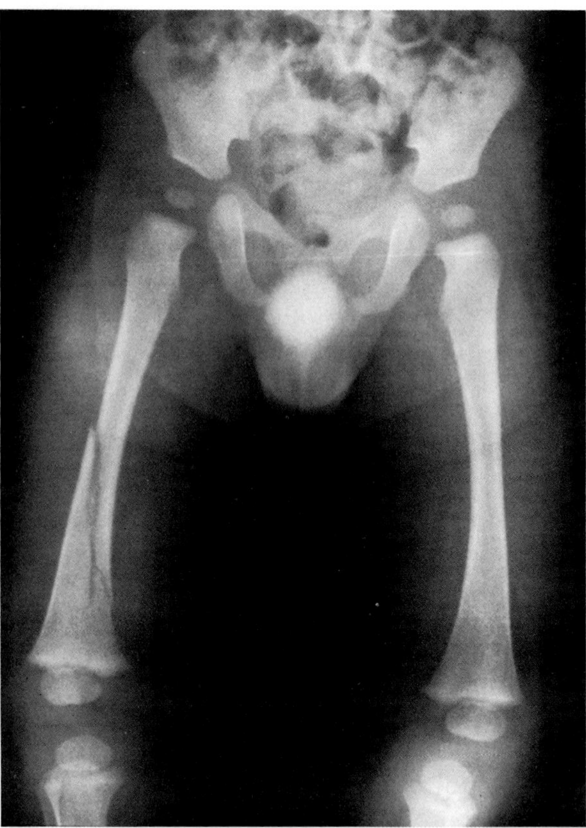

FIG. 28-7. A 13-month-old child sustained spiral fracture of the femur. The history indicated "falling out of bed." Child abuse was suspected and subsequently was confirmed after further questioning.

finally, epiphyseal fractures in smaller children, which are those fractures that should be considered with greater suspicion. Toddlers, as they start walking, might sustain a stress fracture that appears as an oblique lucent line mostly in the tibia. Although there may be a good explanation for this fracture, one should always look into the history very carefully and examine the other clues if available before making this diagnosis.

MANAGEMENT

When child abuse is suspected, an attempt for documentation is the next step. However, indiscriminate requests for full skeletal surveys in all cases of suspected child abuse may contribute to unnecessary radiation exposure and health care costs. Radiographic skeletal survey is more helpful in children younger than 5 years of age with a history of physical abuse.[19] The yield from such examinations in neglected and sexually abused children is extemely low and does not justify radiologic investigation. The survey should include the skull and thoracolumbar spine in anteroposterior and lateral views, as well as anteroposterior views of the thoracic cage and extremities. The extremities should include shoulders and pelvis as well as the hands and feet. A single film of the entire infant is not usually helpful to the radiologists. The use of radionuclide bone scan as a screening procedure for skeletal trauma in suspected victims of abuse is controversial. Some investigators have suggested that radionuclide bone scan is a more sensitive screening test in cases of physical abuse. Haase and associates[13] performed bone scans in 44 children with early trauma, and no child with an initially negative bone scan developed subsequent radiologic changes in long bones, ribs, or vertebrae. Other investigators have found a 12% false-negative result with the skeletal survey compared with only a 0.8% false-negative result in scintigraphy.[25] Bone-seeking radionuclides concentrate in areas of increased blood flow and bone formation so that fractures appear as "hot spots" in the bone scan. These findings, however, are not specific for fractures and may be seen in any

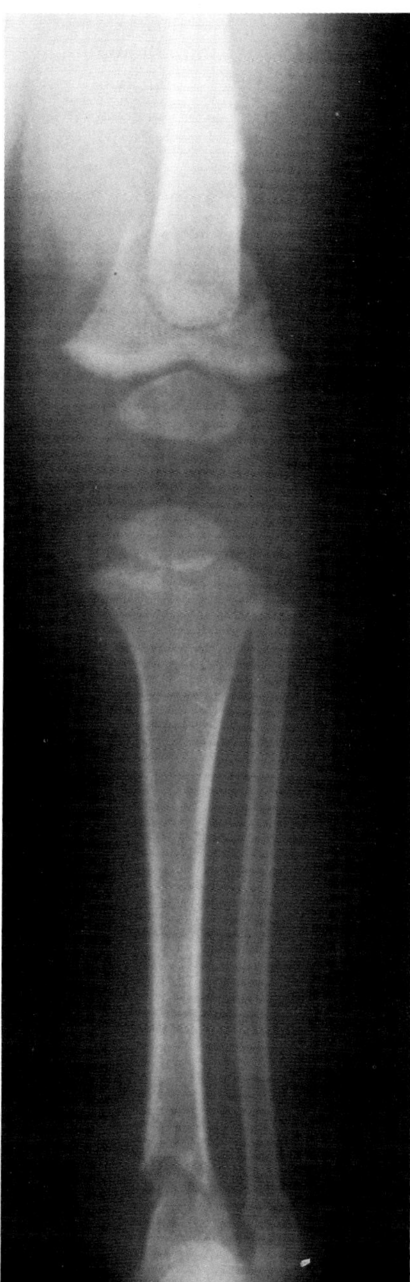

FIG. 28-8. Multiple fractures in various stages of healing are considered to be a pathognomonic finding in physically abused children as seen in this 7-month-old infant with an old fracture of the femur and recent fracture of the tibia. (Courtesy of Dr. Armand Brodeur, Department of Radiology, Cardinal Glennon Children's Hospital, St Louis, Missouri)

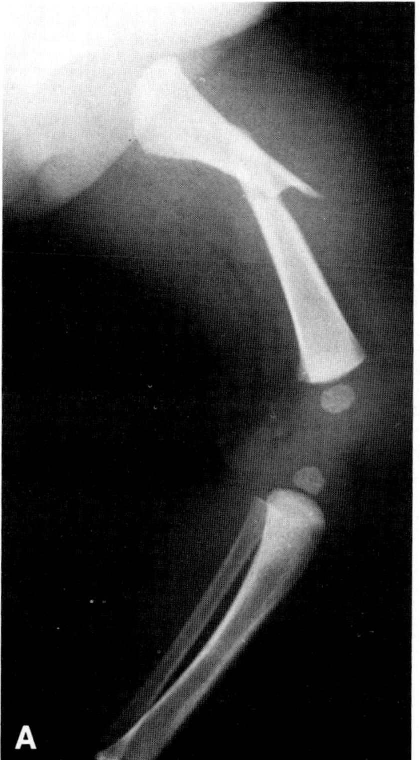

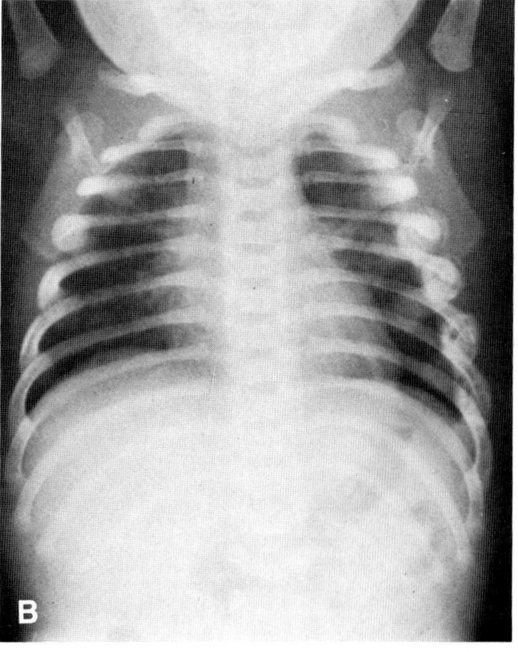

FIG. 28-9. A 2-month-old infant was seen with an acute fracture of the femur. History indicated a "fall from the sofa." *(A)* Spiral fracture of the femur. *(B)* Multiple rib fractures with callus formation. (Courtesy of Dr. Armand Brodeur, Cardinal Glennon Children's Hospital, St Louis, Missouri)

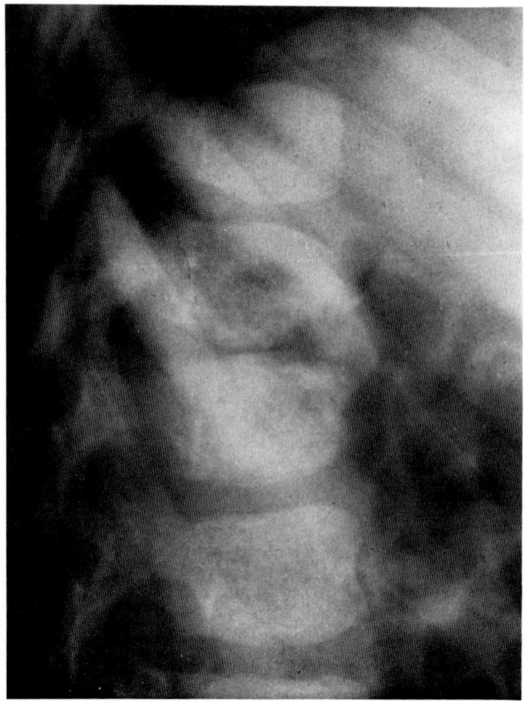

FIG. 28-10. Narrowing of the disc space, anterior vertebral notching, and end-plate irregularities of the vertebra, caused by nonaccidental trauma.

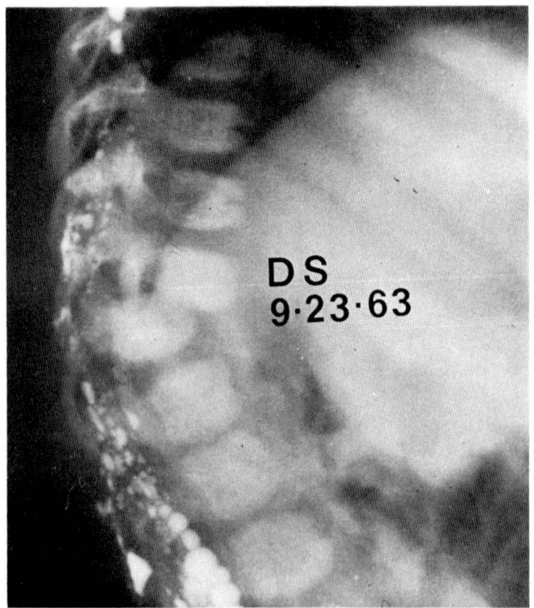

FIG. 28-11. Fracture-dislocation of the spine in a 2-year-old child, victim of abuse, who became paraplegic. (Courtesy of Dr. Robert B. Winter, St Paul, Minnesota)

rapid bone turnover such as osteomyelitis or neoplasm. An additional problem relates to normal increased radionuclide uptake and activity adjacent to the growth plate, making the identification of the epiphyseal metaphyseal fractures more difficult. Limitations to the use of bone scan as an initial skeletal imaging procedure also include the relative lack of nuclear medicine service at all hours in many hospitals, inexperience in performance and interpretation of pediatric bone scan by many general departments, and the relatively high radiation dose delivered to the growth plates.[19] In addition, the bone scan lacks capability in identifying the age and mechanism of trauma. It is thus preferable to examine children suspected of abuse by the radiographic skeletal survey, and, if the initial radiographs do not show any evidence of trauma, the bone scan may prove extremely useful in identifying subtle or occult injuries to the ribs, spine, diaphyses, and, occasionally, the epiphysis. Some of these occult fractures may not be visible in plain radiographs before 7 to 10 days. Thus, there is a place for a bone scan if the plain radiographs are negative or questionable (Fig. 28-12). A coagulation profile (prothrombin time, partial thromboplastin time, platelet count, and bleeding time) will rule out bleeding disorders. Hemoglobinuria and hematuria are known to occur with major trauma.

Skeletal manifestations of child abuse are so characteristic as to be rarely confused with other disorders. They usually speak for the child who is unable or unwilling or too sick to speak for himself. Conditions that might be considered in the differential diagnosis are syphilis, osteogenesis inperfecta, scurvy, Caffey's disease, osteomyelitis, septic arthritis, fatigue fractures, osteoid osteoma and other tumors, rickets, hypophosphatasia, leukemia, metastatic neuroblastoma, fractures in neurogenic disorders, congenital indifference to pain, and osteopetrosis. These conditions all have additional signs of the primary disorder and the history of prior disease to allow for differentiation from nonaccidental trauma.

Fractures in the neonatal period often involve the humerus, clavicle, and femur, and, in these, callus usually appears on radiographs by day 11 of life. In this age group, an unusual site or the absence of callus after 11 days should alert physicians to the possibility of nonaccidental trauma.[9] Pathologic fractures

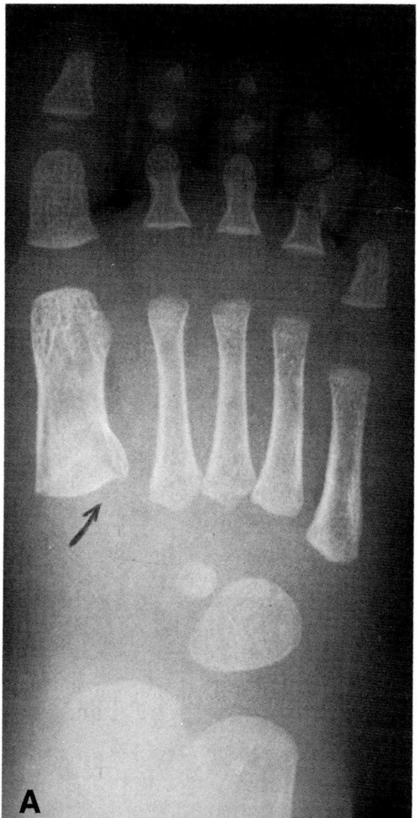

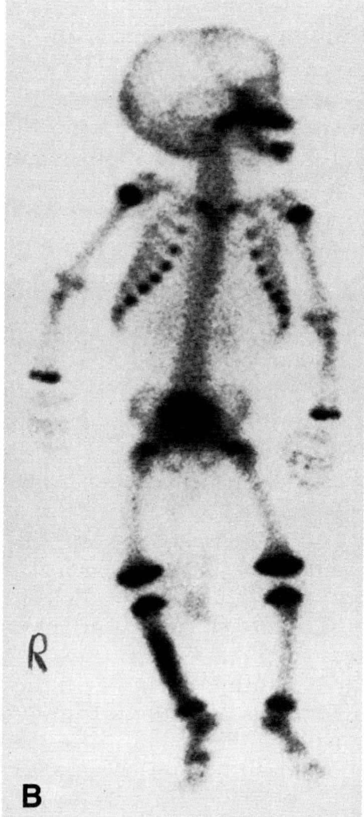

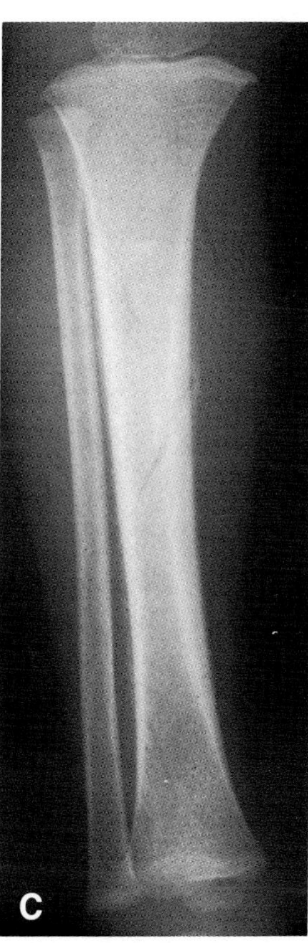

FIG. 28-12. *(A)* Roentgenogram of the right foot showing a fracture at the base of the first metatarsal bone. *(B)* A technetium^{99} bone scan showing increased uptake of the right foot as well as the right tibia. *(C)* Anteroposterior roentgenogram of the right tibia was then obtained, which showed an old fracture of the midshaft of the tibia. (From AAOS Home Syllabus)

due to rickets are also seen in this age group, especially in premature babies.

Falling out of bed is a common excuse frequently related when parents bring the child to the care of a physician. Helfer and associates[15] studied 246 children younger than 5 years of age who fell out of bed. There were only 3 skull fractures, 3 clavicle fractures, and 1 humerus fracture. None developed neurologic impairment from skull fractures. In another prospective study of 436 infants from birth to the age of 1 year there were 101 or 30% falls.[18] There were no limb fractures, and there were only 2 skull fractures. Based on these statistics, falling out of bed is rarely the cause of fractures in very young infants. We believe that any injury to a child younger than the age of 3 years without a clear history must be considered nonaccidental until proved otherwise.

The management of child abuse is divided into two phases: diagnosis and treatment. If child abuse is suspected, every effort should be made to protect the child. Although the statistics and the incidence of child abuse as well as the resulting mortality rate are admittedly inaccurate, it is recognized that an appreciable number of these children eventually die from these injuries. The home environment where child abuse occurs is unquestionably pathologic. To return the child to this home, in most instances, subjects him to repeated abuse and further complications and possible death. Because it is believed that child abuse is a symptom of family distress and a problem with multiple complex origins, it should be managed by a diagnostic interdisciplinary team that includes a pediatrician, a social worker, a nurse, a psychiatrist, and an attorney. When such a diagnostic unit is not avaliable, it is necessary for a physician to work with a social worker and the protective services agencies to which mandated reports are sent for management of these cases. A social worker should be called at the time of the family's presentation to facilitate the social assessment and to form a helping relationship. It is helpful to avoid any confrontations in the emergency room; therefore, admission of the patient into the hospital is desirable.[12] In most cases, this is acceptable to the parents if the need for more study is explained to them. It provides a more relaxing atmosphere in which better evaluation of the child and parents can be carried out. If the parents refuse to admit the child, the law in many states allows the hospital or the physician to assume custody of the child for a limited period of time until a court order can be obtained. A report should be made to the local protective services' agency immediately. This usually is an oral report followed by a written report, which is required within 24 hours. Under the new Child Abuse Prevention and Treatment Act, a central registry of child abuse is required in all states. There are now laws that make the reporting mandatory in all states.

Abuse and neglect must be identified before the child protective agencies can deal with it. Public awareness has increased the number of abuse and neglect incidents reported. However, certain groups of professionals often do not report suspected cases for a variety of reasons. These persons are in unique positions to observe abused and neglected children and are required by law in most states to report such instances. Among these professionals are nurses, social service workers, physicians, teachers, and school personnel. Some of the reasons for hesitation to report among these professionals are (1) lack of knowledge of the responsibility to report, (2) not knowing what type of cases to report and to whom, (3) concern about confidentiality conflicts, (4) pressure by others not to report and possible law suits or reprisal by parents, (5) reluctance to get involved, and (6) belief that reporting would not really help and might aggravate the situation.

It is obvious that education is the most effective way to overcome the above causes of underreporting. There is now a nationwide toll-free hotline to receive reports on a 24-hour basis, and this has caused a sharp increase in reported cases. The physician or any reporter has immunity against any civil or criminal liability.[21] This means that the parent or caretaker cannot bring a successful lawsuit against the physician for defamation or for invasion of the family's right to privacy. Failure to report, however, in many states, may subject the physician to civil or criminal liability.

The most important phase of the management of child abuse cases is the follow-up and rehabilitation of the child and family. In many cases, failure to do this, because of lack of funding or personnel, has caused a higher rate of re-injury or death.

The following seven axioms of child abuse management appear in the literature on child abuse.[5] (1) Once diagnosed, abused children, especially infants younger than 1 year of age, are at great risk of re-injury or continued neglect. (2) In the event that the child is re-injured, it is likely that the parents will seek care at a different medical facility. (3) There is rarely any need to establish precisely who injured the child and if the injury was intentional. The symptoms itself should open the door to a helping alliance and comprehensive service plans for the child and the family. (4) If there is evidence that the child is at major risk, hospitalization is appropriate to allow time for interdisciplinary assessment. The complex origins of the child's injuries are seldom revealed in the crisis atmosphere at the time of presentation. (5) Protection of the child must be the principal goal of intervention, but protection must go hand-in-hand with the development of a family-oriented service plan. (6) Traditional social casework alone may not adequately protect an abused child in the environment in which he received his injuries. Multidisciplinary follow-up is also necessary, and frequent contact by all those involved in the service plan may be needed to encourage the child's healthy development. (7) Problems of public social service agencies in both urban and rural areas, especially in numbers of adequately trained personnel and quality of administrative and supervisory functions, militate against their effective operations in isolation from other care-providing agencies. Simply reporting a case to the public agency mandated to receive child abuse case reports may not be sufficient to protect an abused child or to help the family.

There is no doubt that prevention is the

goal. We are slowly on our way to reaching this ultimate goal through various national and state programs. This can be possible by identifying the high-risk children and helping the families under distress. Orthopaedic surgeons, however, can play an important role in breaking the cycle of child abuse by awareness, early detection, and helping to start therapeutic and rehabilitation measures for the child and his family.

REFERENCES

1. Akbarnia BA, Akbarnia NO: The role of orthopaedist in child abuse and neglect. Orthop Clin North Am 7:773, 1976
2. Akbarnia BA, Torg JS, Kirkpatrick J, *et al:* Manifestations of the battered-child syndrome. J Bone Joint Surg 56:1159, 1974
3. Altman DH, Smith RL: Unrecognized trauma in infants and children. J Bone Joint Surg 42A:407, 1960
4. Anh NT: "Pseudo-battered child" syndrome. JAMA 236:2288, 1976
5. Bittner S, Newberger EH: Pediatric understanding of child abuse and neglect. Pediatr Rev 2, No. 7:197, 1981
6. Caffey J: The whiplash shaken infant syndrome: Manual shaking by the extremities with whiplash-induced intracranial and intraocular bleedings, linked with residual permanent brain damage and mental retardation. Pediatrics 54:396, 1974
7. Caffey J: Multiple fractures in the long bones of infants suffering from chronic subdural hematoma. Am J Roentgenol 56:163, 1946
8. Cullen JC: Spinal lesions in battered babies. J Bone Joint Surg 57B:364, 1975
9. Cumming WA: Neonatal skeletal fractures. Birth trauma or child abuse? J Can Assoc Radiol 30:30, 1979
10. DeLee JC, Wilkins KE, Rogers LF, Rockwood CA: Fracture separation of the distal humeral epiphysis. J Bone Joint Surg 62A:46, 1980
11. Galleno H, Oppenheim WL: The battered-child syndrome revisited. Clin Orthop Rel Res 162:11, 1982
12. Gross RH: Child abuse: Are you recognizing it when you see it? Contemp Orthop 2:676, 1980
13. Haase GM, Ortiz VN, Sfakianakis GN, Morse TS: The value of radionuclide bone scanning in the early recognition of deliberate child abuse. Trauma 20:873, 1980
14. Helfer RE, Kempe CH (eds): The battered child. Chicago, University of Chicago Press, 1968
15. Helfer RE, Slovis TL, Black M: Injuries resulting when small children fall out of bed. Pediatrics 60:533, 1977
16. Holter JC, Friedman SB: Child abuse. Early case finding in the emergency department. Pediatrics 42:128, 1968
17. Kempe CH, Silverman FN, Steele BF, Droegmueller W, Silver HK: The battered child syndrome. JAMA 181:17, 1962
18. Kravitz H, Driessen G, Gomberg R, *et al:* Accidental falls from elevated surfaces in infants from birth to 1 year of age. Pediatrics 44 (Suppl): 869, 1969
19. Leonidas JC: Skeletal trauma in the child abuse syndrome. Pediatr Ann 12:875, 1983
20. McClelland CO, Heiple KG: Fractures in the first year of life. A diagnostic dilemma? Am J Dis Child 136:26, 1982
21. Newberger EH: Child abuse. Boston, Little, Brown & Co, 1982
22. O'Neill JA Jr, Meacham WF, Griffin PP, Sawyers JL: Patterns of injury in the battered child syndrome. J Trauma 13:332, 1973
23. Silverman FN: The roentgen manifestations of unrecognized skeletal trauma in infants. Am J Roentgenol 69:413, 1953
24. Straus MA, Gelles RJ, Steinmetz SK: Behind closed doors: Violence in the American family. New York, Anchor Press, 1980
25. Sty JR, Starshak RJ: The role of scintigraphy in the evaluation of the suspected abused child. Radiology 146:369, 1983
26. Swischuk LE: Spine and spinal cord trauma in the battered-child syndrome. Radiology 92:733, 1969
27. United States Senate. Hearing before the subcommittee on children and youth of the committee on labor and public welfare. United States Senate, 93rd Congress, First Session, On S.1191, Child Abuse Prevention Act. Washington, DC, US Government Printing Office, 1973
28. Wilson EF: Estimation of the age of cutaneous contusions in child abuse. Pediatrics 60:750, 1977

Index

Page numbers followed by f indicate illustrations; t following a page number indicates tabular material.

abductor digiti quinti, 899
abductor hallucis, 899
abuse, child. *See* child abuse
acetabular index, 718–719
acetabular procedures, in congenital dislocation of hip, 724–735
acetabulum, 718
Achilles tendon, lengthening of
  in cerebral palsy, 381–382, 382f, 384, 384f
  in pes cavus, 946
achondroplasia, 45–47
  cell column zone and, 31
  clinical findings in, 45, 46f
  clinical implications of, 47
  genetics in, 45
  roentgenographic findings in, 45–47, 47f
acquired immunodeficiency syndrome (AIDS), 210–211
acrocephalosyndactyly, 679–680, 679f
acrogenesis
  clinical implications of, 44–45
  roentgenographic findings in, 44
adductor
  lengthening and transfer of, 377, 379, 379f–380f
  short, in cerebral palsy, 354
adolescent
  assessment of gait in, 1061–1079
  bunion in, 957–961
  Cushing's syndrome in, 134f
    hallux rigidus of, 964–965
    tibia vara in, 875
Adriamycin, for osteosarcoma, 235–236
adult, anticipated height of, 805
agammaglobulinemia, Swiss-type, 58f, 59
age, skeletal, 802–803, 802f
AIDS (acquired immunodeficiency syndrome), 210–211
alar lamina, 12, 12f
allele(s), 153
Alpert's syndrome, 679–680, 679f
alphafetoprotein (AFP), in myelomeningocele, 404
amelia
  lower limb, 1022, 1024f–1026f, 1025
  upper limb, 1007–1008, 1008f–1009f
amniocentesis, 175–177
  in muscular disorders, 262
amniotic cavity, 2, 4f
amputation
  acquired, 980–998
    complications in, 981–984
      bony spurs, 983
      bursa formation, 983, 984f
      neuromas, 983–984
      phantom limb, 984
      stump scarring, 983, 985f
      terminal overgrowth, 981–983, 983f
    etiology of, 980–981, 980f–981f
    immediate postsurgical prosthetic fitting, 997–998
    lower limb prosthetic fitting, 992–997
      above-knee amputations, 996–997, 999f–1000f
      age considerations, 992–993
      below-knee amputations, 995–996, 995f–997f
      functional development in, 993
      hemipelvectomy, 997
      hip disarticulations in, 997, 1000f–1001f
      knee disarticulations in, 996, 998f–999f
      Syme's-type ankle disarticulation in, 993–995, 994f
    prosthetic management in, 984–998. *See also* prosthesis, surgical principles in
    upper limb prosthetic fitting, 984–992, 986f–987f
      above-elbow amputations, 989, 991, 991f
      age factors in, 987
      below-elbow amputations, 988–989, 989f–990f
      elbow disarticulation in, 989, 990f
      elbow hinges in, 988
      forequarter amputations in, 992, 993f
      hand prostheses in, 985, 986f–987f, 987
      harnessing in, 988

amputation, upper limb prosthetic fitting (*continued*)
shoulder disarticulations in, 991–992, 992f
shoulder joints in, 988
wrist disarticulation in, 988, 988f
age at time of, 980f–981f
congenital, of upper limb, 650–651, 651f
congenital limb deficiencies, 148, 149f, 998–1026
limb loss from malignancy, 998
in osteosarcoma, 233–234
amputee, 979–1026
amyotrophic lateral sclerosis, 329
anatomic malalignment, in overuse injuries, 1105
Anderson principle, 844, 845f, 847
anemia
Cooley's, 193
Mediterranean, 193
sickle cell, 151. *See also* sickle cell disease
anesthesia
in head injury, 487
in muscular disorders, 262–263
aneurysmal bone cyst, 251–252
diagnosis of, 251–252
anhidrosis, familial sensory neuropathy with, 334–335, 334f
ankle
disarticulation of, Syme's-type prosthesis in, 993–995, 994f
foot and. *See* foot and ankle
fusion of, 304
motion of, 1069, 1069f
orthopaedic treatment of, in juvenile arthritis, 472–473, 474f
overuse injuries of, 1118
ankle-foot orthosis (AFO), 1031
ankylosing spondylitis. *See* spondylitis, ankylosing
anterior compartment of foot, 897–900
anterior cord syndrome, 503
anterior horn cell disease, *in utero*, 319
antibiotics, in cerebral contusion, 481–482
antihemophilic globulin, 196
anti-inflammatory drugs
for ankylosing spondylitis, 476
for juvenile arthritis, 463
anti-malarial drugs, for juvenile arthritis, 463
apophysitis, calcaneal, 952, 953f
arachnodactyly, 123, 123f
Arnold-Chiari malformation, 533–534
arteriovenous fistula, 819–820
artho-ophthalmopathy, hereditary, 61
arthritis
juvenile, 457–474. *See also* juvenile arthritis
rheumatoid, torticollis due to, 564
septic, 448–452
clinical features of, 449–450
diagnostic aids in, 450–451, 450f
differential diagnosis of juvenile arthritis and, 461–462
of infancy, 450, 450f
introduction to, 448, 449f
in older child, 450
pathogenesis of, 448–449
bacteriologic phase in, 448–449
immunologic phase in, 449
treatment of, 451–452
arthrochalasis multiplex congenita, 124
arthrodesis
ankle-fusion and pantalar, 304
in congenital talipes varus, 914–915, 915f
extra-articular subtalar, 297–299, 298f–299f
calcaneal osteotomy for, 299, 299f
overcorrection in, 298, 298f
in juvenile arthritis, 467, 467f
pantalar, 300f, 304
in paralytic dislocation of hip, 312
in pes cavus, 950–951
in poliomyelitis of foot and ankle, 297–306
of shoulder, 313–314
triple (foot), 299–303
age in, 299–300
ankle stability in, 299
calcaneal deformity in, 303–304, 304f
complications in, 300–301, 302f
fixed equinus deformity in, 301–302, 302f
goals of, 299
operative technique in, 300, 301f
talipes calcaneus in, 302–303, 303f
types of, 300, 300f
arthrography, in Legg-Calvé-Perthes syndrome, 755
arthrogryposis multiplex congenita, 318–328, 676–678
causes of, 319
clinical features of, 320–321, 322f, 676, 677f
elbow and shoulder joint in, 327–328
etiology and pathogenesis of, 318–319
foot in, 322–324, 323f–324f
hand in, 326–327
hip joint in, 325–326
knee joint in, 324–325, 325f–326f
management of, 321–328
in newborn period, 322
myopathic, 328
pathology of, 319–320
surgical management of extremities, 322–328
treatment of, 676–678, 677f
upper extremity in, 326–328
wrist joint in, 327
arthropathy, hemophilic, 204
pathogenesis of, 205–206, 206f
arthroplasty
Colonna, 723
in juvenile arthritis, 467–468
arthroscopy, 464–465
ascorbic acid, for scurvy, 123
aspiration, in acute hematogenous osteomyelitis, 443–444
aspirin
for ankylosing spondylitis, 476
for juvenile arthritis, 462–463
astragalectomy, for calcaneal deformity, 303, 303f
ataxia
in cerebral palsy, 347
in head injuries, 490–494, 491f–492f
hereditary spinal cerebellar, 328–329, 329f–330f. *See also* Friedreich's ataxia
athetosis, in cerebral palsy, 347
atlantoaxial development, 19
atlantoaxial dislocation, 506

atlantoaxial rotary displacement
  clinical findings in, 562–563, 564f
  classification of, 561–562, 563f
  etiology and mechanism of, 560
  roentgenographic features of, 560–562, 561f–563f
  treatment of, 563–564
atlantoaxial rotary fixation, 559–560
atlantoaxial rotary subluxation, 506
atlanto-occipital dislocation, 505–506, 505f
atlas, occipitalization of, 543–544, 543f–544f
autosomal chromosomal abnormalities, 168–169
autosomal conditions, 153
autosomal dominant conditions, 154–158
  schematic pedigree of, 155f
autosomal dominant muscular dystrophy, 268
autosomal recessive conditions, 158–161
  schematic pedigree of, 158, 158f
autosomal recessive muscular dystrophy, 267–268
autosome(s), 153, 158
avascular necrosis, 750
axonal process, 11

Babinski reflex, 13
back pain, causes of, 637–638, 639f
bacteriologic phase, of septic arthritis, 448–449
Bamberger-Marie syndrome, 120
band(s), constricting, 691–692, 692f
Barlow examination, 707, 707f
Barnes' procedure, 830
basal lamina, 12, 12f
basilar impression, 531–534
  age of onset, 534
  Arnold-Chiari malformation in, 533–534
  Chamberlain's line in, 531, 532f
  clinical findings in, 533–534
  Fischgold-Metzger's line in, 531, 532f, 533
  McGregor's line in, 531–533, 532f–533f
  McRae's line in, 531, 532f, 533
  primary, 531
  roentgenographic findings in, 531–533, 532f–533f
  syringobulbia in, 534
  syringomyelia in, 533–534
  treatment in, 534
  types of, 531
  vertebral artery anomalies in, 534
basilar invagination. *See* basilar impression
battered child syndrome, 1147
Becker type, of sex-linked muscular dystrophy, 267
behavioral changes, in head injuries, 489
biofeedback, in cerebral palsy, 363
biopsy
  in muscular disorders, 261–262
    Dubowitz and Brooke procedure, 261–262
    fiber type nomenclature in, 262
    myopathic changes in, 262
    neuropathic changes in, 262
  of synovium, 464, 464t
bipartite patella, 886–887
birth
  and developmental history in cerebral palsy, 347–348
  growth patterns at, 26
  injury, of brachial plexus, 696–698, 697f
bladder, in spinal cord injury, 523–524
bleeding, abnormal. *See* hemophilia; hemorrhage
blood dyscrasias, 453
blood groups, genetics of, 156
Blount's disease, 869–875. *See also* tibia vara
body segment motion, 1063–1065, 1063f–1064f
bone. *See also specific bones*
  appositional growth of, 29
  architecture of, in foot, 896
  calcium storage in, 85
  crisis, in Gaucher's disease, 184, 184f
  embryonic, development of, 16–17
  in flexible flatfoot, 926
  growth mechanisms of, 29–37
    disorders of, associated with neurofibromatosis, 1134–1135, 1136f
    epiphyseal plate in, 29–33, 30f
    in epiphysis, 35
    remodeling and funnelization of, 33–35, 34f
    in small bones, 35
    in spine, 35, 36f
  infections of. *See* infection(s), of bones and joints
  long, normal growth and behavior of, 781–783, 782f–783f
  maturation, disorders of, 129–135
    fibrous dysplasia, 133–135
    glucocorticoids in, 133
    gonadal abnormalities, 132–133
    hypopituitarism, 129–131
    hypothyroidism, 131–132
    normal variant short stature, 129
  physiology of, 110–111
  resection of, 813–819. *See also* resection, bone
  small, growth of, 35
  tumors. *See* tumors, bone
bone bar, 1083, 1084f, 1085
bone block, posterior, 316
bone bridge, 1083
bone dysplasia. *See* dysplasia, bone
bone graft, and osteoplasty, 747, 749
Bost-Larsen procedure, 829–830, 830f–832f
bowel, in spinal cord injury, 522–523
boys. *See also* children
  growth patterns in, 26, 27f
  normal growth charts of, 127f
brachial plexus, birth injuries of, 696–698, 697f
brachymelia, 53–54
bracing. *See also* orthosis
  in ankylosing spondylitis, 477
  in cerebral palsy, 363
  lumbar, in adolescent idiopathic scoliosis, 591, 593, 594f–595f
  in Marfan's scoliosis, 612, 615
  Marshall-type, 1117f
  Milwaukee
    in adolescent idiopathic scoliosis, 587, 589–591, 591f–592f
    in congenital scoliosis, 610–611
    in infantile idiopathic scoliosis, 581–582

bracing, Milwaukee (*continued*)
in juvenile idiopathic scoliosis, 585
in myelomeningocele, 408, 408f–409f
in Scheuermann's disease, 626–627, 628f–629f
Toronto, 765f
underarm, treatment of thoracic curves with, 593
Brailsford syndrome, 72–73, 74f
brain
in myelomeningocele, 399, 400f
in occipitocervical synostosis, 555
brevicollis, 535–545. *See also* Klippel-Feil syndrome
"Buddha posture," in rickets, 93
bunion, adolescent, 957–961
anatomy of, 958–959
clinical features of, 959
cuneiform variation in, 958
etiology of, 957–958
family history of, 958
introduction, 957
long first metatarsal in, 958
os intermetatarseum in, 958
roentgenographic features of, 959, 960f
treatment of, 959–961
complications of, 959–961
conservative, 959
surgical, 959, 961f–962f
bursa, in amputations, 983, 984f
bursitis, in overuse injuries, 1109
Butler-Albright syndrome, 98

café-au-lait spots, 1124–1125, 1126f
Caffey's disease, 120, 121f
calcaneal apophysitis, 952, 953f
calcaneocuboid joint, wedge resection of, 913–914
calcaneovalgus foot, 924–925
clinical features of, 924, 924f
treatment of, 924–925
calcaneus
congenital short tendo, 918–919
deformity of
arthrodesis in, 300–304, 304f
tendon transfer in, 296, 297f
osteotomy of, 299, 299f
in congenital talipes equinovarus, 913
in pes cavus, 949–950, 951f
calciferol, 87, 88f
calcification, hypertrophic cell zone and, 31
calcitonin, 91–92
calcium, daily requirement of, 89, 89f
calcium homeostasis, 84–90
calcium kinetics, 91, 91f–92f
calf
pseudohypertrophy of, 264, 264f
short, in cerebral palsy, 354–355, 354f
callus, 231
camptodactyly, 680
Camurati-Engelmann disease, 66–67, 67f
CAPP device. *See* child amputee prosthetic project terminal device
capsule, in congenital dislocation of hip, 718
capsulotomy, posterior, knee, in arthrogryposis multiplex congenita, 325, 325f–326f
caput quadratum, in rickets, 93
cardiac anomalies, in congenital scoliosis, 607, 609f
cardiopulmonary disorders, in muscular dystrophy, 273
cardiovascular abnormalities, Klippel-Feil syndrome and, 541
cardiovascular effects, of spinal cord injury, 521
cartilage cell zone, 30
cartilage-hair dysplasia, 57–59, 58f
cartilaginous exostoses, multiple, 61, 63–64, 63f
cartilaginous matrix, calcification of, hypertrophic cell zone and, 31
cartilaginous plates, embryology of, 19
cast(s)
in congenital absence of radius, 653, 654f
in congenital dislocation of hip, 716–717
in congenital talipes equinovarus, 907–908, 908f–909f
correction, in cerebral palsy, 363
in hemophilia, 203
Petrie, 765f
Risser-Cotrel, 603
Catterall classification, of Legg-Calvé-Perthes syndrome, 756–758, 756f–763f
cell column zone, 30–31
cell mass, inner, 2
center-edge angle, 719
central cord syndrome, 503
central core disease, 276–277
central nervous system surgery, in cerebral palsy, 364
cerebral concussion, 481
treatment of, 481–482
cerebral contusion, 481–482
contrecoup, 481
treatment of, 481–482
antibiotics in, 481–482
cerebral edema in, 481
convulsions in, 482
cooling measures in, 482
hypertension in, 482
lumbar puncture in, 481
cerebral edema, 481
cerebral palsy, 345–393
aphorisms about, 392–393
assessment of, 347
associated with neuromuscular scoliosis, 617–618, 619f–621f
basic science in, 355–361
biofeedback in, 363
birth and developmental history in, 347–348
bracing in, 363
cast correction in, 363
central nervous system surgery in, 364
clinical examination in, 350–355
diagnosis of, 347–350
differential, 349–350
diplegia in, 374–392
drugs for, 363–364
equinovalgus foot in, 384–385, 384f
etiologic types of, 347
etiology of, 346
functional electrical stimulation in, 363
gait in, 348
geographical types, 346–347
gross neurologic signs in, 348–349
hemiplegia in, 385–392

hemiplegic foot in, 386f–387f, 391–392, 392f
hip in, 370–373, 370f–373f
incidence of, 345
joint contracture and instability in, 355
joint muscles in, 360
knee in, 382, 383f
kneel walking in, 350–351
lifeskills training in, 364
locomotor generator in, 355–357, 356f–357f
muscle balance in, 360, 368f, 387f
muscle growth in, 357–358, 358f
muscle lengthening in, 376–385
muscles in, 359–360, 359f
short, recognition of, 351–355, 351f–354f
physiologic types, 347
prevalence of, 345
prevention of, 346
problems and options, 368–392, 368t–369t
sitting ability in, 350, 373–374, 374f–375f
spine in, 373–374, 374f–375f
surgery in, 365–368, 365f, 367f, 368f
goals of, 366
problem solving in, 367
repertoire of techniques, 367–368, 367f–368f, 387f
tactics, 365–366, 365f
talking to parents about, 364–365
tendon lengthening in, 360–361, 367, 367f
tendon transfer in, 367, 368f, 387f
therapeutic recreation and fitness in, 364
therapy in, 363
totally involved child, 346
management of, 370–374
treatment in, 361–368
goal setting in, 361
modalities of, 363–368
strategy of, 361–363, 362f
upper limb in, 385–391, 386f–387f, 389f–390f
walking ability in, 350, 351f
cerebral spastic disability, acquired, causes of, 495
cervical burst fracture, 507, 507f
cervical compression fracture, 506–507
cervical fracture-dislocation, 507–508, 508f
cervical spine, orthopaedic treatment of, in juvenile arthritis, 473–474
Chamberlain's line, 531, 532f, 533
Charcot-Marie-Tooth disease, 329–331, 330f–332f
genetics of, 165
chemical synovectomy, in hemophilia, 209
chemotherapy, in osteosarcoma, 234–236
Chiari reconstruction
in congenital dislocation of hip, 732–734, 732f–733f
in Legg-Calvé-Perthes syndrome, 769–770
child abuse
clinical manifestations of, 1149
definition of, 1148
diagnosis of, 1148–1149
head injuries in, 1150
history of, 1147–1148
internal injuries in, 1150–1151
management of, 1154, 1156–1159, 1157f
orthopaedic manifestations of, 1151–1154, 1151f–1156f
prevalence of, 1148
role of orthopaedic surgeon in, 1147–1159
skin lesions in, 1149–1150, 1149f–1150f
child amputee prosthetic project (CAPP) terminal device, 986f, 987
children. *See also* boys; girls
assessment of gait in, 1061–1079
older
arthrogryposis multiplex congenita in, foot surgery for, 323–324, 324f
poliomyelitis in, 285
septic arthritis in, 450
overuse injuries in, 1103–1119
Chinese population, foot deformities in, 965t
cholecalciferol, 87, 88f
chondrification, of axial skeleton, 18
chondroblastoma, 241–242
diagnosis and therapy, 242
chondrodysplasia
hereditary, 78f, 79
metaphyseal
Jansen type, 56–57, 56f
McKusick type, 57–59, 58f
with malabsorption and neutropenia, 59
Schmid type, 57, 58f
with thymolymphopenia, 59
chondrodysplasia fetalis, 45
chondrodysplasia punctata, 47–48
clinical findings in, 48, 48f
clinical implications of, 48
genetics of, 165
roentgenographic findings in, 48, 48f
chondrodystrophia adolescentium Sui-Tarda, 57, 58f
chondrodystrophic dwarfism, 45
chondroectodermal dysplasia, 52–53
chondrolysis, 750, 751f
chondroma, 237–239
chondromatosis, internal, 64–65, 64f
chondromyxoid fibroma, 32, 242
chondrosarcoma, 32, 242–243
juxtacortical, 243
mesenchymal, 243
radiation sarcoma, 243
Christmas disease, 196. *See also* hemophilia
chromosome abnormalities, 166–172
autosomal, 168–169
cri du chat, 169
D trisomy, 168
E trisomy, 168, 168f–169f
G trisomy, 168
Philadelphia chromosome in, 169
trisomy 21, 169
Turner's syndrome and, 171
mongolism determination in, 169, 170f–171f, 171
study techniques in, 167–168
X chromosome and, 171–172
chromosome studies, 167–168
clasped thumb, 683
congenital, 686–687, 687f
clavicle, congenital pseudoarthrosis of, 667–670, 668f–670f
clinical features of, 667, 668f
treatment of, 667–668, 669f
clawtoe, 304–305, 966

cleavage, 1
cleft foot, congenital, 954–955, 954f
cleidocranial dysostosis, 54, 55f, 56, 668, 670, 670f
cleidocranial dysplasia, 54, 55f, 56
cleidocraniodigital dysostosis, 54, 55f, 56
clinodactyly, 681–682, 682f
  treatment of, 682
clubfoot, congenital, 172, 173f
  showing forefoot adduction, 903f
coalition, tarsal, 935–940
  classification of, 935–937, 936f
  clinical features of, 937
  etiology and genetic aspects of, 937
  incidence of, 935
  roentgenographic findings in, 937–940, 938f–939f
  treatment of, 940
Cobb technique, 573, 575f
cognitive reorganization, 489
collagen molecule, 111
Colonna arthroplasty, 723
coma, classification of, 487, 488f
computed tomography (CT), of spine, 575
congenital disorder(s), 148–150
  absence of radius, 652–656, 654f–655f, 657f–658f
  absence of thumb, 664, 665f
  absence of ulna, 656–662, 659f–661f
  angular tibial deformities, 875–878
  bowing, associated with neurofibromatosis, 1135–1138, 1137f, 1139f
  clasped thumb, 686–687, 687f
  cleft foot, 954
  congenital amputation, 148, 149f
    of upper limb, 650–651, 651f
  curly toe, 963
  dislocation of elbow, 673–675, 674f
  dislocation of hip, 703–736. *See also* hip, congenital dislocation of
  dislocation of radial head, 673, 674f
  dislocation of shoulder, 666–667, 668f
  elevation of scapula, 693–696, 694f–695f
  of forefoot, 954–964
  hallux varus, 955, 957
  limb deficiencies, 998–1026
  in lower limb length discrepancy, 784–788, 785f–790f
  mallet toe, 964
  metatarsus varus, 915–918
  multifactorial conditions, 172, 173f
    congenital clubfoot, 172, 173f
    congenital dislocation of hip, 172, 173f
    meningomyelocele with spina bifida, 172
  overriding of fifth toe, 961–963
  pseudarthrosis of clavicle, 667–670, 668f–670f
  radiohumeral synostosis, 672–673, 672f
  radioulnar synostosis, 671–672, 671f
  rubella virus and, 148
  short femur with coxa vara, 739–741, 740f–741f
  short first metatarsal, 961
  short tendo calcaneus, 918–919
  talipes equinovarus, 901–915
  thalidomide and, 148, 149f
  of upper limb, classification of, 649–650
  undetected at birth, 151–153, 152f
  uterine environment and, 148, 149f
  vertical talus, 919–923
  webbing of elbow, 675–676, 676f
  x-ray examination and, 148–150
congenital dystrophy, 269
congruence angle, 880, 880f
connective tissue syndromes, 123–126
Conradi-Hunermann disease, 47–48, 48f
consciousness, level of, 479–480
constitutional growth delay, 129
constricting band(s), 691–692, 692f
constriction band syndrome, 650
containment treatment, in Legg-Calvé-Perthes syndrome, 763–764, 764f
contracture
  equinus, in muscular dystrophy, 270–272, 273f
  extension, knee, in myelomeningocele, 426
  flexion
    in hemophilia, 197–198, 200f
    hip
      in arthrogryposis multiplex congenita, 326
      in muscular dystrophy, 272
    knee, 306, 307f
      in arthrogryposis multiplex congenita, 324
      in muscular dystrophy, 272
      in myelomeningocele, 426
  joint, in cerebral palsy, 355
  pathology of, 361
  in poliomyelitis, 288
  supination, of forearm, 316–317
convulsions, 482
Cooley's anemia, 193
cooling measures, in cerebral contusion, 482
corticosteroids, for juvenile arthritis, 463
costovertebral articulations, embryology of, 18
coxa plana. *See* Legg-Calvé-Perthes syndrome
coxa vara, 736–741
  clinical features of, 736–737
  congenital short femur with, 739–741, 740f–741f
    clinical and radiographic features of, 740, 740f
    prognosis and natural history of, 740
    treatment of, 740–741, 741f
  differential diagnosis of, 737–738
  etiology of, 736, 737f
  prognosis and natural history of, 737f, 738
  radiographic findings in, 737, 738f
  treatment of, 738–739, 739f
cranial nerve function, 480
creatine phosphokinase (CPK), 260–261
cri du chat, 169
cryoprecipitate fraction, 202
crystallysis, 85
cuneiform, osteotomy of, in congenital talipes equinovarus, 914
curly toe, congenital, 963
curvature of spine, measurement in, 573, 575f

Cushing's syndrome, in adolescent, 134f
cutaneous nodules, of neurofibromatosis, 1125, 1126f
cyclophosphamide, for Ewing's sarcoma, 247
cyst(s)
  aneurysmal bone, 251–252
  popliteal, 891
  simple unicameral bone, 248–249

dactylitis, in sickle cell disease, 191
dantrolene sodium, for malignant hyperthermia, 263
deafness, Klippel-Feil syndrome and, 542
7-dehydrocholesterol, 87, 88f
Dejerine-Sottas disease, 329
delta phalanx, 685–686, 685f
deltoid, 313
dens. *See* odontoid
dens bicornis, 545, 545f
deoxyribonucleic acid (DNA), 150f, 151
dermal neurofibroma, 1125
dermatomyositis, 267, 277–279, 278f
  laboratory data in, 278–279
  management of acute stage, 279
  management of chronic stage, 279
development, arrest of, in upper limb, 649–650
Dial osteotomy, in congenital dislocation of hip, 730, 731f, 732
diapers, in congenital dislocation of hip, 714, 715f
diaphragm, embryology of, 15
diaphyseal dysplasia, 66–67, 67f
diaphyseal sclerosis, multiple, hereditary, 67, 68f
diastrophic dwarfism, 50–52
diencephalon, 9
1,25-dihydroxy vitamin D, and vitamin D-resistant rickets, 99–100
diplegia, in cerebral palsy, 346, 374–385
disc
  herniation of, back pain caused by, 638
  intervertebral, embryology of, 18–19
dischondroplasia, 64–65, 64f
discoid meniscus, 887
disease state, associated, in overuse injuries, 1105
dislocation
  atlanto-occipital, 505–506, 505f
  atlantoaxial, 506
  cervical fracture, 507–508, 508f
  congenital
    of elbow, 673–675, 674f
    of patella, 882, 883f
    of radial head, 673
    of shoulder, 666–667
    and subluxation, of knee, 882–886
  habitual, of patella, 882
  hip, 703–736. *See also* hip, congenital dislocation of
    in myelomeningocele, 416, 418–420
  residual deformities from, in head injuries, 489–490, 490f
  thoracolumbar fracture, 509, 510f
DNA. *See* deoxyribonucleic acid
Dorrance hand terminal device, 987, 987f
Dorrance hook terminal device, 986f, 987
dorsiflexor(s), paralysis of, 292
Down's syndrome. *See* mongolism
D-penicillamine, for juvenile arthritis, 463
drop foot, recurrent equinus and, 391–392
drug therapy. *See also specific disorders; specific drugs and classes of drugs*
  in cerebral palsy, 363–364
  in juvenile arthritis, 462–463
Dubowitz and Brooke procedure, 261–262
Duchenne muscular dystrophy, 618–619, 625f
  sex-linked, 263–267
dumbbell lesions, associated with neurofibromatosis, 1133–1134, 1135f
dural ectasia, 1133
dwarfism, 41
  chondrodystrophic, 45
  diastrophic, 50–52, 174, 175f
  mesomelic, 53–54
  metatropic, 48–49
  polydystrophic, 73
  pseudometatropic, 49–50
  thanatophobic, 174
  thanatotrophic, 45
dysautonomia, familial, 334
dyschondrodysplasia fetalis, 45
dyscrasias, blood, 453
dysostosis, cleidocranial, 54, 55f, 56, 668, 670, 670f
dysostosis enchondralis, 57, 58f
dysostosis epiphysealis multiplex, 59–61, 60f
dysostosis tarda, metaphyseal, 57, 58f
dysplasia
  bone, 41–79
    asphyxiating thoracic, 53
    chondroectodermal, 52–53
    classification of, 41–42
    cleidocranial, 54, 55f, 56
    diaphyseal, 66–67, 67f
    multiple epiphyseal, 59–61
    Paris nomenclature of constitutional (intrinsic) diseases of bone, 42–44
    pseudoachrondroplastic spondyloepiphyseal, 77–79, 77f
    spondyloepiphyseal, 75–79
  cartilage-hair, 57–59, 58f
  fibrous. *See* fibrous dysplasia
  hip, 706, 706f
  osteodental, 54, 55f, 56
dysplasia epiphysealis hemimelica, 61, 62f
dysreflexia, autonomic, in spinal cord injury, 521
dystrophia myotonica, 274–275, 276f
  in infancy, 275
dystrophy
  asphyxiating thoracic, 53, 53f
  congenital, 269
  distal, 269
  muscular. *See* muscular dystrophy
  ocular, 268
  oculopharyngeal, 269
  thoracic pelvic pharyngeal, 53, 53f

ectasia, dural, 1133
ectoderm, structures arising from, 3
ectodermal ridge, apical, 20, 20f–21f, 22–23, 24f

ectodermal ring, 19, 20f
Ehlers-Danlos syndrome, 124–125, 125f
elbow
  amputation above, prosthesis in, 989, 991, 991f
  amputation below, prosthesis in, 988–989, 989f–990f
  in arthrogryposis multiplex congenita, 327–328
  congenital dislocation of, 673–675, 675f
    clinical features of, 673–674, 675f
    treatment of, 674–675
  congenital webbing of, 675–676, 676f
  deformity of, orthotics for, 1056–1058
  disarticulation, prosthesis in, 989, 990f
  flexion, in cerebral palsy, 391
  orthopaedic treatment of, in juvenile arthritis, 470, 470f
  osteochondritis dissecans of, 698–699, 699f
  overuse injuries of, 1112–1113
  poliomyelitis of, 314–316
    flexion paralysis in, 314–316
    triceps brachii paralysis in, 316
electrical stimulator(s)
  in adolescent idiopathic scoliosis, 593
  limb lengthening by, 820–821
electrocardiogram, 262
electromyography, 261
elephantiasis, 1125, 1126f, 1127
elephantiasis neuromatosa, 1125
Ellis-van Creveld syndrome, 52–53
Elmslie procedure, for calcaneal deformity, 303–304, 304f
embryo
  7th day, 2
  12th day, 2
  21st day, 4–5, 6f
  22nd day, 5, 7f
  32nd day, 5, 8f
  46th day, 5, 8f
  60th day, 5, 7, 9f
  developing, 2–7
  seven-somite, 5, 7f
embryology
  of axial skeleton, 17–19
  of limbs, 19–24
  of muscular system, 13–16
  of nervous system, 7–13
  of neuromusculoskeletal apparatus, 1–24
  ontogeny in, 1–74
  of skeletal system, 16–17
enchondroma, 32, 237
enchondromatosis, 64–65, 64f
  multiple, 64–65, 64f
enchondrosis, 64–65, 64f
end organ sensitivity, and vitamin D-resistant rickets, 100
endochondral ossification, 16, 781
endocrine abnormalities, of immature skeleton, 81–135
endocrinopathies, with indefinite pathophysiology, 126–135
endoderm, structures arising from, 3
Engelmann disease, 66–67, 67f
ENT examination, 480
eosinophilic granuloma, 250–251
ependymal layer, 10
epidural hematoma, 483, 485
  management of, 485, 486f
  signs and symptoms of, 483, 485
epiphyseal dysplasia, multiple, 59–61, 60f
epiphyseal-metaphyseal injury, 792, 795f
epiphyseal plate, 29–33, 30f
  cell column zone in, 30–31
  closure of, 32–33
  hypertrophic cell zone in, 31
  metaphysis in, 31–32
  partial growth arrest of, 1083–1100
    evaluation of, 1085–1089, 1086f–1088f
    introduction, 1083–1085, 1084f
    treatment of, 1089–1100
      excision of physeal bars in, 1090–1100, 1090t, 1091t, 1092f–1100f
  perichondral groove in, 33
  rate of growth regulation and, 33
  small cartilage cell zone in, 30
  stapling of, 811–813
    advantages of, 812–813
    complications of, 813, 814f–815f
    disadvantages of, 813
    indications for, 812, 812f
epiphysiodesis, 809–811
  advantages and disadvantages of, 811
  complications in, 811
  history of, 809–810, 809f–810f
  indications for, 810
  prerequisites for, 810–811
  technique in, 811
epiphysis. *See also* epiphyseal plate
  growth of, 35
  "ringed," 122
  slipped capital femoral, 741–750
  vertebral arch, 18
equalization of lower limb
  factors in, 784–808
  methods of, 808–853
equinovalgus, in cerebral palsy, 384–385
equinovarus
  congenital metatarsal varus, 915–918
  congenital short tendo calcaneus, 918–919, 919f
  congenital talipes, 901–915
    clinical findings in, 903
    conservative management of, 904–910
      criteria for correction, 905–906
      manipulation of foot, 906–907, 906f–907f
      retentive splints in, 910
      technique of cast application in, 907–908, 908f–909f
    etiology of, 901–902
    genetic implications in, 901
    idiopathic, classification of, 904, 905f
    introduction, 901
    operative management of, 910–915
      derotational osteotomy of tibia and fibula, 914
      forefoot adduction in, 910
      operations on bone in, 913–915
      osteotomy of calcaneus, 913
      osteotomy of medial cuneiform, 914
      osteotomy of metatarsals, 913
      posterior release in, 910–911
      posterior tibial tendon transfer in, 910

soft-tissue release in, 911–913, 912f
tendon transfer in, 910
triple arthrodesis in, 914–915, 915f
wedge rescetion of calcaneocuboid joint, 913–914
pathology of, 902–903
roentgenographic examination in, 903–904, 903f
treatment of, 904–915
deformities of, 901–919
dynamic, 392
equinus
in cerebral palsy, correction of, 381–382, 381f–383f
contractures in muscular dystrophy, 270–272, 273f
dynamic, dorsiflexion insufficiency with orthotics in, 1035, 1035f
recurrent, drop foot and, 391–392
triple arthrodesis in, 301–302, 302f
ergosterol, 87, 88f
Escherichia coli, infection caused by, 438
Eulenburg's disease, 274
Ewing's sarcoma
differential diagnosis of, 245–246
treatment of, 246–248
complications in, 247–248
excessive lateral pressure syndrome (ELPS), 880
treatment of, 882
excision
joint, in juvenile arthritis, 467
of physeal bars, 1090–1100
exercise
for juvenile arthritis, 464
for prevention of contractures, in spinal cord injury, 520–521
exostoses, 239–240
multiple, cartilaginous, 61, 63–64, 63f
extensor digitorum brevis, 897
extensor digitorum longus, 897
extensor hallucis longus, 897
extensors, peroneal and long-toe, paralysis of, 295
extremity(ies)
in arthrogryposis multiplex congenita, surgical management of, 327–328
lower. *See also* limb, lower
surgery for spasticity in, 491, 493–494, 493f–494f
upper. *See also* limb, upper
in arthrogryposis multiplex congenita, 326–328, 327f
cerebral palsy in, 385–391
assessment of, 386–387, 386f
bracing for, 387
elbow flexion, 391
finger flexion deformity, 390
mass movements, 385
mirror movements, 385
sensory poverty, 385
shoulder abduction, 391
surgery for, 387–388
swan neck deformity, 390–391
therapy for, 387
thumb-in-palm deformity, 388, 389f–390f
treatment of, 387
wrist and finger deformity, 388, 390
surgery of, in hemophilia, 209, 209f

Factor VIII
blood levels of, vs. severity of clinical manifestations of defective hemostasis, 196t
inhibitors in, 204–205
Fairbank disease, 59–61, 60f
familial incidence, of Gaucher's disease, 181
fascioscapulohumeral dystrophy, 268, 268f
febrile arthritis, acute, 458–459
femoral neck osteotomy, 749
femoral procedures, in congenital dislocation of hip, 734, 735f
femur
congenital short, coxa vara with, 739–741, 740f–741f
head of
avascular necrosis of, 190, 190f
blood supply to, 753–754
changes in, in Legg-Calvé-Perthes syndrome, 754–755, 754f
in congenital dislocation of hip, 718
necrosis of, 183, 183f
lengthening of, by osteotomy and gradual distraction, 825–838
motion of, 1067–1069, 1068f
osteosarcoma of, 234
proximal, in congenital dislocation of hip, 718
proximal focal deficiency of, 1014–1021
classification of, 1016–1017, 1017f–1018f
clinical picture in, 1016, 1016f
treatment of, 1017–1019, 1019f
surgical, 1019–1021, 1020f–1021f
rotational osteotomy of, 734, 735f
slipped capital epiphysis of, 741–750
acute, 750
classification of, 743
clinical features of, 742, 743f
complications in, 750
epidemiology of, 742
etiology of, 741–742, 742f
pathology of, 744
prognosis and natural history of, 744, 746
radiographic features of, 743, 744f–745f
results of, 749
treatment in, 746–749
bone graft and osteoplasty in, 747, 749
femoral neck osteotomy, 749
fixation in situ, 746–747, 747f–748f
nonoperative, 746
subtrochanteric osteotomy in, 749
varus rotational osteotomy of, 734, 735f
fetus, 7
sexing of, amniocentesis for, 176–177
fiber-type disproportion, 277
fiber-type nomenclature, 262
fibrodysplasia ossificans progressiva, 280–282
clinical features of, 280–281
laboratory data in, 281, 281f
management of, 281–282

fibroma, 249
  chondromyxoid, 242
fibroma molluscum, 1125
fibrous dysplasia, 133–135, 135f
  clinical manifestations of, 134
  endocrinopathies associated with, 134–135
  radiologic findings in, 134
  treatment of, 135
fibula
  derotational osteotomy of, in congenital talipes equinovarus, 914
  fractures of, orthotics for, 1039
finger(s)
  flexion contracture of, 197, 200f
  flexion deformity of, in cerebral palsy, 390
  gigantism of, 690–691, 691f
  loss of function of, orthotics for, 1056, 1056f
  polydactyly of, 689–690
Fischgold-Metzger's line, 531, 532f, 533
fistula, arteriovenous, 819–820
flail knee, 308
flatfoot, 919–942
  accessory navicular, 940–942
  calcaneovalgus foot, 924–925
  congenital vertical talus, 919–923
  flexible, 925–935
    association with congenital pes calcaneovalgus, 926
    clinical features of, 925–926, 925f
    etiology of, 926–928
      bone in, 926
      muscle in, 926–928
    roentgenographic features of, 926, 926f
    treatment in, 928–935
      conservative, 928–929, 930f
      indications for surgery in, 929
      surgical, 929–935
      surgical procedure in adolescents, 932–935, 932f–933f
      types of surgical procedure, 930–932
  spasmodic, 935
  tarsal coalition, 935–940
flexor digitorum brevis, 899
flexor digitorum longus, 898, 899
flexor hallucis longus, 898
floppy baby, 260, 260f
flowing wax bone, 65–66
Fong syndrome, 68–69, 69f
foot, 895–968
  anatomy of, 895–900
    anterior compartment of, 897–900
    bony architecture of, 896
    integument in, 895–896
    muscles of, 897
  and ankle
    dorsiflexion insufficiency of, orthotics in, 1034–1036, 1035f
    dynamic varus deformity during stance phase in, 1036
    flail, 1037, 1037f–1038f
    in limb length discrepancy, 806
    metatarsus adductus, 1033
    orthotics for, 1033–1038
    painful, orthotics for, 1037–1038
    pes calcaneovalgus, 1034
    pes planovalgus, 1033–1034, 1034f
    plantar flexion insufficiency of, 1036–1037, 1036f–1037f
    poliomyelitis of, 291–306
      ankle fusion and pantalar arthrodesis in, 304
      arthrodesis in, 297–306
      bony procedures in, 305
      calcaneal deformity in, 303–304, 304f
      claw-toe deformity in, 304–305
      dorsiflexor paralysis in, 292
      extra-articular subtalar arthrodesis in, 297–299, 298f–299f
      flail foot in, 297, 297f
      peroneal and long-toe extensor paralysis in, 295
      peronei paralysis in, 294, 294f
      pes cavus in, 305
      posterior bone block in, 305–306
      soft-tissue procedures for cavus deformity in, 305, 306f
      soft-tissue surgery of, 292–297
      tibialis anterior, toe flexors and peronei paralysis in, 293–294
      tibialis anterior and tibialis posterior paralysis in, 292–293, 293f
      tibialis anterior paralysis in, 292, 292f
      tibialis posterior paralysis in, 293
      triceps surae paralysis in, 295–296, 295f, 297f
      triple arthrodesis in, 299–303, 300f–303f
    talipes equinovarus and, 1034
  in arthrogryposis multiplex congenita, 324
    congenital convex pes valgus in, 323–324, 324f
    surgery in, 323–324
    talipes equinovarus in, 322, 323f
  biomechanics of, 900–901, 901t
  calcaneovalgus, 924–925, 924f
  in cerebral palsy, equinovalgus in, 384–385
  congenital cleft foot, 954–955, 954f
  embryology of, 895
  equinovarus deformities, 901–919
  flail, 297, 297f
  flatfoot deformities, 919–942
  forefoot deformities, 951–966
  hemiplegic, in cerebral palsy, 391–392
  lobster claw, 954–955, 954f
  manipulation of, in equinovarus deformities, 906–907, 906f–907f
  in myelomeningocele, 426–427
  orthopaedic treatment of, in juvenile arthritis, 472–473, 474f
  osteochondroses in, 951
  overuse injuries of, 1118
  pes cavus, 942–951
  skin and nails of, abnormalities of, 966–968
  structure and function of, 895
footwear, in overuse injuries, 1105
forearm
  embryologic pronation of, 20, 22–23, 23f, 24f
  poliomyelitis of, 316–317
    supination contracture in, 316–317
forefoot, deformities of, 954–966
  acquired, 964–966
  congenital, 954–964

incidence of, in Chinese population, 965t
forequarter, amputation at, prosthesis in, 923f, 992
fracture(s)
bone bar occurrence after, 1083, 1084f, 1085
cervical burst, 507
cervical compression, 506–507
in child abuse, 1151–1154, 1151f–1156f
hangman's, 506
in hemophilia, 201–202, 202f
long bone, in spinal cord injury, 516–517
in myelomeningocele, 427–430, 427f–429f
odontoid, 506
residual deformities from, in head injury, 489–490, 490f
of skull, 483, 484f–486f
stress, in overuse injuries, 1106–1107, 1108f
management of, 1107
thoracolumbar burst, 508–509, 509f
thoracolumbar compression, 508
tibial and fibular, orthotics for, 1039, 1041f
fragilitas ossium, 111–116
freckles, axillary, 1127
Freiberg's infarction, 951–952, 952f
Frejka pillow, 713
Friedreich's ataxia, 328–329, 329f–330f
laboratory data in, 328–329
management of, 329
prognosis in, 329
funnelization, 34, 35f

gait, 1061
assessment of
in children and adolescents, 1061–1079
methods of, 1078–1079
instrument-assisted analysis, 1078–1079
observational analysis, 1078
in cerebral palsy, 348
internal rotation, 382, 384
kinematics in, 1061–1070
kinetics in, 1071–1076
mature, development of, 1076–1077
muscle activity in, 1070–1071
normal, interpretation of, 1077–1078
stance phase, 1062
swing phase, 1062
ganglionectomy, 820
ganglioside, 185
Garceau procedure, in Legg-Calvé-Perthes syndrome, 770, 770f–771f
gargoylism, 70–71, 71f
gastrocnemius, 897–898
gastrointestinal disorders, in rickets and osteomalacia, 97–98, 98f, 99t
gastrosoleus, short, in cerebral palsy, 355
Gaucher's disease, 181–185
bone crisis in, 184, 184f
clinical features of, 182
femoral necrosis in, 183, 183f
general features of, 181
genetics of, 159–161
metaphysis enlargement in, 182, 182f
skeletal manifestations of, 182–185, 182f–185f
spine in, 184, 185f
spleen in, 181, 184
gene(s), 153
dominant
additive effect of, 156, 158
codominance of, 156
sex-linked dominant, 154
sex-linked recessive, 154
variable expressivity of, 155–156, 157f
genetic aspects of orthopaedic conditions, 147–177
genetic counseling, 172, 174–177
amniocentesis in, 175–177, 176f
dwarfism in, 174, 174f–175f
making and explaining diagnosis in, 172, 174, 174f–175f
in muscular dystrophy, 273
risk of recurrence and, 174–175
genetic diseases
chromosome abnormalities, 166–172
Mendelian disorders, 153–166
multifactorial conditions, 172, 173f
noncongenital, 151–153, 152f
age of onset, 153
Maroteaux-Lamy syndrome, 153
phenylketonuria, 151
vitamin D-resistant rickets, 151–152
spectrum of, 147–148
sporadic incidence of, 150
genetics, in myelomeningocele, 403–404
genu recurvatum, 1042
in poliomyelitis, 307–308, 308f
genu valgum, 1041–1042, 1042f
physiologic, 866–868, 867f
post-traumatic, 868–869, 868f
genu valgus, 866–869
genu varum, 1039–1041, 1041f
physiologic, 869, 870f
giant cell tumor(s), 243–245
diagnosis of, 244–245
treatment of, 245
gigantism
of fingers, 690–691, 691f
of upper limb, 650
girls. *See also* children
growth patterns in, 26, 27f
normal growth charts of, 128f
glenoid ligament of Cruveilhier, 899–900
glucocorticoids, 133
gluteus maximus, in poliomyelitis, 311
gluteus medius, in poliomyelitis, 310–311
gold salts, for juvenile arthritis, 463
gonad(s), abnormalities of, 132–133
Gower's maneuver, 265, 265f
graft. *See* bone graft
granuloma, eosinophilic, 250–251
diagnosis of, 250
treatment of, 251
granulomatous infections, of bones and joints, 452–453
Green-Anderson curves, 27, 28f
Green procedure, for Sprengel's deformity, 695
Grice arthrodesis, 298, 298f
ground reaction force, and joint moments, 1073–1076, 1074f–1075f
growing person, spinal injury in, 499–528
growth, 25–38
bone
mechanisms of, 29–37
remodeling and funnelization in, 33–35
small, 35
of epiphysis, 35
of hip, 35–37

growth (*continued*)
of limb, 26–28, 28f–29f. *See also* limb, growth of
normal, of long bone, 781–783, 782f–783f
in overuse injuries, 1105–1106
patterns of, 25–29, 126, 127f–128f
abnormal, 126, 129
at birth, 26
in boys, 26, 27f
in girls, 26, 27f
limbs in, 26–28, 28f–29f
maturation rate in, 25–26
spine in, 28–29
plate, partial arrest of, 1083–1100
rate of, epiphyseal plate in, 29–33
soft-tissue, mechanisms of, 37–38
of spine, 28–29, 35
stimulation of, limb lengthening by, 819–821
growth hormone, cell column zone and, 31
deficiency of, 129–131, 130f
growth hormone assay, 130
growth plate. *See* epiphyseal plate
growth-remaining chart, Green-Anderson, 803, 803f
Guillain-Barré-Strohl syndrome, 317

habilitation, in myelomeningocele, 430–432, 430f–432f
hallux rigidus, adolescent, 964–965
hallux valgus, 384–385
hallux varus, congenital, 955, 957
hammertoe, 964f, 965–966
hamstring
lengthening of, 377, 378f–379f
short, in cerebral palsy, 353, 353f
hand
in arthrogryposis multiplex congenita, 326–327
lobster-claw, 664, 666, 666f–667f
orthopaedic treatment of, in juvenile arthritis, 468, 469f, 470
"trident," 45
and wrist, orthotics for, 1053–1056
Hand-Christian-Schüller disease, 250
hangman's fracture, 506
Harrington instrumentation, 601, 603
head injury(ies), 479–496
acute and long-term orthopaedic measures in, 489–495
admitting orders in, 482
anesthesia in, 487
ataxia and spasticity in, 490–494, 491f–492f
phenol block in, 491, 492f
reconstructive surgery in, 491–494, 493f–494f
cerebral concussion, 481
cerebral contusion, 481–482
cerebral spastic disability in, 495
in child abuse, 1150
classification of depth of coma, 487, 488f
ectopic ossification in, 494
epidural hematoma, 483, 485, 486f
initial evaluation of, 479
intracerebral hemorrhage, 487
late sequelae in, 494–495
long-term neurologic management of, 487–489
neurologic evaluation of, 479–480
cranial nerve function in, 480
ENT examination in, 480
level of consciousness in, 479–480
motor function in, 480
specific diagnostic tests in, 480
rehabilitation in, 487–489
behavioral changes in, 489
cognitive and language deficits, 489
goals of therapy, 489
intellectual impairment in, 489
residual deformities from fractures and dislocations in, 489–490, 490f
scalp injuries in, 483
scoliosis and leg length discrepancy in, 494–495
skull fracture, 483, 484f–486f
subdural hematoma, 485–486
subdural hygroma, 486–487
heavy metal intoxication, 109–110, 110f
height, anticipated adult, 805
hemangiomatosis, 790f, 797
hemarthrosis, in hemophilia, 202–203, 203f
hematoma
epidural, 483, 485
management of, 485, 486f
signs and symptoms of, 483, 485
subdural, 485–486
acute, 486
chronic, 486
subperiosteal calcifying, associated with neurofibromatosis, 1140, 1140f
hematopoietic system, diseases related to, 181–211
hemiballismus, in cerebral palsy, 347
hemihypertrophy cranii, 134
hemimelia
paraxial fibular, 1011–1013, 1012f–1013f
paraxial radial, 1003–1004, 1004f
paraxial tibial, 1013–1014, 1014f–1016f
paraxial ulnar, 1004–1005, 1005f–1006f
hemipelvectomy, in prosthetics, 997
hemiplegia
in cerebral palsy, 346, 385–392
double, 347
hemivertebra, 404, 405f, 606
excision of, 612
hemoglobin C, 188
hemoglobin S, 188
hemoglobin SC disease, 195
hemoglobinopathy(ies), 188–195
genetic variations in, 195
sickle cell disease, 189–193, 189f–191f
thalassemia, 193, 194f, 195
hemophilia, 195–210
A (classic), 196
AIDS and, 210–211
B (Christmas disease), 196
clinical manifestations of, 197–200
deep muscle bleeding in, 197–199
emotional factors in, 200
factor VIII levels in, 196, 196t
flexion contracture of fingers in, 197, 200f
fractures in, 201–202, 202f
history of, 195–196, 196t

iliopsoas muscle in, 198
incidence of, 196
inheritance in, 196
intracranial bleeding in, 199
knee in, 197, 198f–199f
myositis ossificans in, 205, 205f
oral cavity bleeding in, 199
pathogenesis of arthropathy in, 205–206, 206f
phases or cycles in, 199–200
pseudotumor in, 200–201, 201f
respiratory tract bleeding in, 199
soft-tissue hemorrhage in, 197, 199f–200f
surgery for, 206–210
brace after, 206, 207f
flexion contractures and, 207, 207f–208f
synovectomy in, 207, 209
total hip replacement and, 209–210
total knee joint replacement in, 210
upper extremity and, 209, 209f
treatment of, 202–205, 203f–204f
arthropathy and, 204
casts in, 203
cryoprecipitate fraction in, 202
deep muscle bleeding and, 203–204, 204f
Factor VIII inhibitors and, 204–205
hemarthrosis and, 202–203, 203f
urinary tract bleeding in, 199
Hemophilus influenzae, infection caused by, 439
hemorrhage
intracerebral, 487
soft-tissue, 197, 199f–200f
Hessing brace, in hemophilia, 206, 207f
Hilgenreiner's line, 718
hip, 703–773
adduction-abduction control of, orthotics for, 1045–1046, 1046f
in arthrogryposis multiplex congenita, 325–326
in cerebral palsy
screening for, 370–371, 370f–371f
spastic dislocation of, treatment of, 371–373, 371f–373f
congenital dislocation of, 172, 173f
evaluation and treatment after walking age, 717–736
acetabular index in, 717–718, 720f
acetabular procedures in, 724–734
acetabulum in, 717
capsule in, 717
center-edge angle in, 718, 721f
Chiari reconstruction in, 732–734, 732f–733f
closed reduction in, 718–722
Colonna arthroplasty in, 723
combined acetabular and femoral procedures in, 734, 736
complicated reduction in, 723
Dial osteotomy in, 730, 731f, 732
femoral head and proximal femur in, 717
femoral procedures in, 734, 735f
femoral rotational osteotomy in, 734, 735f
innominate osteotomy of Salter in, 726–728, 726f–728f
ligamentum teres in, 717
maintaining reduction by secondary procedures in, 723–736
open reduction in, 722–723
pathology in, 717
Pemberton osteotomy in, 728–730, 729f
realignment techniques in, 724, 725f–726f, 726
reduction in, 718–723
roentgenographic evaluation in, 717–718, 720f–721f
shelf procedure in, 724, 725f–726f, 726
Steel procedure in, 730, 730f
Sutherland procedure in, 730, 731f
varus derotation osteotomy in, 734, 735f
evaluation and treatment before walking age, 703–717
Barlow examination in, 707, 707f
cast application in, 716–717
change of clinical signs in, 710–711, 711f
diagnosis of, 706–711, 707f–711f
diapers in, 714, 715f
early treatment in, 711–717, 712f–716f
embryology and anatomy in, 703–704
etiology of, 704–705
incidence of, 706
open reduction in, 717
orthotic devices in, 711–714, 712f–715f
Ortolani maneuver in, 707, 707f
Pavlik harness in, 712, 712f
residual subluxation in, 717
roentgenographic studies in, 708–710, 708f– 710f
terminolgy in, 706, 706f
traction in, 716, 716f
types of dislocations, 705–706, 705f
congenital disorders of, multifactorial conditions, 172, 173f
disarticulations, prosthesis in, 997, 1000f–1001f
dysplasia, 706, 706f
flexion contracture of, in muscular dystrophy, 272
flexion contractures in muscular dystrophy, 272
growth of, 35–37, 36f–37f
motion of, 1065–1067, 1066f–1067f
in myelomeningocele, 415–426
dislocation in, 416, 418–420
congenital, 418, 418f
functional subluxation and, 418
late, 418, 419f–421f, 420
muscle function in, 415–416, 417t
treatment in, 420, 422–426
at L5 levels, 426
at lower lumbar levels, 420, 422–423, 423f–425f

hip, in myelomeningocele, treatment in (*continued*)
at thoracic and upper lumbar levels, 420
myodesis of, in cerebral palsy, 354
orthopaedic treatment of, in juvenile arthritis, 468
orthotics for, 1045–1052
overuse injuries of, 1113–1114, 1114f
paralytic dislocation in, 311–312
poliomyelitis of, 310–312
gluteus maximus paralysis in, 311
gluteus medius paralysis in, 310–311
paralytic dislocation in, 311–312
snapping, 1113
total replacement of, 209–210
histiocytosis X, 250
history taking, in spinal deformities, 571–572
history taking and physical examination, of bone tumors, 222–224
"hitchhiker" thumb, 50, 51f
HLA. *See* human leukocyte antigen
Hodgkin's disease, 245–246
Hoke's triple arthrodesis, 300, 300f
homeostasis
calcium and phosphorus, 84–92
facts concerning, 85
homocystinuria, 125–126
treatment of, 126
hormone
growth, cell column zone and, 31
sex, 31
epiphyseal plate closure and, 33
human leukocyte antigen (HLA)
in ankylosing spondylitis, 475
associated with arthritis, 459
humerus, in sickle cell disease, 190
Hunter's syndrome, 71–72, 72f
Hurler's syndrome, 70–71, 71f
hydromyelia, 405, 405–406, 406f
curve measurements and treatment of, 409t
hydrotherapy, for juvenile arthritis, 464
25-hydroxy vitamin D, 87, 88f
hydroxyapatite, 85
hypertrophic cell zone and, 31
hydroxychloroquine, for JA, 463
hygroma, subdural, 486–487
hypercalcemia, 109–110
idiopathic, 109
in spinal cord injury, 522
hyperparathyroidism, 106–107
hyperpigmentation, 1125, 1126f
hyperplasias, verrucous, 1126f, 1127
hypertension, 482
hyperthermia, malignant, 262–263
treatment of, 263
hypertrophic cell zone, 31
hypervitaminosis A, 120–122
hypervitaminosis D, 109
hypoparathyroidism, 107–108
hypophosphatasia, 105–106
florid, 107f
hypopituitarism, 129–131, 130f
treatment of, 131
hypoplasia
of thumb, 662–664, 663f
upper limb, 650
hypothyroidism, 131–132, 131f–133f
laboratory studies in, 131–132
treatment of, 132
hypotonia, in cerebral palsy, 347
hysterical scoliosis, 579–580, 582f

idiopathic hypercalcemia, 109
idiopathic scoliosis. *See* scoliosis, idiopathic
"iliac horns," 69f
iliopsoas muscle, 198
iliotibial band, 308–309, 309f
immobilization, in surgical treatment of scoliosis, 603
immunologic phase, of septic arthritis, 449
immunotherapy, in osteosarcoma, 236
indomethacin, for ankylosing spondylitis, 476
infant(s). *See also* children; boys; girls
dystrophia myotonica in, 275
septic arthritis in, 450, 450f
infantile cortical hyperostosis, 120, 121f
infantile thoracic dystrophy, 53
infection(s)
of bones and joints, 437–456
acute hematogenous osteomyelitis in, 439–448
case history, 456
general features of, 437–439
granulomatous, 452–453
inflammatory response in, 437–438, 438f
morbidity and mortality in, 439
problems and pitfalls in, 453–456
blood dyscrasias in, 453
intravenous seeding in, 453, 454f
leg length problems and, 455f, 456
Riley-Day syndrome and sickle cell disease and, 453
sacroiliac joint and, 453
septic arthritis, 448–452
types of infections, 438–439, 439f
in lower limb length discrepancy, 790, 792f–794f
inflammatory myopathy(ies), 277–279
inflammatory response, 437–438, 438f
inheritance
codominant, 156
disorders not detected at birth, 151–153, 152f
molecular basis of, 150–151
DNA, 150f, 151
mRNA, 151
sickle cell anemia, 151
injury. *See also* trauma
in child abuse
head, 1150
internal, 1150–1151
overuse
in children, 1103–1119
etiology and risk factors, 1104–1106
anatomic malalignment, 1105
associated disease state, 1105
footwear and playing surface, 1105
growth, 1105–1106
muscle-tendon imbalance, 1104–1105
training error, 1104
prevention of, 1119
sites of, 1109–1118
ankle and foot, 1118
elbow, 1112–1113
hip and pelvis, 1113–1114, 1114f
knee, 1114–1117, 1115f–1118f

shoulder, 1111–1112, 1112f
spine, 1109, 1110f–1111f, 1111
type of, 1106–1109
bursitis, 1109
joint disorders, 1109
stress fractures, 1106–1107, 1108f
tendonitis, 1107–1109
innominate osteotomy of Salter, in congenital dislocation of hip, 726–728, 726f–728f
integument, of foot, 895–896
intellectual impairment, 489
intelligence, in myelomeningocele, 400, 401f
interossei, 899
intervertebral disc, embryology of, 18–19
intoxication, heavy metal, 109–110, 110f
intracerebral hemorrhage, 487
intracranial bleeding, in hemophilia, 199
intramembranous ossification, 16
intrathoracic meningocele, associated with neurofibromatosis, 1133–1134, 1135f
intravenous seeding, 453
involucrum, 440, 441
iridocyclitis, 458
irradiation sarcoma, 247–248

Jeune syndrome, 53
joint movements, ground reaction force and, 1073–1076, 1074f–1075f
joint motion, 1065–1070, 1065f–1070f
joint necrosis, 888
joints. *See also specific joints*
disorders of, in overuse injuries, 1109
excision of, in juvenile arthritis, 467
infections of. *See* infection(s), of bones and joints
orthopaedic treatment of, 468–474
juvenile arthritis (JA), 457–474
ankle and foot in, 472–473, 474f
cervical spine in, 473–474
classification of, 457–459
acute febrile form in, 458–459
pauci-articular form in, 457–458
polyarthritis form in, 458
diagnostic procedures in, 464–465
arthroscopy and, 464–465
synovial biopsy, 464, 464t
differential diagnosis of, 460–462
foreign body synovitis in, 462
leukemia in, 461
rheumatic fever in, 460–461
septic arthritis in, 461–462
transient synovitis in, 462
drug therapy in, 462–463
anti-inflammatory, 463
anti-malarial, 463
aspirin, 462–463
corticosteroids, 463
gold salts, 463
elbow in, 470, 470f
etiology of, 459
hand and wrist in, 468, 469f, 470
hip in, 468
knee in, 470–472, 471f–473f
orthopaedic management of, 464–474
pathology of, 459–460
physical therapy in, 463–464
reconstructive surgery in, 465–468
arthrodesis in, 467, 467f
arthroplasty in, 467–468, 468f
joint excision in, 467
osteotomy in, 466–467
soft-tissue procedures in, 465–466
synovectomy in, 465–466
contraindications, 466
technique, 466
roentgenographic features of, 460, 460f–461f
shoulder in, 470
treatment of, 462–464
juvenile myasthenia gravis, 283
juvenile osteoporosis, idiopathic, 116–118, 117f–118f
juvenile roundback, 1111
juxtacortical chondrosarcoma, 243
juxtacortical osteosarcoma, 236–237
survival rate in, 237
treatment of, 237

karyotype, normal, 153, 154f
kinematics, 1061–1070
body segment motion, 1063–1065, 1063f–1064f
events in gait cycle, 1061–1063, 1062f–1063f, 1063t
specific joint motion, 1065–1070
ankle motion, 1069, 1069f
femur and tibia motion, 1067–1069, 1068f–1069f
hip motion, 1065–1067, 1066f–1067f
pelvic motion, 1064f–1066f, 1065
shoulder and trunk motion, 1069–1070, 1070f
kinetics, 1071–1076, 1072f–1074f
ground reaction force and joint movements, 1073–1076, 1074f–1075f
Klinefelter's syndrome, 171
Klippel-Feil syndrome, 535–545
abnormalities associated with, 535–536, 535f–536f, 536t
associated conditions in, 540–542
cardiovascular abnormalities in, 541
clinical appearance of, 536–537, 537f, 539
deafness in, 542
of entire cervical spine, 536, 536f
mirror motions (synkinesia) in, 542
neurologic symptoms of, 542–543
patterns of cervical motion in, 543–544, 543f–544f
pterygium colli in, 537
renal abnormalities in, 541
respiratory difficulties in, 541
roentgenographic features of, 538f–541f, 539–540
difficulties with, 538f, 539
flexion extension views in, 540, 540f
hypoplasia of disc space in, 536f, 539
laminae fusion in, 540, 541f
thoracic involvement in, 540
in young child, 538f, 539
scoliosis and, 540–541
Sprengel's deformity in, 537
symptoms of, 542–544
treatment of, 544–545

knee. *See also* patella
  amputation below, prosthesis in, 995–996, 995f–997f
  amputations above, 996–997, 999f–1000f
  in arthrogryposis multiplex congenita, 324–325
    extension deformity of, 325
    flexion contracture of, 324
    posterior capsulotomy in, 325, 325f
  in cerebral palsy, stiff, extended, 382, 383f
  disarticulations, prosthesis in, 996, 998f–999f
  flexion contracture of
    in muscular dystrophy, 272
    orthotics in, 1044, 1045f
  flexion contractures in muscular dystrophy, 272
  in hemophilia, 197, 198f–199f, 210
  in myelomeningocele, 426
  orthopaedic treatment of, in juvenile arthritis, 470–472, 471f–473f
  orthotics for, 1039–1045
  overuse injuries of, 1114–1117, 1115f–1118f
  poliomyelitis of, 306–310
    flail knee in, 308
    flexion contracture of, 306, 307f
    genu recurvatum in, 307, 308f
    iliotibial band in, 308–310, 308f
    pelvic obliquity in, 310
    quadriceps paralysis in, 306–308, 308f
  stiff, 282
knee-ankle-foot orthosis (KAFO), 1031
kneel walking, in cerebral palsy, 350–351
Kniest syndrome, 49–50
Kohler's disease, 952, 953f
Kugelberg-Welander disease, 266, 318, 319f
kyphoscoliosis, 572
  associated with neurofibromatosis; 1131, 1132f
kyphosis
  classification of, 570
  congenital, 631–635
    nonoperative treatment of, 633
    progression of, 631, 632f, 633
    surgical treatment of, 633–635, 634f, 636f
      anterior fusion in, 633
      posterior fusion in, 633, 634f
      thoracic type, 633, 636f
      for type II deformities, 633, 635
    types of, 631, 631f
  measurement of, 573, 575, 576f–577f
  in myelomeningocele, surgical treatment of, 412–415, 413f–417f
  postlaminectomy, 635, 637f
  postural, 619
  Scheuermann's, 1111

labyrinthine reflex, 348
Lambrinudi drop-foot arthrodesis, 301–302, 302f
laminectomy, kyphosis following, 635, 637f
laminography, of spine, 575
language deficits, 489
latissimus dorsi, 315, 316
lead poisoning, 109–110, 110f
leg(s). *See also* limb, lower
  length problems in, 455f, 456
    in head injuries, 494–495
    scoliosis and, 578–579, 581f
  orthotics for, 1038–1039
Legg-Calvé-Perthes syndrome, 750–770
  arthrography in, 755
  blood supply to femoral head, 753–754
  clinical features of, 752
  differential diagnosis of, 759–760
  etiology of, 752–753
  femoral head changes in, 754–755, 754f
  incidence and epidemiology of, 752
  orthotics in, 1049–1051
    nonweightbearing hip-adduction internal rotation orthosis in, 1050
    Scottish Rite Hospital orthosis in, 1051, 1051f
    Toronto orthosis in, 1049–1050, 1050f
    trilateral-socket hip-abduction orthosis in, 1050–1051, 1050f
  pathology of, 753
  prognosis in, 755–759
    Catterall classification in, 756–758, 756f–763f
      group I, 756, 756f
      group II, 756–757, 757f–758f
      group III, 757, 759f–760f
      group IV, 757–758, 761f–763f
    factors influencing, 758–759
  radioactive isotope studies in, 755
  roentgenographic evaluation of, 754–755, 754f
  treatment of, 760–770
    combined procedures in, 770, 772f
    containment methods, 763–764, 764f–765f
    discontinuing, 765–766, 766f
    nonweightbearing methods, 762
    orthosis methods, 765
    plans of management in, 761–762
    plaster method, 764–765, 764f
    principles in, 760–762, 764f
    reconstruction in, 768–770, 769f
      Chiari procedure in, 769–770
      Garceau proedure in, 770, 770f–771f
      Salter osteotomy, 769
      valgus osteotomy, 770
      varus osteotomy, 769
    surgical procedures in, 766–767, 767f–769f
      Salter osteotomy, 767, 769f
      varus osteotomy, 767, 767f–768f
Leri-Weill disease, 53
lesions
  Brown-Sequard, 503
  functional significance of, in spinal cord injury, 526–528
  tumor-like, 248–252
    aneurysmal bone cyst, 251–252
    eosinophilic granuloma, 250–251
    metaphyseal fibrous defects, 249–250
    simple unicameral bone cyst, 248–249
Letterer-Siwe disease, 250
leukemia, 186–188, 187f–188f

differential diagnosis of juvenile arthritis and, 461
growth arrest in, 186, 188f
leukemic lines in, 186, 187f
lymphocytic, 186, 187f
osteolytic lesions in, 186–187, 188f
skeletal changes in, 186, 187f
treatment of, 188
lifeskills training, in cerebral palsy, 364
ligamentun teres, 718
Lignac-Fanconi syndrome, 98
limb
artificial, surgical conversion to, 808–809
bud
embryonic development of, 19–24
apical ectodermal ridge in, 20, 20f–21f, 22–23
in early gestation, 19–20, 20f–21f
ectodermal ring in, 19
experimental deformity of, 22–24, 24f
forearm pronation in, 20, 23f
mesoderm coalescence in, 20, 23f
innervation of, 13
musculature of, 15–16
congenital deficiencies of, 998–1026
classification of, 1001–1002, 1002f
etiology of, 1000–1001
incidence of, 998
medical management of, 1002–1003
terminology in, 1001–1002
growth of, 26–28, 28f–29f
angular and torsional shape in, 28
Green-Anderson curves in, 26–27, 28f
leg measurement, 26
limb growth plates in, 27–28, 29f
orthoroentgenogram in, 26
patterns of, 26–28, 28f–29f
roentgenographic measurements in, 26
scanogram in, 26
teleoroentgenogram in, 26
loss of, from malignancy, 998
lower, 865–891. *See also* extremity, lower; leg(s)
bipartite patella, 886–887
congenital angular deformities of tibia in, 875–878
congenital deficiencies of, 1011–1026
amelia, 1022, 1024f–1026f, 1025
paraxial fibular hemimelia, 1011–1013, 1012f–1013f
paraxial tibial hemimelia, 1013–1014, 1014f–1016f
phocomelia, 1022, 1022f–1024f
proximal femoral focal deficiency, 1014, 1016–1021, 1016f–1021f
congenital dislocation and subluxation of knee, 882–886
congenital dislocation of patella, 882
discoid meniscus, 887
equalization in, 784–808
methods of, 808–860
genu valgum of, 866–869
genu varum of, 869
length discrepancy of, 781–860
anticipated adult height and, 805
cause of, 784–799
congenital and developmental, 784, 785f–790f, 787–788
infectious, 790, 792f–794f
miscellaneous, 790, 797, 797f–798f, 799
paralytic, 788–789, 791f
traumatic, 790, 795f–796f, 797
degree of, 799–802, 799f–801f
etiologies of, 784
foot and ankle status, 806
health factors in, 806–807
localization of inequality in, 806
needs and desires of patient and parent in, 807–808
physiologic factors in, 806–807
progression in, 803–805, 803f–805f
psychological factors in, 807
sex of patient in, 806
skeletal age in, 802–803, 802f
strength and balance of musculature in, 805–806
length equalization in, 808–853
arteriovenous fistula in, 819–820
bone shortening (resection) in, 813, 815–816, 817f–818f, 819
case histories, 853–860
conversion to artificial limb, 808–809
correction by lengthening, 819–853
by electrical stimulation, 820–821
epiphyseal plate stapling in, 811–813, 814f–815f
epiphysiodesis in, 809–811, 809f–810f, 812f
femoral lengthening in, 825–838
ganglionectomy or sympathectomy in, 820
implementation of equalization procedures in, 853
inequality due to angular deformity, 850, 851f, 852
mechanical lengthening in, 821–825
metaphyseal stimulation in, 820
multiple surgical insults in, 820
nonsurgical methods in, 808
normal growth and behavior of, 781–783
osteotomy and gradual distraction in, 822–849. *See also* osteotomy, and gradual distraction
periosteal stripping in, 820
by physeal distraction, 850, 850f
shortening of long side, 809–819
simultaneous femoral and tibial lengthening in, 849–850

limb, lower, length equalization in (*continued*)
by stimulation of growth, 819–821
surgical methods in, 808–853
tibial lengthening in, 838–849
treatment of, 852–853
orthotics for, 1033–1052
Osgood-Schlatter disease, 890–891
osteochondritis dissecans, 887–890
popliteal cyst, 891
prosthetic fitting of, 992–997
recurrent subluxation and dislocation of patella, 878–882
tibia vara of, 869–875
tibial torsion of, 865–866
phantom, 984
upper, 649–699. *See also* extremity, upper
arrest of development of, 649–650
arthrogryposis of, 676–678, 677f
birth injuries of brachial plexus of, 696–698, 697f
camptodactyly of, 680
clinodactyly of, 681–682, 682f
congenital absence, 664, 665f–666f
congenital absence of radius, 625–656, 654f–655f, 657f–658f
congenital absence of ulna, 656–662, 659f–661f
congenital amputations of, 650–651, 651f
congenital clasped thumb, 686–687, 687f
congenital deficiencies of, 1003–1011
amelia, 1007–1008, 1008f–1009f
externally powered upper limb prostheses for, 1008–1011, 1010f–1011f
paraxial radial hemimelia, 1003–1004, 1004f
paraxial ulnar hemimelia, 1004–1005, 1005f–1006f
phocomelia, 1005–1007, 1007f
congenital dislocation of elbow, 673–675, 674f
congenital dislocation of radial head, 673, 674f
congenital dislocation of shoulder, 666–667, 668f
congenital pseudarthrosis of clavicle, 667–670, 668f–670f
congenital radiohumeral synostosis, 672–673, 672f
congenital radioulnar syntostosis, 671–672, 671f
congenital trigger thumb, 683
congenital webbing of elbow, 675–676, 676f
constricting bands of, 691–692, 692f
delta phalanx of, 685–686, 685f
duplication of parts in, 650
failure of differentiation of parts in, 650
gigantism of fingers, 690–691, 691f
hypoplastic thumb, 662–664, 663f
lobster-claw hand, 664, 666, 666f–667f
Madelung's deformity of, 692–693, 693f
malformations of, classification of, 649–650
orthotics for, 1052–1058, 1053–1058
osteochondritis dissecans of elbow, 698–699, 699f
phocomelia in, 651–652, 652f
polydactyly of, 687–690, 688f
prosthetic fitting of, 984–992
Sprengel's deformity of, 693–696, 694f–695f
syndactyly of, 678–680, 678f–679f, 681f
triphalangeal thumb of, 683–685, 683f
lipochondrodystrophy, 70–71, 71f
Little League elbow, 1112
Little League shoulder, 1111
Lobstein's disease, 111–116
lobster-claw, 664, 666, 666f–667f, 954–955, 954f
clinical features of, 664, 666, 666f
treatment of, 666, 667f
locomotion, in myelomeningocele, 401–402, 402f
locomotor generator, 355–357, 356f–357f
longitudinal deficiency(ies), of upper limb, 649–650
Looser's lines, 95–96, 96f
lordosis, measurement of, 573, 575, 576f–577f
Lowe's syndrome, 98
lumbosacral spine orthosis (LSO), 1031
lumbricals, 899
lupus erythematosus, systemic, 279–280
etiology of, 279
laboratory data in, 279
management of, 279–280
Luque instrumentation, 604
lymphoma, non-Hodgkin's, 246
lymphosarcoma, 246
Lyon hypothesis, 164–165
lysis, in osteosarcoma, 230

McGregor's line, 531–533, 532f–533f
McRae's line, 531, 532f, 533
macrodactyly, 690–691, 691f
of toes, 955, 956f
Madelung's deformity, 53, 692–693, 693f
Maffucci's syndrome, 240
malignancy, 116
limb loss from, 998
mallet toe, congenital, 964, 964f
marble bone disease, 118–120, 119f
Marfan's scoliosis, 612–617. *See also* scoliosis, Marfan's
Marfan's syndrome, 123–124, 123f–124f
genetics of, 156
marginal layer, 10
Marie-Sainton disease, 54, 55f, 56
Maroteaux-Lamy syndrome, 73, 153
genetics of, 161, 162f–163f
maturation, rate of, 25–26
mechanical lengthening, of limbs, 821–825
Mediterranean anemia, 193
Melnick-Needles syndrome, 67–68
melorheostosis, 65–66

mendelian disorder(s), 153–166
  autosomal dominant conditions, 154–158
    additive effect of dominant genes, 156
    blood groups in, 156
    codominance of dominant genes, 156
    Marfan's syndrome, 156
    new mutation in, 155
    orthopaedic, 155, 156f
    penetrance in, 154–155
    pleiotropic effect in, 156
    schematic pedigree in, 154, 155f
    variable expressivity, 155–156, 157f
  autosomal recessive conditions, 158–161
    bias of ascertainment in, 159, 160f
    Gaucher's disease, 159–161
    Maroteaux-Lamy syndrome, 161, 162f–163f
    recessive gene load, 158–161
    schematic pedigree of, 158, 158f
    Tay-Sachs disease, 159
    variability of recessive disorders, 161, 162f–163f
  dominant conditions, 154
  normal karyotype, 153, 154f
  recessive conditions, 154
  sex-linked conditions, 154
  various inheritance patterns in
    Charcot-Marie-Tooth disease, 165
    chondrodysplasia punctata, 165
    idiopathic scoliosis, 165–166
    osteogenesis imperfecta, 166, 166f
  X-linked dominant conditions, 161–163
    pedigree in, 162, 164f
    schematic of, 161, 164f
    vitamin D-resistant rickets, 162–163, 164f
  X-linked recessive conditions, 163–165
    Lyon hypothesis in, 164–165
    pedigree in, 163, 165f
    pseudohypertrophic muscular dystrophy, 165
meningocele, 399, 399f
  intrathoracic, associated with neurofibromatosis 1133–1134, 1135f
meningomyelocele, with spina bifida, 172
meninx primitiva, 13
meniscus, discoid, 887
Meryon's sign, 265, 266f
mesencephalon, 9
mesenchymal chondrosarcoma, 243
mesenchyme, tissues arising from, 3
mesoderm
  extraembryonic, 2, 3f
  intraembryonic, 2, 3f
  tissues arising from, 3
mesomelia, 53–54
messenger ribonucleic acid (mRNA), 151
metabolic abnormalities
  connective tissue syndromes, 123–126
  Ehlers-Danlos syndromes, 124–125
  fibrous dysplasia, 133–135
  homocystinuria, 125–126
  hypercalcemia, 109–110
  hypervitaminosis A, 120–122
  hypervitaminosis D, 109
  hypophosphatasia, 105–106
  hypopituitarism, 129–131
  hypothyroidism, 131–132
  idiopathic juvenile osteoporosis, 116–118
  of immature skeleton, 81–135
  Marfan's syndrome, 123–124
  normal variant short stature, 129
  osteogenesis imperfecta, 111–116
  osteopetrosis, 118–120
  parathyroid disorders, 106–109
  periosteal reaction, 120–123
  renal osteodystrophy, 101–105
  rickets and osteomalacia, 92–101
  scurvy, 122
metabolic disorders
  Gaucher's disease, 181–185
  Niemann-Pick disease, 184–185
metaphyseal aclasis, 240
metaphyseal chondrodysplasia. *See* chondrodysplasia, metaphyseal
metaphyseal fibrous defects, 249–250
metaphysis, 31–32
  enlarged, in Gaucher's disease, 182, 182f
  stimulation of, 820
metastability, 85
metatarsal
  congenital short first, 961
  osteotomy of
    in congenital talipes equinovarus, 913
    in pes cavus, 949, 950f
metatarsus adductus, 1033
metatarsus atavicus, 961
metatarsus varus, congenital, 915–918
  clinical appearance of, 915–916, 916f
  incidence of, 916
  roentgenographic findings in, 916, 917f
  treatment of, 916–918
    conservative, 916–918
    surgical, 918
metatropic dwarfism, 48–49
metencephalon, 9
methotrexate, for osteosarcoma, 235
midget, 41
milkman's pseudofractures, 95–96, 96f
Milwaukee brace. *See* bracing, Milwaukee
mineral phase, of metabolic and endocrine abnormalities of skeleton, 84–110
mineralization, 111
mirror motions, in Klippel-Feil syndrome, 542
mitosis, of white cells, 167
MMN syndrome, metaphyseal chondrodysplasia with, 58f, 59
molecular basis, of inheritance, 150–151, 150f
mongolism
  amniocentesis for, 176
  chromosomal nondisjunction in, 169, 170f
  chromosomal translocation in, 169, 170f–171f, 171
  determination of type of, 169, 171
morbidity, in infections of bones and joints, 439
Moro reflex, 348, 349f
Morquio's syndrome, 72–73, 74f
mortality, in infections of bones and joints, 439
morula, 1, 2f

Mosely straight-line graph, 804, 804f
motion
  body segment, 1063–1065, 1063f–1064f
  joint, 1065–1070, 1065f–1070f
motor function, 480
mucopolysaccharidosis, 69–75
  conditions resembling, 75
  differential diagnosis of, 70t
  Hunter's syndrome, 71–72, 72f
  Hurler's syndrome, 70–71, 71f
  Morquio's syndrome, 72–73, 74f
  polydystrophic dwarfism, 73
  Sanfilippo's syndrome, 73–75, 75f
  Scheie's syndrome, 75
muscle(s). *See also specific muscles*
  balance, in cerebral palsy, 360, 368f, 387f
  biomechanics of, 358–359, 359f–360f
  cerebral palsy, 359–360, 359f
  in flexible flatfoot, 926–928
  of foot, 897–899
  function, in myelomeningocele of hip, 415–416, 417t
  joint, in cerebral palsy, 360
  lengthening of, 376–385
  in shortened limb, strength and balance of, 805–806
muscle activity, 1070–1071, 1071f
muscle and peripheral nerves, diseases of, 259–260
  floppy baby and, 260, 260f
  physical examination in, 259–260
muscle biopsy, 261–262
muscle growth, in cerebral palsy, 357–358, 358f
muscle shortening, in cerebral palsy, 351–355, 351f–354f
muscle-tendon imbalance, in overuse injuries, 1104–1105
muscular disorder(s)
  and amniocentesis, 262
  anesthesia in, 262–263
  electrocardiogram in, 262
  electromyography in, 261
  evaluation of, 260–263
  laboratory data in, 260–261
  muscle biopsy in, 261–262
  nerve conduction studies in, 261
  ophthalmologic evaluation in, 262
  pulmonary function studies in, 262
muscular dystrophy. *See also* dystrophy
  autosomal dominant, 268
  autosomal recessive, 267–268
  fascioscapulohumeral, 268, 268f
  limb-girdle types, 267–268
  myotonic disorders, 273–275
  progressive, 263–277
  pseudohypertrophic, 165
  sex-linked, 263–267
    Becker type, 267
    Duchenne type, 263–267
      differential diagnosis of, 266–267
      dorsal shift in, 264, 264f
      Gower's maneuver in, 265, 265f
      laboratory data in, 266
      Meryon's sign in, 265, 266f
      pseudohypertrophy of calf in, 264, 264f
      scoliosis in, 618–619, 625f
      wheelchair-bound patient and, 266, 267f
  treatment of, 269–273
    cardiopulmonary measures in, 273
    functional testing in, 269–270, 270f
    genetic counseling in, 273
    orthosis in, 270, 271f–272f
    physical therapy in, 269
    surgery in, 270–272
      equinus contractures and, 270–272, 273f
      hip flexion contractures and, 272, 274f
      knee flexion contractures and, 272
    wheelchair in, 272–273
muscular system, embryology of, 13–16
  of body wall, 13–14
  cervical region, 15
  epaxial muscle mass in, 14–15, 14f
  hypomeric muscle mass in, 14f, 15
  in limbs, 15–16
mutation, autosomal dominant, 155
myasthenia gravis, 282–283
  juvenile, 283
  neonatal persistent, 282–283
  neonatal transient, 282
Mycobacterium avium intracellulare, infection with, 210
myelencephalon, 9
myelination, 11
myelodysplasia, 397, 398
myelography
  in occipitocervical synostosis, 554
  of spine, 575
myelomeningocele, 397–432
  brain stem anomalies associated with, 399, 400f
  classification and pathology of, 398–400, 399f–400f
  cross-section of, 399, 399f
  developmental sequence and, 402–403
  embryology of, 397–398
  foot in, 426–427
  forme fruste of, 398
  fractures in, 427–430, 427f–429f
  genetics in, 403–404
  hip in, 415–426. *See also* hip, in myelomeningocele
  incidence of, 403
  knee in, 426
  natural history of, 400–402, 401f–402f
    death rate in, 400, 401f
    intelligence in, 400, 401f
    locomotion in, 401–402, 402f
  pathology of, 397
  treatment of, 404–430
    foot, 426–427
    fractures, 427–430
    habilitation in, 430–432
    hip, 415–426
    knee, 426
    selection of, 402
    spine, 404–415. *See also* spine, in myelomeningocele
myodesis, of hip, in cerebral palsy, 354
myoelectric control, 1009
myopathic arthrogryposis, 328
myopathy(ies)
  characteristic changes, 262
  congenital, 275–277
    central core disease, 276–277
    fiber-type disproportion, 277

myotubular, 277
nemaline, 277
inflammatory, 277–279
dermatomyositis, 277–279, 278f
polymyositis, 277–279
myositis ossificans, 280–282
in hemophilia, 205, 205f
progressiva, 280–282
clinical features of, 280–281
laboratory data in, 281, 281f
management of, 281–282
traumatic, 280
myotonia congenita, 273–274, 275f
myotonic disorders, 273–275
myotubular myopathy, 277

nail-patella syndrome, 68–69, 69f
nails, abnormalities of, 966–968
naproxen, for juvenile arthritis, 463
navicular, accessory, 940–942
clinical signs and symptoms of, 941, 941f
treatment of, 941–942
nonoperative, 941–942
surgical, 942
neck reflex, 348
necrosis
avascular, 750
joint, 888
nemaline myopathy, 277
neoplasia, associated with neurofibromatosis, 1140–1141
nerve(s)
conduction studies, 261
lesions, peripheral, 328–335
peripheral, diseases of, 259–260
spinal, 13
nervous system, embryology of, 7–13
brain in, 8–9, 10f
ependymal layer in, 10–11
marginal layer in, 10
myelination in, 11
neural plate in, 8, 9f
neural tube in, 8–12, 9f
neuroblasts in, 10
spinal cord in, 11–13, 12f
spinal nerves in, 13
neural crest, 13
neural injury, classification of, 502–503
neural plate, 4, 8, 9f
neural tube, 8–12, 9f
neurectomy
obturator, 381, 381f
in pes cavus, 949
neuroblastoma, 246
neuroblast(s), 10, 11f
neurofibroma, dermal, 1125
neurofibromatosis, 1121–1142
clinical findings in, 1124–1127
diagnostic problems in, 1122–1124
genetics in, 1124
historical comments, 1121–1122, 1122f
lower limb length discrepancy in, 797, 798f
miscellaneous, 1141–1142
skeletal manifestations in, 1127–1141
neurogenic tumor(s), associated with neurofibromatosis, 1138, 1140
neurologic disorder(s), in congenital scoliosis, 607, 609–610, 610f–611f
neurologic evaluation, in head injury, 479–480
neurologic management, in head injury, 487–489
neurologic signs, in cerebral palsy, 348, 349f
neuroma, 983–984
neuromuscular disorders, 259–334
neuromuscular scoliosis, 617–619
neuromusculoskeletal apparatus, embryology of, 1–24
neuropathy
characteristic changes, 262
congenital sensory, 332, 333f, 334
familial sensory, 334–335
hereditary, 328–335
hereditary and motor sensory, 329–332
management of, 331–332, 332f
type I, 329–330, 330f
type II, 330–331, 331f
type III, 331
type IV (Refsum's disease), 331
hereditary sensory radicular, 334
nevus(i), with neurofibromatosis, 1125, 1126f
newborn. *See also* infant(s)
arthrogryposis multiplex congenita in, 322
asphyxiating thoracic dystrophy of, 53
congenital dislocation of hip in, diagnosis of, 706–711, 707f–711f
growth rate of, 26
spine in, 29
Niemann-Pick disease, 185–186
cell pathology of, 185
incidence and clinical course of, 185
skeletal manifestations and treatment of, 185–186
Nievergelt mesomelic syndrome, 54
nodes of Ranvier, 11
non-Hodgkin's lymphoma, 246
nondisjunction
of chromosomes, 150
in mongolism, 169, 170f
nonweightbearing treatment, in Legg-Calvé-Perthes syndrome, 762
Noonan's syndrome, 171
normal variant short stature, 129
notochordal canal, 4, 6f

obstetric paralysis, of upper limb, 696–698, 697f
occipitocervical synostosis, 552–555, 553f
brain stem compression in, 555
clinical findings in, 554–555
development of, 552–553
developmental errors in, 553, 554t
flexion-extension stress films in, 554
McRae measurements in, 554
myelography in, 554
roentgenographic findings in, 553–554
treatment in, 555
vascular disturbances in, 555
ocular dystrophy, 268
oculopharyngeal dystrophy, 269
odontoid
congenital anomalies of, 545–552
aplasia of, 546, 548
cervical spine fusion in, 551, 552t
clinical findings in, 550–551
definitions in, 546–547
etiology of, 547
frequency of, 547

odontoid, congenital anomalies of (*continued*)
  Gallie fusion in, 551, 552t
  hypoplasia of, 546, 547f, 548, 548f
  normal variations of, 548, 548f
  roentgenographic features of, 547–548
  treatment of, 551–552, 552t
 development of, 545–546, 545f–547f
odontoid fractures, 506
oligodendrocyte, 11
oligophrenia, polydystrophic, 73–75, 75f
Ollier disease, 64–65, 64f
ontogeny, 1–7
 amniotic cavity in, 2, 4f
 cleavage in, 1
 extraembryonic mesoderm in, 2, 3f
 fetal period in, 7
 inner cell mass in, 2
 intraembryonic mesoderm in, 2, 3f
 neural plate in, 4
 notochordal canal in, 4, 6f
 primitive streak in, 2, 5f
 somites in, 4–5, 6f–7f
 trophoblast in, 2
onychoarthrosis, 68–69, 69f
onychomesodysplasia, 68–69, 69f
ophthalmologic evaluation, 262
ophthalmoplegia, progressive external, 268
oral cavity, in hemophilia, 199
organic phase, of metabolic and endocrine abnormalities of skeleton, 110–135
orthopaedic manifestations, of child abuse, 1151–1154, 1151f–1156f
orthoroentgenogram, of limbs, 26
orthosis, 1031. *See also* bracing
 advances in, 1032–1033
 in congenital hip dislocation, 711–714, 712f–715f 1051–1052
 lower limb, 1033–1052
  foot and ankle in, 1033–1038
   dorsiflexion insufficiency of, 1034–1036, 1035f
    with dynamic equinus, 1035, 1035f
    isolated, 1035, 1035f
    with varus, 1035–1036
   dynamic varus deformity during stance phase in, 1036, 1036f
   flail, 1037, 1037f–1038f
   metatarsus adductus of, 1033
   painful, 1037–1038
   pes calcaneovalgus of, 1034
   pes planovalgus of, 1033–1034, 1034f
   plantar flexion insufficiency in, 1036–1037, 1036f–1037f
   talipes equinovarus of, 1034
  hip in, 1045–1052
   adduction-abduction control of, 1045–1046, 1046f
   congenital dislocation of, 1051–1052
   femoral anteversion of, 1048–1049, 1049f
   flexion-extension control in, 1046–1048, 1047f–1048f
   Legg-Calvé-Perthes disease of, 1049–1050, 1050f
   nonweightbearing hip-abduction internal rotation orthosis in, 1050
   rotational control in, 1046
   trilateral-socket hip-abduction orthosis of, 1050–1051, 1050f–1051f
  knee in, 1039–1045
   femoral anteversion of, 1048–1049, 1049f
   flexion contracture of, 1044, 1045f
   genu recurvatum of, 1042
   genu varum of, 1039–1041, 1041f
   joint protection of, 1044–1045
   quadriceps insufficicency in, 1042–1044, 1043f–1044f
  leg in, 1038–1039
   fractures of tibia and fibula of, 1039, 1041f
   protection of, 1039, 1040f
   tibial torsion of, 1038–1039, 1039f–1040f
 management in, 1031–1059
 in muscular dystrophy, 270, 271f
 in myelomeningocele, 406, 408, 408f–409f
 philosophy of prescription in, 1033
 in poliomyelitis
  chronic stage, 289
  convalescent stage, 288
 rationale for prescription in, 1031–1032
 rotational control of, orthotics in, 1046
 in spinal cord injury, 524–526, 526f–527f
 spine in, 1058f–1059f, 1059
 terminology in, 1031
 trilateral-socket hip-abduction, 1050–1051, 1050f–1051f
 upper limb, 1053–1058
  elbow and shoulder in, 1056–1058
   correction of deformity of, 1057
   prevention of deformity of, 1056–1057
   restoration of function of, 1057–1058, 1058f
  hand and wrist in, 1053–1056
   combined loss of function of thumb, fingers and wrist in, 1056, 1057f
   correction of deformity of, 1054–1055, 1055f
   loss of extensor power secondary to radial nerve palsy of, 1054
   loss of function of thumb and fingers in, 1056, 1056f
   loss of thumb opposition and abduction of, 1054, 1054f–1055f
   loss of thumb opposition in, 1054f, 1055–1056
   loss of wrist stability of, 1055
   prevention of deformity of, 1053–1054, 1054f
   restoration of function in, 1055
 weaning from, 593
Ortolani maneuver, 707, 707f
Ortolani sign, 710–711, 711f
os odontoideum, 546, 547f, 548–550, 549f–550f
Osgood-Schlatter disease, 1116
 clinical features of, 891
 etiology of, 890–891
 treatment of, 891

ossiculum terminale, 545–546
ossiculum terminale persistens, 546, 546f
ossification
  ectopic, 494
  endochondral, 16, 781
  heterotopic, in spinal cord injury, 517–519
  intramembranous, 16
osteitis fibrosa, 101, 116
osteitis fibrosa cystica disseminata, 133–135
osteoblastoma, 228–229
  diagnosis of, 228–229
  treatment of, 229
osteochondritis
  of metatarsal head, 951–952, 952f
  of tarsal navicular, 952, 953f
osteochondritis dissecans, 887–890
  clinical features of, 888, 889f, 890
  of elbow, 698–699, 699f
  etiology of, 888
  in sickle cell disease, 190, 191f
  of talus, 953–954
  treatment of, 890
osteochondroma, 239–241
  diagnosis of, 239–240
  treatment of, 240–241
osteochondroses, 951–954
osteodental dysplasia, 54, 55f, 56
osteodysplasty, 67–68
osteodystrophy, renal, 101–105
  biochemical alterations in, 103–104
  chemical and bony changes in, 101, 102f
  pathophysiology of, 101–103
  radiographic changes in, 103–104, 103f–105f
  treatment of, 104–105
osteogenesis imperfecta, 111–116, 231
  biochemical studies in, 114
  classification of, 112, 113t
  clinical features of, 112
  genetics of, 166, 166f
  histologic changes in, 113–114
  inheritance of, 112
  treatment of, 115–116
osteolytic lesions, in leukemia, 186–187, 188f
osteoma, 226
  osteoid, 226–228
    diagnosis of, 227
    lower limb overgrowth in, 797, 797f
    treatment of, 227–228
  parosteal, 226
osteomalacia, 116
  and rickets, 92–101. *See also* rickets, and osteomalacia
osteomalacia congenita, 111–116
osteomyelitis, 32
  acute hematogenous, 439–448
    aspiration in, 443–444
    clinical features of, 440–441
    diagnosis in, 441–444
    laboratory tests in, 439f, 442
    pathology of, 438f, 439–440, 441f
    radioactive bone scanning in, 442–443, 443f
    roentgenographic aids in, 441f, 442
    treatment of, 444–448
      chronic stage, 441f, 446–448
      early stage, 441f, 444
      intermediate stage, 444–446
      intramedullary irrigation technique in, 445–446, 446f
      surgical, 444–445, 446f
  in sickle cell disease, 190–191
osteo-onychodysostosis, 68–69, 69f
osteopathia condensans disseminata, 65, 66f
osteopathia striata, 65
osteopenia, 116
osteopetrosis, 118–120, 119f
  clinical features of, 118
  histology of, 119–120
  radiographic findings in, 118, 119f
  treatment of, 120
osteoplasty, bone graft and, 747, 749
osteopoikilosis, 65, 66f
osteoporosis, 116
  idiopathic juvenile, 116–118, 117f–118f
  secondary to disuse, 117–118, 118f
osteoporosis fetalis, 111–116
osteosarcoma, 229–236
  diagnosis of, 230–232
    confusion in, 232
    histologic difficulties in, 231–232
    histologic dilemma in, 232
    lysis in, 230
    technetium scan in, 231
  incidence of, 230
  juxtacortical, 236–237
    survival rate in, 237
    treatment of, 237
  treatment of, 232–236
    amputation in, 232–234
      level of, 233
      lower femoral lesions and, 234
      preoperative radiation therapy and, 234
      proximal tibial lesions and, 234
    chemotherapy, 234–236
      Adriamycin in, 235–236
      methotrexate in, 235
    immunotherapy, 236
osteosclerosis fragilis generalisata, 118–120, 119f
osteotomy
  of calcaneus, 913
    in pes cavus, 949–950, 951f
  Chiari, 732–734, 732f–733f
  in congenital talipes equinovarus, 913–914
  derotational
    of fibula, 914
    of tibia, 914
  Dial, 730, 731f, 732
  femoral neck, 749
  of femur
    rotational, 734, 735f
    varus derotational, 734, 735f
  and gradual distraction
    distraction device in, 822
    femoral lengthening by, 825–838
      advantages in, 827–828
      anticipated adult height, 826
      Barnes technique of, 830
      bone grafting and plating of Wagner, 835, 836f–837f
      Bost-Larsen technique of, 829–830, 830f–832f
      contraindications in, 827
      degree of discrepancy in, 825
      disadvantages in, 828–829
      etiology of discrepancy in, 825
      indications for, 825–826
      location of discrepancy in, 825–826
      methods in, 829–838
      prerequisites for, 826–827, 826f

osteotomy, and gradual distraction, femoral lengthening by (*continued*)
      technique of plate removal, 835–836
      Wagner technique of, 830–835, 834f
    in limb length equalization, 822–849
    limits of distraction in, 823–824, 824f
    osteotomy in, 822
    program of distraction in, 822–823, 823f
    rate of lengthening in, 824–825
    tibial lengthening by, 838–849
      advantages in, 840
      Anderson technique of, 844, 846–847
      complications of, 840–843, 841f–844f
      contraindications in, 840
      disadvantages in, 840
      indications for, 840
      prerequisites for, 840
      technical aspects of, 844, 845f
      Wagner technique of, 846f–848f, 847–849
  in juvenile arthritis, 466–467
  in Legg-Calvé-Perthes syndrome
    Salter, 769
    valgus, 770
    varus, 769
  of medial cuneiform, 914
  of metatarsals, 913
    in pes cavus, 949, 950f
  pelvic, femoral lengthening by, 838
  Pemberton, 728–730, 729f
  of Salter, 726–728, 726f–728f
  Steel, 730, 730f
  subtrochanteric, 749
  and sudden distraction, femoral lengthening by, 836, 838
  Sutherland, 730, 731f
  tarsal, in pes cavus, 949
Osterreicher-Fong syndrome, 68–69, 69f
overgrowth
  lower limb
    chronic infection of, 790, 794f
    trauma in, 790, 792
  terminal, in amputation, 981–983, 983f
  upper limb, 650
overuse injury. *See* injury, overuse

pachydermatocele, 1125
pain
  back, causes of, 637–638, 639f
  congenital indifference to, 332–335
  congenital insensitivity to, 332, 333f–334f, 333t
  in spinal cord injury, 519
palsy, cerebral. *See* cerebral palsy
panhypopituitarism, 130f
parachute reflex, 348, 349f
paralysis
  of deltoid, 313
  of dorsiflexors, 292
  of elbow flexion, 314–316
  of gluteus maximus, 311
  of gluteus medius, 310–311
  in lower limb length discrepancy, 788–789, 791f
  obstetric, of upper limb, 696–698, 697f
  of peroneal and long-toe extensors, 295
  of peronei, 294, 294f
  of quadriceps muscle, 306–308, 308f
  of steering muscle, 313
  of tibialis anterior, 292, 292f
  of tibialis anterior and posterior, 292–293, 293f
  of tibialis anterior, toe extensors, and peronei, 293–294
  of tibialis posterior, 293
  of triceps brachii, 316
  of triceps surae, 295–296
paramyotonia congenita, 274
paraparesis, 503
paraplegia, 347
  ascending, 503
  associated with congenital kyphosis, 631, 632f, 633
  complete, 503
  incomplete, 503
  pseudocomplete, 503
parathyroid disorder(s), 106–109
  hyperparathyroidism, 106–107
  hypoparathyroidism, 107–108
  pseudohypoparathyroidism, 108–109, 108f
parathyroid hormone (PTH), 101
  action of, in calcium transport, 86, 86f
Paris nomenclature of constitutional (intrinsic) diseases of bone, 42–44
parosteal osteoma, 226
patella. *See also* knee
  bipartite, 886–887
  congenital dislocation and subluxation of, 882–886
    etiology of, 883, 884f
    prognosis of, 886
    treatment of, 883, 885–886, 885f–886f
  congenital dislocation of, 882
  habitual dislocation of, 282
  recurrent subluxation and dislocation of, 878–882
    clinical features and diagnosis of, 879–880, 880f
    etiology of, 878–879
    treatment of, 880–882
patellofemoral congruence angle, 880
patellofemoral stress syndrome, 1114
pauci-articular arthritis, 457–458
Pavlik harness, 712, 712f
pectoralis major muscle, 315
pectoralis major tendon, 315
pectoralis minor muscle, 315
pelvicocleidocranial dysostosis, 54, 55f, 56
pelvis
  motion of, 1065, 1065f–1066f
  obliquity of, 310
  overuse injuries of, 1113–1114, 1114f
Pemberton osteotomy, in congenital dislocation of hip, 728–730, 729f
penetrance, autosomal dominant, 154–155
perichondral groove, 33
periosteal reaction, 120–123
  leukemia associated with, 120
periosteum
  reaction of, 120–123
  stripping of, 820
peroneus, in poliomyelitis, 294, 294f
peroneus brevis, 897–898
peroneus longus, 897
pes calcaneovalgus
  congenital, in flexible flatfoot, 926
  orthotics in, 1034
pes cavus, 305–306, 942–951
  clinical evaluation of, 944–946, 945f–948f
  etiology of, 942–943, 942t

pathogenesis of, 943–944, 943t, 944f
extrinsic and intrinsic imbalance combined, 944, 944f
extrinsic muscle imbalance in, 944
intrinsic muscle weakness in, 943–944
theories of, 943t
in poliomyelitis
bony procedures in, 305
posterior bone block in, 305–306
soft-tissue procedures in, 305, 306f
treatment of, 946, 948–951
procedures in bone, 949–951
metatarsal osteotomy, 949, 950f
osteotomy of calcaneus, 949–950, 951f
tarsal osteotomy, 949
triple arthrodesis, 950–951
soft-tissue procedures, 946, 948–949
plantar release, 946, 948
selective neurectomy, 949
tendo Achilles lengthening in, 946
tendon transfers, 948–949, 949f
pes planovalgus, orthotics in, 1033–1034, 1034f
pes valgus, congenital convex, 323–324, 324f
Petrie cast, 765f
pH, and calcium absorption, 90
phantom limb, 984
phenol block, 491, 492f
phenylbutazone, for ankylosing spondylitis, 476
phenylketonuria, 151
Philadelphia chromosome, 169
phocomelia, upper limb, 651–652, 652f
treatment of, 652
phosphate diabetes, 99
and vitamin D-resistant rickets, 99
phosphorus homeostasis, 90–92
phosphorus kinetics, 90, 90f
phycomelia
lower limb, 1022, 1022f–1024f
upper limb, 1005–1007, 1007f
physeal bars, excision of, 1090–1100
follow-up, 1095, 1097
history in, 1090, 1090t, 1091t
interposition materials, 1091–1092
results of, 1097–1098, 1100
technique of, 1092, 1092f–1100f, 1094–1095
physical examination, in diseases of muscle and peripheral nerves, 259–260
physical therapy
in juvenile arthritis, 463–464
in muscular dystrophy, 269
in poliomyelitis, 287, 289
phytohemagglutinin, 167
plantar aponeurosis, 898
plantar flexion insufficiency, orthotics in, 1036–1037, 1036f–1037f
plantar warts, 966–967
plantaris, 898
plaster treatment, in Legg-Calve-Perthes syndrome, 764–765, 764f
platybasia, 531
playing surface, in overuse injuries, 1105
pleiotropic effect, 156
Pneumocystis carinii pneumonia, 210
poliomyelitis, 283–317
acute stage, 285–287, 286f
anatomic positioning in, 286–287, 286f
assessment in, 285–286
cervical-innervated muscle paresis in, 286
differential diagnosis in, 286
lumbar-innervated muscle involvement in, 286
management of, 286–287
in older children and adults, 285
symptoms in, 285
age of onset, 289
chronic stage, 288–317
muscle balance in, 289, 290f
orthosis in, 289, 289f
physical therapy in, 289
tendon transfer in, 289–291, 290f
convalescent stage, 287–288
contractures in, 288
hydrotherapy in, 288
orthosis in, 288
overactivity in, 287–288
physical therapy in, 287
rate of recovery in, 287
of elbow, 314–316
flexion paralysis of, 314–316, 314f
triceps brachii paralysis in, 316
epidemiology, 283–284
foot and ankle in, 291–306. *See also* foot and ankle, poliomyelitis of
of forearm, 316–317
of hip, 310–312. *See also* hip, poliomyelitis of
of knee, 306–310. *See also* knee, poliomyelitis of
pathology of, 284–285
prognosis for muscle recovery in, 285
of shoulder, 312–314. *See also* shoulder, poliomyelitis of
polyarthitis arthritis, 458
polydactyly, 687–690, 688f
of fingers, 689–690
genetics of, 156, 157f
of thumb, 688–689, 688f
of toes, 955, 956f
polydystrophic dwarfism, 73
polydystrophic oligophrenia, 73–75, 75f
polymyositis, 267, 277–279
polyneuropathy, acute idiopathic postinfectious, 317
popliteal cyst, 891
postural scoliosis, 578
pouce flottant, 662–663, 663f
primitive streak, 2, 5f
prosencephalon, 8
prosthesis
above-elbow amputation, 989, 991, 991f
above-knee amputation, 996–997, 999f–1000f
in amputation, 984–998. *See also* amputation, prosthetic management in
below-elbow amputation, 988–989, 989f–990f
below-knee amputation, 995–996, 995f–997f
CAPP terminal device, 986f, 987
in congenital amputation, 650–651
Dorrance hand terminal device, 987, 987f
Dorrance hook terminal device, 986f, 987
elbow disarticulation, 989, 990f

prosthesis (*continued*)
  externally powered upper limb, 1008–1011, 1010f–1011f
  forequarter amputation, 992, 993f
  hemipelvectomy, 997
  hip disarticulation, 997, 1000f–1001f
  immediate postsurgical fitting of, 997–998
  knee disarticluation, 996, 998f
  shoulder disarticulation, 991–992, 992f
  surgical principles in, 981, 982f
  Syme's-type ankle disarticulation, 993–995, 994f
  wrist disarticulation, 988, 988f
provitamin D, metabolism of, 87, 88f
pseudarthrosis
  associated with neurofibromatosis, 1135–1138, 1137f, 1139f
  in surgical treatment of scoliosis, 604
pseudoachrondroplastic spondyloepiphyseal dysplasia, 77–79, 77f
pseudohypertrophy
  of calf, 264, 264f
  in muscular dystrophy, 165
pseudohypoparathyroidism, 108–109, 108f
pseudometatropic dwarfism, 49–50
pseudotumor, in hemophilia, 200–201, 201f
psoas
  lengthening of, 376–377, 376f
  short, in cerebral palsy, 351–353, 351f–352f
pterygium colli, 537
pterygium cubitale, 675–676, 676f
pulmonary function testing,
  in neuromuscular disorders, 262
  in scoliosis, 576
pulmonary sequelae, in spinal cord injury, 521–522

quadratus plantae, 899
quadriceps
  paralysis of, 306–308, 308f
  insufficiency of, 1042–1044, 1043f–1044f
  progressive contracture of, 282
  short, in cerebral palsy, 354, 354f
quadriplegia
  complete, 502
  incomplete, 503

rachischisis, 399, 399f
radiation sarcoma, 243
radioactive bone scanning, in acute hematogenous osteomyelitis, 442–443, 443f
radioactive isotope studies, in Legg-Calvé-Perthes syndrome, 755
radius
  congenital absence of, 652–656
    clinical features of, 652–653, 654f–655f
    treatment of, 653, 654–656
      casting, 653
      surgery, 653, 655–656, 657f–658f
  congenital dislocation of, 673, 674f
recreation, in spinal cord injury, 528
recreation and fitness, in cerebral palsy, 364
rectus abdominis muscle, origin of, 15
reduction
  complicated, 723
  in congenital dislocation of hip, 719–723
    closed, 719, 721–722
    open, 717, 722–723
  maintaining, by secondary procedures, 723–736
reflex, Babinski, 13
Refsum's disease, 331
rehabilitation
  in head injury, 487–489
  in spinal cord injury, 515–528
remodeling, bone, 33–35, 34f
renal abnormalities, Klippel-Feil syndrome and, 541
renal osteodystrophy. *See* osteodystrophy, renal
renal tubular acidosis, 100
  and vitamin D-resistant rickets, 100
resection
  bone, 813–819
    advantages of, 819
    disadvantages of, 819
    femoral vs. tibial, 816, 817f
    history in, 813, 815
    indications for, 815–816
    technique in, 816, 818f, 819
  wedge, of calcaneocuboid joint, 913–914
respiratory sequela(e), in spinal cord injury, 521–522
respiratory tract, in hemophilia, 199
reticuloendotheliosis, 250
reticulosarcoma, 245
reticulosis, 250
Rheinhardt-Pfeiffer disease, 53
rheumatic fever, differential diagnosis of juvenile arthritis and, 460–461
rheumatoid arthritis, torticollis due to, 564
rhombencephalon, 9
Ribbing-Muller disease, 59–61, 60f
Ribbings disease, 67, 68f
ribonucleic acid (RNA), messenger, 151
rib-vertebral angle difference, 581
rickets
  chemical findings in, 99t
  and osteomalacia, 92–101
    causes of, 96–97, 97t, 99t
    clinical manifestations of, 93
    gastrointestinal disorders and, 97–98, 99t
    histologic changes in, 93–94, 94f–95f
    radiographic changes in, 94–96, 95f–96f
    vitamin D-deficient, 97, 98f
  unusual forms of, 97t, 98f, 100–101
  vitamin D-resistant, 98–100, 98f, 99t, 151–152
Riley-Day syndrome, 334, 453
Risser-Cotrel cast, 603
roentgenographic examination
  of bone tumors, 224–225
  of congenital dislocation of hip, 718–719, 720f–721f
    in newborn, 708–710, 708f–710f
  of juvenile arthritis, 460, 460f–461f
  of Legg-Calvé-Perthes syndrome, 754–755, 754f
  of limbs, 26
rotary displacement, atlantoaxial, 559–564. *See also* atlantoaxial rotary displacement

rotational osteotomy, in congenital dislocation of hip, 734, 735f
rubella virus, 148
Ryerson's triple arthrodesis, 300, 300f

sacrococcygeal development, 19
sacroiliac joint, 453
salicylate therapy. *See* aspirin
Salter innominate procedure, in congenital dislocation of hip, 726–728, 726f–728f
Salter osteotomy, in Legg-Calvé-Perthes syndrome, 769
Sanfilippo's syndrome, 73–75, 75f
sarcoma
  Ewing's, 245–248
    differential diagnosis of, 245–246
    treatment of, 246–248
  irradiation, 247–248
  osteogenic, 32
  radiation, 243
scalp injury, 483
scanogram, of limbs, 26
scapula, congenital elevation of, 693–696, 694f–695f
scarring, of stump, 983, 985f
Scheie's syndrome, 75
Scheuermann's disease, 619, 623–624, 626–631
  back pain caused by, 637–638
  diagnosis of, 623, 626f–627f
  etiology of, 623
  natural history of, 623, 626
  treatment of, 626–631
    exercise in, 626
    Milwaukee brace in, 626–627, 628f–629f
    nonoperative, 626–627, 628f–629f
    surgical, 627, 629–631, 630f
Scheuermann's kyphosis, 1111
Scheuthauer-Marie (-Sainton) syndrome, 54, 55f, 56
Schwachman-Diamond syndrome, with metaphyseal dysostosis, 58f, 59
Schwann cells, 11
scleroderma, 280
sclerosis
  amyotrophic lateral, 329
  hereditary multiple diaphyseal, 67, 68f
sclerotome, 14
scoliosis
  associated with neurofibromatosis, 1127–1131, 1128f–1130f
  classification of, 569–570
  congenital, 605–612
    cardiac anomalies in, 607, 609f
    classification of, 605
    Milwaukee brace in, 610–611
    neurologic disorders in, 607, 609–610, 610f–611f
    nonprogressive curves in, 605, 607f
    orthotic treatment in, 610–611
    patient evaluation in, 606–610, 609f–611f
    surgical treatment of, 611–612, 613f–615f, 613f–616f
      hemivertebra excision in, 612, 613f–616f
    unilateral unsegmented bar in, 605–606, 608f
    urinary anomalies in, 607
  glossary, 571
  growth of spine and, 29
  in head injuries, 494–495
  hysterical, 579–580, 582f
  idiopathic, 580–604
    adolescent, 585–593, 586f–592f, 594f–595f
      electrical stimulators in, 593
      indication for bracing in, 589–590
      lumbar orthosis in, 591, 593, 594f–595f
      Milwaukee brace in, 587, 589–591, 591f–592f
      natural history of, 585
      patient management with bracing, 590–591
      progression of, 585, 587, 589f–590f
      thoracic bracing in, 593
      treatment of, 587, 589–593
      weaning from brace, 593
    genetics of, 165–166
    infantile, 580–582
      treatment of, 581–582, 583f–584f
    juvenile, 582, 585
    surgical treatment of, 593, 596–604
      duration of immobilization in, 603–604, 604f–605f
      fusion area selection in, 596–601, 597f–600f, 602f
      Harrington instrumentation in, 601, 603
      Luque instrumentation in, 604
      patient selection in, 593, 596
      pseudarthrosis in, 604
      technique in, 601, 603–604, 604f–605f
      Zielke device in, 603
  Klippel-Feil syndrome and, 540–541
  leg length discrepancy in, 494–495, 578–579, 581f
  Marfan's, 612–617
    clinical features of, 612
    treatment of, 612, 615, 617
      orthotic, 612, 615
      surgical, 615, 617
  in myelomeningocele, 405–406, 406f–407f
    surgical treatment of, 409–412, 411f–412f
  neuromuscular, 617–619
    Duchenne muscular dystrophy in, 618–619, 625f
    lower motor neuron lesions in, 618, 622f, 624f
    upper motor neuron lesions in, 617–618
      cerebral palsy associated with, 617–618, 619f–621f
  nonstructural, 578–580
  postural, 578
  terminology, 570–571
  untreated, adult sequelae of, 576–578, 579f–580f
Scottish Rite Hospital orthosis, for Legg-Calvé-Perthes syndrome, 1051, 1051f
scurvy, 122–123, 122f
  clinical findings in, 122, 122f
  laboratory studies in, 122–123
  treatment of, 123
seat belt-type injury(ies), 509, 510f
septic arthritis. *See* arthritis, septic
sequela(e), late, in head injury, 494–495
sequestrum, 440

serum creatine phosphokinase (CPK), 260–261
Sever's disease, 952, 953f, 1118
sex hormone
  cell column zone and, 31
  epiphyseal plate closure and, 33
sex-limited conditions, 153
sex-linked genes, 154
sex-linked muscular dystrophy, 263–267
sex steroids, 132–133
sexuality, in spinal cord injury, 528
shelf procedure, in congenital dislocation of hip, 724, 725f–726f, 726
shock, spinal, 502
shoulder
  abduction, in cerebral palsy, 391
  in arthrogryposis multiplex congenita, 327
  congenital dislocation of, 666–667, 668f
    clinical features of, 666–667
    diagnosis of, 667
    treatment of, 667, 668f
  deformity of, orthotics for, 1056–1058, 1058f
  disarticulation, prosthesis in, 991, 991–992, 992f
  motion of, 1069–1070, 1070f
  orthopaedic treatment of, in juvenile arthritis, 470
  overuse injuries of, 1111–1112, 1112f
  poliomyelitis of, 312–314
    arthrodesis in, 313–314
    deltoid paralysis in, 313
    steering muscle paralysis in, 313
sickle cell disease, 151, 189–193, 189f–191f
  in bone and joint infections, 453
  dactylitis in, 191
  femoral head collapse in, 190, 190f
  humeral head collapse in, 190
  osteochondritis dissecans in, 190, 191f
  osteomyelitis in, 190–191
  treatment of, 191–193
  vertebral biconcavity in, 189–190, 189f
sickle thalassemia disease, 195
sitting, in cerebral palsy, 350, 373–374, 374f
skeletal age, 802–803, 802f
skeletal system, embryology of, 16–17
  endochondral ossification in, 16
  intramembranous ossification in, 16
skeletal wryneck, 559
skeleton
  abnormalities of, in upper limb, 650
  axial
    embryology of, 17–19
      sclerotome migration in, 17f, 17–18
    embryology of
      atlantoaxial development in, 19
      cartilaginous plates in, 19
      chondrification in, 18
      costovertebral articulations in, 18
      intervertebral disc in, 18–19
      sacrococcygeal development in, 19
      vertebral arch epiphysis in, 18, 18f
  immature, metabolic and endocrine abnormalities of, 81–135
skewfoot, 915
skin
  abnormalities of, 966–968
  care of, in spinal cord injury, 516, 517f–518f
  lesions, in child abuse, 1149–1150, 1149f–1150f
skull, fractures of, 483, 484f–486f
snapping hip, 1113
soft tissue
  growth mechanisms of, 37–38
  hemorrhage of, 197, 199f–200f
  procedures, in juvenile arthritis, 465–466
  surgery, in poliomyelitis of foot and ankle, 292–297
soleus, 898
somites, 4–5, 6f–7f
spastic crouch, 381f, 382
spasticity
  in cerebral palsy, 347
  in head injury, 490–494, 491f–492f
  in spinal cord injury, 519–520
sphingomyelinase, 185
spina bifida
  amniocentesis for, 176, 176f
  meningomyelocele with, 172
spinal cerebellar ataxia, hereditary, 328–329, 329f, 330f
spinal cerebellar degenerative disease, 328–329, 329f
spinal cord
  embryology of, 11–13, 12f
    alar lamina, 12, 12f
    basal lamina, 12, 12f
    meninx primitiva, 13
    neural crest in, 13
    sulcus limitans in, 12
  injury, 499, 500f–501f, 501
    approach to, 503–504, 504f
    cervical, 504–508, 505f, 507f–508f
    classification of neural injury, 502–503
    etiology of, 499, 500f
    paraplegia, 503
    quadriplegia, 502–503
    rehabilitation in, 515–528
      adaptive equipment in, 524, 525f
      autonomic dysreflexia in, 521
      bladder in, 523–524
      bowel in, 522–523
      cardiovascular effects of, 521
      heterotopic ossification in, 517–519
      hypercalcemia in, 522
      long bone fracture in, 516–517
      orthosis in, 524–526, 526f–527f
      pain in, 519
      pulmonary and respiratory sequelae in, 521–522
      recreation in, 528
      sexuality in, 528
      significance of lesions in, 526–528
      skin care in, 516, 517f–518f
      spasticity in, 519–520
      temperature regulation in, 516
      therapeutic exercise in prevention of contractures in, 520–521
      wheelchair in, 524
    spinal shock in, 502
    spine deformities secondary to, 509, 511, 511f–515f
      treatment of, 511, 513f–515f

thoracolumbar, 508–509, 509f–510f
tumors of, back pain caused by, 638, 639f
spinal dysrhaphism, 399
spinal shock, 502
spine
in cerebral palsy, treatment of deformity of, 373
cervical, 531–564
basilar impression and, 531–534
clinical findings, 533–534
roentgenographic findings, 531–533, 532f–533f
treatment of, 534
congenital anomalies of odontoid in, 545–552
congenital muscular torticollis in, 555–559
disorders of, associated with neurofibromatosis, 1131–1132, 1133f–1134f
injuries to, 504–508, 505f
atlantoaxial dislocation, 506
atlantoaxial rotary subluxation, 506
atlanto-occipital dislocation, 505–506, 505f
burst fractures, 507, 507f
compression fractures, 506–507
fracture-dislocations, 507–508, 508f
hangman's fracture, 506
odontoid fractures, 506
whiplash, 505
juvenile arthritis in, 473– 474
Klippel-Feil syndrome of, 535–545
occipitocervical synostosis in, 552–555
torticollis due to bony anomalies in, 559–564
congenital deformity of, 604–617
adult sequelae of untreated, 576–578, 579f–580f
classification of, 569–570
kyphosis in, 631–635. *See also* kyphosis, congenital
post-radiation, 635
scoliosis in, 605–612. *See also* scoliosis, congenital
Scheuermann's disease, 619, 623, 626–631. *See also* Scheuermann's disease
deformity of
orthotics for, 1058f–1059f, 1059
post-radiation, 637
secondary to spinal cord injury, 509, 511, 511f–515f
treatment of, 511, 513f–515f
examination of, 572
in Gaucher's disease, 184, 185f
growth of, 28–29, 35, 36f
rate of, 28–29
scoliosis in, 29
injuries to
approach to, 503–504, 504f
in growing person, 499–528
rationale for classification of, 501–502, 502f
kyphosis of, 631–635. *See also* kyphosis, congenital
postlaminectomy, 635, 637f
Marfan's scoliosis in, 612, 615, 617
muscular atrophy of, 317–318
classification of, 317–318
group I (Werdnig-Hoffmann disease), 317–318
group II, 318
group III, 318
group IV (Kugelberg-Welander disease), 318, 319f
laboratory data in, 318
orthopaedic deformities in, 318, 320f–321f
in myelomeningocele, 404–415
bony congenital anomalies in, 404, 405f
general considerations, 404–406, 404f–407f
orthotic treatment, 406–408, 408f–409f
scoliosis in, 405, 406f
surgical treatment in, 408–415
kyphosis and, 412–415, 413f–417f
posterior fusion in, 410, 412, 412f
scoliosis and, 409–412, 410f–412f
nerves of, embryology of, 13
neuromuscular deformity of, 617–619
Duchenne muscular dystrophy and, 618–619, 625f
lower motor neuron lesions in, 618, 622f, 624f
upper motor lesions in, 617–618, 619f–621f
neuromuscular scoliosis in, cerebral palsy in, 617–618, 619f–621f
of newborn, 29
overuse injuries of, 1109, 1110f–1111f, 1111
patient evaluation and, 571–576
history taking in, 571–572
physical examination in, 572–573, 574f
pulmonary function testing in, 576
radiologic evaluation in, 573–575
post-radiation deformity of, 635
radiologic evaluation of
CT scans in, 575
curvature measurement in, 573, 575f
kyphosis and lordosis measurement in, 573, 575, 576f–577f
laminography in, 575
myelography in, 575
rotation measurement in, 575
Scheuermann's disease in, 619, 623–624, 626–631
scoliosis of
congenital, 605–612
idiopathic, 580–604
Marfan's, 612–617
neuromuscular, 617–619
nonstructural, 578–580
thoracolumbar, 508–509, 509f–510f
burst fractures, 508–509, 509f
compression fractures, 508
fracture-dislocations, 509, 510f
seat belt-type injury, 509, 510f
untreated deformity of adult sequelae of, 576–578, 579f–580f
spleen, in Gaucher's disease, 181, 184
splints
for congenital absence of radius, 655–656

splints (*continued*)
for congenital absence of ulna, 660
retentive, in congenital talipes equinovarus, 909
spondylodiscitis, 475
spondyloepiphyseal dysplasia, 75–79
spondyloepiphyseal dysplasia congenita, 75–77, 76f
spondyloepiphyseal dysplasia tarda, 78f, 79
spondylolisthesis, 638–646
associated with neurofibromatosis, 1132–1133
back pain caused by, 637
classification of, 638–639
degenerative, 638
dysplastic, 638
evaluation of, 639, 640f
isthmic, 638
treatment of, 639–646
grade I slips, 640
grade II slips, 640–641, 643
grades III and IV slips, 641f, 643
with lumbosacral kyphosis, 644–646, 645f
with nerve root involvement, 642f–644f, 643–644
spondylolysis, 638
back pain caused by, 637
treatment of, without slip, 639–640, 641f
spondylitis, ankylosing, 474–477
clinical features of, 475
laboratory studies in, 475
medical management of, 476
orthopaedic management of, 476–477
roentgenographic features of, 475–476
treatment of, 476–477
spongiosa, 32
sport, injuries associated with, 1103–1119
spotted bones, 65, 66f
Sprengel's deformity, 693–696
clinical evaluation of, 693–694
diagnosis of, 694–695, 694f–695f
Klippel-Feil syndrome and, 537
treatment of, 695–696
spurs, bony, 983
stance phase, of gait cycle, 1062
standing, joint motion in, interrelationships of, 901t
Staphylococcus aureus, infection caused by, 438
stapling, epiphyseal plate, 811–813, 812f
startle reflex, 348, 349f
stature, short, normal variant, 129
Steel procedure, in congenital dislocation of hip, 730, 730f
steering muscle, 313
Steinert's disease, 274–275, 276f
sternocleidomastoid muscle, 315
origin of, 15
steroids, sex, 132–133
Stickler disease, 61
Still's disease, 457
stress fractures, in overuse injuries, 1106–1107, 1108f
management of, 1107
stripping, periosteal, 820
stump, scarring of, 983, 985f
subdural hematoma, 485–486
acute, 486
chronic, 486
subdural hygroma, 486–487
subluxation
atlantoaxial rotary, 506, 559
in congenital dislocation of hip, 717
and congenital dislocation of knee, 882–886
functional, in myelomeningocele of hip, 418
recurrent, of patella, 878–882
subperiosteal bone proliferation, associated with neurofibromatosis, 1140, 1140f
subtrochanteric osteotomy, 749
sulcus limitans, 12
superglycine syndrome, 98
surgical insults, multiple, 820
Sutherland procedure, in congenital dislocation of hip, 730, 731f
swing phase, of gait cycle, 1062
Swiss-type agammaglobulinemia, 58f, 59
sympathectomy, 820
syndactyly, 678–680, 678f–679f
clinical features of, 678
of toes, 955
treatment of, 678–679, 678f–679f
syndrome of pancreatic exocrine disorder, 58f, 59
synkinesia, in Klippel-Feil syndrome, 542
synostosis
congenital, cervical vertebral, 535–545. *See also* Klippel-Feil syndrome
occipitocervical, 552–555, 553f
radiouhumeral, 672–673, 672f
radioulnar, 671–672, 671f
synovectomy
in hemophilia, 207, 209
in juvenile arthritis, 465–466
contraindications, 466
technique, 466
synoviorthesis, 209
synovitis
foreign body, differential diagnosis of juvenile arthritis and, 462
transient, 770–773
clinical features of, 772
differential diagnosis of, 772
differential diagnosis of juvenile arthritis and, 462
etiology of, 770, 772
sequelae of, 773
treatment of, 773
synovium, biopsy of, 464, 464t
syringobulbia, 534
syringomyelia, 533–534
systemic lupus erythematosus, 279–280

talipes calcaneus
in poliomyelitis, 295
tendon transfers in, 296, 297f
triple arthrodesis in, 302–303, 303f
talipes equinovarus
in arthrogryposis multiplex congenita, 322, 323f
congenital, 901–915
orthotics in, 1034
triple arthrodesis in, 300, 301f
talo-first metatarsal (TMT) angle, 904
talus
congenital vertical, 919–923
clinical findings in, 920
differential diagnosis of, 920
pathologic anatomy of, 919–920
roentgenographic features of, 920, 920f
treatment of, 920–923
nonoperative, 920–921
surgical, 921–923, 923f
osteochondritis dissecans of, 953–954

tarsus
  coalition of, 935–940. *See also* coalition, tarsal
  osteotomy of, in pes cavus, 949
Tay-Sachs disease, 159
technetium bone scan, 231
telencephalon, 8
teleoroentgenogram, of limbs, 26
temperature regulation, in spinal cord injury, 516
tendon
  Achilles. *See* Achilles tendon
  lengthening of, in cerebral palsy, 360–361, 367, 367f
  transfers
    in calcaneal deformity, 296, 297f
    in cerebral palsy, 367, 368f, 387f
    in congenital talipes equinovarus, 910
    in pes cavus, 948–949, 949f
    in poliomyelitis, 289–291, 290f
tendonitis, in overuse injuries, 1107–1109
  management of, 1108
tendonosis, in overuse injuries, 1109
thalassemia, 193, 194f, 195
thalidomide, 148, 149f
thanatrophic dwarfism, 45
Thomsen's disease, 273–274, 275f
thoracic dysplasia, asphyxiating, 53
thoracic pelvic phalangeal dystrophy (TPPD), 53
thoracolumbar burst fractures, 508–509, 509f
thoracolumbar compression fractures, 508
thoracolumbar fracture-dislocations, 509, 510f
thumb
  absent, 663–664, 663f
  congenital absence of, 664, 665f
  floating, 662–663, 663f
  "hitchhiker," 50, 51f
  hypoplastic, 662–664, 663f
    abducted, 662, 663f
    adducted, 662, 663f
  loss of function of, orthotics for, 1056, 1056f
  loss of opposition and abduction in, 1054, 1054f–1955f
  loss of opposition of, 1054f, 1055–1056
  polydactyly of, 688–689, 688f
  short, 662, 663f
  trigger, 683
  triphalangeal, 683–685, 683f
thumb-in-palm deformity, in cerebral palsy, 388, 389f–390f
thymolymphopenia, metaphyseal chondrodysplasia with, 58f, 59
tibia
  congenital angular deformities of, 875–878
    anterior bowing in, 876
    clinical features of, 876, 877f
    posterior bowing in, 875–876, 876f
    treatment of, 876, 878
  derotational osteotomy of, in congenital talipes equinovarus, 914
  fractures of, orthotics for, 1039, 1041f
  lengthening of, by osteotomy and gradual distraction, 838–849
  motion of, 1067–1069, 1068f
  osteosarcoma of, 234
  torsion of, 865–866
    orthotics for, 1038–1039, 1039f–1040f
tibia vara, 869–875
  adolescent, 875
  clinical features of, 871–873, 871f
  etiology of, 870–871
  treatment of, 873–875, 873f–874f
tibial muscle, posterior, 898
tibialis anterior
  poliomyelitis of, 292, 292f
  posterior and, poliomyelitis of, 292–293, 293f
  toe extensors, peronei, and poliomyelitis in, 293–294
tibialis posterior, poliomyelitis of, 293
toe
  claw, 304–305, 966
  congenital curly, 963
  congenital mallet, 964, 964f
  extensors, in poliomyelitis, 293–294
  fifth, congenital overriding of, 961–963, 963f
  hammer, 964f, 965–966
  macrodactyly of, 955, 956f
  mallet, 964, 964f
  polydactyly of, 955, 956f
  syndactyly of, 955
  walkers, habitual, 918–919
toenails, ingrown, 967–968, 967f
tolmetin, for juvenile arthritis, 463
Toronto brace, 765f
  in Legg-Calvé-Perthes syndrome, 1049–1050, 1050f
torsion, tibial, 865–866
  orthotics for, 1038–1039, 1039f–1040f
torticollis
  bony anomalies and, 559–564
    atlantoaxial rotary displacement, 559–564
      classification of, 561–562, 563f
      clinical findings of, 564f, 652–563
      etiology and mechanism in, 560
      roentgenographic features of, 560–562, 561f–563f
      treatment of, 563–564
    congenital, 559
  congenital muscular, 555–559, 556f, 558f
    clinical appearance of, 558f
    etiology of, 557
    treatment of, 557–559
      conservative, 557
      postoperative regimen in, 557–559
      surgery in, 557, 558f
  differential diagnosis of, 560
  rheumatoid arthritis and, 564
Touraine syndrome, 68–69, 69f
traction, in congenital dislocation of hip, 715f, 716
training error, in overuse injuries, 1104
translocation, in mongolism, 169, 170f–171f, 171
transverse defects, of upper limb, 649
trapezius muscle, origin of, 15
trauma, in lower limb length discrepancy, 790, 792, 795f–796f, 797
triceps brachii
  anterior transfer of, 315–316
  in poliomyelitis, 316
triceps surae, poliomyelitis of, 295–296
  management of, 295–296
  tendon transfers for calcaneal

triceps surae, poliomyelitis of (*continued*)
deformity in, 296, 297f
trigger thumb, 683
triphalangeal thumb, 683–685, 683f
triplegia, 347
trisomy
21, 169
D, 168
E, 168, 168f–169f
G, 168
trophoblast, 2
tumors, bone, 217–252
chondroblastoma, 241–242
chondroma, 237–239
chondromyxoid fibroma, 242
chondrosarcoma, 242–243
classification of, 217, 218t
critical bibliography in, 220–221
diagnosis of, 221–226
history taking and physical examination in, 222–224
laboratory studies in, 224
pathology in, 225–226
roentgenograms in, 221–222, 224–225
Ewing's sarcoma, 245–248
giant cell, 243–245
juxtacortical osteosarcoma, 236–237
osteoblastoma, 228–229
osteochondroma, 239–241
osteoid osteoma, 226–228
osteosarcoma, 229–236
significance of, 218–220
clinical, 218
interpretive, 219
technical, 218–219
Turner-Kieser syndrome, 68–69, 69f
Turner's syndrome, 171

Ullrich disease, 72–73, 74f
ulna, congenital absence of, 656–662
clinical features of, 656–658, 659f
treatment of, 659–662, 660f–661f
umbauzonen, 95–96, 96f
undergrowth, upper limb, 650
unicameral bone cyst, simple, 248–249
urinary tract
in congenital scoliosis, 607
in hemophilia, 199
uterine environment, congenital disorders and, 148, 149f

valgus deformity, of knee, in myelomeningocele, 426
valgus osteotomy, in Legg-Calvé-Perthes syndrome, 770
van der Hoeve's disease, 111–116
varus deformity
dorsiflexion insufficiency with, orthotics in, 1035–1036
during stance phase, orthotics in, 1036, 1036f
varus derotation osteotomy, in congenital dislocation of hip, 734, 735f
varus osteotomy, in Legg-Calvé-Perthes syndrome, 769
vascular abnormalities, in occipitocervical synostosis, 555
verruca plantaris, 966–967
verrucous hyperplasia, 1126f, 1127
vertebra
biconcave, 189–190, 189f
cervical, congenital synotosis of, 535–545. *See also* Klippel-Feil sydrome
vertebral arch epiphysis, 18
vertebral artery, anomalies of, in basilar impression, 534
vertebral body infections, back pain caused by, 638
vincristine, for Ewing's sarcoma, 247
vitamin C, deficiency of, 122. *See also* scurvy
vitamin D
action of, in calcium transport, 86, 87f
first conversion of, 87, 88f
metabolism of, 86–89, 88f–89f
second conversion of, 87, 89f
vitamin D-deficient rickets, 97, 98f
vitamin D-resistant rickets, 98–100, 99t, 151–152
genetics of, 162–163, 164f
types of, 99–100
von Rosen splint, 713
Voorhoeve's disease, 65
Vrolik's disease, 111–116

Wagner procedure
of femoral lengthening, 830–835, 834f
of tibial lengthening, 847–849, 847f
walkers and nonwalkers, in cerebral palsy, 350, 351f
walking cycle, 1061–1063, 1062f–1063f
muscle activity in, 1070–1071, 1071f
warts, plantar, 966–967
Werdnig-Hoffmann disease, 317–318
wheelchair
in muscular dystrophy, 272–273
in spinal cord injury, 524
whiplash, 505
WHO classification, of bone tumors, 218t
Williams' syndrome, 109
Wimberger's sign, 122
Woodward procedure, for Sprengel's deformity, 695–696
wound(s), penetrating, in skull fractures, 483, 486f
wrist
in arthrogryposis multiplex congenita, 327
disarticulation of, prosthesis in, 988, 988f
and finger deformity, in cerebral palsy, 388, 390
hand and, orthotics for, 1053–1056
loss of stability of, 1055
orthopaedic treatment of, in juvenile arthritis, 468, 469f, 470
prosthesis for, 987–988
wryneck
congenital, 555–559, 556f, 558f
skeletal, 559

X chromosome, 153
abnormalities of, 171–172
X-linked dominant conditions, 161–163
X-linked genes, 153
X-linked recessive conditions, 163–165
x-ray examination, congenital disorders and, 148–150

Y chromosome, 153

Zielke device, 603
zygote, cell division of, 1